Clinical Environmental Medicine

Identification and Natural Treatment of
Diseases Caused by Common Pollutants

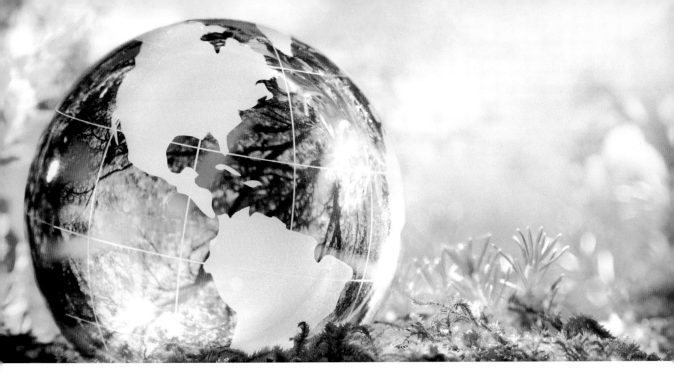

Clinical Environmental Medicine

Identification and Natural Treatment of Diseases Caused by Common Pollutants

WALTER J. CRINNION, ND

President, SpiritMed LLC, CrinnionOpinion
Adjunct Faculty, George Washington University School of Medicine and Health Sciences
Adjunct Faculty, University of Western States
Co-Chair, Environmental Health Symposium
Physician, Naturopathic Specialists
Scottsdale, Arizona

JOSEPH E. PIZZORNO, ND

Editor-in-Chief, *Integrative Medicine, A Clinician's Journal*
President, SaluGenecists, Inc.
Treasurer, Board of Directors, Institute for Functional Medicine
Founding President, Bastyr University
Seattle, Washington

ELSEVIER

ELSEVIER

3251 Riverport Lane
St. Louis, Missouri 63043

Clinical Environmental Medicine: Identification and Natural Treatment of   ISBN: 978-0-323-480864
Diseases Caused by Common Pollutants

Library of Congress Cataloging-in-Publication Data

Names: Crinnion, Walter, 1953- author. | Pizzorno, Joseph E., Jr., author.
Title: Clinical environmental medicine: identification and natural treatment of diseases caused by common
    pollutants / Walter J. Crinnion, Joseph Pizzorno.
Description: St. Louis, Missouri: Elsevier Inc., [2019]
Identifiers: LCCN 2018000841 | ISBN 9780323480864 (pbk.)
Subjects: | MESH: Environmental Medicine–methods | Environmental Pollutants–toxicity
Classification: LCC RA566 | NLM WA 30.5 | DDC 363.738/4–dc23 LC record available at https://lccn.loc.gov/
    2018000841

Director, Private Sector Education: Kristin Wilhelm
Senior Content Strategist: Linda Woodard
Senior Content Development Manager: Luke Held
Senior Content Development Specialist: Diane Chatman
Content Development Specialist: John Tomedi, Spring Hollow Press

To all of the patients I have had the privilege of working with and all the environmentally ill persons who desperately need health care providers who understand environmental illness. This work is also dedicated to my children and their progeny. May they live in a less polluted world.

Walter J. Crinnion, ND

To the courageous pioneers of natural/holistic/functional/integrative medicine who, at great personal cost, kept this medicine alive in the culture despite active persecution by vested interests. Historically, I recognize and thank John Bastyr, DC, ND; Robert Carroll, DC, ND; Lawrence Dicky, MD; Benedict Lust, ND; William Rea, MD; and Theron Randolph, MD. Their work had a profound impact on my understanding of why patients are sick and how to help them become healthy through detoxification.

Joseph E. Pizzorno, ND

CONTRIBUTORS

Lyn Patrick, ND
President, Progressive Medical Education
Co-chair Environmental Health Symposium
President, Naturopathic Academy of Environmental
    Medicine
Irvine, California

ACKNOWLEDGEMENTS

The authors thank Joseph Katzinger, ND; John Nowicki, ND; Michael Rak, ND; and Lyn Patrick, ND for their assistance in providing research for this textbook.

The authors combined have almost a century of experience in environmental medicine: studying, researching, teaching, writing, and caring for patients. We have reviewed several thousand research studies, run thousands of laboratory tests to assess toxic load, and treated thousands of people suffering the effects of toxins and toxicants. We believe the time has come for a definitive textbook focused not on the academician or researcher, but on the needs of the clinician who must care for metal- and chemical-damaged patients.

As "detoxification" is a foundational concept in naturopathic medicine, our interest in this field started early in our careers. In fact, in 1978, the first class ever taught at then-named John Bastyr College of Naturopathic Medicine was "Health Effects of Environmental Pollutants." This was a very challenging class to teach for an institution trying to advance "science-based natural medicine" (a concept promoted by founding president Dr. Pizzorno), as the research support was almost nonexistent. The available textbooks only covered industrial exposure. They strongly asserted that these toxicants only affected highly exposed industrial workers and were not a problem for the general public. As detoxification appeared to be clinically effective in non-industrially exposed populations, there was clearly a disconnect between the available research and clinical experience. Walking the pre-PubMed journal stacks searching for population-based research on how the metals and the new-to-nature chemicals being released into the environment were causing disease was very frustrating as, except for lead, there was virtually no research. The research foundation for damaging effects of environmental pollution has improved dramatically the past 20 years. The time has finally come for a definitive textbook on the practical application of environmental medicine.

In this textbook, we worked to create a useful resource for both students learning this important body of knowledge and the clinician committed to improving their understanding of how to care for environmentally ill patients. While the concepts and approach described here are based on naturopathic medicine principles, the toxicity, assessment, and interventions are fully documented with peer-reviewed research.

While we make a very strong case that environmental, endogenous, and "toxins of choice" are now the primary drivers of chronic disease, we want to be clear that we are not asserting that nutritional deficiencies and excess are not serious and common causes of chronic disease. Rather, we assert that the toxin load has become high enough to become an even bigger cause of the chronic disease epidemic now being suffered virtually throughout the world.

ORGANIZATION OF THE TEXT

The 65 chapters are organized into six sections:

Section I: Introduction to Environmental Medicine, where we lay out foundational principles and provide an overview of the many sources of toxins and toxicants.

Section II: The Toxicants, which covers the toxic damage caused by metals, inorganic chemicals, solvents, pesticides, herbicides, plasticizers, persistent organic pollutants, preservatives, mold, ozone, particulate matter, sulfur and nitrogen oxides, gut-derived toxins, and what we call *toxins of choice*—alcohol, marijuana, and factors that are only toxic at high dosages or when genetically susceptible.

Section III: Systemic Effects of Toxins summarizes impact of toxicants on physiologic system function and their association with virtually every chronic disease in these systems. Each physiologic system is covered in its own chapter.

Section IV: Assessment of Toxic Load reviews the conventional and unconventional laboratory testing available, with special emphasis on clinical application and the limitations of available research.

Section V: Biotransformation and Excretion covers the diverse routes of toxin and toxicant breakdown and elimination from the body and how these are impacted by nutritional status and genomic susceptibility.

Finally, **Section VI: Therapeutics** presents our recommendations for toxicant elimination based on our experience with thousands of patients and a review of the available research.

FOREWORD

With a wealth of literature, it is a herculean task to take on modern Environmental Medicine. In *Clinical Environmental Medicine: Identification and Natural Treatment of Diseases Caused by Common Pollutants*, Dr. Walter Crinnion and Dr. Joseph Pizzorno do a yeoman's job of covering the toxicity of many metals, chemicals, and biological agents. This work can be used as both a learning tome for students and a reference book in the practice of Environmental Medicine. Within these pages, the authors define some of the most common of the 80,000 metals and chemicals and articulate what we as clinicians should do about them.

UNDERSTANDING HOW TO PRACTICE ENVIRONMENTAL MEDICINE

Chemical sensitivity and toxicity are two different entities. Toxicity is in fact poisoning, while sensitivity creates abnormalities at a lowered threshold. The latter appears to be more common today. It can affect the patient at lesser levels and give hypersensitive responses. This hypersensitivity is what is most commonly seen in current society, since the patient is exposed to more frequent and "low levels" of multiple substances, which in combination can make the patient ill.

Coherence Phenomenon

There is a need for all of medicine and biology to understand the coherence phenomenon as well as the sensitivities phenomenon. Society has elected to assault both phenomena and ignore their combined consequences. The coherence phenomenon observed by Professors C. Smith and H. Frohlich—that nature has a phenomenon in which chemicals, food, pollen, dust, mold, and electromagnetic fields can have similar and accumulative responses to their reactions—is often ignored or not perceived in Western medicine. The accumulation of the toxic effects and sensitivities results in a sick or nonoptimum functioning population. Because of this lack of understanding, we now have a population that is fatigued and sluggish, with non-optimal functioning dependent on symptom-suppressing modalities. These treatments (medications, illicit drugs, and many other modalities) provide short-term relief but eventually result in years of misery and poor function that over time progress to chronic disease. Chemical intolerance contributes significantly to this phenomenon, since there are over 80,000 new-to-nature chemicals in our environment—many of which were designed to be difficult to detoxify.

Sensitization and Spreading Phenomena

The sensitization and spreading phenomena are yet another segment of the mystery, and understanding is critically important when caring for environmentally damaged patients.

While level of exposure is a foundational issue, the total actual body pollutant load and clinical response can be different in each individual depending not only on their exposure but also on their genomics, nutrient availability for the detoxifying systems, and their ability to desensitize their exposure.

The body cannot simply detoxify the *total pollutant load*, but also needs to be able to halt the *spreading phenomenon* of the hypersensitivity to other organs and systems. The clinician and the scientist must be able to recognize the possibility of a *bipolar response*, where the patient has a stimulating phase and then a depressed phase. Also, the clinician must always realize there is a *masking* or *adaptive phenomenon* in which the patient gets temporarily used to a substance that can appear harmless but is, in fact, still causing damage due to the exposure as long as the exposure continues. In addition, reconstruction of the *switch phenomenon* must be done where the exposure may cause an alternative set of symptoms like from a runny nose to a headache to a cough at different stages of life. This causes the patients to think they do not have the same triggering agents. The spreading phenomenon is a secondary response to more and more target organs where chemical sensitivity can bring down the individual. Here the sensitivity can go from organ, to organ, where eventually so many organs malfunction that the patient is incapacitated.

Biochemical Individuality

Biochemical individuality also must be considered, because no two patients have the same exact makeup. This also brings up the genetic susceptibility where no two people are alike and therefore respond differently to the total body load and specific body load. Also, the state of nutrition may be different and the patients' respond in an unlikely manner.

Clinical Environmental Medicine: Identification and Natural Treatment of Diseases Caused by Common Pollutants addresses these important issues, and I commend the authors for writing such a volume. The reader will gain a wealth of information and be able to help a great many patients.

William J. Rea, M.D., FA.C.S., F.A.A.E.M.

TABLE OF CONTENTS

SECTION IV Assessment of Toxic Load

SECTION V Biotransformation and Excretion

SECTION VI Therapeutics

1

The Science of Environmental Medicine

Environmental medicine (EM) is a relatively new field distinct from toxicology, occupational and industrial medicine, and public health. Industrial medicine physicians and toxicologists deal almost exclusively with individuals who have been acutely or chronically poisoned by a highly toxic compound with clearly defined toxicological markers. EM, on the other hand, deals with persons exposed daily to small dosages of multiple compounds, none of which are at levels high enough to cause defined toxicity, but cause chronic health problems nonetheless. Yet these chronic health problems are typically not associated with one single compound and may have a host of other causes as well. For example, the literature is replete with studies showing that, within 2 days of a peak in urban air pollution, respiratory and cardiovascular mortality rates increase.[1,2] Although increased levels of pollutants from vehicular exhaust contributed to their deaths, none of those individuals were technically poisoned by the pollutants.

One of the most basic principles of toxicology is that the dose is critical in determining toxicity. We all drink water daily, but few of us die from it. Yet, in the proper dose, water is lethal. Toxicological endpoints are measurable markers specific to poisoning by a certain compound. A high enough dose of organophosphate pesticides (OPs) can cause a measurable change in acetylcholinesterase levels in the body. If someone is exposed to these compounds and has a certain symptom constellation along with reduced acetylcholinesterase levels, he or she would be diagnosed with acute OP poisoning. On the other hand, an individual with the same OP exposure with a

TERMINOLOGY

The field of toxicology provides useful definitions that will be used throughout the body of this text.

Environmental health science specialty (master of public health)—This discipline seeks to translate environmental health research into effective public health practice, promote human health and well-being, and foster safe and healthy environments. (https://publichealth.yale.edu/ehs/curriculum/mph/)

Environmental medicine—The branch of medicine that deals with diagnosing and caring for people exposed to chemical and physical hazards in their homes, communities, and workplaces through such media as contaminated soil, water, and air.

(*Role of the Primary Care Physician in Occupational and Environmental Medicine*, Institute of Medicine, U.S. Division of Health Promotion and Disease Prevention)

Occupational medicine—The branch of medicine that deals with the prevention and treatment of occupational injuries and diseases. (http://www.thefreedictionary.com/occupational+medicine)

Poisons—Toxicants that cause immediate death or illness when experienced in very small amounts.

Toxicants—Substances (not produced by living organisms) that produce adverse biological effects of any nature.

(http://www.merriam-webster.com/dictionary/toxicology)

Toxicology—The science that deals with poisons and their effect and with the problems involved (e.g., clinical, industrial, or legal).

Toxins—Specific proteins produced by living organisms that typically produce immediate effects (amanitin toxin, trichothecene mycotoxin, etc.).

different set of neurological symptoms who does not have reduced acetylcholinesterase levels would not be diagnosed as having OP toxicity. Toxicologists take many factors into consideration when determining a toxic dose, including how much of the total dose was absorbed and how well the normal biotransformation processes are working. Other factors considered include the presence of other compounds that might be additive, antagonistic, potentiating, or synergistic to the toxic damage of the compound in question, as well as the effect other substances can have on detoxification rate (Table 1.1).

Toxicology also takes into account the number of doses of the toxicant, the frequency of the dosing, and the total time period of the exposure.

The diagnosis of toxicity weighs heavily on the detectable levels of the toxicant or its metabolites. Serum or urine levels of compounds below which no indication of toxic endpoint damage is identifiable are listed as no observable adverse effect level (NOAEL). Once the known toxicological effects of a compound become detectable, the level of the toxicant in the blood is considered the lowest observable adverse effect level (LOAEL). NOAEL refers to the highest dose of a compound that has shown no observable toxic or adverse effect. In other words, it is the maximum level of OPs that can be present without any observable reduction in acetylcholinesterase. Another example is how much mercury one can have in one's blood without any of the known symptomatic and physiological markers of mercury toxicity being detectable. LOAEL refers to the lowest dose at which these same markers of toxicity are now detectable for a certain compound (Fig. 1.1).

NOAEL and LOAEL are based upon the defined toxic damage of a single compound leading to acute or chronic poisoning. Using OPs as an example again, NOAEL would be the urinary levels of OP metabolites at which no change in acetylcholinesterase is found. However, persons exposed to OPs have been found to have adverse neurological effects without any depletion in acetylcholinesterase.[3] By toxicology standards, those individuals would not have been affected by OPs, but an EM practitioner would not discard that possibility. The rest of this textbook will elucidate the strong documentation linking common adverse health effects from regularly encountered toxic compounds that are all present below NOAEL levels.

> **NOTE** To download a basic toxicology lecture go to http://www.toxipedia.org/display/toxipedia/Teaching+Resources.

ENVIRONMENTAL HEALTH PROFESSIONS
Industrial and Occupational Medicine
Industrial medicine physicians are employed by industry to provide medical care to workers, whereas occupational medicine doctors focus on environmental and workplace exposures. In 1970, President Richard M. Nixon signed legislation starting the Occupational Safety and Health Administration (OSHA) under the United States Department of Labor. Its purpose is to assure safe and healthful conditions for working men and women by setting and enforcing standards and by providing training, outreach,

TABLE 1.1 Terms Related to the Presence of Other Compounds in Toxicology

Term	Definition
Additivity	A combination of two or more chemicals in the sum of the expected individual responses (rather than being greater than the sum)
Antagonism	Exposure to one chemical reduces the toxic effect of another chemical
Potentiation	Exposure to one chemical results in another chemical having a greater than normal toxic effect when given alone
Synergism	The combination of two or more chemicals results in a greater toxic effect than the sum of the two individually

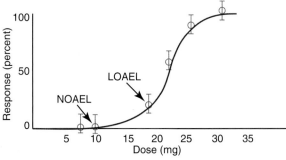

FIG. 1.1 No observable effect level (NOAEL) and lowest observable effect level (LOAEL).

education, and assistance. By 1989, OSHA had established workplace exposure limits for 188 compounds. Exposure to compounds at levels below OSHA standards is considered by many to be "safe."

OCCUPATIONAL HEALTH REGULATORY VALUES

The **threshold limit value (TLV)** of a chemical substance is the level a worker could be exposed to daily for a working lifetime without adverse health effects. TLVs were established by the American Conference of Governmental Industrial Hygienists and adopted by OSHA after its formation.

The **workplace environmental exposure level** was created by a committee of the American Industrial Hygiene Association to provide guidance for protecting most workers from adverse health effects related to occupational chemical **exposures**.

Permissible exposure limits (PELs), set by OSHA and originally based on established TLVs, are the levels of airborne chemicals that workers may be exposed to over an 8-hour work day. Levels above PEL are considered to be toxic; those lower are considered to be safe.

When OSHA received its mandate in 1970 to protect workers' health, it had a Herculean task. One of its first steps was to establish toxic and safe values for exposure to workplace airborne chemicals. Instead of starting from scratch, OSHA adopted the TLVs that were already established by the American Conference of Governmental Industrial Hygienists (ACGIH). The ACGIH, despite its name, is not associated with the U.S. government but does include government officials, academics, and industry representatives. To establish TLVs, the ACGIH used data provided by industry and tried to balance workers' health with cost to industry. A review of the process by which the TLVs were established revealed that both TLVs and PELs are primarily based on industry input rather than any scientific studies.[4] The TLV/PEL values for individual chemicals do not take into account the total load of the individual nor the genetic differences in his or her biotransformation pathways.

NOTE For a basic overview course on occupational health, go to https://www.jhsph.edu/academics/certificate-programs/certificates-for-hopkins-and-non-degree-students/environmental-and-occupational-health.html.

Public Health

Individuals seeking a master's degree in public health (MPH) can specialize in several areas, including biostatistics, epidemiology, health service administration, behavioral science, and environmental health science. Those with an MPH in environmental health science typically utilize their knowledge to
- develop management strategies to reduce environmental hazards;
- make policy recommendations to reduce such hazards;
- pursue research in the field of EM; and
- conceptualize, design, implement, and evaluate programs and policies to protect and promote public health.

Environmental Medicine

Toxicologists and occupational medicine physicians are fully trained to identify individuals acutely or chronically poisoned by toxicants. They receive no training in identifying or treating those who have become ill from low-level daily toxicant exposures in their air, food, and water. This is the void into which EM physicians step. Those in the field recognize that the total body burden of environmental toxins and toxicants can lead to chronic health complaints that typically improve when the total toxic load is reduced. Rarely, if ever, will an environmentally ill person meet the diagnostic criteria for poisoning by a single toxicant. To identify an environmentally induced illness, an EM physician must assess several pieces of information that will be covered in this textbook:
1. Does the patient's case history show the classic signs of environmental overload?
2. Does the patient's presentation reflect the picture of low-level exposure to a certain toxin/toxicant?
3. Did the patient have exposure to the compound matching his or her presenting symptoms?
4. Was the timing of exposure to that pollutant consistent with the onset or worsening of the patient's symptoms?
Laboratory assessments for some of the common toxicants are available to help confirm exposure and assess the success of avoidance techniques.

TOTAL TOXICANT BODY BURDEN

The main principle of EM is to recognize the 'Total Load' of xenobiotic pollutants that are adversely affecting the patient.[5] Many patients want to point to the one chemical exposure that initiated their illness as the only compound that made them ill. This idea fits with the basic tenets of toxicology that focus on a single toxicant at a time, ignoring the fact that all persons have multiple toxicants present. In reality, the symptom-initiating exposure merely overloaded an already taxed homeostatic balance leading to the health crisis. EM takes into account the possible synergism of the total load of toxicants as a causative factor in illness.[6,7]

The Centers for Disease Control and Prevention (CDC) has been conducting ongoing laboratory assessment on samples gathered in the National Health and Nutrition Examination Survey (NHANES) trial to quantify the total load of xenobiotic compounds present in the average U.S. resident.[8] The overall purpose of this work is to "provide unique exposure information to scientists, physicians, and health officials to help prevent exposure to some environmental chemicals."

The goals of this survey include the following:
- To identify chemicals found in the U.S. population and their concentration levels
- For chemicals with known toxicity levels (as defined by the field of toxicology), to determine the prevalence of people with levels that exceed safe limits (e.g., a blood lead level ≥10 mcg/dL)
- To establish reference values that can be used by physicians and scientists to determine whether a person or group has an unusually high exposure. This information is especially helpful for identifying population groups that merit further assessment of exposure sources or health effects

Before the CDC's publication of these reports, the reference values for the compounds used by laboratories reflected industrial workplace standards. The new CDC values give us, instead, a population-based reference range, allowing us to identify those with higher-than-normal burdens of these toxic compounds. Although the report does not provide information on the percentage of the population in which these compounds are found, those toxicants for which mean population values are given can be considered as ubiquitously present.

Samples of urine, blood, and serum collected from NHANES participants have been assessed for the presence of 246 environmental chemicals or their metabolites. Of these 246 compounds, 120 were ubiquitous enough to have mean values assigned (Table 1.2).

HALF-LIFE DEFINITIONS

Half-life—The time it takes for a substance (drug, radioactive nuclide, or other) to lose half of its pharmacological, physiological, or radiological activity. (http://www.ncbi.nlm.nih.gov/mesh?term=half%20life)

Plasma half-life—The time it takes for the blood plasma concentration of a substance to be reduced by 50%.

Note—Five half-lives are required for a compound to be cleared fully from the bloodstream.

Note—Clearance from the plasma does not mean that the compound has left the body, merely that it has left the plasma. The tissue half-lives of compounds may be much longer than the plasma half-lives.

Tissue half-life—The time it takes for the tissue levels of a compound to be reduced by 50%.

Table 1.2 also notes which of the toxicants present are biologically persistent, with longer half-lives, and which are not. With the exception of the persistent metals, the other persistent toxicants all carry a number of halogen molecules (chlorine, bromine, and fluorine). Nonpersistent chemicals have shorter biological half-lives, typically less than 24 hours, yet predominate over other toxicants, with the average person having over 600 µg/L in his or her urine.

Exposure to these persistent, and some nonpersistent, compounds begins during the fetal stage, as all appear to easily cross the placental barrier.[9] To this maternally transferred burden is added daily exposures to xenobiotics in the air, food, water, and personal care products. Many of these compounds are potent toxins to the immune, neurological, and endocrine systems, all of which are going through critical developmental milestones in the fetus. Theo Colburn, PhD, author of *Our Stolen Future,* developed an interactive website showing how exposure to certain toxicants during certain weeks of gestation leads to long-term health problems. It is available for viewing at http://endocrinedisruption.org.

Cord blood samples taken at birth offer an accurate reading of which xenobiotics the fetus is exposed to. The Environmental Working Group (EWG) tested the cord blood of 10 babies born in U.S. hospitals for the presence of 413 toxic compounds.[10] Of those, 287 were detected in the samples, with an average of 200 of these compounds

CHAPTER 1 The Science of Environmental Medicine 5

TABLE 1.2 Ubiquitous Pollutants in the CDC 4th National Exposure Report

Compound	# Tested	# Commonly Found	Persistent	Nonpersistent	Avg. Urine Conc.	Avg. Serum Conc.
Acrylamides	2	2		X		120.5 pmol/g
Benzophenone-3 (sunscreen)	2	1		X	22.9 µg/L	
Bisphenol A	1	1		X	2.64 µg/L	
Chlorinated pesticides	16	5	X		2.85 µg/L	277.27 ng/g lipid
Cotinine, NNAL (smoking)	2	2		X	1.06 pg/mg cr	0.71 ng/mL
Dichlorophenol	3	3		X	7.75 µg/L	
Dioxins/furans	17	2	X			.0425 ng/g lipid
Herbicides	23	2		X	25.17 µg/L	
Metals	26	16	X		146 µg/L	
MTBE	1	1	X		6.16 ng/mL	
Nitrate	1	1	X		40.7 mg/L	
Organophosphate pesticide metabolites	16	4		X	4.1 µg/L	
Parabens	3	3	X		65.3 µg/L	
Perchlorate	1	1		X	3.4 µg/L	
Perflourinated compounds	12	7	X		16.8 µg/L	
Phthalates	16	12		X	288 µg/L	
Polybrominated diphenyl ethers	11	5	X			33.7 ng/g lipid
Polychlorinated biphenyls (PCBs)	40	33	X			113.89 ng/g lipid
Polycyclic aromatic hydrocarbons (exhaust)	10	10		X	3.83 µg/L	
Pyrethroid pesticides	5	1		X	.418 µg/L	
Solvents	28	6		X		.45 ng/mL
Thiocyanate	1	1	X		1.15 mg/L	
Trihalomethanes (chlorine water treatment)	4	2		X		18.27 pg/mL
Triclosan (disinfectant)	1	1		X	13.0 µg/L	

Compiled from Centers for Disease Control and Prevention. (2017). *National Report on Human Exposure to Environmental Chemicals*. Retrieved from www.cdc.gov/exposurereport

present in each infant. Table 1.3 shows the compounds that were looked for in the cord blood samples and how many were found.

A review of studies on levels of certain xenobiotic compounds in meconium samples also revealed multiple compounds in newborns' first bowel movements, indicating fetal exposure (Table 1.4).[11] These compounds include pharmaceutical agents, illegal drugs, heavy metals, and pesticides.

The meconium studies found organophosphate pesticides that were not looked for in the EWG cord blood study. Organophosphate pesticides, along with pyrethroid pesticides, are the most commonly used insecticidal agents at present. This is quite a combined neurotoxic pesticide burden for a child to start out with, especially as the liver, brain, endocrine, and immune systems are all still developing, and many of these compounds are toxic to those tissues.

TABLE 1.3 Xenobiotics Found in the Cord Blood of 10 Children Born in U.S. Hospitals

Compound	# Tested	# Found	How They Are Used, Where They Are Found
Mercury	1 (Hg)	1	Seafood, dental amalgams
Polycyclic aromatic hydrocarbons (PAHs)	18	9	Combustion byproduct (from tailpipes and cigarettes)
Polybrominated dioxins and furans (PBDD/Fs)	12	7	Contaminants of brominated fire retardants
Polychlorinated dioxins and furans (PCDD/Fs)	17	11	Byproducts of polyvinyl chloride production (PVC), industrial bleaching and, incineration
Perfluorinated chemicals (PFCs)	12	9	Teflon, Scotchgard, fabric and carpet protectors, food wrap coatings
Chlorinated pesticides	28	21	Most are now banned from use. Commonly found in animal fat and farmed salmon
Polybrominated diphenyl ethers (PBDEs)	46	32	Flame retardants. High in farmed salmon
Polychlorinated naphthalenes	70	50	Wood preservatives, varnishes
Polychlorinated biphenyls (PCBs)	209	147	Used as lubricants and insulation, but there is now a worldwide ban on production and use. High in farmed salmon

Complied from Body Burden: The Pollution in Newborns. http://www.ewg.org/research/body-burden-pollution-newborns. Copyright © Environmental Working Group, www.ewg.org. Reproduced with permission.

PERSISTENT ORGANIC POLLUTANTS

The United Nations Environment Programme defines persistent organic pollutants as "chemical substances that persist in the environment, bioaccumulate through the food web, and pose a risk of causing adverse effects to human health and the environment." With the evidence of long-range transport of these substances to regions where they have never been used or produced and the consequent threats they pose to the global environment, the international community has now, on several occasions, called for urgent global action to reduce and eliminate release of these chemicals.

They are aldrin, chlordane, chlordecone, dieldrin, endrin, heptachlor, hexabromobiphenyl, hexabromocyclododecane, hexabromodiphenyl ether, hexachlorobenzene, hexachlorobutadiene, α and β hexachlorocyclohexane, lindane, mirex, pentachlorobenzene, pentachlorophenol, PCBs, polychlorinated naphthalenes, endosulphan, tetra- and pentabromodiphenyl ethers, and toxaphene.

Copied from The Stockholm Convention on Persistent Organic Pollutants website http://chm.pops.int/TheConvention/Overview/tabid/3351/

OTHER FACTORS IMPORTANT IN ENVIRONMENTAL MEDICINE

EM physicians also consider many other factors besides toxicant levels as part of the total load on an individual. Many factors can negatively affect the body's ability to clear toxicants and thus protect itself from damage."

- Genetic polymorphisms—Single nucleotide polymorphisms and copy number variations for the genes encoding the phase 1 and phase 2 biotransformation enzymes (see Chapter 56) will reduce the ability of the body to metabolize xenobiotic toxicants.
- Nutrient deficiencies—Deficiencies of nutrients needed for biotransformation (phases 1 and 2), excretion (phase 3), and protection against toxicant damage can result in reduced clearance and increased oxidative damage. Inadequate dietary fiber is also very important, as it plays a critical role in elimination of toxicants excreted by the liver.
- Dietary choices—The amounts and ratios of proteins, fats, and carbohydrates can either speed or inhibit the clearance of toxicants from the bloodstream (see Chapter 56).
- Emotional/mental/spiritual stressors—Stresses from our families, jobs, society, relationships, etc., can

TABLE 1.4 Xenobiotic Compounds Found in Meconium			
Pharmaceuticals	**Drugs of Abuse**	**Heavy Metals**	**Pesticides & PCBs**
Anesthetics	Cocaine	Lead	Arochlor (PCB)
Analgesics	Opiates	Cadmium	Chlordane
Antihistamines	Cannabinoids	Mercury	Chlorpyrifos
Adrenergics	Morphine		Organophosphate metabolites
Expectorants	Methadone		DDT
Antidepressants	Stimulants		Lindane
Anticonvulsants	Cotinine (nicotine)		Malathion
			Parathion

Data from Barr, D. B., Bishop, A., & Needham, L. L. (2007). Concentrations of xenobiotic chemicals in the maternal-fetal unit. *Reproductive Toxicology, 23*(3), 260–266.

directly affect our health and how we clear and react to environmental toxicants.[12]

- Lifestyle choices—How we live our lives can have a direct bearing on our exposures and how well our bodies can handle toxic burden. This includes the amount of sleep and exercise and leisurely time that we get.
- Overall health and wellness.
- Infections, disease, organ function—The health of our organs, tissues, and cells has a profound effect on our ability to clear toxicants efficiently[13] and to resist toxic damage. The presence of pathogenical organisms that release their own toxins can be a decisive contributor to the total load.
- Microbiome makeup, especially if endotoxicity is present.
- EMF exposure. Exposure to electromagnetic fields (EMF).

REFERENCES

1. Zhang, P., Dong, G., Sun, B., Zhang, L., Chen, X., Ma, N., et al. (2011). Long-term exposure to ambient air pollution and mortality due to cardiovascular disease and cerebrovascular disease in Shenyang, China. *PLoS ONE, 6*(6), e20827. PubMed PMID: 21695220.
2. Ito, K., Mathes, R., Ross, Z., Nadas, A., Thurston, G., & Matte, T. (2011). Fine particulate matter constituents associated with cardiovascular hospitalizations and mortality in New York City. *Environmental Health Perspectives, 119*, 467–473. PubMed PMID: 21463978.
3. Srivastava, A. K., Gupta, B. N., Bihari, V., Mathur, N., Srivastava, L. P., Pangtey, B. S., et al. (2000). Clinical, biochemical and neurobehavioral studies of workers engaged in the manufacture of quinalphos. *Food and Chemical Toxicology, 38*, 65–69. PubMed PMID: 10685015.
4. Castleman, B., & Ziem, G. (1988). Corporate influence on threshold limit values. *American Journal of Industrial Medicine, 13*, 51–59. PubMed PMID: 3287906.
5. Rea, W. J. (1992). *Chemical Sensitivity*, Vol. 1 (17–21). Boca Raton, FL: CRC Press.
6. McKinney, J. D. (1997). Interactive hormonal activity of chemical mixtures. *Environmental Health Perspectives, 105*(9), 896. PubMed PMID: 9410738.
7. Rajpakse, N., Silva, E., & Kortenkamp, A. (2002). Combining xenoestrogens at levels below individual no-observed-effect concentrations dramatically enhances steroid hormone action. *Environmental Health Perspectives, 110*(9), 917–921. PubMed PMID: 12204827.
8. From Centers for Disease Control and Prevention. (2017). *National Report on Human Exposure to Environmental Chemicals*. Retrieved from www.cdc.gov/exposurereport (Accessed April 13, 2017.)
9. Myllynen, P., Pasanen, M., & Pelkonen, O. (2005). Human placenta: A human organ for developmental toxicology research and biomonitoring. *Placenta, 26*, 361–371. PubMed PMID: 15850640.
10. http://www.ewg.org/research/body-burden-pollution-newborns. (Accessed April 13, 2017.)
11. Barr, D. B., Bishop, A., & Needham, L. L. (2007). Concentrations of xenobiotic chemicals in the maternal-fetal unit. *Reproductive Toxicology, 23*, 260–266. PubMed PMID: 17386996.
12. Cooney, C. M. (2011). Stress-pollution interactions: An emerging issue in children's health research. *Environmental Health Perspectives, 119*(10), a430–a435. PubMed PMID: 22069778.
13. Blouin, R. A., Farrell, G. C., Ioannides, C., Renton, K., & Watlington, C. O. (1999). Impact of diseases on detoxication. *Journal of Biochemical and Molecular Toxicology, 13*(3,4), 215–218. PubMed PMID: 10098907.

2

Oxidative Damage and Inflammation

SUMMARY

- Presence in population: Ubiquitous
- Major diseases: Cardiovascular disease, diabetes, neurological conditions, cancer
- Primary sources: Air pollution, diet, lifestyle choices, toxic metals, persistent organic pollutants (POPs), pesticides, solvents
- Best measure: 8-hydroxy-2-deoxyquanosine (8-OHdG), F2-isoprotane
- Best intervention: Avoidance of toxicants, antioxidant supplementation

DESCRIPTION

Oxidative damage to cells has long been associated with aging and the development of many chronic diseases, including cancer, heart disease, and diabetes. In fact, virtually every chronic disease is associated with oxidative stress. Reactive oxygen species (ROSs) such as superoxide radicals, hydrogen peroxide, and hydroxyl radicals are produced through normal biochemical processes in the body such as oxidative phosphorylation in the mitochondria during the production of adenosine triphosphate (ATP). They are also produced throughout the body by the cytochrome P450 system active in the production, metabolism, and catabolism of numerous compounds in the body. In addition, ROSs are generated by white blood cells that attack bacterial invaders and by peroxisomes that break down fatty acids. These prooxidants then attack and damage lipids, nucleic acids, and proteins, leading to DNA damage, abnormal protein folding, lipid peroxidation, and mitochondrial membrane damage.

Environmental toxicants significantly increase the oxidant load, some poison antioxidant enzymes, and some induce proinflammatory epigenetic modification. These all heighten total oxidative stress, thereby increasing risk of disease and effects of aging.[1] In fact, a twin study in Denmark revealed that the bulk of oxidative damage is caused by environmental factors, with only 17% to 22% resulting from genetics.[2]

Because these processes go on constantly in the body, there is always a level of ROSs that needs to be addressed. Oxidative stress occurs when the prooxidants are more numerous than the available antioxidants in the body. To handle these prooxidants, the body has a number of ways to protect itself, including enzymes such as superoxide dismutase, catalase (CAT), and glutathione (GSH) peroxidase; antioxidant compounds such as ubiquinone, GSH, bilirubin, and uric acid; and numerous diet-related antioxidant compounds, including tocopherols, ascorbic acid, polyphenols, carotenoids, N-acetyl cysteine (NAC), and other nutrients.

MECHANISMS

Oxygen is required for normal cellular function. When oxygen is lacking, tissue hypoxia causes what has been termed the "oxidative stress paradox." During periods of hypoxia or anoxia, there is an increase in oxidative damage, which is most often characterized by the severe damage of a stroke or myocardial infarction. Much of the damage in anoxia or hypoxia results from an increase in reactive nitrogen species and a smaller increase in ROSs. Increased ROS concentrations reduce the amount of bioactive nitric

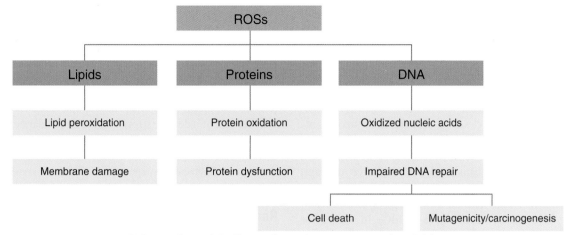

FIG. 2.1 Potential effects of reactive oxygen species (ROSs).

oxide by chemical inactivation to form toxic peroxynitrite. Peroxynitrite both damages cellular enzymes and DNA and upregulates "hypoxia genes," thus changing the cell's function.[3]

Indirectly, free radicals act as secondary messengers in inflammatory and immunological cellular responses, activating transcription factors like nuclear factor kappa-light-chain-enhancer of activated B cells (NF-κB) and activator protein 1 (AP-1) that control genes involved in inflammation.[4] ROSs initiate a variety of toxic reactions, including lipid peroxidation, direct inhibition of mitochondrial respiratory chain enzymes, inactivation of glyceraldehyde-3 phosphate dehydrogenase, inhibition of membrane sodium/potassium ATP-ase activity, and inactivation of membrane sodium channels. Each of these toxic reactions play a role in the pathophysiology of inflammation (Fig. 2.1).[5] Inflammation is also associated with the formation of reactive oxygen intermediates, including cytokines (e.g., IL-1, IL-2, and IL-6), granulocyte-macrophage colony stimulating factor (GM-CSF), and tumor necrosis factor (TNF-α or TNF-β).

SOURCES

Physiological

Under normal physiological conditions, mitochondria generate ROSs. During aerobic respiration, about 5% of oxygen consumed is lost to ROSs.[6] Extreme endurance exercise leads to increased ROSs that cause oxidative DNA damage demonstrated by elevated 8-OHdG levels.[7,8]

Toxic Metals

Arsenic,[9] cadmium,[10,11] mercury,[12] and lead[13,14] have all been shown to cause increased DNA oxidation, measurable by 8-OHdG. Iron, copper, chromium, vanadium, and cobalt undergo redox-cycling reactions producing toxicity, whereas mercury, cadmium, and nickel deplete GSH and bond to the sulfhydryl groups of proteins.[15] Lead not only generates ROSs but also causes a reduction in the activity of ROS-quenching enzymes such as superoxide dismutase, CAT, and GSH peroxidase, resulting in diminished antioxidant defense. At the cellular level, cadmium provokes the generation of ROSs, which indirectly modulates gene expression and signal transduction and reduces activities of proteins involved in antioxidant defenses.[16]

The carcinogenetic effect of arsenic may be related to the activation of redox-sensitive transcription factors involving NF-κβ and AP-1.[17]

Persistent Organic Pollutants

Exposure to organophosphate pesticides will lead to DNA oxidative damage, resulting in an increase in 8-OHdG.[18,19] Malathion, a commonly used organophosphate pesticide, generates free radicals that induce oxidative stress in human erythrocytes through the inhibition of CAT, GSH peroxidase, and superoxide dismutase.[20] Oxidative stress from malathion exposure may also be a result of damage to mitochondrial complexes by inhibiting the activity of Complex IV.[21] A positive correlation between exposure to pesticides and oxidative stress biomarkers has been found in farmers.[22]

Permethrin has been shown to increase superoxide anion production and the activity of the hydrogen peroxide–myeloperoxidase system in rat polymorphonuclear neutrophils.[23] Pyrethroid exposure induces lipid peroxide and protein oxidation and depletes reduced GSH.[24]

Air Pollution

Diesel exhaust particles, probably the most toxic component of urban outdoor air pollutants, are a mixture of carbon particles, organic chemicals, heavy metals, and free radicals, causing DNA oxidative damage, measurable by elevated 8-OHdG levels.[25,26] Persons exposed to traffic in their work (e.g., traffic officers) also have higher levels of 8-OHdG, indicative of increased oxidative damage.[27,28]

Urban air pollution has long been positively associated with respiratory and cardiac problems and increased mortality rates. Particulate matter (PM) is one of the major components of urban air pollution and has been linked to increased levels of 8-OHdG.[29,30] PM causes significant oxidative damage in the tissues and organs to which they are distributed and has been associated with increased mortality, primarily from cardiovascular,[31,32,33,34] respiratory,[35,36] and neoplastic diseases.[37] The powerful prooxidant action of ozone is primarily responsible for respiratory damage, as ozone exposure depletes the normal level of antioxidants in the respiratory tract.[38]

A study in Taiwan demonstrated that exposure to indoor air pollutants causes an increase in oxidative damage, aggravating sick building syndrome–related symptoms.[39] Peruvian women exposed particulate matter from wood smoke generated by indoor cooking fires (PM_{10} and $PM_{2.5}$) also had higher urinary 8-OHdG levels.[40] Asbestos fibers are genotoxic to the lungs and are linked with increased levels of 8-OHdG.[41,42]

Prescription and Over-the-Counter Drugs

Many prescription and over-the-counter (OTC) drugs have been shown to increase oxidative stress and inflammation. These adverse effects are discussed more thoroughly in Chapter 8, Drugs.

Nonsteroidal antiinflammatory drugs (NSAIDs) have been shown to induce ROSs in cardiac and cardiovascular-related cells, which may explain the increased risk of heart attack and stroke associated with NSAID use.[43] Rofecoxib, a cyclooxygenase (COX)-2 inhibitor, was removed from the market, as its extended use increased the risk of atherothrombotic events. It is now known that

the cardiotoxicity of rofecoxib was not related to COX-2 inhibition but rather to the oxidative modification of low-density lipoproteins and cellular membrane lipids, which contributed to plaque instability and thrombus formation.[44]

Doxorubicin, an oncological agent, induced cardiotoxicity through DNA damage and apoptosis in cardiac cells because of oxidative stress, and the antioxidant effect of NAC attenuated these processes.[45] Animal studies have demonstrated neurotoxic and genotoxic side effects from the use of oxcarbazepine, an antiepileptic drug, resulting from toxic metabolites, free radicals, and ROSs.[46,47]

Radiation

Ionizing radiation can cause DNA damage, gene mutation, apoptosis, and cancer. The toxic effects of radiation result from rapid generation of ROSs through radiolysis of water molecules as well as secondary reactions leading to increased levels of ROSs, which can diffuse within the cell and delay the toxic effects.[48]

Solvents

Ethylbenzene exposure results in elevated 8-OHdG levels in workers,[49] as does exposure to benzene[50,51] and styrene,[52] but not toluene.

Toxins of Choice

Alcohol. Alcohol consumption has been shown to facilitate ROS production, release cytokines, reduce antioxidants, and promote an *in vivo* oxidative microenvironment.[53] Hydroxyethyl free radicals, generated during ethanol metabolism by cytochrome P450 2E1 (CYP2E1), react with hepatic proteins, stimulating humoral and cellular immune reactions, which may represent the mechanism by which alcohol-induced oxidative stress contributes to the perpetuation of chronic hepatic inflammation.[54] Induction of CYP2E1 also contributes to increased lipid peroxidation associated with alcoholic liver injury and enhances acetaldehyde production, which in turn impairs defense systems against oxidative stress.[55] See Chapter 36, Alcohol, for a more complete discussion.

Tobacco. Chronic tobacco smoke inhalation induces an intracellular oxidative environment characterized by decreased concentrations of circulating antioxidants, increased oxidation of GSH, and increased levels of DNA damage.[56] Tobacco smoke has long been linked with elevated levels of 8-OHdG in smokers[57,58] and in those exposed to secondhand smoke.[59] One study of smokers showed 50% higher 8-OHdG levels compared with nonsmokers,[60] with cessation of smoking resulting in a 21% drop in 8-OHdG levels after 4 weeks.[61] In a group of lung cancer patients, 8-OHdG levels were significantly positively correlated with not only smoking but also aggressiveness of the cancer.[62] See Chapter 40, Smoking, for a more complete discussion.

ASSESSMENT

Urinary nucleoside metabolites serve as indirect measures of oxidative stress and toxin load. Currently the two most easily accessible laboratory markers for measuring oxidative stress in the body are urinary levels of 8-OHdG and F2-isoprostane.[63,64,65] F2-isoprotane is a prostaglandin-like compound formed *in vivo* involving the free radical–catalyzed peroxidation of arachidonic acid independent of the cyclooxygenase enzyme.[66] F2-isoprostane is an excellent marker for lipid peroxidation and offers the clinician valuable insight into the level of lipid damage. It has also illuminated the role of oxidant injury in association with cancer and with cardiovascular, neurological, hepatic, renal, and pulmonary diseases.[67,68]

In nucleic acid, guanine is the base most prone to oxidative damage. When hydroxyl radicals contact cellular or mitochondrial DNA, they are added to the eighth position of the guanine molecule to form C8-hydroxyguanosine (8-OHGua), 8-OHdG, and 8-oxo-7,8-dihydro-2'0deoxyguanosine (8-oxodG). The hydroxylation of guanine by ROSs leads to the misreading of the modified base, and repair is performed by the cell for survival.[69] In both nuclear and mitochondrial DNA, 8-OHdG is produced as a result of oxidative damage and has been used as a urinary marker for oxidative stress, carcinogenesis, and degenerative diseases.[70] 8-OHdG is found in many tissues in the body and is released into the urine during DNA repair.

Evidence of oxidative damage can also be provided by the presence of malondialdehyde, a byproduct of lipid peroxidation.

BIOTRANSFORMATION AND OXIDATIVE STRESS

The liver protects the body from potential toxic damage via a two-phase detoxification process. During phase I, cytochrome P450 enzymes catalyze the oxidation, reduction, hydrolysis, hydration, or dehalogenation of substances, creating more polar and therefore less lipid-soluble intermediary metabolites for final processing in phase II. The broad substrate specificity of these enzymes allows the liver to handle a wide range of chemical exposure. Phase II uses conjugation reactions (e.g., sulfation, glucuronidation, acetylation, methylation, amino acid conjugation, GSH conjugation) to convert intermediary metabolites into more water-soluble metabolites, which can then be excreted from the body.

In addition to the oxidative metabolites produced by normal biochemical functioning, higher levels of ROSs are produced when inflammation is present.[71,72] Accumulation of intrahepatic fatty acids can promote the formation of reactive oxygen intermediates, which in turn can directly impair liver function or act indirectly by perpetuating the inflammatory response.[73]

Variations in genetics, dietary factors, and nutrient cofactors all affect an individual's ability to metabolize chemicals effectively and efficiently.[74] Although there are 57 genes for cytochrome enzymes, 10 to 15 cytochromes carry out the metabolism for almost all xenobiotics (Box 2.1).[75] When the mixed-function oxidase system is induced, greater levels of ROSs will be produced, along with increased levels of urinary 8-OHdG.[76] Induction of cytochrome P450 enzymes (CYP450) is an epigenetic process that requires constant exposure to an inducer. CYP2E1 has emerged as an important cause of ROS overproduction, and higher hepatic CYP2E1 expression and activity may aggravate liver injury from xenobiotic compounds through the generation of harmful reactive metabolites.[77] This is perhaps most recognized in studies examining acetaminophen (APAP) toxicity. CYP2E1 is a very inducible enzyme, particularly by alcohol, with induction resulting in the bioactivation of many toxins and drugs, as well as increased ROS production. Induction combined with exposure to APAP results in the production of the more toxic metabolite N-acetyl-p-benzoquinone imine, which causes an increase in ROSs and nitrosamines,

BOX 2.1 **Human Cytochrome P450 Enzymes in Xenobiotic Metabolism**		
1A1	2C8	2E1
1A2	2C9	2F1
2A6	2C18	3A4
2A13	2C19	3A5
2B6	2D6	3A7

mitochondrial poisoning, lipid peroxidation, and covalent binding to proteins, with eventual necrosis.[78]

Several other substrates affect CYP450, leading to considerable variations in detoxification capacity. 3-methylcholanthrene and other polycyclic aromatic hydrocarbons (PAHs) from combustion induce the entire 1A series (e.g., CYP1A1, 1A2, 1B1), suggesting that all persons living in an urban area with vehicular exhaust will be induced. In addition to the 1A series, PAHs, including benzopyrene from vehicular exhaust, and tobacco smoke will induce CYP3A4. The drugs hydrocortisone and carbamazepine both produce a dose-dependent increase in CYP3A4 activation.[79] Grapefruit juice, azole antifungals, HIV antivirals, and *Zingiber* (ginger) compounds all significantly inhibit CYP3A4,[80] whereas St. John's wort is a well-known inducer of CYP3A4.[81] CYP induction and inhibition by flavonoids appears to be concentrated in the small intestine rather than the liver.[82,83] In this regard, the flavonoid compounds affect drug uptake far more than drug half-life. Steroid hormones like pregnenolone and dehydroepiandrosterone (DHEA), along with the dioxin 2,3,7,8-tetrachlorodibenzo-p-dioxin (TCDD) will all induce CYP1A1. Interestingly, genistein from soy can block the TCDD-elicited induction of CYP1A1.[84] Drinking alcohol and having type 2 diabetes are both associated with an induction of CYP2E1,[85] and the common morning beverage, coffee, is a fantastic inducer of CYP1A2—in those with the right genetics.

Phase II enzymes are generally much less inducible than phase I. However, a deficit in phase II is often responsible for the accumulation of reactive intermediates. For example, increases in ROSs resulting from low levels of GSH and/or GSH S-transferase are associated with chronic exposure to chemical toxins and alcohol, cadmium exposure, HIV/AIDS, Parkinson's disease, and other neurodegenerative disorders.[86] Quinone reductase detoxifies quinones produced by phase I enzymes, auto exhaust, cigarette smoke, and burned organic materials. Higher enzyme activity resulting from NQO2 gene promoter polymorphisms increases production of ROSs and increases the risk of Parkinson's disease.[87] Methylation of oxygen atoms often inactivates bioactive carboxylates, phenols, or alcohols. Inhibition of methylation enzymes by S-adenosyl-l-homocysteine leads to a buildup of intermediates and radicals, which causes damage to the cardiovascular and central nervous systems.[88]

Because most toxins are metabolized through a combination of phase I and phase II activities, the relationship and balance between the phases is important in determining toxicity. Clinically, the worst situation occurs when phase I is induced, producing more highly reactive intermediates, and phase II conjugation is impaired by genetic factors, nutrient deficiencies, or the conjugating molecule being depleted.

Detoxification and biotransformation are discussed more fully in Chapter 56.

CLINICAL SIGNIFICANCE

Carcinogenesis

Oxidative damage has been associated with the development, progression, and monitoring of several mutagenic and carcinogenic processes. Despite countermeasures enacted by antioxidant mechanisms and repair enzymes, excess generation of ROSs has been shown to induce irreversible damage to a variety of macromolecular components that results in genomic alterations, potentiating a carcinogenic state.[89] Oxidative stress–induced mutations (e.g., point mutations, deletions, insertions, chromosomal translocations) are known to upregulate oncogenes and downregulate tumor-suppressor genes.[90] Chronic inflammation is associated with an increased risk of cancer through production of proinflammatory cytokines and diverse reactive oxygen/nitrogen species, which activates signaling molecules involved in carcinogenesis such as NF-κβ, inducible nitric oxide synthase, and COX-2.[91]

Elevated 8-OHdG levels are found in breast cancer patients and are believed to be predictive of breast cancer risk.[92,93,94] However, urinary F2-isoprostane levels may be a better marker for breast cancer.[95] Higher urinary levels of 8-OHdG are found in men with prostate cancer, and men treated with hormonal therapy for prostate cancer have reduced 8-OHdG levels.[96] Another study found that after 3 weeks of daily consumption of tomato sauce on pasta (providing 30 mg of lycopene, a potent antioxidant, daily), the 8-OHdG levels dropped significantly.[97] 8-OHdG may also be a valuable marker for several other cancers, including cervical cancer,[98] ovarian cancer,[99] non–small cell lung cancer,[100,101] nasopharyngeal cancers,[102] acute myeloid leukemia,[103] gastric adenocarcinoma,[104] and bladder cancer.[105]

Cardiovascular Disease

NADPH oxidase, xanthine oxidase, uncoupled endothelial nitric oxide synthase, and the mitochondrial electron transport chain all produce ROSs in the vascular wall.[106] ROSs promote cell proliferation in atherosclerosis, oxidation of LDL, early plaque formation, and endothelial dysfunction.[107] Persons with coronary artery disease have higher 8-OHdG levels, and increasing 8-OHdG levels are positively correlated with disease progression.[108] Oxidative damage markers are also higher in persons who have had an acute myocardial infarction, a stroke,[109] and/or congestive heart failure.[110] Carotid artery intima media thickness, a marker for atherosclerosis, is positively associated with plasma levels of 8-OHdG.[111] These levels are also significantly correlated with the New York Heart Association functional class of congestive heart failure.[112]

Diabetes and Hyperglycemia

Oxidative stress can play a key role in the pathogenesis of diabetes. Hyperglycemia leads to increased production of ROSs by glucose oxidation, activation of NADPH-oxidase, and stimulation of the polyol pathway.[113] Elevated levels of blood sugar lead to increased levels of 8-OHdG.[114] Higher levels are found in persons with metabolic syndrome,[115] and in those with diabetes, the highest levels are found in individuals with diabetic retinopathy.[116] In hyperglycemic environments, advanced glycation end products increase cytosolic ROSs facilitating the production of mitochondrial superoxide and aggravating diabetic nephropathy.[117] It is hypothesized that in diabetic complications the excessive generation of mitochondrial superoxide, which creates a state of redox imbalance, is the primary initiating event that activates all other pathways of tissue damage.[118]

Musculoskeletal

Oxidative stress is a significant cause of chondrocyte dysfunction and articular cartilage degradation, which leads to the pathogenesis of osteoarthritis and cartilage aging. Free radicals damage hyaluronic acid and degrade the joint cartilage by attacking its proteoglycan and inhibiting its synthesis.[119]

Neurological

Oxidative stress from pesticides, air pollution, tobacco smoke, radiation, toxic metals, and dietary factors has been associated with neurodegenerative diseases.[120] Beta-amyloid, the peptide that constitutes the central core of senile plaques in the brains of Alzheimer's disease patients, is associated with free radical oxidative stress and is toxic to neurons.[121] Oxidative damage combined with an inhibition of antioxidant enzymes may play a significant role in neurodegenerative disease. For example, in Parkinson's disease, although the brain may be able to withstand the effects of individual chemicals toxic to the dopaminergic system, multiple chemicals targeting numerous sites compromise oxidative defense mechanisms and result in neuronal death.[122]

INTERVENTION

Antioxidants—Vitamin C and E

Antioxidants are essential components in the treatment and prevention of oxidative damage. Antioxidants protect the liver from damage, support detoxification processes, and counteract oxidative stress by reducing the formation of free radicals. Dark-colored fruits and vegetables are rich sources of antioxidants, as are several vitamins, minerals, and nutraceuticals.

Antioxidants such as vitamin C and vitamin E (daily dosages of which are 500 mg and 400 IU, respectively) have been shown to protect women smokers from DNA damage,[123] and epicatechins have been shown in mucosal cell cultures to protect against cigarette smoke oxidative DNA damage.[124]

Vitamin E is a combination of eight different fat-soluble compounds: tocopherols (e.g., alpha, beta, gamma, and delta) and tocotrienols. Tocopherols tend to be more biologically active, with alpha-tocopherol being the most active of the group. The primary function of vitamin E is to scavenge free radicals, thereby protecting the body from oxidative damage.[125] Healthy individuals who consumed a balanced diet that supplied adequate vitamin E amounts had decreased oxidative damage when supplemented with vitamin E at 10 times the recommended daily allowance (RDA).[126] Vitamin E supplementation has been shown to enhance immunity,[127] help protect low-density lipoprotein (LDL) from oxidative damage,[128] repair membranes,[129] and decrease platelet aggregation and blood clot formation.[130]

Animal studies have evaluated the benefits of antioxidants after exposure of rats to permethrin. Treatment with 200 mg/kg of vitamins E and C protected erythrocytes against plasma membrane lipid peroxidation and maintained the activity of GSH peroxidase.[131] Vitamin E plus coenzyme Q10 reversed the negative effect of permethrin on the central nervous system, restoring plasma membrane fluidity and preserving GSH levels.[132]

Glutathione

Nutrients that boost GSH are of critical importance in the treatment and prevention of oxidative damage. GSH is the major endogenous antioxidant produced by the cells and participates directly in the neutralization of free radicals. It is involved in metabolic and biochemical reactions such as DNA synthesis and repair, protein synthesis, prostaglandin synthesis, amino acid transport, and enzyme activation. GSH, therefore, affects every system in the body, especially the nervous, gastrointestinal, immune, and respiratory systems. GSH levels decline as conjugation reactions exceed the cells' ability to regenerate GSH. Chemicals such as polychlorinated biphenyls (PCBs) and organochlorine pesticides increase oxidative damage and deplete GSH levels.[133] If GSH is depleted, *de novo* synthesis of GSH is upregulated, as is cysteine synthesis.[134] GSH levels can be increased through supplementation with NAC,[135] whey protein powder,[136] alpha-lipoic acid,[137] S-adenosyl L-methionine (SAMe),[138] *Silybum marianum* (milk thistle); meditation[139]; exercise[140]; and/or direct administration of GSH via IV,[141] nebulized, topical, or intranasal route.[142]

NAC is a precursor to GSH and exhibits direct antioxidant benefits. Studies demonstrate that NAC is effective at attenuating oxidative damage by increasing the activities of superoxide dismutase (SOD), CAT, and glutathione-s-transferase (GST), and by decreasing GSH depletion and MDA levels.[143,144] Polychlorinated-biphenyl–induced oxidative stress and cytotoxicity in cell lines can be mitigated by NAC.[145] Magnesium is necessary for both steps in *de novo* GSH synthesis, and a deficiency of magnesium is associated with low GSH levels[146] whereas magnesium supplementation increases GSH.[147] The use of liposomal GSH supplementation has proven highly effective in humans to increase GSH levels and rebalance cytokine levels.[148]

Resveratrol

Cotreatment of human bronchial epithelial cells with resveratrol protects against arsenic-induced oxidative damage by reducing the levels of ROSs, reducing chromosomal and DNA damage, reducing cell apoptosis, and elevating the concentration of GSH.[149]

Resveratrol has also shown a genoprotective effect from permethrin-induced oxidative damage, as demonstrated by diminishing indices on chromosome aberrations and sister chromatid exchange tests.[150]

Curcumin

Curcumin upregulates several phase II enzymes, including GST, and downregulates some phase I enzymes associated with carcinogenic toxicity.[151] Curcumin protects against cardiovascular dysfunction resulting from oxidative stress associated with cadmium exposure through free radical scavenging, metal chelation, regulation of inflammatory enzymes, and increasing nitric oxide (NO+).[152,153] In human cells, curcumin protects against DNA damage from PAHs,[154] protects against arsenic toxicity, prevents DNA damage, and enhances DNA repair enzymes against arsenic-induced damage.[155]

Mediterranean Diet

Persons with metabolic syndrome who switched to a Mediterranean diet were rewarded with a reduction in their F2-isoprostane and 8-OHdG levels.[156] A diet high in polyphenols has demonstrated effectiveness at lowering 8-OHdG levels.[157] The consumption of brassica family vegetables and flavonoid-containing botanicals, like ginkgo biloba and green tea, has also demonstrated clear anti-oxidant benefit.[158,159]

Quercetin

Onions, which are a major component in Mediterranean diets are the food source with the highest levels of the flavonoid quercetin. In animal studies, quercetin inhibits leukocyte recruitment, TNF-α and IL-1β production, superoxide anion production, decrease of antioxidant levels, and NF-$\kappa\beta$ activation.[160] Quercetin can lower 8-OHdG levels and decrease oxidative stress, even in the face of methylmercury.[161] Quercetin also inhibits histamine release from mast cells and basophils when stimulated by antigens,[162] phospholipase A_2 in neutrophils, lipoxygenase, anaphylactic contractions of smooth muscle, and biosynthesis of slow reacting substance of anaphylaxis.[163] Quercetin has been shown in animal studies to protect against the oxidative stress induced by dioxins and enhances the protective effects of beta-carotene on DNA from PAHs.[164,165] In human cell lines, epigallocatechin gallate (EGCG) and quercetin protect against DNA damage from PCBs.[166]

Melatonin

Melatonin has been shown to be a potent free-radical scavenger and antioxidant. Melatonin reverses mercury-induced oxidative tissue damage by increasing GSH levels and decreasing myeloperoxidase activity, the latter of which can serve as an index of neutrophil infiltration.[167] Melatonin also eliminates the deleterious effects of a high-salt diet on the kidneys via direct antioxidative effects.[168] In rats with renal ablation, melatonin reduced oxidative stress, hypertension, and inflammation.[169]

Ginger

There is ample animal research showing that *Zingiber officinale* (ginger) has protective effects on tissues exposed to toxic compounds and oxidative damage. Ginger specifically increases activity of kidney antioxidant enzymes in obese and diabetic rats.[170] The antiinflammatory benefits of ginger result from its antioxidant properties and the epigenetic downregulation of proinflammatory genes.[171]

Lycopene, Olive Leaf Extract, and Other Factors

Lycopene, another common component in Mediterranean diets, neutralizes the decreased antioxidant enzyme activity and increased ROS formation caused by organophosphate (OP) toxicity.[172,173] After permethrin exposure, olive leaf extract has shown genoprotective effects via inhibition of oxidative stress and scavenging of free radicals.[174,175] Ellagic acid,[176] propolis,[177,178] boron,[179] vitamin C,[180,181] vitamin E combined with selenium,[182] and vitamin E combined with curcumin have also shown protective effects against OP-induced oxidative stress.[183]

REFERENCES

1. Pilger, A., & Rüdiger, H. W. (2006). 8-Hydroxy-2'-deoxyguanosine as a marker of oxidative DNA damage related to occupational and environmental exposures. *International Archives of Occupational and Environmental Health*, 80(1), 1–15. PubMed PMID:16685565.
2. Broedbaek, K., Ribel-Madsen, R., Henriksen, T., Weimann, A., Petersen, M., Andersen, J. T., et al. (2011). Genetic and environmental influences on oxidative damage assessed in elderly Danish twins. *Free Radical Biology & Medicine*, 50(11), 1488–1491. PubMed PMID: 21354303.
3. Poyton, R. O., Castello, P. R., Ball, K. A., Woo, D. K., & Pan, N. (2009). Mitochondria and hypoxic signaling: A new view. *Annals of the New York Academy of Sciences*, 1177, 48–56. PubMed PMID: 19845606.
4. Hitchon, C. A., & El-Gabalawy, H. S. (2004). Oxidation in rheumatoid arthritis. *Arthritis Research and Therapy*, 6(6), 265–278. PubMed PMID: 15535839.
5. Cuzzocrea, S. (2006). Role of nitric oxide and reactive oxygen species in arthritis. *Current Pharmaceutical Design*, 12(27), 3551–3570. PubMed PMID: 17017948.
6. Klaunig, J. E., & Kamendulis, L. M. (2004). The role of oxidative stress in carcinogenesis. *Annual Review of Pharmacology and Toxicology*, 44, 239–267. PubMed PMID: 14744246.
7. Mastaloudis, A., Leonard, S. W., & Traber, M. G. (2001). Oxidative stress in athletes during extreme endurance exercise. *Free Radical Biology & Medicine*, 31, 911–922. PubMed PMID: 11585710.
8. Poulsen, H. E., Loft, S., & Visitsen, K. (1996). Extreme exercise and oxidative DNA modification. *Journal of Sports Sciences*, 14, 343–346. PubMed PMID 8887214.
9. Lin, T. S., Wu, C. C., Wu, J. D., & Wei, C. H. (2012). Oxidative DNA damage estimated by urinary 8-hydroxy-2'-deoxyguanosine and arsenic in glass production workers. *Toxicology and Industrial Health*, 28(6), 513–521. PubMed PMID: 22033425.
10. Huang, M., Choi, S. J., Kim, D. W., Kim, N. Y., Park, C. H., et al. (2009). Risk assessment of low-level cadmium and arsenic on the kidney. *Journal of Toxicology and Environmental Health. Part A*, 72(21–22), 1493–1498. PubMed PMID: 20077223.
11. Mikhailova, M. V., Littlefield, N. A., Hass, B. S., Poirier, L. A., & Chou, M. W. (1997). Cadmium-induced 8-hydroxydeoxyguanosine formation, DNA strand breaks and antioxidant enzyme activities in lymphoblastoid cells. *Cancer Letters*, 115(2), 141–148. PubMed PMID: 9149117.
12. Chen, C., Qu, L., Li, B., Xing, L., Jia, G., et al. (2005). Increased oxidative DNA damage, as assessed by urinary 8-hydroxy-2'-deoxyguanosine concentrations, and serum redox status in persons exposed to mercury. *Clinical Chemistry*, 51(4), 759–767. PubMed PMID: 15695327.
13. Hong, Y. C., Oh, S. Y., Kwon, S. O., Park, M. S., Kim, H., Leem, J. H., et al. (2013). Blood lead level modifies the association between dietary antioxidants and oxidative stress in an urban adult population. *The British Journal of Nutrition*, 109(1), 148–154. PubMed PMID: 22464667.
14. Bolin, C. M., Basha, R., Cox, D., Zawia, N. H., Maloney, B., Lahiri, D. K., et al. (2006). Exposure to lead and the developmental origin of oxidative DNA damage in the aging brain. *FASEB Journal*, 20(6), 788–790. PMID: 16484331.
15. Valko, M., Morris, H., & Cronin, M. T. (2005). Metals, toxicity and oxidative stress. *Current Medicinal Chemistry*, 12(10), 1161–1208. PubMed PMID: 15892631.
16. Bertin, G., & Averbeck, D. (2006). Cadmium: Cellular effects, modifications of biomolecules, modulation of DNA repair and genotoxic consequences (a review). *Biochimie*, 88(11), 1549–1559. PubMed PMID: 17070979.

17. Yang, C., & Frenkel, K. (2002). Arsenic-mediated cellular signal transduction, transcription factor activation, and aberrant gene expression: Implications in carcinogenesis. *Journal of Environmental Pathology, Toxicology and Oncology, 21*(4), 331–342. PubMed PMID: 12510962.

18. Ding, G., Han, S., Wang, P., Gao, Y., Shi, R., Wang, G., et al. (2012). Increased levels of 8-hydroxy-2'-deoxyguanosine are attributable to organophosphate pesticide exposure among young children. *Environmental Pollution, 167*, 110–114. PubMed PMID: 22561897.

19. Atherton, K. M., Williams, F. M., Egea González, F. J., Glass, R., Rushton, S., Blain, P. G., et al. (2009). DNA damage in horticultural farmers: A pilot study showing an association with organophosphate pesticide exposure. *Biomarkers: Biochemical Indicators of Exposure, Response, and Susceptibility to Chemicals, 14*(7), 443–451. PubMed PMID: 19863182.

20. Durak, D., Uzun, F. G., et al. (2009). Malathion-induced oxidative stress in human erythrocytes and the protective effect of vitamins C and E in vitro. *Environmental Toxicology, 24*(3), 235–242. PubMed PMID: 18655177.

21. Delgado, E. H., Streck, E. L., et al. (2006). Mitochondrial respiratory dysfunction and oxidative stress after chronic malathion exposure. *Neurochemical Research, 31*(8), 1021–1025. PubMed PMID: 16865556.

22. Lee, K. M., Park, S. Y., et al. (2017). Pesticide metabolite and oxidative stress in male farmers exposed to pesticide. *Annals of Occupational and Environmental Medicine, 29*, 5. PubMed PMID: 28265414.

23. Gabbianelli, R., Falcioni, M. L., Nasuti, C., Cantalamessa, F., Imada, I., & Inoue, M. (2009). Effect of permethrin insecticide on rat polymorphonuclear neutrophils. *Chemico-Biological Interactions, 182*(2–3), 245–252. PubMed PMID: 19772857.

24. Vontas, J. G., Small, G. J., & Hemingway, J. (2001). Glutathione S-transferases as antioxidant defence agents confer pyrethroid resistance in Nilaparvata lugens. *The Biochemical Journal, 357*(Pt. 1), 65–72. PubMed PMID: 11415437.

25. Harri, M., Svoboda, P., Mori, T., Mutanen, P., Kasai, H., & Savela, K. (2005). Analysis of 8-hydroxydeoxyguanosine among workers exposed to diesel particulate exhaust: Comparison with urinary metabolites and PAH air monitoring. *Free Radical Research, 39*(9), 963–972. PubMed PMID: 16087477.

26. Kuusimäki, L., Peltonen, Y., Mutanen, P., Peltonen, K., & Savela, K. (2004). Urinary hydroxy-metabolites of naphthalene, phenanthrene and pyrene as markers of exposure to diesel exhaust. *International Archives of Occupational and Environmental Health, 77*(1), 23–30. PubMed PMID: 14564527.

27. Lai, C. H., Liou, S. H., Lin, H. C., Shih, T. S., Tsai, P. J., Chen, J. S., et al. (2005). Exposure to traffic exhausts and oxidative DNA damage. *Occupational and Environmental Medicine, 62*(4), 216–222. PubMed PMID: 15778253.

28. Prasad, S. B., Vidyullatha, P., Vani, G. T., Devi, R. P., Rani, U. P., Reddy, P. P., et al. (2013). Association of gene polymorphism in detoxification enzymes and urinary 8-OHdG levels in traffic policemen exposed to vehicular exhaust. *Inhalation Toxicology, 25*(1), 1–8. PubMed PMID: 23293967.

29. Kim, J. Y., Mukherjee, S., Ngo, L. C., & Christiani, D. C. (2004). Urinary 8-hydroxy-2'-deoxyguanosine as a biomarker of oxidative DNA damage in workers exposed to fine particulates. *Environmental Health Perspectives, 112*(6), 666–671. PubMed PMID: 15121508.

30. Song, S., Paek, D., Park, C., Lee, C., Lee, J. H., & Yu, S. D. (2013). Exposure to ambient ultrafine particles and urinary 8-hydroxyl-2-deoxyguanosine in children with and without eczema. *The Science of the Total Environment, 458-460*, 408–413. PubMed PMID: 23685365.

31. Frikke-Schmidt, H., Roursgaard, M., Lykkesfeldt, J., Loft, S., Nøjgaard, J. K., & Møller, P. (2011). Effect of vitamin C and iron chelation on diesel exhaust particle and carbon black induced oxidative damage and cell adhesion molecule expression in human endothelial cells. *Toxicology Letters, 203*(3), 181–189. PubMed PMID: 21421028.

32. Harrison, C. M., Pompilius, M., Pinkerton, K. E., & Ballinger, S. W. (2011). Mitochondrial oxidative stress significantly influences atherogenic risk and cytokine-induced oxidant production. *Environmental Health Perspectives, 119*(5), 676–681. PubMed PMID: 21169125.

33. Zhang, P., Dong, G., Sun, B., Zhang, L., Chen, X., Ma, N., et al. (2011). Long-term exposure to ambient air pollution and mortality due to cardiovascular disease and cerebrovascular disease in Shenyang, China. *PLoS ONE, 6*(6), e20827. PubMed PMID: 21695220.

34. Ito, K., Mathes, R., Ross, Z., Nadas, A., Thurston, G., & Matte, T. (2011). Fine particulate matter constituents associated with cardiovascular hospitalizations and mortality in New York City. *Environmental Health Perspectives, 119*, 467–473. PubMed PMID: 21463978.

35. Oh, S. M., Kim, H. R., Park, Y. J., Lee, S. Y., & Chung, K. H. (2011). Organic extracts of urban air pollution

particulate matter (PM2.5)-induced genotoxicity and oxidative stress in human lung bronchial epithelial cells (BEAS-2B cells). *Mutation Research*, *723*(2), 142–151. PubMed PMID: 21524716.

36. Guaita, R., Pichiule, M., Maté, T., Linares, C., & Díaz, J. (2011). Short-term impact of particulate matter (PM(2.5)) on respiratory mortality in Madrid. *International Journal of Environmental Health Research*, *21*(4), 260–274. PubMed PMID: 21644129.

37. Katanoda, K., Sobue, T., Satoh, H., Tajima, K., Suzuki, T., Nakatsuka, H., et al. (2011). An association between long-term exposure to ambient air pollution and mortality from lung cancer and respiratory diseases in Japan. *Journal of Epidemiology*, *21*(2), 132–143. PubMed PMID: 21325732.

38. Servais, S., Boussouar, A., Molnar, A., Douki, T., Pequignot, J. M., & Favier, R. (2005). Age-related sensitivity to lung oxidative stress during ozone exposure. *Free Radical Research*, *39*(3), 305–316. PubMed PMID: 15788235.

39. Lu, C. Y., Ma, Y. C., Lin, J. M., Li, C. Y., Lin, R. S., & Sung, F. C. (2007). Oxidative stress associated with indoor air pollution and sick building syndrome-related symptoms among office workers in Taiwan. *Inhalation Toxicology*, *19*(1), 57–65. PubMed PMID: 17127643.

40. Commodore, A. A., Zhang, J. J., Chang, Y., Hartinger, S. M., Lanata, C. F., Mäusezahl, D., et al. (2013). Concentrations of urinary 8-hydroxy-2'-deoxyguanosine and 8-isoprostane in women exposed to woodsmoke in a cookstove intervention study in San Marcos, Peru. *Environment International*, *60*, 112–122. PubMed PMID: 24041735.

41. Marczynski, B., Kraus, T., Rozynek, P., Raithel, H. J., & Baur, X. (2000). Association between 8-hydroxy-2'-deoxyguanosine levels in DNA of workers highly exposed to asbestos and their clinical data, occupational and non-occupational confounding factors, and cancer. *Mutation Research*, *468*(2), 203–212. PubMed PMID: 10882897.

42. Yoshida, R., Ogawa, Y., Shioji, I., Yu, X., Shibata, E., Mori, I., et al. (2001). Urinary 8-oxo-7, 8-dihydro-2'-deoxyguanosine and biopyrrins levels among construction workers with asbestos exposure history. *Industrial Health*, *39*(2), 186–188. PubMed PMID: 11341550.

43. Ghosh, R., Alajbegovic, A., & Gomes, A. V. (2015). NSAIDs and cardiovascular diseases: Role of reactive oxygen species. *Oxidative Medicine and Cellular Longevity*, *468*, 536962. PubMed PMID: 26457127.

44. Mason, R. P., Walter, M. F., McNulty, H. P., et al. (2006). Rofecoxib increases susceptibility of human LDL and membrane lipids to oxidative damage: A mechanism of cardiotoxicity. *Journal of Cardiovascular Pharmacology*, *47*(Suppl. 1), S7–S14. PubMed PMID: 16785833.

45. Yoshida, M., Shiojima, I., et al. (2009). Chronic doxorubicin cardiotoxicity is mediated by oxidative DNA damage-ATM-p53-apoptosis pathway and attenuated by pitavastatin through the inhibition of Rac1 activity. *Journal of Molecular and Cellular Cardiology*, *47*(5), 698–705. PubMed PMID: 19660469.

46. Akbar, H., Khan, A., et al. (2017). The genotoxic effect of oxcarbazepine on mice blood lymphocytes. *Drug and Chemical Toxicology*, 1–6. PubMed PMID: 28503984.

47. Araujo, I. M., Ambrosio, A. F., et al. (2004). Neurotoxicity induced by antiepileptic drugs in cultured hippocampal neurons: A comparative study between carbamazepine, oxcarbazepine drugs, BIA 2-024 and BIA 2-093. *Epilepsia*, *45*(12), 1498–1505. PubMed PMID: 15571507.

48. Leach, J. K., Van Tuyle, G., et al. (2001). Ionizing radiation-induced, mitochondria-dependent generation of reactive oxygen/nitrogen. *Cancer Research*, *61*(10), 3894–3901. PubMed PMID: 11358802.

49. Chang, F. K., Mao, I. F., Chen, M. L., & Cheng, S. F. (2011). Urinary 8-hydroxydeoxyguanosine as a biomarker of oxidative DNA damage in workers exposed to ethylbenzene. *The Annals of Occupational Hygiene*, *55*(5), 519–525. PubMed PMID: 21430133.

50. Lagorio, S., Tagesson, C., Forastiere, F., Iavarone, I., Axelson, O., & Carere, A. (1994). Exposure to benzene and 8-hydroxydeoxyguanosine, a biological marker of oxidative DNA damage. *Occupational and Environmental Medicine*, *51*, 739–741. PMID: 7849850.

51. Liu, L., Zhang, Q., Feng, J., Deng, L., Zeng, N., Yang, A., et al. (1996). The study of DNA oxidative damage in benzene-exposed workers. *Mutation Research*, *370*, 145–150. PMID: 8917660.

52. Marczynski, B., Rozynek, P., Elliehausen, H. G., Korn, M., & Baur, X. (1997). Detection of 8-hydroxydeooxyguanosine, a marker of oxidative DNA damage, in white blood cells of workers occupationally exposed to styrene. *Archives of Toxicology*, *71*, 496–500. PMID: 9248627.

53. Wu, D., & Cederbaum, A. I. (2003). Alcohol, oxidative stress, and free radical damage. *Alcohol Research and Health*, *27*(4), 277–284. PubMed PMID: 15540798.

54. Albano, E. (2006). Alcohol, oxidative stress and free radical damage. *The Proceedings of the Nutrition Society*, *65*(3), 278–290. PubMed PMID: 16923312.

55. Lieber, C. S. (1997). Role of oxidative stress and antioxidant therapy in alcoholic and nonalcoholic liver diseases. *Advances in Pharmacology, 38*, 601–628. PubMed PMID: 8895826.

56. Mena, S., Ortega, A., & Estrela, J. M. (2009). Oxidative stress in environmental-induced carcinogenesis. *Mutation Research, 674*(1–2), 36–44. PubMed PMID: 18977455.

57. Kiyosawa, H., Suko, M., Okudaira, H., Murata, K., Miyamoto, T., Chung, M. H., et al. (1990). Cigarette smoking induces formation of 8-hydroxydeoxyguanosine, one of the oxidative DNA damages in human peripheral leukocytes. *Free Radical Research Communications, 11*(1–3), 23–27. PubMed PMID: 2074046.

58. Fujihara, M., Nagai, N., Sussan, T. E., Biswal, S., & Handa, J. T. (2008). Chronic cigarette smoke causes oxidative damage and apoptosis to retinal pigmented epithelial cells in mice. *PLoS ONE, 3*(9), e3119. PubMed PMID: 18769672.

59. Howard, D. J., Ota, R. B., Briggs, L. A., Hampton, M., & Pritsos, C. A. (1998). Environmental tobacco smoke in the workplace induces oxidative stress in employees, including increased production of 8-hydroxy-2'-deoxyguanosine. *Cancer Epidemiology, Biomarkers and Prevention, 7*(2), 141–146. PubMed PMID: 9488589.

60. Loft, S., Vistisen, K., Ewertz, M., Tjonneland, A., Overvad, K., & Poulsen, H. E. (1992). Oxidative DNA damage estimated by 8-hydroxydeoxyguanosine excretion in humans: Influence of smoking, gender and body mass index. *Carcinogenesis, 13*, 2241–2247. PMID: 1473230.

61. Prieme, H., Loft, S., Klarlund, M., Gronbaek, K., Tonnesen, P., & Poulsen, H. E. (1998). Effect of smoking cessation on oxidative DNA modification estimated by 8-oxo-7,8-dihyro-2'-deoxyguanosine excretion. *Carcinogenesis, 19*, 347–351. PMID: 9498287.

62. Yano, T., Shoji, F., Baba, H., Koga, T., Shiraishi, T., Orita, H., et al. (2009). Significance of the urinary 8-OHdG level as an oxidative stress marker in lung cancer patients. *Lung Cancer (Amsterdam, Netherlands), 63*(1), 111–114. PubMed PMID: 18676055.

63. Valavanidis, A., Vlachogianni, T., & Fiotakis, C. (2009). 8-hydroxy-2'-deoxyguanosine(8-OHdG): A critical biomarker of oxidative stress and carcinogenesis. *Journal of Environmental Science and Health. Part C, Environmental Carcinogenesis & Ecotoxicology Reviews, 27*(2), 120–139. PubMed PMID: 19412858.

64. Wu, L. L., Chiou, C. C., Chang, P. Y., & Wu, J. T. (2004). Urinary 8-OHdG: A marker of oxidative stress to DNA and a risk factor for cancer, atherosclerosis and diabetics. *Clinica Chimica Acta, 339*(1–2), 1–9. PubMed PMID: 14687888.

65. Il'yasova, D., Scarbrough, P., & Spasojevic, I. (2012). Urinary biomarkers of oxidative status. *Clinica Chimica Acta, 413*(19–20), 1446–1453. PubMed PMID: 22683781.

66. Milne, G. L., Musiek, E. S., & Morrow, J. D. (2005). F2-isoprotanes as markers of oxidative stress in vivo: An overview. *Biomarkers: Biochemical Indicators of Exposure, Response, and Susceptibility to Chemicals, 1*(Suppl. 10), S10–S23. PubMed PMID: 16298907.

67. Basu, S. (2008). F2-isoprostanes in human health and diseases: From molecular mechanisms to clinical implications. *Antioxidants & Redox Signaling, 10*(8), 1405–1434. PubMed PMID: 18522490.

68. Montuschi, P., Barnes, P. J., & Roberts, L. J., 2nd. (2004). Isoprostanes: Markers and mediators of oxidative stress. *FASEB Journal, 18*(15), 1791–1800. PubMed PMID:15576482.

69. Chiou, C. C., Chang, P. Y., Chan, E. C., et al. (2003). Urinary 8-hydroxydeoxyguanosine and its analogs as DNA marker of oxidative stress: Development of an ELISA and measurement in both bladder and prostate cancers. *Clinica Chimica Acta, 334*(1–2), 87–94. PubMed PMID: 12867278.

70. Kasai, H. (1997). Analysis of a form of oxidative DNA damage, 8-hydroxy-2'-deoxyguanosine, as a marker of cellular oxidative stress during carcinogenesis. *Mutation Research, 387*(3), 147–163. PubMed PMID: 9439711.

71. Wiseman, H., & Halliwell, B. (1996). Damage to DNA by reactive oxygen and nitrogen species: Role in inflammatory disease and progression to cancer. *The Biochemical Journal, 313*(Pt. 1), 17–29. PubMed PMID: 8546679.

72. Roselló-Lletí, E., de Burgos, F. G., Morillas, P., Cortés, R., Martínez-Dolz, L., Almenar, M., et al. (2012). Impact of cardiovascular risk factors and inflammatory status on urinary 8-OHdG in essential hypertension. *American Journal of Hypertension, 25*(2), 236–242. PubMed PMID: 22052073.

73. Gentile, C. L., & Pagliassotti, M. J. (2008). The role of fatty acids in the development and progression of nonalcoholic fatty liver disease. *The Journal of Nutritional Biochemistry, 19*(9), 567–576. PubMed PMID: 18430557.

74. Desta, Z., Zhao, X., et al. (2002). Clinical significance of the cytochrome P450 2C19 genetic polymorphism. *Clinical Pharmacokinetics, 41*(12), 913–958. PubMed PMID: 12222994.

75. Guengerich, F. P. (2008). Cytochrome p450 and chemical toxicology. *Chemical Research in Toxicology*, *21*(1), 70–83. PubMed PMID: 18052394.

76. Yuan, J., Lu, W. Q., Zou, Y. L., Wei, W., Zhang, C., Xie, H., et al. (2009). Influence of aroclor 1254 on benzo(a) pyrene-induced DNA breakage, oxidative DNA damage, and cytochrome P4501A activity in human hepatoma cell line. *Environmental Toxicology*, *24*(4), 327–333. PubMed PMID: 18767135.

77. Aubert, J., Begriche, K., et al. (2011). Increased expression of cytochrome P450 2E1 in nonalcoholic fatty liver disease: Mechanisms and pathophysiological role. *Clinics and Research in Hepatology and Gastroenterology*, *35*(10), 630–637. PubMed PMID: 21664213.

78. Larson, A. M. (2007). Acetaminophen hepatotoxicity. *Clinics in Liver Disease*, *11*(3), 525–548. PubMed PMID: 17723918.

79. El-Sankary, W., Plant, N. J., Gibson, G. G., & Moor, D. J. (2000). Regulation of the CYP3A4 gene by hydrocortisone and xenobiotics: Role of the glucocorticoid and pregnane X receptors. *Drug Metabolism and Disposition: The Biological Fate of Chemicals*, *28*(5), 493–496. PubMed PMID: 10772626.

80. Pelkonen, O., Turpeinen, M., et al. (2008). Inhibition and induction of human cytochrome P450 enzymes: Current status. *Archives of Toxicology*, *82*(10), 667–715. PubMed PMID: 18618097.

81. Di, Y. M., Li, C. G., Xue, C. C., & Zhou, S. F. (2008). Clinical drugs that interact with St. John's Wort and implication in drug development. *Current Pharmaceutical Design*, *14*(17), 1723–1742. PubMed PMID: 18673195.

82. Hanley, M. J., Cancalon, P., Widmer, W. W., & Greenblatt, D. J. (2011). The effect of grapefruit juice on drug disposition. *Expert Opinion on Drug Metabolism and Toxicology*, *7*(3), 267–286. PubMed PMID: 21254874.

83. Veronese, M. L., Gillen, L. P., Burke, J. P., et al. (2003). Exposure-dependent inhibition of intestinal and hepatic CYP3A4 in vivo by grapefruit juice. *Journal of Clinical Pharmacology*, *43*(8), 831–839. PubMed PMID: 12953340.

84. Hukkanen, J., Lassila, A., Paivarinta, K., Valanne, S., Sarpo, S., Hakkola, J., et al. (2000). Induction and regulation of xenobiotic-metabolizing cytochrome P450s in the human A549 lung adenocarcinoma cell line. *American Journal of Respiratory Cell and Molecular Biology*, *22*(3), 360–366. PubMed PMID: 1069073.

85. Hannon-Fletcher, M., O'Kane, M., Moles, K., Barnett, Y., & Barnett, C. (2001). Lymphocyte cytochrome P450-CYP2E1 expression in human IDDM subjects. *Food and Chemical Toxicology*, *39*, 125–132. PubMed PMID: 11267705.

86. Townsend, D. M., Tew, K. D., & Tapiero, H. (2003). The importance of glutathione in human disease. *Biomedicine & Pharmacotherapy*, *57*(3–4), 145–155. PubMed PMID: 12818476.

87. Wang, W., Le, W. D., Pan, T., et al. (2008). Association of NRH: Quinone oxidoreductase 2 gene promoter polymorphism with higher gene expression and increased susceptibility to Parkinson's disease. *The Journals of Gerontology. Series A, Biological Sciences and Medical Sciences*, *63*(2), 127–134. PubMed PMID: 18314446.

88. Zhu, B. T. (2002). Catechol-O-Methyltransferase (COMT)-mediated methylation metabolism of endogenous bioactive catechols and modulation by endobiotics and xenobiotics: Importance in pathophysiology and pathogenesis. *Current Drug Metabolism*, *3*(3), 321–349. PubMed PMID: 12083324.

89. Nakabeppu, Y. (2001). Regulation of intracellular localization of human MTH1, OGG1, and MYH proteins for repair of oxidative DNA damage. *Progress in Nucleic Acid Research and Molecular Biology*, *68*, 75–94. PubMed PMID: 11554314.

90. Ohshima, H., Tatemichi, M., & Sawa, T. (2003). Chemical basis of inflammation-induced carcinogenesis. *Archives of Biochemistry and Biophysics*, *417*(1), 3–11. PubMed PMID: 1291773.

91. Ohshima, H., Tazawa, H., et al. (2005). Prevention of human cancer by modulation of chronic inflammatory processes. *Mutation Research*, *591*(1–2), 110–122. PubMed PMID: 16083916.

92. Pande, D., Negi, R., Karki, K., Khanna, S., Khanna, R. S., & Khanna, H. D. (2012). Oxidative damage markers as possible discriminatory biomarkers in breast carcinoma. *Translational Research*, *160*(6), 411–418. PubMed PMID: 22885175.

93. Li, D., Zhang, W., Zhu, J., Chang, P., Sahin, A., Singletary, E., et al. (2001). Oxidative DNA damage and 8-hydroxy-2-deoxyguanosine DNA glycosylase/ apurinic lyase in human breast cancer. *Molecular Carcinogenesis*, *31*(4), 214–223. PubMed PMID: 11536371.

94. Musarrat, J., Arezina-Wilson, J., & Wani, A. A. (1996). Prognostic and aetiological relevance of 8-hydroxyguanosine in human breast carcinogenesis. *European Journal of Cancer*, *32A*(7), 1209–1214. PubMed PMID: 8758255.

95. Rossner, P., Jr., Gammon, M. D., Terry, M. B., Agrawal, M., Zhang, F. F., Teitelbaum, S. L., et al. (2006). Relationship between urinary 15-F2t-isoprostane and

8-oxodeoxyguanosine levels and breast cancer risk. *Cancer Epidemiology, Biomarkers and Prevention, 15*(4), 639–644. PubMed PMID: 16614103.

96. Miyake, H., Hara, I., Kamidono, S., & Eto, H. (2004). Oxidative DNA damage in patients with prostate cancer and its response to treatment. *The Journal of Urology, 171*(4), 1533–1536. PubMed PMID: 15017214.

97. Chen, L., Stacewicz-Sapuntzakis, M., Duncan, C., Sharifi, R., Ghosh, L., van Breemen, R., et al. (2001). Oxidative DNA damage in prostate cancer patients consuming tomato sauce-based entrees as a whole-food intervention. *Journal of the National Cancer Institute, 93*(24), 1872–1879. PubMed PMID: 11752012.

98. Romano, G., Sgambato, A., Mancini, R., Capelli, G., Giovagnoli, M. R., Flamini, G., et al. (2000). 8-hydroxy-2'-deoxyguanosine in cervical cells: Correlation with grade of dysplasia and human papillomavirus infection. *Carcinogenesis, 21*(6), 1143–1147. PubMed PMID: 10837002.

99. Pylväs, M., Puistola, U., Laatio, L., Kauppila, S., & Karihtala, P. (2011). Elevated serum 8-OHdG is associated with poor prognosis in epithelial ovarian cancer. *Anticancer Research, 31*(4), 1411–1415. PubMed PMID: 21508394.

100. Peddireddy, V., Siva Prasad, B., Gundimeda, S. D., Penagaluru, P. R., & Mundluru, H. P. (2012). Assessment of 8-oxo-7, 8-dihydro-2'-deoxyguanosine and malondialdehyde levels as oxidative stress markers and antioxidant status in non-small cell lung cancer. *Biomarkers: Biochemical Indicators of Exposure, Response, and Susceptibility to Chemicals, 17*(3), 261–268. PubMed PMID: 22397584.

101. Caliṣkan-Can, E., Firat, H., Ardiç, S., Simṣek, B., Torun, M., & Yardim-Akaydin, S. (2008). Increased levels of 8-hydroxydeoxyguanosine and its relationship with lipid peroxidation and antioxidant vitamins in lung cancer. *Clinical Chemistry and Laboratory Medicine, 46*(1), 107–112. PubMed PMID: 18194082.

102. Huang, Y. J., Zhang, B. B., Ma, N., Murata, M., Tang, A. Z., & Huang, G. W. (2011). Nitrative and oxidative DNA damage as potential survival biomarkers for nasopharyngeal carcinoma. *Medical Oncology, 28*(1), 377–384. PubMed PMID: 20339958.

103. Zhou, F. L., Zhang, W. G., Wei, Y. C., Meng, S., Bai, G. G., Wang, B. Y., et al. (2010). Involvement of oxidative stress in the relapse of acute myeloid leukemia. *The Journal of Biological Chemistry, 285*(20), 15010–15015. PubMed PMID: 20233720.

104. Chang, C. S., Chen, W. N., Lin, H. H., Wu, C. C., & Wang, C. J. (2004). Increased oxidative DNA damage, inducible nitric oxide synthase, nuclear factor kappaB expression and enhanced antiapoptosis-related proteins in Helicobacter pylori-infected non-cardiac gastric adenocarcinoma. *World Journal of Gastroenterology, 10*(15), 2232–2240. PubMed PMID: 15259072.

105. Soini, Y., Haapasaari, K. M., Vaarala, M. H., Turpeenniemi-Hujanen, T., Kärjä, V., & Karihtala, P. (2011). 8-hydroxydeguanosine and nitrotyrosine are prognostic factors in urinary bladder carcinoma. *International Journal of Clinical and Experimental Pathology, 4*(3), 267–275. PubMed PMID: 21487522.

106. Li, H., Horke, S., & Forstermann, U. (2014). Vascular oxidative stress, nitric oxide and atherosclerosis. *Atherosclerosis, 237*(1), 208–219. PubMed PMID: 25244505.

107. Warnholtz, A., Nickenig, G., Scholz, E., et al. (1999). Increased NADH-oxidase–mediated superoxide production in the early stages of atherosclerosis: Evidence for involvement of the renin-angiotensin system. *Circulation, 99*(15), 2027–2033. PubMed PMID: 10209008.

108. Xiang, F., Shuanglun, X., Jingfeng, W., Ruqiong, N., Yuan, Z., Yongqing, L., et al. (2011). Association of serum 8-hydroxy-2'-deoxyguanosine levels with the presence and severity of coronary artery disease. *Coronary Artery Disease, 22*(4), 223–227. PubMed PMID: 21407076.

109. Ho, H. Y., Cheng, M. L., Chen, C. M., Gu, P. W., Wang, Y. L., Li, J. M., et al. (2008). Oxidative damage markers and antioxidants in patients with acute myocardial infarction and their clinical significance. *Biofactors, 34*(2), 135–145. PubMed PMID: 19706979.

110. Kobayashi, S., Susa, T., Tanaka, T., Wada, Y., Okuda, S., Doi, M., et al. (2011). Urinary 8-hydroxy-2'-deoxyguanosine reflects symptomatic status and severity of systolic dysfunction in patients with chronic heart failure. *European Journal of Heart Failure, 13*(1), 29–36. PubMed PMID: 20965876.

111. Ari, E., Kaya, Y., Demir, H., Cebi, A., Alp, H. H., Bakan, E., et al. (2011). Oxidative DNA damage correlates with carotid artery atherosclerosis in hemodialysis patients. *Hemodialysis International, 15*(4), 453–459. PubMed PMID: 22111813.

112. Watanabe, E., Matsuda, N., Shiga, T., Kajimoto, K., Ajiro, Y., Kawarai, H., et al. (2006). Significance of 8-hydroxy-2'-deoxyguanosine levels in patients with idiopathic dilated cardiomyopathy. *Journal of Cardiac Failure, 12*(7), 527–532. PubMed PMID: 16952786.

113. Bonnefont-Rousselot, D. (2002). Glucose and reactive oxygen species. *Current Opinion in Clinical Nutrition and Metabolic Care, 5*(5), 561–568. PubMed PMID: 12172481.

114. Chang, C. M., Hsieh, C. J., Huang, J. C., & Huang, I. C. (2012). Acute and chronic fluctuations in blood glucose levels can increase oxidative stress in type 2 diabetes mellitus. *Acta Diabetologica, 49*(Suppl. 1), S171–S177. PubMed PMID: 22547264.

115. Cangemi, R., Angelico, F., Loffredo, L., Del Ben, M., Pignatelli, P., Martini, A., et al. (2007). Oxidative stress–mediated arterial dysfunction in patients with metabolic syndrome: Effect of ascorbic acid. *Free Radical Biology & Medicine, 43*(5), 853–859. PubMed PMID: 17664149.

116. Longo-Mbenza, B., Mvitu Muaka, M., Masamba, W., Muizila Kini, L., Longo Phemba, I., Kibokela Ndembe, D., et al. (2014). Retinopathy in non diabetics, diabetic retinopathy and oxidative stress: A new phenotype in Central Africa? *International Journal of Ophthalmology, 7*(2), 293–301. PubMed PMID: 24790873.

117. Coughlan, M. T., Thorburn, D. R., et al. (2009). RAGE-induced cytosolic ROS promote mitochondrial superoxide generation in diabetes. *Journal of the American Society of Nephrology, 20*(4), 742–752. PubMed PMID: 19158353.

118. Nishikawa, T., Edelstein, D., Du, X. L., et al. (2000). Normalizing mitochondrial superoxide production blocks three pathways of hyperglycaemic damage. *Nature, 404*(6779), 787–790. PubMed PMID: 10783895.

119. Hadjigogos, K. (2003). The role of free radicals in the pathogenesis of rheumatoid arthritis. *Panminerva Medica, 45*(1), 7–13. PubMed PMID: 12682616.

120. Migliore, L., & Coppede, F. (2009). Environmental-induced oxidative stress in neurodegenerative disorders and aging. *Mutation Research, 674*(1–2), 73–84. PubMed PMID: 18952194.

121. Butterfield, D. A., Howard, B., Yatin, S., et al. (1999). Elevated oxidative stress in models of normal brain aging and Alzheimer's disease. *Life Sciences, 65*(18–19), 1883–1892. PubMed PMID: 10576432.

122. Drechsel, D. A., & Patel, M. (2008). Role of reactive oxygen species in the neurotoxicity of environmental agents implicated in Parkinson's disease. *Free Radical Biology & Medicine, 44*(11), 1873–1886. PubMed PMID: 18342017.

123. Mooney, L. A., Madsen, A. M., Tang, D., et al. (2005). Antioxidant vitamin supplementation reduces benzo(a)pyrene-DNA adducts and potential cancer risk in female smokers. *Cancer Epidemiology, Biomarkers and Prevention, 14*(1), 237–242. PubMed PMID: 15668500.

124. Baumeister, P., Reiter, M., Kleinsasser, N., et al. (2009). Epigallocatechin-3-gallate reduces DNA damage induced by benzo[a]pyrene diol epoxide and cigarette smoke condensate in human mucosa tissue cultures. *European Journal of Cancer Prevention, 18*(3), 230–235. PubMed PMID: 19491610.

125. Burton, G. W., & Ingold, K. U. (1989). Vitamin E as an in vitro and in vivo antioxidant. In A. T. Diplock, L. J. Machoin, L. Parker, & W. A. Pryor (Eds.), *Vitamin E: Biochemistry and Health Implications. Ann NY Acad Sci* (Vol. 570, pp. 7–22). PubMed PMID: 2698111.

126. Horwitt, M. K. (1988). Supplementation with vitamin E. *The American Journal of Clinical Nutrition, 47,* 1088–1089. PubMed PMID: 3376907.

127. Prasad, J. S. (1980). Effect of vitamin E supplementation on leukocyte function. *The American Journal of Clinical Nutrition, 33,* 606–608. PubMed PMID: 7355845.

128. Kagan, V. E., Serbinova, E. A., Forte, T., et al. (1992). Recycling of vitamin E in low density lipoproteins. *Journal of Lipid Research, 33,* 385–387. PubMed PMID: 1314881.

129. Gonzalez-Flecha, B. S., Repetto, M., Evalson, P., & Boveris, A. (1991). Inhibition of microsomal lipid peroxidation by alpha tocopherol and alpha tocopherol acetate. *Xenobiotica, 21,* 1013–1022. PubMed PMID: 1776274.

130. Steiner, M. (1991). Influences of vitamin E on platelet function in humans. *Journal of the American College of Nutrition, 10,* 466–473. PubMed PMID: 1955623.

131. Gabbianelli, R., Nasuti, C., Falcioni, G., & Cantalamessa, F. (2004). Lymphocyte DNA damage in rats exposed to pyrethroids: Effect of supplementation with vitamins E and C. *Toxicology, 203*(1–3), 17–26. PubMed PMID: 15363578.

132. Nasuti, C., Falcioni, M. L., Nwankwo, I. E., Cantalamessa, F., & Gabbianelli, R. (2008). Effect of permethrin plus antioxidants on locomotor activity and striatum in adolescent rats. *Toxicology, 251*(1–3), 45–50. PubMed PMID: 18692543.

133. Ludewig, G., et al. (2000). Mechanisms of toxicity of PCB metabolites: Generation of reactive oxygen species and glutathione depletion. *Central European Journal of Public Health, 8*(Suppl.), 15–17. PubMed PMID: 10943438.

134. Townsend, D. M., Tew, K. D., & Tapiero, H. (2003). The importance of glutathione in human disease. *Biomedicine & Pharmacotherapy, 57*(3–4), 145–155. PubMed PMID: 12818476.

135. Soltan-Sharifi, M. S., et al. (2007). Improvement by N-acetylcysteine of acute respiratory distress syndrome through increasing intracellular glutathione. *Human and Experimental Toxicology, 26*(9), 697–703. PubMed PMID: 17984140.

136. Micke, P., et al. (2001). Oral supplementation with whey proteins increases plasma glutathione levels of HIV-infected patients. *European Journal of Clinical Investigation*, 31(2), 171–178. PubMed PMID: 11168457.

137. Jariwalla, R. J., et al. (2008). Restoration of blood total glutathione status and lymphocyte function following alpha-lipoic acid supplementation in patients with HIV infection. *The Journal of Alternative and Complementary Medicine: Research on Paradigm, Practice, and Policy*, 14(2), 139–146. PubMed PMID: 18315507.

138. Lieber, C. S., & Packer, L. (2002). S-Adenosylmethionine: Molecular, biological, and clinical aspects—an introduction. *The American Journal of Clinical Nutrition*, 76(5), 1148S–1150S. PubMed PMID: 12418492.

139. Sharma, H., Datta, P., et al. (2008). Gene expression profiling in practitioners of Sudarshan Kriya. *Journal of Psychosomatic Research*, 64(2), 213–218. PubMed PMID: 18222135.

140. Rundle, A. G., Orjuela, M., et al. (2005). Preliminary studies on the effect of moderate physical activity on blood levels of glutathione. *Biomarkers: Biochemical Indicators of Exposure, Response, and Susceptibility to Chemicals*, 10(5), 390–400. PubMed PMID: 16243723.

141. Háuser, R. A., Lyons, K. E., et al. (2009). Randomized, double-blind, pilot evaluation of intravenous glutathione in Parkinson's disease. *Movement Disorders*, 24(7), 979–983. PubMed PMID: 19230029.

142. Mischley, L. K., et al. (2013). Safety survey of intranasal glutathione. *Journal of Alternative and Complementary Medicine (New York)*, 19(5), 459–463. PubMed PMID: 23240940.

143. Ekor, M., Adesanoye, O. A., & Farombi, E. O. (2010). N-acetylcysteine pretreatment ameliorates mercuric chloride-induced oxidative renal damage in rats. *African Journal of Medicine and Medical Sciences*, 39(Suppl.), 153–160. PubMed PMID: 22416658.

144. Kelly, G. S. (1998). Clinical applications of N-acetylcysteine. *Alternative Medicine Review: A Journal of Clinical Therapeutics*, 3(2), 114–127. PubMed PMID: 9577247.

145. Zhu, Y., Kalen, A. L., Li, L., et al. (2009). Polychlorinated-biphenyl–induced oxidative stress and cytotoxicity can be mitigated by antioxidants after exposure. *Free Radical Biology & Medicine*, 47(12), 1762–1771. PubMed PMID: 19796678.

146. Mills, B. J., Lindeman, R. D., & Lang, C. A. (1986). Magnesium deficiency inhibits biosynthesis of blood glutathione and tumor growth in the rat. *Proceedings of the Society for Experimental Biology and Medicine*, 181(3), 326–332. PubMed PMID: 3945642.

147. Bede, O., Nagy, D., Surányi, A., et al. (2008). Effects of magnesium supplementation on the glutathione redox system in atopic asthmatic children. *Inflammation Research*, 57(6), 279–286. PubMed PMID: 18516713.

148. Ly, J., Lagman, M., Saing, T., et al. (2015). Liposomal glutathione supplementation restores TH1 cytokine response to mycobacterium tuberculosis infection in HIV-infected individuals. *Journal of Interferon and Cytokine Research*, 35(11), 875–887. PubMed PMID: 26133750.

149. Chen, C., Jiang, X., Hu, Y., & Zhang, Z. (2013). The protective role of resveratrol in the sodium arsenite-induced oxidative damage via modulation of intracellular GSH homeostasis. *Biological Trace Element Research*, 155(1), 119–131. PubMed PMID: 23884857.

150. Turkez, H., & Aydin, E. (2013). The genoprotective activity of resveratrol on permethrin-induced genotoxic damage in cultured human lymphocytes. *Brazilian Archives of Biology and Technology*, 56, 405–411.

151. Garg, R., Gupta, S., & Maru, G. B. (2008). Dietary curcumin modulates transcriptional regulators of phase I and phase II enzymes in benzo[a] pyrene-treated mice: Mechanism of its anti-initiating action. *Carcinogenesis*, 29(5), 1022–1032. PubMed PMID: 18321868.

152. Kukongviriyapan, U., Apaijit, K., & Kukongviriyapan, V. (2016). Oxidative stress and cardiovascular dysfunction associated with cadmium exposure: Beneficial effects of curcumin and tetrahydrocurcumin. *The Tohoku Journal of Experimental Medicine*, 239(1), 25–38. PubMed PMID: 27151191.

153. Kukongviriyapan, U., Pannangpetch, P., Kukongviriyapan, V., et al. (2014). Curcumin protects against cadmium-induced vascular dysfunction, hypertension and tissue cadmium accumulation in mice. *Nutrients*, 6(3), 1194–1208. PubMed PMID: 24662163.

154. Zhu, W., Cromie, M. M., Cai, Q., et al. (2014). Curcumin and vitamin E protect against adverse effects of benzo[a]pyrene in lung epithelial cells. *PLoS ONE*, 9(3), e92992. PubMed PMID: 24664296.

155. Mukherjee, S., Roy, M., et al. (2007). A mechanistic approach for modulation of arsenic toxicity in human lymphocytes by curcumin, an active constituent of medicinal herb Curcuma longa Linn. *Journal of Clinical Biochemistry and Nutrition*, 41(1), 32–42. PubMed PMID: 18392098.

156. Mitjavila, M. T., Fandos, M., Salas-Salvadó, J., Covas, M. I., Borrego, S., Estruch, R., et al. (2013). The Mediterranean diet improves the systemic lipid and DNA oxidative damage in metabolic syndrome individuals. A randomized, controlled, trial. *Clinical Nutrition*, *32*(2), 172–178. PubMed PMID: 22999065.

157. Pedret, A., Valls, R. M., Fernández-Castillejo, S., Catalán, Ú., Romeu, M., Giralt, M., et al. (2012). Polyphenol-rich foods exhibit DNA antioxidative properties and protect the glutathione system in healthy subjects. *Molecular Nutrition & Food Research*, *56*(7), 1025–1033. PubMed PMID: 22760977.

158. Qian, G., Xue, K., Tang, L., Wang, F., Song, X., Chyu, M. C., et al. (2012). Mitigation of oxidative damage by green tea polyphenols and Tai Chi exercise in postmenopausal women with osteopenia. *PLoS ONE*, *7*(10), e48090. PubMed PMID: 23118932.

159. He, Y. T., Xing, S. S., Gao, L., Wang, J., Xing, Q. C., & Zhang, W. (2014). Ginkgo biloba attenuates oxidative DNA damage of human umbilical vein endothelial cells induced by intermittent high glucose. *Die Pharmazie*, *69*(3), 203–207. PubMed PMID: 24716410.

160. Ruiz-Miyazawa, K. W., et al. (2017). Quercetin inhibits gout arthritis in mice: Induction of an opioid-dependent regulation of inflammasome. *Inflammopharmacology*, [Epub ahead of print]; PubMed PMID: 28508104.

161. Barcelos, G. R., Grotto, D., Serpeloni, J. M., Angeli, J. P., Rocha, B. A., de Oliveira Souza, V. C., et al. (2011). Protective properties of quercetin against DNA damage and oxidative stress induced by methylmercury in rats. *Archives of Toxicology*, *85*(9), 1151–1157. PubMed PMID: 21286687.

162. Foreman, J. C. (1984). Mast cells and the actions of flavonoids. *The Journal of Allergy and Clinical Immunology*, *73*, 769–774. PubMed PMID: 6202730.

163. Hope, W. C., et al. (1983). In vitro inhibition of the biosynthesis of slow reacting substance of anaphylaxis (SRS-A) and lipoxygenase activity by quercetin. *Biochemical Pharmacology*, *32*, 367–371. PubMed PMID: 6191762.

164. Ciftci, O., Ozdemir, I., Tanyildizi, S., et al. (2011). Antioxidative effects of curcumin, β-myrcene and 1,8-cineole against 2,3,7,8-tetrac hlorodibenzo-p-dioxin–induced oxidative stress in rats liver. *Toxicology and Industrial Health*, *27*(5), 447–453. PubMed PMID: 21245202.

165. Chang, Y. Z., Lin, H. C., Chan, S. T., & Yeh, S. L. (2012). Effects of quercetin metabolites on the enhancing effect of β-carotene on DNA damage and cytochrome P1A1/2 expression in benzo[a]

pyrene-exposed A549 cells. *Food Chemistry*, *133*(2), 445–450. PubMed PMID: 25683418.

166. Ramadass, P., Meerarani, P., Toborek, M., et al. (2003). Dietary flavonoids modulate PCB-induced oxidative stress, CYP1A1 induction, and AhR-DNA binding activity in vascular endothelial cells. *Toxicological Sciences*, *76*(1), 212–219. PubMed PMID: 12970578.

167. Sener, G., Sehirli, A. O., & Ayanoglu-Dulger, G. (2003). Melatonin protects against mercury (II)-induced oxidative tissue damage in rats. *Pharmacology and Toxicology*, *93*(6), 290–296. PubMed PMID: 14675463.

168. Leibowitz, A., Volkov, A., Voloshin, K., Shemesh, C., Barshack, I., & Grossman, E. (2016). Melatonin prevents kidney injury in a high-salt diet-induced hypertension model by decreasing oxidative stress. *Journal of Pineal Research*, *60*(1), 48–54. PubMed PMID: 26465239.

169. Quiroz, Y., Ferrebuz, A., Romero, F., Vaziri, N. D., & Rodriguez-Iturbe, B. (2008). Melatonin ameliorates oxidative stress, inflammation, proteinuria, and progression of renal damage in rats with renal mass reduction. *American Journal of Physiology – Renal Physiology*, *294*(2), F336–F344. PubMed PMID: 18077597.

170. Shalaby, M. A., & Saifan, H. Y. (2014). Some pharmacological effects of cinnamon and ginger herbs in obese diabetic rats. *Journal of Intercultural Ethnopharmacology*, *3*(4), 144–149. PubMed PMID: 26401364.

171. Kim, M. K., Chung, S. W., Kim, D. H., et al. (2010). Modulation of age-related NF-kappaB activation by dietary zingerone via MAPK pathway. *Experimental Gerontology*, *45*(6), 419–426. PubMed PMID: 20211236.

172. Ural, M. S. (2013). Chlorpyrifos-induced changes in oxidant/antioxidant status and haematological parameters of Cyprinus carpio carpio: Ameliorative effect of lycopene. *Chemosphere*, *90*(7), 2059–2064. PubMed PMID: 23312461.

173. Yonar, S. M. (2013). Toxic effects of malathion in carp, Cyprinus carpio carpio: Protective role of lycopene. *Ecotoxicology and Environmental Safety*, *97*, 223–229. PubMed PMID: 23932509.

174. Turkez, H., & Togar, B. (2011). Olive (Olea europaea L.) leaf extract counteracts genotoxicity and oxidative stress of permethrin in human lymphocytes. *The Journal of Toxicological Sciences*, *36*(5), 531–537. PubMed PMID: 22008529.

175. Turkez, H., Togar, B., & Polat, E. (2012). Olive leaf extract modulates permethrin induced genetic and

oxidative damage in rats. *Cytotechnology, 64*(4), 459–464. PubMed PMID: 22262123.

176. Ural, M. S., Yonar, M. E., & Mise Yonar, S. (2015). Protective effect of ellagic acid on oxidative stress and antioxidant status in Cyprinus carpio carpio during malathion exposure. *Cellular and Molecular Biology (Noisy-Le-Grand, France), 61*(5), 58–63. PubMed PMID: 26516111.

177. Enis Yonar, M., Yonar, S. M., Ural, M. S., Silici, S., & Dusukcan, M. (2012). Protective role of propolis in chlorpyrifos-induced changes in the haematological parameters and the oxidative/antioxidative status of Cyprinus carpio carpio. *Food and Chemical Toxicology, 50*(8), 2703–2708. PubMed PMID: 22634289.

178. Yonar, S. M., Ural, M. S., Silici, S., & Yonar, M. E. (2014). Malathion-induced changes in the haematological profile, the immune response, and the oxidative/antioxidant status of Cyprinus carpio carpio: Protective role of propolis. *Ecotoxicology and Environmental Safety, 102*, 202–209. PubMed PMID: 24480596.

179. Coban, F. K., Ince, S., Kucukkurt, I., Demirel, H. H., & Hazman, O. (2015). Boron attenuates malathion-induced oxidative stress and acetylcholinesterase inhibition in rats. *Drug and Chemical Toxicology, 38*(4), 391–399. PubMed PMID: 25342379.

180. Eroglu, S., Pandir, D., Uzun, F. G., & Bas, H. (2013). Protective role of vitamins C and E in dichlorvos-induced oxidative stress in human erythrocytes in vitro. *Biological Research, 46*(1), 33–38. PubMed PMID: 23760412.

181. Ozkan, F., Gunduz, S. G., Berkoz, M., Hunt, A. O., & Yalin, S. (2012). The protective role of ascorbic acid (vitamin C) against chlorpyrifos-induced oxidative stress in Oreochromis niloticus. *Fish Physiology and Biochemistry, 38*(3), 635–643. PubMed PMID: 21818541.

182. Aboul-Soud, M. A., Al-Othman, A. M., El-Desoky, G. E., Al-Othman, Z. A., Yusuf, K., Ahmad, J., et al. (2011). Hepatoprotective effects of vitamin E/selenium against malathion-induced injuries on the antioxidant status and apoptosis-related gene expression in rats. *The Journal of Toxicological Sciences, 36*(3), 285–296. PubMed PMID: 21628957.

183. Hassani, S., Sepand, M. R., Jafari, A., Jaafari, J., et al. (2015). Protective effects of curcumin and vitamin E against chlorpyrifos-induced lung oxidative damage. *Human and Experimental Toxicology, 34*(6), 668–676. PubMed PMID: 25233897.

3

Food Pollution

SUMMARY

- Most common food contaminants: Persistent organic pollutants (POPs), organophosphate and pyrethroid pesticides, plasticizers, bisphenol A, metals
- Most contaminated foods: Sardines, farmed salmon, large carnivorous fish, conventional meats, the "dirty dozen" fruits and vegetables
- Best intervention: Consume certified organic foods, wash produce in acidic or alkaline water, peel produce

INTRODUCTION

All of the food produced before the mid-1940s would now be considered "organically raised." Organophosphate pesticides, first synthesized in 1820, were further developed into warfare nerve gas agents in Germany in the 1930s and since 1941 have primarily been used as agricultural pesticides. Dichloro-diphenyl-trichloroethane (DDT) was first synthesized in 1874, and its pesticide effects were discovered in 1939. DDT was used in wartime to control typhus and malaria, and was first utilized in US agriculture in 1945. DDT was banned from use by the US government in 1972, a decade after Rachel Carson published her landmark book *Silent Spring*.

In 1970, Norman Borlaug was awarded the Nobel Peace Prize for what is now called the "Green Revolution." He developed the F1 hybrid wheat seed that produced greatly increased yields when used with nitrogen fertilizer. After its introduction in Mexico in the 1950s, Mexican wheat yields increased sixfold in 20 years. After the F1 hybrid was introduced into India, the country's wheat production doubled, and India no longer needed to import wheat. Unfortunately, the fertilizers also stimulated weed growth, which necessitated using petrochemical herbicides to provide maximal harvest. Pesticides were then needed to prevent insect-related crop loss as well. Once the pesticides killed off the "primary" pests, their natural prey abounded, resulting in an increase of the total number of insects causing a million dollars of more of crop damage per year from only 10 to 300 individuals insects.[1] Due to the increased use of pesticides, 72% of these secondary pests are now insecticide resistant. In fact, there are now more than 500 species of insects that are resistant to pesticides, and since 1980, the number of herbicide resistant weeds has increased from 12 to 50. Of all the millions of pounds of pesticides that have been used agriculturally since the 1940s, <0.1% actually reach the target pest, leaving the rest in the environment.[2] No one has accounted for where the other 99.9% ends up, but it is known these compounds can travel thousands of miles around the globe.[3,4]

Since the 1950s, the amount of pesticides used agriculturally has more than tripled (Fig. 3.1).[5] Annual world pesticide use exceeded 5.2 billion pounds in both 2006 and 2007 (total cost, $39.4 billion), with the United States accounting for more than 1.2 billion of those pounds per year at an annual cost of $11.8 billion.[6]

The US Food and Drug Administration (FDA) and the US Department of Agriculture (USDA) both have ongoing assays for pesticides and toxicants in the US

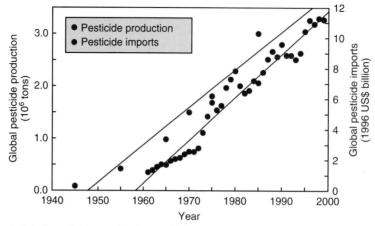

FIG. 3.1 Total global pesticide production and imports 1940 to 2000. (From Tilman, D., Cassman, K.G., Matson, P.A., Naylor, R., & Polasky, S. (2002). Agricultural sustainability and intensive production practices. *Nature*, *418*, 671–677.)

BOX 3.1   Links to Federal Programs Monitoring the US Food Supply

US Food and Drug Administration Total Diet Study: https://www.fda.gov/Food/FoodScienceResearch/TotalDietStudy/ucm184293.htm

US Food and Drug Administration Pesticide Data Program: https://www.ams.usda.gov/datasets/pdp

Environmental Working Group Shopper's Guide: https://www.ewg.org/foodnews/

BOX 3.2   2017 EWG Shopper's Guide

Most Toxic Fruits and Vegetables
1. Strawberries
2. Spinach
3. Nectarines
4. Apples
5. Peaches
6. Pears
7. Cherries
8. Grapes (imported)
9. Celery
10. Tomatoes
11. Sweet bell peppers
12. Potatoes

https://www.ewg.org/foodnews/guide.php Copyright © Environmental Working Group, www.ewg.org. Reproduced with permission.

---

food supply (Box 3.1). The USDA compiles the Pesticide Data Program (PDP), whereas the FDA compiles the Total Diet Study (TDS). The USDA PDP is primarily focused on providing pesticide residue data on foods most commonly consumed by children and is the database used for the "Dirty Dozen" list of the Environmental Working Group (EWG). The USDA PDP assesses the pesticide burden in a very small number of foods. Only 3 samples of 18 foods were assessed in the 2015 study.[7] Some of the foods assayed change yearly, which accounts for foods being added to, or subtracted from, the EWG Shopper's Guide (Box 3.2). The FDA TDS assays about 280 foods for more than 800 substances, making it the most comprehensive ongoing food pollution study. Numerous other countries in Europe, Asia, and the Americas have also begun doing TDSs on their food supplies.

The FDA has published all the TDS data on toxic and nutritional elements for the years 1991 to 2005 and 2006 to 2011 by both foods and chemical contaminants. Two assays of radionucleotides in foods have also been published for the years 1992 to 2005 and 2006 to 2014.

PDFs of each of these reports are available at the FDA website.* According to the TDS data, 50% of the daily US dioxin intake comes from meat and dairy products.[8]

---

*https://www.fda.gov/Food/FoodScienceResearch/TotalDietStudy/ucm184293.htm

TABLE 3.1 POP Exposures in a Typical Daily Western US Diet

POP	Cantaloupe	Carrot	Cheese	Cucumber	Peanut	Radish	Farmed Salmon	Summer Squash
Chlordane				X		X		X
DDE	X	X	X	X	X	X	X	X
DDT		X				X	X	X
Dieldrin	X	X	X	X	X	X	X	X
Endrin	X			X		X		X
Heptachlor	X		X	X	X	X	X	X
HCB			X				X	X
Toxaphene	X			X	X	X		X

Modified from Schafer, K.S., & Kegley, S.E. (2002). Persistent toxic chemicals in the US food supply. *Journal of Epidemiology and Community Health, 56*(11), 813-817.

PERSISTENT ORGANIC POLLUTANTS

- Polychlorinated biphenyls (PCBs)
- Organochlorine pesticides (OCPs)
- Brominated flame retardants

Data on 12 POPs in foods assayed in the FDA TDA and the USDA PDP were used to determine toxicant content of typical meals consumed in the Northeast, Southeast, Western, and Midwest regions of the US.[9] Southeastern meal plans would provide 70 POP exposures daily, Western would have 66, Northeast 64, and Midwest 63, whereas a typical holiday dinner alone would provide 38 POP exposures. Table 3.1 shows the POP exposures from a typical daily Western US diet.

POP residues were found in meat, poultry, and dairy products as well as baked goods, fruits, and vegetables. The total daily amount of DDT that could possibly be ingested by one individual consuming foods currently contaminated by DDT and its breakdown product Dichlorodiphenyldichloroethylene (DDE) was 3154 μg/d (Table 3.2).

Polychlorinated Biphenyls and Organochlorine Pesticides

- Sardines and farmed salmon
- Great Lakes fish
- Meat and dairy

In the 2004 to 2005 FDA TDS, 100% of the salmon samples were found to contain PCBs and DDE. Currently 50% of world fish consumption comes from aquaculture,[10] and two-thirds of all salmon consumed in North America is farmed.[11] It has been estimated that farmed salmon is

TABLE 3.2 Estimated Personal Daily Total DDT Intake from Commonly Consumed Foods

Food	Serving Size, Grams	Total μg Pesticide Ingested
Fish	372	1860
Carrots	125	375
Milk	250	312
Potatoes	250	250
Toast (grains)	250	125
Eggs	125	62
Spinach	125	62
Legumes	250	50

Modified from Schafer, K.S., & Kegley, S.E. (2002). Persistent toxic chemicals in the US food supply. *Journal of Epidemiology and Community Health, 56*(11), 813-817.

responsible for 97% of dietary POP exposure.[12] POP levels were assessed on 700+ salmon (totaling approximately 2 metric tons of farmed and wild salmon) from around the globe.[13] Fourteen persistent chlorinated compounds were found in significantly higher levels in farmed salmon than in wild salmon. The only compound that did not reach statistical significance was lindane, which was still higher in farmed than wild salmon. The four compounds with the greatest differences were PCBs, dioxins, toxaphene, and dieldrin. The PCB content in farmed salmon averaged 42.5 ng/g, whereas wild Alaskan salmon averaged only 3.2 ng/g. Fish samples from farms off the coast of Washington State and Chile had lower PCB concentrations than salmon farmed by Scotland and the Faroe Islands. POP levels in the fish samples paralleled the POP levels in the fish pellets used in those areas.[14] Another study revealed the average PCB content in farm-raised Atlantic salmon to be 28 to 38 ng/g, whereas total PCB content in wild Alaskan salmon averaged 2.8 to 13.7 ng/g.[15] The PCBs found in Atlantic salmon, dominated by highly toxic PCB 138, 153, and 180, are different from those in Alaskan salmon, which have fewer chlorine molecules and greater water solubility, and are far less toxic to humans. Some changes have been made to the fish pellets that are fed to farmed salmon, resulting in a decrease in some of the POPs present in the fish.[16] Unfortunately, the levels of PCBs 135, 153, and 180 have remained about the same. Farmed shrimp and tilapia, along with cod, are relatively free of the POPs found high in farmed salmon, providing less toxic fish alternatives.[12]

Sportfishing in the Great Lakes and other areas of the country remains another exposure source of POPs for those who eat their catch.[17,18,19] Table 3.3 compares PCB content between sardines, wild Alaskan salmon, farmed Atlantic salmon, and hamburger. Sardines had the highest concentration of the highly toxic PCBs 138, 153, and 180, followed closely by farmed salmon and then hamburger.

Brominated Flame Retardants

- Sardines
- Farmed salmon
- Pork sausage
- Hotdogs

Persistent polybrominated diphenyl ethers (PBDEs), often used as flame retardants, are found to be highest in fish, meats, and dairy products, with fish having the highest levels (mean of 1120 pg/g).[20] Sardines topped the chart, with an average PBDE content of 3726 pg/g, again making them the most POP-contaminated fish. Farmed salmon were the next most contaminated, with levels of 1999, 3082, and 1732 pg/g. Wild Alaskan salmon had far lower levels, 141 and 605 pg/g. Although the mean level of PDBEs in all the meats tested was 383 pg/g, levels widely varied from sample to sample in the same food category. For example, three samples of bacon had 39 pg/g, whereas two others contained 105 and 165 pg/g. One pork sausage sample had a whopping 1426 pg/g, yet another only contained 195 pg/g, and some hotdogs had 1348 pg/g.

For Canadians, the two greatest sources of PCB exposure were butter and fish.[21] The average intake of PCBs for Canadians is 5.7 ng/kg/day. Spanish butter has been shown to have average European levels of PCBs (5.4 ng/g wet weight), but elevated levels of hexachloro-benzene (HCB), beta-hexachlorocyclohexane (HCH), and lindane.[22] Mexican butter was tested for compounds other than PCBs and was found to contain organochlo-rines in most samples.[23] Lindane was found in 91%, HCB in 90%, p,p-DDE in 88%, alpha HCH in 63%, p,p-DDT in 42%, beta-HCH in 38%, and o,p-DDT in 17% in all butter samples.

TABLE 3.3   PCB Content (ng/g) and PBDE Content (pg/g) in Fish and Hamburger

POP	Wild Salmon	Farmed Salmon	Sardines	Catfish/Tuna/Tilapia/Cod	Hamburger
PCB 101	0.2	0.51	*	< DL	*
PCB 110	0.1	*	*	< DL	*
PCB 118	0.2	0.43	0.8	< DL	*
PCB 138	0.2	0.93	1.8	< DL	*
PCB 153	0.3	1.21	1.83	< DL	1.2
PCB 180	0.19	0.44	0.49	< DL	0.21
ΣPBDE	373	2253	3726	228.6	168.5

*Denotes that no assessments were done for those PCBs

Data from Schecter, A., Colacino, J., Haffner, D., Patel, K., Opel, M., Päpke, O., Birnbaum, L. (2010). Perfluorinated compounds, polychlorinated biphenyls, and organochlorine pesticide contamination in composite food samples from Dallas, Texas, USA. *Environmental Health Perspectives, 118*(6), 796-802. Hayward, D., Wong, J., & Krynitsky, A.J. (2007). Polybrominated diphenyl ethers and polychlorinated biphenyls in commercially wild caught and farm-raised fish fillets in the United States. *Environmental Research, 103*(1), 46-54. Badia-Vila, M., Ociepa, M., Mateo, R., & Guitart, R. (2000). and Van Leeuwen, S.P., van Velzen, M.J., Swart, C.P., van der Veen, I., Traag, W.A., de Boer, J. (2009). Halogenated contaminants in farmed salmon, trout, tilapia, pangasius, and shrimp. *Environmental Science & Technology, 43*(11), 4009-4015.

Coffee and Tea

As noted in Table 3.5, instant coffee is listed on the pesticide-free list, indicating that all commonly used pesticides are eliminated in the roasting process. A German study of 19 green coffee beans from 11 different countries found, with two exceptions, levels of pesticides to be quite low. In two other coffee bean samples, no pesticides were noted. After roasting, all pesticide residues present were reduced to "insignificance."[24] A more recent Japanese study actually added 0.2 and 1.0 µg/g (parts per million, PPM) concentrations of lindane, two chlordanes, piperonyl butoxide, and atrazine to green coffee beans and then measured for the presence of these compounds after roasting.[25] Their findings confirmed that the roasting process clears 90% to 100% of the pesticides from the beans. Lindane and atrazine were completely removed by roasting; of the heptachlor, less than 99% of the 1.0 µg/g concentration was cleared, whereas the levels of chlordane and piperonyl butoxide were reduced by 90%.

Black tea appeared to contain contaminants that were uniform for their country of origin. Sri Lankan teas had the least amount (in both number and amount) of residues of any of the big tea-producing countries.[26] Some teas contained HCH, lindane, and DDT, but all were in very low amounts. Black tea in Canada was found to have low levels of OCP present (DDE averaged 56 PPM, trans-Nonachlor averaged 2.74 PPM, and oxychlordane 1.94 PPM) and six metabolites of OPs that were already commonly found in the Canadian population.[27] Drinking the tea made no difference in the body levels of these compounds and caused no problems for pregnant women.

NONPERSISTENT POLLUTANTS

- Pesticides (organophosphate and pyrethroid) and herbicides
  - Strawberries, spinach, nectarines, apples, peaches, pears, cherries, imported grapes, celery, tomatoes, sweet bell peppers, potatoes
  - Nonorganic soy protein
- Plasticizers
  - Plastic-wrapped foods
- Bisphenol A (BPA)
  - Canned foods and beverages

In addition to POP residue in foods, there are currently a huge number of commercially applied agricultural chemicals including organophosphate (OP) pesticides, pyrethroid, and neonicotinoid pesticides, along with Roundup (which contains varying combinations of glyphosate and petroleum distillates), atrazine, and other herbicides.

Longitudinal studies that measure pesticide content in meals prepared by families have revealed significant foodborne pesticide exposure.[28] A study in Baltimore revealed malathion in 75.2% of the meals, chlorpyrifos in 38.3%, and DDE in 21.4% of the samples. Malathion and chlorpyrifos were found together 35.4% of the time, malathion and DDE 18.8%, and chlorpyrifos and DDE 8.9% of the time. DDE levels showed no seasonal differences, but the highest concentrations of malathion and chlorpyrifos occurred in the samples taken March through June. A study in Florida revealed common exposure to both organophosphate and pyrethroid pesticides.[29]

Table 3.4 shows the most frequently found chemical contaminants from the 2004 to 2005 FDA TDS. Organophosphates topped the list of the most frequently found pesticides. However, 6 of these top 16 were chlorinated pesticides. OCPs are no longer used agriculturally, but their presence in our food supply attests to their

TABLE 3.4 Most Commonly Found Chemical Toxicants in the 2004 to 2005 FDA TDS

Pesticide	TDS 2004–2005 Total # Findings	Occur, %
Chlorpyrifos-menthyl	311	64
Malathion	370	63
Toxaphene	37	58
p,p-DDE	582	49
Dieldrin	258	36
Lindane	46	36
Methamidophos	60	33
Permethrin	266	30
Diphenyl 2 ethylhexyl phosphate	37	29
Chlorpyrifos	164	27
Heptachlor epoxide	38	25
o-Phenylphenol	36	24
Pirimiphos methyl	41	22
Thiabenzole	75	19
Diazinon	17	15
Endosulfan sulfate	89	12

persistence in the environment. Another interesting finding in this list is diphenyl 2 ethylhexyl phosphate (DPOP). DPOP is a plasticizer found in cellulose films used to package food. DPOP has previously been identified individually or in combination with other plasticizers in confectionery, meat pies, cakes, and sandwiches, at total levels from 0.5 to 53 mg/kg.[30,31] Plastic contamination of food will be discussed later in this section. Foods containing no pesticide residue from two earlier TDS reports are found in Table 3.5.

Residues in repackaged foods are also assessed in the TDS and are presented in Table 3.6.

Glyphosate

• Nonorganic soy protein

Five different combinations of glyphosate and petroleum distillates comprise the bulk of worldwide sales for the herbicide labeled Roundup™. With the development of "Roundup ready" genetically modified organism (GMO) crops, the amount of Roundup that can "safely" be used with each crop has increased by more than 500 million pounds.[32] This allows a more thorough elimination of any "weeds" (unwanted plants growing in the same soil) that might compete with the crop for nutrients and sunlight. High levels of glyphosate residues are found in all Roundup ready soybeans, whereas none are found in organically raised soybeans.[33] All soy protein isolates from GM soy contained residues of glyphosate and its metabolite in levels up to 2.7 µg/g.[34] Fortunately, no residues were found in soy milk or soybean oil, nor were any found in corn oil, cow's milk, whole milk powder, or breast milk. Glyphosate residues have also been found in wheat.[35]

Solvents

• Increased transfer from "microwave safe" food containers and packing material
• Styrofoam food containers

Styrene and ethylbenzene are found in foodstuffs due to migration from polystyrene food containers.[36,37] Styrene migration is dependent on fat content in the food and storage temperature as well as length of exposure.[38,39] Cooking pork in thermoset polyester dishes (microwave safe) for 1.5 hours resulted in a styrene migration range of 6 to 2400 mcg/kg and 6 to 34 mcg/kg for ethylbenzene.[40] Total daily exposure rates for styrene for persons in the US is estimated at 9 mcg/day and 1 to 4 mcg/day for residents of the UK.[41]

TABLE 3.5 **Foods Found with No Organic Pesticide Residues**	
TDS 1984–1986	**TDS 1986–1991**
Avocados, raw	Bananas and pineapple with tapioca
Bananas, raw	Beef bouillon, canned, reconstituted
Beans, navy, boiled from dried	Coffee, instant, decaf
Beans, pinto, boiled from dried	Corn, canned
Beer, canned	Corn, creamed style, canned
Coffee, instant	Corn flakes
Coffee, instant, decaf	Cream substitute, powdered
Corn, canned	Infant formulas, canned, milk-based
Corn, cream style, canned	Margarine, stick type
Corn, fresh/frozen, boiled	Peas, green, canned
Infant formula, canned, milk, with iron	Peas (strained/junior)
Infant formula without iron	Pineapple, canned in juice pack
Milk, skim	Pineapple juice, canned
Onions, raw	Pudding/custard, any flavor
Pineapple, canned in juice pack	Salad dressing, Italian, bottled
Pineapple juice, canned	Soda, sweetened, cola, canned
Prune juice, bottled	Powdered soft drink, cherry, sweet
Soda, low calorie w/ saccharin	Sugar, white, granulated
Soda, cola, sweetened, canned	Syrup, pancake, bottled
Soda, sweetened, lemon lime, can	Water
Soup, vegetable beef, canned	Whiskey, 80 proof
Tea	

Data from Gunderson, E.L. (1995). FDA Total Diet Study, July 1986–April 1991, dietary intakes of pesticides, selected elements, and other chemicals. *Journal of AOAC International*, 78(6), 1353-1363.

TABLE 3.6 Chemical Residues Found in Packaged Foods in FDA TDS		
Food Item	# of Findings	Avg. in µg/g
Tortilla, flour	81	3.5579
Cake, yellow	78	1.328
Cake, chocolate with icing	106	1.220
Cornbread	90	0.6361
Muffins, blueberry or plain	117	0.5961
Coffeecake	13	0.5713
Onion rings	81	0.4880
Margarine	33	0.4227
White sauce	168	0.3964
Fish, cod or haddock	53	0.3308
Fish sticks	100	0.3269

Data from KAN-DO Office and Pesticide Team, US FDA. (1995). Accumulated pesticide and industrial chemical findings from a 10-year study of ready-to-eat foods. *Journal of AOAC International*, *78*(3), 614-631.

TABLE 3.7 DEHP in Commercially Available Foods	
Food	DEHP (ng/g)
Pork bacon, sausage, ham, pork	300
Sliced and shredded cheese, ice cream, butter, yogurt	144
Canola, olive, and vegetable oils	117
Beef and poultry, hotdogs	102
Infant food	75
Bread, cake mix, cereals, rice, cookies	62
Milk	49
Atlantic salmon filets, tuna, shrimp, clams, sardines	32
Pancake syrup, marinade, BBQ sauce, salad dressing, ketchup	30

From Schecter, A., Lorber, M., Guo, Y., Wu, Q., Yun, S.H., Kannan, K., Hommel, M., Imran, N., Hynan, L.S., Cheng, D., Colacino, J.A., Birnbaum, L.S. (2013). Phthalate concentrations and dietary exposure from food purchased in New York State. *Environmental Health Perspectives*, *121*(4), 473-494.

Plasticizers

• Increased transfer to high-fat foods and when heated
• Fast food

Plasticizers can contaminate food from simple contact with plastic food wrap. A total phthalate level of 42.5 µg/g was found in the "top tortilla" in the package of tortillas tested in the previously mentioned TDS. That level of phthalates migrated from the ink on the package to the tortilla, whereas the other tortillas in the package had very little phthalate content, yet the average remained at 3.5 µg/g, as seen in Table 3.6. Numerous articles have documented the transfer of plasticizers from various food wraps into the food.[42,43] Plastic migration increases with the fat content of the food (Table 3.7), time in contact, and temperature, just as is found with styrene and ethylbenzene.[44,45]

Diethylhexyl phthalate (DEHP) contamination in meals also comes from the wearing of disposable polyvinylchloride (PVC) gloves by those preparing the food.[46,47] DEHP levels in lunches packed with the use of PVC gloves ranged from 0.80 to 11.8 mg/kg, whereas they only measured 0.012 to 0.30 mg/kg in lunches made without gloves. Fast food consumption is also positively associated with increased levels of urinary phthalates.[48]

Bisphenol A

• Canned foods and beverages

The daily intake of BPA by US residents is estimated at 12.6 ng/kg/day, of which 12.4 ng/kg/day is from foods.[49] On average, the consumption of one canned food item daily increased urinary BPA by 24%, and consuming two items increased urinary BPA by 54%.[50] However, not all canned foods increased urinary BPA to the same degree. Consumption of one can of soup increased urinary levels by 229%, pasta by 70%, and fruits and vegetables by 41%. Consuming one can of soup daily for 5 days has been shown to increase urinary BPA levels by more than 1000%.[51] In a double-blind trial, 75 volunteers consumed either freshly made (no canned ingredients) or canned soup for 5 days. After a 2-day washout period, they then switched to the other type of soup. Their starting and ending urinary BPA levels are presented in Fig. 3.2.

Those who consumed the fresh soup in the first week and the canned soup in the second week ended up with slightly higher urinary BPA. But those who consumed the canned soup in week 1 still had elevated urinary BPA a week later. Data from the National Health and Nutrition Examination Survey (NHANES) 2005 to 2006 revealed that soda pop, school lunches, and meals prepared outside of the home were the most significant sources of BPA.[52] In that study, bottled water and canned tuna were not

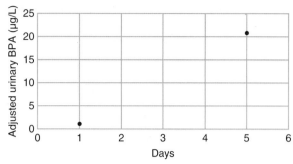

FIG. 3.2 Adjusted average urinary BPA (µg/L) before and after consuming canned soup for 5 days. (Data from Carwile, J.L., Ye, X., Zhou, X., Calafat, A.M., Michels, K.B. (2011). Canned soup consumption and urinary bisphenol A: A randomized crossover trial. *Journal of the American Medical Association, 306*(20), 2218-2220.)

found to be significant sources of this compound. Consumption of two servings of soy milk from glass bottles resulted in an average urinary BPA level of 0.31 µg/L, yet drinking two servings of soy milk from cans increased urinary BPA to an average of 8.22 µg/L.[53]

More information on BPA levels in canned commercial products can be found at: http://www.ewg.org/research/bpa-canned-food.

Metals
Aluminum

- Increased transfer from aluminum cookware in foods that are acidic or salty, or when fluoridated water is used
- Present in some processed foods

Aluminum leaching from cooking utensils is enhanced by both lower food pH and the presence of fluoridated water.[54,55] The mean daily aluminum intake in China is estimated to be 1.79 mg/kg weekly, with maximal exposure going up to 7.6 mg/kg/week, whereas in Hong Kong, it is only 0.60 mg/kg/week.[56,57] This difference appears to be due to the regular consumption in mainland China of a fry-bread called "youtiao," which is heavily contaminated with aluminum.[58] Daily aluminum exposures in Spain are estimated to be between 1.0 and 2.93 mg/d (0.12–0.34 mg/kg/week), whereas the average in Italy is higher (6.3 mg/d).[59,60] The difference is probably due to the fact that acidic foods, like tomato sauce, and salty foods both enhance aluminum migration. When tomatoes were cooked in aluminum pots, the aluminum content went from 1.3 to 31.7 mg/100 g. Leaving the tomato

mixture in the pot overnight increased that level to 52.9 mg/100 g.[61] Cooking black currant juice in aluminum pots also increased the aluminum content, from 0.05 mg/L to 23 to 50 mg/L, and heating stewed rhubarb increased aluminum content from 0.8 mg/kg to 15 to 23 mg/kg after just 12 minutes of cooking.[62] Interestingly, rhubarb stewed in a 30-year-old aluminum pot contained more aluminum than batches cooked in newer pots. Brewing and storing coffee, another acidic compound, in an aluminum percolator (such as the kind found at church or social functions) increased the aluminum content to between 0.88 and 1.18 mg per cup.[63] The aluminum content in soft drinks has also been shown to increase with time of storage.[64]

Arsenic

- Fish
- Rice—arsenic levels can be reduced with washing
- Poultry

The use of tap water still remains the greatest human source of health-damaging arsenic species.[65] Once consumed with water Inorganic arsenic is methylated once to become monomethylarsonic acid (MMA) which can then have a second methyl group added to become dimethylarsinic acid (DMA). MMA is more toxic than inorganic arsenic while DMA is over 200-fold less toxic. But seafood is the greatest food source of total arsenic intake, which, fortunately, predominantly comprises nontoxic arsenobetaine. Arsenic found in shrimp is another nontoxic organic arsenic (arsenocholine). There has been significant focus recently on the role of rice consumption as a source of arsenic exposure. Based on total arsenic levels, it has been estimated that consumption of 0.56 cups of cooked rice daily (the US average) is comparable to drinking 1 liter a day of water containing 10 µg/L of arsenic.[66] Although total arsenic intake may be similar, the composition and potential toxic action are quite different. The rice-consuming group that was studied did have statistically significantly higher levels of both dimethylarsinous acid (DMA) and monomethylarsonous acid (MMA) in their urine. Other studies have confirmed that rice consumers typically have twice the level of urinary DMA than is present in persons who do not regularly consume rice.[67] However, the NHANES data showed that Mexican Americans, for whom rice is commonly present in meals, did not have any noticeable increase in arsenic over other populations.[68]

Both the composition of arsenic species and the total arsenic burden in rice vary greatly based on where and how it is grown, how it is washed, and how it is cooked. The percent of rice contaminated with inorganic arsenic varies from 33% to 89% (the rest of the arsenic being organic) simply based on where and how it is grown.[69] Rice plants absorb arsenic from the water in which they are growing, so rice grown in areas with high groundwater arsenic will have higher arsenic content than rice grown in other areas. Rice grown in the south-central United States (Texas) had an average arsenic concentration of 0.30 μg/g, yet rice grown in California averaged 0.16 μg/g (41% less).[70] The arsenic content in rice can then be either increased or decreased depending on whether the rice is washed with high- or low-arsenic water.[71] Washing rice in low-arsenic water reduces the total arsenic content by 28%, whereas washing rice in high-arsenic water increases the arsenic level. Discarding the cooking water before the rice is done and replacing it with fresh water can reduce the total arsenic content by an additional 57%. And simply cooking rice with excess water can reduce arsenic content by 35% to 45%.[72]

Until 2014 arsenic was fed to commercially raised chickens in the form of 3-nitro-4-hydroxyphenylarsonic acid (roxarsone). Even though arsenic has a short half-life, conventionally raised chickens contained 1.8 μg/kg average total arsenic, whereas organic chickens were found to have an average of 0.6 μg/kg.[73] In roxarsone-fed chickens, arsenite was found along with arsenobetaine, DMA, and MMA in breast meat, and would have provided the average chicken-consuming US resident with only 0.3 (±0.2) μg/day of arsenite.[74]

Cadmium

- Tofu from conventionally grown soy beans
- Sunflower seeds

The greatest source of dietary cadmium is tofu, a food that the FDA TDS has not yet assessed, followed by cooked cereals and green leafy vegetables (both cooked and in salads) (Table 3.8).[75] "Tofu consumption" includes not just tofu, but also tempeh and products such as soy hotdogs, soy cheese, and soy burgers. Once-weekly consumption of any of those products resulted in an average urinary cadmium of 0.11 μg/g (only 0.02 μg/g below levels found in smokers). Ingestion of any of those products twice weekly or more increased the urinary cadmium burden to 0.30 μg/g, more than twice the increase found from smoking. Moderate dietary deficiencies of iron, zinc,

TABLE 3.8   Cadmium Content of Foods in the FDA Total Diet Study (Which Does Not Assess for Contaminants in Tofu)

Food	Frequency Found, %	Cadmium in PPM
Roasted sunflower seeds	100	0.478
Spinach (fresh or frozen)	100	0.144
Beef liver	100	0.58
Potato chips	99.8	0.56
Peanuts/peanut butter	100	0.55
French fries/baked potato	99.8	0.53
Shredded wheat cereal	100	0.52
Pasta	100	0.32
Boiled shrimp	90	0.17 (0.009–0.226)

From US Food and Drug Administration. (April, 2017) *Analytical results.* Retrieved from https://www.fda.gov/Food/FoodScienceResearch/TotalDietStudy/ucm184293.htm.

and calcium also enhance the absorption of cadmium, and abundance of these minerals in the body reduced absorption.[76] Men absorb about 5% of dietary cadmium, and women absorb twice that amount.

Mercury

- Fish

A number of fish have high methyl mercury (MeHg) content, but due to the long half-life of MeHg, regularly consuming even low-mercury fish can lead to elevated blood mercury levels.[77] Due to the increased production of coal-fired power plants in Asia releasing mercury into the air, the mercury level in the Pacific Ocean is expected to increase another 50% by 2050, with an equivalent MeHg increase in fish from those waters.[78] Almost the entire eastern seaboard, much of the Gulf of Mexico, well over 1.2 million miles of freshwater rivers, and more than 16 million acres of freshwater lakes in the US have mercury advisories.[79] The US Environmental Protection Agency (EPA) places such warnings on waters containing fish with levels of mercury exceeding the limit of 1.0 PPM to warn consumers about the danger of eating the fish. MeHg levels for most fish range from < 0.01 PPM to 0.5 PPM, with an average of > 0.3 PPM.[80] Usually only the large predator fish like shark and swordfish will exceed the FDA limit for human consumption of 1 PPM. The

TABLE 3.9 Mercury Levels in Commercial Fish and Shellfish 1990 to 2010

Highest in Mercury	PPM	Lowest in Mercury	PPM
1. Tilefish (Gulf of Mexico)	1.45	1. Scallop	0.003
2. Swordfish	0.995	2. Clam	0.009
3. Shark	0.979	3. Shrimp	0.009
4. King mackerel	0.730	4. Oyster	0.012
5. Tuna (bigeye/ ahi)	0.689	5. Sardine	0.013
6. Orange roughy	0.571	6. Tilapia	0.013
7. Marlin	0.485	7. Salmon, canned	0.014
8. Spanish Mackerel (gulf)	0.454	8. Anchovies	0.016
9. Grouper (all species)	0.448	9. Salmon, fresh, frozen	0.022
10. Tuna (other species)	0.415– 0.391	10. Catfish	0.024
11. Tuna (albacore)	0.358	11. Squid	0.024
12. Chilean sea bass	0.354	12. Pollock	0.031
13. Tuna, yellowfin (ahi)	0.354	13. Crawfish	0.033
14. Croaker, white (Pacific)	0.287	14. Shad	0.038
15. Scorpion fish	0.286	15. American mackerel	0.050
16. Halibut	0.241	16. Haddock	0.055
17. Spanish mackerel (Atlantic)	0.166	17. Flounder/ sole	0.056
18. Snapper	0.182	18. Crab	0.065
19. Lobster	0.166	19. Trout	0.071
20. Canned tuna	0.128	20. Cod	0.111

From US Food and Drug Administration. Mercury Levels in Commercial Fish and Shellfish (1990-2012). Retrieved from http://www.fda.gov/food/foodborneillnesscontaminants/metals/ucm115644.htm

TABLE 3.10 Levels of Mercury (PPM) in Fish by Source Compared with FDA Reported Levels

Fish	FDA Level	Imports	Atlantic	Pacific
Herring	0.4	0.13	0.14	0.04
Crab	0.06	0.10	0.26	0.15
Sea bass	0.22	0.19	0.14	0.22
Lobster	0.17	0.10	0.28	0.17
Mackerel	0.15	0.15	0.22	0.09
Salmon	0.01	0.04	0.13	0.04
Snapper	0.19	0.21	0.28	0.25

From Sunderland, E.M. (2007). Mercury exposure from domestic and imported estuarine and marine fish in the US seafood market. *Environmental Health Perspectives, 115*(2), 235-242.

FDA lists commercially sold fish according to their average mercury content (Table 3.9).

Even though canned tuna has far lower levels of mercury than are found in high-mercury fish such as swordfish and shark, it accounts for approximately 40% of the total MeHg intake because it is the most frequently consumed fish in the US.[81] The next most frequently consumed fish in the US is farmed salmon, which ranks among the lowest of mercury-containing fish yet has also been associated with elevated blood mercury levels because of its regular use.[82] Levels of mercury have been noted in Atlantic salmon that are quite close to levels found in canned tuna (Table 3.10).

INTERVENTION

- Washing in acid or alkaline solution
- Peeling
- Consumption of organic varieties

Rinsing with tap water alone reduced residue levels of captan, chlorothalonil, iprodione, endosulfan, permethrin, methoxychlor, malathion, diazinon, and DDE but did not remove vinclozolin, bifenthrin, or chlorpyrifos.[83] The water solubility of the pesticide appeared to make absolutely no difference in whether levels were reduced with rinsing (15–30 seconds in cold water). The three pesticides with the best removal rates with simple water rinsing were malathion, captan, and chlorothalonil. Similar results with malathion were found in another study in which lettuce was rinsed with deionized water or a surfactant.[84] Both the surfactant and water rinsing lowered the malathion levels by 30% but did not remove it.

Peeling potatoes reduced pesticide content by at least 70% for both chlorinated and organophosphate pesticides.[85] Potato skins contained the highest amounts of DDE, lindane, and HCB of any part of the potato (Table 3.11). Washing with water as well as cooking helped to eliminate most of the rest of the residues.

A Belgian study reported that washing fruits and vegetables with tap water provided no significant reduction in pesticide residues.[86] Washing lettuce reduced propamocarb only 8% and parathion only 12% but was slightly more effective for vinclozolin at 43%. On the other hand, they found that peeling fruits and vegetables removed almost all pesticides

Acid washing may be the most effective means of reducing pesticide residue for produce that lends itself to this method (Tables 3.12 and 3.13).[87] Different acid solutions (e.g., radish [made by cutting the green part of *Raphanus sativus* into small pieces and soaking in water], citric acid, ascorbic acid, acetic acid, and hydrogen peroxide) were tested against neutral and alkaline solutions and tap water. Radish solutions worked the best for organochlorine residues, followed by citric acid and then

TABLE 3.11 Chlorinated and Organophosphate Pesticides in the Skin and Flesh of Potatoes

Class of Pesticide	Skin	Flesh
Organochlorine	3.03	1.60
Organophosphorus	2.61	0.55

Data from Soliman, K.M. (2001). Changes in concentration of pesticide residues in potatoes during washing and home preparation. *Food and Chemical Toxicology*, 39(8):887-891.

TABLE 3.13 Organophosphate Pesticide Reduction With Water, Acid, or Alkaline Washes, %

Solution	Pirimiphos-Methyl	Malathion	Profenofos
Radish–5/10	100	100	100
Acetic–5/10	100	100	100
Citric–5/10	100	94.7/96.9	100
Ascorbic–5/10	100	87.9/92.7	100
H_2O_2–5/10	100	89.9/93	100
Tap water	12.9	11.6	13.5
Na_2CO_3–5	98.5	NA	NA
Na_2CO_3–5	98.8	NA	NA

Zohair, A. (2001). Behavior of some organophosphorus and organochlorine pesticides in potatoes during soaking in different solutions. *Food and Chemical Toxicology*, 39(7), 751-755.

TABLE 3.12 Reduction of Chlorinated Pesticide Residue with Water, Acid, and Alkaline Washes, %

Solution	Lindane	Aldrin	Heptachlor Epoxide	o,p-DDE	p,p-DDE	o,p-DDD
Radish–5 conc.	100	100	100	67.6	100	100
Radish–10 conc.	100	100	100	73.1	100	100
Acetic acid–5 conc.	66.7	72	95.2	75.2	96.1	96
Acetic acid–10	78.3	84	96.6	86.7	97.4	97.4
Citric acid–5	100	76	100	73.1	98	100
Citric acid–10	100	85.2	100	77.5	18.4	100
Ascorbic acid–5	100	84	100	57.5	91.9	100
Ascorbic acid–10	100	90.8	100	67.6	94.9	100
H_2O_2–5	81.2	64	94.5	80.4	100	100
H_2O_2–10	89.1	78	95.9	87	100	100
Tap water	12	10	9.8	2	3.5	3.9
Na_2CO_3–5	89.1	84	93.2	NA	NA	NA
Na_2CO_3–10	92	88	95.2	NA	NA	NA

Modified from Zohair, A. (2001). Behavior of some organophosphorus and organochlorine pesticides in potatoes during soaking in different solutions. *Food and Chemical Toxicology*, 39(7), 751-755.

ascorbic acid. The acidic solutions also worked best for organophosphate insecticide residues (98.5%–100% for pirimiphos-methyl, 87.9%–100% for malathion, and 100% for profenofos), but alkaline washes also were quite effective.

As shown in Table 3.13, malathion residues only decreased by 11.6% after rinsing with water, a level lower than what was previously discussed. We could find no hard data on use of bleach to reduce pesticide exposure, and researchers at a major bleach manufacturer (personal communication, April 2017) were also not aware of any research.

ORGANIC FOODS

Organic foods should not be considered "pesticide free" but are clearly less contaminated than commercially grown food. A review utilizing data from the USDA, the Consumers Union, and the California Department of Pesticide Regulation revealed that organically raised foods had one-third the amount of chemical residues found in conventionally grown foods.[88] Compared with produce grown with integrated pest management techniques, the organic produce had one-half the amount of residue. In addition, organic foods were 10-fold less likely than nonorganic produce to have more than one residue present. Only 2.6% of organic foods had multiple residues detected compared with 26% of conventionally grown foods. On average, 82% of conventional fruits were positive for insecticide residues compared with 23% of organic fruits. Commercially grown potatoes have twice the pesticide and heavy metal contamination as organic potatoes.[89]

A meta-analysis of 343 peer-reviewed articles on organic foods concluded that only 11% of all organic foods tested had pesticide residue present, whereas 46% of commercial foods did.[90] Organically grown foods also had 48% less cadmium, 30% less nitrates, and 87% less nitrites. In addition, organic foods have far higher content of the health-promoting polyphenol compounds.

Children with diets consisting of ≥ 75% organic foods had a ninefold lower mean level (sixfold lower median level) of organophosphate pesticide residues in their urine than those whose diet was ≥ 75% nonorganic.[91] As little as 5 days of replacing conventionally grown foods with organic varieties resulted in the disappearance of urinary malathion and chlorpyrifos metabolites in their urine.[92] Once the subjects returned to eating their normal conventional foods, five different OP metabolites reappeared in their urine.

REFERENCES

1. Ausubel, K. (1994). *Seeds of Change: The Living Treasure: The Passionate Story of the Growing Movement to Restore Biodiversity and Revolutionize the Way We Think About Food*. New York: Harper Collins.
2. Pimental, D. (1995). Amounts of pesticides reaching target pests: environmental impacts and ethics. *Journal of Agricultural and Environmental Ethics, 8*(1), 17–29.
3. Harner, T., Pozo, K., Gouin, T., et al. (2006). Global pilot study for persistent organic pollutants (POPs) using PUF disk passive air samplers. *Environmental Pollution, 144*(2), 445–452. [Epub April 17, 2006]; PubMed PMID: 16616403.
4. Li, J., Zhu, T., Wang, F., et al. (2006). Observation of organochlorine pesticides in the air of the Mt. Everest region. *Ecotoxicology and Environmental Safety, 63*(1), 33–41. PubMed PMID: 15922448.
5. Tilman, D., Cassman, K. G., Matson, P. A., et al. (2002). Agricultural sustainability and intensive production practices. *Nature, 418*(6898), 671–677. PubMed PMID: 12167873.
6. Environmental Protection Agency. *Pesticides Industry Sales and Usage: 2006 and 2007. Market Estimates.* Available from https://www.epa.gov/sites/production/files/2015-10/documents/market_estimates2007.pdf. (Accessed May 1, 2017.)
7. United States Department of Agriculture. *Pesticide Date Program: Annual Summary, Calendar Year 2015.* Available from https://www.ams.usda.gov/sites/default/files/media/2015PDPAnnualSummary.pdf. (Accessed April 28, 2017.)
8. Charnley, G., & Doull, J. (2005). Human exposure to dioxins from food, 1999-2002. *Food and Chemical Toxicology, 43*(5), 671–679. PubMed PMID: 15778006.
9. Schafer, K. S., & Kegley, S. E. (2002). Persistent toxic chemicals in the US food supply. *Journal of Epidemiology and Community Health, 56*(11), 813–817. PubMed PMID: 12388566.
10. NOAA Fisheries. *Basic Questions about Aquaculture.* Available from http://www.nmfs.noaa.gov/aquaculture/faqs/faq_aq_101.html#4howmuch. (Accessed April 29, 2017.)
11. Knapp, G., et al. *The Great Salmon Run: Competition Between Wild and Farmed Salmon.* Available from http://www.iser.uaa.alaska.edu/Publications/2007_0.1-GreatSalmonRun.pdf (Accessed April 29, 2017.)

12. van Leeuwen, S. P., van Velzen, M. J., Swart, C. P., et al. (2009). Halogenated contaminants in farmed salmon, trout, tilapia, pangasius, and shrimp. *Environmental Science & Technology*, 43(11), 4009–4015. PubMed PMID: 19569323.

13. Hites, R. A., Foran, J. A., Carpenter, D. O., et al. (2004). Global assessment of organic contaminant in farmed salmon. *Science*, 303, 226–229. PubMed PMID: 14716013.

14. Carlson, D. L., & Hites, R. A. (2005). Polychlorinated biphenyls in salmon and salmon feed: global differences and bioaccumulation. *Environmental Science & Technology*, 39(19), 7389–7395. PubMed PMID: 16245806.

15. Ikonomou, M. G., Higgs, D. A., Gibbs, M., et al. (2007). Flesh quality of market-size farmed and wild British Columbia salmon. *Environmental Science & Technology*, 41(2), 437–443. PubMed PMID:17310704.

16. Nøstbakken, O. J., Hove, H. T., Duinker, A., et al. (2015). Contaminant levels in Norwegian farmed Atlantic salmon (Salmo salar) in the 13-year period from 1999 to 2011. *Environment International*, 74, 274–280. PubMed PMID: 25454244.

17. Hanrahan, L. P., Falk, C., Anderson, H. A., et al. (1999). Serum PCB and DDE levels of frequent Great Lakes sport fish consumers: a first look. The Great Lakes Consortium. *Environmental Research*, 80(2 Pt. 2), S26–S37. PubMed PMID: 10092417.

18. Newsome, W. H., & Andrews, P. (1993). Organochlorine pesticides and polychlorinated biphenyl cogeners in commercial fish from the Great Lakes. *Journal of AOAC International*, 76(4), 707–710. PubMed PMID: 8374320.

19. He, J. P., Stein, A. D., Humphrey, H. E., et al. (2001). Time trends in sport-caught Great Lakes fish consumption and serum polychlorinated biphenyl levels among Michigan anglers, 1973-1993. *Environmental Science & Technology*, 35(3), 435–440. PubMed PMID: 11351711.

20. Schecter, A., Päpke, O., Harris, T. R., et al. (2006). Polybrominated diphenyl ether (PBDE) levels in an expanded market basket survey of U.S. food and estimated PBDE dietary intake by age and sex. *Environmental Health Perspectives*, 114(10), 1515–1520. PubMed PMID: 17035135.

21. Newsome, W. H., Davies, D. J., & Sun, W. F. (1998). Residues of polychlorinated biphenyls (PCB) in fatty foods of the Canadian diet. *Food Additives and Contaminants*, 15(1), 19–29. PubMed PMID: 9534869.

22. Badia-Vila, M., Ociepa, M., Mateo, R., & Guitart, R. (2000). Comparison of residue levels of persistent organochlorine compounds in butter from Spain and from other European countries. *Journal of Environmental Science and Health. Part. B, Pesticides, Food Contaminants, and Agricultural Wastes*, 35(2), 201–210. PubMed PMID: 10736769.

23. Waliszewski, S. M., Villalobos-Pietrini, R., Gómez-Arroyo, S., & Infanzón, R. M. (2003). Persistent organochlorine pesticides in Mexican butter. *Food Additives and Contaminants*, 20(4), 361–367. PubMed PMID: 12775478.

24. Cetinkaya, M., von Duszeln, J., Thiemann, W., & Silwar, R. (1984). [Organochlorine pesticide residues in raw and roasted coffee and their degradation during the roasting process]. *Zeitschrift fur Lebensmittel-Untersuchung Und -Forschung*, 179(1), 5–8. PubMed PMID: 6485555.

25. Sakamoto, K., Nishizawa, H., & Manabe, N. (2012). Behavior of pesticides in coffee beans during the roasting process. *Shokuhin Eiseigaku Zasshi. Journal of the Food Hygienic Society of Japan*, 53(5), 233–236. PubMed PMID: 23154763.

26. Petersen, J. H., & Jensen, K. G. (1986). Pesticide residues in black tea. *Zeitschrift fur Lebensmittel-Untersuchung Und -Forschung*, 182(6), 489–491.

27. Colapinto, C. K., Arbuckle, T. E., Dubois, L., & Fraser, W. (2015). Tea consumption in pregnancy as a predictor of pesticide exposure and adverse birth outcomes: The MIREC Study. *Environmental Research*, 142, 77–83. PubMed PMID: 26117816.

28. MacIntosh, D., Kabiru, C. W., & Ryan, P. B. (2001). Longitudinal investigation of dietary exposure to selected pesticides. *Environmental Health Perspectives*, 109, 145–501. PubMed PMID: 11266324.

29. Melnyk, L. J., Xue, J., Brown, G. G., et al. (2014). Dietary intakes of pesticides based on community duplicate diet samples. *The Science of the Total Environment*, 468–469. 785-90. PubMed PMID: 24070872.

30. Cao, X. L., Zhao, W., Churchill, R., & Hilts, C. (2014). Occurrence of Di-(2-ethylhexyl) adipate and phthalate plasticizers in samples of meat, fish, and cheese and their packaging films. *Journal of Food Protection*, 77(4), 610–620. PubMed PMID: 24680073.

31. Castle, L., Mercer, A. J., Startin, J. R., & Gilbert, J. (1988). Migration from plasticized films into foods. 3. Migration of phthalate, sebacate, citrate and phosphate esters from films used for retail food packaging. *Food Additives and Contaminants*, 5(1), 9–20. PubMed PMID: 3356285.

32. Benbrook, C. M. (2012). Impacts of genetically engineered crops on pesticide use in the U.S. – the first sixteen years. *Environmental Sciences Europe*, 24, e1600850. PubMed PMID: 5020710.

33. Bøhn, T., Cuhra, M., Traavik, T., et al. (2014). Compositional differences in soybeans on the market: glyphosate accumulates in Roundup ready GM

soybeans. *Food Chemistry*, 153, 207–215. PubMed PMID: 24491722.

34. Ehling, S., & Reddy, T. M. (2015). Analysis of glyphosate and aminomethylphosphonic acid in nutritional ingredients and milk by derivatization with fluorenylmethyloxycarbonyl chloride and liquid chromatography-mass spectrometry. *Journal of Agricultural and Food Chemistry*, 63(48), 10562–10568. PubMed PMID: 26568409.

35. Granby, K., Johannesen, S., & Vahl, M. (2003). Analysis of glyphosate residues in cereals using liquid chromatography-mass spectrometry (LC-MS/MS). *Food Additives and Contaminants*, 20(8), 692–698. PubMed PMID: 13129785.

36. Tang, W., Hemm, I., & Eisenbrand, G. (2000). Estimation of human exposure to styrene and ethylbenzene. *Toxicology*, 144, 39–50. PubMed PMID:10781869.

37. Genualdi, S., Nyman, P., & Begley, T. (2014). Updated evaluation of the migration of styrene monomer and oligomers from polystyrene food contact materials to foods and food simulants. *Food Additives & Contaminants. Part A, Chemistry, Analysis, Control, Exposure & Risk Assessment*, 31(4), 723–733. PubMed PMID: 24383702.

38. Tawfik, M. S., & Huyghebaert, A. (1998). Polystyrene cups and containers: styrene migration. *Food Additives and Contaminants*, 15(5), 592–599. PubMed PMID: 9829045.

39. Lickly, T. D., Lehr, K. M., & Welsh, G. C. (1995). Migration of styrene from polystyrene foam food contact articles. *Food and Chemical Toxicology*, 33(6), 475–481.

40. Gramshaw, J. W., & Vandenburg, H. J. (1995). Compositional analysis of samples of thermoset polyester and migration of ethylbenzene and styrene from thermoset polyester into pork during cooking. *Food Additives and Contaminants*, 12(2), 223–234.

41. Lickly, T. D., Breder, C. V., & Rainey, M. L. (1995). A model for estimating the daily dietary intake of a substance from food contact articles: styrene from polystyrene food contact polymers. *Regulatory Toxicology and Pharmacology*, 21(3), 406–417.

42. Castle, L., Mayo, A., & Gilbert, J. (1989). Migration of plasticizers from printing inks into food. *Food Additives and Contaminants*, 6(4), 437–443.

43. Dastle, L., Mercer, A. J., Startin, J. R., & Gilbert, J. (1988). Migration from plasticized films into foods. 3. Migration of phthalate, sebacate, citrate and phosphate esters from films used for retail food packaging. *Food Additives and Contaminants*, 5(1), 9–20. PubMed PMID: 3356285.

44. Castle, L., Nichol, J., & Gilbert, J. (1992). Migration of polyisobutylene from polyethylene/polyisobutylene films into foods during domestic and microwave oven use. *Food Additives and Contaminants*, 9(4), 315–330.

45. Page, B. D., & Lacroix, G. M. (1995). The occurrence of phthalate ester and di-2-ethylhexyl adipate plasticizers in Canadian packaging and food sampled in 1985-1989: a survey. *Food Additives and Contaminants*, 12(1), 129–151.

46. Tsumura, Y., Ishimitsu, S., Saito, I., et al. (2003). Estimated daily intake of plasticizers in 1-week duplicate diet samples following regulation of DEHP-containing PVC gloves in Japan. *Food Additives and Contaminants*, 20(4), 317–324. PubMed PMID: 12775472.

47. Tsumura, Y., Ishimitsu, S., Kaihara, A., et al. (2001). Di(2-thylhexyl) phthalate contamination of retail packed lunches caused by PVC gloves used in the preparation of foods. *Food Additives and Contaminants*, 18(6), 569–579. PubMed PMID: 11407756.

48. Zota, A. R., Phillips, C. A., & Mitro, S. D. (2016). Recent fast food consumption and bisphenol A and phthalates exposures among the U.S. population in NHANES, 2003-2010. *Environmental Health Perspectives*, 124(10), 1521–1528. PMID: 27072648.

49. Lorber, M., Schecter, A., Paepke, O., et al. (2015). Exposure assessment of adult intake of bisphenol A (BPA) with emphasis on canned food dietary exposures. *Environment International*, 77, 55–62. PubMed PMID: 25645382.

50. Hartle, J. C., Navas-Acien, A., & Lawrence, R. S. (2016). The consumption of canned food and beverages and urinary bisphenol A concentrations in NHANES 2003-2008. *Environmental Research*, 150, 375–382. PubMed PMID: 27362993.

51. Carwile, J. L., Ye, X., Zhou, X., et al. (2011). Canned soup consumption and urinary bisphenol A: a randomized crossover trial. *Journal of the American Medical Association*, 306(20), 2218–2220. PubMed PMID: 22110104.

52. Lakind, J. S., & Naiman, D. Q. (2011). Daily intake of bisphenol A and potential sources of exposure: 2005-2006 National Health and Nutrition Examination Survey. *Journal of Exposure Science and Environmental Epidemiology*, 21(3), 272–279. PubMed PMID: 20237498.

53. Bae, S., & Hong, Y. C. (2015). Exposure to bisphenol A from drinking canned beverages increases blood pressure: randomized crossover trial. *Hypertension*, 65(2), 313–319. PubMed PMID: 25489056.

54. Rao, K. S., & Rao, G. V. (1995). Aluminum leaching from utensils – a kinetic study. *International Journal of Food Sciences and Nutrition*, 46(1), 31–38. PubMed PMID: 7712341.

55. Moody, G. H., Southam, J. C., Buchan, S. A., & Farmer, J. G. (1990). Aluminum leaching and fluoride. *British Dental Journal*, 169(2), 47–50. PubMed PMID: 2390386.

56. Ma, N., Liu, Z. P., Yang, D. J., et al. (2016). Risk assessment of dietary exposure to aluminium in the Chinese population. *Food Additives & Contaminants. Part A, Chemistry, Analysis, Control, Exposure & Risk Assessment*, 33(10), 1557–1562. PubMed PMID: 27595294.

57. Wong, W. W., Chung, S. W., Kwong, K. P., et al. (2010). Dietary exposure to aluminium of the Hong Kong population. *Food Additives & Contaminants. Part A, Chemistry, Analysis, Control, Exposure & Risk Assessment*, 27(4), 457–463. doi:10.1080/19440040903490112. PubMed PMID: 20234962.

58. Li, G., Zhao, X., Wu, S., et al. (2017). Dietary exposure to aluminium in the popular Chinese fried bread youtiao. *Food Additives & Contaminants. Part A, Chemistry, Analysis, Control, Exposure & Risk Assessment*, 1–8. PubMed PMID: 28332421.

59. Cabrera-Vique, C., & Mesías, M. (2013). Content and bioaccessibility of aluminium in duplicate diets from southern Spain. *Journal of Food Science*, 78(8), T1307–T1312. PubMed PMID: 23957422.

60. Gramiccioni, L., Ingrao, G., Milana, M. R., et al. (1996). Aluminium levels in Italian diets and in selected foods from aluminium utensils. *Food Additives and Contaminants*, 13(7), 767–774. PubMed PMID: 8885317.

61. Lione, A. (1984). Aluminum in foods. *Nutrition Reviews*, 42(1), 31. PubMed PMID: 6700843.

62. Fimreite, N., Hansen, O., & Pettersen, H. C. (1997). Aluminum concentrations in selected foods prepared in aluminum cookware, and its implications for human health. *Bulletin of Environmental Contamination and Toxicology*, 58, 1–7. PubMed PMID: 8952918.

63. Lione, A., Allen, P. V., & Smith, J. C. (1984). Aluminium coffee percolators as a source of dietary aluminium. *Food and Chemical Toxicology*, 22(4), 265–268. PubMed PMID: 6539273.

64. Abercrombie, D., & Fowler, R. (1997). Possible aluminum content of canned drinks. *Toxicology and Industrial Health*, 13(5), 649–654. PubMed PMID: 9284535.

65. Focazio, M., Welch, A., Watkins, S., Helsel, D., & Horn, M. *A Retrospective Analysis on the Occurrence of Arsenic in Ground-Water Resources of the United States and Limitations in Drinking-Water-Supply Characterizations.* USGS Water Resources Investigation Report 99-4279. http://pubs.usgs.gov/wri/wri994279/pdf/wri994279.pdf (Accessed August 17, 2016.)

66. Gilbert-Diamond, D., Cottingham, K. L., Gruber, J. F., et al. (2011). Rice consumption contributes to arsenic exposure in US women. *Proceedings of the National Academy of Sciences of the United States of America*, 108(51), 20656–20660. PubMed PMID: 22143778.

67. Davis, M. A., Mackenzie, T. A., Cottingham, K. L., et al. (2012). Rice consumption and urinary arsenic concentrations in U.S. children. *Environmental Health Perspectives*, 120(10), 1418–1424. PMID: 23008276.

68. Centers for Disease Control and Prevention. *National Report on Human Exposure to Environmental Chemicals. Updated Tables, January 2017.* Available at www.cdc.gov/exposurereport/. (Accessed April 17, 2017.)

69. Juhasz, A. L., Smith, E., Weber, J., et al. (2006). In vivo assessment of arsenic bioavailability in rice and its significance for human health risk assessment. *Environmental Health Perspectives*, 114(12), 1826–1831. PubMed PMID: 17185270.

70. Williams, P. N., Raab, A., Feldmann, J., & Meharg, A. A. (2007). Market basket survey shows elevated levels of As in South Central U.S. processed rice compared to California: consequences for human dietary exposure. *Environmental Science & Technology*, 41(7), 2178–2183. PubMed PMID: 17438760.

71. Sengupta, M. K., Hossain, M. A., Mukherjee, A., et al. (2006). Arsenic burden of cooked rice: Traditional and modern methods. *Food and Chemical Toxicology: An International Journal Published for the British Industrial Biological Research Association*, 44(11), 1823–1829. PMID:16876928.

72. Raab, A., Baskaran, C., Feldmann, J., & Meharg, A. A. (2009). Cooking rice in a high water to rice ratio reduces inorganic arsenic content. *Journal of Environmental Monitoring*, 11(1), 41–44. PubMed PMID: 19137137.

73. Nachman, K. E., Baron, P. A., Raber, G., et al. (2013). Roxarsone, inorganic arsenic, and other arsenic species in chicken: a U.S.-based market basket sample. *Environmental Health Perspectives*, 121(7), 818–824. PMID: 23694900.

74. Liu, Q., Peng, H., Lu, X., et al. (2016). Arsenic species in chicken breast: temporal variations of metabolites, elimination kinetics, and residual concentrations. *Environmental Health Perspectives*, 124(8), 1174–1181. PubMed PMID: 26992196.

75. Adams, S. V., Newcomb, P. A., Shafer, M. M., et al. (2011). Sources of cadmium exposure among healthy premenopausal women. *The Science of the Total Environment*, 409(9), 1632–1637. PubMed PMID: 21333327.

76. Reeves, P. G., & Chaney, R. L. (2008). Bioavailability as an issue in risk assessment and management of food cadmium: a review. *The Science of the Total Environment*, 398(1–3), 13–19. PubMed PMID: 18430461.

77. Mahaffey, K. R., Clickner, R. P., & Bodurow, C. C. (2004). Blood organic mercury and dietary mercury intake: National Health and Nutrition Examination Survey, 1999 and 2000. *Environmental Health Perspectives, 112*(5), 562–570. PubMed PMID: 15064162.

78. Sunderland, E. M., Krabbenhoft, D. P., Moreau, J. W., Strode, S. A., & Landing, W. M. (2009). Global Biogeochemical Cycles. *Global Biogeochemical Cycles, 23*, GB2010.

79. Environmental Protection Agency. (2011) *National Listing of Fish Advisories (NLFA)*. Available from https://www.epa.gov/sites/production/files/2015-06/documents/maps-and-graphics-2011.pdf. (Accessed May 1, 2017.)

80. U.S. Food and Drug Administration. Mercury in fish: cause for concern? *FDA Consumer*, September 1994, Revised May 1995. https://www.fda.gov/OHRMS/DOCKETS/ac/02/briefing/3872_Advisory%207.pdf. (Accessed May 1, 2017.)

81. Sunderland, E. M. (2007). Mercury exposure from domestic and imported estuarine and marine fish in the U.S. seafood market. *Environmental Health Perspectives, 115*(2), 235–242. PubMed PMID: 17384771.

82. Nielsen, S. J., Kit, B. K., Aoki, Y., & Ogden, C. L. (2014). Seafood consumption and blood mercury concentrations in adults aged ≥20 y, 2007-2010. *The American Journal of Clinical Nutrition, 99*(5), 1066–1070. PubMed PMID: 24522443.

83. Krol, W. J., Arsenault, T. L., Pylypiw, H. M., & Incorvia Mattina, M. J. (2000). Reduction of pesticide residues on produce by rinsing. *Journal of Agricultural and Food Chemistry, 48*(10), 4666–4670. PubMed PMID: 11052716.

84. Leyva, J., Lee, P., & Goh, K. S. (1998). Removal of malathion residues on lettuce by washing. *Bulletin of Environmental Contamination and Toxicology, 60*, 592–595. PubMed PMID: 9557197.

85. Soliman, K. M. (2001). Changes in concentration of pesticide residues in potatoes during washing and home preparation. *Food and Chemical Toxicology, 39*(8), 887–891. PubMed PMID: 11434996.

86. Dejonckheere, W., Steurbaut, W., Drieghe, S., et al. (1996). Pesticide residue concentrations in the Belgian total diet, 1991-1993. *Journal of AOAC International, 79*(2), 520–528. PubMed PMID: 8920141.

87. Zohair, A. (2001). Behavior of some organophosphorus and organochlorine pesticides in potatoes during soaking in different solutions. *Food and Chemical Toxicology, 39*(7), 751–755. PubMed PMID: 11397522.

88. Baker, B. P., Benbrook, C. M., Groth, E., 3rd, & Lutz Benbrook, K. (2002). Pesticide residues in conventional, integrated pest management (IPM)-grown and organic foods: insights from three US data sets. *Food Additives and Contaminants, 19*(5), 427–446. PubMed PMID: 12028642.

89. Mansour, S. A., Belal, M. H., Abou-Arab, A. A., et al. (2009). Evaluation of some pollutant levels in conventionally and organically farmed potato tubers and their risks to human health. *Food and Chemical Toxicology, 47*(3), 615–624. PubMed PMID: 19138717.

90. Barański, M., Srednicka-Tober, D., Volakakis, N., et al. (2014). Higher antioxidant and lower cadmium concentrations and lower incidence of pesticide residues in organically grown crops: a systematic literature review and meta-analyses. *The British Journal of Nutrition*, 1–18. PubMed PMID: 24968103.

91. Curl, C. L., Fenske, R. A., & Elgethun, K. (2003). Organophosphorus pesticide exposure of urban and suburban preschool children with organic and conventional diets. *Environmental Health Perspectives, 111*(3), 377–382. PubMed PMID: 12611667.

92. Lu, C., Barr, D. B., Pearson, M. A., & Waller, L. A. (2008). Dietary intake and its contribution to longitudinal organophosphorus pesticide exposure in urban/suburban children. *Environmental Health Perspectives, 116*(4), 537–542. PubMed PMID: 18414640.

4

Water Pollution

SUMMARY

- Primary sources: Agricultural, industrial, geological
- Primary toxicants: EPA-governed categories include microorganisms, disinfectants, disinfection by-products, inorganic chemicals, organic chemicals, and radionuclides.

- Primary disease associations: Cancer, brain and nervous system damage, cardiovascular disease, developmental defects, infertility, reproductive dysfunction, and hormone disruption
- Best intervention: Reverse osmosis water filtration

INTRODUCTION

Passed in 1974, the Safe Drinking Water Act (SDWA) was originally designed to regulate public drinking water and its sources, including rivers, lakes, reservoirs, springs, and groundwater wells (excluding private wells). There are currently more than 170,000 public water systems, which supply 85% of the drinking water in the United States. Current US Environmental Protection Agency (EPA) regulations apply to only 91 contaminants, with no contaminants having been added to the list of regulated pollutants since 1996. Additionally, the allowable limits have very rarely changed, despite extensive research indicating lower thresholds are more appropriate, particularly to more sensitive populations such as children, older adults, and those with chronic diseases. Even at existing (inadequate) standards, tens of millions of Americans are exposed to toxicant levels that exceed EPA guidelines. Additionally, the source water (e.g., the surface water [streams, rivers, and lakes] and groundwater [aquifers]) that provides water to both public and private systems has become increasingly contaminated.

MAJOR POLLUTANTS AND ADVERSE HEALTH EFFECTS

Table 4.1 shows contaminants and regulatory limits for chemicals in drinking water set by the World Health Organization (WHO), the EPA, and the European Union Council. The categories include microorganisms, disinfectants, disinfection by-products, inorganic chemicals, organic chemicals, and radionuclides. The SDWA requires that three criteria must be met for a contaminant to be regulated: 1) the contaminant may have an adverse effect on the health of persons; 2) the contaminant is known to occur or there is a substantial likelihood the contaminant will occur in drinking water with a frequency and at levels of public health concern; and 3) in the sole judgment of the EPA administrator, regulation of the contaminant presents a meaningful opportunity for reducing health risks for persons served by public water systems.

Microorganisms

Although not the primary focus of this chapter, microorganisms still remain a potential threat despite the effectiveness of water treatment for reducing pathogen levels. For example, a 2008 analysis of US drinking water found that more than 10 million infections (and 5.4 million illnesses, assuming 1/2 of all infections lead to illness) occur each year as a result of community groundwater system contamination, and another 26 million infections (13 million illnesses) occur from municipal surface water systems; the total estimated waterborne illnesses in the United States are estimated to be nearly 20 million per year.[1]

TABLE 4.1 National Primary Drinking Water Regulations

Contaminant	MCLG (mg/L)	MCL or TT (mg/L)	Potential Health Effects from Long-Term Exposure Above the MCL (Unless Specified as Short-Term)	Sources of Contaminant in Drinking Water
MICROORGANISMS				
Cryptosporidium	0.00	TT	Gastrointestinal illness (such as diarrhea, vomiting, and cramps)	Human and animal fecal waste
Giardia lamblia	0.00	TT	Gastrointestinal illness (such as diarrhea, vomiting, and cramps)	Human and animal fecal waste
Heterotrophic plate count (HPC)	n/a	TT	HPC has no health effects; it is an analytic method used to measure the variety of bacteria common in water. The lower the concentration of bacteria in drinking water, the better maintained the water system is.	HPC measures a range of bacteria that are naturally present in the environment
Legionella	0.00	TT	Legionnaire's Disease, a type of pneumonia	Found naturally in water; multiplies in heating systems
Total Coliforms (including fecal coliform and *Escherichia Coli*)	0.00	5.0%	Not a health threat in itself; it is used to indicate whether other potentially harmful bacteria may be present	Coliforms are naturally present in the environment; as well as feces; fecal coliforms and E. coli only come from human and animal fecal waste.
Turbidity	n/a	TT	Turbidity is a measure of the cloudiness of water. It is used to indicate water quality and filtration effectiveness (such as whether disease-causing organisms are present). Higher turbidity levels are often associated with higher levels of disease-causing microorganisms such as viruses, parasites and some bacteria. These organisms can cause symptoms such as nausea, cramps, diarrhea, and associated headaches.	Soil runoff
Viruses (enteric)	0.00	TT	Gastrointestinal illness (such as diarrhea, vomiting, and cramps)	Human and animal fecal waste

Continued

TABLE 4.1 National Primary Drinking Water Regulations—cont'd

Contaminant	MCLG (mg/L)	MCL or TT (mg/L)	Potential Health Effects from Long-Term Exposure Above the MCL (Unless Specified as Short-Term)	Sources of Contaminant in Drinking Water
DISINFECTION BY-PRODUCTS				
Bromate	0.00	0.01	Increased risk of cancer	By-product of drinking water disinfection
Chlorite	0.8	1	Anemia; infants and young children: nervous system effects	By-product of drinking water disinfection
Haloacetic acids (HAA5)	n/a	0.06	Increased risk of cancer	By-product of drinking water disinfection
Total Trihalomethanes (TTHMs)	n/a	>0.080	Liver, kidney or central nervous system problems; increased risk of cancer	By-product of drinking water disinfection
DISINFECTANTS				
Chloramines (as Cl2)	MRDLG = 4	MRDL = 4.0	Eye/nose irritation; stomach discomfort, anemia	Water additive used to control microbes
Chlorine (as Cl2)	MRDLG = 4	MRDL = 4.0	Eye/nose irritation; stomach discomfort	Water additive used to control microbes
Chlorine dioxide (as ClO2)	MRDLG = 0.8	MRDL = 0.8	Anemia; infants and young children: nervous system effects	Water additive used to control microbes
INORGANIC CHEMICALS AND METALS				
Antimony	0.006	0.006	Increase in blood cholesterol; decrease in blood sugar	Discharge from petroleum refineries; fire retardants; ceramics; electronics; solder
Arsenic	0	0.010	Skin damage, problems with circulatory system, increased risk of many cancers	Erosion of natural deposits; runoff from orchards, runoff from glass and electronic production wastes
Asbestos (fiber > 10 micrometers)	7 million fibers per liter (MFL)	7 MFL	Increased risk of developing benign intestinal polyps	Decay of asbestos cement in water mains; erosion of natural deposits
Barium	2	2	Increase in blood pressure	Discharge of drilling wastes; discharge from metal refineries; erosion of natural deposits

Continued

TABLE 4.1   **National Primary Drinking Water Regulations—cont'd**

Contaminant	MCLG (mg/L)	MCL or TT (mg/L)	Potential Health Effects from Long-Term Exposure Above the MCL (Unless Specified as Short-Term)	Sources of Contaminant in Drinking Water
Beryllium	0.004	0.004	Intestinal lesions	Discharge from metal refineries and coal-burning factories; discharge from electrical, aerospace, and defense industries
Cadmium	0.005	0.005	Kidney damage	Corrosion of galvanized pipes; erosion of natural deposits; discharge from metal refineries; runoff from waste batteries and paints
Chromium (total)	0.1	0.1	Allergic dermatitis	Discharge from steel and pulp mills; erosion of natural deposits
Copper	1.3	TT; Action Level = 1.3	Short-term exposure: Gastrointestinal distress. Long-term exposure: Liver or kidney damage. People with Wilson's Disease should consult their personal doctor if the amount of copper in their water exceeds the action level	Corrosion of household plumbing systems; erosion of natural deposits
Cyanide (as free cyanide)	0.2	0.2	Nerve damage or thyroid problems	Discharge from steel/metal factories; discharge from plastic and fertilizer factories
Fluoride	4	4	Bone disease (pain and tenderness of the bones); Children may get mottled teeth	Water additive that promotes strong teeth; erosion of natural deposits; discharge from fertilizer and aluminum factories
Lead	0.00	TT; Action Level = 0.015	Infants and children: Delays in physical or mental development; children could show slight deficits in attention span and learning abilities. Adults: Kidney problems; high blood pressure	Corrosion of household plumbing systems; erosion of natural deposits

Continued

TABLE 4.1   National Primary Drinking Water Regulations—cont'd

Contaminant	MCLG (mg/L)	MCL or TT (mg/L)	Potential Health Effects from Long-Term Exposure Above the MCL (Unless Specified as Short-Term)	Sources of Contaminant in Drinking Water
Mercury (inorganic)	0.002	0.002	Kidney damage	Erosion of natural deposits; discharge from refineries and factories; runoff from landfills and croplands
Nitrate (measured as nitrogen)	10	10	Infants below the age of 6 months who drink water containing nitrate in excess of the MCL could become seriously ill and, if untreated, may die. Symptoms include shortness of breath and blue-baby syndrome.	Runoff from fertilizer use; leaking from septic tanks, sewage; erosion of natural deposits
Nitrite (measured as nitrogen)	1	1	Infants below the age of 6 months who drink water containing nitrite in excess of the MCL could become seriously ill and, if untreated, may die. Symptoms include shortness of breath and blue-baby syndrome.	Runoff from fertilizer use; leaking from septic tanks, sewage; erosion of natural deposits
Selenium	0.05	0.05	Hair or fingernail loss; numbness in fingers or toes; circulatory problems	Discharge from petroleum refineries; erosion of natural deposits; discharge from mines
Thallium	0.0005	0.002	Hair loss; changes in blood; kidney, intestine, or liver problems	Leaching from ore-processing sites; discharge from electronics, glass, and drug factories
ORGANIC CHEMICALS				
Acrylamide	0.00	TT	Nervous system or blood problems; increased risk of cancer	Added to water during sewage/wastewater treatment
Alachlor	0.00	0.002	Eye, liver, kidney or spleen problems; anemia; increased risk of cancer	Runoff from herbicide used on row crops
Atrazine	0.003	0.003	Cardiovascular system or reproductive problems	Runoff from herbicide used on row crops
Benzene	0.00	0.005	Anemia; decrease in blood platelets; increased risk of cancer	Discharge from factories; leaching from gas storage tanks and landfills

Continued

TABLE 4.1   National Primary Drinking Water Regulations—cont'd

Contaminant	MCLG (mg/L)	MCL or TT (mg/L)	Potential Health Effects from Long-Term Exposure Above the MCL (Unless Specified as Short-Term)	Sources of Contaminant in Drinking Water
Benzo(a)pyrene (PAHs)	0.00	0.0002	Reproductive difficulties; increased risk of cancer	Leaching from linings of water storage tanks and distribution lines
Carbofuran	0.04	0.04	Problems with blood, nervous system, or reproductive system	Leaching of soil fumigant used on rice and alfalfa
Carbon tetrachloride	0.00	0.005	Liver problems; increased risk of cancer	Discharge from chemical plants and other industrial activities
Chlordane	0.00	0.002	Liver or nervous system problems; increased risk of cancer	Residue of banned termiticide
Chlorobenzene	0.1	0.1	Liver or kidney problems	Discharge from chemical and agricultural chemical factories
2,4-D	0.07	0.07	Kidney, liver, or adrenal gland problems	Runoff from herbicide used on row crops
Dalapon	0.2	0.2	Minor kidney changes	Runoff from herbicide used on rights of way
1,2-Dibromo-3-chloropropane (DBCP)	0.00	0.0002	Reproductive difficulties; increased risk of cancer	Runoff/leaching from soil fumigant used on soybeans, cotton, pineapples, and orchards
o-Dichlorobenzene	0.6	0.6	Liver, kidney, or circulatory system problems	Discharge from industrial chemical factories
p-Dichlorobenzene	0.075	0.075	Anemia; liver, kidney or spleen damage; changes in blood	Discharge from industrial chemical factories
1,2-Dichloroethane	0.00	0.005	Increased risk of cancer	Discharge from industrial chemical factories
1,1-Dichloroethylene	0.007	0.007	Liver problems	Discharge from industrial chemical factories
cis-1,2-Dichloroethylene	0.07	0.07	Liver problems	Discharge from industrial chemical factories
trans-1,2-Dichloroethylene	0.1	0.1	Liver problems	Discharge from industrial chemical factories
Dichloromethane	0.00	0.005	Liver problems; increased risk of cancer	Discharge from drug and chemical factories
1,2-Dichloropropane	0.00	0.005	Increased risk of cancer	Discharge from industrial chemical factories
Di(2-ethylhexyl) adipate	0.4	0.4	Weight loss; liver problems; possible reproductive difficulties	Discharge from chemical factories
Di(2-ethylhexyl) phthalate	0.00	0.006	Reproductive difficulties; liver problems; increased risk of cancer	Discharge from rubber and chemical factories

Continued

TABLE 4.1 National Primary Drinking Water Regulations—cont'd

Contaminant	MCLG (mg/L)	MCL or TT (mg/L)	Potential Health Effects from Long-Term Exposure Above the MCL (Unless Specified as Short-Term)	Sources of Contaminant in Drinking Water
Dinoseb	0.007	0.007	Reproductive difficulties	Runoff from herbicide used on soybeans and vegetables
Dioxin (2,3,7,8-TCDD)	0.00	0.00000003	Reproductive difficulties; increased risk of cancer	Emissions from waste incineration and other combustion; discharge from chemical factories
Diquat	0.02	0.02	Cataracts	Runoff from herbicide use
Endothall	0.1	0.1	Stomach and intestinal problems	Runoff from herbicide use
Endrin	0.002	0.002	Liver problems	Residue of banned insecticide
Epichlorohydrin	0.00	TT	Increased cancer risk, and over a long period of time, stomach problems	Discharge from industrial chemical factories; an impurity of some water treatment chemicals
Ethylbenzene	0.7	0.7	Liver or kidney problems	Discharge from petroleum refineries
Ethylene dibromide	0.00	0.00005	Problems with liver, stomach, reproductive system, or kidneys; increased risk of cancer	Discharge from petroleum refineries
Glyphosate	0.7	0.7	Kidney problems; reproductive difficulties	Runoff from herbicide use
Heptachlor	0.00	0.0004	Liver damage; increased risk of cancer	Residue of banned termiticide
Heptachlor epoxide	0.00	0.0002	Liver damage; increased risk of cancer	Breakdown of heptachlor
Hexachlorobenzene	0.00	0.001	Liver or kidney problems; reproductive difficulties; increased risk of cancer	Discharge from metal refineries and agricultural chemical factories
Hexachlorocyclopentadiene	0.05	0.05	Kidney or stomach problems	Discharge from chemical factories
Lindane	0.0002	0.0002	Liver or kidney problems	Runoff/leaching from insecticide used on cattle, lumber, gardens
Methoxychlor	0.04	0.04	Reproductive difficulties	Runoff/leaching from insecticide used on fruits, vegetables, alfalfa, livestock
Oxamyl (Vydate)	0.2	0.2	Slight nervous system effects	Runoff/leaching from insecticide used on apples, potatoes, and tomatoes

Continued

TABLE 4.1	National Primary Drinking Water Regulations—cont'd			
Contaminant	MCLG (mg/L)	MCL or TT (mg/L)	Potential Health Effects from Long-Term Exposure Above the MCL (Unless Specified as Short-Term)	Sources of Contaminant in Drinking Water
Polychlorinated biphenyls (PCBs)	0.00	0.0005	Skin changes; thymus gland problems; immune deficiencies; reproductive or nervous system difficulties; increased risk of cancer	Runoff from landfills; discharge of waste chemicals
Pentachlorophenol	0.00	0.001	Liver or kidney problems; increased cancer risk	Discharge from wood preserving factories
Picloram	0.5	0.5	Liver problems	Herbicide runoff
Simazine	0.004	0.004	Problems with blood	Herbicide runoff
Styrene	0.1	0.1	Liver, kidney, or circulatory system problems	Discharge from rubber and plastic factories; leaching from landfills
Tetrachloroethylene	0.00	0.005	Liver problems; increased risk of cancer	Discharge from factories and dry cleaners
Toluene	1	1	Nervous system, kidney, or liver problems	Discharge from petroleum factories
Toxaphene	0.00	0.003	Kidney, liver, or thyroid problems; increased risk of cancer	Runoff/leaching from insecticide used on cotton and cattle
2,4,5-TP (Silvex)	0.05	0.05	Liver problems	Residue of banned herbicide
1,2,4-Trichlorobenzene	0.07	0.07	Changes in adrenal glands	Discharge from textile finishing factories
1,1,1-Trichloroethane	0.2	0.2	Liver, nervous system, or circulatory problems	Discharge from metal degreasing sites and other factories
1,1,2-Trichloroethane	0.003	0.005	Liver, kidney, or immune system problems	Discharge from industrial chemical factories
Trichloroethylene	0.00	0.005	Liver problems; increased risk of cancer	Discharge from metal degreasing sites and other factories
Vinyl chloride	0.00	0.002	Increased risk of cancer	Leaching from PVC pipes; discharge from plastic factories
Xylenes (total)	10	10	Nervous system damage	Discharge from petroleum factories; discharge from chemical factories
RADIONUCLIDES				
Alpha particles	0.00	15 picocuries per Liter (pCi/L)	Increased risk of cancer	Erosion of natural deposits of certain minerals that are radioactive and may emit a form of radiation known as alpha radiation

Continued

TABLE 4.1 National Primary Drinking Water Regulations—cont'd

Contaminant	MCLG (mg/L)	MCL or TT (mg/L)	Potential Health Effects from Long-Term Exposure Above the MCL (Unless Specified as Short-Term)	Sources of Contaminant in Drinking Water
Beta particles and photon emitters	0.00	4 millirems per year	Increased risk of cancer	Decay of natural and man-made deposits of certain minerals that are radioactive and may emit forms of radiation known as photons and beta radiation
Radium 226 and Radium 228 (combined)	0.00	5 pCi/L	Increased risk of cancer	Erosion of natural deposits
Uranium	0.00	30 µg/L	Increased risk of cancer, kidney toxicity	Erosion of natural deposits

MCL, Maximum contaminant level, the highest level of a contaminant allowed in drinking water. MCLs are set as close to MCLGs as feasible using the best available treatment technology and taking cost into consideration. MCLs are enforceable standards. MCLG, Maximum contaminant level goal, the level of a contaminant in drinking water below which there is no known or expected risk to health. MCLGs allow for a margin of safety and are nonenforceable public health goals. MRDL, Maximum residual disinfectant level, the highest level of a disinfectant allowed in drinking water. There is convincing evidence that addition of a disinfectant is necessary for control of microbial contaminants. MRDLG, Maximum residual disinfectant level goal, the level of a drinking water disinfectant below which there is no known or expected risk to health. MRDLGs do not reflect the benefits of the use of disinfectants to control microbial contaminants. TT, Treatment technique, a required process intended to reduce the level of a contaminant in drinking water.
From Environmental Protection Agency. (2017). National primary drinking water regulations. Retrieved from www.epa.gov/ground-water-and-drinking-water/national-primary-drinking-water-regulations

In 2015, there were more than 10,000 violations (2574 health-based) just for coliform contaminants in community water systems, serving nearly 18 million people (10,118,586 health based violations), yet formal enforcement was taken in only 8.8% of cases. A similar number of people were exposed to pathogens such as *Cryptosporidium* or *Giardia* in this same period.[2] In 2015, roughly one-third of the approximately 52,000 community water systems, serving more than 75 million people in the United States (one-fourth of the US population), had a reported violation. See Table 4.2 for a full list of violations. It should also be noted that this is likely a gross underestimate for a variety of reasons. For example, atrazine levels in the Delaware River (Kansas) were more than 100-fold higher in July than in February; depending on when the sample was taken and reported, a violation of the atrazine level may or may not be detected.[3]

Disinfectants and Disinfection By-products

Used to reduce exposure to pathogens, exposure to disinfectants and disinfectant by-products (DBPs, formed when chemical disinfectants such as chlorine and chloramine react with natural organic matter and anthropogenic pollutants) has been linked to cancer and potentially to reproductive effects such as miscarriages and birth defects.[4,5] Although the EPA currently regulates 11 DBPs, it has been estimated that as many as 600 to 700 are formed by treatment.[6] As noted in Table 4.2, the greatest number of health-based violations occurred in this category of contaminants, affecting more than 12 million people in 2015.

Among the most well-studied DBPs are the trihalomethanes (THMs, which includes chloroform, bromoform, and dibromochloromethane [DBCM]). Human exposure depends not only on direct ingestion

TABLE 4.2 **Health-Based Violations of the Safe Drinking Water Act in 2015, Ranked by Population Served**

Rule Name	Population Served	Number of Violations	Number of Systems
All violations	76,922,570	80,834	18,094
Combined disinfectants and disinfection by-products rules	25,173,431	11,311	4,433
Lead and copper rule	18,350,633	8,044	5,367
Total coliform rule	17,768,807	10,261	5,233
Combined surface, groundwater, and filter backwash rules	17,312,604	5,979	2,697
Right-to-know ("Consumer Confidence") rule	14,422,712	7,906	5,030
Public notification rule	8,381,050	13,202	3,394
Nitrates and nitrites rule	3,867,431	1,529	971
Volatile organic contaminants rule	3,451,072	10,383	406
Synthetic organic contaminants rule	2,669,594	6,864	311
Arsenic rule	1,842,594	1,537	573
Radionuclides rule	1,471,364	2,297	523
Inorganic contaminants rule	1,312,643	1,505	224
Miscellaneous rules	3,718	16	10

From Natural Resources Defense Council. (2017). *Threats on tap*. Retrieved from www.nrdc.org/sites/default/files/threats-on-tap-water-infrastructure-protections-report.pdf Republished with permission from the Natural Resources Defense Council.

of drinking water but also occurs due to volatilization of DBPs during showering, bathing, and cooking. A study in Texas revealed that serum THM levels were high in women right after showering.[7] Dietary factors also have an effect, as consumption of raw cruciferous vegetables has been inversely associated with THM levels in the National Health and Nutritional Examination Survey (NHANES).[8] Additionally, *in vitro* studies show that brominated THMs (bromoform, Bromodichloromethane (BDCM), DBCM) are activated to mutagenic intermediates by glutathione S-transferase-theta-1 (GSTT1), and polymorphisms in this gene are linked to greater bladder cancer risk.[9] THMs in drinking water have also been linked to altered genomic methylation patterns, with 29 CpGs located in 11 genes associated with cancer development affected.[10]

Exposure has been associated with adverse reproductive outcomes, as well as cancers of the digestive and genitourinary systems, and more recently with hepatic injury (evidenced by elevated serum alanine aminotransferase (ALT)).[11] For example, a recent NHANES analysis found participants with elevated ALT activity were 1.35 times more likely to have been exposed to high DBCM concentrations. Those with high ALT and no alcohol consumption (who are more likely to have nonalcoholic fatty liver disease [NAFLD]) were 1.6 to 4.0 times more likely to have had elevated exposure to THMs.[12] Bladder cancer remains the strongest link; in one study of participants living in New York, a nearly sixfold increase in risk was observed, with the highest risk found among those who consumed the greatest amount of water that went through disinfection 10 days before use (rather than 3 days postdisinfection).[13] Exposure to DBPs is also more common in specific communities, such as those near hydraulic fracturing (fracking) oil and gas sites.[14]

Inorganic Chemicals, Metals, Organic Chemicals, and Radionuclides

By far roughly 80% of all contaminants regulated by EPA are classified as either an organic or inorganic, which include metals such as arsenic, lead, and mercury, and organics, including pesticides, solvents, and industrial run-off. A small number of radionuclides, including uranium and radium, also may affect the water supply, largely due to erosion of natural deposits.

Lead. Perhaps the most public attention has been given to lead, which enters drinking water from lead-containing service pipes when they corrode, as well as from brass- and chrome-plated faucets and fixtures with lead solder; this is much more likely in homes built before 1986. The EPA has set the maximum contaminant level goal (MCLG) for lead in drinking water at zero, however the MCL has been set to 0.015 mg/L (15 parts per billion (PPB)). Currently, more than 2000 water systems and 4 to 6 million individuals in the United States were exposed to levels exceeding this MCL (see Fig. 4.1). Among those sites affected are schools and day care centers. A water sample at a Maine elementary school

was 42 times higher than the EPA limit of 15 parts per billion, whereas a Pennsylvania preschool was 14 times higher, records show. At an elementary school in Ithaca, N.Y., one sample tested stunningly contained 5000 PPB of lead, the EPA's threshold for "hazardous waste."[15]

Arsenic. Other toxic metals, including arsenic and chromium, are equally concerning with contamination of US water apparently widespread (Figs. 4.2 and 4.3). Even in populations with low arsenic drinking water exposure, water consumption has been shown to predict urinary arsenic levels.[16] Indeed, even in communities with water levels under the EPA's new maximum contaminant level

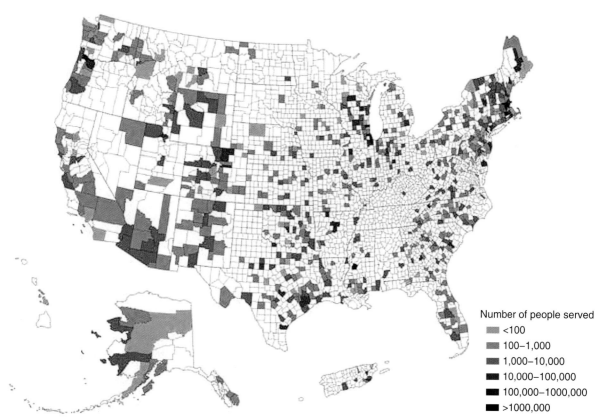

Number of people served
- <100
- 100–1,000
- 1,000–10,000
- 10,000–100,000
- 100,000–1000,000
- >1000,000

FIG. 4.1 Community water systems with action level exceedances (lead): populations served by community water systems that exceeded the 15 PPB action level for lead in 2013 through 2015. In all, 1110 community water systems exceeded the lead action level. These systems serve nearly 4 million people. (From Natural Resources Defense Council. [2017]. *What's in your water? Flint and beyond.* Retrieved from www.nrdc.org/sites/default/files/whats-in-your-water-flint-beyond-report.pdf) Republished with permission from the Natural Resources Defense Council.

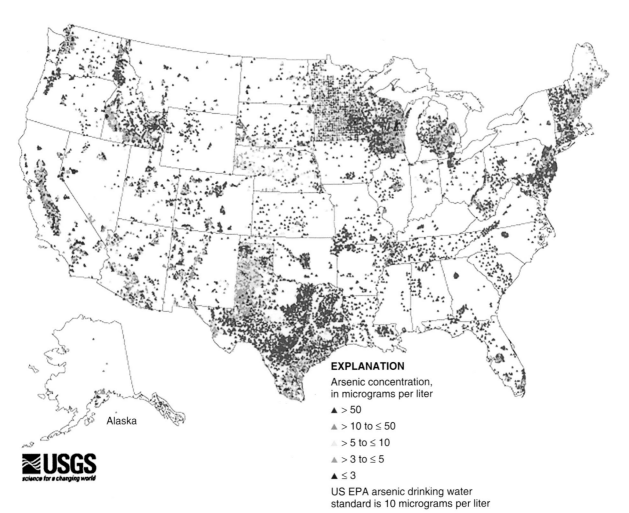

FIG. 4.2 Arsenic in US groundwater. (From U.S. Geological Survey. [2017]. *Trace elements national synthesis project.* Retrieved from https://water.usgs.gov/nawqa/trace/arsenic)

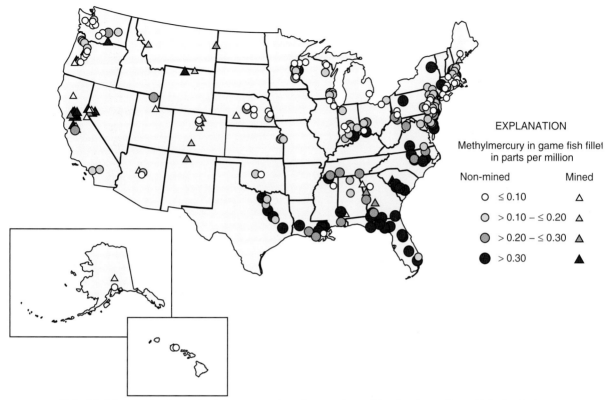

FIG. 4.3 Mercury in the nation's streams—Levels, trends, and implications. (From U.S. Geological Survey. [2017]. *Mercury in the nation's streams—levels, trends, and implications.* Retrieved from https://water.usgs.gov/nawqa/home_maps/circ_1395.html)

of 10 μg/L, drinking water arsenic levels were associated with an increase in risk for very low birth weight and preterm birth.[17] Even at "low" arsenic concentrations, water levels of arsenic have also been associated with bladder cancer among men and women, as well as lung cancer among women.[18] An increase in prostate cancer risk has also been observed at very low arsenic drinking water levels; a 23% increase in risk was found comparing men drinking water at 2.07 to 2.98 PPB versus 1.08 to 2.06 PPB. Aggressive prostate cancer had an even greater relative risk (RR) in the high arsenic drinking water group (RR 1.36 for arsenic 2.99–18.6 PPB).[19] Lifetime exposure to low-level arsenic via drinking water has also been associated with an increased risk for coronary heart disease in a population of more than 500 Colorado residents.[20]

Hexavalent Chromium. Hexavalent chromium is also a widespread water pollutant (Fig. 4.4). For instance, from 2013 to 2015, utilities tested 60,000 samples of drinking water and found hexavalent chromium, a known carcinogen, in more than 75% of the samples, potentially affecting more than 200 million individuals in the United States.[21] Widely used in numerous industrial processes (including chrome pigment production, chrome plating, stainless steel manufacturing, and leather tanning), proximity to industrial sites increases soil, groundwater, and air chromium levels. Current EPA regulations apply only to total chromium, with no specific standard for hexavalent chromium, though the California EPA has proposed 0.02 parts per billion as a cut-off.

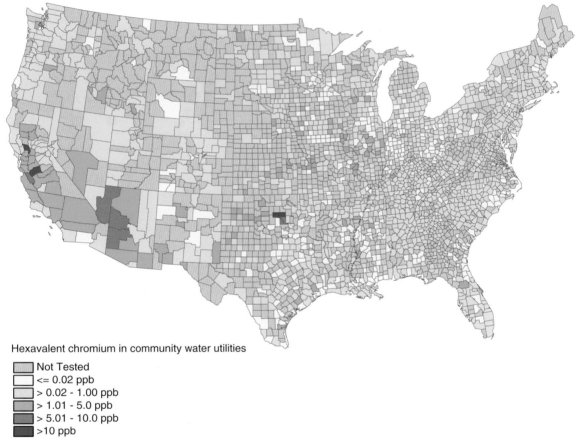

Hexavalent chromium in community water utilities

Not Tested
<= 0.02 ppb
> 0.02 - 1.00 ppb
> 1.01 - 5.0 ppb
> 5.01 - 10.0 ppb
>10 ppb

FIG. 4.4 Average level of Chromium-6 Contamination in Community Water Utilities testing for Chromium-6 in EPA's *UCMR-3,* the third Unregulated Contaminant Monitoring Rule. (From Environmental Working Group. [2017]. *Hexavalent chromium in community water utilities.* Retrieved from www.ewg.org/interactive-maps/2016-chromium6-lower-48.php) Copyright © Environmental Working Group, www.ewg.org. Reproduced with permission.

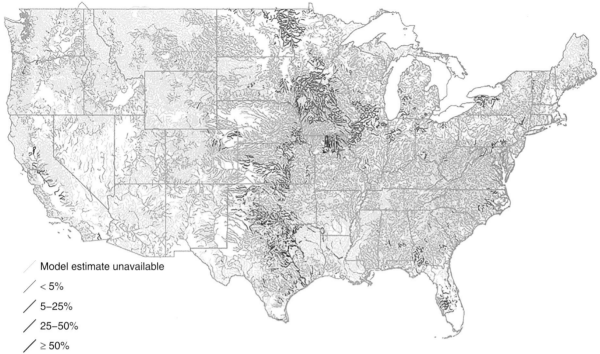

Model estimate unavailable

< 5%

5–25%

25–50%

≥ 50%

FIG. 4.5 Probability that chlorpyrifos exceeds the 4-day moving average acute fish aquatic life benchmark. (From U.S. Geological Survey. [2017]. *Predicting pesticides in streams and rivers: Where is water-quality at risk?* Retrieved from https://water.usgs.gov/nawqa/home_maps/predicting_pesticides.html)

Pesticides and Herbicides. Many organic pesticides, such as chlorpyrifos and atrazine, are also common drinking water contaminants. Chlorpyrifos is the most commonly used organophosphate insecticide, primarily applied to cotton, corn, citrus, and almond crops (Fig. 4.5). It has shown to be damaging to the nervous system of developing humans. Prenatal exposure has been linked to childhood tremor, as well as inversely associated with childhood IQ and memory.[22,23] No limit is set on drinking water, and in 2017 the EPA overturned a proposed ban on this neurotoxin.

Atrazine is also used in large amounts, particularly in the Midwest United States. Nearly 80 million pounds of this herbicide are applied annually, primarily for broadleaf and grassy weeds, on crops such as corn, sorghum grass, sugar cane, and wheat. As can be seen from Figs. 4.6 and 4.7, the likelihood that atrazine (and its breakdown product) will exceed drinking water standards near areas of application is fairly likely. Prenatal exposure has been linked to both preterm and very-preterm delivery.[24] It has been shown to affect the hypothalamic-pituitary-gonadal axis, with adult exposure studies reporting "robust alterations in reproductive hormones including GnRH, LH, FSH, P4, and PRL" (see Fig. 4.8).[25]

Unregulated Contaminants

Many other contaminants not regulated by the EPA are also quite concerning.

Iodinated or Nitrogenated DBPs. Iodinated or nitrogenated DBPs may occur in water supplies at very low concentrations and may be more toxic than their chlorinated analogs.[26]

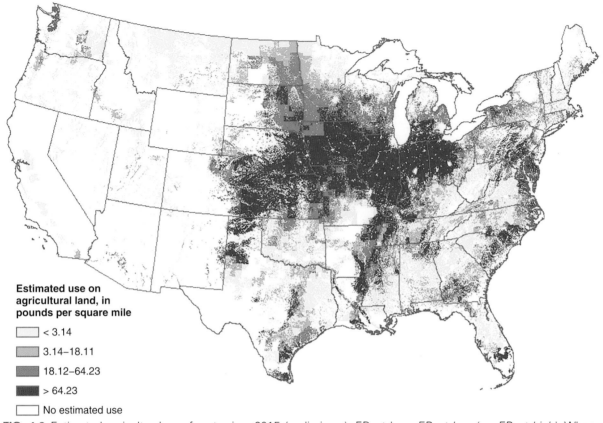

FIG. 4.6 Estimated agricultural use for atrazine, 2015 (preliminary), EPest low. *EPest low (vs. EPest high),* When a crop reporting district (CRP) was surveyed and pesticide use was not reported for a particular crop, EPest-low assumes zero use for that pesticide-by- crop combination. ... EPest-high, however, treats the unreported use for that pesticide-by- crop combination in the CRD as missing data. (From U.S. Geological Survey. [2017]. Retrieved from https://water.usgs.gov/nawqa/pnsp/usage/maps/show_map.php?year=2015&map=ATRAZINE&hilo=L&disp=Atrazine)

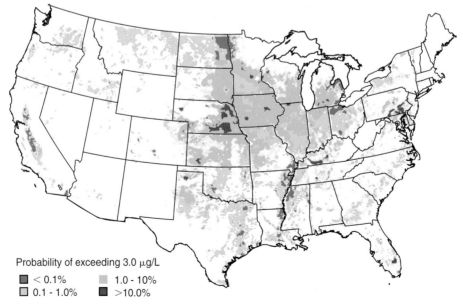

FIG. 4.7 Likelihood that atrazine plus deethylatrazine will exceed drinking-water standard in shallow groundwater underlying agricultural areas. (From U.S. Geological Survey. [2017]. *Pesticide national synthesis project.* Retrieved from https://water.usgs.gov/nawqa/pnsp)

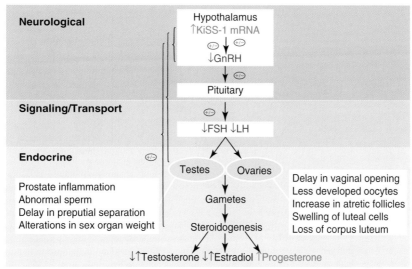

FIG. 4.8 Working conceptual model of atrazine toxicity on the hypothalamus-pituitary-gonadal (HPG) axis across mammalian, anuran, and fish species. *VO,* vaginal opening. (Modified from Wirbisky, S. E., & Freeman, J. L. [2015]. Atrazine exposure and reproductive dysfunction through the hypothalamus-pituitary-gonadal [HPG] axis. *Toxics, 3*[4], 414–450.)

Perchlorate. Perchlorate is well known to inhibit thyroid uptake of iodine; an analysis of NHANES data found tap water, as well as diet, to be the most important predictors of urinary levels.[27] Pregnant women with the highest levels of perchlorate (top 10%) had more than a threefold risk for offspring with an IQ in the lowest 10%. Importantly, levothyroxine treatment did not mitigate this effect.[28]

Perfluorinated Compounds. Perfluorinated chemical exposure from drinking water may be as important dietary intake, with carcinogenic, immune, and endocrine adverse effects. Unlike most other drinking water contaminants, "the human dose-response curve for several effects appears to be steepest at the lower exposure levels, including the general population range, with no apparent threshold for some endpoints."[29] Harvard researchers recently determined that more than 6 million US residents exceed the EPA's lifetime health advisory (70 ng/L) for perfluorooctanesulfonic acid (PFOS) and perfluorooctanoic acid (PFOAs). As seen in Fig. 4.9, exposure is heightened in proximity to military, fire, and industrial sites. Among samples with detectable PFAS (perfluoroalkyl substance) levels, each additional military site within a watershed's eight-digit hydrologic unit is associated with a 20% increase in PFHxS, a 10% increase in both perfluoroheptanoic acid (PFHpA) and PFOA, and a 35% increase in PFOS.[30]

Other Contaminants. Other potentially toxic contaminants, including 1,4-Dioxane, polybrominated diphenyl ether (PBDE) flame retardants, sunscreens/UV filters, pesticide degradation products, and chemical warfare agents are reviewed elsewhere.[31] Furthermore, the combined effects of multiple contaminants, although nearly universally encountered, has not been evaluated. For example, in Midwestern streams, weekly water samples showed 94 pesticides and 89 degradates, with a median of 25 compounds detected per sample and 54 detected per site, with likely toxicity to nontarget aquatic life.[32]

INTERVENTION

Residents in areas with high groundwater arsenic levels can utilize reverse-osmosis (RO) filters to reduce up to 80% of their water arsenic.[33,34] RO units are also effective at removing chromate and perchlorate from tap water.[35] In fact, RO units remove 95% of all toxic compounds, making this form of water purification far more effective than charcoal alone.

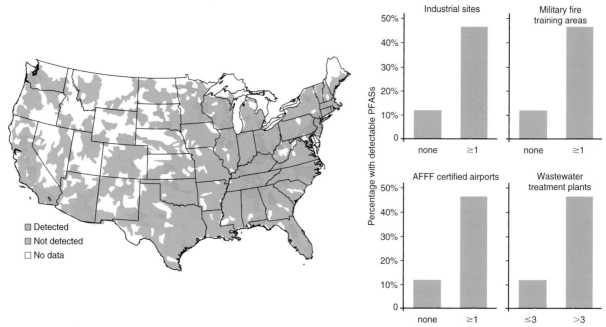

FIG. 4.9 Hydrological units with detectable PFASs. (From Hu, X. C., Andrews, D. Q., Lindstrom, A. B., Burton, T. A., Schaider, L. A., Grandjean, P., Lohmann, R., Carignan, C. C., Blum, A., Balan, S. A., Higgins, C. P., Sunderland, E. M. [2016]. Detection of poly- and perfluoroalkyl substances (PFASs) in U.S. drinking water linked to industrial sites, military fire training areas, and wastewater treatment plants. *Environmental Science & Technology Letters*, *3*[10], 344–350. Copyright © 2016 American Chemical Societ)

REFERENCES

1. Reynolds, K. A., Mena, K. D., & Gerba, C. P. (2008). Risk of waterborne illness via drinking water in the United States. *Reviews of Environmental Contamination and Toxicology*, *192*, 117–158.

2. Fedinick, K. P., Wu, M., & Olson, E. D. (2017). *Threats on Tap: Widespread Violations Highlight Need for Investment in Water Infrastructure and Protections. Natural Resources Defense Council website.* Available at https://www.nrdc.org/resources/threats-tap-widespread-violations-water-infrastructure. (Accessed September 2017).

3. John, K. S., Kathryn, D. G., & Barbara, J. R. (April 1995). *Atrazine Concentrations in the Delaware River, Kansas,* USGS Fact Sheet 001-94. http://ks.water.usgs.gov/pubs/fact-sheets/fs.001-94.stamer.html.

4. Colman, J., Rice, G. E., Wright, J. M., Hunter, E. S. 3rd, Teuschler, L. K., Lipscomb, J. C., Hertzberg, R. C., Simmons, J. E., Fransen, M., Osier, M., Narotsky, M. G. (2011). Identification of developmentally toxic drinking water disinfection byproducts and evaluation of data relevant to mode of action. *Toxicology and Applied Pharmacology*, *254*(2), 100–126. PMID: 21296098.

5. Bove, F., Shim, Y., & Zeitz, P. (2002). Drinking water contaminants and adverse pregnancy outcomes: A review. *Environmental Health Perspectives*, *110*(Suppl. 1), 61–74. PMID: 11834464.

6. Richardson, S. D., Plewa, M. J., Wagner, E. D., Schoeny, R., Demarini, D. M. (2007). Occurrence, genotoxicity, and carcinogenicity of regulated and emerging disinfection by-products in drinking water: A review and roadmap for research. *Mutation Research*, *636*(1–3), 178–242. PMID: 17980649.

7. Lynberg, M., Nuckols, J. R., Langlois, P., Ashley, D., Singer, P., Mendola, P., Wilkes, C., Krapfl, H., Miles, E., Speight, V., Lin, B., Small, L., Miles, A., Bonin, M., Zeitz, P., Tadkod, A., Henry, J., Forrester, M. B. (2001). Assessing exposure to disinfection by-products in women of reproductive age living in Corpus Christi, Texans, and Cobb Count, Georgia: Descriptive results and methods. *Environmental Health Perspectives*, *109*(6), 597–604.

8. Riederer, A. M., Dhingra, R., Blount, B. C., & Steenland, K. (2014). Predictors of blood trihalomethane concentrations in NHANES 1999-2006. *Environmental Health Perspectives*, *122*(7), 695–702. PMID: 24647036.

9. Cantor, K. P., Villanueva, C. M., Silverman, D. T., Figueroa, J. D., Real, F. X., Garcia-Closas, M., Malats, N., Chanock, S., Yeager, M., Tardon, A., Garcia-Closas, R., Serra, C., Carrato, A., Castaño-Vinyals, G., Samanic, C., Rothman, N., Kogevinas, M. (2010). Polymorphisms in GSTT1, GSTZ1, and CYP2E1, disinfection by-products, and risk of bladder cancer in Spain. *Environmental Health Perspectives*, *118*(11), 1545–1550. PMID: 20675267.

10. Salas, L. A., Bustamante, M., Gonzalez, J. R., Gracia-Lavedan, E., Moreno, V., Kogevinas, M., Villanueva, C. M. (2015). DNA methylation levels and long-term trihalomethane exposure in drinking water: An epigenome-wide association study. *Epigenetics*, *10*(7), 650–661. PMID: 26039576.

11. Rahman, M. B., Driscoll, T., Cowie, C., & Armstrong, B. K. (2010). Disinfection by-products in drinking water and colorectal cancer: A meta-analysis. *International Journal of Epidemiology*, *39*, 733–745. PMID: 20139236.

12. Burch, J. B., Everson, T. M., Seth, R. K., Wirth, M. D., Chatterjee, S. (2015). Trihalomethane exposure and biomonitoring for the liver injury indicator, alanine aminotransferase, in the United States population (NHANES 1999-2006). *The Science of the Total Environment*, *521-522*, 226–234. PMID: 25847167.

13. Bove, G. E., Jr., Rogerson, P. A., & Vena, J. E. (2007). Case-control study of the effects of trihalomethanes on urinary bladder cancer risk. *Archives of Environmental and Occupational Health*, *62*(1), 39–47. PMID: 18171646.

14. Parker, K. M., Zeng, T., Harkness, J., Vengosh, A., Mitch, W. A. (2014). Enhanced formation of disinfection byproducts in shale gas wastewater-impacted drinking water supplies. *Environmental Science & Technology*, *48*(19), 11161–11169.

15. Young, A., & Nichols, M. (2016). *Beyond Flint: Excessive lead levels found in almost 2,000 water systems across all 50 states*. Available at https://www.usatoday.com/story/news/2016/03/11/nearly-2000-water-systems-fail-lead-tests/81220466/. (Accessed September 2017).

16. Rivera-Núñez, Z., Meliker, J. R., Slotnick, M. J., Nriagu, J. O. (2012). Urinary arsenic species, toenail arsenic, and arsenic intake estimates in a Michigan population with low levels of arsenic in drinking water. *Journal of Exposure Science and Environmental Epidemiology*, *22*(2), 182–190. PMID: 21878987.

17. Almberg, K. S., Turyk, M. E., Jones, R. M., Rankin, K., Freels, S., Graber, J. M., Stayner, L. T. (2017). Arsenic in drinking water and adverse birth outcomes in Ohio. *Environmental Research*, *157*, 52–59. PMID: 28521257.

18. Mendez, W. M., Jr., Eftim, S., Cohen, J., Warren, I., Cowden, J., Lee, J. S., Sams, R. (2017). Relationships between arsenic concentrations in drinking water and lung and bladder cancer incidence in U.S. counties. *Journal of Exposure Science and Environmental Epidemiology*, *27*(3), 235–243. PMID: 27901016.

19. Roh, T., Lynch, C. F., Weyer, P., Wang, K., Kelly, K. M., Ludewig, G. (2017). Low-level arsenic exposure from drinking water is associated with prostate cancer in Iowa. *Environmental Research*, *159*, 338–343. PMID: 28841521.

20. James, K. A., Byers, T., Hokanson, J. E., Meliker, J. R., Zerbe, G. O., Marshall, J. A. (2015). Association between lifetime exposure to inorganic arsenic in drinking water and coronary heart disease in Colorado residents. *Environmental Health Perspectives*, *123*(2), 128–134. PMID: 25350952.

21. Andrews, D., & Walker, B. (2016). *'Erin Brockovich' Carcinogen in Tap Water of More Than 200 Million Americans. Environmental Working Group website*. Available at http://www.ewg.org/research/chromium-six-found-in-us-tap-water#ref6. (Accessed September 2017).

22. Rauh, V. A., Garcia, W. E., Whyatt, R. M., Horton, M. K., Barr, D. B., Louis, E. D. (2015). Prenatal exposure to the organophosphate pesticide chlorpyrifos and childhood tremor. *Neurotoxicology*, *51*, 80–86. PMID: 26385760.

23. Rauh, V., Arunajadai, S., Horton, M., Perera, F., Hoepner, L., Barr, D. B., Whyatt, R. (2011). Seven-year neurodevelopmental scores and prenatal exposure to chlorpyrifos, a common agricultural pesticide. *Environmental Health Perspectives*, *119*(8), 1196–1201. PMID: 21507777.

24. Stayner, L. T., Almberg, K., Jones, R., Graber, J., Pedersen, M., Turyk, M. (2017). Atrazine and nitrate in drinking water and the risk of preterm delivery and low birth weight in four Midwestern states. *Environmental Research*, *152*, 294–303.

25. Wirbisky, S. E., & Freeman, J. L. (2015). Atrazine exposure and reproductive dysfunction through the hypothalamus-pituitary-gonadal (HPG) axis. *Toxics*, *3*(4), 414–450. PMID: 28713818.

26. Plewa, M. J., Muellner, M. G., Richardson, S. D., Fasano, F., Buettner, K. M., Woo, Y. T., McKague, A. B., Wagner, E. D. (2008a). Occurrence, synthesis, and mammalian cell cytotoxicity and genotoxicity of haloacetamides: An emerging class of nitrogenous drinking water

disinfection byproducts. *Environmental Science & Technology*, 42, 955–961. PMID: 18323128.

27. Lau, F. K., deCastro, B. R., Mills-Herring, L., Tao, L., Valentin-Blasini, L., Alwis, K. U., Blount, B. C. (2013). Urinary perchlorate as a measure of dietary and drinking water exposure in a representative sample of the United States population 2001-2008. *Journal of Exposure Science and Environmental Epidemiology*, 23(2), 207–214. PMID: 23188482.

28. Taylor, P. N., Okosieme, O. E., Murphy, R., Hales, C., Chiusano, E., Maina, A., Joomun, M., Bestwick, J. P., Smyth, P., Paradice, R., Channon, S., Braverman, L. E., Dayan, C. M., Lazarus, J. H., Pearce, E. N. (2014). Maternal perchlorate levels in women with borderline thyroid function during pregnancy and the cognitive development of their offspring: Data from the Controlled Antenatal Thyroid Study. *The Journal of Clinical Endocrinology and Metabolism*, 99(11), 4291–4298. PMID: 25057878.

29. Post, G. B., Cohn, P. D., & Cooper, K. R. (2012). Perfluorooctanoic acid (PFOA), an emerging drinking water contaminant: A critical review of recent literature. *Environmental Research*, 116, 93–117. PMID: 22560884.

30. Hu, X. C., Andrews, D. Q., Lindstrom, A. B., Burton, T. A., Schaider, L. A., Grandjean, P., Lohmann, R., Carignan, C. C., Blum, A., Balan, S. A., Higgins, C. P., Sunderland, E. M. (2016). Detection of poly- and perfluoroalkyl substances (PFASs) in U.S. drinking water linked to industrial sites, military fire training areas, and wastewater treatment plants. *Environmental*

Science and Technology Letters, 3(10), 344–350. PMID: 27752509.

31. Richardson, S. D., & Kimura, S. Y. (2016). Water Analysis: Emerging Contaminants and Current Issues. *Analytical Chemistry*, 88(1), 546–582. PMID: 26616267.

32. Nowell, L. H., Moran, P. W., Schmidt, T. S., Norman, J. E., Nakagaki, N., Shoda, M. E., Mahler, B. J., Van Metre, P. C., Stone, W. W., Sandstrom, M. W., Hladik, M. L. (2017 Aug 4). Complex mixtures of dissolved pesticides show potential aquatic toxicity in a synoptic study of Midwestern U.S. streams. *The Science of the Total Environment*, pii: S0048-9697(17)31573-5. PMID: 28802893.

33. George, C. M., Smith, A. H., Kalman, D. A., & Steinmaus, C. M. (2006). Reverse osmosis filter use and high arsenic levels in private well water. *Archives of Environmental and Occupational Health*, 61(4), 171–175. PubMed PMID: 17867571.

34. Walker, M., Seiler, R. L., & Meinert, M. (2008). Effectiveness of household reverse-osmosis systems in a Western U.S. region with high arsenic in groundwater. *The Science of the Total Environment*, 389(2–3), 245–252. PubMed PMID: 17919687.

35. Yoon, J., Amy, G., Chung, J., Sohn, J., & Yoon, Y. (2009). Removal of toxic ions (chromate, arsenate, and perchlorate) using reverse osmosis, nanofiltration, and ultrafiltration membranes. *Chemosphere*, 77(2), 228–235. PubMed PMID: 19679331.

5

Indoor Air Pollution

SUMMARY

- Most common indoor air pollutants: Molds and mycotoxins, polycyclic aromatic hydrocarbons (PAHs), perfluorocarbons (PFCs), volatile organic compounds (VOCs), polybrominated diphenyl ether (PBDE), trihalomethanes, phthalates
- Most common sources: Building materials, fabric and carpeting, teflon pans, air fresheners, water-damaged buildings, dust

- Best interventions: Not wearing shoes indoors, removal of offgassing sources, no carpeting, high-quality furnace filters, indoor air purification units, proper mold prevention and remediation, indoor plants

OVERVIEW

The majority of urban dwellers spend at least 90% of their time inside, breathing indoor air. Indoor air pollution is ranked at the eighth major global burden of disease risk, whereas ambient particulate matter (PM) is listed as the sixth cause.[1] A portion of the total load of PM, PAHs, VOCs, molds, and all other contaminants in outdoor air is transferred to indoor air.[2] The level of outdoor air pollutants found indoors primarily depends on the type of ventilation system as well as the outdoor concentration of pollutants. To this base of pollution are added offgassing chemicals from building materials, solvents, PAHs from indoor cooking and combustion, trihalomethanes from water disinfection, molds, metals, radon, VOCs, and semivolatile organic compounds (SVOCs), along with other pollutants.

SOLVENTS

- VOCs
- Chlorinated solvents

It has long been recognized that the greatest personal exposure to VOCs occurs from indoor rather than outdoor air.[3,4] In Elizabeth and Bayonne, New Jersey, home to multiple chemical plants, indoor levels of 11 VOCs (Box 5.1) were up to 10 times higher than outdoor concentrations.

Table 5.1 lists the activities and household goods associated with personal and breath levels of VOCs. The compounds found most commonly indoors were: paradichlorobenzene (air fresheners and from mothballs—replacement for the more flammable naphthalene); styrene (plastics, foam rubber, and insulation); tetrachloroethylene (dry cleaning); vinylidene chloride, styrene, and xylene (paints); and benzene, ethylbenzene, and xylene (gasoline). Higher levels of benzene, xylene, and tetrachloroethylene were recorded in personal sample cartridges after the individuals went to the dry cleaner or a gas station (even though New Jersey is one of two states that do not allow customers to pump their own gas). Levels of VOCs were also naturally higher in smokers than in nonsmokers. In fact, smoking is the highest source of benzene, toluene, ethylbenzene, and xylene (BTEX) in home air.[5] Other common causes of elevated BTEX include an attached garage, recent renovations, and paint remover and fragrances. Smoking also increases indoor levels of PAHs and lead.

61

BOX 5.1 Volatile Organic Compounds Found Consistently in Breath Samples in TEAM Study

- Chloroform
- 1,1,1-Trichloroethane
- Benzene
- Carbon tetrachloride
- Trichloroethylene
- Tetrachloroethylene
- Styrene
- m,p-Dichlorobenzene
- Ethylbenzene
- o-Xylene
- m,p-Xylene

Wallace, L., Pellizzari, E., Hartwell, T., et al. (1986). Concentrations of 20 volatile organic compounds in the air and drinking water of 350 residents of New Jersey compared with concentrations in their exhaled breath. *Journal of Occupational Medicine, 28*(8), 603–608. PubMed PMID: 3746480.
Wallace, L. A., Pellizzari, E. D., Hartwell, T. D., et al. *Personal Exposures, Outdoor Concentrations, and Breath Levels of Toxic Air Pollutants Measured for 425 Persons in Urban, Suburban and Rural Areas. EPA 0589.* Presented at the annual meeting of the Air Pollution Control Association, June 25, 1984. San Francisco, CA.

TABLE 5.1 Activities and Household Goods Associated with Personal and Breath Levels of VOCs

Activities Associated with Higher Personal Exposure and Breath Levels	
Smoking	Benzene, xylene, styrene, ethylbenzene
Visiting a gasoline station	Benzene
Driving	Benzene
Visiting a dry cleaner	Tetrachloroethylene
Working in a chemical plant	Ethylbenzene, styrene, xylene
Working as a painter	Ethylbenzene, styrene, xylene
Working in a plastic plant	Ethylbenzene, styrene, xylene

Home Products Associated with Personal Exposure and Breath Levels	
Moth balls, deodorants	Paradichlorobenzene
Plastics, foam rubber	Styrene
Insulation	Styrene
Dry cleaning	Tetrachloroethylene
Paints	Vinylidene chloride, styrene, xylene
Gasoline	Benzene, ethylbenzene, xylene
Tap water	Chloroform, bromodichloromethane
Cigarettes	Benzene (double of nonsmokers), styrene

Indoor chloroform levels originate from chlorine-based water disinfectants that are released as vapor from hot water. Increases in serum trihalomethane (chloroform, bromodichloromethane, dibromochloromethane, and bromoform) levels are found after showering.[6]

Studies of more than 800 homes showed that every one of the 40 or more VOCs measured had higher levels indoors than outdoors, often 10 times higher.[3,4,7,8] The sources for these compounds were numerous and included building materials, furnishings, dry-cleaned clothes, cigarettes, gasoline, cleansers, moth balls, hot showers, and printed materials. Table 5.2 shows the differences in personal and outdoor samples of various solvents during the nighttime and the daytime.[9]

In an effort to determine the role that dry-cleaned clothes has in indoor solvent levels, nine homes had dry-cleaned clothing introduced, while two homes functioned as controls.[10] After introduction of the clothing, elevated levels of tetrachloroethylene were found in seven of the nine homes, with concentrations reaching 300 μg/m³ and persisting for 48 hours. Breath levels of tetrachloroethylene increased two- to sixfold for those living in the homes. Tetrachloroethylene levels in the indoor air, personal air,

and breath were significantly related to the number of garments brought into the home.

Elevated levels of tetrachloroethylene were also found in the homes of dry cleaning workers, due primarily to their exhalation while at home.[11]

Air Fresheners

Numerous solvents are present in air fresheners (Table 5.3) in addition to diethyl phthalate (DEP), which will increase indoor ozone levels.[12,13] Exposure of mice for 1 hour to a commercially available air freshener resulted in increased sensory and pulmonary irritation, decreased airflow velocity, and abnormalities in behavior.[14]

Semivolatile Organic Compounds

- Pesticides
- Brominated and organophosphorus flame retardants

TABLE 5.2 Personal and Outdoor Air Pollutant Levels During the Day and Night, µg/mg³

Toxicant	Personal Night	Personal Day	Outside Night	Outside Day
1,1,1 trichloroethylene	120	870	5.3	9.1
Benzene	31	27	8.6	9.5
Carbon tetrachloride	14	4.3	1.1	1.0
Chloroform	10	7.8	1.2	1.6
Dichlorobenzene	55	35	1.5	1.8
Ethylbenzene	13	26	3.8	4.3
Styrene	2.7	16	0.9	0.8
Tetrachloroethylene	11	83	3.6	8.1
Trichloroethylene	7.7	19	2.1	2.3
Xylene	72	67	15	16

Data from Lioy, P. J., Wallace, L., & Pellizzari, E. (1991). Indoor/outdoor, and personal monitor and breath analysis relationships for selected volatile organic compounds measured at three homes during New Jersey TEAM-1987. *Journal of Exposure Analysis and Environmental Epidemiology, 1*(1), 45–61.

TABLE 5.3 Compounds Present in Air Fresheners

Compound	Min. mg/kg	Max. mg/kg
α-pinene	0.03	596.3
Linalool	93	228
Formaldehyde	4.9	96
Benzyl alcohol	7.8	46.4
Toluene	0.04	11.9
Xylene	0.003	0.7
Benzene	0.005	0.7
d-limonene	0.15	1.5
Diethyl phthalate	Unknown	Unknown

- Polychlorinated biphenyls (PCBs)
- PAHs
- Phthalates
- PFCs

SVOCs include flame retardants (organophosphorus and brominated), pesticides, plasticizers, PCBs, PAHs, PFCs, dioxins, and furans. As the name implies, these compounds are not as volatile and, as such, tend to be found in greater levels in dust or attached to fabric than the VOCs, which tend to stay airborne. A review of SVOCs in house dust reported several PAHs, PCBs, and brominated flame retardants (Table 5.4).[15]

Indoor levels of pesticides were measured at homes in Springfield and Chicopee, Massachusetts (a region with relatively little indoor pesticide use), as well as homes in Jacksonville, Florida (an area with relatively high household pesticide use).[16] Concentrations of indoor pesticides were usually higher indoors and tended to be higher in the summer, lower in spring, and lowest in the winter. In homes in Jacksonville, an average of 12 pesticides were found in the carpet dust compared with 7.5 in the air samples of the same residences (Table 5.5). Table 5.6 lists pesticide levels in the air before and after pesticide application.

The finding of higher pesticides levels in indoor dust rather than the air has been confirmed in other studies.[17] It is estimated that if a child ingested 100 mg per day of dust from contact with carpet and breathed 6.3 m³ of air per day (inside the home for 24 hours), then >50% of their pesticide exposure would still come from indoor air, not dust. Pesticides in indoor dust are typically found in the smallest dust particles (0–100 µm) and account for <4% of total adult pesticide exposure, but up to 24% of a child's total exposure.[18]

A group of researchers at the University of Washington realized that infant and adult breathing zones were different and attempted to determine whether the pesticide content closer to the floor was similar to that found several feet higher. After an indoor application of chlorpyrifos, peak concentrations in the infant breathing zone were 94 µg/m³ in nonventilated rooms and 61 µg/m³ in ventilated rooms, both higher than levels found in adult breathing zones.[19] Depending on time after application and ventilation, contamination at infant breathing levels was 50% to 500% higher than air at the elevation typically found for seated adults. Using the data, it was estimated that infants absorbed 0.08 to 0.16 mg/kg on the day of application and 0.04 to 0.06 mg/kg the day

TABLE 5.4 **SVOC Compounds in House Dust**	
Geographical Area	**SVOC**
West Midlands, UK (25 residences)	α-HBCD
	β-HBCD
	γ-HBCD
Kuwait (24 residences)	Phenanthrene
	Pyrene
	Fluorenone
	Chrysene
	Benzo(a)anthracene
	Benzo(a)pyrene
	Benzo(b)fluoranthene
	Benzo(k)fluoranthene
Toronto, Canada (10 residences)	PCB 28 and 31
	PCB 52
	PCB 101
	PCB 118
	PCB 138
	PCB 153
	PCB 180
Wisconsin, USA (38 residences)	BDE-47
	BDE-99
	BDE-100
Ottawa, Canada (59 residences)	MeFOSE
	EtFOSE
Brisbane, Australia (10 residences)	BDE-47
	BDE-99
Ottawa, Canada (62 residences)	BDE-17
	BDE-28
	BDE-47
	BDE-99
	BDE-100

α–, β–, & γ–hexa-bromocyclododecane (HBCD), polychlorinated biphenyl (PCB), brominated diphenyl ethers (BDE), N-methylperflouro-octane sulfonamidoethanol (MeFOSE), N-ethyl perflouro-octane sulfonamidoethanol (EtFOSE)
Modified from Weschler, C. J., & Nazaroff, W. W. (2010). SVOC partitioning between gas phase and settled dust indoors. *Atmospheric Environment, 44,* 3609–3620.

following application (1.2–5.2 times the no observable effect level).

With the exception of the brominated flame retardant BDE 209, it appears that household dust is the primary source of polybrominated diphenyl ethers (PBDEs) found in human serum (Fig. 5.1).[20]

At least 10 different organophosphorus flame retardants are also present in house dust.[21] Levels of these compounds are found in higher levels proximal to electronic equipment and appear to be higher in homes with more electronic gear.

Phthalates are also commonly found in the dust of homes, schools, and workplaces.[21,22] High-molecular-weight phthalates like di(2-ethylhexyl) phthalate (DEHP) are found to be higher in the presence of polyvinyl flooring, foam mattresses, shower curtains, and other plastic material in the home.[23,24] Plastic-coated wallpaper, often found in bathrooms, puts out higher levels of DEHP with higher ambient moisture content.[25] As previously mentioned, low-molecular-weight DEP is released into the air from all fragrances and from plug-in air fresheners.[12]

PAHs are present in the home due to outdoor PAH concentration, PAHs tracked into the home on shoes and retained in carpet dust, smoking, and indoor combustion.[26] Many areas of the world still use solid fuel for indoor cooking, which results in exceptionally high levels of indoor PAH and PM. Natural gas appliances, candles, indoor smoking, and the burning of incense all contribute to indoor PAH levels.[27] Women cooking on gas stoves have an increased odds ratio (OR) for wheezing (OR 2.07), waking with shortness of breath (OR 2.32), and asthma attacks (OR 2.6).[28]

PFCs are used in Teflon cookware, Scotchgard, and other consumer products. Of the five PFCs found in all persons in the Centers for Disease Control and Prevention (CDC) report on human exposure (www.cdc.gov/exposurereport/), the two found in the highest amounts were PFOA (Teflon) and PFOS (Scotchgard). Both of these and other PFCs are found routinely in home air samples and are primarily found in dust.[29,30,31,32]

Biologicals

- Mycotoxins
- Endotoxins

Mold contamination is a common occurrence in water-damaged or humid residential and nonresidential buildings, with estimates as high as 50% of buildings in North America showing such damage. Mold and bacterial presence contaminates these structures with VOCs, mycotoxins, and endotoxins. The most common mycotoxins present in buildings include aflatoxin B1 from species of *Aspergillus;* ochratoxin from *Aspergillus* and *Penicillium,* and trichothecene are primarily from *Stachybotrys chartarum* (toxic black mold), but are also produced by *Fusarium* and *Myrothecium.* Endotoxins,

TABLE 5.5 Pesticides Found in Carpet Dust				
Analyte	# Detected in Dust	Median in Dust µg/g	Mean in Dust µg/g	Mean in Air µg/m³
Heptachlor	10	0.3	1.3	0.11
Chlorpyrifos	11	4.7	5.8	0.31
Aldrin	10	0.4	0.4	<0.01
Dieldrin	10	0.5	2.2	0.23
Chlordane	10	6.3	14.9	0.45
Total DDT	9	0.7	1.2	<0.01
o-Phenylphenol	10	1.3	0.8	0.02
Propoxur	9	0.6	1.6	0.03
Diazinon	9	0.4	1.7	0.01
Carbaryl	5	1.6	1.4	ND
Atrazine	2	0.7	0.7	ND

ND – non-detectable

From Whitmore, R. W., Immerman, F. W., & Camann, D. E., et al. (1994). Nonoccupational exposures to pesticides for residents of two U.S. cities. *Archives of Environmental Contamination and Toxicology, 26,* 47–59.

TABLE 5.6 Residential Pesticides Favoring Air or Dust Immediately and 8 Weeks After Application				
	AIR (ng/m³)		DUST (ng/g)	
Pesticide	Post Appl	8 Wks Post Appl	Post Appl	8 Wks Post Appl
Chlorpyrifos	ND	ND	655	700
Cis-permethrin	ND	ND	2550	550
Transpermethrin	ND	ND	3850	675
Propoxur	434.3	5.8	215	235
0-Phenyphenol	63.0	35.8	ND	ND
Dichlorvos	354.7	ND	ND	ND

Data from Roinestad, K. S., Louis, J. B., & Rosen, J. D. (1993). Determination of pesticides in indoor air and dust. *Journal of AOAC International, 76*(5), 1121–1126.

lipopolysaccharides from gram-negative bacterial cell walls, are commonly found in most buildings, whether water-damaged or not.[33] However, they are found in higher levels in water-damaged structures. *Stachybotrys chartum* requires both cellulose (abundant in wall board and lumber) and a constant moisture source to grow; it is often found in bathrooms, laundry rooms, and kitchens. The most frequently reported symptoms by individuals with *Stachybotrys* exposure were cough (79%), shortness of breath (70%), and chest tightness (64%).[34] In addition, those with *Stachybotrys* exposure were more likely to report heightened symptoms when walking into a carpeted room and to complain of experiencing a chemical or metallic taste. The Environmental Relative Moldiness Index (ERMI) test has been developed to identify homes with higher mold presence, which poses an increased risk of asthma for residents.[35,36,37]

Construction and Furnishing

Energy-efficient practices entered the home building trade in the early 1980s as a result of the desire to reduce oil and natural gas consumption. Energy-efficient building methods emphasize a reduction in incidental exchange of inside and outside air so the internal home climate will not diffuse, and therefore less energy will be needed to maintain its temperature. As a consequence of reducing the inside air exchange, these homes retain greater levels of all chemical compounds introduced into them. The historical home design that allowed cross-ventilation through windows was abandoned in favor of heating/

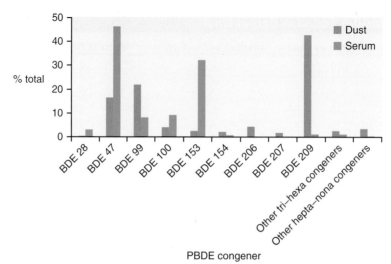

FIG. 5.1 PBDE in dust and serum. (From Johnson, P. I., Stapleton, H. M., Sjodin, A., & Meeker, J. D. (2010). Relationships between PBDE concentrations in house dust and serum. *Environmental Science & Technology, 44*(14), 5627–5632.)

ventilating/air conditioning (HVAC) systems. Homes with natural ventilation via windows and doors have lower levels of indoor air pollutants than homes with HVAC systems.[2] Standard energy-efficient "tight" homes built in areas with radon emissions have higher indoor radon levels.[38]

During the same time frame, there has been a tremendous increase in the use of VOC- and SVOC-containing compounds in building materials, fabrics, and home furnishings. Polyurethane foam and polyester fiberfill replaced traditional upholstery fillers in sofas and chairs, and synthetic fabrics replaced cotton, rayon (although synthesized, it is almost entirely cellulose), and silk in draperies and upholstery. Benzene- and styrene-containing memory foam mattresses, mattress toppers, and pillows are now commonplace. Plastic items offgassing phthalates are now found throughout the home. The presence of many "home offices" with computers, fax machines, and copiers also increases the amount of pollutants present in homes. These items, in addition to paints, glues, gas heating, gas appliances, attached garages, stored paint, paint thinner, gasoline, pesticides, herbicides, and biological contaminants of molds and bacteria, contribute to a very toxic home environment.

Sick Buildings

The change in building practices in the 1970s and 1980s preceded the appearance of myriad health

> ### BOX 5.2   Common SBS Symptoms
>
> **Mucus Membrane Irritation**
> Eye and throat irritation, cough
>
> **Respiratory Symptoms**
> Shortness of breath, cough, wheeze
>
> **Neurological Symptoms**
> Headaches, fatigue, lack of concentration
>
> **Skin Symptoms**
> Rash, pruritus, dryness
>
> **Chemosensory Changes**
> Chemical sensitivity

complaints occurring in persons working in new office buildings, which came to be called sick building syndrome (SBS).[39] SBS is often defined as a set of chronic symptoms occurring when individuals are at their place of work that often improve when away from work. The most common presenting symptoms of SBS are headache; eye, nose, and throat irritation; dizziness; disorientation; difficulty concentrating; and fatigue (Box 5.2).[40] SBS is most often associated with the type of ventilation system, SVOC and VOC levels in the building, moldiness, and stressors.[41,42,43,44] The levels of SBS symptoms present are significantly associated with higher levels of urinary 8-OHdG, a measurement of oxidative stress.[45]

Carpeting in homes, schools, and workplaces has been repeatedly associated with SBS.[46,47,48] Not surprisingly, providing a carpet-free environment led to a reduction of symptoms. Four specific groups of VOCs were significantly associated with the prevalence of chronic SBS symptoms: terpenes, VOCs, SVOCs, and butanols.[48] Household items linked to increased asthma rates were wall-to-wall carpeting, formaldehyde, VOCs, and CO_2.[49]

Next to indoor smoking, carpeting is probably the single largest source of and reservoir for SVOC in the home. The new carpet smell is familiar to all and is composed of a host of offgassing compounds that differ depending on the type of carpeting and the way it is installed. Organotins, pyrethroid pesticides, formaldehyde, and brominated flame retardants have all been identified in carpet samples.[50] PBDEs are also found in the most commonly used types of carpet padding.[51] Two different rubber-backed (styrene-butadiene rubber) carpet samples showed high emission levels of styrene and 4-phenylcyclohexene (4-PCH), which is the "new carpet" odor.[52] Carpet with a polyvinyl chloride backing emitted formaldehyde, vinyl acetate, isooctane, 1,2-propanediol, and 2-ethyl-1-hexanol. Carpet with polyurethane backing primarily emitted butylated hydroxytoluene. Four other carpet samples consistently emitted high levels of the VOCs 4-PCH and 2,2-butyxyethoxy-ethanol (up to 170 and 320 $\mu g/m^3$) and lower levels of benzene, toluene, ethylbenzene, xylene, styrene, formaldehyde, and other carbonyl compounds.[53]

Green Buildings. The U.S. Green Building Council (USGBC; http://www.usgbc.org) has established the Leadership in Energy and Environmental Design (LEED) certification program for constructing sustainable buildings (Box 5.3). LEED provides a set of guidelines to be followed for buildings to receive different levels of certification.

Green building design tends to result in improved health for those living in houses that use it.[54] However, it appears that rigorous adherence to green building practices is needed for this to occur. Low-income senior housing units that underwent a retrofit/remodel minimally conforming to LEED standards found reduced indoor formaldehyde levels but increased $PM_{2.5}$ (1.4 to 2-fold higher than outdoors for nonsmoker apartments).[55] Those residing in smoker apartments (not allowed in LEED

BOX 5.3 Leadership in Energy and Environmental Design (LEED) Certification Criteria

LEED requirements include the following:
- High-efficiency gas hydronic heat and hot water
- Heat-recovery ventilation that continuously exhausts air from bathrooms to capture and reuse heat loss for kitchen, bathroom, stairs, hallways
- Green envelope (walls, insulation, doors, windows, etc.)
- Low-VOC interior materials
- Nonsmoking policy

---

certification) had $PM_{2.5}$ levels five to eight times higher than outdoors. In new housing constructed to be more adherent to LEED standards, $PM_{2.5}$ levels indoors were reduced by 57%, and NO_2 dropped 65% compared with conventional housing.[56] Those in green homes also reported greater overall health and had dramatic reductions in SBS symptoms. Lower-respiratory symptoms were reduced by 48%, mucosal symptoms by 58%, neurological symptoms by 55%, and fatigue by 48%. Seniors who moved into green-renovated public housing scored better on the mental health index and reported more days of better mental health.[57] Seniors who moved into green rather than conventional renovated units also had a 50% decrease in falls.

Bau Biologie (Building Biology) is a German initiative that goes beyond LEED and is used to construct buildings that encourage health (https://buildingbiology.com). Building Biology adheres to 25 principles of building (Box 5.4). Training is available for those interested in certification in this profession.

INTERVENTION

- Elimination of offgassing sources
- Removal of carpeting
- Dust control
  - Clear HVAC ducts of dust and debris buildup
  - Replace HVAC filters with electrostatic pleated filters with a minimum efficiency reporting value (MERV) rating of 7 or higher
- High-quality HEPA and charcoal air purifier units
- Indoor plants that clear VOCs
  - Mother-in-law's tongue
  - Spider plant

BOX 5.4   Principles of Building Biology

Building Materials and Noise Control

1. Use natural and unadulterated building materials.
2. A building shall have a pleasant or neutral smell, not releasing any toxins.
3. Use building materials with the lowest possible level of radioactivity.
4. Protective measures against noise and vibration pollution need to be based on human needs.

Indoor Climate

5. Regulate indoor air humidity naturally by using humidity-buffering materials.
6. The total moisture content of a new building shall be low and dry out quickly.
7. Strive for a well-balanced ratio between thermal insulation and heat retention.
8. Optimize indoor surface and air temperatures of a given space.
9. Promote good indoor air quality through natural ventilation.
10. Use radiant heat for heating.
11. Interfere as little as possible with the natural balance of nature's own background radiation.
12. Prevent exposures to human-made sources of electromagnetic fields and radio-frequency radiation.
13. Minimize exposures to mold, bacteria, dust, and allergens.

The Environment, Energy, and Water

14. Minimize energy consumption while using renewable energy whenever possible.
15. Prefer regional building materials, not promoting the exploitation of scarce and hazardous resources.
16. Building activities shall cause no environmental problems.
17. Choose the best possible drinking water quality.

Interior Design

18. Take harmonic measures, proportions, and shapes into consideration.
19. Select light exposures, lighting systems, and color schemes following natural conditions.
20. Base interior and furniture design on physiological and ergonomic findings.

Building Site

21. Site buildings on land free from geological and human-made disturbances.
22. Locate residential homes away from pollutant and noise sources.
23. Provide low-density housing with sufficient green space.
24. Develop individualized housing and settlements in harmony with nature in ways that support human and family needs.
25. Building activities shall cause no social problems.

From Institute of Building Biology + Sustainability: 25 Principles of Building Biology. Available at https://buildingbiology.com/principles-of-baubiologie/. Accessed January 23, 2018.

- Janet Craig
- Gerbera daisy

The first step in all environmental medicine is *avoidance*, which in this case would be removing the sources of indoor air pollution. For homes with wall-to-wall carpeting, the best intervention would be carpet removal. Although an extremely dirty job (ask anyone who has done it), it is often one of the last steps taken because of the investment in the carpeting and the cost of installing new flooring. Discontinuing the wearing of shoes indoors and the use of fragrances, scented laundry sheets, aerosol sprays, Teflon pans, and perfumes will reduce airborne pollutants.

Dust is the primary repository of SVOCs in the home, so proper dust control will help to reduce exposure. This is a three-step process, beginning with using one of several companies that will vacuum the dust out of the existing HVAC system in the home. The second step is to replace the furnace filters regularly with pleated electrostatic filters

rated MERV 7 or higher. These filters effectively reduce the levels of small PM in the indoor air,[58] but cost more than inefficient nonpleated filters. These will deny entry of a great deal of dust into the ventilation system. The final step, which also removes VOCs from the air, is to use a high-quality air purifier unit. This unit will force the air through a series of filters, including HEPA and charcoal, to eliminate over 90% of $PM_{2.5}$ in the home air. Even moderate quality HEPA filters can have a dramatic effect in reducing indoor PM levels and improving health.[59,60,61,62]

Certain indoor plants can reduce the level of VOCs in the air. Two species of mother-in-law's tongue, *Sansevieria trifasciata* and *S. hyacinthoides*, clear toluene and ethylbenzene from the air.[63] *Chlorophytum comosum* (spider plant) is also effective at decreasing ethylbenzene levels. Three or more *Dracaena deremensis* (Janet Craig) plants in an office setting reduced total VOC levels by 50% to 70%.[64] *Spathiphyllum* (sweet chico) is also effective at lowering VOCs. In offices with high formaldehyde offgassing, 20 plants are needed to begin to reduce airborne formaldehyde levels. Using up to 15 plants in that setting made no difference.

REFERENCES

1. GBD 2015 Risk Factors Collaborators. (2016). Global, regional, and national comparative risk assessment of 79 behavioural, environmental and occupational, and metabolic risks or clusters of risks, 1990-2015: A systematic analysis for the Global Burden of Disease Study 2015. *Lancet*, 388(10053), 1659–1724. PubMed PMID: 27733284.
2. Kumar, P., & Morawska, L. (2013). Energy-pollution nexus for urban buildings. *Environmental Science & Technology*, 47(14), 7591–7592. PubMed PMID: 23805849.
3. Wallace, L., Pellizzari, E., Hartwell, T., et al. (1986). Concentrations of 20 volatile organic compounds in the air and drinking water of 350 residents of New Jersey compared with concentrations in their exhaled breath. *Journal of Occupational Medicine*, 28(8), 603–608. PubMed PMID: 3746480.
4. Wallace, L. A., Pellizzari, E. D., Hartwell, T. D., et al. *Personal Exposures, Outdoor Concentrations, and Breath Levels of Toxic Air Pollutants Measured for 425 Persons in Urban, Suburban and Rural Areas. EPA 0589.* Presented at the annual meeting of the Air Pollution Control Association, June 25, 1984. San Francisco, CA.
5. Wheeler, A. J., Wong, S. L., Khouri, C., & Zhu, J. (2013). Predictors of indoor BTEX concentrations in Canadian residences. *Health Reports*, 24(5), 11–17. PubMed PMID: 24258095.
6. Lynberg, M., Nuckols, J. R., Langlois, P., et al. (2001). Assessing exposure to disinfection by-products in women of reproductive age living in Corpus Christi, Texans, and Cobb County, Georgia: Descriptive results and methods. *Environmental Health Perspectives*, 109(6), 597–604.
7. Wallace, L. A., Pellizzari, E. D., Hartwell, T. D., et al. (1987). The TEAM (Total Exposure Assessment Methodology) Study: Personal exposures to toxic substances in air, drinking water, and breath of 400 residents of New Jersey, North Carolina, and North Dakota. *Environmental Research*, 43(2), 290–307. PubMed PMID: 3608934.
8. Wallace, L., Nelson, W., Ziegenfus, R., et al. (1991). The Los Angeles TEAM Study: Personal exposures, indoor-outdoor air concentrations, and breath concentrations of 25 volatile organic compounds.
9. Lioy, P. J., Wallace, L., & Pellizzari, E. (1991). Indoor/outdoor, and personal monitor and breath analysis relationships for selected volatile organic compounds measured at three homes during New Jersey TEAM-1987. *Journal of Exposure Analysis and Environmental Epidemiology*, 1(1), 45–61. PubMed PMID: 1824311.
10. Thomas, K. W., Pellizzari, E. D., Perritt, R. L., & Nelson, W. C. (1991). Effect of dry-cleaned clothes on tetrachloroethylene levels in indoor air, personal air and breath for residents of several New Jersey homes. *Journal of Exposure Analysis and Environmental Epidemiology*, 1(4), 475–490. PMID: 1824329.
11. Aggazzotti, G., Fantuzzi, G., Righi, E., et al. (1994). Occupational and environmental exposure to perchloroethylene in dry cleaners and their family members. *Archives of Environmental Health*, 49(6), 487–493.
12. Kim, S., Hong, S. H., Bong, C. K., & Cho, M. H. (2015). Characterization of air freshener emission: The potential health effects. *The Journal of Toxicological Sciences*, 40(5), 535–550. PubMed PMID: 26354370.
13. Nørgaard, A. W., Kudal, J. D., Kofoed-Sørensen, V., et al. (2014). Ozone-initiated VOC and particle emissions from a cleaning agent and an air freshener: Risk assessment of acute airway effects. *Environment International*, 68, 209–218. PubMed PMID: 24769411.
14. Anderson, R. C., & Anderson, J. H. (1997). Toxic effects of air freshener emissions. *Archives of Environmental Health*, 52(6), 433–441. PubMed PMID: 9541364.
15. Weschler, C. J., & Nazaroff, W. W. (2010). SVOC partitioning between gas phase and settled dust indoors. *Atmospheric Environment*, 44, 3609–3620.
16. Whitmore, R. W., Immerman, F. W., Camann, D. E., et al. (1994). Non-occupational exposures to pesticides for residents of two US cities. *Archives of Environmental Contamination and Toxicology*, 26, 47–59. PubMed PMID: 8110023.
17. Roinestad, K. S., Louis, J. B., & Rosen, J. D. (1993). Determination of pesticides in indoor air and dust. *Journal of AOAC International*, 76(5), 1121–1126. PubMed PMID: 8241815.
18. Wang, W., Huang, M.-H., Wu, F.-Y., et al. (2013). Risk assessment of bioaccessible organochlorine pesticides exposure via indoor and outdoor dust. *Atmospheric Environment*, 77, 525–533.
19. Fenske, R. A., Black, K. G., Elkner, K. P., Lee, C. L., Methner, M. M., & Soto, R. (1990). Potential exposure and health risks of infants following indoor residential pesticide applications. *American Journal of Public Health*, 80(6), 689–693. PubMed PMID: 1693041.

20. Johnson, P. I., Stapleton, H. M., Sjodin, A., & Meeker, J. D. (2010). Relationships between polybrominated diphenyl ether concentrations in house dust and serum. *Environmental Science & Technology*, *44*(14), 5627–5632. PubMed PMID: 20521814.

21. Brandsma, S. H., de Boer, J., van Velzen, M. J., & Leonards, P. E. (2014). Organophosphorus flame retardants (PFRs) and plasticizers in house and car dust and the influence of electronic equipment. *Chemosphere*, *116*, 3–9. PubMed PMID: 24703013.

22. Larsson, K., Lindh, C. H., Jönsson, B. A., et al. (2017). Phthalates, non-phthalate plasticizers and bisphenols in Swedish preschool dust in relation to children's exposure. *Environment International*, *102*, 114–124. PubMed PMID: 28274486.

23. Jeon, S., Kim, K. T., & Choi, K. (2016). Migration of DEHP and DINP into dust from PVC flooring products at different surface temperature. *The Science of the Total Environment*, *547*, 441–446. PubMed PMID: 26824397.

24. Sukiene, V., Gerecke, A. C., Park, Y. M., et al. (2016). Tracking SVOCs' transfer from products to indoor air and settled dust with deuterium-labeled substances. *Environmental Science & Technology*, *50*(8), 4296–4303. PubMed PMID: 27019300.

25. Hsu, N. Y., Liu, Y. C., Lee, C. W., et al. (2017). Higher moisture content is associated with greater emissions of DEHP from PVC wallpaper. *Environmental Research*, *152*, 1–6. PubMed PMID: 27736685.

26. Cattaneo, A., Fermo, P., Urso, P., et al. (2016). Particulate-bound polycyclic aromatic hydrocarbon sources and determinants in residential homes. *Environmental Pollution*, *218*, 16–25. PubMed PMID: 27543903.

27. Roberts, D., & Pontin, D. (2016). The health risks of incense use in the home: An underestimated source of indoor air pollution? *Community Practitioner*, *89*(3), 36–41. Review. PubMed PMID: 27111977.

28. Jarvis, D., Chinn, S., Luczynska, C., & Burney, P. (1996). Association of respiratory symptoms and lung function in young adults with use of domestic gas appliances. *Lancet*, *347*(8999), 426–431. PubMed PMID: 8618483.

29. Winkens, K., Koponen, J., Schuster, J., et al. (2017). Perfluoroalkyl acids and their precursors in indoor air sampled in children's bedrooms. *Environmental Pollution*, *222*, 423–432. PubMed PMID: 28012670.

30. Fromme, H., Dreyer, A., Dietrich, S., et al. (2015). Neutral polyfluorinated compounds in indoor air in Germany–the LUPE 4 study. *Chemosphere*, *139*, 572–578. PubMed PMID: 26340371.

31. Ericson Jogsten, I., Nadal, M., van Bavel, B., et al. (2012). Per- and polyfluorinated compounds (PFCs) in house dust and indoor air in Catalonia, Spain: Implications for human exposure. *Environment International*, *39*(1), 172–180. PubMed PMID: 22208757.

32. Huber, S., Haug, L. S., & Schlabach, M. (2011). Per- and polyfluorinated compounds in house dust and indoor air from northern Norway: a pilot study. *Chemosphere*, *84*(11), 1686–1693. PubMed PMID: 21632089.

33. Salonen, H., Duchaine, C., Létourneau, V., et al. (2013). Endotoxins in indoor air and settled dust in primary schools in a subtropical climate. *Environmental Science & Technology*, *47*(17), 9882–9890. PubMed PMID: 23927534.

34. Al-Ahmad, M., Manno, M., Ng, V., et al. (2010). Symptoms after mould exposure including Stachybotrys chartarum, and comparison with darkroom disease. *Allergy*, *65*(2), 245–255. PubMed PMID: 19796210.

35. Vesper, S., McKinstry, C., Haugland, R., et al. (2007). Development of an Environmental Relative Moldiness index for US homes. *Journal of Occupational and Environmental Medicine*, *49*(8), 829–833. PubMed PMID: 17693779.

36. Reponen, T., Singh, U., Schaffer, C., et al. (2010). Visually observed mold and moldy odor versus quantitatively measured microbial exposure in homes. *The Science of the Total Environment*, *408*(22), 5565–5574. PubMed PMID: 20810150.

37. Vesper, S., & Wymer, L. (2016). The relationship between environmental relative moldiness index values and asthma. *International Journal of Hygiene and Environmental Health*, *219*(3), 233–238. PubMed PMID: 26861576.

38. Arvela, H., Holmgren, O., Reisbacka, H., & Vinha, J. (2014). Review of low-energy construction, air tightness, ventilation strategies and indoor radon: Results from Finnish houses and apartments. *Radiation Protection Dosimetry*, *162*(3), 351–363. PubMed PMID: 24243314.

39. Redlich, C. A., Sparer, J., & Cullen, M. R. (1997). Sick-building syndrome. *Lancet*, *349*(9057), 1013–1016. PubMed PMID: 9100639.

40. Middaugh, D. A., Pinney, S. M., & Linz, D. H. (1992). Sick building syndrome. Medical evaluation of two work forces. *Journal of Occupational Medicine*, *34*(12), 1197–1203. PubMed PMID: 1464788.

41. Seppänen, O., & Fisk, W. J. (2002). Association of ventilation system type with SBS symptoms in office workers. *Indoor Air*, *12*(2), 98–112. Review. PubMed PMID: 12216473.

42. Wolkoff, P., Wilkins, C. K., Clausen, P. A., & Nielsen, G. D. (2006). Organic compounds in office environments: sensory irritation, odor, measurements and the role of reactive chemistry. *Indoor Air*, *16*(1), 7–19. Review. PubMed PMID: 16420493.

43. Straus, D. C. (2009). Molds, mycotoxins, and sick building syndrome. *Toxicology and Industrial Health*, *25*(9–10), 617–635. Review. PubMed PMID: 19854820.

44. Ten Brinke, J., Selvin, S., Hodgson, A. T., et al. (1998). Development of new volatile organic compound (VOC) exposure metrics and their relationship to "sick building syndrome" symptoms. *Indoor Air*, *8*, 140–152.

45. Lu, C. Y., Ma, Y. C., Lin, J. M., et al. (2007). Oxidative stress associated with indoor air pollution and sick building syndrome–related symptoms among office workers in Taiwan. *Inhalation Toxicology*, *19*(1), 57–65. PubMed PMID: 17127643.

46. Kielb, C., Lin, S., Muscatiello, N., et al. (2015). Building-related health symptoms and classroom indoor air quality: A survey of school teachers in New York State. *Indoor Air*, *25*(4), 371–380. PubMed PMID: 25196499.

47. Azuma, K., Ikeda, K., Kagi, N., Yanagi, U., & Osawa, H. (2015). Prevalence and risk factors associated with nonspecific building-related symptoms in office employees in Japan: Relationships between work environment, indoor air quality, and occupational stress. *Indoor Air*, *25*(5), 499–511. PubMed PMID: 25244340.

48. Norbäck, D., Torgén, M., & Edling, C. (1990). Volatile organic compounds, respirable dust, and personal factors related to prevalence and incidence of sick building syndrome in primary schools. *British Journal of Industrial Medicine*, *47*(11), 733–741. PubMed PMID: 2123116.

49. Norbäck, D., Björnsson, E., Janson, C., et al. (1995). Asthmatic symptoms and volatile organic compounds, formaldehyde, and carbon dioxide in dwellings. *Occupational and Environmental Medicine*, *52*(6), 388–395. PubMed PMID: 7627316.

50. Allsopp, M., Santillo, D., & Johnson, P. Hazardous chemicals in carpets. Greenpeace Research Laboratories, 2001. http://www.greenpeace.to/publications/carpet.pdf. (Accessed April 27, 2017.)

51. DiGangi, J., & Strakova, J. A survey of PBDEs in recycled carpet padding. IPEN. 2011. http://ipen.org/sites/default/files/t/2011/04/POPs-in-recycled-carpet-padding-23-April-20111.pdf. (Accessed April 27, 2017.)

52. Hodgson, A. T., Wooley, J. D., & Daisey, J. M. (1993). Emissions of volatile organic compounds from new carpets measured in a large-scale environmental chamber. *Journal of the Air and Waste Management Association*, *43*(3), 316–324. PubMed PMID: 8457318.

53. Katsoyiannis, A., Leva, P., & Kotzias, D. (2008). VOC and carbonyl emissions from carpets: A comparative study using four types of environmental chambers. *Journal of Hazardous Materials*, *152*(2), 669–676. PubMed PMID: 17854990.

54. Allen, J. G., MacNaughton, P., Laurent, J. G., et al. (2015). Green buildings and health. *Current Environmental Health Reports*, *2*(3), 250–258. PubMed PMID: 26231502.

55. Frey, S. E., Destaillats, H., Cohn, S., et al. (2015). The effects of an energy efficiency retrofit on indoor air quality. *Indoor Air*, *25*(2), 210–219. PubMed PMID: 24920242.

56. Colton, M. D., MacNaughton, P., Vallarino, J., et al. (2014). Indoor air quality in green vs conventional multifamily low-income housing. *Environmental Science & Technology*, *48*(14), 7833–7841. PubMed PMID: 24941256.

57. Breysse, J., Dixon, S. L., Jacobs, D. E., Lopez, J., & Weber, W. (2015). Self-reported health outcomes associated with green-renovated public housing among primarily elderly residents. *Journal of Public Health Management and Practice*, *21*(4), 355–367. PubMed PMID: 25679773.

58. Stephens, B., & Siegel, J. A. (2013). Ultrafine particle removal by residential heating, ventilating, and air-conditioning filters. *Indoor Air*, *23*(6), 488–497. PubMed PMID: 23590456.

59. Weichenthal, S., Mallach, G., Kulka, R., et al. (2013). A randomized double-blind crossover study of indoor air filtration and acute changes in cardiorespiratory health in a First Nations community. *Indoor Air*, *23*(3), 175–184. PubMed PMID: 23210563.

60. Chen, R., Zhao, A., Chen, H., et al. (2015). Cardiopulmonary benefits of reducing indoor particles of outdoor origin: A randomized, double-blind crossover trial of air purifiers. *Journal of the American College of Cardiology*, *65*(21), 2279–2287. PubMed PMID: 26022815.

61. McNamara, M. L., Thornburg, J., Semmens, E. O., et al. (2017). Reducing indoor air pollutants with air filtration units in wood stove homes. *The Science of the Total Environment*, *592*, 488–494. PubMed PMID: 28320525.

62. Allen, R. W., Carlsten, C., Karlen, B., et al. (2011). An air filter intervention study of endothelial function among healthy adults in a woodsmoke-impacted community. *American Journal of Respiratory and Critical Care Medicine*, *183*(9), 1222–1230. PubMed PMID: 21257787.

63. Sriprapat, W., Suksabye, P., Areephak, S., et al. (2014). Uptake of toluene and ethylbenzene by plants: Removal of volatile indoor air contaminants. *Ecotoxicology and Environmental Safety*, *102*, 147–151. PubMed PMID: 24530730.

64. Dela Cruz, M., Christensen, J. H., Thomsen, J. D., & Müller, R. (2014). Can ornamental potted plants remove volatile organic compounds from indoor air? A review. *Environmental Science and Pollution Research International*, *21*(24), 13909–13928. PubMed PMID: 25056742.

6

Outdoor Air Pollution

SUMMARY

- Primary sources: Vehicular exhaust, gas and oil production, industry, agriculture
- Primary toxicants: Particulate matter (PM) with adsorbed polycyclic aromatic hydrocarbons (PAHs), volatile organic compounds (VOCs), and metals; ozone; carbon monoxide (CO); sulfur and nitrogen oxides; lead
- Primary disease associations: Cardiovascular, neoplastic, respiratory, immune, neurological, endocrine

OVERVIEW

According to the World Health Organization (WHO), outdoor air pollution accounts for 3 million premature deaths worldwide every year.[1] With the exception of diarrheal diseases, HIV/AIDS, tuberculosis, and traffic accidents, air pollution contributes to all of the WHO's major top 10 causes of death, as listed in Table 6.1.[2] Once those associations are taken into account, it would appear that outdoor air pollution is likely to be an even greater cause of mortality across the globe than is currently recognized.

MAJOR POLLUTANTS

Outdoor air is contaminated with a host of pollutants from combustion (vehicular, industrial, stationary, and natural sources), evaporation, and spraying, along with particulates that are picked up and carried by wind (Table 6.2).

Urban Air Pollution

The major population centers have the greatest amounts of air pollutants due to traffic congestion and industry. Because of the multiple health problems posed by such pollution, the United States Congress passed the Clean Air Act in 1970, which set limits for emissions from stationary and mobile sources of pollution. In May of the following year, the Environmental Protection Agency (EPA) was established to implement the mandates of the Clean Air Act. Since 1970, the Clean Air Act has been amended twice (in 1977 and 1990).[3] As part of the original 1970 mandate, it allowed the newly formed EPA to set national ambient air quality standards for various pollutants. The EPA chose the six most common and most damaging pollutants: particle pollution (often referred to as PM), ground-level ozone, CO, sulfur oxides, nitrogen oxides, and lead. Of the six pollutants, particle pollution and ground-level ozone are the most widespread health threats. These six are called "criteria" air pollutants (CAPs) because their permissible levels are derived from either human health–based or environmentally based criteria (science-based guidelines). These criteria are referred to as "primary" when they are based on human health outcomes and "secondary" when they are associated with environmental or property damage.[4]

> **NOTE The Six EPA Criteria Air Pollutants**
> - PM
> - Ozone
> - CO
> - Sulfur oxides
> - Nitrogen oxides
> - Lead

EPA's Six Criteria Air Pollutants

Particulate matter. PM (also referred to as particulate pollution) is a combination of liquid droplets (aerosols) and solid particles like dust, soot, smoke, and dirt. PM carries a number of chemicals including multiple PAHs and VOCs, which account for some of its toxic health effects.[5]

PM is differentiated according to particle size, with "coarse" particles that are less than 10 micrometers but larger than 2.5 micrometers having the designation of PM_{10}. PM_{10} is often encountered near dusty roadways and industries. Fine particles are between 2.5 and 0.1 micrometers in diameter and are designated as $PM_{2.5}$. Ultrafine particles (UFPs), also called nanoparticles, are less than 0.1 micrometer in size and are more soluble than their larger counterparts. These can also be referred to as $PM_{0.1}$.

> **NOTE** To check on the levels of air pollution in your local area go to:
> http://ephtracking.cdc.gov/showAirLanding.action
> https://www3.epa.gov/enviro/myenviro/
> http://aqicn.org/map/world/

Any PM less than 10 micrometers is readily absorbed in the lungs and then distributed throughout the body. Ultrafine PM levels in the livers of rats 18 to 24 hours after exposure were found to be five times higher than the PM levels in their lungs.[6] PM has also shown the ability to travel from the nose to the brain via the olfactory nerve.[7] PM of iron oxide, India ink, and titanium dioxide that was initially identified in alveolar macrophages was found a day later not only in the lung (highest concentration), but also in the liver, kidney, heart, tracheobronchial and mediastinal lymph nodes, anterior and posterior nasal cavity, brain, and blood. At 7 days postexposure, PM was still found in the lungs, liver, and blood.[8] Rats exposed once to UFP and then sacrificed after 3 weeks, 2 months, or 6 months showed that the PM concentrations in the brain, heart, spleen, liver, and lungs from the single exposure slowly reduced over time, with the lungs retaining the most.[9] Individuals with constant daily exposure would be expected to have these particles with their adsorbed toxicants throughout their bodies.

PM causes significant oxidative damage in the tissues and organs that it is distributed to[10,11,12] and has been

TABLE 6.1 Top 10 Causes of Death Worldwide

World	Deaths in Millions	% of Deaths
Ischemic heart disease	7.25	12.8%
Stroke (CVA)	6.15	1.8%
Lower respiratory infection	3.46	6.1%
COPD	3.28	5.8%
Diarrheal diseases	2.46	4.3%
HIV/AIDS	1.78	3.1%
Respiratory tract cancers	1.39	2.4%
Tuberculosis	1.34	2.4%
Diabetes mellitus	1.26	2.2%
Traffic accidents	1.21	2.1%

Data from http://www.who.int/mediacentre/factsheets/fs310/en/. (Accessed April 24, 2017.)

TABLE 6.2 Major Outdoor Air Pollutants by Source Category

Combustion	Evaporation	Spraying	Particulate/Windborne
Aromatic hydrocarbons	Solvents	Solvents	Dust
Sulfur dioxide	Pesticides	Pesticides	Bacteria/viruses
Nitrogen dioxide	Heavy metals	Particulate matter	Mold
Ozone	Particulate matter		Radioactive matter
Particulate matter			Plastics
Plastics			Heavy metals
Heavy metals			Particulate matter
Diesel exhaust particles			
Solvents			

associated with increased mortality, primarily from cardiovascular,[13,14] respiratory,[15] and neoplastic diseases.[16]

Ozone. Ozone can be "bad" or "good" depending on where in the atmosphere it is. Ozone between 10 to 30 miles above the earth forms a layer that protects the earth from the harmful ultraviolet (UV) rays of the sun. In contrast, ground-level ozone causes damage to mammalian respiratory tracts, crops, and other plants. In the United States, ozone is responsible for $500 million in crop damage per year.[17] Ground-level ozone is produced from the interaction of sunlight with solvents (VOCs) or nitrogen dioxide. Sunlight and hot weather will combine with vehicular and industrial emissions to form high levels of ozone, which is one of the primary constituents of smog. Nitrogen dioxide is one of the criteria pollutants and is discussed later.

Because of the known adverse health effects of ozone, ozone monitoring stations are now maintained in every county in the United States.

> **NOTE** To find the level of ozone (and other pollutants) in your area go to: http://www.airnow.gov/
> Or go to your county website (typically www .yourcountyname.gov) and search for "ozone" or "ozone map."

During the Clinton administration, the EPA proposed new rules reducing allowable ozone levels from 0.12 PPM over a 1-hour period to 0.08 PPM. The U.S. Chamber of Commerce then brought suit against the EPA over this ruling. The court ruled against the EPA, and the new lower standard then became unenforceable.[18] Yet effects on lung function have been found in subjects exercising outdoors exposed to 1-hour maximum levels below 120 ug/m3 (PPB).[19] One study suggested adverse effects at only 100 PPM. But on March 12, 2008, the EPA successfully strengthened the 8-hour "primary" ozone standard to 0.075 PPM. Ozone from East Asia, at levels of 0.085 PPM (higher than current unenforceable EPA standards), has been recorded off the Olympic Peninsula (Washington State) within a few days of release from Asia.[20]

The following are the most common respiratory problems related to ozone exposure:
- Airway irritation and inflammation
- Aggravation of asthma and coughing
- Wheezing and breathing difficulties during exercise or outdoor activities
- Increased susceptibility to respiratory illnesses like pneumonia and bronchitis

Urban joggers exposed to ozone exhibited increased markers of chronic respiratory inflammation.[21] Adverse respiratory function with ozone exposure was also found in hikers (ages 18–64) in New Hampshire. With each 50 PPB (not PPM) incremental increase in ambient ozone level, the hikers experienced a 2.6% decline in forced expiratory volume (FEV) and a 2.2% decline in forced vital capacity (FVC).[22] Those hikers with a history of asthma or wheezing had a fourfold greater response to ozone than the others. Children exposed to higher levels of ground-level ozone have greater rates of asthma and rhinitis than children in areas with less ozone.[23] College students exposed to high ambient ozone had statistically significantly poorer lung function, as exhibited by lower FEV_1 and forced expiratory flow at 25% to 75% (FEF25-75).[24] They also exhibited more respiratory symptoms of cough, phlegm, and wheezing that were not due to colds. Acute ambient ozone exposure in children resulted in marked reduction of FVC and FEV_1 the day after exposure to elevated ozone (<80 PPB).[25] Hospital admissions for pneumonia are higher when the ambient ozone levels increase.[26] A large study of 36 U.S. cities showed that a 5 PPB increase in ground-level ozone leads to an increase in hospital admissions for pneumonia.[27]

The powerful prooxidant action of ozone is primarily responsible for the respiratory damage it causes.[28] Ozone exposure depletes the normal level of antioxidants in the respiratory tract. Cyclists supplemented with 15 mg beta carotene, 75 mg vitamin E, and 650 mg vitamin C experienced none of the adverse effects of ozone in any of the respiratory parameters tested, whereas all of those without supplementation did.[29] Ascorbic acid levels in bronchial lavage of nine persons exposed to 0.2 PPM of ozone for 2 hours were found to drop.[30] In addition, macrophage levels dropped 6 hours after ozone exposure.

Health damage from ozone goes beyond the respiratory tract, to the cardiovascular system as well. Animals exposed to 0.5 PPM of ozone for 8 hours a day exhibited altered blood pressure and heart rate, endothelial-dependent vascular function, oxidative stress, mitochondrial damage, and development of atherosclerotic plaque.[31] Ozone exposure is also associated with increased mortality for city dwellers.[32]

Carbon monoxide. CO is a colorless and odorless gas produced by combustion, typically along with PAHs. The EPA has established an 8-hour exposure limit of 9 PPM for CO and 35 PPM over a 1-hour period.[33] The main health problem from CO is displacement of oxygen from hemoglobin, resulting in reduced oxygenation throughout the body. At high levels that can only be attained in an indoor situation, death can occur.

Sulfur oxides. If contaminated with sulfur, combustion of fossil fuels produces a number of sulfur oxide gasses, the most common of which is sulfur dioxide (SO_2). Seventy-three percent of all SO_2 emissions come from coal-fired power plants, with another 20% from industrial facilities. Volcanoes are the only natural source of SO_2. The EPA first set a 24-hour standard of 140 PPB for SO_2 in 1971. The 3-hour average was set at 500 PPB and an annual average was set at 30 PPB.[34] Sulfur oxides in the atmosphere can be transformed into H_2SO_4, the primary component of acid rain. Outdoor air levels of SO_2 have been associated with increased rates of asthma in French children,[35] and industrial exposure to SO_2 was associated with bronchial hyperresponsiveness and a reduced FEV_1/FVC ratio.[36] In Taiwanese children, SO_2 levels were associated with increased incidence of contracting the flu as well as asthma.[37] Maternal exposure to SO_2 has also been associated with a greater risk of preterm delivery[38] and having a low-birth-weight baby.[39]

Nitrogen oxides. There are two major nitrogen oxide air pollutants, nitrogen dioxide (NO_2) and nitric oxide (NO), both of which are produced by combustion from vehicles, stationary sources, appliances, and smoking. NO_2 is a powerful respiratory irritant that can lead to asthma, decreased lung function, pulmonary edema, and diffuse lung injury.[40] https://www.epa.gov/no2-pollution/basic-information-about-no2#Effects. Emergency room visits for asthma are increased 1 to 5 days after outdoor levels of NO_2 spike.[41,42] NO_2 exposure in individuals with allergic tendencies increases their reactivity to airborne pollens.[43,44] These individuals will then react allergically to levels of pollen that would previously not have induced a reaction. At least part of this allergic sensitization occurs because NO_2 increases eosinophil activation.[45]

Lead. Starting in the 1920s, tetraethyl lead was added to gasoline to reduce engine knock. In January of 1996, the Clean Air Act stopped the sale of leaded gasoline for regular use on all roadways in the United States. Leaded gas is still sold for use in marine engines, racing cars (NASCAR), farm equipment, and propeller-driven aircraft.

Since the ban on leaded gasoline, average lead levels in U.S. residents has dropped dramatically—more than 80%.[46] Since lead's elimination from gasoline, its primary sources of exposure include indoor air, dust, consumer products, and foods. This will be covered in more depth in Chapter 13. Lead is associated with a drop in IQ in children,[47] attention deficit–hyperactivity disorder,[48] reduced cognition in adults,[49] elevated blood pressure,[50] parkinsonism,[51] and increased mortality.[52]

Mercury. Those living near plants using coal for electricity, cement manufacturing, and other purposes are exposed to mercury in the air. This can easily be seen in Fig. 6.1.

As most coal is contaminated with mercury, countries such as China, which are highly dependent on coal burning for electrical energy, are heavily contaminated. In fact, as can be seen in Table 6.3, China releases more than 50% of the total mercury contamination in the world.[53]

Sources

Vehicular exhaust comprises the single greatest source of health-damaging air pollutants (Table 6.4). Among vehicle types, diesel exhaust is the largest single source of PM, contributing up to 100 times more than gasoline engines emit and being responsible for up to 90% of the total outdoor PM.[54] Diesel engines (both stationary and vehicular) also produce significant levels of CO, sulfur and nitrogen oxides, and other ozone-forming compounds. Diesel exhaust is a combination of gaseous compounds and diesel exhaust particles (DEPs) (Table 6.5). DEPs are built around a carbon core with a large surface area to which hundreds of chemicals and metals are attached. DEPs are either $PM_{2.5}$ "fine particles" or $PM_{0.1}$.

Numerous chemical compounds are adsorbed to PM, including PAHs. PAHs are highly lipophilic and are found naturally in oil, coal, and tar deposits, and are also formed during the incomplete burning of coal, oil, and gas for fuels, incineration of garbage, smoking of tobacco, and charbroiling of meat. In short, burning anything will produce PAHs.

Comparing Emissions from Diesel and Biodiesel. Low-sulfur diesel fuels put out less sulfur oxides and approximately 26% less total PM, whereas 100% biodiesel (from waste cooking oil) only reduced total PM by 9%.[55] But, although the total mass of PM from the biodiesel fuels is lower than for diesel itself, more of the total PM is composed of ultrafine nanosized particles, which are

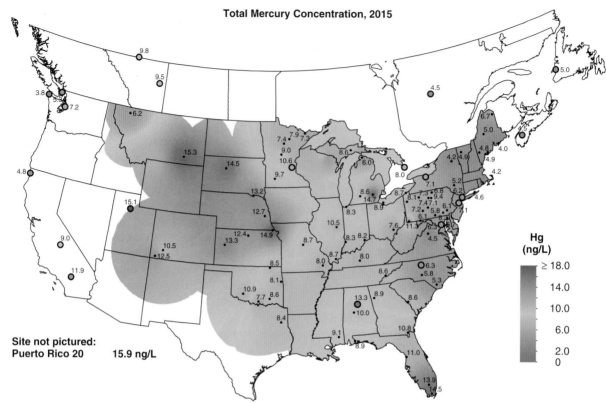

FIG. 6.1 Mercury levels in air reflect coal burning. (From United States Environmental Protection Agency. Mercury Study: Report to Congress. By Office of Air Quality Planning and Standards and Office of Research and Development. Available at https://www3.epa.gov/airtoxics/112nmerc/volume1.pdf. December 1997. (EPA-452/R-97-003).)

TABLE 6.3	Leaders in Anthropogenic Hg Emission Globally in 2000
Country	Tons of Hg Released in 2000
China	604.7
South Africa	256.7
India	149.9
Japan	143.5
Australia	123.5
USA	109.2

Pacyna, E. G., Pacyna, J. M., Steenhisenc, F., & Wilson, S. (2006). Global anthropogenic mercury emission inventory for 2000. *Atmospheric Environment. 40*:4048–4063.

TABLE 6.4	Major Sources of Air Pollutants
Air Pollution Source	Classes of Pollutant
1. Transportation: autos, buses, trucks	PAH, VOC, particulate, CO, ozone
2. Fuel consumption in stationary sources: refineries, factories, and power plants.	PAH, VOC, particulate, CO, ozone
3. Industrial processes (zinc, nickel, and electronics)	Heavy metals, particulate, CO, ozone
4. Forest fires	PAH, particulate
5. Solid waste disposal	VOC
6. Chemical dumps	VOC
7. Aerial spraying of farms	Pesticides, herbicides
8. Active volcanoes	PAH, particulate

more damaging to health.[56] Biodiesel exhaust also has lower sulfates but higher levels of nitrogen oxides than regular diesel exhaust.[57] Biodiesel blends ranging from 20% to 80% cooking oil (mixed with regular diesel fuel) did produce lower emissions of formaldehyde, 1,3-butadiene, toluene, and xylene but had higher emissions of acetaldehyde and benzene.[58] Overall, biodiesel does not make a positive impact on reducing total outdoor air pollution from diesel engines.

Table 6.6 shows the different emissions measured in filtered air, exhaust from standard diesel fuel, a mixture of 50% diesel fuel and 50% biodiesel, and 100% biodiesel.[59] Unfortunately, this study did not measure the differences in ultrafine PM or NO_2.

From the data in Table 6.6, it can be clearly seen that biodiesel blends produce far fewer PAHs and VOCs than standard diesel fuel, but the 50% biodiesel mix had the highest levels of PM, CO, and sulfur compounds. These researchers also carefully studied animals that were exposed to each type of exhaust as well as filtered air to see which exposure resulted in greater physiological changes. Surprisingly, they found that biodiesel resulted in greater adverse cardiovascular, hematological, and proinflammatory changes.

The EPA has determined that benz[a]anthracene, benzo[a]pyrene, benzo[b]fluoranthene, benzo[k]fluoranthene, chrysene, dibenz[a,h]anthracene, and indeno[1,2,3- c,d]pyrene are probable human carcinogens.[60] Benzo[a]pyrene is the main lung carcinogen in cigarette smoke[61] and vehicular exhaust.[62] Both PM and PAHs are known to damage mitochondria and suppress their proper functioning.[11,63,64] Table 6.7 lists the 17 most common PAHs as well as their carcinogenic rating by the EPA and their presence in diesel exhaust. As shown, diesel exhaust is the major source of the most common PAHs, including those that are absolute (benzo[a]pyrene) or probable carcinogens.

TABLE 6.5 Major Chemical Components of Diesel Exhaust

Compounds	Atmospheric Reaction Products
Carbon dioxide	
Carbon monoxide	
Nitrogen oxides	Nitric acid, ozone
Sulfur dioxide	Sulfuric acid – acid rain
Alkanes (C5 – C18)	Aldehydes, alkyl nitrates, ketones
Alkenes (<C4) – 1,3-butadiene	Aldehydes, ketones
Formaldehyde	CO, hydroperoxyl radicals
Acetaldehyde and acrolein	Peroxyacyl nitrates
VOCs – benzene, toluene, etc.	
PAHs	Nitro-PAHs
Nitro-PAH	Quinones and hydroxylated nitro products
Pb, S, Fe, Cu, Cr, etc.	

Data from Betha, R., & Balasubramanian, R. (2011). Particulate emissions from a stationary engine fueled with ultralow-sulfur diesel and waste-cooking-oil-derived biodiesel. *Journal of Air & Waste Management Association.* *61*(10):1063–1069. PubMed PMID: 22070039.

TABLE 6.6 Air Pollutants From Different Forms of Diesel Fuel Compared with Filtered Air

Emission	Filtered Air	Diesel Exhaust	50% Biodiesel	100% Biodiesel
PM	33 ug/m3	424 ug/m3	517 ug/m3	229 ug/m3
CO	0	10	12	4
Black carbon	1 ug/m3	43 ug/m3	69 ug/m3	27 ug/m3
Sulfur	0.128 ng/m3	0.464 ng/m3	0.591 ng/m3	0.218 ng/m3
Lead	0.005 ng/m3	0.015 ng/m3	0.005 ng/m3	0.010 ng/m3
Copper	0.017 ng/m3	0.018 ng/m3	0.085 ng/m3	0.073 ng/m3
Iron	0.009 ng/m3	0.047 ng/m3	0.073 ng/m3	0.048 ng/m3
VOCs	767 ug/m3	10,717 ug/m3	2251 ug/m3	4211 ug/m3
PAHs	19–150 ng/m3	861–8020 ng/m3	55–645 ng/m3	28–96 ng/m3

Modified from Brito, J. M., Belotti, L., Toledo, A. C., Antonangelo, L., Silva, F. S., & Alvim, D. S., et al. (2010). Acute cardiovascular and inflammatory toxicity induced by inhalation of diesel and biodiesel exhaust particles. *Toxicological Sciences.* *116*(1):67–78. PMID: 20385657.

TABLE 6.7 Major PAH Compounds in the Air, Along with Their Status as Carcinogens and Presence in Diesel Exhaust

Most Common PAHs	EPA-Listed Probable Carcinogens	Present in Diesel Exhaust
Acenapthene		
Acenapthylene		X
Anthracene		X
Benz-anthracene	X	X
Benzo-a-pyrene	X	X
Benzo-e-pyrene		X
Benzo-b-flouranthene	X	X
Benzo-j-flouranthene		X
Benzo-k-flouranthene	X	X
Benzo-g,h,i-perylene		X
Chrysene	X	X
Dibenzo-anthracene	X	
Flouranthene		X
Flourene		X
Indenol-pyrene	X	X
Phenanthrene		X
Pyrene		X

Data from Betha, R., & Balasubramanian, R. (2011). Particulate emissions from a stationary engine fueled with ultralow-sulfur diesel and waste-cooking-oil-derived biodiesel. *Journal of Air & Waste Management Association.* 61(10):1063–1069. PubMed PMID: 22070039.

TABLE 6.8 Solvent Levels in Rural and Urban Cyclists Before and After a Ride

	Rural Rides (blood ng/L)		Urban Rides (blood ng/L)	
	Pre	Post	Pre	Post
Benzene	190.0	188.9	186.1	224.2
Toluene	310.1	320.2	310.3	436.3
Ethylbenzene	232.0	237.0	239.0	292.5
Xylenes	735.0	697.3	831.4	1190.0

	Rural Rides (urine ng/L)		Urban Rides (urine ng/L)	
	Pre	Post	Pre	Post
Benzene	127.6	112.4	104.2	120.5
Toluene	282.0	280.1	295.1	338.3
Ethylbenzene	82.8	86.1	70.1	74.5
Xylenes	210.4	219.0	220.3	251.1

Modified from Bergamaschi, E., Burstolin, A., De Palma, G., Manini, P., Mozzoni, P., & Andreoli, R., et al. (1999). Biomarkers of dose and susceptibility in cyclists exposed to monoaromatic hydrocarbons. *Toxicology Letters. 108*:241–247. PubMed PMID: 10511268.

Industrial- and Vehicle-Generated Volatile Organic Compounds. VOCs, also referred to as solvents, are typically short-chain hydrocarbons that form ozone when activated by sunlight. VOCs are used in paints, glues, inks, fragrances, and building materials, and are found in cigarette smoke, gasoline, and vehicular exhaust. The four most common VOC compounds—benzene, toluene, ethylbenzene, and xylene—are often referred to simply as BTEX and can account for up to 27% of every gallon of gasoline dispensed at the pump for every vehicle. For the United States as a whole, vehicular emissions are the greatest source of these compounds found in urban and rural air. But in areas of the country where refineries and chemical plants are located, these nonmobile sources far surpass those emissions put out by transport vehicles. At the EPA website (https://www.epa.gov/air-emissions-inventories), information on total VOC emissions for the entire U.S. or by state or county can be found.

The 1990 U.S. EPA Cumulative Exposure Project assessed 148 toxic air contaminants for each of the 30,803 census tracts in the contiguous United States.[65] Concentrations of benzene, formaldehyde, and 1,3-butadiene exceeded cancer benchmark concentrations in more than 90% of the census tracts. Approximately 10% of the census tracts had one or more carcinogenic hazardous air pollutants in concentrations higher than the 1-in-10,000 risk level. In Minnesota, 10 pollutants were found to exceed cancer benchmarks: acrolein, arsenic, benzene, 1,3-butadiene, carbon tetrachloride, chromium, chloroform, ethylene dibromide, formaldehyde, and nickel.[66]

The Brookhaven Medical Unit, an environmentally controlled clinic, has filters of activated charcoal and aluminum oxide impregnated with potassium permanganate to rapidly eliminate fumes and provide less-polluted air for those in the clinic. Yet even in such a tightly controlled unit, at times of peak traffic flow, levels of hydrocarbons and other exhaust components (CO, chlorine dioxide, hydrogen cyanide, NO_2, and ozone) were detected inside the unit.[67]

A study of cyclists in an urban area showed elevated serum benzene and toluene, and elevated toluene and xylenes in the urine after a 2-hour ride. These levels were higher than after the same duration of ride in rural areas (Table 6.8).[68]

Industrial Pollution. Refineries and chemical plants are major sources of many of the CAPs, along with VOCs, PAHs, and other compounds. It is fortunate that government regulations in the United States have resulted in a reduction of overall pollution from petroleum refineries (Fig. 6.2).[69] However, there are still tens of thousands of pounds of VOCs and CAPs released annually by these facilities. Industry is required to report all emissions into the air, water, and soil to the EPA, which compiles the data into the annual Toxic Release Inventory (TRI).[70] Data from the 2002 TRI has been made available in an easy-to-access way at www.scorecard.org.

Table 6.9 contrasts the national sources of VOC emissions to those of the state of Texas, home to 29 oil refineries and 67 chemical companies.[71] It is interesting to see that the VOC releases from Texas comprise a significant portion of the total U.S. industrial emissions.

Fracking. Unconventional natural gas (UNG) well-drilling, often referred to as "fracking," is a relatively new and alarming source of air and water emissions. There are more than 1 million active gas and oil wells, compressors, and processing stations in the United States.[72] Tens of thousands of those are fracking wells that emit tons of PAHs and VOCs daily into the air.[73]

Fig. 6.3 shows the concentrations of total PAHs along with phenathrene and the carcinogenic benzo[a]pyrene that are produced by UNG wells. Both total PAH and phenathrene concentrations are still elevated more than a mile away from each site. The areas that contain UNG sites typically have a high number within each county, making the levels of these toxic pollutants quite high. This will result in rural dwellers being exposed to PAH levels that would regularly be experienced by their urban

TABLE 6.9 Texas VOC Emissions, by Tons Annually, Compared With Total U.S. Emissions		
Source	Total U.S.	Texas
Mobile	6,229,268	362,987
Solvent	3,162,230	258,487
Industrial processes	2,523,796	1,467,247
Miscellaneous	1,173,494	95,507
Fuel combustion	518,145	25,183
Agricultural	83,438	
Fires	83,438	
Dust		3

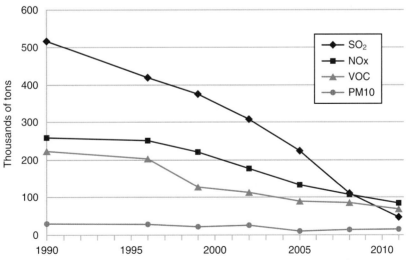

FIG. 6.2 U.S. petroleum refinery emissions 1990 to 2011. (From Nelson, T., & Nguyen, B. (2015). Historical air emissions from United States petroleum refineries. Sage Environmental Consulting. Available at https://www.afpm.org/uploadedFiles/Content/documents/Sage-Report.pdf. (Accessed June 16, 2017.))

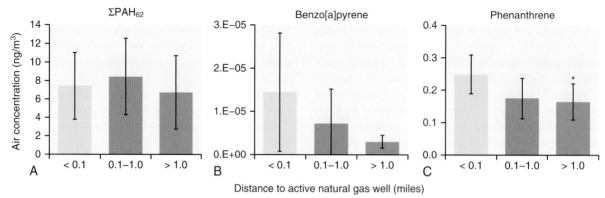

FIG. 6.3 PAH emissions from UNG sites. Average PAH concentrations grouped by distance to the closest active natural gas well: (A) sum of 62 PAHs, (B) benzo(a)pyrene, and (C) phenanthrene. The three groups are close < 0.1 mile (n = 5), middle 0.1–1.0 mile (n = 12), and far >1.0 miles (n = 6). Error bars represent one standard deviation. The asterisk indicates a significant difference between the close and far groups for pheneanthrene ($p < 0.05$). (From Paulik, L. B., Donald, C. E., Smith, B. W., Tidwell, L. G., Hobbie, K. A., & Kincl, L. et al. (2016). Emissions of polycyclic aromatic hydrocarbons from natural gas extraction into air. *Environmental Science & Technology*. 50(14):7921–7929. PubMed PMID: 27400263.)

counterparts. Fig. 6.4 shows the relative levels of VOCs from traffic and roadsides, background levels, and compared with levels at two UNG sites.[74]

Agricultural Chemicals. Pesticides and herbicides have been detected in air, rain, snow, and fog across the U.S. Levels of these compounds are typically highest in spring and summer, and lowest in winter and fall, according to their spraying schedules (Fig. 6.5). When the types of agricultural chemicals in air and rain samples were quantified, air had higher levels of chlorinated pesticides, whereas rain held more herbicides (Fig. 6.6).

Because of low volatility and low solubility in water, long-distance atmospheric pesticide movement was thought not to occur. However, detection of DDT and other organochlorine compounds in Arctic and Antarctic snow, ice, fish, and mammals corrected that idea. It now appears that, unless pesticides get trapped in the soil, tree bark, or other stable materials, persistent volatile pesticides—including DDT and toxaphene—begin a wind-driven leapfrog around the globe.

> **NOTE** For information on deposition of pollutants in the Arctic go to:
> http://www.amap.no

The more volatile the chemical, the faster it hops and the less readily it enters the fat of any plant or animal it contacts. Volatile chemicals applied in tropical regions evaporate into the atmosphere and then condense in cooler climates. As the ambient temperature falls, the compound becomes less volatile, so the rest periods between when a compound hops from one place to another tend to lengthen. So, if two forests were exposed to identical amounts of a volatile pesticide, trees in the colder climate forest would become more heavily contaminated.[75] DDT is less volatile and doesn't leapfrog as well, so it tends to get stuck where it lands and may be there for a year or longer before jumping again.

ADVERSE HEALTH EFFECTS

Mortality

Increased mortality has been associated with elevated levels of PM_{10}. Persons living in larger cities are 15% to 17% more likely to die a premature death than people living in cities with cleaner air. In Phoenix, Arizona, total mortality was significantly associated with ambient SO_2 and NO_2 levels. Cardiovascular mortality was significantly associated with CO, NO_2, SO_2, $PM_{2.5}$, PM_{10}, and elemental carbon.[76] In Sao Paulo, Brazil, 15% of deaths were attributable to CO, 13% to SO_2, and 7% to PM_{10}.[77] In Sydney, Australia, increased mortality has been found with

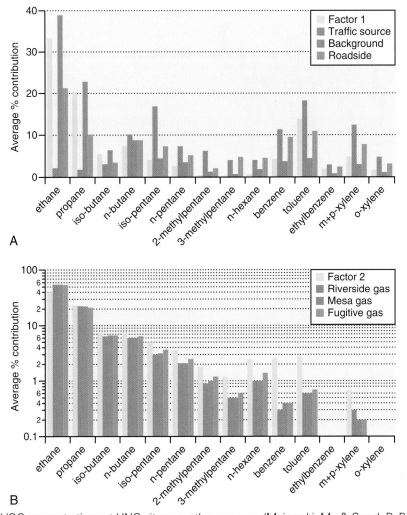

FIG. 6.4 VOC concentrations at UNG sites vs. other sources. (Majewski, M., & Capel, P. Pesticides in the atmosphere: distribution, trends and governing factors. U.S. Geological Survey Open File Report 94 to 506. National water quality assessment program. https://coast.noaa.gov/czm/pollutioncontrol/media/Technical/D52%20-%20Majewski%20and%20Capel.%201996.%20Pesticides%20in%20the%20Atmosphere.pdf (Accessed April 23, 2017.))

exposures to PM, ozone, and NO_2.[78] When levels of the daily mean of individual pollutants increased from the 10th to the 90th percentile, all-cause mortality increased 2.63% for PM, 2.04% for ozone, and 2.66% for NO_2. A rise in the daily mean of each of these pollutants was accompanied by increases in cardiovascular mortality of 2.68% for PM, 2.52% for ozone, and 2.34 for NO_2. Respiratory mortality similarly increased by 3.24% for PM and 7.71% for NO_2.

Cardiovascular

PM_{10} was found to lead to increased levels of platelets and fibrinogen,[79] and of C reactive protein.[80] PM exposure has been associated with indicators of autonomic function of the heart, including increased heart rate, increased cardiac arrhythmias, and decreased heart rate variability (Fig. 6.7). Several markers of increased risk for sudden cardiac death have also been associated with PM exposure.[81]

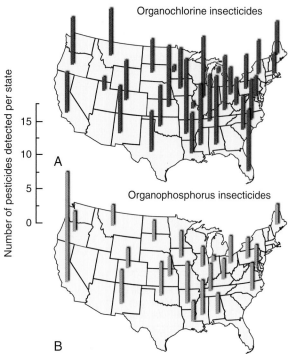

Number of pesticides detected per state

Organochlorine insecticides

A

Organophosphorus insecticides

B

FIG. 6.5 Organochlorine and organophosphorous pesticides and herbicides in air, rain, snow, and fog. (From U.S. Geological Survey. Pesticides in the Atmosphere. Fact Sheet FS-152-95. By Pesticide National Synthesis Project. Available at https://water.usgs.gov/nawqa/pnsp/pubs/fs152-95/atmos_4.html. (Accessed June 16, 2017.))

CO has been linked to the development of ventricular ectopic beats[82] and increased hospital admissions for congestive heart failure.[83,84] In older (>65 years of age) residents of Tokyo, ambient levels of NO_2 and PM_{10} were positively associated with hospital admissions for angina, cardiac insufficiency, hypertension, myocardial infarction, asthma, chronic bronchitis, and pneumonia.[85]

Living close to a major roadway alone confers increased risk of dying from an acute heart attack. By collecting data on home location/proximity data from 3886 persons presenting to hospitals with an acute myocardial infarction (MI), it was found that those living between 200 and 1000 meters from a major roadway were 13% more likely to have a fatal heart attack than those living more than 1000 meters away. If they lived 100 to 200 meters from a major roadway, they were 19% more likely to die from the heart attack. Those who lived closest to high traffic

(within 100 meters) had the highest risk of dying from the MI, with an odds ratio of 1.27.[86]

Neoplasia

The California State EPA's Office of Environmental Health Hazard Assessment, in conjunction with the American Lung Association of California, published a fact sheet on the health effects of diesel exhaust.[87] In it, they state: "In fact, long-term exposure to diesel exhaust particles poses the highest cancer risk of any toxic air contaminant evaluated by OEKKA. ARB estimates that about 70% of cancer risk that the average Californian faces from breathing toxic air pollutants stems from diesel exhaust particles." Lung cancer risk for persons occupationally exposed to diesel exhaust is 19% to 68% higher than for those nonexposed, yet gasoline exhaust had only a weakly positive and nonsignificant association with lung cancer.[88] Squamous cell and large cell carcinomas were higher in those exposed to diesel exhaust. Similar risk values were found in a Canadian study of 857 men with lung cancer, 533 population controls, and 1349 cancer (nonlung) controls.[89] Compared with the population controls, those who had moderate exposure to diesel exhaust showed a 20% increased risk, and those with greater diesel exposure showed a 60% risk. Various components of air pollution have been closely linked to increased rates of and increased mortality from lung cancer.[90,91,92] Ambient air pollution has also been linked to increased risk of lung cancer in nonsmoking adults in California. Both males and females had higher rates of lung cancer with increasing levels of PM_{10} (5.21 for males and 1.21 for females) and SO_2 (2.66 for males and 2.14 for females). The second highest risk for developing lung cancer, after PM_{10}, was found in males exposed to 100 PPB of ozone (RR 3.56).[93]

Respiratory

Children exposed to industrial air pollution have more respiratory symptoms and diseases, including frequent colds (three or more per year), bronchitis, asthma, and other respiratory diseases. These were more common among children who lived in communities with industrial pollution. This study was done on 8000 second- and fifth-grade children in three Israeli coastal towns: one town with no heavy industry, one with relatively heavy industry, one with very heavy industrialization.[94] Children living in areas with high SO_2 and NO_2 were found to have higher rates of asthma, rhinitis, eczema, and conjunctivitis.[95]

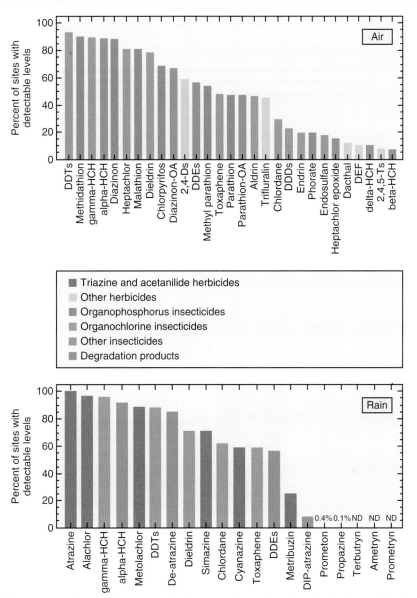

FIG. 6.6 Percentage of pesticides and herbicides found most in air and rain. (From U.S. Geological Survey. Pesticides in the Atmosphere. Fact Sheet FS-152-95. By Pesticide National Synthesis Project. Available at https://water.usgs.gov/nawqa/pnsp/pubs/fs152-95/atmos_4.html. (Accessed June 16, 2017.))

Several studies have explored the relationship between childhood asthma and respiratory problems with exposure to vehicle exhaust. Children in the Netherlands living within 100 m of a freeway had significantly more cough, wheeze, rhinitis, and diagnosed asthma than those living farther away.[96] Both the intensity of truck traffic and the concentration of black smoke measured in the schools were significantly associated with chronic respiratory symptoms. Italian researchers found that the amount of truck traffic on the street where the children resided was significantly associated with increased risk of bronchitis (OR 1.69), bronchiolitis (OR 1.74), and

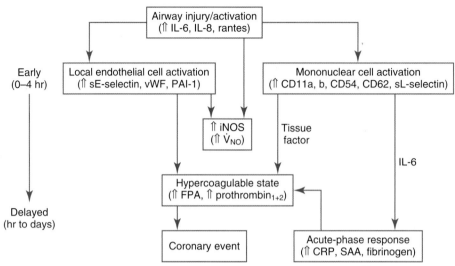

FIG. 6.7 Relationship between airway and cardiovascular responses to UFP and inducible nitric oxide synthase. (From Frampton, M. W. (2001). Systemic and cardiovascular effects of airway injury and inflammation: ultrafine particle exposure in humans. *Environmental Health Perspectives.* *109*(suppl 4):529–532. PubMed PMID: 11544158.)

	Boys (Adjusted OR)	Girls (Adjusted OR)
TABLE 6.10 Adjusted Odds Ratio for Boys and Girls Aged 0 to 15 Years Old Living on Busy Roadways		
Respiratory Problem	Boys (Adjusted OR)	Girls (Adjusted OR)
Wheeze – ever	1.2	4.4
Wheeze – past year	0.7	5.3
Dyspnea – ever	0.9	4.8
Dyspnea – past year	0.4	15.8
Respiratory meds	1.7	2.9
Diagnosed allergy	1.1	2.5

From Weisel CP, Cody RP, & Lioy PJ. (1995). Relationship between summertime ambient ozone levels and emergency department visits for asthma in central New Jersey. *Environmental Health Perspectives.* *103*(suppl 2):97–102. PubMed PMID: 7614954.

pneumonia (OR 1.84), as well as persistent phlegm (OR 1.68) and wheezing (OR 1.86) that was severe enough to limit speech.[97] Another Netherlands study of families living on busy roadways found that girls had significantly higher risk of wheezing and using respiratory medication (Table 6.10).[98] In the same study, adults living on busy

streets were 80% more likely to have dyspnea (95% CI 1.1–3.0).

Both men and women living in downtown Marseilles had significantly altered baseline lung function than those living in the suburbs.[99] Males living downtown also showed higher rates of bronchial hyperreactivity and symptoms of asthma. All the differences persisted regardless of the season when the study occurred. The greatest associations to specific air pollutants were shown with NO_2 and PM_{10}. Seasonal differences are seen in Fig. 6.8.

Exposure to SO_2 after ozone exposure (0.120 PPM for 45 min) resulted in a significant decrease in forced expiratory volume and Vmax50 (compared with FEV and Vmax50 without ozone preexposure).[100] This study was done with adolescents who were asthmatic. But asthma-related visits to the emergency room are themselves associated with ozone levels. A study in New Jersey reported that ER visits for asthma occurred 28% more frequently when the mean ozone levels were >0.06 PPM than when they were <0.06 PPM.[101] Men with chronic obstructive pulmonary disease (COPD) and healthy controls were both exposed to "worst case" ambient levels of ozone at 0.24 PPM, and both groups showed lung dysfunction as a result of exposure. Those with COPD who exercised during ozone exposure exhibited the worst respiratory response.[102]

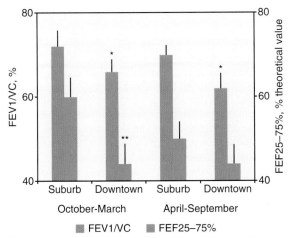

FIG. 6.8 Lung function of suburban and urban dwellers according to time of year. (From Gong, H., Shamoo, D., Anderson, K., & Linn, W. (1997). Responses of older men with and without chronic obstructive pulmonary disease to prolonged ozone exposure. *Archives Environmental Health.* 52(1):18–25. PubMed PMID: 9039853.)

Immunological

Exposing mice to a mixture of ozone and NO_2 reduced cell-mediated immune response (CMI). Daily 3-hour exposure to 0.5 PPM of NO_2 and 0.1 PPM of ozone resulted in the highest drop in CMI, as evidenced by increased mortality rates and shortened survival time after exposure to streptococcal pneumonia.[103] Exposing rat alveolar macrophages to diesel exhaust particles caused a decreased production of IL-1 and TNF-alpha, resulting in reduced Th1 CMI function.[104] Because this was not seen with the carbon black portion of DEP, it was thought to be due to the organic chemical constituents of the emission.

Pollutants Acting as Allergic Adjuvants. Direct exposure to diesel exhaust has been linked to the development of asthma that persists even after exposure ceases.[105] Animal models have revealed that exposure to diesel emission particles increases IgE responsiveness to ovalbumin.[106] The authors state: "The possibility cannot be excluded that diesel emission particles, which are kept buoyant in the environmental atmosphere of urban districts, may exert an adjuvant activity for IgE antibody production after being inhaled into the human body and have some relation to the mechanism of the outbreak of allergic rhinitis caused by pollens in Japan." Before the Second World War, pollen allergies were virtually nonexistent in Japan; since then, it has become a common disorder. Individuals living along main roads lined with older cedar trees (heavier pollen count) that have heavy traffic (heavier DEP exposure) had higher rates of cedar pollen allergy (13.2%) than those living in cedar forest areas with low traffic (5.1%).[107]

Researchers in Germany looked at the prevalence of allergies in two different areas of Germany. One area had high industrial pollution, the other had no local sources of industrial pollution. Children from the area with high industrial pollution sources had a 50% increased lifetime prevalence of allergies, eczema, and bronchitis. They also had twice the number of respiratory symptoms of wheezing, shortness of breath (SOB), and coughs without colds than their nonpolluted neighbors.[108] The children in the polluted county also had higher rates of positive skin-prick testing and higher specific IgE levels.

Neurological

Exposure to PM less than 2.5 micrometers in diameter ($PM_{2.5}$) from vehicular exhaust is one of the great threats to cognitive function for all ages. Computerized testing for working memory and attentiveness of a group of Spanish school children revealed a clear negative association between cognitive development and traffic-related $PM_{2.5}$.[109] The $PM_{2.5}$ readings were taken both inside and outside of their schools rather than in their homes, allowing the study to focus on the effect of classroom air quality on learning. Children in Mexico City with no clear risk factors for cognitive deficits living in polluted areas exhibited clear cognitive deficiencies.[110] A study on the effects of traffic-related pollution on the cognitive function of older men (with an average age of 71) used black carbon (BC) as a marker for vehicular exhaust instead of $PM_{2.5}$.[111] The findings were consistent with the studies on children: the greater the exposure to vehicular exhaust (either inside or outside), the lower the scores on mental functioning. Those men with the highest levels of BC exposure had a mental decline that equaled 1.9 years of aging. A study of older women showed almost the same results, although $PM_{2.5}$ was measured instead of BC. Women between the ages of 70 and 81 with higher long-term exposure to $PM_{2.5}$ and $PM_{2.5-10}$ exhibited a cognitive decline equivalent to 2 years of aging.[112]

Reproductive and Other Health Effects

Maternal exposure to outdoor air pollution, specifically to SO_2 and total suspended particles, during the third trimester led to significantly lower birth weights.[113] Exposure to CO (>5.5 PPM 3 month avg.) during the last trimester was associated with a significantly increased risk of low birth weight (OR 1.22).[114] Maternal hydrocarbon exposure has also been linked to DNA damage in their offspring.[115] Children raised in suburbs that were polluted by a lead smelter or waste incinerator also showed effects. Those children who had higher levels of hydrocarbon urinary metabolites also showed greater DNA damage.[116] The children who lived near the waste incinerators showed delayed sexual maturity, and the boys had lower testicular volume than controls. Those with higher serum levels of lead also showed glomerular or tubular renal dysfunction. Urban air pollution reduces sperm counts and viability, and may cause a reduction in male fertility.[117]

REFERENCES

1. World Health Organization. *Ambient (outdoor) air quality and health.* Available at http://www.who.int/mediacentre/factsheets/fs313/en/. (Accessed April 23, 2017.)
2. World Health Organization. *The top 10 causes of death.* Available at http://www.who.int/mediacentre/factsheets/fs310/en/. (Accessed April 24, 2017.)
3. U.S. Environmental Protection Agency. *Clean Air Act Overview: Clean Air Act Requirements and History.* Available at https://www.epa.gov/clean-air-act-overview/clean-air-act-requirements-and-history. (Accessed April 24, 2017.)
4. U.S. Environmental Protection Agency. *Criteria Air Pollutants.* Available at https://www.epa.gov/criteria-air-pollutants. (Accessed April 24, 2017.)
5. Yu, J. Z., Huang, X. H., Ho, S. S., & Bian, Q. (2011). Nonpolar organic compounds in fine particles: Quantification by thermal desorption-GC/MS and evidence for their significant oxidation in ambient aerosols in Hong Kong. *Analytical and Bioanalytical Chemistry, 401*(10), 3125–3139. PubMed PMID: 21983947.
6. Oberdorster, G., Sharp, Z., Atudorel, V., et al. (2002). Extrapulmonary translocation of ultrafine carbon particles following whole-body inhalation exposure of rats. *Journal of Toxicology and Environmental Health. Part A, 65*(20), 1531–1543. PubMed PMID: 12396867.
7. Oberdorster, G., Sharp, Z., Atudorel, V., et al. (2004). Translocation of inhaled ultrafine particles to the brain. *Inhalation Toxicology, 16*(607), 437–445. PubMed PMID: 15204759.
8. Takenaka, S., Karg, E., Roth, C., et al. (2001). Pulmonary and systemic distribution of inhaled ultrafine silver particles in rats. *Environmental Health Perspectives, 109*(Suppl. 4), 547–551. PubMed PMID: 11544161.
9. Semmler, M., Seitz, J., Erbe, R., et al. (2004). Long-term clearance kinetics of inhaled untrafine insoluble iridium particles from the rat lung, including transient translocation into secondary organs. *Inhalation Toxicology, 16*(6–7), 453–459. PubMed PMID: 15204761.
10. Oh, S. M., Kim, H. R., Park, Y. J., et al. (2011). Organic extracts of urban air pollution particulate matter (PM2.5)-induced genotoxicity and oxidative stress in human lung bronchial epithelial cells (BEAS-2B cells). *Mutation Research, 723*(2), 142–151. PubMed PMID: 21524716.
11. Frikke-Schmidt, H., Roursgaard, M., Lykkesfeldt, J., et al. (2011). Effect of vitamin C and iron chelation on diesel exhaust particle and carbon black induced oxidative damage and cell adhesion molecule expression in human endothelial cells. *Toxicology Letters, 203*(3), 181–189. PubMed PMID: 21421028.
12. Harrison, C. M., Pompilius, M., Pinkerton, K. E., & Ballinger, S. W. (2011). Mitochondrial oxidative stress significantly influences atherogenic risk and cytokine-induced oxidant production. *Environmental Health Perspectives, 119*(5), 676–681. PubMed PMID: 21169125.
13. Zhang, P., Dong, G., Sun, B., et al. (2011). Long-term exposure to ambient air pollution and mortality due to cardiovascular disease and cerebrovascular disease in Shenyang, China. *PLoS ONE, 6*(6), e20827. PubMed PMID: 21695220.
14. Ito, K., Mathes, R., Ross, Z., et al. (2011). Fine particulate matter constituents associated with cardiovascular hospitalizations and mortality in New York City. *Environmental Health Perspectives, 119*, 467–473. PubMed PMID: 21463978.
15. Guaita, R., Pichiule, M., Maté, T., Linares, C., & Díaz, J. (2011). Short-term impact of particulate matter (PM(2.5)) on respiratory mortality in Madrid. *International Journal of Environmental Health Research, 21*(4), 260–274. PubMed PMID: 21644129.
16. Katanoda, K., Sobue, T., Satoh, H., et al. (2011). An association between long-term exposure to ambient air pollution and mortality from lung cancer and respiratory diseases in Japan. *Journal of Epidemiology, 21*(2), 132–143. PubMed PMID: 21325732.
17. U. S. Environmental Protection Agency. Ozone Pollution. https://www.epa.gov/ozone-pollution. (Accessed April 23, 2017.)

18. Breslin, K. (2000). EPA: airing on the side of caution or pulling standards out of thin air? *Environmental Health Perspectives, 108*(9), A176, 7. PubMed PMID: 10753106.

19. Brunekreef, B., Dockery, D. W., & Krzyzanowski, M. (1995). Epidemiologic studies on short-term effects of low levels of major ambient air pollution components. *Environmental Health Perspectives, 103*(Suppl. 2), 3–13. PubMed PMID: 7614944.

20. Sorensen, E. (1999). 'Asian Express' blows Northwest and ill wind, UW scientist finds. *The Seattle Times* 12/4/99.

21. Kinney, P. L., Nilsen, D. M., Lippmann, M., et al. (1996). Biomarkers of lung inflammation in recreational joggers exposed to ozone. *American Journal of Respiratory and Critical Care Medicine, 154*(5), 1430–1435. PubMed PMID:8912760.

22. Korrick, S., Neas, L., Dockery, D., et al. (1998). Effects of ozone and other pollutants on the pulmonary function of adult hikers. *Environmental Health Perspectives, 106*(2), 93–99. PubMed PMID: 9435151.

23. Kim, B. J., Kwon, J. W., Seo, J. H., et al. (2011). Association of ozone exposure with asthma, allergic rhinitis, and allergic sensitization. *Annals of Allergy, Asthma and Immunology, 107*(3), 214–9.e1. PubMed PMID: 21875539.

24. Glizia, A., & Kinney, P. L. (1999). Long-term residence in areas of high ozone: Associations with respiratory health in a nationwide sample of nonsmoking young adults. *Environmental Health Perspectives, 107*(8), 675–679. PubMed PMID: 10417367.

25. Chen, P. C., Lai, Y. M., Chan, C. C., et al. (1999). Short-term effect of ozone on the pulmonary function of children in primary school. *Environmental Health Perspectives, 107*(11), 921–925. PubMed PMID: 10544161.

26. Tsai, S. S., & Yang, C. Y. (2014). Fine particulate air pollution and hospital admissions for pneumonia in a subtropical city: Taipei, Taiwan. *Journal of Toxicology and Environmental Health. Part A, 77*(4), 192–201. PubMed PMID: 24555678.

27. Medina-Ramon, M., Zanobetti, A., & Schwartz, J. (2006). The effect of ozone and PM10 on hospital admissions for pneumonia and chronic obstructive pulmonary disease: A national multicity study. *American Journal of Epidemiology, 163*(6), 579–588. PubMed PMID: 16443803.

28. Servais, S., Boussouar, A., Molnar, A., et al. (2005). Age-related sensitivity to lung oxidative stress during ozone exposure. *Free Radical Research, 39*(3), 305–316. PubMed PMID: 15788235.

29. Grievink, L., Jansen, S., van't Veer, P., & Brunekreef, B. (1998). Acute effects of ozone on pulmonary function of cyclists receiving antioxidant supplements. *Occupational and Environmental Medicine, 55*, 13–17. PubMed PMID: 9536157.

30. Mudway, I., Krishna, M., Frew, A., et al. (1999). Compromised concentrations of ascorbate in fluid lining the respiratory tract in human subjects after exposure to ozone. *Occupational and Environmental Medicine, 56*, 473–481. PubMed PMID: 10472319.

31. Chuang, G. C., Yang, Z., Westbrook, D. G., et al. (2009). Pulmonary ozone exposure induces vascular dysfunction, mitochondrial damage, and atherogenesis. *American Journal of Physiology. Lung Cellular and Molecular Physiology, 297*(2), L209–L216. PubMed PMID: 19395667.

32. Chen, C., Zhao, B., & Weschler, C. J. (2012). Assessing the influence of indoor exposure to "outdoor ozone" on the relationship between ozone and short-term mortality in U.S. communities. *Environmental Health Perspectives, 120*(2), 235–240. PubMed PMID: 22100611.

33. U.S. Environmental Protection Agency. *Carbon Monoxide (CO) Pollution in Outdoor Air*. Available at https://www.epa.gov/co-pollution. (Accessed April 23, 2017.)

34. U.S. Environmental Protection Agency. *Reviewing National Ambient Air Quality Standards (NAAQS): Scientific and Technical Information*. Available at https://www.epa.gov/naaqs. (Accessed April 23, 2017.)

35. Penard-Morand, C., Charpin, D., Raherison, C., et al. (2005). Long-term exposure to background air pollution related to respiratory and allergic health in schoolchildren. *Clinical and Experimental Allergy, 35*(10), 1279–1287. PubMed PMID: 16238786.

36. Abramson, M. J., Benke, G. P., Cui, J., et al. (2010). Is potroom asthma due more to sulphur dioxide than fluoride? An inception cohort study in the Australian aluminium industry. *Occupational and Environmental Medicine, 67*(10), 679–685. PubMed PMID: 20798006.

37. Liao, C. M., Hsieh, N. H., & Chio, C. P. (2011). Fluctuation analysis-based risk assessment for respiratory virus activity and air pollution associated asthma incidence. *The Science of the Total Environment, 409*(18), 3325–3333. PubMed PMID: 21663946.

38. Sagiv, S. K., Mendola, P., Loomis, D., et al. (2005). A time-series analysis of air pollution and preterm birth in Pennsylvania, 1997-2001. *Environmental Health Perspectives, 113*(5), 602–606. PubMed PMID: 15866770.

39. Dugandzic, R., Dodds, L., Steib, D., & Smith-Doiron, M. (2006). The association between low level

exposures to ambient air pollution and term low birth weight: A retrospective cohort study. *Environmental Health: A Global Access Science Source, 5*, 3. PubMed PMID: 16503975.

40. U.S. Environmental Protection Agency. *Indoor Air Quality (IAQ)*. Available at https://www.epa.gov/no2-pollution/basic-information-about-no2#Effects. (Accessed December 8, 2011.)

41. Pereira, G., Cook, A., De Vos, A. J., & Holman, C. D. (2010). A case-crossover analysis of traffic-related air pollution and emergency department presentations for asthma in Perth, Western Australia. *The Medical Journal of Australia, 193*(9), 511–514. PubMed PMID: 21034384.

42. Krmpoti, D., Luzar-Stiffler, V., Rakusic, N., et al. (2011). Effects of traffic air pollution and hornbeam pollen on adult asthma hospitalizations in Zagreb. *International Archives of Allergy and Immunology, 156*(1), 62–68. PubMed PMID: 21447960.

43. Strand, V., Svartengren, M., Rak, S., Barck, C., & Bylin, G. (1998). Repeated exposure to an ambient level of NO2 enhances asthmatic response to a nonsymptomatic allergen dose. *The European Respiratory Journal, 12*(1), 6–12. PubMed PMID: 9701406.

44. Wang, J. H., Devalia, J. L., Duddle, J. M., et al. (1995). Effects of six-hour exposure to nitrogen dioxide on early phase nasal response to allergen challenge in patients with a history of seasonal allergic rhinitis. *The Journal of Allergy and Clinical Immunology, 96*(5 Pt. 1), 669–676. PubMed PMID: 7599684.

45. Wang, J. H., Duddle, J., Devalia, J. L., & Davies, R. J. (1995). Nitrogen dioxide increases eosinophil activation in the early-phase response to nasal allergen provocation. *International Archives of Allergy and Immunology, 107*(1–3), 103–105. PubMed PMID: 7613114.

46. Centers for Disease Control and Prevention (CDC). (1994, August 5). *Blood Lead Levels – United States, 1988-1991*. Morbidity and Mortality Weekly Reports. Retrieved from http://www.cdc.gov/mmwr/preview/mmwrhtml/00032080.htm. (Accessed April 23, 2017.)

47. Canfield, R. L., Henderson, C. R., Cory-Slechta, D. A., et al. (2003). Intellectual impairment in children with blood lead concentrations below 10ug per deciliter. *The New England Journal Medicine, 348*(16), 1517–1526. PubMed PMID: 12700371.

48. Wang, H. L., Chen, X. T., Yang, B., et al. (2008). Case-control study of blood lead levels and attention deficit hyperactivity disorder in Chinese children. *Environmental Health Perspectives, 116*, 1401–1406. PubMed PMID: 18941585.

49. Bandeen-Roche, K., Glass, T. A., Bolla, K. I., et al. (2009). Cumulative lead dose and cognitive function in older adults. *Epidemiology, 20*, 831–839. PubMed PMID: 19752734.

50. Yazbeck, C., Thiebaugeorges, O., Moreau, T., et al. (2009). Maternal blood lead levels and the risk of pregnancy-induced hypertension: The EDEN cohort study. *Environmental Health Perspectives, 117*(10), 1526–1530. PubMed PMID: 20019901.

51. Weisskopf, M. G., Weuve, J., Nie, H., et al. (2010). Association of cumulative lead exposure with Parkinson's disease. *Environmental Health Perspectives, 118*(11), 1609–1613. PubMed PMID: 20807691.

52. Khalil, N., Wilson, J. W., Talbott, E. O., et al. (2009). Association of blood lead concentrations with mortality in older women: A prospective cohort study. *Environmental Health: A Global Access Science Source, 8*, 15. PubMed PMID: 19344498.

53. Pacyna, E. G., Pacyna, J. M., Steenhuisenc, F., & Wilson, S. (2006). Global anthropogenic mercury emission inventory for 2000. *Atmospheric Environment, 40*, 4048–4063.

54. Air Quality Expert Group. *Particulate matter in the United Kingdom*. London; Defra: 2005. http://webarchive.nationalarchives.gov.uk/20130402151656/http://archive.defra.gov.uk/environment/quality/air/airquality/publications/particulate-matter/index.htm. (Accessed April 23, 2017.)

55. Betha, R., & Balasubramanian, R. (2011). Particulate emissions from a stationary engine fueled with ultra-low-sulfur diesel and waste-cooking-oil-derived biodiesel. *Journal of the Air and Waste Management Association (1995), 61*(10), 1063–1069. PubMed PMID: 22070039.

56. Jayaram, V., Agrawal, H., Welch, W. A., et al. (2011). Real-time gaseous, PM and ultrafine particle emissions from a modern marine engine operating on biodiesel. *Environmental Science & Technology, 45*(6), 2286–2292. PubMed PMID: 21344849.

57. Zhu, L., Zhang, W., Liu, W., & Huang, Z. (2010). Experimental study on particulate and NOx emissions of a diesel engine fueled with ultra low sulfur diesel, RME-diesel blends and PME-diesel blends. *The Science of the Total Environment, 408*(5), 1050–1058. PubMed PMID: 19913283.

58. Di, Y., Cheung, C. S., & Huang, Z. (2009). Experimental investigation of regulated and unregulated emissions of a diesel engine fueled with ultra low sulfur diesel fuel blended with biodiesel from waste cooking oil. *The Science of the Total Environment, 407*(2), 835–846. PubMed PMID: 18947856.

59. Brito, J. M., Belotti, L., Toledo, A. C., et al. (2010). Acute cardiovascular and inflammatory toxicity induced by inhalation of diesel and biodiesel exhaust particles. *Toxicological Sciences*, *116*(1), 67–78. PMID: 20385657.

60. Department of Health ond Human Services, Public Health Service, Agency for Toxic Substances and Disease Registry. *Toxic Substances Portal—Polycyclic Aromatic Hydrocarbons (PAHs)*. Available at http://www.atsdr.cdc.gov/PHS/PHS.asp?id=120&tid=25. (Accessed April 23, 2017.)

61. Alexandrov, K., Rojas, M., & Satarug, S. (2010). The critical DNA damage by benzo(a)pyrene in lung tissues of smokers and approaches to preventing its formation. *Toxicology Letters*, *198*(1), 63–68. PubMed PMID: 20399842.

62. Armstrong, B., Hutchinson, E., Unwin, J., & Fletcher, T. (2004). Lung cancer risk after exposure to polycyclic aromatic hydrocarbons: A review and meta-analysis. *Environmental Health Perspectives*, *112*(9), 970–978. PubMed PMID: 15198916.

63. Xia, T., Kovochich, M., & Nel, A. E. (2007). Impairment of mitochondrial function by particulate matter (PM) and their toxic components: Implications for PM-induced cardiovascular and lung disease. *Frontiers in Bioscience*, *12*, 1238–1246. PubMed PMID: 17127377.

64. Jiang, Y., Zhou, X., Chen, X., et al. (2011). Benzo(a) pyrene-induced mitochondrial dysfunction and cell death in p53-null Hep3B cells. *Mutation Research*, *726*(1), 75–83. PubMed PMID: 21911080.

65. Woodruff, T. J., Axelrod, D. A., Caldwell, J., et al. (1998). Public health implications of the 1990 toxics concentrations across the United States. *Environmental Health Perspectives*, *106*(95), 245–251. PubMed PMID: 9518474.

66. Pratt, G. C., Palmer, K., Wu, C. Y., et al. (2000). An assessment of air toxics in Minnesota. *Environmental Health Perspectives*, *108*(9), 815–825. PubMed PMID: 11017885.

67. Edgar, R. T., Fenyves, E. J., & Rea, W. J. (1979). Air pollution analysis used in operating an environmental control unit. *Annals of Allergy*, *42*(3), 166–173. PubMed PMID: 426326.

68. Bergamaschi, E., Burstolin, A., De Palma, G., et al. (1999). Biomarkers of dose and susceptibility in cyclists exposed to monoaromatic hydrocarbons. *Toxicology Letters*, *108*, 241–247. PubMed PMID: 10511268.

69. Nelson, T., & Nguyen, B. *Historical air emissions from United States petroleum refineries*. 2015. https://www.afpm.org/uploadedFiles/Content/ documents/Sage-Report.pdf. (Accessed April 24, 2017.)

70. U.S. Environmental Protection Agency. *Toxics Release Inventory (TRI) Program*. Available at https://www.epa.gov/toxics-release-inventory-tri-program. (Accessed April 24, 2017.)

71. U.S. Energy Information Administration. *Petroleum and other liquids*. Available at http://www.eia.gov/dnav/pet/pet_pnp_cap1_dcu_STX_a.htm. (Accessed April 24, 2017.)

72. Fracktracker Alliance. Oil and gas exploration by location. https://www.fracktracker.org/map/. (Accessed 19 March 2018)

73. Swarthout, R. F., Russo, R. S., Zhou, Y., et al. (2015). Impact of Marcellus Shale natural gas development in southwest Pennsylvania on volatile organic compound emissions and regional air quality. *Environmental Science & Technology*, *49*(5), 3175–3184. PubMed PMID: 25594231.

74. Field, R., Soltis, J., McCarthy, M., et al. (2015). Influence of oil and gas field operations on spatial and temporal distributions of atmospheric non-methane hydrocarbons and their effect on ozone formation in winter. *Atmospheric Chemistry and Physics*, *15*, 3527–3542. www.atmos-chem-phys.net/15/3527/2015/.

75. Raloff, J. (1996). The pesticide shuffle. *Science News*, *149*, 174–176.

76. Mar, T. F., Norris, G. A., Koenig, J. Q., & Larson, T. V. (2000). Associations between air pollution and mortality in Phoenix, 1995-1997. *Environmental Health Perspectives*, *108*(4), 347–353. PubMed PMID: 10753094.

77. Coneicao, G. M. S., Miraglia, S. G. E. K., Kishi, H. S., et al. (2001). Air pollution and child mortality: A time-series study in Sao Paulo, Brazil. *Environmental Health Perspectives*, *109*(Suppl. 3), 347–350. PubMed PMID: 11427383.

78. Morgan, G., Corbett, S., Wlodarczyk, J., & Lewis, P. (1998). Air pollution and daily mortality in Sydney, Australia, 1989 through 1993. *American Journal of Public Health*, *88*, 759–764. PubMed PMID: 9585741.

79. Schwartz, J. (2001). Air pollution and blood markers of cardiovascular risk. *Environmental Health Perspectives*, *109*(Suppl. 3), 405–409. PubMed PMID: 11427390.

80. Donaldson, K., Stone, V., Seaton, A., & MacNee, W. (2001). Ambient particle inhalation and cardiovascular system: Potential mechanisms. *Environmental Health Perspectives*, *109*(Suppl. 40), 523–527. PubMed PMID: 11544157.

81. Dockery, D. W. (2001). Epidemiologic evidence of cardiovascular effects of particulate air pollution.

Environmental Health Perspectives, 109(Suppl. 4), 483–486. PubMed PMID: 11544151.

82. Leaf, D., & Kleinman, M. (1996). Urban ectopy in the mountains: Carbon monoxide exposure at high altitude. *Archives of Environmental Health, 51*(4), 283–285. PubMed PMID: 8757408.

83. Morris, R. D., & Naumova, E. N. (1998). Carbon monoxide and hospital admissions for congestive heart failure: Evidence of an increased effect at low temperature. *Environmental Health Perspectives, 106*(10), 649–653. PubMed PMID: 9755140.

84. Morris, R., Naumova, E., & Munasinghe, R. (1995). Ambient air pollution and hospitalization for congestive heart failure among elderly people in seven large US cities. *American Journal of Public Health, 85*(10), 1361–1365. PubMed PMID: 7573618.

85. Ye, F., Piver, W. T., Ando, M., & Portier, C. J. (2001). Effects of temperature and air pollutants on cardiovascular and respiratory diseases for males and females older than 65 years of age in Tokyo, July and August 1980-1995. *Environmental Health Perspectives, 109*(4), 355–359. PubMed PMID: 11335183.

86. Rosenbloom, J. I., Wilker, E. H., Mukamal, K. J., et al. (2012). Residential proximity to major roadway and 10-year all-cause mortality after myocardial infarction. *Circulation, 125*(18), 2197–2203. PubMed PMID: 22566348.

87. Office of Environmental Health Hazard Assessment (OEHHA). *Health Effects of Diesel Exhaust.* Available from http://oehha.ca.gov/public_info/facts/dieselfacts.html. (Accessed April 23, 2017.)

88. Velleneuve, P. J., Parent, M. E., Sahni, V., & Johnson, K. C.; Canadian Cancer Registries Epidemiology Research Group. (2011). Occupational exposure to diesel and gasoline exhaust emissions and lung cancer in Canadian men. *Environmental Research, 111*(5), 727–735. PubMed PMID: 2156265.

89. Parent, M. E., Rousseau, M. C., Boffetta, P., Cohen, A., & Siemiatycki, J. (2007). Exposure to diesel and gasoline engine emissions and the risk of lung cancer. *American Journal of Epidemiology, 165*(1), 53–62. PubMed PMID: 17062632.

90. Reymão, M. S., Cury, P. M., Lichtenfels, A. J., et al. (1997). Urban air pollution enhances the formation of urethane-induced lung tumors in mice. *Environmental Research, 74*(2), 150–158. PubMed PMID: 9339228.

91. Tokiwa, H., Nakanishi, Y., Sera, N., Hara, N., & Inuzuka, S. (1998). Analysis of environmental carcinogens associated with the incidence of lung cancer. *Toxicology Letters, 99*, 33–41. PubMed PMID: 9801028.

92. Biggeri, A., Barbone, F., Lagazio, C., et al. (1996). Air pollution and lung cancer in Trieste, Italy: Spatial analysis of risk as a function of distance from sources. *Environmental Health Perspectives, 104*, 750–754. PubMed PMID: 8841761.

93. Beeson, W. L., Abbey, D. E., & Knutsen, S. F. (1998). Long-term concentrations of ambient air pollutants and incident lung cancer in California adults: Results from the AHSMOG study. Adventist Health Study on Smog. *Environmental Health Perspectives, 106*(12), 813–822. PubMed PMID: 9831542.

94. Goren, A. I. (1995). Respiratory conditions among schoolchildren and their relationship to environmental tobacco smoke and other combustion products. *Archives of Environmental Health, 50*(2), 112–118. PubMed PMID: 7786047.

95. Kim, Y. K., Baek, D., Koh, Y. I., et al. (2001). Outdoor air pollutants derived from industrial processes may be causally related to the development of asthma in children. *Annals of Allergy, Asthma and Immunology, 86*(4), 456–460. PubMed PMID: 11345292.

96. Van Vliet, P., Knape, M., de Hartog, J., et al. (1977). Motor vehicle exhaust and chronic respiratory symptoms in children living near freeways. *Environmental Research, 74*, 122–132. PubMed PMID: 9339225.

97. Ciccone, G., Forastiere, F., Agabiti, N., et al. (1998). Road traffic and adverse respiratory effects in children. SIDRIA Collaborative Group. *Occupational and Environmental Medicine, 55*(11), 771–778. PubMed PMID: 9924455.

98. Oosterlee, A., Drijver, M., Lebret, E., & Brunekreef, B. (1966). Chronic respiratory symptoms in children and adults living along streets with high traffic density. *Occupational and Environmental Medicine, 53*, 241–247. PubMed PMID: 8664961.

99. Jammes, Y., Delpierre, S., Delvolgo, M. J., et al. (1998). Long-term exposure of adults to outdoor air pollution is associated with increased airway obstruction and higher prevalence of bronchial hyper responsiveness. *Archives of Environmental Health, 53*(6), 372–377. PubMed PMID: 9886154.

100. Koenig, J. Q., Covert, D. S., Hanley, W. S., et al. (1990). Prior exposure to ozone potentiates subsequent response to sulfur dioxide in adolescent asthmatic subjects. *The American Review of Respiratory Disease, 141*, 377–380. PubMed PMID: 2301855.

101. Weisel, C. P., Cody, R. P., & Lioy, P. J. (1995). Relationship between summertime ambient ozone levels and emergency department visits for asthma in central New Jersey. *Environmental Health Perspectives, 103*(Suppl. 2), 97–102. PubMed PMID: 7614954.

102. Gong, H., Shamoo, D., Anderson, K., & Linn, W. (1997). Responses of older men with and without chronic obstructive pulmonary disease to prolonged ozone exposure. *Archives of Environmental Health, 52*(1), 18–25. PubMed PMID: 9039853.

103. Ehrlich, R., & Findlay, J. C. (1979). Effects of repeated exposures to peak concentrations of nitrogen dioxide and ozone on resistance to streptococcal pneumonia. *Journal of Toxicology and Environmental Health, 5,* 621–642. PubMed PMID: 385895.

104. Castranova, V., Ma, J. Y. C., Yang, H. M., et al. (2001). Effect of exposure to diesel exhaust particles on susceptibility of the lung to infection. *Environmental Health Perspectives, 109*(Suppl. 4), 609–612. PubMed PMID: 11544172.

105. Wade, J. F., & Newman, L. S. (1993). Diesel asthma, reactive airway disease following overexposure to locomotive exhaust. *Journal of Occupational Medicine, 35*(2), 149–154. PubMed PMID: 8433186.

106. Takafuji, S., Suzuki, S., Koizumi, K., et al. (1987). Diesel-exhaust particulates inoculated by the intranasal route have and adjuvant activity for IgE production in mice. *The Journal of Allergy and Clinical Immunology, 79,* 639–645. PubMed PMID 2435776.

107. Ishizaki, T., Koizumi, K., Ikemori, R., et al. (1987). Studies of prevalence of Japanese cedar pollinosis among residents in a densely cultivated area. *Annals of Allergy, 58,* 265–270. PubMed PMID: 3565861.

108. Heinrich, J., Hoelscher, B., Wjst, M., Ritz, B., Cyrys, J., & Wichmann, H. (1999). Respiratory disease and allergies in two polluted areas in East Germany. *Archives of Environmental Health, 107*(1), 53–62. PubMed PMID: 9872717.

109. Basagaña, X., Esnaola, M., Rivas, I., et al. (2016). Neurodevelopmental deceleration by urban fine particles from different emission sources: a longitudinal observational study. *Environmental Health Perspectives, 124*(10), 1630–1636. PubMed PMID: 27128166.

110. Calderón-Garcidueñas, L., Mora-Tiscareño, A., Ontiveros, E., et al. (2008). Air pollution, cognitive deficits and brain abnormalities: A pilot study with children and dogs. *Brain and Cognition, 68*(2), 117–127. PubMed PMID: 18550243.

111. Power, M. C., Weisskopf, M. G., Alexeeff, S. E., et al. (2011). Traffic-related air pollution and cognitive function in a cohort of older men. *Environmental Health Perspectives, 119*(5), 682–687. PubMed PMID: 21172758.

112. Weuve, J., Puett, R. C., Schwartz, J., et al. (2012). Exposure to particulate air pollution and cognitive decline in older women. *Archives of Internal Medicine, 172*(3), 219–227. PubMed PMID: 22332151.

113. Wang, X., Ding, H., Ryan, L., & Xu, X. (1997). Association between air pollution and low birth weight: A community based study. *Environmental Health Perspectives, 105,* 514–520. PubMed PMID: 9222137.

114. Ritz, B., & Yu, F. (1999). The effect of ambient carbon monoxide on low birth weight among children born in Southern California between 1989 and 1993. *Environmental Health Perspectives, 107*(1), 17–25. PubMed PMID: 9872713.

115. Whyatt, R. M., Santella, R. M., Jedrychowski, W., et al. (1998). Relationship between ambient air pollution and DNA damage in Polish mothers and newborns. *Environmental Health Perspectives, 106*(Suppl. 3), 821–826. PubMed PMID: 9646044.

116. Staessen, J. A., Nawrot, T., Hond, E. D., et al. (2001). Renal function, cytogenetic measurements, and sexual development in adolescents in relation to environmental pollutants: A feasibility study of biomarkers. *Lancet, 357*(9269), 1660–1669. PubMed PMID: 11425371.

117. Radwan, M., Jurewicz, J., Polańska, K., et al. (2016). Exposure to ambient air pollution–does it affect semen quality and the level of reproductive hormones? *Annals of Human Biology, 43*(1), 50–56. PubMed PMID: 26211899.

7

Health and Beauty Products

SUMMARY

- Presence in population: Exposure is ubiquitous
- Major diseases: Endocrine and reproductive disruption

- Best measure: Urinary metabolites
- Best intervention: Avoidance

DESCRIPTION

A cosmetic product is defined by The Polish Act on cosmetics as "any chemical substance or mixture intended for external contact with the human body whose sole or main purpose is to keep it clean, nurture, protect, perfume, change the appearance, or improve its scent." An estimated 95% of women and 75% of men have daily multiple contacts with cosmetics.[1] Despite the widespread usage of personal care products (PCPs), little is known about concentrations and profiles of or human exposure to compounds in PCPs. Phthalates and other chemical constituents are seldom listed on product labels because U.S. regulations require only limited labeling. For example, the U.S. Food and Drug Administration (FDA) regulates sunscreens, antiperspirant deodorants, and antibacterial hand soaps as over-the-counter drugs, and only "active" ingredients must be labeled.[2,3] Cleaning products only require labeling for compounds, such as antimicrobials, that are regulated by the U.S. Environmental Protection Agency (EPA).[4] For cosmetics, the FDA requires ingredients to be labeled in order of predominance, *except* chemical constituents of fragrances and incidental ingredients, as they are protected as "proprietary trade secrets."[2,3]

It can be difficult to assess the toxicity of any given substance because many studies assume, albeit incorrectly, that no one is exposed to more than one toxicant at a time, and that the subjects involved are completely free from any toxicants before the exposure being considered.

Cumulative exposure certainly poses greater risk. Complex mixtures, dose additivity, and synergism between and among hormones and chemicals complicate toxicity studies. For example, multiple xenoestrogens can alter estrogen action even when each of the xenoestrogens is present in a concentration below that which will produce an observed effect alone, and there is no obvious threshold for this effect.[5]

The lack of transparency regarding ingredients, along with the multitude of chemicals included in PCPs, not only makes it difficult for consumers to make educated choices but also hinders research on the true toxic effects of PCPs. In cases of toxicity, source identification can be hampered by lack of information regarding product ingredients as well as chemicals that may be present as byproducts, residual starting materials, processing aids, and/or contaminants. There are potentially thousands of chemicals used in PCPs and cosmetics, and estimating exposure to all of these chemicals is not possible.[6] Nonetheless, there is increasing evidence linking the use of PCPs, and more specifically a subset of individual chemicals contained in them, to a variety of adverse health effects.

SOURCES

The use of health and beauty products is ubiquitous, and human exposure to known or suspected endocrine disrupting chemicals (EDCs) in these products has been documented in the United States and worldwide.[7] These include phthalates, parabens, triclosan (TCS), ultraviolet (UV) filters (e.g., benzophenone-3 [BP-3]), and toxic metals. Mechanisms by which EDCs act in the body include direct and indirect actions on estrogen receptors; antiandrogenic effects; thyroid effects; disruption of enzymes and nuclear and membrane receptors involved in steroidogenesis, steroid metabolism and protein/peptide synthesis; and molecular epigenetic changes.[8-10] Toxic metals cause damage in a variety of ways, including increased free radical production, enzyme poisoning, direct DNA damage, endocrine disruption, and mitochondrial or cell wall damage[11] (details can be found in corresponding chapters).

Parabens

Methyl-, ethyl-, propyl-, butyl-, and benzylparabens, all esters of p-hydroxybenzoic acid, are widely used in cosmetics, pharmaceuticals, foods, and beverages as antimicrobial agents and preservatives. Because of their low cost, inertness, broad spectrum of activity, and low toxicity, parabens are commonly used throughout the world. Paraben exposure comes mainly from the use of PCPs containing propylparaben and/or methylparaben.[12] Besides water, parabens are considered the most common ingredient in cosmetics and are present in approximately 80% of PCPs. Products found to contain parabens include hand soap, body lotion, shampoo, conditioner, face lotion, facial cleansers, foundation, lipstick, mascara, hairspray, mousse, hair gel, toothpaste, and sunscreen.[13] Therefore, parabens can contact the skin, hair and scalp, lips, mucosae (oral, ocular, and vaginal), axillae, and nails. PCPs can be used on an occasional to a daily basis and their use can extend over a period of years, leading to nearly continuous application. A 1995 study showed that nearly all (99%) leave-on cosmetics and more than 75% of rinse-off cosmetics contained parabens.[14]

The potential estrogenicity and tissue presence of parabens are causes for concern regarding breast cancer. Although the exact health effects of parabens are currently unknown, they do possess some estrogenic activity, can adversely affect the breakdown of endogenous estrogens, and may cause mitochondrial dysfunction. An *in vitro* yeast-based estrogen assay found that the four most widely used parabens (methyl-, ethyl-, propyl-, and butylparaben) were all weakly estrogenic, with the magnitude of the estrogenic response increasing with alkyl group size.[15] Specifically, methylparaben produced the weakest response

(2,500,000-fold less potent than 17β-estradiol), followed by ethylparaben (150,000-fold less potent), propylparaben (30,000-fold less potent), and butylparaben (10,000-fold less potent).

In addition, parabens and their common metabolite, p-hydroxybenzoic acid, have been shown to possess androgen antagonist activity, to act as inhibitors of sulfotransferase enzymes, and to possess genotoxic activity.[16] Parabens can indirectly affect estrogen levels via inhibition of sulfotransferase activity inside the cytosol of human skin cells, causing estrogen levels to remain higher than normal.[17] Methyl- and propylparabens are also potent inhibitors of mitochondrial function.[18,19] This effect on mitochondrial function has been proposed as a mechanism for the role of parabens in male infertility.[20]

Phthalates

Phthalates are synthetic aromatic chemicals that can be used as plasticizers in polyvinyl chloride plastics, to hold scent and as solvents in PCPs, and in food packaging and processing materials. Di-2-ethylhexyl phthalate (DEHP), di-n-octyl phthalate (DnOP), diisononyl phthalate (DiNP), and diisodecyl phthalate (DiDP) belong to the high-molecular-weight phthalates and are used as plasticizers in building materials and furniture. Low-molecular-weight (LMW) phthalates include di-*n*-butyl phthalate (DnBP), diisobutyl phthalate (DiBP), dimethyl phthalate (DMP), and diethyl phthalate (DEP), and are used in PCPs (e.g., nail polish, fragrance, hairspray), lacquers, varnishes, and coatings. A variety of other metabolites including monoisobutyl phthalate (MiBP), mono-*n*-butyl phthalate (MnBP), and monoethyl phthalate (MEP) are also commonly found in cosmetics and PCPs.

A report from the Environmental Working Group and Healthcare Without Harm revealed that DEP and dibutyl phthalate (DBP) were the two phthalates most prevalent in cosmetics.[21] DEP was found in 71% of all cosmetics tested, including deodorant, hair mousse, hairspray, and hand and body lotions; it was found in 100% of all fragrances and 86% of all hair gels. The fragrances carried the highest concentrations (in parts per million [PPM]) of DEP, with five products having 20,000 to 28,000 PPM. DBP was also found in 67% of the nail polishes tested.

A study of baby care products revealed that most infants (81%) had seven or more urinary phthalate metabolites above the limit of detection, and urinary concentrations of metabolites increased with the number of products (e.g., lotions, powders, and shampoos) used.[22]

Recent use of hairspray or hair gel (within 48 hours) was found to be associated with a 63% increase in urinary MEP concentrations (95% confidence interval (CI): 7–148) among 5-year-olds.[23] A study of 8- to 13-year-olds reported sex-specific positive associations between urinary MEP concentrations and use of deodorant, cologne or perfume, and hair conditioner.[24] Similar positive trends with urinary MEP concentration and number of PCPs used in the past 24 to 48 hours have also been reported in adults. Men who used cologne or aftershave within 48 hours before urine collection had higher median levels of MEP (265 and 266 ng/mL, respectively) than those who did not use cologne or aftershave (108 and 133 ng/mL, respectively), and for each additional type of PCP used, MEP increased 33% (95% CI: 14–53%).[25] As can be seen in Fig. 7.1, phthalate levels in the blood directly correlate with use of health and beauty aids.

Phthalates have various mechanisms of action on thyroid homeostasis, including interfering with the activity of the sodium/iodide symporter (NIS),[26] inhibiting T3 uptake in cells,[27] and competitively binding to trans-thyretin (TTR), a major thyroid hormone transporter in serum.[28] Significant mild negative correlations were found between total T4 (TT4) and free T4 (FT4) and urinary phthalate monoesters in pregnant women exposed to DnBP.[29] Phthalates have been found in significantly higher levels in infertile men, where they are linked with mitochondrial depolarization along with increased levels of reactive oxygen species and lipid peroxidases.[30]

DnBT, di-mono-*n*-butyl phthalate (DMBT) and DnBP also inhibit mitochondrial activity.[31,32] This mitochondrial inhibition, along with hypoandrogenism, undoubtedly plays a role in phthalates increasing rates of obesity and diabetes.[33] Phthalate inhibition of mitochondrial function (decreased activity of succinate dehydrogenase) is also responsible for the adverse effect on Sertoli cells, leading to male infertility.[34]

Triclosan

TCS is a chlorinated phenolic bactericide used as an active ingredient in PCPs including soaps, acne cream, shaving cream, underarm deodorants, shower gels, and toothpastes, as well as toys and clothing.[35] The effectiveness of TCS as an antibacterial agent has led to its extensive use, and TCS can now be found in nearly all body fluids (e.g., urine, breast milk, serum), placenta, fat tissue, and nails.[36] In the United States, 76% of all liquid commercial soaps examined contained TCS.[37] TCS concentrations have been shown to be higher in both the plasma and milk of nursing mothers who used PCPs, suggesting that PCPs may be

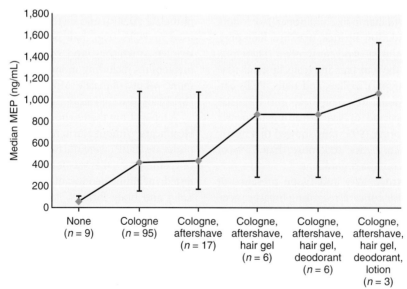

FIG. 7.1 Cosmetic use increases monoethyl phthalate levels in the blood. (From Duty, S. M., Ackerman, R. M., Calafat, A. M., & Hauser, R. [2005]. Personal care product use predicts urinary concentrations of some phthalate monoesters. *Environmental Health Perspectives, 113*(11), 1530–1535.)

the principal source of exposure in humans.[38] Single spot urine samples of more than 2500 individuals involved in the 2003 to 2004 National Health and Nutrition Examination Survey (NHANES) detected concentrations of total (free plus conjugated) TCS in nearly three-quarters of the samples tested at geometrical mean and 95th percentile concentrations of 13.0 μg/L (12.7 μg/g creatinine) and 459.0 μg/L (363.8 μg/g creatinine), respectively.[39]

In animal studies, TCS has been shown to alter thyroid hormone, disrupt testosterone concentrations, and have estrogenic effects.[40] TCS may be an antagonist or weak agonist to the estrogen receptor and/or a weak antagonist of the androgen receptor.[41,42] Although still being researched, adverse effects of TCS on thyroid hormone may include upregulation of hepatic catabolism, interference with thyroid hormone sulfation, and altered expression of cellular transport.[43] Determining clinical endocrine significance is challenging, as doses of TCS reported to produce significant thyroid dysfunction or adverse effects in male and female reproduction, gestation, and animal offspring are several orders of magnitude greater than the estimated exposure levels in humans.[44]

TCS interference with detoxification appears more clinically significant. It can interact with UDP-glucuronosyltransferases as a selective inhibitor of the glucuronidation and sulfonation of phenol xenobiotics[45] and as an activator of the human pregnane X receptor altering PXR-regulated steroid hormone metabolism.[46] In addition, low molecular concentrations of TCS lead to mitochondrial dysfunction, inhibiting the activity of succinate dehydrogenase and accelerating the production of superoxide anion, enhancing the production of reactive oxygen species [ROS (i.e., free radicals)].[47]

Ultraviolet Filters

UV filters are a class of chemicals that absorb or reflect UVA and UVB light and can protect human skin against the deleterious effects of UV radiation.[48] There are 16 UV filters permitted for use in cosmetics (e.g., sunscreen, lip balm, facial moisturizer) in the United States, and 9 of the 16 are used in more than 98% of products.[49] Box 7.1 lists the 16 approved UV filters. As a result of their persistence, stability, and lipophilicity, UV filters can bioaccumulate in organisms and have been reported in human placenta tissue,[50] breast milk, plasma, feces, and urine.[51] The most commonly used UV filters can be divided into three main groups: benzophenones, camphor derivatives, and cinnamate derivatives. Although general toxicity of

---

BOX 7.1 FDA-Approved UV Filters

- Aminobenzoic acid
- Homosalate
- Octyl salicylate
- Sulisobenzone
- Avobenzone
- Menthyl anthranilate
- Oxybenzone
- Titanium dioxide
- Cinoxate
- Octocrylene
- Octyl dimethyl PABA
- Trolamine salicylate
- Dioxybenzone
- Octyl methoxycinnamate
- Phenylbenzimidazole sulfonic acid
- Zinc oxide

PABA, para-aminobenzoic acid.
From Nash, J. F. (2006). Human safety and efficacy of ultraviolet filters and sunscreen products. *Dermatologic Clinics, 24*(1), 35–51.

UV filters is discussed, some sections primarily focus on the effects of oxybenzone, also known as benzophenone-3 (BP-3), as this agent has been more thoroughly studied.

A variety of animal studies have reported endocrine disruption effects of UV filters resulting in developmental and reproductive toxicities.[52] BP-3 is associated with increased uterine weight in rat studies and increased proliferation of human breast cells *in vitro*.[53] Considering that 60% of skin sunscreen products specifically marketed for babies contain two to six UV-absorbing chemicals,[54] the concern of endocrine disruption is paramount. Table 7.1 describes a summary of the endocrine disrupting effects and mechanisms of toxicity of the commonly used UV filters.

A good example of the sometimes-subtle effects of toxicants is the lack of consideration of the clinical effect of blocking UV, the mechanism for producing vitamin D in the skin. Researchers more than 30 years ago demonstrated a greater than 50% decrease in elevation of vitamin D during summer, with resultant even lower levels in winter.[55]

Toxic Metals

Aluminum. PCPs are potential contributors to the body's burden of aluminum through the use of aluminum-containing antiperspirants, lipsticks, and sunscreens.

TABLE 7.1	**Endocrine Disrupting Effects of UV Filters**	
UV Filter	**Endocrine Receptor Involved**	**Endocrine Disrupting Effects**
Benzophenones	Estrogen	• Activation of ERα, ERβ • Inhibition of activity of 17β-estradiol • Induction of proliferation of MCF-7 cell • Induction of VTG in fathead minnows • Reduction of uterine weight in immature Long-Evans rats
	Androgen	• Antagonist of human AR transactivation • Repression of 4,5-dihydrotestosterone-induced transactivational activity • Inhibition of testosterone formation in mice and rats
	Thyroid	• Inhibition of human recombinant TPO • Interference with THR • Inhibition of TPO activity in rats
	Progesterone	• Antagonist of PR
Camphor derivatives	Estrogen	• Activation of ERα, ERβ • Inhibition of activity of 17β-estradiol • Induction of proliferation of MCF-7 cell • Induction of pS2 protein in MCF-7 cells • Induction of VTG in fish • Reduction of uterine weight in rats
	Androgen	• Repression of 4,5-dihydrotestosterone-induced transactivational activity • Inhibition of testosterone formation in HEK-293 cells • Antagonist of human AR
	Progesterone	• Antagonist of PR • Increase of PR mRNA levels in rats • Inhibition of expression of PR protein in rats • Disturbance of expression of membrane-associated PR in insects
Cinnamate derivatives	Estrogen	• Activation of ERα • Inhibition of activity of 17β-estradiol • Induction of proliferation of MCF-7 cells • Induction of VTG in fish • Reduction of uterine weight in rats
	Androgen	• Antagonist of AR • Inhibition of 4,5-dihydrotestosterone activity • Reduction of prostate and testicular weight in rats
	Thyroid	• Decrease of T4 level • Inhibition of conversion of T4 to T3 in rats
	Progesterone	• Antagonist of PR

AR, Androgen receptor; *ER,* estrogen receptor; *ERα,* estrogen receptor alpha; *ERβ,* estrogen receptor beta; *PR,* progesterone receptor; *T4,* thyroxine; *T3,* triiodothyronine; *THR,* thyroid hormone receptor; *TPO,* thyroid peroxidase; *VTG,* vitellogenin.
From Wang, J., Pan, L., Wu, S., Lu, L., Xu, Y., Zhu, Y., Guo, M., Zhuang, S. (2016). Recent advances on endocrine disrupting effects of UV filters. *International Journal of Environmental Research and Public Health, 13*(8), pii:E782. Reprinted under the terms and conditions of the Creative Commons Attribution (CC-BY) license (http://creativecommons.org/licenses/by/4.0/)

Aluminum is a metalloestrogen, genotoxic, bound by DNA, and prooxidant, and has been shown to be carcinogenic in animal studies.[56] There is evidence that skin is permeable to aluminum when it is applied in an antiperspirant.[57]

Mercury. Inorganic mercury poisoning following the use of skin-lightening creams has been reported from Africa, Europe, the U.S., Mexico, Australia, and Hong Kong.[58] Mercury vapor concentrations as high as 50 µg/m³ have been detected in household locations of individuals using skin-lightening creams.[59] A population-based biomonitoring study confirmed that exposure to inorganic mercury from the use of imported mercury-containing skin lightening creams occurred in Dominican and possibly Caribbean groups in New York City.[60] Thirteen individuals (all women) had urine mercury concentrations that equaled or exceeded the New York State reportable level of 20 μg/L, and four Dominican women had mercury levels > 50 μg/L.

BODY BURDEN

In adult women in the U.S., total dermal intake doses (the sum of all phthalates or parabens) have been calculated to be 0.37 and 31.0 μg/kg-bw/day for phthalates and parabens, respectively, and although dermal intake of phthalates for PCPs was lower for infants and toddlers, the calculated maximum daily exposure dose was determined to be three times higher than that calculated for adult women (range = 58.6–766 μg/kg-bw/day).[61] Although phthalates are not believed to accumulate in the body and some temporal variability exists, it is possible to use a single spot urine sample to estimate mean exposure up to 6 months in children,[62] 3 months in men,[63] and 1 month in women.[64] In other words, most people's exposure is so consistent that single samples are good measures of average body load.

The average daily personal paraben exposure resulting from cosmetics and PCPs is estimated to be 50 mg. Although in vitro skin penetration studies have suggested that parabens penetrate human skin at a rate of > 20%,[65] a Cosmetic Ingredient Review (CIR) Expert Panel estimated that, because of their hydrolysis by skin esterases, as little as 1% of topically applied parabens is available for absorption into the body intact.[66]

Detoxification/Excretion Processes

Parabens. Animal studies have shown that parabens are quickly absorbed from the gastrointestinal tract and metabolized. Parabens are lipophilic, can be absorbed through the skin, and are found intact in tissue. In fact, these compounds have been found in breast cancer tissue in levels ranging from 20 ng/g tissue to 100 ng/g tissue.[67] Once in the bloodstream, parabens are conjugated in the liver with glycine, sulfate, or glucuronate for excretion in the urine. Almost 80% to 85% of parabens are excreted in urine predominantly in their conjugated forms within the first 24 hours of administration,[68] and p-hydroxyhippuric

acid has been identified as the major but nonspecific metabolite.[69]

Phthalates. After entering the body via ingestion, dermal absorption, or inhalation, phthalates can be metabolized to their hydrolytic monoesters, and some monoesters are further transformed into oxidative metabolites after enzymatic oxidation.[70] Phthalates are quickly metabolized and excreted in urine, with elimination half-lives of less than 24 hours.[71] Although urinary measurements may underestimate some phthalate exposure, studies show that urine is the most reliable method of quantifying overall exposure, as phthalate metabolites are unlikely to be biased by external contamination.[72]

Triclosan. TCS is readily absorbed from the gastrointestinal tract and oral mucosa and has rapid turnover in humans, with maximum plasma concentration being reached within 1 to 3 hours and a terminal plasma half-life of 21 hours.[73] TCS has been detected in human breast milk at levels ranging from 0 to 2100 μg/kg lipid,[74] in serum,[75] and as metabolites in urine.[76]

Benzophenone-3. BP-3 has been found to be readily absorbed from the gastrointestinal tract, and BP-3 along with its metabolite 2,4-dihydroxybenzophenone have been detected in human urine as soon as 4 hours after topical application of sunscreen products.[77] Conjugation of BP-3 with glucuronic acid is the major systemic elimination route, and the elimination pattern is biphasic, with alpha and beta half-lives of 0.88 and 15.90 hours, respectively.[78] BP-3 has been detected in urine, serum, and breast milk samples, suggesting bioaccumulation in humans.[79] There is evidence that low levels of BP-3 may remain in the body for up to 5 days after dermal exposure.[80]

Clinical Significance
Endocrine
Parabens. Parabens have weak estrogenic activity and have been shown to induce the growth of MCF-7 human breast cancer cells in vitro,[81] leading some researchers to suggest their potential as initiators or promoters of breast cancer. Part of the concern arises from an increasing number of breast cancers that occur in the upper outer quadrant of the breast, where paraben-containing antiperspirant is applied.[82] Parabens demonstrate multiple cancer hallmarks and characteristics, including: 1) Parabens have been measured as present in 99% of human

breast tissue samples; 2) Parabens possess estrogenic activity and can stimulate sustained proliferation of human breast cancer cells at concentrations measurable in the breast; 3) Parabens can inhibit the suppression of breast cancer cell growth by hydroxytamoxifen; 4) Long-term exposure (> 20 weeks) to parabens leads to increased migratory and invasive activity in human breast cancer cells; 5) Methylparaben increases mTOR, a key regulator of energy metabolism; and 6) Parabens can cause DNA damage at high concentrations in a short term.[83]

Phthalates. Maternal levels of phthalates during pregnancy have been associated with long-term hormonal imbalance in their male children up to 14 years later, and maternal levels of the LMW MiBP (often found in fingernail polish) are inversely associated with testosterone levels.[84] Boys exposed to higher levels of phthalates in utero also experienced delayed puberty. The clear inverse relationship between phthalates and testosterone levels has been repeatedly established across the globe.[85-87] Urinary phthalate metabolites in pregnant women have been found to correlate with genital changes in their infant males (Odds Ratio (OR) for MEP and MiBP = 4.7 and 9.1, respectively),[88] and breast-milk phthalate metabolites have been correlated with higher serum sex hormone binding globulin levels and LH:free testosterone ratios in infant males.[89]

Phthalate presence in young girls has been associated with both delayed menarche and premature breast development (thelarche).[90] Young Puerto Rican girls with thelarche had serum DEHP levels averaging 450 parts per billion (ppb), while those without thelarche averaged only 70 ppb.[91]

In the 2007 to 2010 NHANES trial, LMW phthalates (MnBP, MEP, and MiBP) were significantly associated with obesity in boys and adolescents.[92] MEP was also found to be positively associated with waist circumference in adolescent girls.[93] In 70-year-old Swedish women, MiBP and MMP were positively related to waist circumference and truncal fat mass.[94]

An increased risk of developing metabolic syndrome (MetS) has been associated with higher concentrations of certain phthalate metabolites.[95] Phthalates, including diethyl phthalate, dibutyl phthalate, dimethyl phthalate, and dibenzyl phthalate, are associated with the development of type 2 diabetes and obesity by interfering with various cell-signaling pathways involved in weight and glucose homeostasis.[96]

Neurological

Phthalates. Women's phthalate urine levels in late pregnancy are associated with reduced scores on both the Mental Development Index and Psychomotor Index for their daughters by age 2.[97] The most significant correlations were found for maternal levels of the LMW phthalate metabolites mono-*n*-butyl, monoisobutyl, and monobenzyl phthalates that are commonly used in nail polish and other PCPs. Levels of these phthalates in women were also associated with a 6.7- to 7.6-point drop in IQ in their offspring by age 7.[98] The presence of LMW phthalate metabolites in a mother's urine during her third trimester of pregnancy has been significantly correlated with the child having greater problems with social cognition, social awareness, and social communication by the age of 7.[99]

LMW phthalates, commonly found in liquid PCPs, have also been linked to depression. U.S. residents over the age of 60 who participated in the 2006 to 2012 NHANES trial and had higher urine levels of two common phthalates (mono-carboxypropyl-phthalate and mono-*n*-butyl phthalate) were more than twice as likely to be depressed as those with lower phthalate levels.[100]

Toxic metals. Aluminum is certainly a potential contributor to the onset, progression, and aggressiveness of neurological disease,[101] and a potential link has been observed between aluminum and Alzheimer's disease, amyotrophic lateral sclerosis (ALS), and autism spectrum disorders.[102]

Mercury is a ubiquitous environmental pollutant and is toxic at any level. Methylmercury (MeHg) is a potent neurotoxin via several mechanisms including demyelination, oxidative stress, and autonomic dysfunction.[103] Metallic mercury interrupts the normal uptake and release of neurotransmitters and can result in excitability and irritability.

Reproductive

Parabens. Butyl paraben has been reported to affect reproductive tract development in rats, causing significant decreases in sperm count and sperm motility in the epididymis.[104] The addition of parabens to the diet of postweaning male rats resulted in decreased daily sperm production and its efficiency in the testes, and the exposure level at which this disruption was observed is the same as the upper-limit acceptable daily intake (10 mg/kg body weight/day) of parabens.[105] Male partners in infertile couples with higher than average levels of methylparaben were 81% more likely to experience failure of *in vitro* fertilization (IVF) with their partners.[106]

Phthalates. The male reproductive system is a major target organ of phthalates, leading to embryotoxic and teratogenic effects including reduced anogenital distance, hypospadias, nipple retention, malformed epididymis, Leydig cell hyperplasia, deterioration of semen quality, and decreased fertility index.[107] Multiple studies have demonstrated a statistically positive association between urinary MEP levels and altered DNA integrity in sperm.[108,109] In 234 Swedish men undergoing their military conscript medical examination, subjects in the highest quartile for MEP had fewer motile sperm (mean difference = 8.8%; 95% CI, 0.8–17), more immotile sperm (8.9%; 0.3–18), and lower luteinizing hormone values (0.7 IU/L; 0.1–1.2).[110] Elevated urinary levels of LMW phthalates found in fragrances are significantly associated with a 20% reduction in male fertility.[111]

Atopy. Allergenic ingredients of cosmetics/PCPs include fragrances, hair dyes, preservatives, emollients, surfactants, UV filters, pigments, antioxidants, and/or resins. Fragrances are the most common cause of allergies to cosmetics, followed by preservatives and hair dyes.[112] Fragrances from magazine scent strips have been shown to exacerbate asthma symptoms, producing significant declines in forced expiratory volume (FEV_1) in asthmatic patients compared with controls.[113] Exposure to fragrances has also been associated with allergic contact dermatitis, headaches, and mucosal symptoms.[114] Hair dyes containing phenylenediamines have a potential to induce and elicit contact allergic sensitization.[115] Photoallergy can occur with the use of some UV filters (para-aminobenzoic acid [PABA] derivatives, cinnamates, benzophenones, and octocrylene), which should be used with caution on lesional skin and in pediatric settings.[116]

INTERVENTION

Choosing PCPs that are labeled to be free of phthalates, parabens, TCS, and BP-3 can significantly reduce personal exposure to these harmful toxicants. A study of female Latina teens showed that after only 3 days of avoidance, urinary concentrations of monoethyl phthalate decreased by 27.4%; methyl- and propylparaben concentrations decreased by 43.9% and 45.4%, respectively; TCS concentrations decreased by 35.7%; and BP-3 concentrations decreased by 36.0%.[117] Use reduction targeted at EDCs

in consumer products has the potential to significantly decrease occupational and residential exposures. However, the lack of transparency regarding ingredients along with the multitude of chemicals included in PCPs not only makes it difficult for consumers to make educated choices, but also hinders research on the true toxic effects of PCPs. Apps like ThinkDirty are now available to quickly assess the level of toxic constituents in health and beauty aids. Some websites are good resources to help navigate product labels and reduce exposure to toxicants contained in PCPs:

- Good Guide: http://www.goodguide.com
- Green Seal: http://www.greenseal.org/
- EPA's Design for the Environment program: https://www.epa.gov/saferchoice/design-environment-programs-initiatives-and-projects
- Environmental Working Group: http://www.ewg.org/skindeep

REFERENCES

1. Zukiewicz-Sobczak, W. A., Adamczuk, P., et al. (2013). Allergy to selected cosmetic ingredients. *Postepy Dermatologii i Alergologii, 30*(5), 307–310. PubMed PMID: 24353491.
2. *Fair Packaging and Labeling Act.* (1967). https://www.ftc.gov/enforcement/rules/rulemaking-regulatory-reform-proceedings/fair-packaging-labeling-act. (Last accessed June 20, 2017.)
3. *Federal Food, Drug, and Cosmetic Act.* (1938). https://www.fda.gov/aboutfda/whatwedo/history/centennialoffda/centennialeditionoffdaconsumer/ucm093787.htm. (Last accessed June 20, 2017.)
4. *FIFRA (Federal Insecticide, Fungicide, and Rodenticide Act).* (1972). https://www.epa.gov/laws-regulations/summary-federal-insecticide-fungicide-and-rodenticide-act. (Last accessed June 20, 2017.)
5. Rajapakse, N., Silva, E., & Kortenkamp, A. (2002). Combining xenoestrogens at levels below individual no-observed-effect concentrations dramatically enhances steroid hormone action. *Environmental Health Perspectives, 110*(9), 917–921. PubMed PMID: 12204827.
6. Egeghy, P. P., Judson, R., et al. (2012). The exposure data landscape for manufactured chemicals. *The Science of the Total Environment, 414*, 159–166. PubMed PMID: 22104386.
7. Gore, A. C., Chappell, V. A., et al. (2015). Executive summary to EDC-2: The Endocrine Society's second scientific statement on endocrine-disrupting chemicals. *Endocrine Reviews, 36*(6), 593–602. PubMed PMID: 26414233.

8. Waring, R. H., & Harris, R. M. (2005). Endocrine disruptors: A human risk? *Molecular and Cellular Endocrinology, 244*(1–2), 2–9. PubMed PMID: 16271281.

9. Buck Louis, G. M., Gray, L. E., Jr., et al. (2008). Environmental factors and puberty timing: Expert panel research needs. *Pediatrics, 121*(Suppl. 3), S192–S207. PubMed PMID: 18245512.

10. Anway, M. D., & Skinner, M. K. (2006). Epigenetic transgenerational actions of endocrine disruptors. *Endocrinology, 147*(Suppl. 6), S43–S49. PubMed PMID: 16690803.

11. Flora, S. J., Mittal, M., & Mehta, A. (2008). Heavy metal induced oxidative stress & its possible reversal by chelation therapy. *The Indian Journal of Medical Research, 128*(4), 501–523. PubMed PMID: 19106443.

12. Msagati, T. A., Barri, T., et al. (2008). Analysis and quantification of parabens in cosmetic products by utilizing hollow fibre-supported liquid membrane and high performance liquid chromatography with ultraviolet detection. *International Journal of Cosmetic Science, 30*(4), 297–307. PubMed PMID: 18713076.

13. Kirchhof, M. G., & de Gannes, G. C. (2013). The health controversies of parabens. *Skin Therapy Letter, 18*(2), 5–7. PubMed PMID: 23508773.

14. Rastogi, S. C., Schouten, A., et al. (1995). Contents of methyl-, ethyl-, propyl-, butyl-, and benzylparaben in cosmetic products. *Contact Dermatitis, 32*(1), 28–30. PubMed PMID: 7720367.

15. Routledge, E. J., Parker, J., et al. (1998). Some alkyl hydroxyl benzoate preservatives (parabens) are estrogenic. *Toxicology and Applied Pharmacology, 153*(1), 12–19. PubMed PMID: 9875295.

16. Darbre, P. D., & Harvey, P. W. (2008). Paraben esters: Review of recent studies of endocrine toxicity, absorption, esterase and human exposure, and discussion of potential human health risks. *Journal of Applied Toxicology, 28*(5), 561–578. PubMed PMID: 18484575.

17. Prusakiewicz, J. J., Harville, H. M., Zhang, Y., et al. (2007). Parabens inhibit human skin estrogen sulfotransferase activity: Possible link to paraben estrogenic effects. *Toxicology, 232*, 248–256.

18. Soni, M. G., Taylor, S. L., Greenberg, N. A., & Burdock, G. A. (2002). Evaluation of the health aspects of methyl paraben: A review of the published literature. *Food and Chemical Toxicology, 40*, 1335–1373.

19. Soni, M. G., Burdock, G. A., Taylor, S. L., & Greenberg, N. A. (2001). Safety assessment of propyl paraben: A review of the published literature. *Food and Chemical Toxicology, 39*, 513–532.

20. Tavares, R. S., Martins, F. C., Oliveira, P. J., et al. (2009). Parabens in male infertility – is there a mitochondrial connection? *Reproductive Toxicology, 27*, 1–7.

21. Houlihan, J., Brody, C., & Schwan, B. *Not too pretty: Phthalates, beauty products & the FDA.* https://www.ewg.org/research/not-too-pretty#.WrLYikFICaM. (Last accessed June 22, 2017.)

22. Sathyanarayana, S., Karr, C. J., et al. (2008). Baby care products: Possible sources of infant phthalate exposure. *Pediatrics, 121*(2), e260–e268. PubMed PMID: 18245401.

23. Watkins, D. J., Eliot, M., et al. (2014). Variability and predictors of urinary concentrations of phthalate metabolites during early childhood. *Environmental Science & Technology, 48*(15), 8881–8890. PubMed PMID: 24977926.

24. Lewis, R. C., Meeker, J. D., et al. (2013). Predictors of urinary bisphenol A and phthalate metabolite concentrations in Mexican children. *Chemosphere, 93*(10), 2390–2398. PubMed PMID: 24041567.

25. Duty, S. M., Ackerman, R. M., Calafat, A. M., & Hauser, R. (2005). Personal care product use predicts urinary concentrations of some phthalate monoesters. *Environmental Health Perspectives, 113*(11), 1530–1535. PubMed PMID: 16263507.

26. Breous, E., Wenzel, A., & Loos, U. (2005). The promotor of the human sodium/iodide symporter responds to certain phthalate plasticisers. *Molecular and Cellular Endocrinology, 244*(1–2), 75–78. PubMed PMID: 16257484.

27. Shimada, N., & Yamauchi, K. (2004). Characteristics of 3,5,3'-triiodothyronine (T3)-uptake system of tadpole red blood cells: Effect of endocrine-disrupting chemicals on cellular T3 response. *The Journal of Endocrinology, 183*(3), 627–637. PubMed PMID: 15590988.

28. Ishihara, A., Nishiyama, N., Sugiyama, S., & Yamauchi, K. (2003). The effect of endocrine disrupting chemicals on thyroid hormone binding to Japanese quail transthyretin and thyroid hormone receptor. *General and Comparative Endocrinology, 134*(1), 36–43. PubMed PMID: 13129501.

29. Huang, P. C., Kuo, P. L., Guo, Y. L., Liao, P. C., & Lee, C. C. (2007). Associations between urinary phthalate monoesters and thyroid hormones in pregnant women. *Human Reproduction, 22*(10), 2715–2722. PubMed PMID: 17704099.

30. Pant, N., Shukla, M., Kumar Patel, D., Shukla, Y., Mathur, N., Kumar Gupta, Y., et al. (2008). Correlation of phthalate exposures with semen quality. *Toxicology and Applied Pharmacology, 231*(1), 112–116. PubMed PMID: 18513777.

31. Melnick, R. L., & Schiller, C. M. (1982). Mitochondrial toxicity of phthalate esters. *Environmental Health Perspectives*, 45, 51–56. PubMed PMID: 7140696.
32. Ohyama, T. (1977). Effects of phthalate esters on the latent ATPase and swelling of mitochondria. *Journal of Biochemistry*, 82(1), 9–15. PubMed PMID: 19458.
33. Stahlhut, R. W., van Wijngaarden, E., Dye, T. D., Cook, S., & Swan, S. H. (2007). Concentrations of urinary phthalate metabolites are associated with increased waist circumference and insulin resistance in adult US males. *Environmental Health Perspectives*, 115, 876–882. PubMed PMID: 17589594.
34. Zhou, Y., Fukuoka, M., & Tanaka, A. (1990). Mechanisms of testicular atrophy induced in di-*n*-butyl phthalate in rats. Part 3. Changes in the activity of some enzymes in the Sertoli and germ cells, and in the levels of metal ions. *Journal of Applied Toxicology*, 10(6), 447–453. PubMed PMID: 2128091.
35. Bhargava, H. N., & Leonard, P. A. (1996). Triclosan: Applications and safety. *American Journal of Infection Control*, 24(3), 209–218. PubMed PMID: 8807001.
36. Krishnan, K., Gagne, M., Nong, A., Aylward, L. L., & Hays, S. M. (2010). Biomonitoring equivalents for triclosan. *Regulatory Toxicology and Pharmacology*, 58(1), 10–17. PubMed PMID: 20541577.
37. Perencevich, E. N., Wong, M. T., & Harris, A. D. (2001). National and regional assessment of the antimicrobial soap market: A step toward determining the impact of prevalent antibacterial soaps. *American Journal of Infection Control*, 29(5), 281–283. PubMed PMID: 11584251.
38. Allmyr, M., Adolfsson-Erici, M., et al. (2006). Triclosan in plasma and milk from Swedish nursing mothers and their exposure via personal care products. *The Science of the Total Environment*, 372(1), 87–93. PubMed PMID: 17007908.
39. Calafat, A. M., Ye, X., Wong, L. Y., et al. (2008). Urinary concentrations of triclosan in the U.S. population: 2003–2004. *Environmental Health Perspectives*, 116(3), 303–307. PubMed PMID: 18335095.
40. Stoker, T. E., Gibson, E. K., & Zorilla, L. M. (2010). Triclosan exposure modulates estrogen-dependent responses in the female Wistar rat. *Toxicological Sciences*, 117(1), 45–53. PubMed PMID: 20562219.
41. Ahn, K. C., Zhao, B., Chen, J., et al. (2008). In vitro biologic activities of the antimicrobials, its analogs, and triclosan in bioassay screens: Receptor-based bioassay screens. *Environmental Health Perspectives*, 116(9), 1203–1210. PubMed PMID: 18795164.
42. Chen, J., Ahn, K. C., et al. (2007). Antiandrogenic properties of parabens and other phenolic containing small molecules in personal care products. *Toxicology*

and Applied Pharmacology*, 221(3), 278–284. PubMed PMID: 17481686.
43. Paul, K. B., Hedge, J. M., et al. (2010). Short-term exposure to triclosan decreases thyroxine in vivo via upregulation of hepatic catabolism in Young-Long Evans rats. *Toxicological Sciences*, 113(2), 367–379. PubMed PMID: 19910387.
44. Witorsch, R. J. (2014). Critical analysis of endocrine disruptive activity of triclosan and its relevance to human exposure through the use of personal care products. *Critical Reviews in Toxicology*, 44(6), 535–555. PubMed PMID: 24897554.
45. Wang, L. Q., Falany, C. N., & James, M. O. (2004). Triclosan as a substrate and inhibitor of 3'-phosphoadenosine 5'-phosphosulfate-sul fotransferase and UDP-glucuronosyl transferase in human liver fractions. *Drug Metabolism and Disposition: The Biological Fate of Chemicals*, 32(10), 1162–1169. PubMed PMID: 15269185.
46. Jacobs, M. N., Nolan, G. T., & Hood, S. R. (2005). Lignans, bacteriocides, and organochlorine compounds activate the human pregnane X receptor (PXR). *Toxicology and Applied Pharmacology*, 209(2), 123–133. PubMed PMID: 15885729.
47. Teplova, V. V., Belosludtsev, K. N., & Kruglov, A. G. (2017). Mechanism of triclosan: Mitochondrial dysfunction including complex II inhibition, superoxide releases and uncoupling of oxidative phosphorylation. *Toxicology Letters*, 275, 108–117. PubMed PMID: 28478158.
48. Ohnaka, T. (1993). Health effects of ultraviolet radiation. *The Annals of Physiological Anthropology*, 12(1), 1–10. PubMed PMID: 8507288.
49. Nash, J. F. (2006). Human safety and efficacy of ultraviolet filters and sunscreen products. *Dermatologic Clinics*, 24(1), 35–51. PubMed PMID: 16311166.
50. Valle-Sistac, J., Moilins-Delgado, D., et al. (2016). Determination of parabens and benzophenone-type UV filters in human placenta. First description of the existence of benzyl paraben and benzophenone-4. *Environment International*, 88, 243–249. PubMed PMID: 26773395.
51. Janjua, N. R., Kongshoj, B., et al. (2008). Sunscreens in human plasma and urine after repeated whole-body topical application. *Journal of the European Academy of Dermatology and Venereology*, 22(4), 456–461. PubMed PMID: 18221342.
52. Schlumpf, M., Schmid, P., et al. (2004). Endocrine activity and developmental toxicity of cosmetic UV filters – an update. *Toxicology*, 205(1–2), 113–122. PubMed PMID: 15458796.

53. Schlumpf, M., Cotton, B., et al. (2001). In vitro and in vivo estrogenicity of UV screens. *Environmental Health Perspectives, 109*(3), 239–244. PubMed PMID: 11333184.

54. Wahie, S., Lloyd, J. J., & Farr, P. M. (2007). Sunscreen ingredients and labelling: A survey of products available in the UK. *Clinical and Experimental Dermatology, 32*(4), 359–364. PubMed PMID: 17376206.

55. Matsuoka, L. Y., Ide, L., Wortsman, J., MacLaughlin, J. A., & Holick, M. F. (1987). Sunscreens suppress cutaneous vitamin D3 synthesis. *The Journal of Clinical Endocrinology and Metabolism, 64*(6), 1165–1168.

56. Exley, C., Charles, C. M., et al. (2007). Aluminum in human breast tissue. *Journal of Inorganic Biochemistry, 101*(9), 1344–1346. PubMed PMID: 176299949.

57. Flarend, R., Bin, T., et al. (2001). A preliminary study of the dermal absorption of aluminum from antiperspirants using aluminum-26. *Food and Chemical Toxicology, 39*(2), 163–168. PubMed PMID: 11267710.

58. Chan, T. Y. (2011). Inorganic mercury poisoning associated with skin-lightening cosmetic products. *Clinical Toxicology, 49*(10), 886–891. PubMed PMID: 22070559.

59. Centers for Disease Control and Prevention (CDC). (2012). Mercury exposure among household users and nonusers of skin-lightening creams produced in Mexico – California and Virginia, 2010. *Morbidity and Mortality Weekly Report, 61*(2), 33–36. PubMed PMID: 22258417.

60. McKelvey, W., Jeffery, N., et al. (2011). Population-based inorganic mercury biomonitoring and the identification of skin care products as a source of exposure in New York City. *Environmental Health Perspectives, 119*(2), 203–209. PubMed PMID: 20923743.

61. Guo, Y., & Kannan, K. (2013). A survey of phthalates and parabens in personal care products from the United States and its implications for human exposure. *Environmental Science & Technology, 47*(24), 14442–14449. PubMed PMID: 24261694.

62. Teitelbaum, S. L., Britton, J. A., Calafat, A. M., Ye, X., et al. (2008). Temporal variability in urinary concentrations of phthalate metabolites, phytoestrogens and phenols among minority children in the United States. *Environmental Research, 106*(2), 257–269. PubMed PMID: 17976571.

63. Hauser, R., Meeker, J. D., et al. (2004). Temporal variability of urinary phthalate metabolite levels in men of reproductive age. *Environmental Health Perspectives, 112*(17), 1734–1740. PubMed PMID: 15579421.

64. Peck, J. D., Sweeney, A. M., et al. (2010). Intra- and inter-individual variability of urinary phthalate metabolite concentrations in Hmong women of reproductive age. *Journal of Exposure Science and Environmental Epidemiology, 20*(1), 90–100. PubMed PMID: 19223940.

65. Jewell, C., Prusakiewicz, J. J., et al. (2007). Hydrolysis of a series of parabens by skin microsomes and cytosol from human and minipigs and in whole skin in short-term culture. *Toxicology and Applied Pharmacology, 225*(2), 221–228. PubMed PMID: 17889094.

66. [No authors listed]. (2008). Final amended report on the safety assessment of methylparaben, ethylparaben, propylparaben, isopropylparaben, butylparaben, isobutylparaben, and benzylparaben as used in cosmetic products. *International Journal of Toxicology, 27*(Suppl. 4), 1–82. PubMed PMID: 19101832.

67. Darbre, P. D., Aljarrah, A., Miller, W. R., et al. (2004). Concentrations of parabens in human breast tumours. *Journal of Applied Toxicology, 24*, 5–13.

68. Ye, X., Bishop, A. M., et al. (2006). Parabens as urinary biomarkers of exposure in humans. *Environmental Health Perspectives, 114*(12), 1843–1846. PubMed PMID: 17185273.

69. Moos, R. K., Angerer, J., et al. (2016). Metabolism and elimination of methyl-, iso-, and *n*-butyl paraben in human urine after single oral dosage. *Archives of Toxicology, 90*(11), 2699–2709. PubMed PMID: 26608183.

70. Gao, C. J., Liu, L. Y., Ma, W. L., et al. (2016). Phthalate metabolites in urine of Chinese young adults: Concentration, profile, exposure, and cumulative risk assessment. *The Science of the Total Environment, 543*(Pt. A), 19–27. PubMed PMID: 26575634.

71. Koch, H. M., Bolt, H. M., Preuss, R., & Angerer, J. (2005). New metabolites of di(2-ethylhexyl) phthalate in human urine and serum after single oral doses of deuterium-labelled DEHP. *Archives of Toxicology, 79*(7), 367–376. PubMed PMID: 15700144.

72. Chang, J. W., Lee, C. C., et al. (2017). Estimated daily intake and cumulative risk assessment of phthalates in the general Taiwanese after the 2011 DEHP food scandal. *Scientific Reports, 7*, 45009. PubMed PMID: 28327585.

73. Sandborgh-Englund, G., Adolfsson-Erici, M., et al. (2006). Pharmacokinetics of triclosan following oral ingestion in humans. *Journal of Toxicology and Environmental Health. Part A, 69*(20), 1861–1873. PubMed PMID: 16952905.

74. Dayan, A. D. (2007). Risk assessment of triclosan (Irgasan) in human breast milk. *Food and Chemical Toxicology, 45*(1), 125–129. PubMed PMID: 17011099.

75. Bedoux, G., Roig, B., et al. (2012). Occurrence and toxicity of antimicrobial triclosan and by-products in the environment. *Environmental Science and Pollution Research International, 19*(4), 1044–1065. PubMed PMID: 22057832.

76. Ye, X., Kuklenyik, Z., et al. (2005). Automated on-line column-switching HPLC-MS/MS method with peak focusing for the determination of nine environmental phenols in urine. *Analytical Chemistry, 77*(16), 5407–5413. PubMed PMID: 16097788.

77. Jiang, R., Roberts, M. S., et al. (1999). Absorption of sunscreens across human skin: An evaluation of commercial products for children and adults. *British Journal of Clinical Pharmacology, 48*(4), 635–637. PubMed PMID: 10583038.

78. Kadry, A. M., Okereke, C. S., et al. (1995). Pharmacokinetics of benzophenone-3 after oral exposure in male rats. *Journal of Applied Toxicology, 15*(2), 97–102. PubMed PMID: 7782565.

79. Kim, S., & Choi, K. (2014). Occurrences, toxicities, and ecological risks of benzophenone-3, a common component of organic sunscreen products: A mini-review. *Environment International, 70*, 143–157. PubMed PMID: 24934855.

80. Gonzalez, H., Farbrot, A., Larko, O., & Wennberg, A. M. (2006). Percutaneous absorption of the sunscreen benzophenone-3 after repeated whole-body applications, with and without ultraviolet irradiation. *The British Journal of Dermatology, 154*(2), 337–340. PubMed PMID: 16433806.

81. Byford, J. R., Shaw, L. E., Drew, M. G., et al. (2002). Oestrogenic activity of parabens in MCF7 human breast cancer cells. *The Journal of Steroid Biochemistry and Molecular Biology, 80*, 49–60.

82. Darbre, P. D., & Harvey, P. W. (2008). Paraben esters: Review of recent studies on endocrine toxicity, absorption, esterase and human exposure, and discussion of potential human health risks. *Journal of Applied Toxicology, 28*, 561–578.

83. Darbre, P. D., & Harvey, P. W. (2014). Parabens can enable hallmarks and characteristics of cancer in human breast epithelial cells: A review of the literature with reference to new exposure data and regulatory status. *Journal of Applied Toxicology, 34*(9), 925–938. PubMed PMID: 25047802.

84. Ferguson, K. K., Peterson, K. E., Lee, J. M., Mercado-García, A., Blank-Goldenberg, C., Téllez-Rojo, M. M., et al. (2014). Prenatal and peripubertal phthalates and bisphenol A in relation to sex hormones and puberty in boys. *Reproductive Toxicology, 47*, 70–76. PubMed PMID: 24945889.

85. Joensen, U. N., Frederiksen, H., Blomberg Jensen, M., Lauritsen, M. P., Olesen, I. A., Lassen, T. H., et al. (2012). Phthalate excretion pattern and testicular function: A study of 881 healthy Danish men. *Environmental Health Perspectives, 120*(10), 1397–1403. PubMed PMID: 22832070.

86. Meeker, J. D., Calafat, A. M., & Hauser, R. (2009). Urinary metabolites of di(2-ethylhexyl) phthalate are associated with decreased steroid hormone levels in adult men. *Journal of Andrology, 30*(3), 287–297. PubMed PMID: 19059903.

87. Specht, I. O., Toft, G., Hougaard, K. S., Lindh, C. H., Lenters, V., Jönsson, B. A., et al. (2014). Associations between serum phthalates and biomarkers of reproductive function in 589 adult men. *Environment International, 66*, 146–156. PubMed PMID: 24583187.

88. Swan, S. H., Main, K. M., et al. (2005). Decrease in anogenital distance among male infants with prenatal phthalate exposure. *Environmental Health Perspectives, 113*(8), 1056–1061. PubMed PMID: 16079079.

89. Main, K. M., Mortensen, G. K., et al. (2006). Human breast milk contamination with phthalates and alterations of endogenous reproductive hormones in infants three months of age. *Environmental Health Perspectives, 114*(2), 270–276. PubMed PMID: 16451866.

90. Wolff, M. S., Pajak, A., Pinney, S. M., Windham, G. C., Galvez, M., Rybak, M., et al. (2017). Associations of urinary phthalate and phenol biomarkers with menarche in a multiethnic cohort of young girls. *Reproductive Toxicology, 67*, 56–64. PubMed PMID: 27851993.

91. Colon, I., Caro, D., Bourdony, C. J., & Rosario, O. (2000). Identification of phthalate esters in the serum of young Puerto Rican girls with premature breast development. *Environmental Health Perspectives, 108*, 895–900. PubMed PMID: 11017896.

92. Buser, M. C., Murray, H. E., & Scinicariello, F. (2014). Age and sex differences in childhood and adulthood obesity association with phthalates: Analyses of NHANES 2007-2010. *International Journal of Hygiene and Environmental Health, 217*(6), 687–694. PubMed PMID: 24657244.

93. Hatch, E. E., Nelson, J. W., Qureshi, M. M., Weinberg, J., Moore, L. L., Singer, M., et al. (2008). Association of urinary phthalate metabolite concentrations with body mass index and waist circumference: A cross-sectional study of NHANES data, 1999-2002. *Environmental Health: A Global Access Science Source, 7*, 27. PubMed PMID: 18522739.

94. Lind, P. M., Roos, V., Rönn, M., Johansson, L., Ahlström, H., Kullberg, J., et al. (2012). Serum concentrations of phthalate metabolites are related to abdominal fat distribution two years later in elderly women. *Environmental Health: A Global Access Science Source, 11*, 21. PubMed PMID: 22472124.

95. James-Todd, T. M., Huang, T., Seely, E. W., & Saxena, A. R. (2016). The association between phthalates and metabolic syndrome: The National Health and Nutrition Examination Survey 2001-2010. *Environmental Health: A Global Access Science Source, 15*, 52. PubMed PMID: 27079661.

96. Stojanoska, M. M., Milosevic, N., Milic, N., & Abenavoli, L. (2016). The influence of phthalates and bisphenol A on the obesity development and glucose metabolism disorders. *Endocrine* [Epub ahead of print]. PubMed PMID: 27822670.

97. Doherty, B. T., Engel, S. M., Buckley, J. P., Silva, M. J., Calafat, A. M., & Wolff, M. S. (2016). Prenatal phthalate biomarker concentrations and performance on the Bayley Scales of Infant Development-II in a population of young urban children. *Environmental Research, 152*, 51–58. PubMed PMID: 27741448.

98. Factor-Litvak, P., Insel, B., Calafat, A. M., Liu, X., Perera, F., Rauh, V. A., et al. (2014). Persistent associations between maternal prenatal exposure to phthalates on child IQ at age 7 years. *PLoS ONE, 9*(12), e114003. PubMed PMID: 25493564.

99. Miodovnik, A., Engel, S. M., Zhu, C., Ye, X., Soorya, L. V., Silva, M. J., et al. (2011). Endocrine disruptors and childhood social impairment. *Neurotoxicology, 32*(2), 261–267. PubMed PMID: 21182865.

100. Kim, K. N., Choi, Y. H., Lim, Y. H., & Hong, Y. C. (2016). Urinary phthalate metabolites and depression in an elderly population: National Health and Nutrition Examination Survey 2005-2012. *Environmental Research, 145*, 61–67. PubMed PMID: 26624239.

101. Exley, C. (2014). What is the risk of aluminum as a neurotoxin? *Expert Review of Neurotherapeutics, 14*(6), 589–591. PubMed PMID: 24779346.

102. Shaw, C. A., & Tomljenovic, L. (2013). Aluminum in the central nervous system (CNS): Toxicity in humans and animals, vaccine adjuvants, and autoimmunity. *Immunologic Research, 56*(2–3), 304–316. PubMed PMID: 23609067.

103. Farina, M., Rocha, J. B., & Aschner, M. (2011). Mechanisms of methylmercury-induced neurotoxicity: Evidence from experimental studies. *Life Sciences, 89*(15–16), 555–563. PubMed PMID: 21683713.

104. Kang, K. S., Che, J. H., Ryu, D. Y., et al. (2002). Decreased sperm number and motile activity on the F1 offspring maternally exposed to butyl p-hydroxybenzoic acid (butyl paraben). *The Journal of Veterinary Medical Science / The Japanese Society of Veterinary Science, 64*(3), 227–235. PubMed PMID: 11999442.

105. Oishi, S. (2002). Effects of propyl paraben on the male reproductive system. *Food and Chemical Toxicology: An International Journal Published for the British Industrial Biological Research Association, 40*(12), 1807–1813. PubMed PMID: 12419695.

106. Dodge, L. E., Williams, P. L., Williams, M. A., Missmer, S. A., Toth, T. L., Calafat, A. M., et al. (2015). Paternal urinary concentrations of parabens and other phenols in relation to reproductive outcomes among couples from a fertility clinic. *Environmental Health Perspectives, 123*(7), 665–671. PubMed PMID: 25767892.

107. Pant, N., Shukla, M., et al. (2008). Correlation of phthalate exposures with semen quality. *Toxicology and Applied Pharmacology, 231*(1), 112–116. PubMed PMID: 18513777.

108. Duty, S. M., Singh, N. P., et al. (2003). The relationship between environmental exposures to phthalates and DNA damage in human sperm using the neutral comet assay. *Environmental Health Perspectives, 111*(9), 1164–1169. PubMed PMID: 12842768.

109. Hauser, R., Meeker, J. D., et al. (2007). DNA damage in human sperm is related to urinary levels of phthalate monoester and oxidative metabolites. *Human Reproduction, 22*(3), 688–695. PubMed PMID: 17090632.

110. Jonsson, B. A., Richthoff, J., et al. (2005). Urinary phthalate metabolites and biomarkers of reproductive function in young men. *Epidemiology, 16*(4), 487–493. PubMed PMID: 15951666.

111. Buck Louis, G. M., Sundaram, R., Sweeney, A. M., Schisterman, E. F., Maisog, J., & Kannan, K. (2014). Urinary bisphenol A, phthalates, and couple fecundity: The Longitudinal Investigation of Fertility and the Environment (LIFE) Study. *Fertility and Sterility, 101*(5), 1359–1366. PubMed PMID: 24534276.

112. Gonzalez-Munoz, P., Conde-Salazar, L., & Vano-Galvan, S. (2014). Allergic contact dermatitis caused by cosmetic products. *Actas Dermo-Sifiliograficas, 105*(9), 822–832. PubMed PMID: 24656778.

113. Kumar, P., Caradonna-Graham, V. M., et al. (1995). Inhalation challenge effects of perfume scent strips in patients with asthma. *Annals of Allergy, Asthma and Immunology, 75*(5), 429–433. PubMed PMID: 7583865.

114. Heydorn, S., Johansen, J. D., et al. (2003). Fragrance allergy in patients with hand eczema – a clinical study.

Contact Dermatitis, 48(6), 317–323. PubMed PMID: 14531870.

115. Sosted, H., Basketter, D. A., et al. (2004). Ranking of hair dye substances according to predicted sensitization potency: Quantitative structure-activity relationships. *Contact Dermatitis, 51*(5–6), 241–254. PubMed PMID: 15606648.

116. Bens, G. (2014). Sunscreens. *Advances in Experimental Medicine and Biology, 810*, 429–463. PubMed PMID: 25207381.

117. Harley, K. G., Kogut, K., et al. (2016). Reducing phthalate, paraben, and phenol exposure from personal care products in adolescent girls: Findings from the HERMOSA Intervention study. *Environmental Health Perspectives, 124*(10), 1600–1607. PubMed PMID: 26947464.

8

Drugs

SUMMARY

- Presence in population: Approximately 59% of adults report current use of at least one prescription medication and 15% use five or more
- Major diseases: Hepatotoxicity, cardiotoxicity, renal disease

- Best measure: Liver enzymes, kidney function, 8-OHdG
- Best intervention: Avoidance

DESCRIPTION

An adverse drug reaction (ADR) has been defined as "an appreciably harmful or unpleasant reaction, resulting from an intervention related to the use of a medicinal product, which predicts hazard from future administration and warrants prevention or specific treatment, or alteration of the dosage regimen, or withdrawal of the product."[1] In principle, the risk-benefit ratio for an agent must be interpreted in the context of the nature and severity of the disease. For example, acetylsalicylic acid and warfarin prevent cardiovascular events when used appropriately.[2,3] Too often, however, pharmaceuticals are used, either prescribed by a physician or purchased over the counter without fully evaluating this ratio. In previous studies, the prevalence of hospital admissions due to ADRs ranged from 3.0% to 13.8%.[4,5,6] Although the number of fatal ADRs is unknown, a large meta-analysis of hospitalized patients in the United States estimated that ADRs accounted for 4.6% of all fatalities.[7]

Between 1999/2000 and 2011/2012 the percentage of adults reporting use of any prescription medication increased from an estimated 51% to 59%, and polypharmacy (≥ five prescriptions) increased from an estimated 8.2% to 15%.[8] Table 8.1 shows the estimated percentage of U.S. adults reporting use of any prescription medication in 2011 to 2012 overall and by population characteristics. Disconcertingly, 39% of adults over 65

are being prescribed polypharmacy, though there are virtually no studies of interactions in patients taking five or more drugs. This likely helps explain why ADRs account for 4.9% of all hospital admissions, increasing to a worrisome 16.6% for the elderly.[9]

Even those not willingly taking doctor-prescribed or over-the-counter medications may still be exposed. A study conducted by the Environmental Working Group released in 2008 found that at least 40 million Americans drink tap water with detectable levels of prescription medications such as antibiotics, hormones, and drugs used to treat epilepsy and depression.[10] All pharmaceuticals reported in drinking water supplies are unregulated in treated tap water, and any level is legal.

Many readily available medications have long-term side effects that are not adequately appreciated. Virtually all safety studies are short term. Therefore, many toxic effects are not detected during the research and development stages and arise later in population studies. In addition, several major drug safety studies utilized questionable exclusion criteria and other ruses to dramatically understate ADRs.[11]

TOXICITY

Medications have a variety of toxic mechanisms, most of which, as previously described, are dependent on the inherent properties of the drug involved as well as the

TABLE 8.1 Prevalence of Prescription Drug Use in Prior 30 Days Among U.S. Adults (Age ≥ 20 years), 2011 to 2012

	OVERALL	ANY PRESCRIPTIONS			POLYPHARMACY (≥ FIVE PRESCRIPTIONS)		
	n	n	%	95% CI	n	%	95% CI
Overall	5558	3144	59	55–62	917	15	13–17
Age group (years)							
20–39	1957	596	35	32–39	47	3.1	2.1–4.6
40–64	2352	1428	65	62–67	372	15	13–17
≥ 65	1249	1120	90	87–93	498	39	35–44
Sex							
Male	2739	1398	52	48–57	418	13	10–16
Female	2819	1746	65	62–67	499	16	14–19
Race/ethnicity							
Non-Hispanic white	2040	1377	66	63–69	440	17	15–20
Non-Hispanic black	1455	835	52	49–55	266	14	12–17
Non-Hispanic Asian	794	335	41	36–45	54	6.0	4.0–8.7
Mexican American	539	214	33	28–38	56	6.8	4.2–10
Other Hispanic	578	305	41	36–45	77	8.5	6.0–12
Other	152	78	51	38–63	24	17	8.6–32

CI: confidence interval.
Data from Kantor, E. D., Rehm, C. D., Haas, J. S., Chan, A. T., Giovannucci, E. L. (2015). Trends in prescription drug use among adults in the United States from 1999 to 2012. *Journal of the American Medical Association, 314*(17), 1818–1831.

individual's ability to absorb, detoxify, and respond to the medication. Although dependent on several factors, including nutrition, age, gender, drug use, diet, and environment, 20% to 95% of the variability in drug response is also due to genetic factors.[12] For example, higher hepatic Cytochrome P450 2E1 (CYP2E1) expression and activity may aggravate liver injury from xenobiotic compounds through the generation of harmful reactive metabolites at a rate too high for phase II conjugation.[13] Drugs are considered to be foreign substances by the body, to be eliminated similarly to any other exogenous pollutant. Therefore, understanding genetic variations in enzyme activity among patients, along with the effects of drug interactions that change the systemic exposure of medications due to alterations in metabolism and excretion, is essential to safely and effectively using medications while avoiding excessive toxicity.

CLINICAL SIGNIFICANCE

Cardiovascular

Nonsteroidal anti-inflammatory drugs. Nonsteroidal anti-inflammatory drugs (NSAIDs) have been shown to induce reactive oxygen species (ROS) in cardiac and cardiovascular related cells, which may explain the increased risk of heart attack and stroke associated with NSAID use.[14] Rofecoxib, a COX-2 inhibitor, was removed from the market, as its extended use increased the risk of atherothrombotic events. It is now known that the cardiotoxicity of rofecoxib was not related to COX-2 inhibition, but to the oxidative modification of low-density lipoproteins and cellular membrane lipids, which contributed to plaque instability and thrombus formation.[15] NSAIDs also cause renal damage and elevated blood pressure, which may precipitate heart failure in vulnerable individuals.[16]

Chemotherapy. Cardiovascular toxicity is a potential short- or long-term complication of anticancer therapy. Doxorubicin, an oncological agent, induces cardiotoxicity through oxidative DNA damage and apoptosis in cardiac cells.[17] The cumulative probability of doxorubicin-induced heart failure has shown dose-dependent rates of 3% to 5% at 400 mg/m^2; 7% to 26% at 550 mg/m^2; and 18% to 48% at 700 mg/m^2.[18] The use of vascular endothelial growth factor tyrosine-kinase inhibitors (VEGFR-TKIs)

TABLE 8.2   Potential Cardiac Toxicity Induced by Chemotherapeutic Agents

Drug	Toxic Dose Range	Cardiac Toxicity	Incidence (%)
Doxorubicin	>450 mg/m^2	Left ventricular dysfunction (LVD)	3–12
Epirubicin	>720 mg/m^2		0.9–3.3
Idarubicin			
Paclitaxel	Conventional dose	LVD	5–15
Docetaxel			2.3–8
Cyclophosphamide	>100–120 mg/kg	LVD	3–5
Ifosfamide			
Capecitabine	Conventional dose	Cardiac ischemia	3–9
5-FU			1–68
Paclitaxel	Conventional dose	Cardiac ischemia	<1–5
Docetaxel			1.7
Trabectedin	Conventional dose	Cardiac ischemia	1
Arsenic trioxide (ATO)	Conventional dose	QTc prolongation	26–93
Paclitaxel	Conventional dose	QTc prolongation	0.1–31
Bevacizumab	Conventional dose	Hypertension	7–36
Sunitinib	Conventional dose	Hypertension	3–8
Cediranib	Conventional dose	Hypertension	35–42

From Curigliano, G., Mayer, E. L., Burstein, H. J., Winer, E. P., Goldhirsch, A. (2010). Cardiac toxicity from systemic cancer therapy: A comprehensive review. *Progress in Cardiovascular Diseases, 53*(2), 94–104.

significantly increased the risk of all-grade (Odds ratio (OR) = 2.37, 95% confidence interval (CI): 1.76–3.20, p<0.001) and high-grade (OR = 3.51, 95% CI: 1.74–7.05, p<0.001) congestive heart failure.[19] Table 8.2 shows a variety of other chemotherapeutic agents and their associated potential cardiac toxicities.[20]

Interferons. Cardiac adverse effects of the interferons— interferon-alpha, interferon-beta, and interferon-gamma— are cardiac arrhythmias, cardiomyopathy, and symptoms of ischemic heart disease.[21] Interferon-alpha has been associated with hypotension and tachycardia during the first days of treatment in 5% to 15% of treated patients.[22]

Antidepressants. Tricyclic antidepressants (TCAs) are highly concentrated in myocardial tissue, which may explain their interference with heart rate, cardiac rhythm, and myocardial contractility. TCAs (e.g., amitriptyline, imipramine, nortriptyline, doxepin) have shown anticholinergic and quinidine-like action, interference with the reuptake of adrenergic amines, alterations of membrane permeability, and direct myocardial depression.[23] TCAs can cause hypotension or orthostatic hypotension,[24] tachycardia,[25] and prolongation of the QRS complex on ECG.[26]

Citalopram and escitalopram, both selective serotonin reuptake inhibitors (SSRIs), are known to cause dose-dependent QT prolongation.[27] Lithium may be associated with complete heart block, impaired atrioventricular conduction, and interstitial myocarditis in high concentrations.[28]

Endocrine

Antipsychotics. Concerns have been raised regarding an association between second-generation antipsychotics and increased rates of diabetes, ketoacidosis, hyperglycemia, and lipid dysregulation. Clozapine and olanzapine have been associated with the greatest risk of metabolic disturbance, including clinical weight gain, increased risk of diabetes, and dyslipidemia.[29] A meta-analysis examined the association of diabetes incidence among patients treated with atypical antipsychotics compared with conventional or no antipsychotic treatment.[30] Analyses indicated that clozapine was consistently associated with an increased risk of diabetes (versus conventionals: OR = 1.37; 95% CI: 1.25–1.52; versus no antipsychotic: OR = 7.44; 95% CI: 1.59–34.75), and olanzapine was also associated with an increased risk of diabetes (versus conventionals: OR = 1.26; 95% CI: 1.10–1.46; versus no antipsychotic: OR = 2.31; 95% CI: 0.98–5.46).

Antihypertensives. In patients with hypertension, the use of conventional antihypertensive compounds (e.g., diuretics and beta-blockers), especially when combined, decreases insulin sensitivity and may amplify the development of new-onset diabetes.[31] The diabetes incidence in the course of treatment with thiazide diuretics is estimated to be 2.4%, and for beta-blockers is 1.7% to 3.0%.[32] However, calcium channel blockers (OR = 0.81, 95% CI: 0.73–0.90)[33] as well as angiotensin-converting enzyme (ACE) inhibitors (OR = 0.78, 95% CI: 0.73–0.83) and angiotensin receptor blockers (OR = 0.76, 95% CI: 0.70–0.82)[34] may decrease the odds of developing new-onset type 2 diabetes, but does not reduce the odds of mortality, cardiovascular, or cerebrovascular outcomes.

Glucocorticoids. Glucocorticoids (e.g., prednisolone, hydrocortisone, budesonide, dexamethasone) are believed to increase insulin resistance, decrease glucose tolerance, reduce β-cell mass, increase hepatic insulin resistance, and enhance protein breakdown, adipose tissue lipolysis, and hepatic gluconeogenesis, elevating circulating glucose concentrations.[35] For example, in healthy individuals, prednisolone administration for 7 days led to a 50% reduction in insulin sensitivity.[36] The odds ratio for presenting with new-onset diabetes after taking glucocorticoids in various studies has been reported to range from 1.36 to 2.31.[37,38]

Acute Pancreatitis. Although rare, more than 500 drugs have been implicated in causing acute pancreatitis. Medications with the best evidence linking usage to acute pancreatitis include mesalamine, Dipentum, Azodisalicylate, azathioprine, bezafibrate, cannabis, carbimazole, codeine, enalapril, isoniazid, metronidazole, pravastatin, Premarin, procainamide, pyritinol, simvastatin, stibogluconate, sulfamethoxazole, sulindac, tetracycline, and valproic acid.[39] Epidemiological evidence suggests the risk of pancreatitis is highest for mesalamine (HR = 3.5), azathioprine (HR = 2.5), and simvastatin (HR = 1.8).[40]

Gastrointestinal

Aspirin. Low-dose aspirin therapy is often recommended as the basis of antiplatelet therapy for almost all patients who have had a primary cardiovascular disease event.[41] However, long-term low-dose (≤325 mg) aspirin therapy has been shown to increase the risk of major gastrointestinal (GI) bleeding[42] as well as a number of other adverse GI events, including heartburn/acid reflux, excess stomach acid, gastritis, abdominal pain, epigastric burning, stomach ulcer, and duodenal ulcer.[43] A review of randomized controlled trials on the GI toxicity of aspirin revealed that the pooled odds ratio for categories of GI bleeding is between 1.5 and 2.0.[44]

Olmesartan. Olmesartan, an angiotensin II receptor blocker, has been associated with the development of sprue-like enteropathy characterized by severe diarrhea and histopathological changes in the intestine.[45,46] A study from the Mayo Clinic first reported the association between olmesartan and enteropathy.[47] Twenty-two patients presented with severe diarrhea, weight loss, and biopsies consistent with celiac sprue. However, serological testing for celiac disease was negative, and no patient responded to a gluten-free diet. After cessation of the medication, clinical symptoms resolved quickly and the histological changes disappeared.

Hematological

Drug-induced immune hemolytic anemia (DIIHA) is a rare but important condition in patients with unexplained hemolysis. DIIHA occurs primarily as a result of drug-induced antibodies, and about 130 drugs have been implicated in the development of DIIHA: 42% of these drugs are antimicrobials,16% are nonsteroidal antiinflammatory agents, 13% are antineoplastics, and 6% are antihypertensive/diuretics.[48] The most common drugs associated with DIIHA are cefotetan (53%), ceftriaxone (16%), and piperacillin (9%).[49] Case reports of DIIHA present associations with several common medications, including trimethoprim/sulfamethoxazole (TMP/SMX),[50] metformin,[51] ibuprofen,[52] omeprazole,[53] and levofloxacin.[54]

Hepatic

Drug-induced liver injury (DILI) is the most common cause of acute liver failure in the United States, accounting for nearly 50% of cases and 10% of acute hepatitis cases.[55,56] Several events are believed to be involved in the development of DILI, including reactive metabolite formation, oxidative stress, signaling pathway induction, and innate and adaptive immune responses.[57] DILI can be divided into two classes of medication-related hepatotoxicity: intrinsic and idiosyncratic.[58] Intrinsic is often dose-dependent, with predictable liver injury at hepatotoxic doses. Idiosyncratic DILI is traditionally believed to be unrelated to dose and may affect individuals with underlying susceptibility or predisposition. Both genetic and environmental factors likely play a role in determining the occurrence of idiosyncratic DILI. For example, individuals with the HLA-I and HLA-II genotypes have an increased susceptibility to DILI when taking amoxicillin-clavulanate.[59] It has been reported that compounds with more than 50% hepatic metabolism given at doses higher than 50 mg/day presented the highest risk of hepatotoxicity.[60]

Although acetaminophen overdoses dominate, a significant portion of DILI is related to prescription and over-the-counter drugs and complementary and alternative medications. Offending agents include antimicrobials (e.g., antibacterial agents, antiviral agents, antituberculosis agents), central nervous system agents (e.g., antiepileptic agents, antidepressants, antipsychotics), immunomodulatory agents, analgesics (especially those containing acetaminophen), antineoplastic agents, antihypertensive agents, and lipid-lowering agents.[61] Table 8.3 lists some of the drugs that have been implicated in the development of acute liver failure.[62]

Acetaminophen. Acetaminophen alone is responsible for 50% to 60% of cases of acute liver failure in the United States.[63] Acetaminophen dose-dependently decreases hepatic glutathione (GSH) levels, which would otherwise prevent hepatic necrosis.[64] Reduction of hepatic GSH through acute or chronic use of acetaminophen will deplete not only the antioxidant activity of GSH, but also the functioning of GSH conjugation, resulting in diminished toxicant excretion.

Musculoskeletal

Several medications have demonstrated adverse effects on bone tissue, and many are linked to the development of osteoporosis.

Glucocorticoids and Goserelin. Glucocorticoids inhibit bone formation by impairing the replication, differentiation, and function of osteoblasts and induce apoptosis of mature osteoblasts and osteocytes,[65] resulting in a 17-fold increase in vertebral fracture incidence with glucocorticoid therapy.[66] In patients treated with goserelin, a gonadotropin-releasing hormone (GNRH) analog, bone mineral density at the lumbar spine decreased by 10.5%.[67]

Heparin. Heparin decreases bone formation, inhibits the differentiation and function of osteoblasts, increases bone resorption,[68] and is associated with a 2.2% to 5% incidence of fracture.[69]

Proton Pump Inhibitors. Proton pump inhibitors (PPIs) interfere with calcium absorption through the induction of hypochlorhydria and decrease intestinal absorption of calcium. In postmenopausal women, omeprazole use was a significant and independent predictor of vertebral fractures (Risk Ratio (RR) = 3.50, 95% CI 1.14–8.44).[70] Patients prescribed long-term high-dose PPI therapy showed a significantly increased risk of hip fracture (Adjusted Odds Ratio (AOR), 2.65; 95% CI, 1.80–3.90; $P = .001$).[71]

TABLE 8.3   Drugs Implicated in Causing Acute Liver Failure

Antimicrobials	Anticonvulsants	Complementary and Alternative Medicines	Other
Isoniazid	Phenytoin	LipoKinetix (usnic acid)	Diclofenac
Trimethoprim/sulfamethoxazole	Valproic acid	Herbalife (unspecified)	Etodolac
Nitrofurantoin	Carbamazepine	Mahuang and other Chinese herbs	Disulfiram
Terbinafine		Hydroxycut (unspecified)	Propylthiouracil
Itraconazole			Methyldopa
Ketoconazole			Gemtuzumab
Amoxicillin			Acetaminophen
Ciprofloxacin			
Azithromycin			
Telithromycin			

Data from Reuben, A., Koch, D. G., Lee, W. M.; Acute Liver Failure Study Group. (2010). Drug-induced acute liver failure: results of a U.S. multicenter, prospective study. *Hepatology, 52*(6), 2065–2076.

Selective Serotonin Reuptake Inhibitors. Serotonin inhibits the proliferation of osteoblasts, decreasing bone formation.[72] A dose-dependent relationship exists between daily SSRI use and lower bone mineral density at the hip and the spine.[73]

Thiazolidinediones. Thiazolidinediones interfere with insulin-like growth factor 1 (IGF-1) and may decrease bone formation, as IGF-1 enhances the differentiated function of osteoblasts and bone formation.[74]

Thyroid. Thyroid hormones induce the production of bone-resorbing cytokines,[75] and the suppression of thyroid stimulating hormone (TSH) itself may cause bone loss.[76]

Aromatase Inhibitors. Aromatase inhibitors, such as exemestane, letrozole, and anastrozole, are associated with joint and muscular symptoms, commonly referred to as aromatase inhibitor–associated musculoskeletal syndrome (AIMSS).[77] AIMSS typically presents as symmetrical pain or soreness in the hands, knees, hips, lower back, shoulders, and/or feet and may include additional extra-articular symptoms such as myalgia, fibromyalgia, neuropathy, and carpal tunnel syndrome.[78] The reported incidence of arthralgia and/or bone pain in breast cancer patients receiving aromatase inhibitors varies from 4% to 35.6%.[79] Bone loss and fracture risk are also associated with long-term aromatase inhibitor therapy, as the depletion of estrogen increases the rate of bone turnover and decreases bone mineral density.[80]

Statins. Approximately 25% of the United States population older than 40 years have reported taking a cholesterol-lowering medication, with the majority (90%) involving a statin, for prevention of cardiovascular diseases.[81] Statins may produce myotoxicity (statin-induced myotoxicity, or SIM) that manifests as muscle weakness, myalgia, stiffness, muscle tenderness, cramps, and/or arthralgia.[82] In a cross-sectional analysis using data from the National Health and Nutrition Examination Survey (NHANES) 1999 to 2002, individuals who used statins had 50% greater odds of having any musculoskeletal pain and 50% to 60% greater odds of having musculoskeletal pain in the lower back and lower extremities compared with adults who did not use statins.[83] Although the exact mechanism of SIM is unknown, theories include impaired cholesterol synthesis leading to abnormal cell membrane stability, impaired ubiquinone (CoQ_{10}) synthesis leading to decreased mitochondrial enzyme activity, or prenylated protein synthesis abnormalities causing altered intracellular messaging.[84] Underlying genetic or metabolic muscle abnormalities may predispose individuals to statin intolerance.[85,86]

Neurological

Oxcarbazepine. Animal studies have demonstrated neurotoxic and genotoxic side effects from the use of oxcarbazepine, an antiepileptic drug, resulting from toxic metabolites, free radicals, and ROS.[87,88] In rodent models of chemotherapy-induced peripheral neuropathy, evidence suggests the involvement of innate immune cells, glial cells, and cytokine and chemokine signaling in the development of neuropathic symptoms (e.g., numbness, pain, paresthesia, loss of vibration sensation, and reduced proprioception).[89]

Beta-Lactam Antibiotics. Beta-lactam antibiotics, such as penicillin and amoxicillin, have also demonstrated central nervous system toxicity, including epileptogenic properties.[90,91] The epileptic effect of beta-lactams is believed to result from an inhibitory effect on gamma-aminobutyric acid transmission of cortical pyramidal cells.[92]

Renal

The kidney is exposed to a larger proportion and higher concentration of xenobiotics than other organs through the secretion and reabsorption of toxicants in the renal tubules.[93] Medications are a common cause of acute kidney injury (AKI), commonly resulting in acute tubular necrosis (ATN) or acute interstitial nephritis (AIN). Among hospitalized patients, drug-induced kidney injury is a serious problem, accounting for 19% to 26% of AKI cases.[94] The renal proximal tubule is commonly damaged by drugs such as cisplatin,[95] aminoglycosides (e.g., gentamycin, kanamycin, streptomycin, tobramycin),[96] amphotericin B,[97] antiviral agents (e.g., adefovir, cidofovir, tenofovir),[98] radiocontrast dye,[99] and bisphosphonate.[100] Antibiotics (e.g., penicillins, cephalosporins, quinolones, rifampicin),[101,102] PPIs,[103] NSAIDs,[104] and immunotherapy agents (e.g., ipilimumab, nivolumab)[105] have all been shown to be involved in the development of AIN. A study of 133 patients with biopsy-proven AIN showed that the top three drug causes were omeprazole (12%), amoxicillin (8%), and ciprofloxacin (8%).[106] In a large nested cohort study, the unadjusted odds ratio for AIN was 5.16 (95% CI: 2.21–12.05; p<0.001) for current versus past PPI use.[107]

NSAIDs. Acetaminophen, aspirin, ibuprofen, naproxen, indomethacin, and cyclooxygenase (COX)-2 inhibitors have all been shown to cause kidney damage when used chronically.[108,109,110] Consumption for > 3 years of single and/or combinations of NSAIDs led to irreversible analgesic nephropathy, particularly chronic interstitial nephritis and renal papillary necrosis.[111]

Reproductive

In a large study that utilized NHANES data, high levels of mono-butyl phthalate (MBP), the main dibutyl phthalate (DBP) metabolite, were found in persons taking mesalamine, didanosine, omeprazole, and theophylline.[112] Animal studies exploring prenatal exposure to DBP demonstrate decreased fetal testosterone biosynthesis by Leydig cells and increased incidence of cryptorchidism and hypospadias in male offspring.[113,114]

Respiratory

NSAIDs. Aspirin-exacerbated respiratory disease (AERD) is an asthma phenotype with a prevalence of 2% to 25% of the asthma population.[115] Aspirin and other NSAIDs inhibit cyclooxygenase and promote lipoxygenase.[116] The net result is a shunting of arachidonic acid toward the lipoxygenase pathway and the production of excessive levels of leukotrienes.[117] Bronchoscopy performed 15 minutes after exposure to aspirin revealed elevations of leukotrienes (LTC_4, LTD_4, and LTE_4) in AERD patients.[118] Precipitation of asthma attacks by ingestion of aspirin and other NSAIDs is considered a hallmark of this syndrome. AERD is chronic, and the respiratory mucosal inflammatory disease persists even with avoidance of COX-1 inhibitors.[119,120]

Beta-Blockers. In almost all asthmatics, nonselective beta-blockers cause bronchoconstriction and increase bronchial hyperresponsiveness to methacholine and histamine.[121,122] Regular use of noncardioselective beta-blockers was demonstrated to cause a 13.5% decrease in FEV_1.[123]

Other Drugs. Several other medications have been shown to cause bronchospasm or mimic asthma, including ACE inhibitors, cholinergic agonists, cholinomimetic alkaloids, chemotherapeutic agents, diuretics, corticosteroids, antibiotics, and radiocontrast dyes.[124]

DETOXIFICATION/EXCRETION PROCESSES

Pharmacokinetics involves the study of the time and course of drug absorption, distribution, metabolism, and excretion. The liver is the principal site of drug metabolism and uses oxidation, reduction, hydrolysis, hydration, conjugation, condensation, and/or isomerization to process and detoxify medications. Phase I reactions involve formation of a new or modified functional group or cleavage (oxidation, reduction, hydrolysis), and phase II reactions involve conjugation with an endogenous substance (glucuronic acid, sulfate, glycine, GSH, amino acids, etc.). Approximately 65% of drugs used as medications are metabolized by CYP enzymes.[125] The cytochrome enzyme CYP2D6 metabolizes 20% to 25% of all drugs, at least partially, and has a wide range of functions, extending from poor to ultrarapid metabolic activity. However, 1% of Asians and 10% of Caucasians have two null alleles, resulting in completely absent CYP2D6 activity.[126]

CYP3A enzymes influence circulating steroid levels and responses to half of all oxidatively metabolized drugs. CYP3A members mediate the metabolism of immunosuppressants (e.g., cyclosporine A, tacrolimus), calcium blockers (e.g., nifedipine), chemotherapeutics (e.g., doxorubicin, vincristine, tamoxifen, sunitinib), azole antifungals, macrolides (e.g., erythromycin), tricyclic antidepressants (e.g., amitriptyline, imipramine), SSRIs (e.g., citalopram, sertraline), antipsychotics (e.g., haloperidol, risperidone), opioids, benzodiazepines (e.g., alprazolam, diazepam, triazolam), statins, warfarin, omeprazole, and several other clinically important drugs.[127] Approximately 60% of African Americans and 33% of Caucasians do not possess CYP3A5 activity, which may explain the interindividual and interracial differences in CYP3A-dependent drug clearance and medication responses.[128] Polymorphic phase I enzymes are responsible for approximately 56% of ADRs.[129]

In addition to genetic variability, numerous inducers and inhibitors influence the metabolism of medications. Grapefruit juice, azole antifungals, HIV antivirals, and *Zingiber* (ginger) compounds all significantly inhibit CYP3A4,[130] and St. John's wort is a well-known inducer of CYP3A4.[131] CYP induction and inhibition by flavonoids appears to be concentrated in the small intestine, rather than the liver.[132,133] Because of this, flavonoids mainly affect drug absorption rather drug half-life. CYP2E1 is a very inducible enzyme, particularly by alcohol, with induction resulting in the bioactivation of many toxins and drugs, as well as increased ROS production. This is perhaps most recognized in studies examining acetaminophen (APAP) toxicity. Induction combined with exposure to APAP results in the production of the more toxic metabolite N-acetyl-p-benzoquinone imine, which causes an increase in ROS and nitrosamines, mitochondrial poisoning, lipid peroxidation, and covalent binding to proteins, with eventual necrosis.[134]

The primary route of excretion for most drugs is through the kidney. However, excretion can also occur through the liver (bile), gut (fecal matter), lungs (exhaled air), and skin (sweat). For example, medications including amphetamines (and metabolites),[135] methadone and its metabolites,[136] and antiepileptic drugs have been documented to be excreted in sweat.[137] In fact, the antiepileptic drugs phenytoin, phenobarbital, and carbamazepine were measured in one study after it was noted that a number of hospitalized patients had lower serum levels of phenytoin during a particularly hot summer.[138]

INTERVENTION

Recognition of a drug-induced etiology and withdrawal of the offending agent provide the best hope for recovery. In some cases, the use of nutraceuticals to increase GSH levels, such as N-acetylcysteine (NAC),[139] whey protein powder,[140] alpha-lipoic-acid,[141] S-adenosyl L-methionine (SAMe),[142] and/or direct administration of GSH through an intravenous route,[143] anebulizer, or the intranasal route,[144] may be of benefit. NAC is considered to be a potent antidote to acute acetaminophen toxicity.[145] In addition, the use of *Silybum marianum* (milk thistle) may provide benefit in the prevention of drug-induced toxicity.[146,147]

REFERENCES

1. Edwards, I. R., & Aronson, J. K. (2000). Adverse drug reactions: definitions, diagnosis, and management. *Lancet, 356*(9237), 1255–1259. PubMed PMID: 11072960.
2. Antithrombotic Trialists' Collaboration. (2002). Collaborative meta-analysis of randomized trials of antiplatelet therapy for prevention of death, myocardial infarction, and stroke in high risk patients. *BMJ (Clinical Research Ed.), 324*(7329), 71–86. PubMed PMID: 11786451.
3. Hart, R. G., Benavente, O., et al. (1999). Antithrombotic therapy to prevent stroke in patients with atrial fibrillation: a meta-analysis. *Annals of Internal Medicine, 131*(7), 492–501. PubMed PMID: 10507957.
4. Moore, N., Lecointre, D., Noblet, C., & Mabille, M. (1998). Frequency and cost of serious drug reactions in a department of general medicine. *British Journal of Clinical Pharmacology, 45*(3), 301–308. PubMed PMID: 9517375.
5. Pirmohamed, M., James, S., et al. (2004). Adverse drug reactions as cause of admission to hospital: prospective analysis of 18,820 patients. *BMJ (Clinical Research Ed.), 329*(7456), 15–19. PubMed PMID: 15231615.
6. Mjorndal, T., Boman, M. D., Hagg, S., et al. (2002). Adverse drug reactions as a cause for admissions to a department of internal medicine. *Pharmacoepidemiology and Drug Safety, 11*(1), 65–72. PubMed PMID: 11998554.
7. Lazarou, J., Pomeranz, B. H., & Corey, P. N. (1998). Incidence of adverse drug reactions in hospitalized patients: a meta-analysis of prospective studies. *The Journal of the American Medical Association, 279*(15), 1200–1205. PubMed PMID: 9555760.
8. Kantor, E. D., Rehm, C. D., et al. (2015). Trends in prescription drug use among adults in the United States from 1999-2012. *The Journal of the American Medical Association, 314*(17), 1818–1831. PubMed PMID: 26529160.
9. Beijer, H. J., & de Blaey, C. J. (2002). Hospitalizations caused by adverse drug reactions (ADR): a meta-analysis of observational studies. *Pharmacy World and Science, 24*(2), 46–54. PMID 12061133.
10. Environmental Working Group. *EWG calls on EPA to protect the health of Americans and set standards for pollutants in tap water.* http://www.ewg.org/news/testimony-official-correspondence/ewg-calls-epa-protect-health-americans-and-set-standards. (Accessed June 12, 2017.)
11. Pizzorno, J. (2014). The vilification of cholesterol (for profit?). *Integrative Medicine, 13*(3), 8–14. PMID 6770094.
12. Belle, D. J., & Singh, H. (2008). Genetic factors in drug metabolism. *American Family Physician, 77*(11), 1553–1560. PubMed PMID: 18581835.
13. Aubert, J., Begriche, K., et al. (2011). Increased expression of cytochrome P450 2E1 in nonalcoholic fatty liver disease: mechanisms and pathophysiological

role. *Clinics and Research in Hepatology and Gastroenterology, 35*(10), 630–637. PubMed PMID: 21664213.

14. Ghosh, R., Alajbegovic, A., & Gomes, A. V. (2015). NSAIDs and cardiovascular diseases: role of reactive oxygen species. *Oxidative Medicine and Cellular Longevity, 536962*. PubMed PMID: 26457127.

15. Mason, R. P., Walter, M. F., McNulty, H. P., et al. (2006). Rofecoxib increases susceptibility of human LDL and membrane lipids to oxidative damage: a mechanism of cardiotoxicity. *Journal of Cardiovascular Pharmacology, 47*(Suppl. 1), S7–S14. PubMed PMID: 16785833.

16. Slordal, L., & Spigset, O. (2006). Heart failure induced by non-cardiac drugs. *Drug Safety, 29*(7), 567–586. PubMed PMID: 16808550.

17. Yoshida, M., Shiojima, I., et al. (2009). Chronic doxorubicin cardiotoxicity is mediated by oxidative DNA damage-ATM-p53-apoptosis pathway and attenuated by pitavastatin through the inhibition of Rac1 activity. *Journal of Molecular and Cellular Cardiology, 47*(5), 698–705. PubMed PMID: 19660469.

18. Von Hoff, D. D., Layard, M. W., et al. (1979). Risk factors for doxorubicin-induced congestive heart failure. *Annals of Internal Medicine, 91*(5), 710–717. PubMed PMID: 496103.

19. Qi, W. X., Shen, Z., Tang, L. N., & Yao, Y. (2014). Congestive heart failure risk in cancer patients treated with vascular endothelial growth factor tyrosine kinase inhibitors: a systematic review and meta-analysis of 36 clinical trials. *British Journal of Clinical Pharmacology, 78*(4), 748–762. PubMed PMID: 24661224.

20. Curigliano, G., Mayer, E. L., et al. (2010). Cardiac toxicity from systemic cancer therapy: a comprehensive review. *Progress in Cardiovascular Diseases, 53*(2), 94–104. PubMed PMID: 20728696.

21. Sonnenblick, M., & Rosin, A. (1991). Cardiotoxicity of interferon. A review of 44 cases. *Chest, 99*(3), 557–561. PubMed PMID: 1704826.

22. Vial, T., & Descotes, J. (1994). Clinical toxicity of the interferons. *Drug Safety, 10*(2), 115–150. PubMed PMID: 7516663.

23. Waring, W. S. (2012). Clinical use of antidepressant therapy and associated cardiovascular risk. *Drug, Healthcare and Patient Safety, 4*, 93–101. PubMed PMID: 22936860.

24. Lee, M. Y., Kim, S. J., et al. (2010). Imipramine-induced cardiac depression is responsible for the increase 1/2 in intracellular magnesium and the activation of ERK in rats. *Journal of Cardiovascular Pharmacology and Therapeutics, 15*(3), 303–310. PubMed PMID: 20484120.

25. Thanacoody, H. K., & Thomas, S. H. (2005). Tricyclic antidepressant poisoning: cardiovascular toxicity. *Toxicological Reviews, 24*(3), 205–214. PubMed PMID: 16390222.

26. Roos, J. C. (1983). Cardiac effects of antidepressant drugs. A comparison of the tricyclic antidepressants and fluvoxamine. *British Journal of Clinical Pharmacology, 15*(Suppl. 3), 439S–445S. PubMed PMID: 6407505.

27. Medicines and Healthcare Products Regulatory Authority. *Citalopram and escitalopram: QT interval prolongation: new maximum daily dose restrictions (including in elderly patients), contraindications, and warnings.* http://www.mhra.gov.uk/Safetyinformation/DrugSafetyUpdate/CON137769. (Accessed June 16, 2017.)

28. Talati, S. N., Aslam, A. F., & Vasavada, B. (2009). Sinus node dysfunction in association with chronic lithium therapy: a case report and review of literature. *American Journal of Therapeutics, 16*(3), 274–278. PubMed PMID: 19352146.

29. Newcomer, J. W. (2007). Metabolic considerations in the use of antipsychotic medications: a review of recent evidence. *The Journal of Clinical Psychiatry, 68*(Suppl. 1), 20–27. PubMed PMID: 17286524.

30. Newcomer, J. W. (2007). Metabolic syndrome and mental illness. *The American Journal of Managed Care, 13*(Suppl. 7), S170–S177. PubMed PMID: 18041878.

31. Mancia, G., Grassi, G., & Zanchetti, A. (2006). New-onset diabetes and antihypertensive drugs. *Journal of Hypertension, 24*(1), 3–10. PubMed PMID: 16331092.

32. Grimm, C., Koberlein, J., et al. (2010). New-onset diabetes and antihypertensive treatment. *GMS Health Technology Assessment, 6*, Doc03. PubMed PMID: 21289876.

33. Kuti, E. L., Baker, W. L., & White, C. M. (2007). The development of new-onset type 2 diabetes associated with choosing a calcium channel blocker compared to a diuretic or beta-blocker. *Current Medical Research and Opinion, 23*(6), 1239–1244. PubMed PMID: 17559720.

34. Gillespie, E. L., White, C. M., et al. (2005). The impact of ACE inhibitors on angiotensin II type 1 receptor blockers on the development of new-onset type 3 diabetes. *Diabetes Care, 28*(9), 2261–2266. PubMed PMID: 16123505.

35. Geer, E. B., Islam, J., & Buettner, C. (2014). Mechanisms of glucocorticoid-induced insulin resistance: focus on adipose tissue function and lipid metabolism. *Endocrinology and Metabolism Clinics*

of North America, 43(1), 75–102. PubMed PMID: 24582093.

36. Pagano, G., Cavallo-Perin, P., et al. (1983). An in vivo and in vitro study of the mechanism of prednisone-induced insulin resistance in healthy subjects. *The Journal of Clinical Investigation*, 72(5), 1814–1820. PubMed PMID: 6355186.

37. Gulliford, M. C., Charlton, J., & Latinovic, R. (2006). Risk of diabetes associated with prescribed glucocorticoids in a large population. *Diabetes Care*, 29(12), 2728–2729. PubMed PMID: 17130214.

38. Kwon, S., & Hermayer, K. L. (2013). Glucocorticoid-induced hyperglycemia. *The American Journal of the Medical Sciences*, 345(4), 274–277. PubMed PMID: 23531958.

39. Badalov, N., Baradarian, R., et al. (2007). Drug-induced acute pancreatitis: an evidence-based review. *Clinical Gastroenterology and Hepatology*, 5(6), 648–661. PubMed PMID: 17395548.

40. Nitsche, C. J., Jamieson, N., et al. (2010). Drug induced pancreatitis. *Best Practice & Research. Clinical Gastroenterology*, 24(2), 143–155. PubMed PMID: 20227028.

41. Smith, S. C., Jr., Benjamin, E. J., et al. (2011). AHA/ACCF secondary prevention and risk reduction therapy for patients with coronary and other atherosclerotic vascular disease: 2011 update: a guideline from the American Heart Association and American College of Cardiology Foundation. *Circulation*, 124(22), 2458–2473. PubMed PMID: 22052934.

42. De Berardis, G., Lucisano, G., et al. (2012). Association of aspirin use with major bleeding in patients with and without diabetes. *The Journal of the American Medical Association*, 307(21), 2286–2294. PubMed PMID: 22706834.

43. Tournoij, E., Peters, R. J., et al. (2009). The prevalence of intolerance for low-dose acetylsalicylacid in the secondary prevention of atherothrombosis. *European Journal of Vascular and Endovascular Surgery*, 37(5), 597–603. PubMed PMID: 19297216.

44. Roderick, P. J., Wilkes, H. C., & Meade, T. W. (1993). The gastrointestinal toxicity of aspirin: an overview of randomized controlled trials. *British Journal of Clinical Pharmacology*, 35(3), 219–226. PubMed PMID: 8471398.

45. Campos Ruiz, A., Urtasun Arlegui, L., et al. (2016). Sprue-like enteropathy linked to olmesartan. *Revista Espanola de Enfermedades Digestivas*, 108(5), 292–293. PubMed PMID: 26925975.

46. Ianiro, G., Bibbo, S., et al. (2014). Systematic review: sprue-like enteropathy associated with olmesartan.

Alimentary Pharmacology and Therapeutics, 40(1), 16–23. PubMed PMID: 24805127.

47. Rubio-Tapia, A., Herman, M. L., et al. (2012). Severe spruelike enteropathy associated with olmesartan. *Mayo Clinic Proceedings*, 87(8), 732–738. PubMed PMID: 22728033.

48. Garratty, G. (2010). Immune hemolytic anemia associated with drug therapy. *Blood Reviews*, 24(4–5), 143–150. PubMed PMID: 20650555.

49. Garratty, G. (2009). Drug-induced immune hemolytic anemia. *Hematology*, 73–79. PubMed PMID: 20008184.

50. Frieder, J., Mouabbi, J. A., et al. (2017). Autoimmune hemolytic anemia associated with trimethoprim-sulfamethoxazole use. *American Journal of Health-System Pharmacy*, 74(12), 894–897. PubMed PMID: 28596226.

51. Kirkiz, S., Yarali, N., et al. (2014). Metformin-induced hemolytic anemia. *Medical Principles and Practice*, 23(2), 183–185. PubMed PMID: 24296614.

52. Barbaryan, A., Iyinagoro, C., et al. (2013). Ibuprofen-induced hemolytic anemia. *Case Reports in Hematology [electronic resource]*, 142865. PubMed PMID: 23710383.

53. Marks, D. R., Joy, J. V., & Bonheim, N. A. (1991). Hemolytic anemia associated with the use of omeprazole. *The American Journal of Gastroenterology*, 86(2), 217–218. PubMed PMID: 1992636.

54. Sheikh-Taha, M., & Frenn, P. (2014). Autoimmune hemolytic anemia induced by levofloxacin. *Case Reports in Infectious Diseases*, 201015. PubMed PMID: 25024854.

55. Zimmerman, H. J. (2000). Drug-induced liver disease. *Clinics in Liver Disease*, 4(1), 73–96. PubMed PMID: 11232192.

56. Ostapowicz, G., Fontana, R. J., et al. (2002). Results of a prospective study of acute liver failure at 17 tertiary care centers in the United states. *Annals of Internal Medicine*, 137(12), 947–954. PubMed PMID: 12484709.

57. Liu, Z. X., & Kaplowitz, N. (2006). Role of innate immunity in acetaminophen-induced hepatotoxicity. *Expert Opinion on Drug Metabolism and Toxicology*, 2(4), 493–503. PubMed PMID: 16859400.

58. Roth, R. A., & Ganey, P. E. (2010). Intrinsic versus idiosyncratic drug-induced hepatotoxicity – two villains or one? *The Journal of Pharmacology and Experimental Therapeutics*, 332(3), 692–697. PubMed PMID: 20019161.

59. Daly, A. K., & Day, C. P. (2009). Genetic association studies in drug-induced liver injury. *Seminars in Liver Disease*, 29(4), 400–411. PubMed PMID: 19826974.

60. Lammert, C., Einarsson, S., et al. (2008). Relationship between daily dose of oral medications and

idiosyncratic drug-induced liver injury: search for signals. *Hepatology*, *47*(6), 2003–2009. PubMed PMID: 18454504.

61. Chalasani, N., Fontana, R. J., et al. (2008). Causes, clinical features, and outcomes from a prospective study of drug-induced liver injury in the United States. *Gastroenterology*, *135*(6), 1924–1934. PubMed PMID: 18955056.

62. Reuben, A., Koch, D. G., Lee, W. M., & Acute Liver Failure Study Group. (2010). Drug-induced acute liver failure: results of a U.S. multicenter, prospective study. *Hepatology*, *52*(6), 2065–2076. PubMed PMID: 20949552.

63. Lee, W. M. (2013). Drug-induced acute liver failure. *Clinics in Liver Disease*, *17*(4), 575–586. PubMed PMID: 24099019.

64. Mitchell, J. R., Jollow, D. J., Potter, W. Z., Gillette, J. R., & Brodie, B. B. (1973). Acetaminophen-induced hepatic necrosis. IV. Protective role of glutathione. *The Journal of Pharmacology and Experimental Therapeutics*, *187*(1), 211–217. PubMed PMID: 4746329.

65. Canalis, E., Mazziotti, G., Giustina, A., & Bilezikian, J. P. (2007). Glucocorticoid-induced osteoporosis: pathophysiology and therapy. *Osteoporosis International*, *18*(10), 1319–1328. PubMed PMID: 17566815.

66. Van Staa, T. P., Laan, R. F., et al. (2003). Bone density threshold and other predictors of vertebral fracture in patients receiving oral glucocorticoid therapy. *Arthritis and Rheumatism*, *48*(11), 3224–3229. PubMed PMID: 14613287.

67. Jonat, W., Kaufmann, M., Sauerbrei, W., et al. (2002). Goserelin versus cyclophosphamide, methotrexate, and fluorouracil as adjuvant therapy in premenopausal patients with node positive breast cancer: the Zoladex Early Breast Cancer Research Association Study. *Journal of Clinical Oncology*, *20*(24), 4628–4635. PubMed PMID: 12488406.

68. Rajgopal, R., Bear, M., Butcher, M. K., & Shaughnessy, S. G. (2008). The effects of heparin and low molecular weight heparins on bone. *Thrombosis Research*, *122*(3), 293–298. PubMed PMID: 17716711.

69. Lefkou, E., Khamashta, M., Hampson, G., & Hunt, B. J. (2010). Review: low-molecular-weight heparin-induced osteoporosis and osteoporotic fractures: a myth or an existing entity? *Lupus*, *19*(1), 3–12. PubMed PMID: 19934178.

70. Roux, C., Briot, K., Gossec, L., et al. (2009). Increase in vertebral fracture risk in postmenopausal women using omeprazole. *Calcified Tissue International*, *84*(1), 13–19. PubMed PMID: 19023510.

71. Yang, Y. X., Lewis, J. D., Epstein, S., & Metz, D. C. (2006). Long-term proton pump inhibitor therapy and risk of hip fracture. *The Journal of the American Medical Association*, *296*(24), 2947–2953. PubMed PMID: 17190895.

72. Yadav, V. K., Ryu, J. H., Suda, N., et al. (2008). Lrp5 controls bone formation by inhibiting serotonin synthesis in the duodenum. *Cell*, *135*(5), 825–837. PubMed PMID: 19041748.

73. Richards, J. B., Papaioannou, A., et al. (2007). Effect of selective serotonin reuptake inhibitors on the risk of fracture. *Archives of Internal Medicine*, *167*(2), 188–194. PubMed PMID: 17242321.

74. Giustina, A., Mazziotti, G., & Canalis, E. (2008). Growth hormone, insulin-like growth factors, and the skeleton. *Endocrine Reviews*, *29*(5), 535–559. PubMed PMID: 18436706.

75. Lakatos, P. (2003). Thyroid hormones: beneficial or deleterious for bone? *Calcified Tissue International*, *73*(3), 205–209. PubMed PMID: 14667131.

76. Mazziotti, G., Porcelli, T., Patelli, I., et al. (2010). Serum TSH values and risk of vertebral fractures in euthyroid postmenopausal women with low bone mineral density. *Bone*, *46*(3), 747–751. PubMed PMID: 19892039.

77. Lintermans, A., Laenen, A., et al. (2013). Prospective study to assess fluid accumulation and tenosynovial changes in the aromatase inhibitor-induced musculoskeletal syndrome: 2 year follow-up data. *Annals of Oncology*, *24*(2), 350–355. PubMed PMID: 23038762.

78. Shi, Q., Giordano, S. H., et al. (2013). Anastrozole-associated joint pain and other symptoms in patients with breast cancer. *The Journal of Pain*, *14*(3), 290–296. PubMed PMID: 23452648.

79. Altundag, K., Dede, D., et al. (2007). Aromatase inhibitor-associated arthralgias: pathogenesis, frequency and management. *Joint, Bone, Spine: Revue Du Rhumatisme*, *74*(6), 662–663. PubMed PMID: 17913550.

80. Khan, M. N., & Khan, A. A. (2008). Cancer treatment-related bone loss: a review and synthesis of the literature. *Current Oncology*, *15*(Suppl. 1), S30–S40. PubMed PMID: 18231646.

81. Gu, Q., Paulose-Ram, R., Burt, V. L., & Kit, B. K. (2014). Prescription cholesterol-lowering medication use in adults aged 40 and over: United States, 2003-2012. *National Center for Health Statistics Data Brief*, (177), 1–8. PubMed PMID: 25536410.

82. Thompson, P. D., Clarkson, P. M., et al. (2006). An assessment of statin safety by muscle experts. *The American Journal of Cardiology*, *97*(8A), 69C–76C. PubMed PMID: 16581332.

83. Buettner, C., Davis, R. B., et al. (2008). Prevalence of musculoskeletal pain and stain use. *Journal of General Internal Medicine, 23*(8), 1182–1186. PubMed PMID: 18449611.

84. Antons, K. A., Williams, C. D., Baker, S. K., & Phillips, P. S. (2006). Clinical perspectives of stain-induced rhabdomyolysis. *The American Journal of Medicine, 119*(5), 400–409. PubMed PMID: 16651050.

85. Vladutiu, G. D. (2008). Genetic predisposition to statin myopathy. *Current Opinion in Rheumatology, 20*(6), 648–655. PubMed PMID: 18946323.

86. Oh, J., Ban, M. R., et al. (2007). Genetic determinants of statin intolerance. *Lipids in Health and Disease, 6*, 7. PubMed PMID: 17376224.

87. Akbar, H., Khan, A., et al. (2017). The genotoxic effect of oxcarbazepine on mice blood lymphocytes. *Drug and Chemical Toxicology*, 1–6. PubMed PMID: 28503984.

88. Araujo, I. M., Ambrosio, A. F., et al. (2004). Neurotoxicity induced by antiepileptic drugs in cultured hippocampal neurons: a comparative study between carbamazepine, oxcarbazepine drugs, BIA 2-024 and BIA 2-093. *Epilepsia, 45*(12), 1498–1505. PubMed PMID: 15571507.

89. Lees, J. G., Makker, P. G., et al. (2017). Immune-mediated processes implicated in chemotherapy-induced peripheral neuropathy. *European Journal of Cancer, 73*, 22–29. PubMed PMID: 28104535.

90. Chow, K. M., Hui, A. C., & Szeto, C. C. (2005). Neurotoxicity induced by beta-lactam antibiotics: from bench to bedside. *European Journal of Clinical Microbiology & Infectious Diseases: Official Publication of the European Society of Clinical Microbiology, 24*(10), 649–653. PubMed PMID: 16261307.

91. De Sarro, A., Ammendola, D., et al. (1995). Relationship between structure and convulsant properties of some beta-lactam antibiotics following intracerebroventricular microinjection in rats. *Antimicrobial Agents and Chemotherapy, 39*(1), 232–237. PubMed PMID: 7695312.

92. Raposo, J., Teotonio, R., et al. (2016). Amoxicillin, a potential epileptogenic drug. *Epileptic Disorders, 18*(4), 454–457. PubMed PMID: 27900944.

93. Inui, K. I., Masuda, S., & Saito, H. (2000). Cellular and molecular aspects of drug transport in the kidney. *Kidney International, 58*(3), 944–958. PubMed PMID: 10972658.

94. Mehta, R. L., Pascual, M. T., Soroko, S., et al. (2004). Spectrum of acute renal failure in the intensive care unit: the PICARD experience. *Kidney International, 66*(4), 1613–1621. PubMed PMID: 15458458.

95. Pabla, N., & Dong, Z. (2008). Cisplatin nephrotoxicity: mechanisms and renoprotective strategies. *Kidney International, 73*(9), 994–1007. PubMed PMID: 18272962.

96. Rougier, F., Ducher, M., Maurin, M., et al. (2003). Aminoglycoside dosages and nephrotoxicity: quantitative relationships. *Clinical Pharmacokinetics, 42*(5), 493–500. PubMed PMID: 12739987.

97. Sawaya, B. P., Briggs, J. P., & Schnermann, J. (1995). Amphotericin B nephrotoxicity: the adverse consequences of altered membrane properties. *Journal of the American Society of Nephrology, 6*(2), 154–164. PubMed PMID: 7579079.

98. Izzedine, H., Launay-Vacher, V., & Deray, G. (2005). Antiviral drug-induced nephrotoxicity. *American Journal of Kidney Diseases, 45*(5), 804–817. PubMed PMID: 15861345.

99. Mc Cullough, P. A. (2008). Contrast-induced acute kidney injury. *Journal of the American College of Cardiology, 51*(15), 1419–1428. PubMed PMID: 18402894.

100. Markowitz, G. S., Fine, P. L., Stack, J. I., et al. (2003). Toxic acute tubular necrosis following treatment with zoledronate (Zometa). *Kidney International, 64*(1), 281–289. PubMed PMID: 12787420.

101. De Vriese, A. S., Robbrecht, D. L., Vanholder, R. C., et al. (1998). Rifampicin-associated acute renal failure: pathophysiologic, immunologic, and clinical features. *American Journal of Kidney Diseases, 31*(1), 108–115. PubMed PMID: 9428460.

102. Kleinknecht, D., Vanhille, P., Morel-Maroger, L., et al. (1983). Acute interstitial nephritis due to drug hypersensitivity. An up-to-date review with a report of 19 cases. *Advances in Nephrology from the Necker Hospital, 12*, 277–308. PubMed PMID: 6404139.

103. Härmark, L., van der Wiel, H. E., de Groot, M. C., & van Grootheest, A. C. (2007). Proton pump inhibitor-induced acute interstitial nephritis. *British Journal of Clinical Pharmacology, 64*(6), 819–823. PubMed PMID: 17635502.

104. Bender, W. L., Whelton, A., Beschomer, W. E., et al. (1984). Interstitial nephritis, proteinuria, and renal failure caused by nonsteroidal anti-inflammatory drugs. Immunological characterization of the inflammatory infiltrate. *The American Journal of Medicine, 76*(6), 1006–1012. PubMed PMID: 6375363.

105. Cortazar, F. B., Marrone, K. A., Troxell, M. L., et al. (2016). Clinicopathological features of acute kidney injury associated with immune checkpoint inhibitors. *Kidney International, 90*(3), 638–647. PubMed PMID: 27282937.

106. Murithi, A. K., Leung, N., Valeri, A. M., et al. (2014). Biopsy-proven acute interstitial nephritis, 1993-2011: a case series. *American Journal of Kidney Diseases, 64*(4), 558–566. PubMed PMID: 24927897.

107. Blank, M. L., Parkin, L., Paul, C., & Herbison, P. (2014). A nationwide nested case-control study indicates an increased risk of acute interstitial nephritis with proton pump inhibitor use. *Kidney International, 86*(4), 837–844. PubMed PMID: 24646856.

108. Pan, Y., Zhang, L., Wang, F., Li, X., Wang, H., & China National Survey of Chronic Kidney Disease Working Group. (2014). Status of non-steroidal anti-inflammatory drugs use and its association with chronic kidney disease: a cross-sectional survey in China. *Nephrology, 19*(10), 655–660. PubMed PMID: 25196389.

109. Gooch, K., Culleton, B. F., Manns, B. J., et al. (2007). NSAID use and progression of chronic kidney disease. *The American Journal of Medicine, 120*(3), 280.e1–280.e7. PubMed PMID: 17349452.

110. Ungprasert, P., Cheungpasitporn, W., Crowson, C. S., & Matteson, E. L. (2015). Individual non-steroidal anti-inflammatory drugs and risk of acute kidney injury: a systematic review and meta-analysis of observational studies. *European Journal of Internal Medicine, 26*(4), 285–291. PubMed PMID: 25862494.

111. De Broe, M. E., & Elseviers, M. M. (2009). Over-the-counter analgesic use. *Journal of the American Society of Nephrology, 20*(10), 2098–2103. PubMed PMID: 19423685.

112. Hernandez-Diaz, S., Mitchell, A. A., Kelley, K. E., et al. (2009). Medications as a potential source of exposure to phthalates in the U.S. population. *Environmental Health Perspectives, 117*, 185–189. PubMed PMID: 19270786.

113. Mylchreest, E., Sar, M., Cattley, R. C., & Foster, P. M. (1999). Disruption of androgen-regulated male reproductive development by di(n-butyl) phthalate during late gestation in rats is different from flutamide. *Toxicology and Applied Pharmacology, 156*(2), 81–95. PubMed PMID: 10198273.

114. Foster, P. M. (2006). Disruption of reproductive development in male rat offspring following in utero exposure to phthalate esters. *International Journal of Andrology, 29*(1), 140–147. PubMed PMID: 16102138.

115. Ledford, D. K., Wenzel, S. E., & Lockey, R. F. (2014). Aspirin or other nonsteroidal inflammatory agent exacerbated asthma. *The Journal of Allergy and Clinical Immunology, 2*(6), 653–657. PubMed PMID: 25439353.

116. Tan, Y., & Collins-Williams, C. (1982). Aspirin-induced asthma in children. *Annals of Allergy, 48*(1), 1–5. PubMed PMID: 7055340.

117. Vanderhoek, J. Y., Ekborg, S. L., & Bailey, J. M. (1984). Nonsteroidal anti-inflammatory drugs stimulate 15-lipoxygenase/leukotriene pathway in human polymorphonuclear leukocytes. *The Journal of Allergy and Clinical Immunology, 74*(3 Pt. 2), 412–417. PubMed PMID: 6432882.

118. Szczeklik, A., Sladek, K., Dworski, R., et al. (1996). Bronchial aspirin challenge causes specific eicosanoid response in aspirin-sensitive asthmatics. *American Journal of Respiratory and Critical Care Medicine, 154*(6 Pt. 1), 1608–1614. PubMed PMID: 8970343.

119. Simon, R. A. (2004). Adverse respiratory reactions to aspirin and nonsteroidal anti-inflammatory drugs. *Current Allergy and Asthma Reports, 4*(1), 17–24. PubMed PMID: 14680616.

120. Fahrenholz, J. M. (2003). Natural history and clinical features of aspirin-exacerbated respiratory disease. *Clinical Reviews in Allergy and Immunology, 24*(2), 113–124. PubMed PMID: 12668892.

121. Zaid, G., & Beall, G. N. (1966). Bronchial response to beta-adrenergic blockade. *The New England Journal of Medicine, 275*(11), 580–584. PubMed PMID: 5920412.

122. Okayama, M., Yafuso, N., Nogami, H., et al. (1987). A new method of inhalation challenge with propranolol: comparison with methacholine-induced bronchoconstriction and role of vagal nerve activity. *The Journal of Allergy and Clinical Immunology, 80*(3 Pt. 1), 291–299. PubMed PMID: 3305663.

123. Salpeter, S. R., Ormiston, T. M., & Salpeter, E. E. (2002). Cardioselective beta-blockers in patients with reactive airway disease: a meta-analysis. *Annals of Internal Medicine, 137*(9), 715–725. PubMed PMID: 12416945.

124. Covar, R. A., Macomber, B. A., & Szefler, S. J. (2005). Medications as asthma triggers. *Immunology and Allergy Clinics of North America, 25*(1), 169–190. PubMed PMID: 15579370.

125. Evans, W. E., & Relling, M. V. (1999). Pharmacogenomics: translating functional genomics into rational therapeutics. *Science, 286*(5439), 487–491. PubMed PMID: 10521338.

126. Zanger, U. M., Raimundo, S., & Eichelbaum, M. (2004). Cytochrome P450 2D6: overview and update on pharmacology, genetics, biochemistry. *Naunyn-Schmiedeberg's Archives of Pharmacology, 369*(1), 23–37. PubMed PMID: 14618296.

127. Li, A. P., Kaminski, D. L., & Rasmussen, A. (1995). Substrates of human hepatic cytochrome P450 3A4. *Toxicology, 104*(1–3), 1–8. PubMed PMID: 8560487.

128. Kuehl, P., Zhang, J., Lin, Y., et al. (2001). Sequence diversity in CYP3A promoters and characterization of the genetic basis of polymorphic CYP3A5 expression.

Nature Genetics, 27(4), 383–391. PubMed PMID: 11279519.

129. Ingelman-Sundberg, M. (2005). The human genome project and novel aspects of cytochrome P450 research. *Toxicology and Applied Pharmacology, 207*(Suppl. 2), 52–56. PubMed PMID: 15993453.

130. Pelkonen, O., Turpeinen, M., Hakkola, J., et al. (2008). Inhibition and induction of human cytochrome P450 enzymes: current status. *Archives of Toxicology, 82*(10), 667–715. PubMed PMID: 18618097.

131. Di, Y. M., Li, C. G., Xue, C. C., & Zhou, S. F. (2008). Clinical drugs that interact with St. John's wort and implication in drug development. *Current Pharmaceutical Design, 14*(17), 1723–1742. PubMed PMID: 18673195.

132. Hanley, M. J., Cancalon, P., Widmer, W. W., & Greenblatt, D. J. (2011). The effect of grapefruit juice on drug disposition. *Expert Opinion on Drug Metabolism and Toxicology, 7*(3), 267–286. PubMed PMID: 21254874.

133. Veronese, M. L., Gillen, L. P., Burke, J. P., et al. (2003). Exposure-dependent inhibition of intestinal and hepatic CYP3A4 in vivo by grapefruit juice. *Journal of Clinical Pharmacology, 43*(8), 831–839. PubMed PMID: 12953340.

134. Larson, A. M. (2007). Acetaminophen hepatotoxicity. *Clinics in Liver Disease, 11*(3), 525–548. PubMed PMID: 17723918.

135. Vree, T. B., Muskens, J. M., & Van Rossum, J. M. (1972). Excretion of amphetamines in human sweat. *Archives Internationales de Pharmacodynamie et de Thérapie, 199*, 311–317.

136. Henderson, G. L., & Wilson, K. B. (1973). Excretion of methadone and metabolites in human sweat. *Research Communications in Chemical Pathology and Pharmacology, 5*(1), 1–8.

137. Johnson, H. L., & Maaibach, H. I. (1971). Drug excretion in human eccrine sweat. *The Journal of Investigative Dermatology, 56*(3), 182–188.

138. Parnas, J., Flachs, H., Gram, L., & Wurtz-Jorgensen, A. (1978). Excretion of antiepileptic drugs in sweat. *Acta Neurologica Scandinavica, 58*, 197–204.

139. Soltan-Sharifi, M. S., Mojtahedzadeh, M., Najafi, A., et al. (2007). Improvement by N-acetylcysteine of acute respiratory distress syndrome through increasing intracellular glutathione. *Human and Experimental Toxicology, 26*(9), 697–703. PubMed PMID: 17984140.

140. Micke, P., Beeh, K. M., Schlaak, J. F., & Buhl, R. (2001). Oral supplementation with whey proteins increases plasma glutathione levels of HIV-infected patients. *European Journal of Clinical Investigation, 31*(2), 171–178. PubMed PMID: 11168457.

141. Jariwalla, R. J., Lalezari, J., Cenko, D., et al. (2008). Restoration of blood total glutathione status and lymphocyte function following alpha-lipoic acid supplementation in patients with HIV infection. *The Journal of Alternative and Complementary Medicine: Research on Paradigm, Practice, and Policy, 14*(2), 139–146. PubMed PMID: 18315507.

142. Lieber, C. S., & Packer, L. (2002). S-Adenosylmethionine: molecular, biological, and clinical aspects—an introduction. *The American Journal of Clinical Nutrition, 76*(5), 1148S–1150S. PubMed PMID: 12418492.

143. Hauser, R. A., Lyons, K. E., McCain, T., et al. (2009). Randomized, double-blind, pilot evaluation of intravenous glutathione in Parkinson's disease. *Movement Disorders, 24*(7), 979–983. PubMed PMID: 19230029.

144. Mischley, L. K., Vespignani, M. F., Finnell, J. S., et al. (2013). Safety survey of intranasal glutathione. *Journal of Alternative and Complementary Medicine (New York, N.Y.), 19*(5), 459–463. PubMed PMID: 23240940.

145. Darweesh, S. K., Ibrahim, M. F., & El-Tahawy, M. A. (2017). Effect of N-acetylcysteine on mortality and liver transplantation rate in non-acetaminophen-induced acute liver failure: a multicenter study. *Clinical Drug Investigation, 37*(5), 473–482. PubMed PMID: 28205121.

146. Mooiman, K. D., Maas-Bakker, R. F., Moret, E. E., et al. (2013). Milk thistle's active components silybin and isosilybin: novel inhibitors of PXR-mediated CYP3A4 induction. *Drug Metabolism and Disposition: The Biological Fate of Chemicals, 41*(8), 1494–1504. PubMed PMID: 23674609.

147. Raskovic, A., Stilinovic, N., Kolarovic, J., et al. (2011). The protective effects of silymarin against doxorubicin-induced cardiotoxicity and hepatotoxicity in rats. *Molecules [electronic resource], 16*(10), 8601–8613. PubMed PMID: 21993249.

9

Arsenic

SUMMARY

- Portion of population with body burden increasing risk of disease: >50%
- Major diseases: Diabetes, lung and prostate cancers, cardiovascular diseases (CVDs), chronic obstructive pulmonary disease (COPD), shingles, cognitive decline

- Primary sources: Water, fish, rice
- Best measure: First morning urine
- Best intervention: Avoidance and methylation support

DESCRIPTION AND TOXICITY

Arsenic is a ubiquitous metalloid in our food, air, and water that is the number one substance on the Comprehensive, Environmental, Response, Compensation, and Liability Act (CERCLA) Priority List of Hazardous Substances by the Agency for Toxic Substances and Disease Registry (ATSDR).[1] Toxicants present at Superfund sites are placed on this list based on their potential threat to human health.

Arsenic is found in both inorganic forms (as trivalent or pentavalent states) and organic forms. Groundwater provides a continuous source of inorganic arsenic, whereas foods provided more of the organic arsenicals, along with the metabolites of inorganic arsenic. Each different form of arsenic has a different median lethal dose LD 50 as well as a different half-life, although none of the arsenic species are persistent toxicants (Table 9.1).

Arsenic is well absorbed by both the gastrointestinal and respiratory tracts, and then widely distributed through the body, where it is reduced to arsenite (III)

to be methylated. A single pass through this methylation pathway produces monomethylarsonous acid (+ 3) (MMA). MMA can then pass through the pathway a second time to produce dimethylarsinous acid (+ 3) (DMA).[2] The difference in toxicity, as assessed by LD_{50}, between the single and double methylated forms, is more than 300-fold, as seen in Table 9.1. Methylation primarily occurs enzymatically through the action of arsenic (+ 3 oxidation) methyltransferases (AS3MT) but can also occur nonenzymatically in the presence of either methylcobalamine or glutathione.[3] This nonenzymatic methylation by methylcobalamine is enhanced with the presence of sodium selenite or 2,3-dimercapto-1-propanesulfonic acid (DMPS). Single nucleotide polymorphisms of AS3MT, methyltetrahydrafolate reductase (MTHFR), and glutathione transferase omega 1 (GSTO1) have all been shown to reduce the production of DMA, increasing the levels of MMA, resulting in greater toxicity from inorganic arsenic.[4] S-adenosylmethionine, folate, methionine, and choline all enhance double methylation of inorganic arsenic,[2] whereas deficiencies in those compounds lead to greater

TABLE 9.1	Summary of Arsenic Species			
Species	Type	Half-Life	Primary Source	LD$_{50}$
Arsenate (V)	Inorganic	2–4 days	Water	8 mg/kg
Arsenite (III)	Inorganic	2–4 days	Water	26 mg/kg
MMA	Inorganic	10–20 hours	Food	2 mg/kg
DMA	Inorganic	10–20 hours	Food	648 mg/kg
Arsenobetaine	Organic	4–6 hours	Seafood	>4000 mg/kg

levels of MMA and lower DMA. Proper bowel flora will also methylate inorganic arsenic.[5] Higher levels of MMA have also been linked to elevated homocysteine levels, possibly due to overall methylation defects.[6]

The main mechanism by which MMA and inorganic arsenicals are found to cause cellular and tissue damage is through oxidative stress.[7] Some health effects, primarily cancers, are thought to also be promoted via DNA methylation defects.[8] Oxidative damage to the DNA results in increased urinary excretion of 8-hydroxy-2'-deoxy-quanosine (8-OHdG), which is a valuable marker for both oxidative stress and chronic disease risk.[9] Increases in urinary 8-OHdG levels have been found in those drinking groundwater high in arsenic,[10,11] as well as those occupationally exposed to arsenic.[12]

SOURCES

Groundwater

Groundwater is the most common source of arsenic exposure. In the United States, groundwater arsenic (arsenite [ASIII] and arsenate [ASV]) levels range from <1 µg/L to >30 µg/L, with the average being 1 µg/L.[13] The United States Environmental Protection Agency (EPA) set the date of January 23, 2006, for all municipal water supplies to be in compliance with a new maximum contaminant level of 10 µg/L (10 parts per billion (PPB)).[14] Yet the infrastructure to reduce arsenic in drinking water from 50 µg/L to 10 µg/L in the areas where groundwater arsenic is higher than 10 parts per million (PPM) is still not fully in place.[15] Arsenic levels up to 3100 µg/L have been found in well water samples in Maine, where wells from the entire state were sampled.[16] Bangladesh, Taiwan, Chile, Argentina, China, and India have far higher levels of groundwater arsenic that are typically >300 µg/L (ranging up to 7550 in Argentina). Chronic arsenic poisoning is found in these areas in persons drinking an average of 3.3 liters of water daily, whereas those consuming ≤1.9

liters have not exhibited poisoning.[17] However, current research that will be covered later in this chapter has revealed valid health concerns for persons drinking water with far lower arsenic levels commonly encountered in the United States.

INFORMATION SOURCES FOR GROUNDWATER ARSENIC LEVELS

- World arsenic groundwater map: https://phys.org/news/2016-04-milestone-arsenic-fluoride-contaminated.html
- U.S. arsenic groundwater map: http://water.usgs.gov/nawqa/trace/arsenic/
- U.S. state-by-state groundwater map: http://www.atsdr.cdc.gov/substances/SubstanceMap.asp

The mean daily intake of arsenic for U.S. residents has been estimated to be 3.2 µg/day, with a range of 1 to 20 µg/day.[3] However, arsenic intake far above this average has already been found in certain areas in the United States. A study in southeastern Michigan, where groundwater arsenic levels are far lower than what is found in the southwestern part of the state, revealed that 55% of the total daily arsenic intake comes from drinking water, with an additional 37% due to food intake, with rice being the largest dietary source.[18] In this study, the 95th percentile of arsenic intake ranged from 11 to 24 µg/day, which would obviously be higher in geographical areas with higher groundwater arsenic concentrations.

Food

Food sources of arsenic contain high percentages of the organic arsenicals (arsenobetaine, arsenocholine, arsenosugars, and arsenolipids) that have very short half-lives and are considered virtually nontoxic. Foods also contain DMA and small amounts of MMA but are relatively free of arsenite and arsenate. Table 9.2 lists foods containing the highest total levels of arsenic according to the most

TABLE 9.2 **Arsenic in Food**		
Food	Frequency Found	Mean mg/kg (PPM)
Haddock, pan-cooked	100%	5.54
Tuna, canned in water	100%	0.878
Shrimp, boiled	100%	0.678
Fast food fish sandwich on bun	100%	0.501
Salmon steak	99%	0.469
New England clam chowder	99%	0.141
Tuna noodle casserole	95%	0.112
Mushrooms, raw	95%	0.081
Fried rice, meatless, Chinese takeout	100%	0.072
Infant rice cereal with whole milk	80%	0.042
Chicken leg, fried, fast food	100%	0.023
Granola bar with raisins	90%	0.027
Fruit juice blend	75%	0.013

Compiled from U.S. Food and Drug Administration: Total Diet Study Statistics on Element Results. Available at http://www.fda.gov/downloads/Food/FoodScienceResearch/TotalDietStudy/UCM243059.pdf.

recent Food and Drug Administration (FDA) Total Diet Study.[19]

From the data summarized in Table 9.2, it is clear that fish comprises the greatest food source of arsenic, which is predominantly arsenobetaine. The arsenic found in shrimp is predominantly arsenocholine, which was nondetectable in the National Health and Nutritional Examination Survey (NHANES) data.[20] There has been significant focus recently on the role of rice consumption as a source of arsenic exposure. Based on total arsenic levels, it has been estimated that the consumption of 0.56 cups of cooked rice daily (the U.S. average) is comparable to drinking 1 liter a day of water containing 10 µg/L of arsenic.[21] Although total arsenic intake may be similar, the composition and potential toxic action will be quite different. In this study, the rice-consuming group did have statistically significantly higher levels of both DMA and MMA in their urine. Other studies have confirmed that rice consumers typically have twice the level of urinary DMA than is present in persons who do not regularly consume rice.[22]

Both the composition of arsenic species and the total arsenic burden in rice vary greatly based on where and how it is grown, how it is washed, and how it is cooked.

The levels of inorganic arsenic in rice can vary from 33% to 89% (the rest being organic) simply based on where and how it is grown.[23] Rice plants absorb arsenic from the water in which they are grown, so rice grown in areas with high groundwater arsenic will have far higher arsenic content than plants grown in other areas. Rice grown in the south central United States (Texas) had an average arsenic concentration of 0.30 µg/gram, whereas rice grown in California averaged 0.16 µg/gram (41% less).[24] The arsenic content in rice can then be either increased or decreased depending on whether the rice is washed with high- or low-arsenic water.[25] Washing rice in low-arsenic water reduces the total arsenic content by 28%, and washing rice in high-arsenic water increases arsenic levels. Discarding the cooking water before the rice is done and replacing it with fresh water can reduce the total arsenic content by an additional 57%. And simply cooking rice with excess water can reduce arsenic content by 39% to 45%.[26]

Arsenic was fed to commercially raised poultry in the form of 3-nitro-4-hydroxyphenylarsonic acid (roxarsone and nitarsone) until FDA approval was withdrawn in 2013 (roxarsone) and 2015 (nitarsone). Before their removal from poultry farming, conventionally raised chickens were found to have 1.8 µg/kg total average arsenic in a U.S. market-basket study, whereas organic chickens were found to have an average of 0.6 µg/kg.[27] In roxarsone-fed chickens, arsenite was found (along with arsenobetaine, DMA, and MMA) in breast meat and would have provided the average chicken-consuming U.S. resident with only 0.3 (±0.2) µg/day of arsenite.[12] To date, no studies have shown arsenic-related health problems with the consumption of chicken, and U.S. poultry is now free of this extra arsenic burden.

Other Sources

Arsenic is present in cigarette smoke and is found in higher levels in smokers.[28,29] Arsenic is a component of certain pigments used in glassmaking, so individuals working with those colors may have greater exposure.[30,31] Arsenicals have been used for centuries as pesticides, initially as lead arsenate and more recently as monosodium methanearsonate (MSMA) and dimethylarsinic acids (DMAs). Lead arsenate was a primary pesticide used in orchards for more than a century. It has not been used for the last 50 years, yet this compound is still present in the soil. As orchard land is transformed into housing developments, lead arsenate exposure from the soil and air now occurs in those communities.[32] However, water and foods remain the bulk of exposure sources.[33]

Body Burden

Levels of the various arsenical compounds in residents of the United States have been studied as part of the ongoing NHANES trial and published by the Centers for Disease Control and Prevention (CDC) in their Exposure Report.[20] Table 9.3 summarizes the arsenic findings published in the February 2015 updated tables to the Fourth Report.

These data reveal that, as the total urinary arsenic level rises above 13.7 µg/g creatinine, the greatest

contribution to this increase comes from nontoxic arsenobetaine. It should also be noted that levels of toxic MMA are not detectable until the total urinary arsenic average is >30.8 µg/g creatinine. The CDC has provided average levels of the various arsenic species for the broad ethnic categories of Mexican Americans, non-Hispanic whites, non-Hispanic blacks, and Asian Americans. They also provide the averages for males, females, and three different age groupings (6–11 years, 12–19 years, and 20 years and older). Although rice is a common staple in the Mexican American diet, the highest rice and fish intake is found among Asian Americans. Asian Americans have an average daily intake of >2 cups of rice, whereas the average total U.S. consumption is approximately 0.5 cups daily.[34] Table 9.4 shows the ethnic breakdowns for total arsenic intake, arsenobetaine, MMA, and DMA.

One can see that traditionally higher rice consumption among Mexican Americans did not result in greatly elevated levels of total urinary arsenic, arsenobetaine, or DMA, and only a small increase in MMA levels. However, the averages of the individual arsenicals were far higher for Asian Americans than for any of the other ethnic groups. The mean total arsenic level in Asian

TABLE 9.3 CDC Fourth Report February 2015 Update Tables—Urinary Arsenic µg/g Creatinine

Metal	Mean	75th%	90th%	95th%
Arsenic total	7.77	13.7	30.8	50.4
Arsenobetaine	<LOD	5.63	18.0	36.9
DMA	3.92	5.92	9.86	13.1
MMA	<LOD	<LOD	2.21	2.86
Inorganic arsenic	6.31	9.46	15.1	19.6

LOD = Level of detection

TABLE 9.4 Arsenic by Species and Ethnicity

Arsenic Species	Population	Mean	75th%	90th%	95th%
Total arsenic—µg/g creatinine	Total	7.77	13.7	30.8	50.4
	Mexican Americans	8.00	11.9	26.1	40.8
	Non-Hispanic whites	7.13	12.4	28.4	55.4
	Non-Hispanic blacks	7.24	13.5	28.8	55.4
	Asian Americans	22.3	39.4	100	162
Arsenobetaine—µg/g creatinine	Total	<LOD	5.63	18.0	36.9
	Mexican Americans	<LOD	3.87	12.6	25.9
	Non-Hispanic whites	<LOD	5.0	16.8	35.7
	Non-Hispanic blacks	1.50	6.0	20.3	38.7
	Asian Americans	6.90	21.5	60.4	95.7
DMA—µg/g creatinine	Total	3.92	5.92	9.86	13.1
	Mexican Americans	4.12	5.77	8.06	10.5
	Non-Hispanic whites	3.68	5.32	9.07	11.5
	Non-Hispanic blacks	3.16	4.98	8.27	11.3
	Asian Americans	9.89	15.6	28.6	45.1
MMA—µg/g creatinine	Total	<LOD	<LOD	2.21	2.86
	Mexican Americans	<LOD	<LOD	1.95	2.63
	Non-Hispanic whites	<LOD	<LOD	2.33	2.86
	Non-Hispanic blacks	<LOD	<LOD	1.38	1.97
	Asian Americans	<LOD	2.06	3.07	4.50

Americans was 22.3, compared with a range of 7.13 to 8.00 in the other ethnic groups, with the 90th percentile level of total urinary arsenic levels for Asian Americans being twice the 95th percentile for the combined totals. Correspondingly, the arsenobetaine levels in the North American Asian population were also far higher than in any other ethnic group, indicating that the majority of total urinary arsenicals came from consumption of fish rather than rice. Detectable levels of MMA were present in the 75th percentile in the North American Asian population, but the total arsenic level for that percentile averaged 39.4 µg/g. This confirms that the very toxic MMA form of arsenic only reaches detectable levels in persons whose total arsenic urinary level is ≥30 µg/g creatinine.

Clinical Significance

With one exception, all of the published human studies on the adverse health effects of daily arsenic exposure are based on groundwater consumption rather than food. The sole exception was a study on arsenic-induced genotoxicity done in West Bengal, India.[35] The water arsenic content in this area only averaged 3 to 6 PPM, whereas the rice arsenic content averaged >200 PPB. With an average daily intake of rice of 540 to 640 grams (1.3 pounds) per day, the range of urinary arsenic content went from 32 to 90 µg/L, with an average of 50 µg/L. Although no elevated disease states were found in this group, a genotoxic effect on their urothelial cells were identified. With urinary levels of arsenic in excess of 30 µg/L, MMA would certainly be present, with resultant cellular and tissue damage, and would clearly indicate that daily arsenic intake levels were too high.

This *in vitro* study must be balanced with studies on the use of brown rice in a macrobiotic diet for individuals with diabetes (a disease clearly associated with arsenic). Several articles have recently been published from the MADIAB trial in Italy, where a modified macrobiotic diet is being used. This modified diet still requires the intake of 350 grams of brown rice daily (approximately 1.75 cups) as the major grain source. Yet persons utilizing this diet in a controlled setting are achieving reductions in their HbA1c and other markers of diabetic disease activity.[36,37,38]

Cancer. A cohort of more than 165,000 adults from 17 municipalities in the Viterbo region of Italy were followed for 20 years to observe the influence of groundwater

arsenic on chronic disease conditions.[39] The groundwater arsenic levels in this region varied from 0.5 µg/L to 80.4 µg/L, with a mean level of 19.3 µg/L. Each participant's residential history over the 39.5 years of the study was tracked to insure that the proper data on water arsenic exposure levels were gathered. Tables 9.5 and 9.6 show the disease risks found to be associated with groundwater arsenic exposure for both males and females in this study. Unfortunately, this study did not measure urinary arsenic levels for further comparison.

Lung cancer has been associated with chronic arsenic poisoning and in this study was also found more frequently in persons consuming water with low arsenic content. After adjusting for all the appropriate confounders, persons consuming groundwater arsenic at levels higher than 20 µg/L (PPM) had an 83% increased risk of lung cancer, yet those consuming water with arsenic

TABLE 9.5   Hazard Ratios for Italian Males per Groundwater Arsenic Levels

Cause of Death	As 10–20 µg/L	>20 µg/L	P
Natural causes	1.27	1.51	<0.001
Myocardial infarction	1.32	1.74	<0.001
Ischemic heart disease	1.42	1.70	<0.001
Lung cancer	1.47	1.83	<0.001
Coronary atherosclerosis	1.50	1.58	<0.001
COPD	1.84	2.04	<0.001

TABLE 9.6   Hazard Ratios for Italian Females per Groundwater Arsenic Levels

Cause of Death	As 10–20 µg/L	>20 µg/L	P
Natural causes	1.14	1.19	0.001
Cardiovascular Disease	1.17	1.20	0.020
Stroke	1.23	1.28	0.030
Myocardial infarction	1.32	1.74	<0.001
Lung cancer	1.80	1.69	0.015
Diabetes mellitus	2.12	2.08	<0.001

levels just above the new EPA standards for the United States (10 µg/L) had a 47% increased risk. The women in this study (Table 9.6) showed a similarly elevated risk of lung cancer, although for some reason, the risk was higher in those with lower groundwater arsenic. Increased risk of lung cancer from low levels of groundwater arsenic has also been found in a study done in California and Nevada.[40]

The STRONG heart study followed 3575 Native Americans from Arizona, Oklahoma, North Dakota, and South Dakota between 1989 and 2008 with groundwater arsenic levels ranging from <1 µg/L (Dakotas) to 61 µg/L (Arizona). The data collected were reviewed to see if there was an association between groundwater arsenic, urinary arsenic, and cancer risk.[41] These data revealed that that those with urinary arsenic levels <6.91 µg/g creatinine were protected from increased cancer risk. Comparing individuals with urinary arsenic <6.91 to those >13.22 µg/g creatinine revealed a 14% to 3.3-fold increased hazard ratio for various cancers (Box 9.1).

The findings on lung cancer risk in this study were in line with those seen in the Italian study but lower than those seen in the California and Nevada study. However, this study also revealed a huge risk for prostate cancer, something that no other study had even looked for. Long-term groundwater arsenic exposure among residents in Maine was strongly associated with bladder cancer.[42] Water intake was significantly associated with arsenic levels, and those with the highest arsenic exposure had more than twice

the risk of developing bladder cancer. This association was only significant after consuming high arsenic groundwater for 40 years. A study in New Hampshire reported that increased risk for both basal cell and squamous cell carcinoma (SCC), a common cancer in arsenic poisoning, can occur in persons consuming low levels of groundwater arsenic.[43] This study reported that, for each log-transformed 1 µg/l increase in urinary MMA levels, the risk for SCC increased by 33%, with persons in the third tertile of urinary MMA having a 76% greater risk for SCC than those in the first tertile. The average groundwater arsenic level in this study was quite low (0.32 µg/L), as were the apparent averages for urinary arsenic (controls, 10.27 µg arsenic/L; cases, 12.59 µg arsenic/L).

Respiratory and Cardiovascular Disease. The data on Italian men show that COPD risk doubles in men with higher arsenic intake. Chronic upper respiratory problems, including dyspnea, asthma, and cough, were noted in a study from India with persons consuming groundwater with arsenic levels between 11 and 50 PPM.[44] The Italian study also showed that the risk for various aspects of cardiovascular disease (CVD) increased from 32% to 74% in males. Italian women also had 32% to 74% increased risk for heart attacks but did not have increased risk for stroke or other circulatory disease issues.

Low-level arsenic exposure has been clearly linked in other studies to increasing risk for CVD, including hypertension.[45] The Strong heart study (SHS) subjects had urinary arsenic levels ranging from a low mean of 5.8 µg/g creatinine to 15.7 µg/g creatinine.[46] Those individuals with higher urinary arsenic levels were 65% more likely to have CVD, 71% more likely to have coronary heart disease (CHD), and more than three times more likely to have a fatal stroke. The associations were strongest among those living in Arizona, where the groundwater arsenic was the highest. Comparing their findings to the U.S. averages reported by the CDC (Tables 9.2, 9.3, and 9.7) indicates that 25% of all U.S. residents (those at and higher than the 75th percentile of arsenic, 13.7 µg/g creatinine) would have increased risk for CVD, CHD, and stroke simply due to their daily intake of groundwater arsenic.

Diabetes and Prediabetes Risk. The Italian study reported that women drinking water with >10 µg/L of arsenic had a double the risk for developing diabetes

---

BOX 9.1 Cancer Hazard Ratios

Comparing Urinary Arsenic >13.32 µg/g creatinine (cr) to <6.91 µg/g cr
- Kidney cancer = 0.44
- Overall cancer = 1.14
- Liver cancer = 1.34
- Lung cancer = 1.56
- Prostate cancer = 3.30

Data from García-Esquinas, E., Pollán, M., Umans, J. G., Francesconi, K. A., Goessler, W., & Guallar, E., et al. (2013). Arsenic exposure and cancer mortality in a U.S.-based prospective cohort: the STRONG heart study. *Cancer Epidemiology, Biomarkers and Prevention, 22*(11):1944–1953. Erratum in: *Cancer Epidemiology, Biomarkers and Prevention*, 2013;*22*(8):1479.

TABLE 9.7 **Odds Ratios for Prediabetes and Diabetes Based on Urinary (U) Arsenic Levels (µg/L)[a]**

CDC µg/L	U Arsenic µg/L	Prediabetes	Diabetes
	<5.71	1.00	1.00
(50th) 8.10	5.71–11.20	1.37	1.20
(75th) 14.9	11.21–22.98	1.46	1.55
(90th) 33.3	22.99	2.14	1.81
	P value for trend	0.43	0.17

[a]The CDC values in this table are in µg/L, which differs slightly from the previous values given in Tables 9.3 and 9.4, where the unit of measurement is µg/g creatinine.
Feseke, S. K., St-Laurent, J., Anassour-Sidi, E., Ayotte, P., Bouchard, M., & Levallois, P. (2015). Arsenic exposure and type 2 diabetes: Results from the 2007–2009 Canadian Health Measures Survey. *Health Promotion and Chronic Disease Prevention in Canada: Research, Policy and Practice, 35*(4), 63–72. PubMed PMID: 26083521.

mellitus. The Canadian Health Measures Study also found an association between arsenic intake, blood sugar problems, and diabetes.[47] This study of more than 2000 adult Canadians specifically excluded any seafood eaters and only monitored urinary arsenic levels rather than the levels of arsenic in drinking water. In this study, any urinary arsenic finding higher than 5.71 µg arsenic/L was associated with an increased risk for both prediabetes and diabetes. Table 9.7 shows their findings and compares their levels with the 50th, 75th, and 90th, percentiles.

The data from the STRONG heart study showed that persons with urinary arsenic levels <5.8 µg/g creatinine did not have elevated risk of heart disease. In this study, a similar cutoff value of urinary arsenic (<5.71 µg/g creatinine) was protective against diabetes as well. If the data from this Canadian study are applicable to the residents of the United States, then more than 50% of the U.S. population whose urinary arsenic levels are >8.10 µg/g creatinine have increased risk for developing diabetes just from the water they are drinking. When the data collected from the STRONG heart study were reviewed for noncardiovascular chronic diseases, a positive association was also found for diabetes, although with lower risk values than those found in Canada.[48] The researchers of the STRONG heart study differed from the Canadian study, as they found no association between urinary arsenic levels and hemoglobin A1c levels. Arsenic-related cardiovascular and diabetes risks

were confirmed in another study in Michigan comparing well water arsenic levels (averaging 11 µg/L) with mortality statistics.[49] This study also reported a 28% increased risk for kidney disease from groundwater arsenic consumption.

Other Health Risks. In addition to increasing the risk for various cancers, heart disease, diabetes, and COPD, low-level groundwater arsenic exposure has also been linked to increased risk for herpes zoster, diminished cognitive function, and reduced lung function.

Increased incidence of herpes zoster is common in persons with diabetes, which we now know is associated with chronic low-level arsenic exposure. A review of the data from NHANES (2003–2004 and 2009–2010) was undertaken to find out if there was an association between urinary arsenic levels and seronegativity for herpes zoster, indicating a lack of immunity.[50] The average urinary arsenic level for those with normal immunity to zoster was 6.57 µg arsenic/L, whereas those whose level was >7.5 µg/L had increasing risk of seronegativity that reached 87% for individuals with the highest urinary arsenic content.

SUMMARY OF LOW-LEVEL ARSENIC HEALTH EFFECTS

- Cardiovascular disease (including myocardial infarction [MI], stroke, hypertension [HTN])
- Diabetes and hyperglycemia
- COPD and upper and lower respiratory problems
- Cancers of the prostate, lung, liver, and skin
- Shingles
- Diminished cognition and neurological functioning

Residents in Cochran and Palmer counties, Texas, where the groundwater arsenic averaged 6.32 µg/L, were assessed for neuropsychological functioning as part of an ongoing epidemiological study on cognitive aging among rural inhabitants.[51] A mini–mental status examination along with multiple computer-based tests of cognitive function (attention, language, visuospatial, constructive ability, delayed recall, word association, and verbal fluency) were performed on the study subjects. The test results of individuals from areas with higher groundwater arsenic were then compared with those with lower groundwater arsenic levels.

Both current and long-term exposure to groundwater arsenic were significantly related to poorer scores in language, visuospatial skills, and executive functioning. Long-term exposure (but not current exposure) to low-level groundwater arsenic was also associated with poorer scores in global cognition, processing speeds, and immediate memory.

INTERVENTION

A number of natural compounds and supplements have been shown to improve the methylation of inorganic arsenic, increase the excretion of arsenic, and prevent or reverse arsenic-related tissue damage. As previously mentioned, S-adenosyl methionine, folate, methylfolate, methylcobalamin, and l-methionine have all been shown to enhance the methylation of inorganic arsenic.[5,7] Methylcobalamin and glutathione are able to nonenzymatically enhance double methylation of inorganic arsenic.[4] Daily folic acid supplementation at a dose of 800 µg daily has been shown in volunteers to significantly lower blood arsenic levels.[10]

Several common dietary components have also demonstrated benefit in dealing with arsenic, including protein, brassica-family vegetables, and some botanical agents. A good quality protein level in the diet demonstrated effectiveness at increasing the excretion of inorganic arsenicals.[5] Members of the brassica family of vegetables, rich sources of sulforaphane compounds, appear to prevent cellular damage from arsenic.[52,53] One of the most commonly used dietary spices is turmeric (*Curcuma longa*), containing the flavonoid curcumin. Curcumin has multiple beneficial effects with regard to arsenic, including enhancing both the methylation and excretion of inorganic arsenic and reversing arsenic-induced cellular damage.[54,55] DNA damage from arsenic is a marker of genotoxicity and results in elevated urinary levels of 8-OHdG. The consumption of high-arsenic groundwater has been directly linked to an increase in urinary 8-OHdG levels in a population in West Bengal, India. But when individuals from this area supplemented with 1 gram of curcumin daily for 3 months, the 8-OHdG level dropped, indicating a dramatic reduction in arsenic-induced DNA oxidative damage.[56] Daily intake of green and black teas has also been shown to reverse arsenic-induced cytotoxicity and genotoxicity.[57,58] This benefit seems to be related to both the epigallocatechin gallate (EGCG) and theaflavin content of these teas.

Testing

Random or first-morning urine can be submitted to various laboratories for measurement of arsenic levels. To get a reading free of arsenobetaine, it is recommended that no seafood be consumed for 48 hours before sample collection. Levels <7 µg arsenic/g creatinine would be considered optimal. Levels >12 µg arsenic/g creatinine would be considered higher risk for CVD, diabetes, respiratory problems, cancers, and neurological dysfunction.

Total arsenic levels >30 µg/g creatinine indicate the likelihood that MMA is present in levels high enough to cause genotoxicity.

Assessments

1. Measure urine arsenic level.
2. Test tap water for arsenic content.
   a. https://www.epa.gov/dwlabcert—for a list of state certified testing laboratories
   b. https://www.doctorsdata.com/comprehensive-drinking-water-analysis/
3. Test for functioning AS3MT with a genetic test kit.
   a. http://www.mybiosource.com/prods/ELISA-Kit/Human/Arsenic-3-oxidation-state-methyltransterase/AS3MT/datasheet.php?products_id=753400
4. Urinary 8-OHdG can be elevated from arsenic exposure.[23]
5. Homocysteine levels elevated with higher MMA.[6]

Treatment

1. Avoidance:
   a. Utilize arsenic-removing water filtration units for the home and workplace.
      i. http://www.oregon.gov/oha/ph/HealthyEnvironments/DrinkingWater/SourceWater/Documents/gw/arsenicremoval.pdf
      ii. For consumers of brown rice:
         1. Wash the rice in water that has been run through one of the previously discussed filters; continue to wash the rice until the water is clear.
         2. Strain off the wash water about halfway through cooking time and replace with fresh arsenic-free water.
   b. Avoid cigarette smoke.
2. Supplementation:
   a. Methyl donors: S-adenosyl methionine, methylfolate, methylcobalamin, methionine

   b. Folic acid—800 µg/day

   c. Glutathione (liposomal)

   d. Adequate protein—30 grams of lean protein daily

   e. Consume brassica family vegetables daily

   f. Green or black tea daily—minimum 1 cup

   g. Curcumin—up to 1 gram daily

REFERENCES

1. Agency for Toxic Substances and Disease Registry. *Substance priority list.* Available at https://www.atsdr.cdc.gov/spl/. (Accessed August 17, 2016.)

2. Heck, J. E., Nieves, J. W., Chen, Y., Parvez, F., Brandt-Rauf, P. W., Graziano, J. H., et al. (2009). Dietary intake of methionine, cysteine, and protein and urinary arsenic excretion in Bangladesh. *Environmental Health Perspectives, 117*(1), 99–104. PubMed PMID:19165394.

3. Zahkaryan, R., & Aposhian, V. (1999). Arsenite methylation by methylvitamin B12 and glutathione does not require an enzyme. *Toxicology and Applied Pharmacology, 154,* 287–291. PMID: 9931288.

4. Lindberg, A. L., Kumar, R., Goessler, W., Thirumaran, R., Gurzau, E., Koppova, K., et al. (2007). Metabolism of low-dose inorganic arsenic in a central European population: Influence of sex and genetic polymorphisms. *Environmental Health Perspectives, 115*(7), 1081–1086. PubMed PMID: 17637926.

5. Hall, L. L., George, S. E., Kohan, M. J., Styblo, M., & Thomas, D. J. (1997). In vitro methylation of inorganic arsenic in mouse intestinal cecum. *Toxicology and Applied Pharmacology, 147*(1), 101–109. PubMed PMID: 9356312.

6. Hall, M., Gamble, M., Slavkovich, V., Liu, X., Levy, D., Cheng, Z., et al. (2007). Determinants of arsenic metabolism: Blood arsenic metabolites, plasma folate, cobalamin, and homocysteine concentrations in maternal-newborn pairs. *Environmental Health Perspectives, 115*(10), 1503–1509. PubMed PMID: 17938743.

7. Bernstam, L., & Nriagu, J. (2000). Molecular aspects of arsenic stress. *Journal of Toxicology and Environmental Health. Part B, Critical Reviews, 3*(4), 293–322. Review. PubMed PMID: 11055208.

8. Lambrou, A., Baccarelli, A., Wright, R. O., Weisskopf, M., Bollati, V., Amarasiriwardena, C., et al. (2012). Arsenic exposure and DNA methylation among elderly men. *Epidemiology, 23*(5), 668–676. PubMed PMID: 22833016.

9. Valavanidis, A., Vlachogianni, T., & Fiotakis, C. (2009). 8-hydroxy-2'-deoxyguanosine(8-OHdG): A critical biomarker of oxidative stress and carcinogenesis. *Journal of Environmental Science and Health. Part C, Environmental Carcinogenesis Reviews, 27*(2), 120–139. PubMed PMID: 19412858.

10. Fujino, Y., Guo, X., Liu, J., Matthews, I. P., Shirane, K., Wu, K., et al. (2005). Japan Inner Mongolia Arsenic Pollution Study Group. Chronic arsenic exposure and urinary 8-hydroxy-2'-deoxyguanosine in an arsenic-affected area in Inner Mongolia, China. *Journal of Exposure Analysis and Environmental Epidemiology, 15*(2), 147–152. PubMed PMID: 15150536.

11. Peters, B. A., Hall, M. N., Liu, X., Parvez, F., Sanchez, T. R., van Geen, A., et al. (2015). Folic acid and creatine as therapeutic approaches to lower blood arsenic: a randomized controlled trial. *Environmental Health Perspectives, 123*(12), 1294–1301. PubMed PMID:25978852.

12. Liu, Q., Peng, H., Lu, X., Zuidhof, M. J., Li, X. F., & Le, X. C. (2016). Arsenic species in chicken breast: temporal variations of metabolites, elimination kinetics, and residual concentrations. *Environmental Health Perspectives, 124*(8), 1174–1181. PubMed PMID: 26992196.

13. Focazio, M., Welch, A., Watkins, S., Helsel, D., & Horn, M. *A Retrospective Analysis on the Occurrence of Arsenic in Ground-Water Resources of the United States and Limitations in Drinking-Water-Supply Characterizations.* USGS Water Resources Investigation Report 99-4279. http://pubs.usgs.gov/wri/wri994279/pdf/wri994279.pdf. (Accessed August 17, 2016.)

14. United States Environmental Protection Agency. *Drinking Water Requirements for States and Public Water Systems: Chemical Contaminant Rules.* Available at https://www.epa.gov/dwreginfo/chemical-contaminant-rules. (Accessed August 22, 2016.)

15. Walton, B. (2011). *American Arsenic: After a Decade, Small Communities Still Struggle to Meet Federal Drinking Water Standards.* Circle of Blue. Available at http://www.circleofblue.org/2011/world/american-arsenic-after-a-decade-small-communities-still-struggle-to-meet-federal-drinking-water-standards/. (Accessed August 22, 2016.).

16. Neilsen, M. G., Lombard, P. J., & Schalk, L. F. *Assessment of arsenic concentrations in domestic well water, by town, in Maine, 2009-2009.* U.S. Geological Survey Scientific Investigations Report 2010-5199. http://pubs.usgs.gov/sir/2010/5199/. (Accessed August 21, 2016.)

17. Sinha, S. K., Misbahuddin, M., & Ahmed, A. N. (2003). Factors involved in the development of chronic arsenic poisoning in Bangladesh. *Archives of Environmental Health, 58*(11), 699–700. PubMed PMID: 15702894.

18. Meliker, J. R., Franzblau, A., Slotnick, M. J., & Nriagu, J. O. (2006). Major contributors to inorganic arsenic intake in southeastern Michigan. *International Journal of Hygiene and Environmental Health, 209*(5), 399–411. PubMed PMID: 16731038.

19. U.S. Food and Drug Administration Center for Food Safety and Applied Nutrition. *Total Diet Study Statistics on Element Results.* Available at http://www.fda.gov/downloads/Food/FoodScienceResearch/TotalDietStudy/UCM243059.pdf. (Accessed August 17, 2016.)

20. Centers for Disease Control and Prevention. *National Report on Human Exposure to Environmental Chemicals: Updated tables*, 2017. Available at www.cdc.gov/exposurereport/. (Accessed August 17, 2017.)

21. Gilbert-Diamond, D., Cottingham, K. L., Gruber, J. F., Punshon, T., Sayarath, V., Gandolfi, A. J., et al. (2011). Rice consumption contributes to arsenic exposure in US women. *Proceedings of the National Academy of Sciences of the United States of America, 108*(51), 20656–20660. PubMed PMID: 22143778.

22. Davis, M. A., Mackenzie, T. A., Cottingham, K. L., Gilbert-Diamond, D., Punshon, T., & Karagas, M. R. (2012). Rice consumption and urinary arsenic concentrations in U.S. children. *Environmental Health Perspectives, 120*(10), 1418–1424. PMID: 23008276.

23. Juhasz, A. L., Smith, E., Weber, J., Rees, M., Rofe, A., Kuchel, T., et al. (2006). In vivo assessment of arsenic bioavailability in rice and its significance for human health risk assessment. *Environmental Health Perspectives, 114*(12), 1826–1831. PubMed PMID: 17185270.

24. Williams, P. N., Raab, A., Feldmann, J., & Meharg, A. A. (2007). Market basket survey shows elevated levels of As in South Central U.S. processed rice compared to California: Consequences for human dietary exposure. *Environmental Science & Technology, 41*(7), 2178–2183. PubMed PMID: 17438760.

25. Sengupta, M. K., Hossain, M. A., Mukherjee, A., Ahamed, S., Das, B., Nayak, B., et al. (2006). Arsenic burden of cooked rice: Traditional and modern methods. *Food and Chemical Toxicology, 44*(11), 1823–1829. PMID:16876928.

26. Raab, A., Baskaran, C., Feldmann, J., & Meharg, A. A. (2009). Cooking rice in a high water to rice ratio reduces inorganic arsenic content. *Journal of Environmental Monitoring, 11*(1), 41–44. PubMed PMID: 19137137.

27. Nachman, K. E., Baron, P. A., Raber, G., Francesconi, K. A., Navas-Acien, A., & Love, D. C. (2013). Roxarsone, inorganic arsenic, and other arsenic species in chicken: A U.S.-based market basket sample. *Environmental Health Perspectives, 121*(7), 818–824. PMID: 23694900.

28. Wu, C. C., Chen, M. C., Huang, Y. K., Huang, C. Y., Lai, L. A., Chung, C. J., et al. (2013). Environmental tobacco smoke and arsenic methylation capacity are associated with urothelial carcinoma. *Journal of the Formosan Medical Association, 112*(9), 554–560. PubMed PMID: 23871550.

29. Feki-Tounsi, M., Olmedo, P., Gil, F., Khlifi, R., Mhiri, M. N., Rebai, A., et al. (2013). Low-level arsenic exposure is associated with bladder cancer risk and cigarette smoking: A case-control study among men in Tunisia. *Environmental Science and Pollution Research International, 20*(6), 3923–3931. PubMed PMID: 23184132.

30. National Institute of Health National Library of Medicine. *Haz-Map.* Available at https://hazmap.nlm.nih.gov/category-details?id=260&table=tblprocesses. (Accessed August 17, 2016.)

31. Lin, T. S., Wu, C. C., Wu, J. D., & Wei, C. H. (2012). Oxidative DNA damage estimated by urinary 8-hydroxy-2'-deoxyguanosine and arsenic in glass production workers. *Toxicology and Industrial Health, 28*(6), 513–521. PubMed PMID: 22033425.

32. Hood, E. (2006). The apple bites back: Claiming old orchards for residential development. *Environmental Health Perspectives, 114*(8), A470–A476. PubMed PMID:16882511.

33. Boyce, C. P., Lewis, A. S., Sax, S. N., Eldan, M., Cohen, S. M., & Beck, B. D. (2008). Probabilistic analysis of human health risks associated with background concentrations of inorganic arsenic: Use of a margin of exposure approach. *Human and Ecological Risk Assessment, 14*, 1159–1201.

34. Gilbert-Diamond, D., Cottingham, K. L., Gruber, J. F., Punshon, T., Sayarath, V., Gandolfi, A. J., et al. (2011). Rice consumption contributes to arsenic exposure in US women. *Proceedings of the National Academy of Sciences of the United States of America, 108*(51), 20656–20660. PubMed PMID:22143778.

35. Banerjee, M., Banerjee, N., Bhattacharjee, P., Mondal, D., Lythgoe, P. R., et al. (2013). High arsenic in rice is associated with elevated genotoxic effects in humans. *Scientific Reports, 3*, 2195. PMID: 23873074.

36. Soare, A., Del Toro, R., Khazrai, Y. M., Di Mauro, A., Fallucca, S., Angeletti, S., et al. (2016). A 6-month follow-up study of the randomized controlled Ma-Pi macrobiotic dietary intervention (MADIAB trial) in type 2 diabetes. *Nutrition & Diabetes [electronic resource], 6*(8), e222. PubMed PMID: 27525817.

37. Soare, A., Del Toro, R., Roncella, E., Khazrai, Y. M., Angeletti, S., Dugo, L., et al; MADIAB Group. (2015). The effect of macrobiotic Ma-Pi 2 diet on systemic inflammation in patients with type 2 diabetes: A post

hoc analysis of the MADIAB trial. *BMJ Open Diabetes Research & Care [electronic resource]*, *3*(1), e000079. PubMed PMID: 25852946.

38. Candela, M., Biagi, E., Soverini, M., Consolandi, C., Quercia, S., Severgnini, M., et al. (2016). Modulation of gut microbiota dysbioses in type 2 diabetic patients by macrobiotic Ma-Pi 2 diet. *The British Journal of Nutrition*, *116*(1), 80–93. PubMed PMID: 27151248.

39. D'Ippoliti, D., Santelli, E., De Sario, M., Scortichini, M., Davoli, M., & Michelozzi, P. (2015). Arsenic in drinking water and mortality for cancer and chronic diseases in central Italy, 1990-2010. *PLoS ONE*, *10*(9), e0138182. PubMed PMID: 26383851.

40. Dauphiné, D. C., Smith, A. H., Yuan, Y., Balmes, J. R., Bates, M. N., & Steinmaus, C. (2013). Case-control study of arsenic in drinking water and lung cancer in California and Nevada. *International Journal of Environmental Research and Public Health*, *10*(8), 3310–3324. PubMed PMID: 23917816.

41. García-Esquinas, E., Pollán, M., Umans, J. G., Francesconi, K. A., Goessler, W., Guallar, E., et al. (2013). Arsenic exposure and cancer mortality in a US-based prospective cohort: The strong heart study, *22*(11), 1944–1953. PubMed PMID: 23800676. Erratum in: *Cancer Epidemiology, Biomarkers and Prevention*, 2013;*22*(8):1479.

42. Baris, D., Waddell, R., Beane Freeman, L. E., Schwenn, M., Colt, J. S., Ayotte, J. D., et al. (2016). Elevated bladder cancer in northern New England: The role of drinking water and arsenic. *Journal of the National Cancer Institute*, *108*(9). pii: djw099. PubMed PMID: 27140955.

43. Gilbert-Diamond, D., Li, Z., Perry, A. E., Spencer, S. K., Gandolfi, A. J., & Karagas, M. R. (2013). A population-based case-control study of urinary arsenic species and squamous cell carcinoma in New Hampshire, USA. *Environmental Health Perspectives*, *121*(10), 1154–1160. PubMed PMID: 23872349. Erratum in: *Environmental Health Perspectives*. 2013;*121*(10): 1159.

44. Das, D., Bindhani, B., Mukherjee, B., Saha, H., Biswas, P., Dutta, K., et al. (2014). Chronic low-level arsenic exposure reduces lung function in male population without skin lesions. *International Journal of Public Health*, *59*(4), 659–663. PubMed PMID: 24879317.

45. Abhyankar, L. N., Jones, M. R., Guallar, E., & Navas-Acien, A. (2012). Arsenic exposure and hypertension: A systematic review. *Environmental Health Perspectives*, *120*(4), 494–500. PMID: 22138666.

46. Moon, K. A., Guallar, E., Umans, J. G., Devereux, R. B., Best, L. G., Francesconi, K. A., et al. (2013). Association between exposure to low to moderate arsenic levels and incident cardiovascular disease: A prospective cohort study. *Annals of Internal Medicine*, *159*, 649. PubMed PMID:24061511.

47. Feseke, S. K., St-Laurent, J., Anassour-Sidi, E., Ayotte, P., Bouchard, M., & Levallois, P. (2015). Arsenic exposure and type 2 diabetes: Results from the 2007-2009 Canadian Health Measures Survey. *Health Promotion and Chronic Disease Prevention in Canada: Research, Policy and Practice*, *35*(4), 63–72. PubMed PMID: 26083521.

48. Gribble, M. O., Howard, B. V., Umans, J. G., Shara, N. M., Francesconi, K. A., Goessler, W., et al. (2012). Arsenic exposure, diabetes prevalence, and diabetes control in the Strong Heart Study. *American Journal of Epidemiology*, *176*(10), 869–874. PubMed PMID: 23097256.

49. Meliker, J. R., Wahl, R. L., Cameron, L. L., & Nriagu, J. O. (2007). Arsenic in drinking water and cerebrovascular disease, diabetes mellitus, and kidney disease in Michigan: A standardized mortality ratio analysis. *Environmental Health: A Global Access Science Source*, *6*, 4. PubMed PMID: 17274811.

50. Cardenas, A., Smit, E., Houseman, E. A., Kerkvliet, N. I., Bethel, J. W., & Kile, M. L. (2015). Arsenic exposure and prevalence of the varicella zoster virus in the United States: NHANES (2003-2004 and 2009-2010). *Environmental Health Perspectives*, *123*(6), 590–596. PubMed PMID: 25636148.

51. O'Bryant, S. E., Edwards, M., Menon, C. V., Gong, G., & Barber, R. (2011). Long-term low-level arsenic exposure is associated with poorer neuropsychological functioning: A Project FRONTIER study. *International Journal of Environmental Research and Public Health*, *8*(3), 861–874. PubMed PMID: 21556183.

52. Zheng, Y., Tao, S., Lian, F., Chau, B. T., Chen, J., Sun, G., et al. (2012). Sulforaphane prevents pulmonary damage in response to inhaled arsenic by activating the Nrf2-defense response. *Toxicology and Applied Pharmacology*, *265*(3), 292–299. PubMed PMID: 22975029.

53. Shinkai, Y., Sumi, D., Fukami, I., Ishii, T., & Kumagai, Y. (2006). Sulforaphane, an activator of Nrf2, suppresses cellular accumulation of arsenic and its cytotoxicity in primary mouse hepatocytes. *FEBS Letters*, *580*(7), 1771–1774. PubMed PMID: 16516206.

54. Biswas, J., Sinha, D., Mukherjee, S., Roy, S., Siddiqi, M., & Roy, M. (2010). Curcumin protects DNA damage in a chronically arsenic-exposed population of West Bengal. *Human and Experimental Toxicology*, *29*(6), 513–524. PubMed PMID: 20056736.

55. Gao, S., Duan, X., Wang, X., Dong, D., Liu, D., Li, X., et al. (2013). Curcumin attenuates arsenic-induced

hepatic injuries and oxidative stress in experimental mice through activation of Nrf2 pathway, promotion of arsenic methylation and urinary excretion. *Food and Chemical Toxicology, 59*, 739–747. PubMed PMID: 23871787.

56. Roy, M., Sinha, D., Mukherjee, S., & Biswas, J. (2011). Curcumin prevents DNA damage and enhances the repair potential in a chronically arsenic-exposed human population in West Bengal, India. *European Journal of Cancer Prevention, 20*(2), 123–131. PubMed PMID: 21332098.

57. Sinha, D., Roy, M., Dey, S., Siddiqi, M., & Bhattacharya, R. K. (2003). Modulation of arsenic induced cytotoxicity by tea. *Asian Pacific Journal of Cancer Prevention, 4*(3), 233–237. PubMed PMID; 14507244.

58. Sinha, D., Roy, M., Siddiqi, M., & Bhattacharya, R. K. (2005). Arsenic-induced micronuclei formation in mammalian cells and its counteraction by tea. *Journal of Environmental Pathology, Toxicology and Oncology, 24*(1), 49–56. PubMed PMID: 15715508.

10

Cadmium

SUMMARY

- Portion of population with body load increasing risk of disease: >50%
- Major diseases: Renal disease, osteoporosis, lung, prostate, and pancreatic cancers; reduced cognition, diabetes, and reproductive difficulties
- Primary sources: Smoking and consumption of tofu

- Best measure: First morning urine level for total body burden
- Best intervention: Calcium disodium EDTA chelation with glutathione, diet high in polyphenolic compounds

Description

Cadmium (Cd) is a toxic heavy metal that is widely distributed throughout the world. Environmental and human contamination by industry has occurred primarily through metal smelting and more recently battery manufacturing. It is also used industrially in the manufacturing of pigments, coatings, plastics, and in metal plating processes. It has been found in fertilizers produced from industrial waste that are then applied to agricultural land, where the cadmium content increases in both soil[1] and crops.[2] Nonoccupational exposure occurs mainly through tobacco smoke. Food and tobacco have elevated cadmium levels when grown with high-phosphate fertilizers that are contaminated with cadmium.[3]

Occupational medicine studies consistently report severe renal toxic effects from cadmium, leading to chronic kidney disease along with serious demineralization of the bones in those exposed to high levels of cadmium.

Cadmium causes increased oxidative damage to any cell or tissue it encounters. Enhanced oxidative stress and mitochondrial dysfunction from cadmium exposure have been documented along with an increased level of urinary 8-hydroxy-2'-deoxyquanosine. Cadmium also alters DNA methylation[4] and has demonstrated estrogenic

activity.[5] Cadmium is classified as a category 1 human carcinogen by the International Agency for Research on Cancer as well as other organizations.[6]

SOURCES

Nonoccupational exposure to cadmium occurs for individuals living in areas industrially contaminated by cadmium. This includes those living in reclaimed industrial areas proximal to former smelting facilities. Persons living close to municipal waste incinerators as well as those downwind of coal-burning facilities are also exposed. However, nonobvious industrial exposure must also be considered, such as living or working near a corporation producing colored glass, as can be seen in Fig. 10.1.

For most of the population, the single greatest nonoccupational exposure source of cadmium is cigarette smoke, followed by dietary sources.[7,8] Cadmium is readily absorbed through the respiratory tract and, to a far lower extent, in the gastrointestinal tract. Cadmium is absorbed in the intestines via divalent metal transporter 1 (DMT-1) that transports Fe, Cd, Ni, Pb, Co, Mn, Zn, and Cu in the bloodstream.[9] This accounts for its increased absorption in those who are iron deficient.[10] Moderate dietary

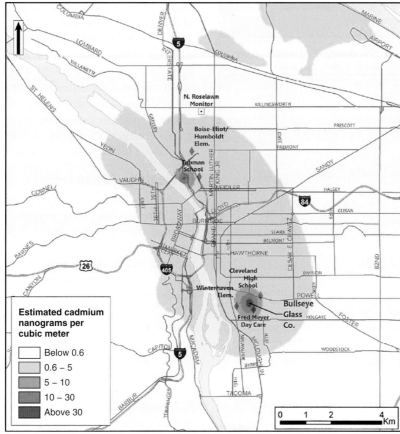

FIG. 10.1 Cadmium exposure in Portland, Oregon, from colored glass manufacturing. http://www.oregonlive.com/environment/index.ssf/2016/02/second_portland_glass_company.html (accessed 1/10/2017)

deficiencies of iron, zinc, and calcium also enhance the absorption of cadmium, whereas an abundance of these minerals in the body reduces absorption.[11] Men absorb about 5% of dietary cadmium, whereas women absorb twice that amount. This is likely due to women's need to absorb more calcium. Table 10.1 lists the cadmium content of selected foods.

A study from the Fred Hutchison Cancer Research center in Seattle, Washington, confirmed the contribution of cooked cereals and green leafy vegetables (both cooked and in salads) to the cadmium burden of healthy premenopausal women.[12] This study also discovered that the greatest dietary contributor was tofu, a food category that the U.S. Food and Drug Administration (FDA) Total Diet Study did not include in its study. This category includes tofu, tempeh, and products such as tofu hotdogs,

tofu cheese, and soy burgers. In fact, the data revealed that once-weekly consumption of tofu increased urinary cadmium by 0.11 μg/g, only 0.02 μg/g less than the increase attributed to smoking. In women who ingested any of those tofu products twice weekly or more, the urinary cadmium burden increased by 0.30 μg/g, more than twice the increase found from smoking in this study.

A study in Spain also gave additional insights revealing that fish and shellfish both provide the greatest sources of dietary cadmium.[13] Interestingly, alcohol consumption has been associated with reduced cadmium absorption.[6]

BODY BURDEN

After entry into the body (via the respiratory or gastrointestinal tract), cadmium binds to serum albumin and

TABLE 10.1   Cadmium Content of Foods in the FDA Total Diet Study

Food	Frequency Found, %	Cadmium in PPM
Roasted sunflower seeds	100	0.478
Spinach (fresh or frozen)	100	0.144
Beef liver	100	0.58
Potato chips	99.8	0.56
Peanuts/peanut butter	100	0.55
French fries/baked potato	99.8	0.53
Shredded wheat cereal	100	0.52
Pasta	100	0.32
Boiled shrimp	90	0.17 (0.009–0.226)

Modified from U.S. Food and Drug Administration. (December 11, 2007). Total Diet Study Statistics on Element Results. By Center for Food Safety and Applied Nutrition. Retrieved from http://www.fda.gov/downloads/Food/FoodScienceResearch/TotalDietStudy/UCM243059.pdf

TABLE 10.2   Cadmium Tissue Distribution and Half-life

Body Distribution	Half-life (persistence)	Representing
Blood	3–4 months	Current exposure
Kidney	10–40 years	Body burden

accumulates in the liver, where it is complexed with metallothionein-1.[14] The blood then carries this cadmium-metallothionein complex to the kidneys, where it is absorbed in the proximal tubules and then stored in the renal cortex. The blood half-life of cadmium is 3 to 4 months and represents a combination of body burden and current exposure. Close to 50% of the total body cadmium burden resides in the kidneys, where it has a much longer half-life of 10 to 40 years (Table 10.2). The urinary cadmium content has been shown to be directly related to the kidney burden and is considered the best measurement of total body cadmium burden.[15] Approximately 0.007% of the total body burden of cadmium is excreted daily in urine, with an additional 0.009% excreted fecally.

Cadmium is found ubiquitously in all human studies in all parts of the world. The January 2017 updated tables in the United States Centers for Disease Control (CDC) Fourth National Report on Human Exposure expanded the reporting and gave averages for both smokers and nonsmokers.[16] The findings were consistent with other studies from across the globe showing that women typically have a higher cadmium burden than men.

Clinical Significance

Chronic, low-level cadmium exposure has been associated with increased risk for the same health problems found in those occupationally exposed to far higher levels. Diseases associated with nonoccupational low-level exposure include osteoporosis, kidney damage, hypertension, insulin resistance, diabetes, cancers, and increased rates of miscarriage.

Cardiovascular Mortality Risk.   Approximately 14,000 adults who participated in the National Health and Nutritional Examination Survey (NHANES) trial (1988–1994) were followed through the end of 2001 to see what association, if any, urinary cadmium had with all-cause and specific-cause mortality.[17] In this sampling of North American residents, the mean urinary cadmium level was 0.40 µg/g creatinine. When that level doubled to 0.80 µg/g creatinine, significant mortality associations were noted. The hazard ratio (HR) for cardiovascular mortality increased by 21%, and all-cause mortality increased by 28%. Death risk from coronary heart disease increased by 36%, whereas overall risk of cancer mortality increased by 55%. NHANES data from 1999 to 2004 confirmed those findings but reported greater HR. When persons with urinary cadmium levels >0.57 µg/g (the 80th percentile for this group) were compared with those with levels <0.14 µg/g, the HR for all-cause mortality was 1.54, cardiovascular disease mortality was 1.74, and coronary heart disease mortality ratio was 2.09.[18] Other studies have reported both increasing blood pressure[19] and increasing stroke risk linked to elevations in cadmium levels.[20]

Cancer Risk.   In the first mortality risk study, mentioned earlier,[17] urinary cadmium levels >0.80 µg/g creatinine were associated with a 55% increase in overall cancer mortality. The STRONG heart study research group

TABLE 10.3   CDC 2017 Fourth Report Cadmium Levels

	50th Percentile	75th Percentile	90th Percentile	95th Percentile
Urinary[a]				
2009 total averages (μg/g)	0.208	0.412	0.678	0.940
2014 total averages (μg/g)	0.138	0.288	0.563	0.800
Nonsmoker 2011–2014	0.160	0.298	0.549	0.753
Smoker 2011–2014	0.259	0.528	0.910	1.48
Blood[b]				
2011–2014 (μg/L)	0.210	0.410	0.840	1.22

[a]Note: OSHA – Industrial standards for urinary cadmium: <3 μg/g cr
[b]Note: OSHA – Industrial standards for blood cadmium: <5 μg/L

reviewed their data to specifically look at the relationship between cadmium burden in their subjects and cancer mortality.[21] The STRONG heart study group was composed of more than 4500 adult Native Americans from four states (Arizona, Oklahoma, North Dakota, and South Dakota). Smoking was the main source of cadmium exposure in the participants whose creatinine-corrected median urinary cadmium burden was 0.93 μg/g (levels almost three times that found in smokers in the CDC Fourth Report [Table 10.3]). In this study, a urinary cadmium level of 0.55 μg/g comprised the 20th percentile, whereas those in the 80th percentile averaged 1.62 μg/g. After numerous adjustments, comparing those with an average urine cadmium of 0.55 μg/g to those with 1.62 μg/g revealed dramatically increased cancer HRs. The adjusted HR for total cancer was 1.30, lung cancer 2.27, and prostate cancer 2.40.

A study of persons living in southern Louisiana specifically focused on pancreatic cancer risk in relation to cadmium burden.[22] In this study, urinary cadmium levels were presented in four quartiles with the following ranges: <0.5 μg/g, 0.5 to <1 μg/g, 1 to <1.5 μg/g, and >1.5 μg/g creatinine. Persons with urinary cadmium levels in the second quartile (0.5 to <1.0 μg/g) had a 3.34 increased risk for pancreatic cancer, whereas those in the third quartile had an odds ratio (OR) of 5.58 and those in the fourth quartile had a 7.70-fold increase in risk. A Taiwanese study revealed that increased risk for urothelial cancers was found in persons with higher urinary cadmium levels.[23]

Renal Disorders. The concentration of cadmium in the renal tissue of smokers is twice that of nonsmokers (40 μg/g versus 20 μg/g).[24] Cadmium damages the renal cortex and proximal tubules, resulting in increased urinary excretion of proteins and tubular enzymes. The released markers include alpha-1 microglobulin (A1M) and N-acetyl-beta-D-glucosaminidase (NAG), both of which have been used as markers for cadmium-induced renal dysfunction. A study of Korean adults showed a positive correlation between urinary cadmium levels and both NAG and 8-hydroxy-2'-deoxyquanosine (8-OHdG). In this study, urinary cadmium levels higher than 0.91 μg/g creatinine were associated with renal damage.[25] Swedish women with a mean urinary cadmium level of 0.80 μg/g creatinine showed significant elevation of markers for renal damage.[26] Renal damage with urinary cadmium levels as low as 0.6 μg/g creatinine was found in Japanese men,[27] whereas urinary cadmium levels as low as 0.52 μg/g creatinine were associated with increased urinary A1M and albumin readings in a different Swedish study.[28] A study of healthy kidney donors whose first morning urine cadmium ranged from 0.04 to 1.12 μg/g (with a mean of 0.29) also showed associations. In this study, kidney tissue burden of cadmium and urinary cadmium levels were both positively and significantly associated with A1M levels.[29] This group of researchers felt that A1M was the most sensitive biomarker for kidney damage from cadmium.

Bone Disorders. The combination of osteoporosis, osteomalacia, and kidney damage was first noted in Japan in areas with high cadmium contamination.[24,30] An increase in urinary calcium is positively associated with cadmium burden and may be related to reduced activation of $25(OH)D_3$ to the more active $1,25(OH)_2D_3$ by the kidney. In a nonindustrially exposed population with relatively low kidney levels of cadmium, simply having cadmium tissue levels higher than the mean significantly increased urinary calcium excretion and decreased bone density.[31] Further, a doubling of urinary cadmium (in a nonoccupationally exposed group) increased the risk of bone fractures in women by 73% and loss of height in men by 60%.[32] Data from the 1988 to 1994 and 1999 to 2004 NHANES revealed that women over 50 with urinary cadmium levels higher than 0.50 µg/g creatinine had a 43% increased risk of being diagnosed with osteoporosis.[33] In children, a doubling of urinary cadmium increased risk of bone resorption by 1.72 times.[34]

Persons with periodontal disease, another form of bone loss, also tend to have higher urinary cadmium levels.[35] Individuals with a urinary cadmium level of only 0.63 µg/g were 54% more likely to have this health problem.

Endocrine (Diabetes and Reproduction). A review of the data from NHANES (1988–1994) for 8772 adults revealed an association between urinary cadmium levels and both elevated fasting blood glucose and type 2 diabetes mellitus (T2DM) (Table 10.4).[36] Elevated fasting glucose and T2DM risk increased dose-dependently with the cadmium levels. Persons with urinary cadmium levels higher than 0.99 µg/g creatinine were 24% more likely to have T2DM and 48% more likely to have elevated fasting glucose. When urine cadmium was higher than 2.0 µg/g, the risk for elevated blood glucose doubled, whereas diabetes risk increased to 45%. The risk for gestational diabetes was found to be elevated in pregnant women from Seattle with far lower urinary cadmium levels than what was found to increase fasting glucose in the study utilizing NHANES data.[37] A 64% increase

in the risk for gestational diabetes (defined by two or more 3-hour glucose tolerance test results exceeding the American Diabetes Association guidelines) was found in women with urinary cadmium levels higher than 0.29 µg/g. When the urinary cadmium content went above 0.43, the risk for gestational diabetes doubled (OR 2.07).

Women with a history of miscarriage, uterine fibroids, and hirsutism have demonstrated evidence of higher kidney cadmium burden.[38] In women participating in the 1999–2002 NHANES, blood cadmium levels were positively associated with higher rates of endometriosis.[39] Those with endometriosis had an average blood cadmium level of 0.53 µg/L, whereas those without endometriosis had a lower average, 0.42 µg/L. Women in the highest tertile of blood cadmium level had more than three times the risk of endometriosis as those in the first tertile (OR 3.39). Higher cadmium levels in girls have been associated with delayed puberty,[40] and in pregnant women with lower-birth-weight infants.[41] Higher cadmium levels have also been associated with high follicle-stimulating hormone (FSH) levels and infertility in men.[42]

Neurological Functioning. Cadmium exposure in children has been associated with a variety of neurological problems. A cohort of mother–child pairs were followed from pregnancy through the child's fifth birthday, comparing urinary cadmium levels with measurements of the children's IQ.[43] The urinary cadmium levels in the mothers ranged from 0.13 to 2.0 µg/L, with a mean of 0.63 µg/L. A doubling of the mother's urinary cadmium level caused a reduction in her child's verbal IQ, performance IQ, and full-scale IQ. The urinary cadmium level of children age 5 was associated with reduced performance IQ and behavior problems. Data on children ages 6 to 15 from NHANES were used to assess neurodevelopmental associations with urinary cadmium levels.[44] When the researchers compared those children in the highest NHANES quartile for urinary cadmium with those in the lowest, it revealed a threefold increased risk that the child would require special education and a 3.21-fold risk that the child would have learning disabilities. When the NHANES data on adults were used to assess the association of cadmium and neuroperformance, it was found that higher urinary cadmium was associated with a reduction in attention and perception.[45] NHANES data also revealed that adults in the highest quintile of blood cadmium were 13% more likely to have a reduction in hearing acuity.[46]

TABLE 10.4 **Blood Sugar and Diabetes Risk (OR) According to Urinary Cadmium Levels**		
Urinary Cadmium (µg/g cr)	High Fasting Glucose	Type 2 Diabetes Mellitus
0–0.99	1	1
1.00–1.99	1.48	1.24
>2	2.05	1.45

Data from Schwartz, G. G., Il'yasova, D., & Ivanova, A. (2003). Urinary cadmium, impaired fasting glucose, and diabetes in the NHANES III. *Diabetes Care, 26*(2), 468–470.

TABLE 10.5 Odds Ratios for Diseases by CDC Fourth Report Percentile

Disease	CDC Percentile	Odds and Hazard Ratios
Pancreatic cancer	≥50th	OR 3.34[22]
Gestational diabetes	≥50th	OR 1.64[37]
Pancreatic cancer	≥75th	OR 3.34[22]
Gestational diabetes	≥75th	OR 2.07[37]
Bone resorption	≥75th	In children, OR 1.72[34]
Fracture risk	≥75th	OR 1.73[32]
Height loss	≥75th	OR 1.62[32]
Osteoporosis	≥75th	For women 50+ = OR 1.43[33]
Cancer mortality	≥75th	HR 1.55[17]
Cardiovascular mortality	≥75th	HR 1.74[17,18]
Hepatic inflammation	>75th	OR 2.21[48]
Nonalcoholic steatohepatitis	>75th	OR 1.95[48]
Reduced FEV/FVC	>75th	Significant reduction in lung function[49]
Late puberty	>75th	Delayed development in girls[40]
Endometriosis	>75th	OR 3.34 [39]
Pancreatic cancer	≥95th	OR 5.58–7.70[22]
Neurocognition	≥95th	1 µg/L increase = 93% decrease in performance[45]
Learning disability	>95th	Child has 3.21-fold risk of learning disability[44]
Special education	>95th	Child has threefold risk of needing special ed[44]
Diabetes	>95th	Above 0.99 = OR 1.48; above 2.0 = OR 2.05[36]
Kidney damage	>95th	Above 1.0 = OR 1.63 for albuminuria 25–29

Other health effects associated with low-level cadmium include hypomethylation of DNA in Argentinian women (whose urinary cadmium averaged only 0.230),[47] nonalcoholic fatty liver disease (OR 2.21) and nonalcoholic steatohepatitis (OR 1.30) with urinary cadmium of 0.65–0.83,[48] and a reduction in pulmonary function forced expiratory volume in 1 second (FEV_1) (FEV_1 and forced vital capacity (FVC)).[49] With all the chronic health problems associated with cadmium, it is not surprising to find that those with the highest blood and urine cadmium levels have shorter leukocyte telomere lengths.[50] Table 10.5 lists the odds ratios for various diseases and conditions.

INTERVENTION

Reducing Cadmium Burden

The most effective agent for the removal of cadmium from the tissues is the polyamino-polycarboxylate compound agent DPTA,[51] which is currently unavailable for use. Intravenous ethylenediaminetetraacetic acid (EDTA), which is readily available, has also demonstrated effectiveness at reducing the kidney burden of cadmium.[52] This agent was successfully used for a year on a rheumatoid arthritis patient to reduce body levels of cadmium and lead and improve her oxidative stress and disease picture.[53] A different study revealed that the use of 50 mg/kg of reduced glutathione in conjunction with intravenous CaEDTA increased the postchelation urinary release of cadmium almost fourfold.[54]

Meso-2,3-dimercaptosuccinic acid (DMSA) has also shown the ability to increase urinary excretion of cadmium, but not to the extent of EDTA.[55] Although DMSA has a higher affinity for cadmium than for any other metal, at a pH of 5.5 (commonly found in the proximal tubules), the majority of the cadmium is released from its DMSA binding. Only at a urinary pH of 7.4 is the cadmium completely DMSA-bound and carried out of the body.[56] This phenomenon could account for the relatively small increase in urinary cadmium noted on post-DMSA urine catches and may further explain its failure to alleviate cadmium burden in children treated with DMSA.[57]

The compound 2,3-dimercaptopropane-1 sulfonate (DMPS) also has an affinity to bind cadmium, but typically DMPS does not move a large amount of cadmium.[58] This is thought to be due to the difficulty that DMPS has in entering a cell to bind with cadmium. However, the addition of L-methionine to DMPS does significantly enhance both renal and fecal clearance of cadmium and reverses cadmium-induced oxidative stress.[59]

Interestingly, the iron-chelating agents deferasirox and deferiprone have both recently been shown to enhance cadmium clearance from rat tissues,[60] but no human studies have been published. In mice, the use of magnesium at 20 mg/kg before cadmium exposure resulted in a significant reduction in renal cadmium burden.[61] In a small human study of cadmium-burdened individuals in China, daily use of 150 µg of selenium resulted in a significant reduction in red blood cell cadmium levels. The researchers concluded that selenium supplementation helped to enhance fecal cadmium excretion.[62]

N-acetyl cysteine (NAC) plays a double role of protecting tissues from cadmium-induced oxidative damage[63] and reducing hepatic and renal levels of cadmium.[64] However, the results of this animal trial revealed that either DMPS or NAC should be used separately for cadmium burden, not together (Table 10.6). A synergistic cadmium mobilization effect was found in a trial using the monoisoamyl form of DMSA (MiADMS) along with NAC.[65] Not only did the use of NAC reverse the cadmium-induced reduction of glutathione, blood catalase, and superoxide dismutase (SOD), but its combination with MiADMS successfully reduced blood and tissue cadmium levels.

Use of low-temperature saunas is another means of enhancing the clearance of cadmium and other heavy metals from the body, as these toxicants are typically found in greater µg/mL of sweat than per mL of urine.[66] The benefit of sweating to greatly reduce the total body load of cadmium is only limited by the total milliliters of sweat that can be produced.

TABLE 10.6   Rat Tissue Cadmium Levels After Treatment with NAC, DMPS, or Both

Treatment	Liver (µg/g)	Kidney (µg/g)	Blood (µg/mL)
Cadmium control	80.24	57.93	0.37
Cd/NAC	55.36	31.82	0.25
Cd/ DMPS	39.79	27.08	0.29
Cd/ DMPS and NAC	37.13	45.72	0.39

From Fatemi, S. J., Saljooghi, A. S., Balooch, F. D., Iranmanesh, M., & Golbafan, M. R. (2012). Removal of cadmium by combining deferasirox and desferrioxamine chelators in rats. *Toxicology and Industrial Health*, *28*(1), 35–41.

Ameliorating Cadmium Toxicity

NAC is joined by alpha lipoic acid (ALA) in reversing cadmium-induced oxidative damage. ALA restores cadmium depletion of glutathione in the liver and throughout the body by enhancing gamma-glutamylcysteine ligase, the enzyme primarily responsible for making glutathione.[67] ALA shows equal effectiveness as intravenous glutathione in restoring cadmium-induced hematological imbalances[68] and oxidative damage in renal tissues.[69] ALA and selenium were both effective at reversing testicular damage from cadmium and restoring testosterone levels.[70] Further, the combination of ALA and melatonin exerts a synergistic effect against cadmium-induced cardiotoxicity.[71]

Both magnesium and carnosine have demonstrated effectiveness at preventing and reversing cadmium-induced cellular and tissue damage. In addition to the previously discussed cadmium tissue reduction, magnesium also demonstrated the ability to restore cadmium-induced glutathione loss.[72] Carnosine prevented hepatotoxicity from cadmium in mice by also preventing glutathione depletion and reversing the cadmium-induced increase in myeloperoxidase and caspace-3 activities.[73]

Numerous botanical agents, especially those high in flavonoid and phenol structures, have demonstrated protective activity against cadmium toxicity. Chief among these compounds are grape skins and grape juice, which are protective against multiple parameters of cadmium toxicity.[74,75,76,77] Blueberries are also quite high in polyphenolic compounds and have also demonstrated effectiveness against cadmium-induced cytotoxicity.[78] When given concurrently with cadmium exposure, blueberry extract prevented any increase in oxidative stress and maintained antioxidant enzyme activity in a dose-dependent manner. Onion extract along with quercetin (onions are the highest dietary source of this flavonoid) have demonstrated the ability to reverse cadmium-induced toxicity and dyslipidemia.[79,80] More recently, a spice mixture containing garlic, ginger, and nutmeg at levels used in cooking was able to protect rats from cadmium-induced hepatic and renal damage.[81]

Assessment

1. Compare the patient's case history to the known presentation of cadmium burden. Does the patient fit the picture of cadmium burden?
   a. In a woman, was there gestational diabetes?

2. Is there known cadmium exposure?
   a. History of smoking
   b. Regular tofu intake
   c. Consumption of sunflower seeds
   d. Use of Ayurvedic medicines
3. First morning nonchallenged urine cadmium
   a. Compare to CDC values and levels associated with cadmium-related health disorders previously listed.
4. Urinary 8-OHdG

Treatment

1. Identify and stop all current cadmium exposures.
2. Enhance normal clearance of cadmium by decreasing hepatic and renal recycling.
   a. NAC: 1000 to 2000 mg daily
   b. Magnesium: up to 500 mg daily
   c. Alkalinize the urine through diet and supplementation.
3. Increase mobilization of cadmium with chelation.
   a. Intravenous CaEDTA: 50 mg/kg with saline or sterile water for proper osmolarity; best given with 50 mg/kg glutathione.
   b. DMSA: 30 mg/kg
      i. Must have urine alkalinized to at least 7.4 during the day while taking DMSA.
      ii. L-methionine: 1 or 2 grams daily during the course of DMSA.
4. Block and reverse cadmium-induced tissue damage.
   a. Green or black teas daily
   b. NAC: 1000 to 2000 mg daily
   c. ALA: 300 to 600 mg
   d. Liposomal glutathione: 500 mg daily
   e. Blueberries, onions, and spices in diet

REFERENCES

1. Brännvall, E., Wolters, M., Sjöblom, R., & Kumpiene, J. (2015). Elements availability in soil fertilized with pelletized fly ash and biosolids. *Journal of Environmental Management, 159*, 27–36. PubMed PMID: 26042629.
2. Abril, J. M., García-Tenorio, R., Enamorado, S. M., Hurtado, M. D., Andreu, L., & Delgado, A. (2008). The cumulative effect of three decades of phosphogypsum amendments in reclaimed marsh soils from SW Spain: (226)Ra, (238)U and Cd contents in soils and tomato fruit. *The Science of the Total Environment, 403*(1–3), 80–88. PubMed PMID: 18602676.
3. Lugon-Moulin, N., Martin, F., Krauss, M. R., Ramey, P. B., & Rossi, L. (2006). Cadmium concentration in tobacco (Nicotiana tabacum L.) from different countries and its relationship with other elements. *Chemosphere, 63*(7), 1074–1086. PMID: 16310829.
4. Jiang, G., Xu, L., Song, S., Zhu, C., Wu, Q., Zhang, L., et al. (2008). Effects of long-term low-dose cadmium exposure on genomic DNA methylation in human embryo lung fibroblast cells. *Toxicology, 244*(1), 49–55. PubMed PMID: 18077075.
5. Johnson, M. D., Kenney, N., Stoica, A., Hilakivi-Clarke, L., Singh, B., Chepko, G., et al. (2003). Cadmium mimics the in vivo effects of estrogen in the uterus and mammary gland. *Nature Medicine, 9*(8), 1081–1084. PubMed PMID: 12858169.
6. Waalkes, M. P. (2003). Cadmium carcinogenesis. *Mutation Research, 533*(1–2), 107–120. PubMed PMID: 14643415.
7. *US Centers for Disease Control and Prevention, Department of Health and Human Services.* (2009). Fourth National Report on Human Exposure to Environmental Chemicals. CAS No. 7440-43-9. www.cdc.gov/exposurereport. (Accessed August 24, 2016.)
8. Gunier, R. B., Horn-Ross, P. L., Canchola, A. J., Duffy, C. N., Reynolds, P., Hertz, A., et al. (2013). Determinants and within-person variability of urinary cadmium concentrations among women in northern California. *Environmental Health Perspectives, 121*(6), 643–649. PubMed PMID: 23552363.
9. Garrick, M. D., Dolan, K. G., Horbinshy, C., Ghio, A. J., Higgins, D., Porubcin, M., et al. (2003). DMT1: A mammalian transporter for multiple metals. *BioMetals, 16*, 41–54. PubMed PMID: 12572663.
10. Kippler, M., Ekström, E. C., Lönnerdal, B., Goessler, W., Akesson, A., El Arifeen, S., et al. (2007). Influence of iron and zinc status on cadmium accumulation in Bangladeshi women. *Toxicology and Applied Pharmacology, 222*(2), 221–226. PubMed PMID: 17543360.
11. Reeves, P. G., & Chaney, R. L. (2008). Bioavailability as an issue in risk assessment and management of food cadmium: A review. *The Science of the Total Environment, 398*(1–3), 13–19. PubMed PMID: 18430461.
12. Adams, S. V., Newcomb, P. A., Shafer, M. M., Atkinson, C., Bowles, E. J., Newton, K. M., et al. (2011). Sources of cadmium exposure among healthy premenopausal women. *The Science of the Total Environment, 409*(9), 1632–1637. PubMed PMID: 21333327.
13. Llobet, J. M., Falcó, G., Casas, C., Teixidó, A., & Domingo, J. L. (2003). Concentrations of arsenic, cadmium, mercury, and lead in common foods and estimated daily intake by children, adolescents, adults, and seniors

of Catalonia, Spain. *Journal of Agricultural and Food Chemistry, 51*(3), 838–842. PubMed PMID: 12537467.

14. Ferraro, P. M., Costanzi, S., Naticchia, A., Sturniolo, A., & Gambaro, G. (2010). Low level exposure to cadmium increases the risk of chronic kidney disease: Analysis of the NHANES 1999-2006. *BMC Public Health, 10*, 304. PubMed PMID: 20525263.

15. Orlowski, C., Piotrowski, J. K., Subdys, J. K., & Gross, A. (1998). Urinary cadmium as indicator of renal cadmium in humans: An autopsy study. *Human and Experimental Toxicology, 17*(6), 302–306. PubMed PMID: 9688352.

16. Centers for Disease Control and Prevention. (January 2017). *National Report on Human Exposure to Environmental Chemicals: Updated Tables.* Available at www.cdc.gov/exposurereport/. (Accessed October 25, 2017.)

17. Menke, A., Muntner, P., Silbergeld, E. K., Platz, E. A., & Guallar, E. (2009). Cadmium levels in urine and mortality among U.S. adults. *Environmental Health Perspectives, 117*(2), 190–196. PubMed PMID: 19270787.

18. Tellez-Plaza, M., Navas-Acien, A., Menke, A., Crainiceanu, C. M., Pastor-Barriuso, R., & Guallar, E. (2012). Cadmium exposure and all-cause and cardiovascular mortality in the U.S. general population. *Environmental Health Perspectives, 120*(7), 1017–1022. PubMed PMID: 22472185.

19. Gallagher, C. M., & Meliker, J. R. (2010). Blood and urine cadmium, blood pressure, and hypertension: A systematic review and meta-analysis. *Environmental Health Perspectives, 118*(12), 1676–1684. PubMed PMID: 20716508.

20. Peters, J. L., Perlstein, T. S., Perry, M. J., McNeely, E., & Weuve, J. (2010). Cadmium exposure in association with history of stroke and heart failure. *Environmental Research, 110*(2), 199–206. PubMed PMID: 20060521.

21. García-Esquinas, E., Pollan, M., Tellez-Plaza, M., Francesconi, K. A., Goessler, W., Guallar, E., et al. (2014). Cadmium exposure and cancer mortality in a prospective cohort: The strong heart study. *Environmental Health Perspectives, 122*(4), 363–370. PubMed PMID: 24531129.

22. Luckett, B. G., Su, L. J., Rood, J. C., & Fontham, E. T. (2012). Cadmium exposure and pancreatic cancer in south Louisiana. *Journal of Environmental and Public Health, 2012*, 180186. PubMed PMID: 23319964.

23. Chang, C. H., Liu, C. S., Liu, H. J., Huang, C. P., Huang, C. Y., Hsu, H. T., et al. (2016). Association between levels of urinary heavy metals and increased risk of urothelial carcinoma. *International Journal of Urology, 23*(3), 233–239. PubMed PMID: 26663353.

24. Järup, L., Berglund, M., Elinder, C. G., Nordberg, G., & Vahter, M. (1998). Health effects of cadmium

exposure—a review of the literature and a risk estimate. *Scandinavian Journal of Work, Environment and Health, 24*(Suppl. 1), 1–51. PubMed PMID: 9569444.

25. Huang, M., Choi, S. J., Kim, D. W., Kim, N. Y., Park, C. H., Yu, S. D., et al. (2009). Risk assessment of low-level cadmium and arsenic on the kidney. *Journal of Toxicology and Environmental Health. Part A, 72*(21–22), 1493–1498. PubMed PMID: 20077223.

26. Akesson, A., Lundh, T., Vahter, M., Bjellerup, P., Lidfeldt, J., Nerbrand, C., et al. (2005). Tubular and glomerular kidney effects in Swedish women with low environmental cadmium exposure. *Environmental Health Perspectives, 113*(11), 1627–1631. PubMed PMID: 16263522.

27. Uno, T., Kobayashi, E., Suwazono, Y., Okubo, Y., Miura, K., Sakata, K., et al. (2005). Health effects of cadmium exposure in the general environment in Japan with special reference to the lower limit of the benchmark dose as the threshold level of urinary cadmium. *Scandinavian Journal of Work, Environment and Health, 31*(4), 307–315. PubMed PMID: 16161714.

28. Akerstrom, M., Sallsten, G., Lundh, T., & Barregard, L. (2013). Associations between urinary excretion of cadmium and proteins in a nonsmoking population: Renal toxicity or normal physiology? *Environmental Health Perspectives, 121*(2), 187–191. PubMed PMID: 23128055.

29. Wallin, M., Sallsten, G., Lundh, T., & Barregard, L. (2014). Low-level cadmium exposure and effects on kidney function. *Occupational and Environmental Medicine, 71*(12), 848–854. Erratum in: *Occupational and Environmental Medicine*, 2015. 72(12), 898. PubMed PMID: 25286916.

30. Emmerson, B. T. (1970). "Ouch-ouch" disease: The osteomalacia of cadmium nephropathy. *Annals of Internal Medicine, 73*(5), 854–855. PubMed PMID: 5476215.

31. Wallin, M., Sallsten, G., Fabricius-Lagging, E., Öhrn, C., Lundh, T., & Barregard, L. (2013). Kidney cadmium levels and associations with urinary calcium and bone mineral density: A cross-sectional study in Sweden. *Environmental Health: A Global Access Science Source, 12*, 22. PubMed PMID: 23497059.

32. Staessen, J. A., Roels, H. A., Emelianov, D., Kuznetsova, T., Thijs, L., Vangronsveld, J., et al. (1999). Environmental exposure to cadmium, forearm bone density, and risk of fractures: Prospective population study. Public Health and Environmental Exposure to Cadmium (PheeCad) Study Group. *Lancet, 353*(9159), 1140–1144. PubMed PMID: 10209978.

33. Gallagher, C. M., Meliker JR. & Kovach, J. S. (2008). Urinary cadmium and osteoporosis in U.S. women >or=

50 years of age: NHANES 1988-1994 and 1999-2004. *Environmental Health Perspectives*, *116*(10), 1338–1343. PubMed PMID: 18941575.

34. Sughis, M., Penders, J., Haufroid, V., Nemery, B., & Nawrot, T. S. (2011). Bone resorption and environmental exposure to cadmium in children: A cross–sectional study. *Environmental Health: A Global Access Science Source*, *10*, 104. PubMed PMID: 22151692.

35. Arora, M., Weuve, J., Schwartz, J., & Wright, R. O. (2009). Association of environmental cadmium exposure with periodontal disease in U.S. adults. *Environmental Health Perspectives*, *117*(5), 739–744. PubMed PMID: 19479015.

36. Schwartz, G. G., Il'yasova, D., & Ivanova, A. (2003). Urinary cadmium, impaired fasting glucose, and diabetes in the NHANES III. *Diabetes Care*, *26*(2), 468–470. PubMed PMID: 12547882.

37. Romano, M. E., Enquobahrie, D. A., Simpson, C. D., Checkoway, H., & Williams, M. A. (2015). A case-cohort study of cadmium body burden and gestational diabetes mellitus in American women. *Environmental Health Perspectives*, *123*(10), 993–998. PubMed PMID: 25712731.

38. Gerhard, I., Monga, B., Waldbrenner, A., & Runnebaum, B. (1998). Heavy metals and fertility. *Journal of Toxicology and Environmental Health. Part A*, *54*(8), 593–661. Erratum in: *Journal of Toxicology Environmental Health*, 1999. 56(5), 371. PubMed PMID: 9726782.

39. Jackson, L. W., Zullo, M. D., & Goldberg, J. M. (2008). The association between heavy metals, endometriosis and uterine myomas among premenopausal women: National Health and Nutrition Examination Survey 1999-2002. *Human Reproduction*, *23*(3), 679–687. PubMed PMID: 18192673.

40. Gollenberg, A. L., Hediger, M. L., Lee, P. A., Himes, J. H., & Louis, G. M. (2010). Association between lead and cadmium and reproductive hormones in peripubertal U.S. girls. *Environmental Health Perspectives*, *118*(12), 1782–1787. PubMed PMID: 20675266.

41. Johnston, J. E., Valentiner, E., Maxson, P., Miranda, M. L., & Fry, R. C. (2014). Maternal cadmium levels during pregnancy associated with lower birth weight in infants in a North Carolina cohort. *PLoS ONE*, *9*(10), e109661. PubMed PMID: 25285731.

42. Akinloye, O., Arowojolu, A. O., Shittu, O. B., & Anetor, J. I. (2006). Cadmium toxicity: A possible cause of male infertility in Nigeria. *Reproductive Biology*, *6*(1), 17–30. PubMed PMID: 16604149.

43. Kippler, M., Tofail, F., Hamadani, J. D., Gardner, R. M., Grantham-McGregor, S. M., Bottai, M., et al. (2012).

Early-life cadmium exposure and child development in 5-year-old girls and boys: A cohort study in rural Bangladesh. *Environmental Health Perspectives*, *120*(10), 1462–1468. PubMed PMID: 22759600.

44. Ciesielski, T., Weuve, J., Bellinger, D. C., Schwartz, J., Lanphear, B., & Wright, R. O. (2012). Cadmium exposure and neurodevelopmental outcomes in U.S. children. *Environmental Health Perspectives*, *120*(5), 758–763. PubMed PMID: 22289429.

45. Ciesielski, T., Bellinger, D. C., Schwartz, J., Hauser, R., & Wright, R. O. (2013). Associations between cadmium exposure and neurocognitive test scores in a cross-sectional study of US adults. *Environmental Health: A Global Access Science Source*, *12*, 13. PubMed PMID: 23379984.

46. Choi, Y. H., Hu, H., Mukherjee, B., Miller, J., & Park, S. K. (2012). Environmental cadmium and lead exposures and hearing loss in U.S. adults: The National Health and Nutrition Examination Survey, 1999 to 2004. *Environmental Health Perspectives*, *120*(11), 1544–1550. PubMed PMID: 22851306.

47. Hossain, M. B., Vahter, M., Concha, G., & Broberg, K. (2012). Low-level environmental cadmium exposure is associated with DNA hypomethylation in Argentinean women. *Environmental Health Perspectives*, *120*(6), 879–884. PubMed PMID: 22382075.

48. Hyder, O., Chung, M., Cosgrove, D., et al. (2013). Cadmium exposure and liver disease among US adults. *Journal of Gastrointestinal Surgery*, *17*(7), 1265–1273. PubMed PMID: 23636881.

49. Lampe, B. J., Park, S. K., Robins, T., Mukherjee, B., et al. (2008). Association between 24-hour urinary cadmium and pulmonary function among community-exposed men: The VA Normative Aging Study. *Environmental Health Perspectives*, *116*(9), 1226–1230. PubMed PMID: 18795167.

50. Zota, A. R., Needham, B. L., Blackburn, E. H., Lin, J., Park, S. K., Rehkopf, D. H., et al. (2015). Associations of cadmium and lead exposure with leukocyte telomere length: Findings from National Health and Nutrition Examination Survey, 1999-2002. *American Journal of Epidemiology*, *181*(2), 127–136. PubMed PMID: 25504027.

51. Andersen, O. (1984). Chelation of cadmium. *Environmental Health Perspectives*, *54*, 249–266. PubMed PMID: 6734560.

52. Waters, R. S., Bryden, N. A., Patterson, K. Y., Veillon, C., & Anderson, R. A. (2001). EDTA chelation effects on urinary losses of cadmium, calcium, chromium, cobalt, copper, lead, magnesium, and zinc. *Biological Trace Element Research*, *83*(3), 207–221. PubMed PMID:11794513.

53. Bamonti, F., Fulgenzi, A., Novembrino, C., & Ferrero, M. E. (2011). Metal chelation therapy in rheumatoid arthritis: A case report. Successful management of rheumatoid arthritis by metal chelation therapy. *BioMetals*, *24*(6), 1093–1098. PubMed PMID: 21655943.

54. Gil, H. W., Kang, E. J., Lee, K. H., Yang, J. O., Lee, E. Y., & Hong, S. Y. (2011). Effect of glutathione on the cadmium chelation of EDTA in a patient with cadmium intoxication. *Human and Experimental Toxicology*, *30*(1), 79–83. PubMed PMID: 20413561.

55. Andersen, O., & Nielsen, J. B. (1988). Oral cadmium chloride intoxication in mice: Effects of penicillamine, dimercaptosuccinic acid and related compounds. *Pharmacology and Toxicology*, *63*(5), 386–389. PubMed PMID: 2853341.

56. Fang, X., Hua, F., & Fernando, Q. (1996). Comparison of rac- and meso-2,3-dimercaptosuccinic acids for chelation of mercury and cadmium using chemical speciation models. *Chemical Research in Toxicology*, *9*(1), 284–290. PubMed PMID: 8924605.

57. Cao, Y., Chen, A., Bottai, M., Caldwell, K. L., & Rogan, W. J. (2013). The impact of succimer chelation on blood cadmium in children with background exposures: A randomized trial. *The Journal of Pediatrics*, *163*(2), 598–600. PubMed PMID: 23601497.

58. Ruprecht, J. (1997). *Dimaval (DMPS): Scientific Product Monograph* (6th ed.). Berlin: HEYL Chem-pharm Fabrik GmbH & Co.

59. Tandon, S. K., Singh, S., & Prasad, S. (1997). Influence of methionine administration during chelation of cadmium by CaNa(3)DTPA and DMPS in the rat. *Environmental Toxicology and Pharmacology*, *3*(3), 159–165. PubMed PMID: 21781774.

60. Fatemi, S. J., Saljooghi, A. S., Balooch, F. D., Golbafan MR. & Iranmanesh, M. (2012). Removal of cadmium by combining deferasirox and desferrioxamine chelators in rats. *Toxicology and Industrial Health*, *28*(1), 35–41. PubMed PMID: 22134990.

61. Djukić-Cosić, D., Ninković, M. Malicević Z, Plamenac-Bulat Z, & Matović V. (2006). Effect of supplemental magnesium on the kidney levels of cadmium, zinc, and copper of mice exposed to toxic levels of cadmium. *Biological Trace Element Research*, *114*(1–3), 281–291. PubMed PMID: 17206009.

62. Wei, H. J. (1989). [Influence of selenium supplement on cadmium metabolism in human]. *Zhongguo Yi Xue Ke Xue Yuan Xue Bao. Acta Academiae Medicinae Sinicae*, *11*(3), 185–189. PubMed PMID: 2529986.

63. Khanna, S., Mitra, S., Lakhera, P. C., & Khandelwal, S. (2016). N-acetylcysteine effectively mitigates cadmium-induced oxidative damage and cell death in

Leydig cells in vitro. *Drug and Chemical Toxicology*, *39*(1), 74–80. PubMed PMID: 25885549.

64. Tandon, S. K., Prasad, S., & Singh, S. (2002). Chelation in metal intoxication: Influence of cysteine or N-acetyl cysteine on the efficacy of 2,3-dimercaptopropane-1-sulphonate in the treatment of cadmium toxicity. *Journal of Applied Toxicology*, *22*(1), 67–71. PubMed PMID: 11807931.

65. Tandon, S. K., Singh, S., Prasad, S., Khandekar, K., Dwivedi, V. K., Chatterjee, M., et al. (2003). Reversal of cadmium induced oxidative stress by chelating agent, antioxidant or their combination in rat. *Toxicology Letters*, *145*(3), 211–217. PubMed PMID:14580892.

66. Sears, M. E., Kerr, K. J., & Bray, R. I. (2012). Arsenic, cadmium, lead, and mercury in sweat: A systematic review. *Journal of Environmental and Public Health*, *2012*, 184745. PubMed PMID: 22505948.

67. Xu, Y., Zhou, X., Shi, C., Wang, J., & Wu, Z. (2015). α-Lipoic acid protects against the oxidative stress and cytotoxicity induced by cadmium in HepG2 cells through regenerating glutathione regulated by glutamate-cysteine ligase. *Toxicology Mechanisms and Methods*, *25*(8), 596–603. PubMed PMID: 26365678.

68. Nikolić, R., Krstić, N., Jovanović, J., Kocić, G., Cvetković, T. P., & Radosavljević-Stevanović, N. (2015). Monitoring the toxic effects of Pb, Cd and Cu on hematological parameters of Wistar rats and potential protective role of lipoic acid and glutathione. *Toxicology and Industrial Health*, *31*(3), 239–246. PubMed PMID: 23293128.

69. Veljkovic, A. R., Nikolic, R. S., Kocic, G. M., Pavlovic, D. D., Cvetkovic, T. P., Sokolovic, D. T., et al. (2012). Protective effects of glutathione and lipoic acid against cadmium-induced oxidative stress in rat's kidney. *Renal Failure*, *34*(10), 1281–1287. PubMed PMID: 23009295.

70. El-Maraghy, S. A., & Nassar, N. N. (2011). Modulatory effects of lipoic acid and selenium against cadmium-induced biochemical alterations in testicular steroidogenesis. *Journal of Biochemical and Molecular Toxicology*, *25*(1), 15–25. PubMed PMID: 20957662.

71. Mukherjee, R., Banerjee, S., Joshi, N., Singh, P. K., Baxi, D., & Ramachandran, A. V. (2011). A combination of melatonin and alpha lipoic acid has greater cardioprotective effect than either of them singly against cadmium-induced oxidative damage. *Cardiovascular Toxicology*, *11*(1), 78–88. Erratum in: *Cardiovascular Toxicology*, 2011. 11(1),89–90. PubMed PMID: 21046280.

72. Djukić-Cosić, D., Ninković, M., Malicević, Z., Matović, V., & Soldatović, D. (2007). Effect of magnesium pretreatment on reduced glutathione levels in tissues of mice exposed to acute and subacute cadmium intoxication: A time course study. *Magnesium Research*, *20*(3), 177–186. PubMed PMID: 17972460.

73. Fouad, A. A., Qureshi, H. A., Yacoubi, M. T., & Al-Melhim, W. N. (2009). Protective role of carnosine in mice with cadmium-induced acute hepatotoxicity. *Food and Chemical Toxicology*, 47(11), 2863–2870. PubMed PMID: 19748544.

74. Pires, V. C., Gollücke, A. P., Ribeiro, D. A., Lungato, L., D'Almeida, V., & Aguiar, O., Jr. (2013). Grape juice concentrate protects reproductive parameters of male rats against cadmium-induced damage: A chronic assay. *The British Journal of Nutrition*, 110(11), 2020–2029. PubMed PMID: 23656754.

75. de Moura, C. F., Ribeiro, F. A., Handan, B. A., Aguiar, O., Oshima, C. T., & Ribeiro, D. A. (2016). Grape juice concentrate protects rat liver against cadmium intoxication: Histopathology, cytochrome C and metalloproteinases expression. *Drug Research*, 66(7), 339–344. PubMed PMID: 27056637.

76. de Moura, C. F., Ribeiro, F. A., de Jesus, G. P., da Silva, V. H., Oshima, C. T., Gollücke, A. P., et al. (2014). Antimutagenic and antigenotoxic potential of grape juice concentrate in blood and liver of rats exposed to cadmium. *Environmental Science and Pollution Research International*, 21(22), 13118–13126. PubMed PMID: 24996944.

77. Lamas, C. A., Gollücke, A. P., & Dolder, H. (2015). Grape juice concentrate (G8000®) intake mitigates testicular morphological and ultrastructural damage following cadmium intoxication. *International Journal of Experimental Pathology*, 96(5), 301–310. PubMed PMID: 26515339.

78. Gong, P., Chen, F. X., Wang, L., Wang, J., Jin, S., & Ma, Y. M. (2014). Protective effects of blueberries (Vaccinium corymbosum L.) extract against cadmium-induced hepatotoxicity in mice. *Environmental Toxicology and Pharmacology*, 37(3), 1015–1027. PubMed PMID: 24751684.

79. Ige, S. F., & Akhigbe, R. E. (2013). Common onion (Allium cepa) extract reverses cadmium-induced organ toxicity and dyslipidaemia via redox alteration in rats. *Pathophysiology*, 20(4), 269–274. PubMed PMID: 23727273.

80. Morales, A. I., Vicente-Sánchez, C., Sandoval, J. M., Egido, J., Mayoral, P., Arévalo, M. A., et al. (2006). Protective effect of quercetin on experimental chronic cadmium nephrotoxicity in rats is based on its antioxidant properties. *Food and Chemical Toxicology*, 44(12), 2092–2100. PubMed PMID: 16962696.

81. Ugwuja, E. I., Erejuwa, O. O., & Ugwu, N. C. (2016). Spices mixture containing garlic, ginger and nutmeg has protective effects on the kidneys and liver of cadmium exposed rats. *Advanced Pharmaceutical Bulletin*, 6(2), 271–274. PubMed PMID: 27478792.

11

Hexavalent Chromium

Dr. Lyn Patrick

SUMMARY

- Presence in population: 4401 public water systems in the U.S. have been found to have levels of hexavalent chromium exceeding the Environmental Protection Agency (EPA) minimum reportable level (MRL) of 0.03 μg/L
- Major diseases: Lung cancer, reproductive and developmental problems, stomach and intestinal
- inflammation, neonatal death, spontaneous abortion, stillbirth and preterm birth
- Primary sources: Contaminated drinking water, airborne contamination in industrial facilities
- Best measure: Red blood cell chromium
- Best intervention: Avoidance through point-of-use drinking water filtration technologies

DESCRIPTION

Hexavalent chromium is commonly referred to as chromium 6, chromium (VI), chrome 6, Cr(VI), Cr + 6, or hexchrome. Hexavalent chromium is also popularly known as the "Erin Brockovich chemical" after the famous case in Hinkley, California, in 1993. The resulting case led to the largest settlement in a direct action lawsuit in U.S. history. The verdict was based on the decision that a local cancer cluster and other significant health problems were the result of hexavalent chromium exposure through drinking water.[1] Recent analyses have revealed that 38% of municipal sources of drinking water in California have detectable levels of hexavalent chromium.[2]

Cr(VI) is a naturally occurring substance that is found, along with its benign counterpart trivalent chromium Cr(III), in the Earth's crust's igneous geological formations. Chromium naturally exists in different oxidation states from −2 to + 6 but is the most stable as either elemental (+ 0), trivalent (+ 3), or hexavalent (+ 6) chromium.[3]

TOXICITY

Hexavalent chromium is considered about 1000 times more toxic than the relatively benign trivalent form that is an essential mineral.[4] Oral exposure to Cr(VI) in drinking water results in increased intracellular levels of Cr(VI) that can act as a carcinogen.[5] This report from the National Toxicology Program included research showing that exposure to chromium(VI) may "present greater risks to certain groups, including infants and children, people who take antacids, and people with poorly functioning livers." When Cr(VI) enters the cell, it binds to glutathione and can be reduced by ascorbate, cysteine, glutathione, hydrogen peroxide (H_2O_2), or glutathione reductase to produce reactive intermediates, including Cr(V), Cr(IV), thiyl radicals, hydroxyl radicals, and the final product, Cr(III).[6] This process generates significant levels of oxygen radicals that initiate mutagenic and oncogenic changes through DNA single stand breaks, DNA adduct formation, and DNA mismatch repair.[7,8] Cr(VI) also decreases the ratio to oxidized glutathione duodenum, indicating oxidative stress locally. It is considered a carcinogen through inhalation and ingestion and has long been defined as an occupational toxicant known to cause lung and nasopharyngeal cancers in workers who inhale chromium fumes or dust.[9]

SOURCES

- Groundwater
- Smoking
- Hip replacements

Hexavalent chromium is used in wood preservation (52%), leather tanning (13%), metal finishing (13%), paint pigments (12%), and the production and use of corrosion inhibitors (the source of contaminated drinking water in Hinkley, California). It is also used in smaller amounts in drilling muds and photographic chemicals. Other industries where hexavalent chromium exposure is a risk include production of antialgae agents, antifreeze, and chrome alloys, chrome electroplating, copier servicing, glassmaking, production of paints/pigments, photoengraving, porcelain and ceramics manufacturing, production of high-fidelity magnetic audio tapes, tattooing, textile manufacturing, and alloy or steel welding.[10] At least 386 of the hazardous waste sites on the National Priority List (Superfund sites) have been shown to be contaminated with a total of 90,000,000 pounds of Cr(VI).[11,12]

Environmental hexavalent chromium also enters the air through the burning of fossil fuels, incineration of waste, and disposal from industrial cooling towers, and may be discharged into water from chromium-containing waste sites. Incineration and automobile emissions create pollution that can contribute to surface water contamination and low-level inhalation exposure in large segments of the general population.[7] Hexavalent chromium is also found in coal ash piles and chromium mining slag piles. Chromium waste slag containing potentially hazardous levels of Cr(VI) was used as fill material in New Jersey at more than 160 residential, industrial, and recreational sites. Before remediation, persons living or working in the vicinity of the sites may have been exposed to elevated levels of hexavalent chromium through inhalation, ingestion, or skin contact with contaminated soils and dust.[13]

Drinking water is considered a significant source of hexavalent chromium exposure, with industrial contamination the leading source in groundwater and subsurface aquifers. Recent published research identifying coal ash as the source of hexavalent chromium contamination in the Piedmont aquifers of North Carolina concludes, "the occurrence of Cr(VI) in shallow drinking water wells is much more widespread than previously thought, with possibly millions in the eastern United States and other parts of the world directly exposed to detectable Cr(VI) from drinking water wells."[14] Detectable hexavalent chromium levels have been found in aquifers in California, Arizona, Mexico, Argentina, Brazil, Italy, and Greece.

In January 2017, the EPA monitoring database for unregulated water contaminants found 4401 public water systems contaminated by hexavalent chromium.[15] These drinking water supplies had levels of hexavalent chromium exceeding the EPA's MRL of 0.03 µg/L (0.03 parts per billion (PPB)). According to an analysis of EPA data for 2009 performed by the Environmental Working Group, approximately 74 million people in nearly 7000 communities had access to drinking water that exceeded the EPA standards for total chromium.[16,17] Because the federal standard does not differentiate between trivalent and hexavalent, it is not possible to identify levels of hexavalent chromium contamination by looking at national data for enforceable standards.

Currently California is the only state that has both a regulatory level, known as the maximum contaminant level (MCL), and a public health goal (PHG) for hexavalent chromium. These two levels determine a regulatory level and a risk level. The PHG was set in 2011 at 0.02 PPB (0.0002 µg/L) by the California Office of Environmental Health Hazard Assessment as a level that was determined to define a lack of public health risk and that would result in no risk for cancer, and is legally defined as a level that would predict a risk of no more than 1 case of cancer/1 million individuals.[18]

One cigarette produces up to 0.5 µg of airborne hexavalent chromium, so a pack-a-day smoker could be inhaling as much as 1.5 µg of hexavalent chromium daily.[19] The current Occupational Safety and Health Administration (OSHA) standard for hexavalent chromium inhalation is 5 µg/m^3 in any given 8-hour period.[20]

Cobalt-chromium metal-on-metal hip replacements have been documented to erode, leading to increased blood and urine chromium levels in some individuals with arthroplasties.[21] Hexavalent chromium is the predominant species released during corrosion of stainless steel and cobalt chrome alloy in these hip replacements, and monitoring both red blood cell and urine levels of total chromium is suggested for long-term management of metal arthroplasty.[22]

BODY BURDEN

Chromium(VI) is more water-soluble than Cr(III) and does have a greater capacity to be absorbed both across the intestinal lining and into the intracellular environment. Unlike Cr(III), it easily enters the cellular environment and concentrates in the liver, kidney, spleen, soft tissue, and bone.[11] However, no data on body burden of Cr(VI) is available.

Detoxification/Excretion Processes

Human gastric juice (in vitro) is capable of reducing approximately 70% of hexavalent chromium to trivalent chromium after 30 minutes, but as the pH rises from 1.4 to 7.0, that reduction capacity decreases and at 7.0 is no longer measurable.[23] So, as stomach pH rises, less hexavalent chromium is reduced and more would theoretically be absorbed intact. For this reason, infants, children, people who take antacids, and people with poor hepatic function are more at risk for hexavalent chromium toxicity. Approximately 10% to 20% of ingested hexavalent chromium escapes gastric detoxification (by reduction) in the human gut and results in its absorption into cells of target tissues, even at very low concentrations.[24]

Excretion of absorbed hexavalent chromium occurs primarily via urine as trivalent chromium; 60% is excreted within 8 hours of ingestion, although red blood cell levels can remain elevated for weeks as a result of hexavalent exposure.[25] Chromium is mainly excreted through urine, with an initial half-life of 2 to 3 days, followed by a terminal half-life of about 1 month. Approximately 10% of an absorbed dose is eliminated in bile, and the remaining amount is excreted in hair, nails, milk, and sweat.

Clearance from plasma is generally rapid (within hours), but elimination from red blood cells and tissues is slower, with a half-life of several days to weeks.[11] Plasma and urinary chromium concentrations will correlate with relatively recent exposure, so exposures that occurred several weeks prior may not be detected by these measurements.[26]

Clinical Significance

Neoplasia. Hexavalent chromium is recognized as a genotoxic carcinogen by the International Agency for Research in Cancer (IARC) and classified as a Group 1 carcinogen (carcinogenic to humans) based on sufficient evidence in industrial exposures, through airborne chromium inhalation and resulting lung cancers.[27] The EPA has also classified hexavalent chromium as Group A: known human carcinogen via inhalation.[28] Hexavalent chromium is known to cause cellular damage and carcinogenic changes through multiple mechanisms: DNA damage, chromosomal aberrations, epigenetic changes, and genetic hypermutability caused by damaged DNA repair mechanisms.[29]

In Greece, where water was contaminated with Cr(VI) (41–156 µg/L), there was significantly increased incidence of lung, liver, and kidney cancer mortality as well as genitourinary cancer mortality in women.[12,30] In a Chinese cohort, an increased risk for lung cancer was also found in those drinking contaminated water.[30,31] Inhalant exposure to hexavalent chromium is also a known risk factor for both lung and sinonasal cancer.

Renal. Although acute poisonings and occupational exposures have been shown to cause gastritis, hepatitis, and cardiopulmonary arrest, there is no conclusive evidence that low-dose oral exposure can cause direct organ damage other than known genotoxic effects. Low-dose chronic Cr(VI) exposure typically results only in transient renal effects, whereas occupational injury can lead to tubular damage.[11] A possible threshold for renal damage has been indicated at exposure levels resulting in 15 µg chromium/g creatinine in urine.[31,32]

Reproduction. Although no human studies have examined developmental endpoints, animal studies have consistently shown that chromium, particularly chromium(VI), is a developmental toxicant.[32-34]

INTERVENTION
Laboratory Testing

According to the Agency for Toxic Substances and Disease Registry Case Studies in Environmental Medicine (CSEM): Chromium Toxicity, the following laboratory testing should be performed on anyone who has been exposed to hexavalent chromium: complete blood count (CBC), liver function tests, blood urea nitrogen (BUN), creatinine, and urine analysis.[34,35] Renal function should be tested (urinalysis, BUN, creatinine, and β2-microglobulin) to determine whether renal tubular damage has occurred. Assuming no source of excessive exposure, urinary chromium values are typically less than 10 µg/L for a

24-hour period and reflect a combination of trivalent and hexavalent chromium.

Distribution of total chromium in the blood appears to be divided evenly between plasma and erythrocytes. In the absence of known exposure, whole blood chromium concentrations are in the range of 2.0 to 3.0 μg/100 mL; lower levels occur in rural areas, and higher levels occur in large urban centers.[35,36] Chromium bound within red blood cells remains there for the life of the cell and indicates an exposure to Cr(Vl) at any point within 120 days. Urine measurement, if it is elevated, will indicate more recent exposure of either detoxified hexavalent or nontoxic trivalent chromium metal.

Chelation

Deferoxamine (DFO) was able to prevent damage from hexchrome in a preexposure animal model, but post-exposure chelation was ineffective.[36,37] 2,3-Dimercapto-1-propanesulfonic acid (DMPS) was successfully used in a 22-year-old male who received severe chromic acid burns over 15% of his body from a 10-minute dermal exposure to Cr(VI). He was treated with intravenous (IV) DMPS 125 mg every 12 hours along with IV N-acetyl cysteine NAC (50 mg/kg every 4 hours) and ascorbic acid (100 mg every 12 hours) for 10 days.[37,38] His initial urine chromium was 88,208 μg/L, which decreased rapidly to 292 μg/L on day 4 and 61 μg/L by day 8. He developed acute renal failure and pulmonary edema on day 3 and required dialysis and plasmapheresis. He was treated with DMPS, NAC, and ascorbate for 10 days in addition to plasmapheresis and continued dialysis until 3 days before discharge 1 month later. His urine chromium levels remained elevated 3 months after exposure, indicating that cellular stores of chromium were excreted at least for that long. His long-term follow-up showed complete recovery with no permanent renal damage.

Oral chelation therapy with high-dose NAC (300 mg/kg/day for 10 days) was used in two patients with metal-on-metal hip implants with positive results, lowering blood chromium levels 85% in one individual.[38,39] The blood chromium levels were stable 6 months later, with no adverse events for the following 3 years. NAC, when given orally, has also reduced chromium hypersensitivity dermatological reactions due to its ability to attenuate inflammation and sensitization in the skin caused by reactive oxygen species.[39,40]

Ascorbate appears to be protective when given before or shortly after Cr(VI) administration, but it increased the toxic effects of hexchrome when given 3 hours postexposure.[40,41] Researchers indicated that this may reflect the difference between reduction of hexavalent chromium extracellularly early on, reducing the ability of Cr(VI) to get into the cells, compared with increased reduction of Cr(VI) intracellularly later on, which would increase DNA-adduct formation.

Avoidance

The most effective intervention for hexavalent chromium appears to be preventing exposure. In areas with water contamination, this would include both point-of-use and whole-house water filtration, because dermal absorption is a route of exposure. The EPA recommends either coagulation/filtration, ion exchange, reverse osmosis, or lime softening to treat water contaminated with chromium. Of these, reverse osmosis is the most economical and commonly available whole-house and point-of-use filtration system available to the public.

Antioxidant Support

Because hexavalent chromium exposure lowers the level of antioxidant-reducing agents in the body (ascorbate, glutathione, cysteine), every effort should be made to address these deficiencies. Green tea has protective effects in animals, preventing the genotoxicity induced by hexavalent chromium.[41,42] Epigallocatechin gallate (EGCG) the main catechin in Green tea EGCG has been shown to aid the process of repairing DNA lesions, termed nucleotide excision repair (NER), reversing a type of damage that appears to be central to chromium-induced mutations. EGCG, quercetin, and rutin have shown protective effects against Cr(VI) toxicity in animals, preventing micronuclei formation in red blood cells, where rutin and quercetin have a stronger effect than EGCG.[42,43]

REFERENCES

1. Egilman, D., & Scout (2006). Corporate corruption of science—the case of chromium(VI). *International Journal of Occupational and Environmental Health*, 12(2), 169–176. PubMed PMID: 16722197.
2. Sedman, R. M., Beaumont, J., McDonald, T. A., et al. (2006). Review of the evidence regarding the carcinogenicity of hexavalent chromium in drinking water. *Journal of Environment Science and Health.Part C, Environmental Carcinogenesis & Ecotoxicology Reviews*, 24(1), 155–182. Review. PubMed PMID: 16690539.

3. Daoud, W., Ebadi, T., & Fahimifar, A. (2015). Removal of hexavalent chromium from aqueous solutions using micro zero-valent iron supported by bentonite layer. *Water Science and Technology, 71*(5), 667–674. PubMed PMID: 25768212.

4. Behari, J., Chandra, S. V., & Tandon, S. K. (1978). Comparative toxicity of trivalent and hexavalent chromium to rabbits. III. Biochemical and histological changes in testicular tissue. *Acta Biologica et Medica Germanica, 37*(3), 463–468. PubMed PMID: 153692.

5. National Toxicology Program. (2008). Toxicology and carcinogenesis studies of sodium dichromate dihydrate (CAS No. 7789-12-0) in F344/N rats and B6C3F1 mice (drinking water studies). *National Toxicology Program Technical Report Series, 546,* 1–192. PubMed PMID: 18716633.

6. Caglieri, A., Goldoni, M., De Palma, G., Mozzoni, P., Gemma, S., Vichi, S., et al. (2008). Exposure to low levels of hexavalent chromium: Target doses and comparative effects on two human pulmonary cell lines. *Acta Bio-Medica, 79*(Suppl. 1), 104–115. PubMed PMID: 18924316.

7. Zhitkovich, A. (2005). Importance of chromium-DNA adducts in mutagenicity and toxicity of chromium(VI). *Chemical Research in Toxicology, 18*(1), 3–11. Review. PubMed PMID: 15651842.

8. Messer, J., Reynolds, M., Stoddard, L., & Zhitkovich, A. (2006). Causes of DNA single-strand breaks during reduction of chromate by glutathione in vitro and in cells. *Free Radical Biology & Medicine, 40*(11), 1981–1992. PubMed PMID:16716899.

9. van Wijngaarden, E., Mundt, K. A., & Luippold, R. S. (2004). Evaluation of the exposure-response relationship of lung cancer mortality and occupational exposure to hexavalent chromium based on published epidemiological data. *Nonlinearity in Biology, Toxicology, Medicine, 2*(1), 27–34. PubMed PMID: 19330106.

10. Pellerin, C., & Booker, S. M. (2000). Reflections on hexavalent chromium: Health hazards of an industrial heavyweight. *Environmental Health Perspectives, 108*(9), A402–A407. PubMed PMID: 11017901.

11. U.S. Department of Health and Human Services. ATSDR. *Toxicological profile for chromium.* Available from https://www.atsdr.cdc.gov/toxprofiles/tp7.pdf. (Accessed August 7, 2017.)

12. Linos, A., Petralias, A., Christophi, C. A., et al. (2011). Oral ingestion of hexavalent chromium through drinking water and cancer mortality in an industrial area of Greece—an ecological study. *Environmental Health: A Global Access Science Source, 10,* 50. PubMed PMID: 21609468.

13. Stern, A. H., Fagliano, J. A., Savrin, J. E., et al. (1998). The association of chromium in household dust with urinary chromium in residences adjacent to chromate production waste sites. *Environmental Health Perspectives, 106*(12), 833–839. PubMed PMID: 9831544.

14. Vengosh, A. C. R., Karr, J., Karr, J., et al. (2016). Origin of hexavalent chromium in drinking water wells from the Piedmont aquifers of North Carolina. *Environmental Science & Technology Letters, 3,* 409–414.

15. US Environmental Protection Agency. *The Third Unregulated Contaminant Monitoring Rule (UCMR 3): Data Summary, January 2017.* https://www.epa.gov/dwucmr/data-summary-third-unregulated-contaminant-monitoring-rule. (Accessed June 30, 2017.)

16. United States Environmental Protection Agency EEP. (2009). *Six-Year Review 2 Health Effects Assessment: Summary Report.* EPA 822-R-09-006. U.S. Environmental Protection Agency, Office of Water.

17. Environmental Working Group. (2010). *Chromium-6 Is Widespread in US Tap Water.* http://www.ewg.org/chromium6-in-tap-water. (Accessed June 30, 2017.)

18. California Environmental Protection Agency. *Public Health Goal for Hexavalent Chromium (Cr VI) in Drinking Water.* (2011). https://clu-in.org/download/contaminantfocus/chromium/Chromium-CA-PHG-2011.pdf. (Accessed August 7, 2017.)

19. Nickens, K. P., Patierno, S. R., & Ceryak, S. (2010). Chromium genotoxicity: A double-edged sword. *Chemico-Biological Interactions, 188,* 276–288. PubMed PMID: 20430016.

20. OSHA. (2006). Occupational exposure to hexavalent chromium. Final rule. https://www.osha.gov/pls/oshaweb/owadisp.show_document?p_id=18599&p_table=federal_register. (Accessed June 30, 2017.)

21. Afolaranmi, G. A., Tettey, J., Meek, R. M., & Grant, M. H. (2008). Release of chromium from orthopaedic arthroplasties. *The Open Orthopaedics Journal, 2,* 10–18. PubMed PMID: 19461924.

22. Merritt, K., & Brown, S. A. (1995). Release of hexavalent chromium from corrosion of stainless steel and cobalt-chromium alloys. *Journal of Biomedical Materials Research, 29*(5), 627–633. PubMed PMID: 7622548.

23. Donaldson, R. M., Jr., & Barreras, R. F. (1966). Intestinal absorption of trace quantities of chromium. *The Journal of Laboratory and Clinical Medicine, 68*(3), 484–493. PubMed PMID: 5922758.

24. Stern, A. H. (2010). A quantitative assessment of the carcinogenicity of hexavalent chromium by the oral route and its relevance to human exposure. *Environmental Research, 110*(8), 798–807. PubMed PMID: 20843510.

25. Kiilunen, M., Kivistö, H., Ala-Laurila, P., Tossavainen, A., & Aitio, A. (1983). Exceptional pharmacokinetics of trivalent chromium during occupational exposure to chromium lignosulfonate dust. *Scandinavian Journal of Work, Environment and Health*, 9(3), 265–271. PubMed PMID: 6612268.

26. Minoia, C., & Cavalleri, A. (1988). Chromium in urine, serum and red blood cells in the biological monitoring of workers exposed to different chromium valency states. *The Science of the Total Environment*, 71(3), 323–327. PubMed PMID: 3406705.

27. IARC. (1990). *Chromium, Nickel and Welding. IARC Monographs on the Evaluation of Carcinogenic Risks to Humans*. Vol 49. Lyon: International Agency for Research on Cancer, 49–256.

28. US. Environmental Protection Agency. *Chromium (VI) CASRN 1850-29-9 IRIS*. https://cfpub.epa.gov/ncea/iris2/chemicallanding.cfm?substance_nmbr=144. (Accessed August 7, 2017.)

29. Pritchard, D. E., Ceryak, S., Ramsey, K. E., et al. (2005). Resistance to apoptosis, increased growth potential, and altered gene expression in cells that survived genotoxic hexavalent chromium [Cr(VI)] exposure. *Molecular and Cellular Biochemistry*, 279(1–2), 169–181. PubMed PMID: 16283527.

30. Beaumont, J. J., Sedman, R. M., Reynolds, S. D., et al. (2008). Cancer mortality in a Chinese population exposed to hexavalent chromium in drinking water. *Epidemiology*, 19(1), 12–23. PubMed PMID: 18091413.

31. Franchini, I., & Mutti, A. (1988). Selected toxicological aspects of chromium(VI) compounds. *The Science of the Total Environment*, 71(3), 379–387. PubMed PMID: 3406707.

32. Marouani, N., Tebourbi, O., Mokni, M., et al. (2011). Embryotoxicity and fetotoxicity following intraperitoneal administrations of hexavalent chromium to pregnant rats. *Zygote*, 19(3), 229–235. PubMed PMID: 21205386.

33. Yoisungnern, T., Das, J., Choi, Y. J., et al. (2016). Effect of hexavalent chromium-treated sperm on in vitro fertilization and embryo development. *Toxicology and Industrial Health*, 32(9), 1700–1710. PubMed PMID: 25903088.

34. ATSDR. (2008). Case studies in environmental medicine- chromium toxicity. (pp. 1–67). Atlanta, GA: Agency for Toxic Substances and Disease Registry. https://www.atsdr.cdc.gov/hec/csem/chromium/docs/chromium.pdf (Accessed November 1, 2017.)

35. Miksche, L. W., & Lewalter, J. (1997). Health surveillance and biological effect monitoring for chromium-exposed workers. *Regulatory Toxicology and Pharmacology*, 26(1 Pt. 2), S94–S99. Review. PubMed PMID: 9380843.

36. Molina-Jijón, E., Zarco-Márquez, G., Medina-Campos, O. N., et al. (2012). Deferoxamine pretreatment prevents Cr(VI)-induced nephrotoxicity and oxidant stress: Role of Cr(VI) chelation. *Toxicology*, 291(1–3), 93–101. PubMed PMID: 22115772.

37. Lin, C. C., Wu, M. L., Yang, C. C., et al. (2009). Acute severe chromium poisoning after dermal exposure to hexavalent chromium. *Journal of the Chinese Medical Association* 2009 Apr; 72(4), 219–221. PubMed PMID: 19372081.

38. Giampreti, A., Lonati, D., Ragghianti, B., et al. (2016). N-acetyl-cysteine as effective and safe chelating agent in metal-on-metal hip-implanted patients: two cases. *Case Reports in Orthopedics*, 2016, 8682737. PubMed PMID:27148463.

39. Lee, Y. H., Su, S. B., Huang, C. C., et al. (2014). N-acetylcysteine attenuates hexavalent chromium-induced hypersensitivity through inhibition of cell death, ROS-related signaling and cytokine expression. *PLoS ONE*, 9(9), e108317. PubMed PMID: 25248126.

40. Bradberry, S. M., & Vale, J. A. (1999). Therapeutic review: Is ascorbic acid of value in chromium poisoning and chromium dermatitis? *Journal of Toxicology Clinical Toxicology*, 37(2), 195–200. Review. PubMed PMID: 10382555.

41. García-Rodríguez, M. C., Vilches-Larrea, R. E., Nicolás-Méndez, T., & Altamirano-Lozano, M. A. (2012). [Green tea and its role on chemoprevention in vivo of genotoxic damage induced by carcinogenic metals (chromium [VI])]. *Nutrición Hospitalaria*, 27(4), 1204–1212. PubMed PMID: 23165563.

42. García-Rodríguez Mdel, C., Nicolás-Méndez, T., Montaño-Rodríguez, A. R., & Altamirano-Lozano, M. A. (2014). Antigenotoxic effects of (-)-epigallocatechin-3-gallate (EGCG), quercetin, and rutin on chromium trioxide-induced micronuclei in the polychromatic erythrocytes of mouse peripheral blood. *Journal of Toxicology and Environmental Health. Part A*, 77(6), 324–336. PubMed PMID: 24593145.

12

Cobalt

SUMMARY

- Presence in population: In 2006, approximately 113,000 hip replacements occurred in the United States, and 35% of these cases involved cobalt-containing metal-on-metal (MoM) prosthetics[1]
- Major diseases: Metal hypersensitivity, sensorineural hearing impairment, vision loss, cognitive impairment, cardiac failure, neuropathy, and hypothyroidism
- Primary sources: Food supply, cobalt-containing hip prostheses

- Best measure: Serum or whole blood levels, urine
- Best intervention: Avoidance of industrial exposure; revision or removal of the cobalt-containing prosthesis to eliminate further exposure; chelation therapy with N-acetyl-cysteine (NAC), ethylenediaminetetraacetic acid (EDTA), glutathione, 2,3-dimercaptosuccinic acid (DMSA), or diethylenetriamepentaacetic acid (DTPA)

DESCRIPTION

Cobalt is the 33rd most abundant element and is a silvery-gray solid metal at room temperature. There is only one stable isotope of cobalt (59Co) and 26 known radioactive isotopes. Cobalt is a naturally occurring element found in food, water, and the environment. Cobalt compounds are used in industrial applications such as aircraft engines and drill tips, as colorants in glass and paints, and in the medical field in hip and joint prostheses.[2] Cobalt is also an essential nutrient for the formation of vitamin B$_{12}$ (cobalamin).

Although cobalt exposure has generally decreased over the years, there has been a recent upsurge with the use of MoM joint prostheses. Cobalt-chromium alloy is used for most MoM implants, and elevated levels of cobalt and chromium are toxic. Although the general toxicity of cobalt is discussed, this chapter will primarily focus on the toxic effects of elevated cobalt resulting from MoM hip prostheses.

TOXICITY

Guidelines have been published with respect to the risk of toxicity from inhaled and ingested cobalt.[3] However, no guidelines exist regarding the toxicity of cobalt from MoM prosthetics. There is significant variability in the analysis of metal ions, including collection techniques, analyses, statistical methodologies, and reporting of results.[4,5] The Medicines and Healthcare products Regulatory Agency (MHRA) has suggested a serum cobalt cutoff level of 7 µg/L and stated that levels greater than this are associated with significant soft-tissue reactions and failed MoM implants.[6] However, studies have shown that this level may be too high and failure can be detected at lower levels.[5,7] These levels are more predictive of failure of the implant rather than cobalt toxicity. Currently, the United States Food and Drug Administration does not recommend routine testing for cobalt metal or ion levels at any time.[8]

The release of cobalt from MoM prostheses is due to the mechanical and oxidative stresses placed on the prosthetic joint, and cobalt exerts its pathological effects through direct cellular toxicity.[9] Cobalt is acutely toxic in larger doses, and *in vitro* tests show that cobalt ions and cobalt metal are cytotoxic, induce apoptosis, and cause necrosis with inflammatory response.[10] Cobalt is also genotoxic as a result of oxidative DNA damage by reactive oxygen species.

SOURCES

The food supply is the largest source of exposure to cobalt for the general population, with estimated intake of 5 to 40 µg/day.[11] Cobalt is often produced as a byproduct of copper and silver production and is widely used in the making of hardened metals in industry (e.g., drill bits, gas turbine blades). It has also been used medically as a treatment for anemia, an antidote for cyanide poisoning, and a potentiator of the action of antibiotics and hydrocortisone.[2] The use of cobalt in these conditions has decreased dramatically, as the adverse effects are numerous and can be severe. In recent years, cobalt has resurfaced as a performance-enhancing agent for athletes, as it stimulates erythropoiesis, providing a potential advantage in aerobic sports.[12,13]

Vitallium, a metal alloy consisting of 65% cobalt, 30% chromium, 5% molybdenum, and 5% other substances, is often used for prostheses in joint replacement surgery because it is strong and corrosion-resistant.[14] It is estimated that one in eight of all total hip replacements requires revision within 10 years, and that 60% of these are because of wear-related complications. The release of metal ions from the bearing couple and/or head-neck taper corrosion leads to an increased risk of early failure due to adverse local tissue reaction to metal debris. Interestingly, it appears that the greatest risk of systemic cobalt toxicity results from accelerated wear of a cobalt-containing revision of a failed ceramic prosthesis and not from primary failure of an MoM prosthesis.[15]

BODY LOAD

In individuals who have had initial MoM total hip arthroplasty, studies show significant increases in serum levels of cobalt at 3 months (1.4 µg/L) and 1 year (2.1 µg/L), but no additional significant increases afterward.[16,17,18] One study showed a mean serum cobalt concentration of 0.7 µg/L at 5 years postsurgery.[19] A

TABLE 12.1 CDC Fourth Report January 2017 Update—Urinary Cobalt µg/g Creatinine

Toxicant	Gender	Mean	75th%	90th%	95th%
Cobalt	Total	0.452	0.656	0.969	1.31
	Male	0.379	0.529	0.758	1.02
	Female	0.534	0.774	1.12	1.48

long-term study of eight individuals with well-functioning MoM total hip replacements showed a mean serum cobalt level of 1.0 µg/L 20 years after implantation.[20] However, in each of these studies, all of the participants had well-functioning MoM prostheses. Failure of the implant causes levels of cobalt to increase rapidly and dramatically, leading to acute toxicity.

Cobalt is absorbed primarily from the pulmonary and gastrointestinal tracts. The liver, kidney, pancreas, and heart accumulate cobalt to the greatest extent. With time, cobalt content increases in the skeleton and skeletal muscle as well.[2] Total body burden is estimated to be 1.1 to 1.5 mg, with 0.11 mg in the liver.[21]

Levels of cobalt in residents of the United States have been studied as part of the ongoing National Health and Nutritional Examination Survey (NHANES) trial and published by the Centers for Disease Control and Prevention (CDC) in its Exposure Report.[22] Table 12.1 summarizes the cobalt findings published in the January 2017 updated tables to the Fourth Report.

The increased urinary levels seen in women may be reflective of men tolerating MoM hip surfaces better than women because women tend to be more sensitive to MoM implants.

Detoxification/Excretion Processes

Oral doses of 33.3 mg Co(II)/kg fed to rats show that blood cobalt concentration peaks at 3.2 hours, with an absorptive half-life of 0.9 hours, an elimination phase half-life of 3.9 hours, and a terminal elimination half-life of 22.9 hours.[23] By 36 hours, approximately 75% of the oral dose is excreted in the feces. Renal excretion shows a triphasic pattern with initial excretion being rapid, followed by a slow phase that lasts several weeks, and then a third long-term phase involving retention in tissues for several years.[2]

Clinical Significance

To eliminate the subjectivity of vague or difficult-to-identify complaints associated with prosthetic hip–associated systemic cobalt toxicity, a more consistent, comprehensive, and objective approach to making the diagnosis is suggested. This would include: 1) elevated serum or whole blood cobalt levels due to a prosthetic hip, 2) at least two test-confirmed findings consistent with cobalt toxicity, and 3) exclusion of other etiologies.[24] The following tests are also recommended to aid in the diagnosis: comprehensive neurocognitive testing, echocardiography, audiometry, nerve conduction, electromyography, and formal ophthalmological evaluation.

Elevated metal ions such as cobalt have carcinogenic and biological concerns as well as concerns regarding hypersensitivity, chromosomal mutation, and fetal exposure to high ion levels.[25,26] Several studies show that severe cobalt intoxication leads to hypothyroidism, peripheral neuropathy, and cardiomyopathy.[27,28] Adverse reactions to cobalt include anorexia, nausea and vomiting, diarrhea, cardiomyopathy, skin reactions, nerve deafness, renal damage, hypothyroidism, asthma, and visual problems.

Allergic Dermatitis

A relatively common complication associated with MoM total hip arthroplasty is hypersensitivity to the metal. Metal sensitivity should be considered in individuals presenting with persistent pain, marked joint effusion, and the development of early osteolysis in the absence of infection. Reactivity to the metal appears to involve the adaptive (macrophage-recruiting) immune system with elevated proliferation and production of interferon [IFN]-gamma indicating a Th1-type response.[29] Tissue samples have shown ulceration associated with perivascular infiltration of lymphocytes and an accumulation of plasma cells with macrophages that contain metallic wear-debris particles.[30] Other histological features include high endothelial venules, massive fibrin exudation, and infiltrates of eosinophilic granulocytes and necrosis.[31]

Pain is often the initial symptom and may be associated with local or systemic dermatitis, urticaria, and/or vasculitis.[32,33] Metal sensitivity should be considered if cutaneous symptoms develop after implantation of a metal device.[34] One unusual presentation of cobalt hypersensitivity occurred in a patient who was diagnosed with a delayed type IV reaction several years after use of cobalt in the contralateral hip.[35]

Cardiomyopathy

In the 1960s, one of the more common causes of cobalt-related cardiomyopathy involved chronic beer drinkers, as cobalt was typically added to beer to stabilize and improve the appearance of its foam.[36,37,38,39,40] Cobalt-related cardiomyopathy has decreased significantly over the years, as cobalt was removed from beer (in the late 1960s), the medicinal uses of cobalt have diminished, and measures have been taken to reduce industrial exposure. The recent increase in the use of MoM hip replacements has produced a relative increase in the failure rate of those implants, and thus an increase in the number of reports of subacute cobalt-related cardiomyopathy.[41,42]

Patients with cobalt-related cardiomyopathy typically present with subacute onset of severe heart failure accompanied by hypotension and cyanosis, pericardial effusion, low voltage on an electrocardiogram, marked elevation of serum enzymes, and lactic acidosis.[43] Although there is no single test that can be used to diagnose cobalt cardiomyopathy, the combination of pathological and biological findings, blood levels, imaging, and surgery together indicate a diagnosis.[44] Complete resolution of symptoms and recovery of cardiac function is possible in those who survive and completely avoid further cobalt exposure.

Hypothyroidism

During the 1950s and 1960s, hypothyroidism was often observed as a side effect of cobalt therapy used in the treatment of anemia.[45,46,47] It was shown that cobalt depresses the uptake of iodine by the thyroid gland and inhibits the tyrosine iodinase system.[48] Low-level cobalt exposure showed an increase in the ratio between T4 and T3, indicating that low levels of cobalt may have an effect on the conversion of T4 to T3.[49] Almost all cases of cobalt toxicity resulting from MoM implant failure have hypothyroidism as a consequence.[25,26,46,50,51,52] However, with reduction of cobalt levels, thyroid function returns to normal.

Pseudotumors

Periarticular soft-tissue masses or pseudotumors have been discovered after MoM resurfacing of the hip and total hip replacement. It is estimated that 1% of patients who have MoM hip resurfacing will develop a pseudotumor within 5 years.[53] The incidence may be higher with longer follow-up and in patients with bilateral implants.[54] Pseudotumors have been characterized histologically by extensive coagulate necrosis, a heavy macrophage infiltrate, and the presence of granulomas containing macrophages and giant cells, which are all suggestive of a delayed type IV immune response, likely to the metal particles.[55,56,57] Patients with elevated serum metal ion levels have a quadrupled risk of developing a pseudotumor.[58] However, a randomized controlled trial showed that elevated cobalt levels (≥ 5 µg/L) were only associated with pseudotumors in women.[59] Pseudotumors may also present as neuropathy, with one study showing irreversible pathological changes in nerve function and neurohistopathological evidence of complete nerve destruction that appeared toxic in nature.[60]

Respiratory Effects

Respiratory effects from work-related cobalt inhalation are well documented. Asthma, pneumonia, wheezing, respiratory irritation, and fibrosis have all been reported as occupational health hazards, especially in workers exposed to cobalt metal powder, cobalt salts, and cobalt-containing dusts.[61,62,63,64] It has been estimated that the concentrations of cobalt in the air of hard metal manufacturing, welding, and grinding factories may range from 1 to 300 µg/m^3,[65] and respiratory effects have been reported at exposure levels ranging from 15 to 130 µg/m^3.

A chronic lung parenchymal condition termed "hard metal disease" has been associated with industrial exposure to cobalt and is characterized by alveolitis resembling multinucleated giant cell pneumonitis and later interstitial pulmonary fibrosis.[66,67] However, it should be noted that workers in these industries are exposed to several substances in addition to cobalt, such as tungsten carbide, iron, and diamond, which may modulate the reactivity of cobalt.[68] Exposure to cobalt alone does not seem to produce the same effects but does produce an allergic-like asthmatic condition.[69]

Vision Loss

Although there are reports of visual problems secondary to elevated serum cobalt levels, little is known about the exact effects on the vision system in humans. Animal studies have shown photoreceptor degeneration associated with toxic levels of cobalt,[70,71] and one study showed a possible similar toxic effect on the human retina.[72] In rabbits, cobalt intoxication caused edema and atrophy of nerve fibers, lesions on retinal neurons, and damage to the nuclei of photoreceptors.[31] Human cases of irreversible and reversible vision loss, optic neuropathy and atrophy, and evidence of abnormal retinal and retinal pigment epithelial function have all been reported.[73,74,75]

INTERVENTION

A multifactorial approach is recommended in the treatment of cobalt toxicity due to MoM hip implants. Because arthroprosthetic cobaltism may result in several comorbid conditions (e.g., hypothyroidism, cardiomyopathy, hypersensitivity), clinical management is complex and further management is often required. Often these conditions will resolve with removal of the MoM prosthesis and reduction of cobalt levels. If removal is not an option, continued surveillance and additional therapy are needed. Even in cases in which the prosthesis is removed, chelation therapy may be used to reduce persistent elevated cobalt blood levels.[50]

Surgery

The primary and most definitive treatment for cobalt toxicity secondary to MoM implants is removal or revision of the prosthesis.[51] Revision with metal-on-polyethylene or ceramic-on-polyethylene is most often recommended.[52] Components that minimize the generation of cobalt debris (e.g., decreased modularity, avoidance of MoM bearings, use of titanium alloy components and ceramic heads) are also suggested.[76] Although cobalt levels have been shown to decrease (in one study from 20.8 µg/L preoperatively to 1.8 µg/L 1 year after revision), complications such as pseudotumor and bone loss may persist.[77]

Chelation Therapy

Clinical management of elevated cobalt levels associated with MoM hip prosthesis, particularly surrounding chelation therapy, is greatly debated. Current medical literature provides no consensus on chelation regarding the levels of cobalt at which chelation should be initiated, which agents to use, the timing of administration, the mode of administration, and the efficacy of treatment.[78,79] However, animal studies as well as human case studies have shown some benefit.

NAC, glutathione, EDTA, DMSA, and DTPA have shown the most benefit as chelating agents in acute cobalt toxicity.[80] In rats, glutathione, NAC, and DTPA have been shown to significantly increase the excretion of cobalt into urine, whereas EDTA, NAC, and DMSA were most effective at increasing fecal elimination of cobalt.[81] NAC (liver and spleen) and glutathione (spleen) have also been shown to be the most effective at reducing the concentration of cobalt in various tissues.[82]

Few human studies exist demonstrating the use of chelating agents in the treatment of MoM cobalt toxicity. Two promising case studies demonstrated the use of NAC to reduce elevated blood metal levels in MoM patients.[83] The first involved a 67-year-old male who presented with elevated cobalt levels (16.06 µg/L) 3 years following MoM hip implantation. He was given chelation therapy with oral high-dose NAC (300 mg/kg/day for 10 days). Cobalt blood concentration immediately dropped by 86% and persisted at the lower level during the following 6 months. The second case involved an 81-year-old female who presented with elevated blood levels of cobalt (20.24 µg/L) 6 years after undergoing MoM total hip arthroplasty. Chelation therapy with oral high-dose NAC (300 mg/kg/day for 9 days) was performed and blood concentrations of cobalt decreased 45%. Considering the safety of NAC, this may be an effective option for treatment at any elevated blood cobalt level. Table 12.2 provides a comprehensive view from the available literature of chelation therapy in metal hip–implanted patients.

TABLE 12.2   Chelation Therapy in Metal Hip–Implanted Patients

Age/Sex	Comorbidity	Hip Type	Latency from Implant to Symptoms or Blood Metals	Clinical Manifestations — Local	Clinical Manifestations — Systemic	Implant Revision	Co/Cr Blood Levels Before Chelation	Chelating Therapy	Co/Cr Blood Level After Chelation
58/F	Type 2 D, HTN	MOP[a]	6–9 mos	Prosthesis wear and local metallosis	Visual/hearing loss, II-VII cranial nerve disorders, sensorimotor disorders, mild hypothyroidism	Yes	Co 549 µg/L Cr 54 µg/L	EDTA IV (25 1-day cycles)	Reduced (not specified)[84]
56/M	Type 2 D	MOM[a]	14–20 mos	Prosthesis wear and hip dislocation	Hearing loss, sensorimotor disorders, walking difficulties, pericardial effusion, cardiomegaly, subclinical hypothyroidism	Yes	Co 506 µg/L Cr 14.3 µg/L	DMPS oral (14 mg/kg/day for 6 days, 4 mg/kg for 5 days, and 4 mg/kg for 4 days)	Reduced (not specified)[46]
52/M	————	MOP[a]	Not specified	Periarticular painful fluctuant mass with black fluid at aspiration	Dilated cardiomyopathy, pericardial effusion, liver failure, hypothyroidism	No	Co 1085 µg/L Cr not reported	Dimercaprol (1 3-day cycle)	Co decrease by 33%[85]

TABLE 12.2 Chelation Therapy in Metal Hip–Implanted Patients—cont'd

Age/Sex	Comorbidity	Hip Type	Latency trom Implant to Symptoms or Blood Metals	Clinical Manifestations Local	Systemic	Implant Revision	Co/Cr Blood Levels Before Chelation	Chelating Therapy	Co/Cr Blood Level After Chelation
55/M	———	MOP[a]	24 mos	Myositis ossificans–like picture	Visual/hearing loss., cardiomyopathy, hypothyroidism	Yes	Co 885 µg/L Cr 48.8 µg/L	DMPS (not specified)	Not specified[86]
75/M	———	MOM[a]	60 mos	Prosthesis wear and local metallosis	Asthenia, dilated cardiomyopathy, pericardial effusion	Yes	Co 46.5 µg/L Cr 76.1 µg/L	NAC oral + IV (IV: 150 mg/kg bolus + 300 mg/kg/d for 10 days) (Oral: two 7-day cycles at 100 mg/kg/d for each cycle)	Co/Cr decrease (by 51% and 40%)[87]
67/M	Cochlear implant, HTN	MOM	30 mos	Little fluid collection near the acetabular cup	No	No	Co 22.5 µg/L Cr 7.4 µg/L	NAC oral (Oral 300 mg/kg/day for 10 days)	Co/Cr decrease (by 86% and 87%) Case 1
81/F	COPD, SLE, mitral/aort reg., renal imp., euthyr goiter, HTN, cataracts	MOM	65 mos	Fluid collection near hip prosthesis	No	No	Co 21.1 µg/L Cr 11.8 µg/L	NAC oral (Oral 300 mg/kg/day for 9 days)	Co/Cr decrease (by 45% and 24%) Case 2

Co, cobalt; COPD, chronic obstructive pulmonary disease; Cr, chromium; DMPS, sodium 2,3-dimercaptopropane sulfonate; EDTA, edetate calcium disodium; euthyr. goiter, euthyroid multinodular goiter; IV, intravenous; HTN, hypertension; M/F, Male/female; mitral/aort. reg., moderate mitral and aortic valve regurgitation; MOM, metal-on-metal; MOP, metal on polyethylene; NAC, N-acetyl-cysteine; Renal imp, mild renal impairment; SLE, systemic lupus erythematosus; Type 2 D, type 2 diabetes.
[a]The prosthesis was implanted after the rupture of a previous ceramic hip implant.
Modified from Harvie, P., Giele, H., Fang, C., Ansorge, O., Ostlere, S., Gibbons, M., Whitwell, D. The treatment of femoral neuropathy due to pseudotumour caused by metal-on-metal resurfacing arthroplasty. Hip International: The Journal of Clinical and Experimental Research on Hip Pathology and Therapy. (2008). 18(4):313-20.

REFERENCES

1. Bozic, K. J., Kurtz, S., Lau, E., et al. (2009). The epidemiology of bearing surface usage in total hip arthroplasty in the United States. *The Journal of Bone and Joint Surgery. American Volume, 91-A*, 1614–1620. PubMed PMID: 19571083.

2. Agency for Toxic Substances and Disease Registry. (2001). *Toxic Substances Portal: Cobalt.* Chemical, physical, and radiological information. https://www.atsdr.cdc.gov/toxprofiles/tp33-c4.pdf. (Accessed March 27, 2017.)

3. Agency for Toxic Substances and Disease Registry. (2011). *Toxic Substances Portal: Cobalt.* Relevance to public health. http://www.atsdr.cdc.gov/toxprofiles/tp33-c2.pdf. (Accessed March 27, 2017).

4. De Smet, K., De Haan, R., Calistri, A., Campbell, P. A., Ebramzadeh, E., Pattyn, C., et al. (2008). Metal ion measurement as a diagnostic tool to identify problems with metal-on-metal hip resurfacing. *The Journal of Bone and Joint Surgery. American Volume, 90*(Suppl. 4), 202–208. PubMed PMID: 18984732.

5. Hart, A. J., Sabah, S. A., Bandi, A. S., et al. (2011). Sensitivity and specificity of blood cobalt and chromium metal ions for predicting failure of metal-on-metal hip replacement. *The Journal of Bone and Joint Surgery. British Volume, 93*(10), 1308–1313. PubMed PMID: 21969427.

6. Medicines and Healthcare Products Regulatory Agency. (2015). *Medical Device Alert: Metal-on-metal (MoM) hip replacements – guidance on implantation and patient management.* https://www.gov.uk/drug-device-alerts/metal-on-metal-mom-hip-replacements-guidance-on-implantation-and-patient-management. (Accessed March 27, 2017.)

7. Hart, A. J., Sabah, S., Henckel, J., Lewis, A., et al. (2009). The painful metal-on-metal hip resurfacing. *The Journal of Bone and Joint Surgery. British Volume, 91*(6), 738–744. PubMed PMID: 19483225.

8. US Food and Drug Administration (2015). *Metal-on-metal hip implants.* US Department of Health and Human Services. https://www.fda.gov/MedicalDevices/ProductsandMedicalProcedures/ImplantsandProsthetics/MetalonMetalHipImplants/ucm241604.htm. (Accessed March 27, 2017.)

9. Cheung, A. C., Banerjee, S., Cherian, J. J., Wong, F., Butany, J., et al. (2016). Systemic cobalt toxicity from total hip arthroplasties: review of a rare condition Part 1 – history, mechanism, measurements, and pathophysiology. *The Bone & Joint Journal, 98-B*(1), 6–13. PubMed PMID: 26733509.

10. Simonsen, L. O., Harbak, H., & Bennekou, P. (2012). Cobalt metabolism and toxicology – a brief update. *The Science of the Total Environment, 432*, 210–215. PubMed PMID: 22732165.

11. Jenkins, D. W. (1980). *Biological monitoring of toxic trace metals: Vol 1.* Biological monitoring and surveillance. Washington, DC: US Environmental Protection Agency.

12. Lippi, G., Franchini, M., & Guidi, G. C. (2005). Cobalt chloride administration in athletes: a new perspective in blood doping? *British Journal of Sports Medicine, 39*(11), 872–873. PubMed PMID: 16244201.

13. Ebert, B., & Jelkmann, W. (2014). Intolerability of cobalt salt as erythropoietic agent. *Drug Testing and Analysis, 6*(3), 185–189. PubMed PMID: 24039233.

14. Payne, L. R. (1977). The hazards of cobalt. *The Journal of the Society of Occupational Medicine, 27*(1), 20–25. PubMed PMID: 834025.

15. Bradberry, S. M., Wilkinson, J. M., & Ferner, R. E. (2014). Systemic toxicity related to metal hip prostheses. *Clinical Toxicology (Philadelphia, Pa.), 52*(8), 837–847. PubMed PMID: 25132471.

16. Hasegawa, M., Yoshida, K., Wakabayashi, H., & Sudo, A. (2012). Cobalt and chromium ion release after large-diameter metal-on-metal total hip arthroplasty. *The Journal of Arthroplasty, 27*(6), 990–996. PubMed PMID: 22325959.

17. Skipor, A. K., Campbell, P. A., Patterson, L. M., Anstutz, H. C., Schmalzried, T. P., & Jacobs, J. J. (2002). Serum and urine metal levels in patients with metal-on-metal surface arthroplasty. *Journal of Materials Science: Materials in Medicine, 13*(12), 1227–1234. PubMed PMID: 15348670.

18. Back, D. L., Young, D. A., & Shimmin, A. J. (2005). How do serum cobalt and chromium levels change after metal-on-metal hip resurfacing? *Clinical Orthopaedics and Related Research, 438*, 177–181. PubMed PMID: 16131888.

19. Brodner, W., Bitzan, P., Meisinger, V., Kaider, A., Gottsauner-Wolf, F., & Kotz, R. (2003). Serum cobalt levels after metal-on-metal total hip arthroplasty. *The Journal of Bone and Joint Surgery. American Volume, 85-A*(11), 2168–2173. PubMed PMID: 14630848.

20. Jacobs, J. J., Skipor, A. K., Doom, P. F., Campbell, P., Schmalzried, T. P., Black, J., et al. (1996). Cobalt and chromium concentrations in patients with metal-on-metal total hip replacements. *Clinical Orthopaedics and Related Research, 329*(Suppl.), S256–S263. PubMed PMID: 8769339.

21. Kim, J., Gibb, H., & Howe, P. (2006). *Cobalt and Inorganic Cobalt Compounds.* Geneva: World Health Organization. http://www.inchem.org/documents/cicads/cicads/cicad69.htm#11.2.1. (Accessed March 27, 2017.)

22. Centers for Disease Control and Prevention. *Fourth National Report on Human Exposure to Environmental Chemicals: Updated Tables*, January 2017, Volume One. Available at https://www.cdc.gov/biomonitoring/pdf/FourthReport_UpdatedTables_Volume1_Jan2017.pdf. (Accessed April 30, 2017.)

23. Ayala-Fierro, F., Firriolo, J. M., & Carter, D. E. (1999). Disposition, toxicity, and intestinal absorption of cobaltous chloride in male Fischer 344 rats. *Journal of Toxicology and Environmental Health. Part A*, 56(8), 571–591. PubMed PMID: 10321386.

24. Pizon, A. F., Abesamis, M., King, A. M., & Menke, N. (2013). Prosthetic hip-associated cobalt toxicity. *Journal of Medical Toxicology*, 9(4), 416–417. PubMed PMID: 24258006.

25. MacDonald, S. J. (2004). Metal-on-metal total hip arthroplasty: the concerns. *Clinical Orthopaedics and Related Research*, 429, 86–93. PubMed PMID: 15577471.

26. Visuri, T., Pukkala, E., Paavolainen, P., Pulkkinen, P., & Riska, E. B. (1996). Cancer risk after metal-on-metal and polyethylene-on-metal total hip arthroplasty. *Clinical Orthopaedics*, 329(Suppl.), 280–289.

27. Oldenburg, M., Wegner, R., & Baur, X. (2009). Severe cobalt intoxication due to prosthesis wear in repeated total hip arthroplasty. *The Journal of Arthroplasty*, 24(5), 825.e15–825.e20. PubMed PMID: 18835128.

28. Dijkman, M. A., de Vries, I., Mulder-Spijkerboer, H., & Meulenbelt, J. (2012). Cobalt poisoning due to metal-on-metal hip implants. *Nederlands Tijdschrift Voor Geneeskunde*, 156(42), A4983. PubMed PMID: 23075776.

29. Hallab, N. J., Caicedo, M., Finnegan, A., & Jacobs, J. J. (2008). Th1 type lymphocyte reactivity to metals in patients with total hip arthroplasty. *Journal of Orthopaedic Surgery and Research*, 3, 6. Feb 13, PubMed PMID: 18271968.

30. Davies, A. P., Willert, H. G., Campbell, P. A., Learmonth, I. D., & Case, C. P. (2005). An unusual lymphocytic perivascular infiltration in tissues around contemporary metal-on-metal joint replacements. *The Journal of Bone and Joint Surgery. American Volume*, 87(1), 18–27. PubMed PMID: 15634811.

31. Willert, H. G., Buchhorn, G. H., Fayyazi, A., Flury, R., Windler, M., Koster, G., et al. (2005). Metal-on-metal bearings and hypersensitivity in patients with artificial hip joints. A clinical and histomorphological study. *The Journal of Bone and Joint Surgery. American Volume*, 87(1), 28–36. PubMed PMID: 15637030.

32. Wong, C. C., & Nixon, R. L. (2014). Systemic allergic dermatitis caused by cobalt and cobalt toxicity from a metal on a metal hip replacement. *Contact Dermatitis*, 71(2), 113–114. PubMed PMID: 25040712.

33. Campbell, P., Shimmin, A., Walter, L., & Solomon, M. (2008). Metal sensitivity as a cause of groin pain in metal-on-metal hip resurfacing. *The Journal of Arthroplasty*, 23(7), 1080 1085. PubMed PMID: 18534479.

34. Hallab, N., Merritt, K., & Jacobs, J. J. (2001). Metal sensitivity in patients with orthopaedic implants. *The Journal of Bone and Joint Surgery. American Volume*, 83-A(3), 428–436. PubMed PMID: 11263649.

35. Perumal, V., Alkire, M., & Swank, M. L. (2010). Unusual presentation of cobalt hypersensitivity in a patient with a metal-on-metal bearing in total hip arthroplasty. *American Journal of Orthopedics*, 39(5), E39–E41. PubMed PMID: 20567745.

36. Kesteloot, H., Roelandt, J., Williams, J., Claes, J. H., & Joossens, J. V. (1968). An enquiry into the role of cobalt in the heart disease of chronic beer drinkers. *Circulation*, 37(5), 854–864. PubMed PMID: 5646867.

37. Sullivan, J. F., George, R., Bluvas, R., & Egan, J. D. (1969). Myocardiopathy of beer drinkers: subsequent course. *Annals of Internal Medicine*, 70(2), 277–282. PubMed PMID: 5764504.

38. Alexander, C. S. (1968). The concept of alcoholic myocardiopathy. *The Medical Clinics of North America*, 52(5), 1183–1191. PubMed PMID: 4876833.

39. Alexander, C. S. (1972). Cobalt-beer cardiomyopathy. A clinical and pathologic study of twenty-eight cases. *The American Journal of Medicine*, 53(4), 395–417. PubMed PMID: 4263183.

40. Health Quality Ontario. (2006). Metal-on-metal total hip resurfacing arthroplasty: an evidence-based analysis. *Ontario Health Technology Assessment Series*, 6(4), 1–57. PubMed PMID: 23074495.

41. Gilbert, C. J., Cheung, A., Butany, J., Zywiel, M. G., Syed, K., et al. (2013). Hip pain and heart failure: the missing link. *The Canadian Journal of Cardiology*, 29(5), 639.e1–639.e2. PubMed PMID: 23313008.

42. Zywiel, M. G., Brandt, J. M., Overgaard, C. B., Cheung, A. C., Turgeon, T. R., & Syed, K. A. (2013). Fatal cardiomyopathy after revision total hip replacement for fracture of a ceramic liner. *The Bone & Joint Journal*, 95-B(1), 31–37. PubMed PMID: 23307670.

43. Packer, M. (2016). Cobalt cardiomyopathy: a critical reappraisal in light of a recent resurgence. *Circulation Heart Failure*, 9(12), Pii: e003604. PubMed PMID: 27852654.

44. Mosier, B. A., Maynard, L., Sotereanos, N. G., & Sewecke, J. J. (2016). Progressive cardiomyopathy in a patient with elevated cobalt ion levels and bilateral metal-on-metal hip arthroplasties. *American Journal of Orthopedics*, 45(3), E132–E135. PubMed PMID: 26991580.

45. Sederholm, T., Kouvalainen, K., & Lamberg, B. A. (1968).
Cobalt-induced hypothyroidism and polycythemia in
lipoid nephrosis. *Acta Medica Scandinavica, 184*(4),
301–306. PubMed PMID: 5710037.

46. Lysaught, J. N. (1955). Goiter occurring during cobalt
therapy. *The Journal of the Oklahoma State Medical
Association, 48*(11), 333–335. PubMed PMID: 13263992.

47. Schirrmacher, U. O. (1967). Case of cobalt poisoning.
British Medical Journal, 1(5539), 544–545. PubMed
PMID: 6017158.

48. Kriss, J. P., Carnes, W. H., & Gross, R. T. (1955).
Hypothyroidism and thyroid hyperplasia in patients
treated with cobalt. *Journal of the American Medical
Association, 157*(2), 117–121. PubMed PMID: 13211322.

49. Prescott, E., Netterstrom, B., Faber, J., Hegedus, L.,
Suadicani, P., & Christensen, J. M. (1992). Effect of
occupational exposure to cobalt blue dyes on the
thyroid volume and function of female plate painters.
*Scandinavian Journal of Work, Environment and Health,
18*(2), 101–104. PubMed PMID: 1604269.

50. Pelclova, D., Sklensky, M., Janicek, P., & Lach, K. (2012).
Severe cobalt intoxication following hip replacement
revision: clinical features and outcome. *Clinical
Toxicology, 50*(4), 262–265. PubMed PMID: 22455358.

51. Kwon, Y. M., Lombardi, A. V., Jacobs, J. J., Fehring,
T. K., Lewis, C. G., & Cabenela, M. E. (2014). Risk
stratification algorithm for management of patients with
metal-on-metal hip arthroplasty: consensus statement
of the American Association of Hip and Knee Surgeons,
the American Academy of Orthopaedic Surgeons, and
the Hip Society. *The Journal of Bone and Joint Surgery.
American Volume, 96*(1), e4. Jan 1, PubMed PMID:
24382732.

52. Lombardi, A. V., Jr., Barrack, R. L., Berend, K. R.,
Cuckler, J. M., Jacobs, J. J., Mont, M. A., et al. (2012).
The Hip Society: algorithmic approach to diagnosis
and management of metal-on-metal arthroplasty. *The
Journal of Bone and Joint Surgery. British Volume, 94*(11
Suppl. A), 14–18. PubMed PMID: 23118373.

53. Pandit, H., Glyn-Jones, S., McLardy-Smith, P., Gundle,
R., Whitwell, D., et al. (2008). Pseudotumours associated
with metal-on-metal hip resurfacings. *The Journal of
Bone and Joint Surgery. British Volume, 90*(7), 847–851.
PubMed PMID: 18591590.

54. Mabilleau, G., Kwon, Y. M., Pandit, H., Murray, D. W.,
& Sabokbar, A. (2008). Metal-on-metal hip resurfacing
arthroplasty: a review of periprosthetic biological
reactions. *Acta Orthopaedica, 79*(6), 734–747. PubMed
PMID: 19085489.

55. Pandit, H., Vlychou, M., Whitwell, D., Crook, D.,
Lugmani, R., Ostlere, S., et al. (2008). Necrotic
granulomatous pseudotumors in bilateral resurfacing

hip arthroplasties: evidence for a type IV immune
response. *Virchows Archiv: European Journal
of Pathology, 453*(5), 529–534. PubMed PMID:
18769936.

56. Mahendra, G., Pandit, H., Kliskey, K., Murray, D.,
Gill, H. S., & Athanasou, N. (2009). Necrotic and
inflammatory changes in metal-on-metal resurfacing
hip arthroplasties. *Acta Orthopaedica, 80*(6), 653–659.
PubMed PMID: 19995315.

57. Campbell, P., Ebramzadeh, E., Nelson, S., Takamura,
K., De Smet, K., & Amstutz, H. C. (2010). Histological
features of pseudotumor-like tissues from metal-on-
metal hips. *Clinical Orthopaedics and Related Research,
468*(9), 2321–2327. PubMed PMID: 20458645.

58. Bosker, B. H., Ettema, H. B., Boomsma, M. F., Kollen,
B. J., Maas, M., & Verheyen, C. C. (2012). High incidence
of pseudotumour formation after large-diameter
metal-on-metal total hip replacement: a prospective
cohort study. *The Journal of Bone and Joint Surgery.
British Volume, 94*(6), 755–761. PubMed PMID:
22628588.

59. Van der Veen, H. C., Reininga, I. H., Zijlstra, W.
P., Boomsma, M. F., Bulstra, S. K., & van Raay, J. J.
(2015). Pseudotumour incidence, cobalt levels and
clinical outcome after large head metal-on-metal
and conventional metal-on-polyethylene total hip
arthroplasty: mid-term results of a randomized
controlled trial. *The Bone & Joint Journal, 97-B*(11),
1481–1487. PubMed PMID: 26530649.

60. Harvie, P., Giele, H., Fang, C., Ansorge, O., Ostlere, S.,
Gibbons, M., et al. (2008). The treatment of femoral
neuropathy due to pseudotumour caused by metal-on-
metal resurfacing arthroplasty. *Hip International, 18*(4),
313–320. PubMed PMID: 19097010.

61. Cugell, D. W. (1992). The hard metal diseases. *Clinics
in Chest Medicine, 13*(2), 269–279. PubMed PMID:
1511554.

62. Cugell, D. W., Morgan, W. K., Perkins, D. G., & Rubin,
A. (1990). The respiratory effects of cobalt. *Archives of
Internal Medicine, 150*(1), 177–183. PubMed PMID:
2297286.

63. Migliori, M., Mosconi, G., Michetti, G., Belotti, L.,
et al. (1994). Hard metal disease: eight workers with
interstitial lung fibrosis due to cobalt exposure. *The
Science of the Total Environment, 150*(1–3), 187–196.
PubMed PMID: 7939595.

64. Davison, A. G., Haslam, P. L., Corrin, B., Coutts, I.
I., et al. (1983). Interstitial lung disease and asthma
in hard-metal workers: bronchoalveolar lavage,
ultrastructural, and analytical findings and results of
bronchial provocation tests. *Thorax, 38*(2), 119–128.
PubMed PMID: 6857569.

65. Barceloux, D. G. (1999). Cobalt. *Journal of Toxicology. Clinical Toxicology*, *37*(2), 201–206. PubMed PMID: 10382556.

66. Cullen, M. R. (1984). Respiratory diseases from hard metal exposure. A continuing enigma. *Chest*, *86*(4), 513–514. PubMed PMID: 6478888.

67. Dai, J. H., Miao, L. Y., Xiao, Y. L., Meng, F. Q., & Cai, H. R. (2009). Giant cell interstitial pneumonia associated with hard metals: a case report and review of the literature. *Zhonghua Jie He He Hu Xi Za Zhi.*, *32*(7), 493–496. PubMed PMID: 19954001.

68. Van den Eeckhout, A. V., Verbeken, E., & Demedts, M. (1989). Pulmonary pathology due to cobalt and hard metals. *Revue Des Maladies Respiratoires*, *6*(3), 201–207. PubMed PMID: 2662276.

69. Shirakawa, T., Kusaka, Y., Fujimura, N., Goto, S., & Morimoto, K. (1988). The existence of specific antibodies to cobalt in hard metal asthma. *Clinical Allergy*, *18*(5), 451–460. PubMed PMID: 3233723.

70. Monies, A., & Prost, M. (1994). Experimental studies on lesions of eye tissues in cobalt intoxication. *Klinika Oczna*, *96*(4–5), 135–139. PubMed PMID: 7990329.

71. Hara, A., Niwa, M., Aoki, H., Kumada, M., et al. (2006). A new model of retinal photoreceptor cell degeneration induced by a chemical hypoxia-mimicking agent, cobalt chloride. *Brain Research*, *1109*(1), 192–200. PubMed PMID: 16863645.

72. Ng, S. K., Ebneter, A., & Gilhotra, J. S. (2013). Hip-implant related chorio-retinal cobalt toxicity. *Indian Journal of Ophthalmology*, *61*(1), 35–37. PubMed PMID: 23275221.

73. Meecham, H. M., & Humphrey, P. (1991). Industrial exposure to cobalt causing optic atrophy and nerve deafness: a case report. *Journal of Neurology, Neurosurgery, and Psychiatry*, *54*(4), 374–375. PubMed PMID: 2056332.

74. Lim, C. A., Khan, J., Chelva, E., Khaan, R., & Unsworth-Smith, T. (2015). The effect of cobalt on the human eye. *Documenta Ophthalmologica. Advances in Ophthalmology*, *130*(1), 43–48. PubMed PMID: 25380579.

75. Steens, W., von Foerster, G., & Katzer, A. (2006). Severe cobalt poisoning with loss of sight after ceramic-metal pairing in a hip – a case report. *Acta Orthopaedica*, *77*(5), 830–832. PubMed PMID: 17068719.

76. Zywiel, M. G., Cherian, J. J., Banerjee, S., Cheung, A. C., et al. (2016). Systemic cobalt toxicity from total hip arthroplasties: review of a rare condition Part 2. Measurement, risk factors, and step-wise approach to treatment. *The Bone & Joint Journal*, *98-B*(1), 14–20. PubMed PMID: 26733510.

77. Van Lingen, C. P., Eyyema, H. B., Bosker, B. H., & Verheyen, C. C. (2015). Revision of a single type of large metal head metal-on-metal hip prosthesis. *Hip International*, *25*(3), 221–226. PubMed PMID: 25907389.

78. Devlin, J. J., Schwartz, M., & Brent, J. (2013). Chelation in suspected prosthetic hip-associated cobalt toxicity. *The Canadian Journal of Cardiology*, *29*(11), 1533.e7. PubMed PMID: 23773894.

79. Hannemann, F., Hartmann, A., Schmitt, J., Lutzner, J., Seidler, A., et al. (2013). European multidisciplinary consensus statement on the use an monitoring of metal-on-metal bearings for total hip replacement and hip resurfacing. *Orthopaedics & Traumatology, Surgery & Research*, *99*(3), 263–271. PubMed PMID: 23507457.

80. Llobet, J. M., Domingo, J. L., & Corbella, J. (1985). Comparison of antidotal efficacy of chelating agents upon acute toxicity of Co(II) in mice. *Research Communications in Chemical Pathology and Pharmacology*, *50*(2), 305–308. PubMed PMID: 4081320.

81. Llobet, J. M., Domingo, J. L., & Corbella, J. (1988). Comparative effects of repeated parenteral administration of several chelators on the distribution and excretion of cobalt. *Research Communications in Chemical Pathology and Pharmacology*, *60*(2), 225–233. PubMed PMID: 2839877.

82. Llobet, J. M., Domingo, J. L., & Corbella, J. (1986). Comparison of the effectiveness of several chelators after single administration on the toxicity, excretion and distribution of cobalt. *Archives of Toxicology*, *58*(4), 278–281. PubMed PMID: 3087329.

83. Giampreti, A., Lonati, D., Ragghianti, B., Ronchi, A., et al. (2016). N-acetyl-cysteine as effective and safe chelating agent in metal-on-metal hip-implanted patients: two cases. *Case Reports in Orthopedics*, *2016*, 8682737. PubMed PMID: 27148463.

84. Pazzaglia, U. E., Apostoli, P., Congiu, T., Catalini, S., Marchese, M., & Zarattini, G. (2011). Cobalt, chromium and molybdenum ions kinetics in the human body: data gained from a total hip replacement with massive third body wear of the head and neuropathy by cobalt intoxication. *Archives of Orthopaedic and Trauma Surgery*, *131*(9), 1299–1308. PubMed PMID: 21298277.

85. Gilbert, C. J., Cheung, A., Butany, J., Zywiel, M. G., Syed, K., McDonald, M., et al. (2013). Hip pain and heart failure: the missing link. *The Canadian Journal of Cardiology*, *29*(5), 639.e1–639.e2. PubMed PMID: 23313008.

86. Dahms, K., Sharkova, Y., Heitland, P., Pankuweit, S., & Schaefer, J. R. (2014). Cobalt intoxication diagnosed with the help of Dr. House. *Lancet, 383*(9916), 574. PubMed PMID: 24506908.

87. Giampreti, A., Lonati, D., & Locatelli, C. A. (2014). Chelation in suspected prosthetic hip-associated cobalt toxicity. *The Canadian Journal of Cardiology, 30*(4), 465. e13. PubMed PMID: 24518658.

13

Lead

SUMMARY

- Presence in population: 50% of the population has lead blood levels associated with disease
- Major disease: Cognitive decline, mood disorder, parkinsonism, cardiovascular disease, renal disease, respiratory and reproductive issues
- Primary sources: Water and dust, maternal–fetal exchange, lead-containing dishes

- Best measure: Blood lead for recent exposures, lead mobilization test for body burden
- Best intervention: Avoidance, chelation with either sodium calcium edetate (CaEDTA) or dimercaptosuccinic acid (DMSA), N-acetyl cysteine, curcumin, and other antioxidants

DESCRIPTION

Lead has been utilized for centuries, resulting in wide distribution throughout the environment, including in all animals and humans. It is a highly persistent heavy metal, because at least 50% of all absorbed lead becomes stored in the bones, where it has a half-life of decades. The two greatest sources of nonoccupational environmental lead contamination were the addition of tetraethyl lead to commercial gasoline (from 1920 until the late 1970s) and its use as a color-enhancing additive in paint (from colonial times through 1978). Upon the government-mandated end of these two industrial uses, blood lead levels (BLLs) in the United States have been consistently dropping over the last few decades.[1] While the U.S. government was taking steps to ban the most common uses of lead, Herbert Needleman, MD, began publishing articles in medical literature on the adverse effects of lead on children raised in urban settings.[2] His numerous publications formed the basic understanding among the public and the medical community about the serious cognitive decline in children due to nonoccupational lead exposure.

The gradual reduction of BLLs in the average U.S. resident since the 1990s has been viewed as a great "win" for public health officials. In addition to the many diseases caused or aggravated by lead, it has also been directly linked to increased rates of homicide and other violent crimes.[3,4] Beginning in the late 1990s, the rates of homicides and societal violence began a dramatic decline that corresponded with dropping BLLs.[5,6] If the present decline of BLLs in the United States were to continue, then rates of violent crime may continue to drop, along with the other problems associated with lead, even at low levels. Unfortunately, changes in the use of disinfectant but corrosive chemicals from chlorine to chloramine in municipal water systems where lead service lines are still in use have resulted in widespread lead exposure in millions of U.S. residents, including highly publicized Flint, Michigan, and numerous other municipalities.[7,8] This alarming new source of lead exposure to millions of North American residents may carry serious public health implications for decades to come.

TOXICITY/METABOLISM

Lead is readily absorbed through both the respiratory and gastrointestinal tracts. Gastrointestinal absorption of lead in children can be up to five times greater than in adults exposed to the same sources.[9] Once absorbed, lead is bound to the red blood cells and transported into soft tissue and bones, with some excretion via the urine. Up to 70% of lead in the blood comes from trabecular bone, with the rest coming from current external exposures. More than 90% of the adult total body lead burden is stored in bones, where it is held for decades. Lead crosses both the blood–brain and placental barriers in adults and, once in the placenta, can easily enter into the fetal brain. In children, more than 80% of total body lead is found in the bones. The half-life of lead in blood and soft tissue averages 35 days, and in trabecular bone with greater bone turnover, the half-life of lead averages 8 years, whereas the half-life in cortical bone is up to 40 years.[10]

Lead is a powerful prooxidant compound, causing a tremendous amount of damage to cells and tissues.[11,12,13] Lead not only generates reactive oxygen species (ROS), but also causes a reduction in the activity of ROS-quenching enzymes such as superoxide dismutase, catalase, and glutathione peroxidase, resulting in diminished antioxidant defense. Cellular levels of reduced glutathione (GSH) also drop secondary to lead exposure. In adults, lead-associated oxidative stress is associated with an increase in urinary 8-hydroxy-2'-deoxyguanosine (8-OHdG) levels,[14] but such an increase has not been seen in children with similar BLLs.[15] Lead also appears to inactivate paraoxonase-1, a potent antioxidant enzyme that protects against organophosphate pesticide-induced neurotoxicity and cardiovascular disorders.[16]

In persons with BLLs higher than 35 µg/dL, the heme enzyme delta-aminolevulinic acid dehydratase (ALAD) is inhibited, leading to anemia, resulting in higher urinary levels of aminolevulinic acid. High BLLs also impair the functioning of ferrochelase, resulting in increased levels of zinc protoporphyrin (ZPP), but ALAD and ZPP levels are not useful in low-level lead burden.[17] Lead is also highly neurotoxic, resulting in severe toxic encephalopathy in those with very high lead burden. Part of its neurotoxic action includes a disruption of dopaminergic, cholinergic, and glutaminergic neurotransmitters, resulting in a host of neurotransmitter-related problems.[18]

SOURCES

As lead-containing paint ages, the lead is released as a very fine dust and reaches the indoor air through cracks in the subsequent layers of latex paint. It is also released in high amounts when older homes are restored and the

paint is removed by various means. Once in the indoor air, lead becomes bound to house dust and to fabrics in the home.[19] Household dust lead levels are positively correlated with BLLs in children.[20] Lead is also present in cigarette smoke and is found in higher levels in smokers and those exposed to secondhand smoke. Children raised in smoking households are found to have higher BLLs as well.[21] Lead has also been found in marijuana sold in Germany.[22]

During pregnancy, women undergo increased bone turnover, which results in greater BLLs for the woman and therefore greater lead exposure to the infant.[23] Women with higher bone lead burden will provide their growing child with a greater burden of lead at birth.[24,25] Bone turnover is also a source of elevated BLLs in menopausal women and must be considered when working up those women with lead-related health problems.[26] BLLs are typically 25% to 30% higher in women who have gone through menopause (and who are not on hormonal replacement) than women who have not experienced menopause.

Because bones are the storehouse of lead, concern has been raised recently about the potential risk of lead exposure for persons consuming bone broth as a regular part of their Paleolithic diet. Bone broth made from chicken bones has been found to contain up to 9.5 µg/L of lead, equivalent to groundwater lead levels associated with adverse health problems.[27] Dinnerware has been repeatedly found to be contaminated with lead, which is readily leached into acidic foods.[28,29] The migration of lead into such foods can be greatly increased when the food is then microwaved on the contaminated dishware.[30] Lead levels in excess of U.S. Food and Drug Administration (FDA) standards have been identified in hot sauces imported to the U.S. from Mexico.[31]

Ayurvedic and patented Chinese medicines can be sources of lead exposure for persons who utilize those therapies.[32,33] Lead is found to a lesser extent in some foods and in plastic products in the home. Lead is used in the manufacturing of polyvinyl chloride (PVC) and has been found in a number of PVC-containing consumer products in the home, including vinyl miniblinds, electrical power cords, artificial Christmas trees, lunchboxes, and toys.[34,35,36] Many of those consumer items are now sold with yellow labels to alert consumers that those items contain lead. Lead exposure in children has also occurred from costume jewelry[37] and tamarind candy.[38] Individuals who melt lead to make bullets, fishing weights, or toy soldiers, as well as those firing lead bullets in indoor shooting ranges also have greater lead exposure.[39] Individuals who have retained bullet fragments from gunshot wounds often have elevated BLLs as a result and must be monitored.[129] Persons who use lead to glaze pottery and who utilize lead-glazed pottery for culinary purposes are also at risk.[40]

However, the greatest source of lead exposure for children appears to come from living in pre-1951 homes. Children living in municipalities where chloramine is now being used in place of chlorine to disinfect the water get additional short-term exposure.[7,8] Children in Wayne County, North Carolina, who were routinely tested for blood lead were assessed based on the water service to their residence.[41] One water system (GWS) switched to chloramine in March 2002, whereas the other (WWS) continued to use chlorine. Fig. 13.1 shows the difference in blood lead between the two water supplies based on the age of the residence. Interestingly, children from both water districts had a jump in blood lead in March 2000, but the blood lead values in GWS district children were significantly higher than those living in the WWS district (4.93 µg/dL vs. 4.19 µg/dL, p < 0.00001). However, children living in homes built before 1950 in either water district had higher BLLs than those living in homes built

after 1951; those in homes built after 1975 had the lowest. The largest difference in blood lead was seen between GWS district children living in homes built after 1975 and those in homes built before 1926, indicating that a large portion of the BLLs in children whose lead values were > 4 µg/dL came from lead dust in the homes.

BODY BURDEN

Lead is found ubiquitously in the North American population and all other populations throughout the world. Table 13.1 summarizes the findings from the most recent update to the Centers for Disease Control and Prevention (CDC) Fourth Report on Human Exposure, based on data collected from the ongoing National Heath and Nutritional Examination Survey (NHANES). This table also contains the average BLLs from the 1999 to 2000 NHANES trial, so the drop in the national averages in BLLs over just the last decade can be clearly seen.

In adults, BLLs >30 µg/dL or two readings >20 µg/dL over a period of 4 weeks are the current maximum allowable level for industrial settings. Pregnant women are advised to have BLLs <5 µg/dL and all adults to have BLLs <10 µg/dL to prevent long-term health problems.[42] Childhood BLLs >40 µg/dL are considered in the toxic

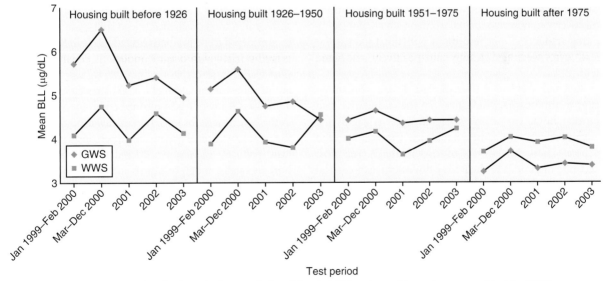

FIG. 13.1 Blood lead values before and after March 2002, when chloramine was added to GWS water treatment, according to age of the home. (From Miranda, M. L., Kim, D., Hull, A. P., Paul, C. J., & Galeano, M. A. (2007). Changes in blood lead levels associated with use of chloramines in water treatment systems. *Environmental Health Perspectives, 115*(2), 221-225. PubMed PMID: 17384768.)

TABLE 13.1   Blood and Urine Lead in the CDC Fourth National Report

CDC Fourth Report	Mean	50th	75th	90th	95th
Blood Lead (µg/dL)					
NHANES 1999/2000	1.66	1.60	2.50	3.80	5.00
NHANES 2011/2012	0.973	0.93	1.52	2.38	3.16
NHANES 2011/2014	0.858	0.830	0.410	0.840	1.22
Urine lead (µg/g cr) NHANES 2011/12	0.409	0.396	0.634	1.00	1.51
NHANES 2011/14	0.320	0.313	0.519	0.823	1.16

From Centers for Disease Control and Prevention, National Report on Human Exposure to Environmental Chemicals. Updated Tables, January 2017. Retrieved from www.cdc.gov/exposurereport/

range; however, the CDC recently established the level of ≥5 µg/dL as being "elevated" (the previous term used was "level of concern").[43] However, there is currently no CDC-approved protocol for children with BLLs <10 µg/dL beyond education and avoidance techniques.[44]

BLLs are utilized primarily to assess current exposure, with 70% of the total BLL coming from the trabecular bones. Correspondingly, postmenopausal women who were born in the post-WWII era are often found to have blood lead values that fall in the higher CDC percentiles due to the release of lead from their bones.[45,46] These findings are due to both the higher bone lead burden carried by this generation and the elevated rate of bone turnover.[47] In postmenopausal women who are not taking estrogen to retard bone resorption, both tibial and patellar lead levels were significantly and positively associated with BLLs.[48]

Research published over the last decade (presented later in this chapter) indicates that the cumulative lead burden holds the strongest significance in predicting adverse health outcomes in adults. Cumulative lead exposure is assessed by one of three methods. The most accurate method is K-shell x-ray fluorescence of cortical (tibia) or trabecular (patella) bones. K-shell x-ray fluorescence is currently only available at seven institutions in North America for research purposes and is not available to clinicians for use on their clients. It has been proposed that repeated BLL measures over time would provide a reasonable assessment of cumulative lead exposure; however, it is impossible to use this method for patients currently seeking help.[10]

The only method available to clinicians to assess the cumulative lead burden in patients is the lead mobilization test.[49,50,51] This protocol utilizes urinary lead values before and after a dose of a chelating agent to mobilize lead from body stores. calcium disodium ethylenediaminetetraacetate (CaEDTA) and DMSA are the two primary agents used for this test. CaEDTA and DMSA have been shown to mobilize lead from different compartments, with EDTA primarily mobilizing it from the trabecular bone and DMSA primarily mobilizing it from soft tissue (primarily the kidneys).[52] The CaEDTA mobilization test typically uses a 1-gram dose of intravenous sodium CaEDTA (35 mg/kg with saline for proper osmolarity) followed by either an 8- or 24-hour urine collection. Because 75% of the intravenous dose of CaEDTA is known to be excreted into the urine within 2.5 hours, a 4-hour collection may be sufficient. A total prechallenge lead spill ≥1 µg in children is considered to be predictive of a high lead burden.[53] In ongoing trials with adult nondiabetic renal patients, a post-CaEDTA lead spill totaling >80 µg was used as the cutoff value for initiation of CaEDTA chelation,[54,55] while a previous study of lead-poisoned children used >200 µg as the benchmark for initiation of chelation therapy.[49] In the nondiabetic renal patient study, persons with a urinary lead level <60 µg were considered to have a body lead burden small enough to not require chelation.

The use of DMSA for the lead mobilization test only requires a 4-hour urinary collection.[56] The bladder is emptied to provide the preprovoked sample, then a 1-gram challenge dose of DMSA (approximately one-half the standard body-weight dose for a 70-kg adult) is used to mobilize soft tissue lead stores. Total lead spills are then measured in the pre-DMSA urine and the 4-hour post-DMSA urine. Published studies have used this basic method to identify "DMSA-chelatable" lead stores in lead workers.[57,58] The conclusion in one of the articles that utilized this method on lead workers stated: "DMSA-chelatable lead was found to be the best predictor of lead-related symptoms, particularly of both total symptoms scores and neuromuscular symptoms, than were the other lead biomarkers."[59] The most common symptoms associated with lead excretion in this group of workers were paresthesias of the arms and legs, muscle pain, and a feeling of irritation at the slightest disturbance. Two recent studies have presented data from this method on nonoccupationally exposed controls that provide insight into normal values for those with "low-level" lead burden. The Belgian study control group had a mean BLL of 2.5 µg/dL, which is more than twice the current CDC mean for U.S. residents and would indicate that current exposure to lead was occurring.[58] The mean baseline urine lead value for this control group was 0.63 µg/4 hours with a range of 0.02 to 2.43. The post-DMSA lead spill for this control group ranged from 1.73 to 23.1 with a mean of 8.6 µg (± 4.5). The lead-exposed persons had baseline levels 13-fold higher than the control group, with a mean BLL of 36.7 and a pre-DMSA mean urine lead of 8.7 µg (Table 13.2). The authors of this study cited the control group's 97.5th percentile urinary lead level of 22 µg/4 hours as the upper reference value for the Belgian population. The second study also appears to have lead-burdened persons in the control group, as their mean BLL was 11.7 µg/dL with a pre-DMSA urine lead of 2.4 µg/4 hours, both values far higher than the CDC 95th percentile.[60] In comparison, the industrial lead–exposed group had a mean BLL of 29.9 µg/dL and a pre-DMSA mean urine lead of 4.8 µg/4 hours, double the level seen in the controls. The post-DMSA mean urine lead for the control group was 7.7 µg (± 5.9) (with a range of 1–25), whereas the lead-exposed group had a mean of 45.3 µg (with a range of 1.7–268 µg). These studies also show that BLLs and urinary lead levels were significantly correlated in lead workers.

A DMSA mobilization test benchmark value for nonoccupationally exposed persons could be derived by utilizing the value of one standard deviation above mean for both groups of controls, which is <14 µg. Utilizing one standard deviation above mean for the pre-DMSA lead total would provide a baseline benchmark of 1.13 µg for the Belgian study.

Clinical Significance

Neurological Disorders. BLLs commonly found in the general population as well as cumulative lifetime exposure to lead have both been associated with a number of common chronic health complaints and diseases. With the initial reports of lead toxicity centered on the cognitive decline of exposed children, it is not surprising that the nervous system shows the most lead-induced problems.

It has been clearly shown that even BLLs in children under the current CDC level of <5 µg/dL are capable of reducing their IQ levels. In 2003, *The New England Journal of Medicine* published an article showing that children with BLLs between 1 and 10 µg/dL had greater IQ point loss with a given increase in BLL than children with BLLs >10 µg/dL.[61] This resulted in a loss of 7.4 IQ points in children with BLLs <10 µg/dL, versus a loss of 4.6 IQ points in those with BLLs >10 µg/dL for the same BLL increase. The IQ loss with BLLs <10 µg/dL was confirmed in a subsequent study of 6-year-old children[62] and children in seven international population studies.[63] IQ loss with BLLs higher than 1.71 µg/dL was also found in a study of Italian adolescents. In this study, a doubling of the BLL equated to a 2.4 point reduction in IQ. The researchers stated that, for each 0.19 µg/dL increase in BLL, one IQ point was lost.[64] In a North Carolina study, BLLs as low as 2 µg/dL were associated with poorer performance in the classroom for school-aged children.[65] Among Hispanic children in Chicago public schools with BLLs <10 µg/dL, increasing BLL values were inversely associated with math and reading scores.[66] Children with BLLs 0 to 4 µg/dL did not exhibit math and reading problems, but children with BLLs of 5 to 9 µg/dL did. Lead-associated

TABLE 13.2 **Blood and Urine Levels in DMSA Lead Mobilization Test Studies**

Group	BLL µg/dL	Lead µg	DMSA Lead µg
Control 1	2.8	0.63 (0.5)	8.6 (4.5)
Lead workers	36.7	8.7 (10.9)	377.6 (538)
Control 2	11.7	2.4 (2.5)	7.7 (5.9)
Lead workers	29.9	4.8 (5.3)	45.3 (56.4)

Data from Bradberry, S., & Vale, A. (2009). A comparison of sodium calcium edetate (edetate calcium disodium) and succimer (DMSA) in the treatment of inorganic lead poisoning. *Clinical Toxicology, 47*(9), 841-858, and Canfield, R. L., Henderson, C. R., Jr., Cory-Slechta, D. A., Cox, C., Jusko, T. A., & Lanphear, B. P. (2003). Intellectual impairment in children with blood lead concentrations below 10 microg per deciliter. *The New England Journal of Medicine, 348*(16), 1517-1526.

decline of cognitive function in children has been shown to persist into adulthood,[67] giving the current state of municipal water lead contamination the potential for grave consequences among future adults in those areas.

BLLs higher than 1.6 µg/dL in children have also been strongly linked to increased risk of attention deficit hyperactive disorder (ADHD), oppositional defiant disorder (ODD), and conduct disorder (CD).[68] Children with BLLs between 1.6 and 2.7 µg/dL (the CDC 50th percentile) were 52% more likely to have inattentive ADHD, 86% more likely to have ODD or CD, and five times more likely to have hyperactive/impulsive ADHD. When the BLLs reached 2.7 µg/dL (CDC 90th percentile for children ages 6–11years), the risk for hyperactive/impulsive ADHD shot up more than sevenfold.

Cumulative lead burden in adults by bone lead assessment has been associated with decreased cognition,[69] whereas BLLs have shown no association.[70] Increasing levels of tibial lead were inversely related to impaired language, processing speed, eye-hand coordination, executive functioning, verbal memory, verbal learning, and visual memory.[71] As the tibial lead concentration rose, hand-eye coordination diminished. Women in the Nurses' Health Study also showed increased cognitive decline with increasing tibial lead.[72] Every 1-standard deviation(SD) jump in tibial lead was associated with a functional decline equivalent to 0.33 years of aging. Patellar lead was associated in the Normative Aging Study with poorer scores on the mini–mental status examination (MMSE) by men.[73] This lead-related decline was more pronounced among those men who also had GSTP1 alleles that reduced the functioning of that particular GSH transferase enzyme.[74] Although presence of the GSTP1 variant was not associated with cognitive decline itself, when found in those with higher patellar lead, its presence accelerated cognitive decline equivalent to 3 years of aging. Computerized neurobehavioral testing, easily done in a clinical setting, shows clear cognitive declines associated with bone lead burden[75] but no correlation with BLLs.[76]

Cumulative lead burden, as assessed by bone lead levels, is also associated with a risk of developing both parkinsonism[77,78] and Alzheimer's disease.[79] And as the tibial lead burden increased in Parkinson's patients, the cognitive functioning of these individuals significantly declined.[80] Higher levels of lead in the patella can also increase the risk of cataracts more than threefold, yet this risk is not associated with BLLs.[81]

Although BLL does not predict the risk of either Parkinson's disease or cognitive decline, it does predict the risk for other neurological dysfunctions in adults, including walking speed, balance, hearing, and mood. Walking speed, which reflects functional mobility and motor performance, declines with increased BLL.[82] Reduced walking speed is associated with increased risk of falls, late-life disability, increased hospital admissions, and mortality. Positive rombergism, long used to monitor acute toxic encephalopathy in impaired motorists, has also been shown to be present in adults with BLLs in the CDC 95th percentile.[83] BLLs ≤ 1.49 showed no increased risk for diminished hearing in adults in the NHANES trial, but higher levels were clearly associated with hearing loss.[84]

BLL also has validity in predicting problems with mood disorders in adults. Adults with BLLs >1.7 µg/dL (the current CDC 50th percentile) were more likely to have problems with depression and panic.[85] When the BLLs reached 3.0 µg/dL, the risk for depression increased 2.3-fold, while the risk for panic quintupled. Interestingly, tibial lead burden has also been associated with increased risk for both depression and phobic anxiety in women participating in the Nurses' Health Study.[86]

Cardiovascular Disorders. Studies utilizing both bone and blood lead levels have shown correlation with cardiovascular disease. Lead is a potent inactivator of nitric oxide and is therefore associated with increased blood pressure.[87] The NHANES data has revealed that adults with BLLs averaging 3.62 µg/dL (>CDC 95th percentile) are 55% more likely to die of a heart attack than those with BLLs <2.58 µg/dL.[88] Increased levels of tibial bone lead also correlate with increased risk for hypertension.[89,90] Higher bone lead levels have also been positively correlated with greater ECG abnormalities and other markers consistent with cardiac disease.[91,92] Lead levels have also been positively correlated with serum levels of homocysteine,[93] which is clearly associated with increased cardiovascular risk.

Renal Disorders. Renal damage is a common finding among lead workers and is also found in persons with nonoccupational low-level lead exposure. The progression to end-stage renal disease increases in direct proportion to the amount of lead in the kidneys.[94] Erythrocyte lead levels have been found to be reflective of kidney lead burden, whereas BLLs were positively associated with increasing serum creatinine levels in the Normative Aging

Study.[95] However, it must be kept in mind that the data for the Normative Aging Study was gathered between 1961 and 1994, when BLLs were at their highest points in the U.S.. Lead damages the kidneys both from direct oxidative damage to renal cells and from lead-induced hypertension. Cumulative lead burden, assessed both via bone lead levels and the CaEDTA lead mobilization test, has demonstrated a clear association between elevated body lead and renal disease (Tsaih – 76). Greater risk for lead-associated renal damage was noted in persons with diabetes. (Lin NEJM 2003) Reducing the total body lead burden via long-term chelation with CaEDTA has proven successful in slowing the renal damage and delaying the need for dialysis. (Lin NEJM 2003)

Respiratory Disorders. BLLs have been inversely associated with lung function, leading to obstructive lung disease (OLD). OLD is defined as having an forced expiratory volume in 1 second (FEV_1)/forced vital capacity (FVC) ratio of <0.7 on spirometry testing. Korean adults whose BLLs were >2.81 µg/dL exhibited significantly lower FEV_1/FVC ratios than those with BLLs <2.03 µg/dL.[96] Another study utilizing the data from the Korean NHANES (KNHANES) IV-V revealed that persons with BLL >3.17 µg/dL had the lowest FEV_1/FVC ratios.[97] Participants with OLD in the 2007 to 2010 NHANES in the United States were also found to have significantly higher BLLs than persons without this respiratory problem.[98] Those with OLD had mean BLLs of only 1.73 while those without OLD averaged 1.18.

Reproductive Disorders. Pregnant Japanese women with an average BLL of 4.52 µg/dL were far more likely to have a preterm delivery than women with only 0.80 µg/dL lower average BLL.[99] Those who were able to carry their babies to term had an average BLL of 3.72 µg/dL. Participants in the Nurses' Health Study with higher cumulative lead burden, assessed by tibial lead levels, experienced menopause earlier than their counterparts with lower lifetime lead burdens.[100] Menopause was advanced by 1.2 years for those women with the highest tibial lead counts. Unfortunately, this will result in an earlier release of the high bone lead stores into the bloodstream and soft tissues of those women.

Infertility is well documented in male lead workers with BLLs >50 µg/dL.[101] However, a study of nonoccupationally exposed couples wishing to conceive found that men's BLLs in the highest tertile were a major factor in failing to conceive a child.[102] The authors of this study noted that the BLLs found in their participants were strikingly similar to those found in NHANES. The presence of lead in seminal fluid has also been associated with failure of both artificial insemination[103] and *in vitro* fertilization attempts.[104]

INTERVENTION

Interventions focus on reduction of lead burden and reversal of lead-induced cellular and tissue damage.

Avoidance

The first step in the reduction of total lead burden is, of course, to identify and stop any current exposure. A BLL or urine lead value higher than the CDC 75th percentile would indicate current lead exposure. All of the previously discussed sources should be checked. With 70% of blood lead coming from bone, osteoporosis is a common source of BLL in higher percentiles. In postmenopausal women, BLL increases with increasing markers of bone turnover (bone-specific alkaline phosphatase and urinary cross-linked N-telopeptides).[105] In such women, the intake of supplemental calcium and vitamin D independently reduces the level of lead in the blood. For household lead exposure, various methods are available to identify lead levels in house dust and dishware. High-efficiency air purification units are also available that can clear toxicant-laden dust particles from home air.

Chelation to Reduce Body Lead Burden

After clearly identifying and stopping external sources of lead exposure, the next step is to begin reducing the body burden of lead. But with more than 90% of the adult lead burden residing in the bones, complete reduction of total body lead stores is simply not possible. Primary strategies for reducing lead burden must then be focused on reducing the soft tissue burden of lead. This will include both reducing trabecular bone stores, in hopes of lowering the amounts of lead that will be released in the future, and preventing increased bone turnover.

DMSA appears to be most effective at reducing soft tissue (primarily renal) levels of lead burden, which may be most relevant to the adverse health effects of lead.[55] DMSA has proven to be safe and highly effective for children with lead-induced encephalopathy in appropriate body weight or body size doses.[106] Coadministration of N-acetyl cysteine with DMSA provides greater lead excretion, possibly due to the fact that cysteine-conjugated DMSA carries the greatest amount of lead from the body.[107] CaEDTA primarily pulls lead from trabecular bone and secondarily from the kidneys, but while doing so may temporarily increase soft-tissue stores of lead in persons with a very high lead burden.[42,108]

Blood levels of lead drop with the use of either CaEDTA or DMSA; however, studies utilizing DMSA have repeatedly shown that the BLLs rise within 2 weeks of DMSA cessation.[109] For this reason, short-term intermittent use of DMSA is ineffective at reversing neurological dysfunction.[110] The regular release of bone lead into the bloodstream from normal bone turnover on a daily basis restores both blood and soft tissue lead levels. Based on this homeostatic balance, it would appear that the most effective means of achieving long-term reduction of both blood and soft tissue lead levels would include ongoing, rather than intermittent, DMSA therapy. For individuals with increased bone turnover, therapy to reduce bone demineralization would be critical in maintaining lower soft tissue and BLLs.[111] (*NB:* The authors do not recommend bisphosphonates for osteoporosis. Rather, this study was quoted to show that decreasing bone turnover decreases blood lead.)

There is no single established protocol for DMSA in treatment for lead that is universally accepted and followed. The dosing is based either on body weight or body surface area. The following protocols have all been utilized:

- 10 mg/kg every 8 hours for a total of 30 mg/kg/day for 5 days, followed by 10 mg/kg twice daily for another 14 days
- 1050 mg/M^2(body size)/day for 7 days, then 700 mg/M^2/day for 19 days
- 10 mg/kg every other day for a month
- 30 mg/kg divided into 3 daily doses (during waking hours) for 5 days, wait 9 days, then repeat
- 30 mg/kg divided into 3 daily doses (during waking hours) for 2 days, wait 5 days, then repeat

A study of Chinese children with BLLs between 10 and 25 µg/dL utilized DMSA at the 10/mg/kg level every other day for a month.[112] One of the treatment groups received concurrent daily doses of 1250 mg calcium and 200 mg of ascorbic acid during their DMSA regimen. The combination of DMSA and nutrients dramatically improved the reduction of BLLs and did a better job at rebalancing ALAD levels (delta-aminolevulinic acid dehydratase, which is inhibited

by lead) and reducing bone lead levels. Multiple studies have consistently shown that the addition of various antioxidant nutrients along with DMSA dramatically improves the outcome over DMSA alone. The use of vitamins E and C, melatonin, alpha lipoic acid, and N-acetyl cysteine concurrently with DMSA not only provides greater reversal of lead-induced biochemical and physiological damage, but significantly increases the excretion of lead itself.[106,113,114,115] Unfortunately, most of the data on the benefit of these antioxidants in tandem with DMSA were from animal studies, where the antioxidant substances were injected into the animals. Because of this, no good data exists on the most beneficial doses of these agents for humans.

Long-term use of CaEDTA for patients with renal failure has clearly revealed the benefit of ongoing chelation while monitoring total urinary lead excretion to determine the total body lead burden. Taiwanese researchers have refined the EDTA lead mobilization test and have shown that renal patients benefit the most by continuous CaEDTA therapy until their lead mobilization test results are <60 µg.[53] Nondiabetic individuals with renal disease who had a high body lead burden (>80 µg Pb and <600 µg) received intravenously either CaEDTA or a placebo weekly for up to 48 months.[116] After the first 3 months of weekly CaEDTA, it was noted that both BLLs and total body lead levels dramatically dropped. As body lead burden levels dropped, renal function improved, as evidenced by reduced serum creatinine and improved glomerular filtration rate. It was estimated that ongoing chelation therapy could delay the need for dialysis by several years. To date, no ongoing protocols with DMSA for lead-burdened persons has been published.

Amelioration of Lead-Induced Damage

In addition to the benefit of reducing total body lead burden, CaEDTA therapy has also been shown to reverse the prooxidant effects of lead.[117] These effects include a restoration of super oxide dismutase (SOD) and catalase levels, a reduction of malondialdehyde levels, improved PON1 function, and a reversal of the depression of acetylcholinesterase activity.

The use of antioxidant compounds as stand-alone agents (not in conjunction with DMSA or CaEDTA) has demonstrated effectiveness in reversing lead-induced damage.[118] Because lead can never be completely cleared from the body, the ability to prevent and reverse cellular and tissue damage from lead becomes a critical point for persons with lead-associated health problems. Both dietary-based antioxidants and antioxidant supplementation appear to be effective in this regard.[119] The best documented of these nutrients is N-acetyl cysteine, which powerfully reverses the oxidative stress following lead exposure. This compound has repeatedly shown benefit in improving biochemical and physiological markers in lead workers.[120,121] Other antioxidants that have shown effectiveness at helping to reverse cellular and tissue damage from lead include the previously mentioned vitamins C and E, l-methionine, zinc, melatonin, and ALA. The most impressive results were found with S-adenosyl methionine, which was able to improve cognition and learning in lead-poisoned animals.[122]

Common dietary components have also demonstrated benefit against lead burden. In animal models, both garlic (*Allium sativum*) and black cumin (*Nigella sativa*) were shown to significantly reduce tissue lead levels.[123,124] Turmeric (*Curcuma longa*), a major component of curry, a spice used by millions worldwide, appears to be one of the most powerful botanical therapies for lead exposure. Turmeric contains the flavonoid curcumin, which has demonstrated the ability to bind lead and other heavy metals,[125] reduce lead levels in animals, and reverse lead-induced oxidative stress.[126] The lead reduction activity of curcumin appears to be dose related, with more bioavailable forms of curcumin providing greater reduction of lead tissue burden.[127] In animal studies, lead levels in the liver, kidneys, and brain were all reduced with curcumin, along with a dramatic reversal of the oxidative stress caused by lead. Curcumin also reversed cognitive defects in lead-poisoned animals that were challenged to find their way through a water maze. The animals given curcumin not only had higher levels of GSH in their brains, but they retained better special memory and had faster escape times from the maze.[128]

Based on this information, the most prudent treatment approach for persons with higher lead burdens and lead-related neurological deficits might include DMSA to reduce BLLs along with antioxidants to reduce oxidative damage and neuroinflammation.

Assessment

1. Presence of symptoms of low-level lead exposure
2. Lead exposure coinciding with onset and aggravation of lead-related health problems
3. BLLs to assess current exposure with comparison to CDC values
4. Lead mobilization test for body burden
   a. Empty bladder and use this for a baseline reading on urinary lead
   b. Administration of lead-mobilizing agent
      i. 1 gram CaEDTA with 200 mL saline delivered over 1 hour
      OR
      ii. Oral DMSA–30 mg/kg
   c. Collect urine for 4 to 6 hours
   d. Estimate total µg/lead per collection time (µg/g creatinine of lead × creatinine level / 100,000 × total volume of urine collected = total µg of lead)
5. Markers of lead-associated damage
   a. Urinary 8-OHdG
6. Markers of increased bone turnover
   a. Urinary cross-linked N-telopeptides
7. Neurobehavioral/neurocognitive testing to identify defects in cognition and executive function

Treatment

1. Identification and avoidance of exposure sources
   a. If urinary telopeptides NTX is elevated, provide support to reduce rate of bone turnover
      i. Bisphosphonates
      ii. Calcium
      iii. Vitamin C
2. Antioxidant support
   a. Nutrients
      i. N-acetyl cysteine
      ii. S-adenosyl methionine
      iii. Vitamin C
      iv. Vitamin E
      v. Alpha lipoic acid
      vi. Melatonin
      vii. L-methionine
   b. Botanicals
      i. Curcumin
3. Chelation if appropriate
   a. Intravenous CaEDTA
      i. 50 mg/kg with saline to proper osmolarity delivered over 20 minutes
      ii. With supportive oral nutrients
   b. Oral DMSA
      i. According to one of the listed protocols

REFERENCES

1. Pirkle, J. L., Brody, D. J., Gunter, E. W., Kramer, R. A., Paschal, D. C., Flegal, K. M., et al. (1994). The decline in blood lead levels in the United States. The National Health and Nutrition Examination Surveys (NHANES). *The Journal of the American Medical Association, 272*(4), 284–291. PubMed PMID: 8028141.

2. Needleman, H. L., Gunnoe, C., Leviton, A., Reed, R., Peresie, H., Maher, C., et al. (1979). Deficits in psychologic and classroom performance of children with elevated dentine lead levels. *The New England Journal of Medicine, 300*(13), 689–695. Erratum in: *The New England Journal of Medicine.* (1994). 331(9):616-617. PubMed PMID: 763299.

3. Stretesky, P. B., & Lynch, M. J. (2004). The relationship between lead and crime. *Journal of Health and Social Behavior, 45*(2), 214–229. PubMed PMID: 15305761.

4. Stretesky, P. B., & Lynch, M. J. (2001). The relationship between lead exposure and homicide. *Archives of Pediatrics and Adolescent Medicine, 155*(5), 579–582. PubMed PMID: 11343501.

5. Mielke, H. W., & Zahran, S. (2012). The urban rise and fall of air lead (Pb) and the latent surge and retreat of societal violence. *Environment International, 43*, 48–55. PubMed PMID: 22484219.

6. Wolf, L. K. (2014). The crimes of lead: Research on the toxic metal's effects on the brain bolsters the hypothesis that childhood exposure is linked to criminal acts. *Chemical & Engineering News, 92*(5), 27–29. Available at http://cen.acs.org/articles/92/i5/Crimes-Lead.html. (Accessed September 2, 2016.)

7. Brown, M. J., Raymond, J., Homa, D., Kennedy, C., & Sinks, T. (2011). Association between children's blood lead levels, lead service lines, and water disinfection, Washington, DC, 1998-2006. *Environmental Research, 111*(1), 67–74. PubMed PMID: 21112052.

8. Young, A., & Nichols, M. *Beyond Flint: Excessive lead levels found in almost 2,000 water systems across all 50 states.* Available at http://www.usatoday.com/story/news/2016/03/11/nearly-2000-water-systems-fail-lead-tests/81220466/. (Accessed August 31, 2016.)

9. Centers for Disease Control and Prevention. (2009). *Fourth national report on human exposure to environmental chemicals.* www.cdc.gov/exposurereport. (Accessed March 22, 2018.)

10. Hu, H., Shih, R., Rothenberg, S., & Schwartz, B. S. (2007). The epidemiology of lead toxicity in adults: Measuring dose and consideration of other methodologic issues. *Environmental Health Perspectives, 115*(3), 455–462. PubMed PMID: 17431499.

11. Lopes, A. C., Peixe, T. S., Mesas, A. E., & Paoliello, M. M. (2016). Lead exposure and oxidative stress: A systematic review. *Reviews of Environmental Contamination and Toxicology, 236*, 193–238. PubMed PMID: 26423075.

12. Kasperczyk, A., Dobrakowski, M., Czuba, Z. P., Horak, S., & Kasperczyk, S. (2015). Environmental exposure to lead induces oxidative stress and modulates the function of the antioxidant defense system and the immune system in the semen of males with normal semen profile. *Toxicology and Applied Pharmacology, 284*(3), 339–344. PubMed PMID: 25771126.

13. Hsu, P. C., & Guo, Y. L. (2002). Antioxidant nutrients and lead toxicity. *Toxicology, 180*(1), 33–44, Review. PubMed PMID: 12324198.

14. Hong, Y. C., Oh, S. Y., Kwon, S. O., Park, M. S., Kim, H., Leem, J. H., et al. (2013). Blood lead level modifies the association between dietary antioxidants and oxidative stress in an urban adult population. *The British Journal of Nutrition, 109*(1), 148–154. PubMed PMID: 22464667.

15. Roy, A., Queirolo, E., Peregalli, F., Mañay, N., Martínez, G., & Kordas, K. (2015). Association of blood lead levels with urinary F_2-8α isoprostane and 8-hydroxy-2-deoxy-guanosine concentrations in first-grade Uruguayan children. *Environmental Research, 140*, 127–135. PubMed PMID: 25863186.

16. Permpongpaiboon, T., Nagila, A., Pidetcha, P., Tuangmungsakulchai, K., Tantrarongroj, S., & Porntadavity, S. (2011). Decreased paraoxonase 1 activity and increased oxidative stress in low lead-exposed workers. *Human and Experimental Toxicology, 30*(9), 1196–1203. PubMed PMID: 21296834.

17. Somashekaraiah, B. V., Venkaiah, B., & Prasad, A. R. (1990). Biochemical diagnosis of occupational exposure to lead toxicity. *Bulletin of Environmental Contamination and Toxicology, 44*(2), 268–275. PubMed PMID: 2322668.

18. Andrade, V. M., Mateus, M. L., Batoréu, M. C., Aschner, M., & Marreilha dos Santos, A. P. (2015). Lead, arsenic, and manganese metal mixture exposures: Focus on biomarkers of effect. *Biological Trace Element Research, 166*(1), 13–23. PubMed PMID: 25693681.

19. Dewalt, F. G., Cox, D. C., O'Haver, R., Salatino, B., Holmes, D., Ashley, P. J., et al. (2015). Prevalence of lead hazards and soil arsenic in U.S. housing. *Journal of Environmental Health, 78*(5), 22–29, quiz 52. PubMed PMID: 26738315.

20. Etchevers, A., Le Tertre, A., Lucas, J. P., Bretin, P., Oulhote, Y., Le Bot, B., et al. (2015). Environmental

determinants of different blood lead levels in children: A quantile analysis from a nationwide survey. *Environment International, 74*, 152–159. PubMed PMID: 25454232.

21. Richter, P. A., Bishop, E. E., Wang, J., & Kaufmann, R. (2013). Trends in tobacco smoke exposure and blood lead levels among youths and adults in the United States: The National Health and Nutrition Examination Survey, 1999-2008. *Preventing Chronic Disease, 10*, E213. PubMed PMID: 24355106.

22. Busse, F., Omidi, L., Timper, K., et al. (2008). Lead poisoning due to adulterated marijuana. *The New England Journal of Medicine, 358*(15), 1641–1642.

23. Gulson, B. L., Mizon, K. J., Korsch, M. J., Palmer, J. M., & Donnelly, J. B. (2003). Mobilization of lead from human bone tissue during pregnancy and lactation—a summary of long-term research. *The Science of the Total Environment, 303*(1–2), 79–104. PubMed PMID: 12568766.

24. García-Esquinas, E., Pérez-Gómez, B., Fernández-Navarro, P., Fernández, M. A., de Paz, C., Pérez-Meixeira, A. M., et al. (2013). Lead, mercury and cadmium in umbilical cord blood and its association with parental epidemiological variables and birth factors. *BMC Public Health, 13*, 841. PubMed PMID: 24028648.

25. Chen, Z., Myers, R., Wei, T., Bind, E., Kassim, P., Wang, G., et al. (2014). Placental transfer and concentrations of cadmium, mercury, lead, and selenium in mothers, newborns, and young children. *Journal of Exposure Science and Environmental Epidemiology, 24*(5), 537–544. PubMed PMID: 24756102.

26. Nash, D., Magder, L. S., Sherwin, R., Rubin, R. J., & Silbergeld, E. K. (2004). Bone density-related predictors of blood lead level among peri- and postmenopausal women in the United States: The Third National Health and Nutrition Examination Survey, 1988-1994. *American Journal of Epidemiology, 160*(9), 901–911. PubMed PMID: 15496543.

27. Monro, J. A., Leon, R., & Puri, B. K. (2013). The risk of lead contamination in bone broth diets. *Medical Hypotheses, 80*(4), 389–390. PubMed PMID: 23375414.

28. Sheets, R. W. (1999). Acid extraction of lead and cadmium from newly-purchased ceramic and melamine dinnerware. *The Science of the Total Environment, 234*(1–3), 233–237. PubMed PMID: 10507162.

29. Sheets, R. W. (1997). Extraction of lead, cadmium and zinc from overglaze decorations on ceramic dinnerware by acidic and basic food substances. *The Science of the Total Environment, 197*(1–3), 167–175. PubMed PMID: 9151439.

30. Sheets, R. W., Turpen, S. L., & Hill, P. (1996). Effect of microwave heating on leaching of lead from old ceramic dinnerware. *The Science of the Total Environment, 182*(1–3), 187–191. PubMed PMID: 8854945.

31. Berger Ritchie, J. A., & Gerstenberger, S. L. (2013). An evaluation of lead concentrations in imported hot sauces. *Journal of Environmental Science and Health. Part. B, Pesticides, Food Contaminants, and Agricultural Wastes, 48*(7), 530–538. PubMed PMID: 23581685.

32. Mathee, A., Naicker, N., & Teare, J. (2015). Retrospective investigation of a lead poisoning outbreak from the consumption of an Ayurvedic medicine: Durban, South Africa. *International Journal of Environmental Research and Public Health, 12*(7), 7804–7813. PubMed PMID: 26184256.

33. Crinnion, W. J. (2011). EDTA redistribution of lead and cadmium into the soft tissues in a human with a high lead burden—should DMSA always be used to follow EDTA in such cases? *Alternative Medicine Review: A Journal of Clinical Therapeutics, 16*(2), 109–112. PubMed PMID: 21649453.

34. Greenway, J. A., & Gerstenberger, S. (2010). An evaluation of lead contamination in plastic toys collected from day care centers in the Las Vegas Valley, Nevada, USA. *Bulletin of Environmental Contamination and Toxicology, 85*(4), 363–366. PubMed PMID: 20721658.

35. Maas, R. P., Patch, S. C., & Pandolfo, T. J. (2004). Artificial Christmas trees: How real are the lead exposure risks? *Journal of Environmental Health, 67*(5), 20–24, 32. PubMed PMID: 15628192.

36. Daluga, M., & Miller, K. (2007). Lead in your child's lunch box. *Clinical Pediatrics, 46*(2), 151–153. PubMed PMID: 17325088.

37. Maas, R. P., Patch, S. C., Pandolfo, T. J., Druhan, J. L., & Gandy, N. F. (2005). Lead content and exposure from children's and adult's jewelry products. *Bulletin of Environmental Contamination and Toxicology, 74*(3), 437–444. PubMed PMID: 15903176.

38. Lynch, R. A., Boatright, D. T., & Moss, S. K. (2000). Lead-contaminated imported tamarind candy and children's blood lead levels. *Public Health Reports, 115*(6), 537–543. PubMed PMID: 11354337.

39. Svensson, B. G., Schütz, A., Nilsson, A., & Skerfving, S. (1992). Lead exposure in indoor firing ranges. *International Archives of Occupational and Environmental Health, 64*(4), 219–221. PubMed PMID: 1468789.

40. Hughes, J. T., Horan, J. J., & Powles, C. P. (1976). Lead poisoning caused by glazed pottery: Case report.

The New Zealand Medical Journal, 84(573), 266–268. PubMed PMID: 1069941.

41. Miranda, M. L., Kim, D., Hull, A. P., Paul, C. J., & Galeano, M. A. (2007). Changes in blood lead levels associated with use of chloramines in water treatment systems. *Environmental Health Perspectives, 115*(2), 221–225. PubMed PMID: 17384768.

42. Kosnett, M. J., Wedeen, R. P., Rothenberg, S. J., Hipkins, K. L., Materna, B. L., Schwartz, B. S., et al. (2007). Recommendations for medical management of adult lead exposure. *Environmental Health Perspectives, 115*(3), 463–471. PubMed PMID: 17431500.

43. Centers for Disease Control and Prevention. *Standard Surveillance Definitions and Classifications.* Available at http://www.cdc.gov/nceh/lead/data/definitions.htm. (Accessed September 29, 2015.)

44. Burke, M. G., & Miller, M. D. (2011). Practical guidelines for evaluating lead exposure in children with mental health conditions: Molecular effects and clinical implications. *Postgraduate Medicine, 123*(1), 160–168. PubMed PMID: 21293095.

45. Krieg, E. F., Jr. (2007). The relationships between blood lead levels and serum follicle stimulating hormone and luteinizing hormone in the third National Health and Nutrition Examination Survey. *Environmental Research, 104*(3), 374–382. PubMed PMID: 17084837.

46. Jurczak, A., Brodowski, J., Grochans, E., Karakiewicz, B., Szkup-Jabłońska, M., Wieder-Huszla, S., et al. (2013). Effect of menopausal hormone therapy on the levels of magnesium, zinc, lead and cadmium in post-menopausal women. *Annals of Agricultural and Environmental Medicine, 20*(1), 147–151. PubMed PMID: 23540229.

47. Jackson, L. W., Cromer, B. A., & Panneerselvamm, A. (2010). Association between bone turnover, micronutrient intake, and blood lead levels in pre- and postmenopausal women, NHANES 1999-2002. *Environmental Health Perspectives, 118*(11), 1590–1596. PubMed PMID: 20688594.

48. Korrick, S. A., Schwartz, J., Tsaih, S. W., Hunter, D. J., Aro, A., Rosner, B., et al. (2002). Correlates of bone and blood lead levels among middle-aged and elderly women. *American Journal of Epidemiology, 156*(4), 335–343. PubMed PMID: 12181103.

49. Wedeen, R. P., Batuman, V., & Landy, E. (1983). The safety of the EDTA lead-mobilization test. *Environmental Research, 30*(1), 58–62. PubMed PMID: 6403349.

50. Markowitz, M. E., & Rosen, J. F. (1991). Need for the lead mobilization test in children with lead poisoning. *The Journal of Pediatrics, 119*(2), 305–310. PubMed PMID: 1907320.

51. Wedeen, R. P. (1985). Use of the CaNa2 EDTA Pb-mobilization test to detect occult lead nephropathy. *Uremia Investigation, 9*(2), 127–130. PubMed PMID: 3939486.

52. Hoet, P., Buchet, J. P., Decerf, L., Lavalleye, B., Haufroid, V., & Lison, D. (2006). Clinical evaluation of a lead mobilization test using the chelating agent dimercaptosuccinic acid. *Clinical Chemistry, 52*(1), 88–96. PubMed PMID: 16239340.

53. Shannon, M., Grace, A., & Graef, J. (1989). Use of urinary lead concentration in interpretation of the EDTA mobilization test. *Veterinary and Human Toxicology, 31*(2), 140–142. PubMed PMID: 2494797.

54. Lin, J. L., Lin-Tan, D. T., Hsu, K. H., & Yu, C. C. (2003). Environmental lead exposure and progression of chronic renal diseases in patients without diabetes. *The New England Journal of Medicine, 348*(4), 277–286. PubMed PMID: 12540640.

55. Chen, K. H., Lin, J. L., Lin-Tan, D. T., Hsu, H. H., Hsu, C. W., Hsu, K. H., et al. (2012). Effect of chelation therapy on progressive diabetic nephropathy in patients with type 2 diabetes and high-normal body lead burdens. *American Journal of Kidney Diseases, 60*(4), 530–538. PubMed PMID: 22721929.

56. Bradberry, S., & Vale, A. (2009). A comparison of sodium calcium edetate (edetate calcium disodium) and succimer (DMSA) in the treatment of inorganic lead poisoning. *Clinical Toxicology (Philadelphia, Pa.), 47*(9), 841–858. PubMed PMID: 19852620.

57. Tassler, P. L., Schwartz, B. S., Coresh, J., Stewart, W. F., & Todd, A. C. (2001). Associations of tibia lead, DMSA-chelatable lead, and blood lead with measures of peripheral nervous system function in former organolead manufacturing workers. *American Journal of Industrial Medicine, 39*(3), 254–261. PubMed PMID: 11241558.

58. Schwartz, B. S., Lee, B. K., Lee, G. S., Stewart, W. F., Lee, S. S., Hwang, K. Y., et al. (2001). Associations of blood lead, dimercaptosuccinic acid-chelatable lead, and tibia lead with neurobehavioral test scores in South Korean lead workers. *American Journal of Epidemiology, 153*(5), 453–464. PubMed PMID: 11226977.

59. Lee, B. K., Ahn, K. D., Lee, S. S., Lee, G. S., Kim, Y. B., & Schwartz, B. S. (2000). A comparison of different lead biomarkers in their associations with lead-related symptoms. *International Archives of Occupational and Environmental Health, 73*(5), 298–304. PubMed PMID: 10963412.

60. Khan, D. A., Qayyum, S., Saleem, S., & Khan, F. A. (2009). Evaluation of lead body burden in occupational workers by lead mobilization test. *Journal*

of the Pakistan Medical Association, 59(6), 350–354. PubMed PMID: 19534366.

61. Canfield, R. L., Henderson, C. R., Jr., Cory-Slechta, D. A., Cox, C., Jusko, T. A., & Lanphear, B. P. (2003). Intellectual impairment in children with blood lead concentrations below 10 microg per deciliter. The New England Journal of Medicine, 348(16), 1517–1526. PubMed PMID:12700371.

62. Jusko, T. A., Henderson, C. R., Lanphear, B. P., Cory-Slechta, D. A., Parsons, P. J., & Canfield, R. L. (2008). Blood lead concentrations < 10 microg/dL and child intelligence at 6 years of age. Environmental Health Perspectives, 116(2), 243–248. PubMed PMID: 18288325.

63. Lanphear, B. P., Hornung, R., Khoury, J., Yolton, K., Baghurst, P., Bellinger, D. C., et al. (2005). Low-level environmental lead exposure and children's intellectual function: An international pooled analysis. Environmental Health Perspectives, 113(7), 894–899. PubMed PMID: 16002379.

64. Lucchini, R. G., Zoni, S., Guazzetti, S., Bontempi, E., Micheletti, S., Broberg, K., et al. (2012). Inverse association of intellectual function with very low blood lead but not with manganese exposure in Italian adolescents. Environmental Research, 118, 65–71. PubMed PMID: 22925625.

65. Miranda, M. L., Kim, D., Galeano, M. A., Paul, C. J., Hull, A. P., & Morgan, S. P. (2007). The relationship between early childhood blood lead levels and performance on end-of-grade tests. Environmental Health Perspectives, 115(8), 1242–1247. PubMed PMID: 17687454.

66. Blackowicz, M. J., Hryhorczuk, D. O., Rankin, K. M., Lewis, D. A., Haider, D., Lanphear, B. P., et al. (2016). The impact of low-level lead toxicity on school performance among Hispanic subgroups in the Chicago public schools. International Journal of Environmental Research and Public Health, 13(8), PubMed PMID: 27490560.

67. Mazumdar, M., Bellinger, D. C., Gregas, M., Abanilla, K., Bacic, J., & Needleman, H. L. (2011). Low-level environmental lead exposure in childhood and adult intellectual function: A follow-up study. Environmental Health: A Global Access Science Source, 10, 24. PubMed PMID: 21450073.

68. Boucher, O., Jacobson, S. W., Plusquellec, P., Dewailly, E., Ayotte, P., Forget-Dubois, N., et al. (2012). Prenatal methylmercury, postnatal lead exposure, and evidence of attention deficit/hyperactivity disorder among Inuit children in Arctic Québec. Environmental Health Perspectives, 120(10), 1456–1461. PubMed PMID: 23008274.

69. Shih, R. A., Glass, T. A., Bandeen-Roche, K., Carlson, M. C., Bolla, K. I., Todd, A. C., et al. (2006). Environmental lead exposure and cognitive function in community-dwelling older adults. Neurology, 67(9), 1556–1562. PubMed PMID: 16971698.

70. van Wijngaarden, E., Winters, P. C., & Cory-Slechta, D. A. (2011). Blood lead levels in relation to cognitive function in older U.S. adults. Neurotoxicology, 32(1), 110–115. PubMed PMID: 21093481.

71. Bandeen-Roche, K., Glass, T. A., Bolla, K. I., Todd, A. C., & Schwartz, B. S. (2009). Cumulative lead dose and cognitive function in older adults. Epidemiology, 20(6), 831–839. PubMed PMID: 19752734.

72. Power, M. C., Korrick, S., Tchetgen Tchetgen, E. J., Nie, L. H., Grodstein, F., Hu, H., et al. (2014). Lead exposure and rate of change in cognitive function in older women. Environmental Research, 129, 69–75. PubMed PMID: 24529005.

73. Wright, R. O., Tsaih, S. W., Schwartz, J., Spiro, A., 3rd, McDonald, K., Weiss, S. T., et al. (2003). Lead exposure biomarkers and mini-mental status exam scores in older men. Epidemiology, 14(6), 713–718. PubMed PMID: 14569188.

74. Eum, K. D., Wang, F. T., Schwartz, J., Hersh, C. P., Kelsey, K., Wright, R. O., et al. (2013). Modifying roles of glutathione S-transferase polymorphisms on the association between cumulative lead exposure and cognitive function. Neurotoxicology, 39, 65–71. PubMed PMID: 2395864.

75. Dorsey, C. D., Lee, B. K., Bolla, K. I., Weaver, V. M., Lee, S. S., Lee, G. S., et al. (2006). Comparison of patella lead with blood lead and tibia lead and their associations with neurobehavioral test scores. Journal of Occupational and Environmental Medicine, 48(5), 489–496. PubMed PMID: 16688005.

76. Krieg, E. F., Jr., Chrislip, D. W., Crespo, C. J., Brightwell, W. S., Ehrenberg, R. L., & Otto, D. A. (2005). The relationship between blood lead levels and neurobehavioral test performance in NHANES III and related occupational studies. Public Health Reports, 120(3), 240–251. PubMed PMID: 16134563.

77. Coon, S., Stark, A., Peterson, E., Gloi, A., Kortsha, G., Pounds, J., et al. (2006). Whole-body lifetime occupational lead exposure and risk of Parkinson's disease. Environmental Health Perspectives, 114(12), 1872–1876. PubMed PMID: 17185278.

78. Weisskopf, M. G., Weuve, J., Nie, H., Saint-Hilaire, M. H., Sudarsky, L., Simon, D. K., et al. (2010). Association of cumulative lead exposure with Parkinson's disease. Environmental Health Perspectives, 118(11), 1609–1613. PubMed PMID: 20807691.

79. Bakulski, K. M., Rozek, L. S., Dolinoy, D. C., Paulson, H. L., & Hu, H. (2012). Alzheimer's disease and environmental exposure to lead: The epidemiologic evidence and potential role of epigenetics. *Current Alzheimer Research, 9*(5), 563–573. PubMed PMID: 22272628.

80. Weuve, J., Press, D. Z., Grodstein, F., Wright, R. O., Hu, H., & Weisskopf, M. G. (2013). Cumulative exposure to lead and cognition in persons with Parkinson's disease. *Movement Disorders: Official Journal of the Movement Disorder Society, 28*(2), 176–182. PubMed PMID: 23143985.

81. Schaumberg, D. A., Mendes, F., Balaram, M., Dana, M. R., Sparrow, D., & Hu, H. (2004). Accumulated lead exposure and risk of age-related cataract in men. *The Journal of the American Medical Association, 292*(22), 2750–2754. Erratum in: *The Journal of the American Medical Association.* (2005). 293(4):425. PubMed PMID: 15585735

82. Ji, J. S., Elbaz, A., & Weisskopf, M. G. (2013). Association between blood lead and walking speed in the National Health and Nutrition Examination Survey (NHANES 1999-2002). *Environmental Health Perspectives, 121*(6), 711–716. PubMed PMID: 23603014.

83. Min, K. B., Lee, K. J., Park, J. B., & Min, J. Y. (2012). Lead and cadmium levels and balance and vestibular dysfunction among adult participants in the National Health and Nutrition Examination Survey (NHANES) 1999-2004. *Environmental Health Perspectives, 120*(3), 413–417. PubMed PMID: 22214670.

84. Choi, Y. H., Hu, H., Mukherjee, B., Miller, J., & Park, S. K. (2012). Environmental cadmium and lead exposures and hearing loss in U.S. adults: The National Health and Nutrition Examination Survey, 1999 to 2004. *Environmental Health Perspectives, 120*(11), 1544–1550. PubMed PMID: 22851306.

85. Bouchard, M. F., Bellinger, D. C., Weuve, J., Matthews-Bellinger, J., Gilman, S. E., Wright, R. O., et al. (2009). Blood lead levels and major depressive disorder, panic disorder, and generalized anxiety disorder in US young adults. *Archives of General Psychiatry, 66*(12), 1313–1319. PubMed PMID: 19996036.

86. Eum, K. D., Korrick, S. A., Weuve, J., Okereke, O., Kubzansky, L. D., Hu, H., et al. (2012). Relation of cumulative low-level lead exposure to depressive and phobic anxiety symptom scores in middle-age and elderly women. *Environmental Health Perspectives, 120*(6), 817–823. PubMed PMID: 22538241.

87. Vaziri, N. D., & Ding, Y. (2001). Effect of lead on nitric oxide synthase expression in coronary endothelial cells: Role of superoxide. *Hypertension, 37*(2), 223–226. PubMed PMID: 11230275.

88. Menke, A., Muntner, P., Batuman, V., Silbergeld, E. K., & Guallar, E. (2006). Blood lead below 0.48 micromol/L (10 microg/dL) and mortality among US adults. *Circulation, 114*(13), 1388–1394. PubMed PMID: 16982939.

89. Tsaih, S. W., Korrick, S., Schwartz, J., Amarasiriwardena, C., Aro, A., Sparrow, D., et al. (2004). Lead, diabetes, hypertension, and renal function: The normative aging study. *Environmental Health Perspectives, 112*(11), 1178–1182. PubMed PMID: 15289163.

90. Park, S. K., Mukherjee, B., Xia, X., Sparrow, D., Weisskopf, M. G., Nie, H., et al. (2009). Bone lead level prediction models and their application to examine the relationship of lead exposure and hypertension in the third National Health and Nutrition Examination Survey. *Journal of Occupational and Environmental Medicine, 51*(12), 1422–1436. PubMed PMID: 19952788.

91. Peters, J. L., Kubzansky, L. D., Ikeda, A., Fang, S. C., Sparrow, D., Weisskopf, M. G., et al. (2012). Lead concentrations in relation to multiple biomarkers of cardiovascular disease: The Normative Aging Study. *Environmental Health Perspectives, 120*(3), 361–366. PubMed PMID: 22142875.

92. Eum, K. D., Nie, L. H., Schwartz, J., Vokonas, P. S., Sparrow, D., Hu, H., et al. (2011). Prospective cohort study of lead exposure and electrocardiographic conduction disturbances in the Department of Veterans Affairs Normative Aging Study. *Environmental Health Perspectives, 119*(7), 940–944. PubMed PMID: 21414889.

93. Schafer, J. H., Glass, T. A., Bressler, J., Todd, A. C., & Schwartz, B. S. (2005). Blood lead is a predictor of homocysteine levels in a population-based study of older adults. *Environmental Health Perspectives, 113*(1), 31–35. PubMed PMID: 15626644.

94. Sommar, J. N., Svensson, M. K., Björ, B. M., Elmståhl, S. I., Hallmans, G., Lundh, T., et al. (2013). End-stage renal disease and low level exposure to lead, cadmium and mercury; a population-based, prospective nested case-referent study in Sweden. *Environmental Health: A Global Access Science Source, 12*, 9. PubMed PMID: 23343055.

95. Kim, R., Rotnitsky, A., Sparrow, D., Weiss, S., Wager, C., & Hu, H. (1996). A longitudinal study of low-level lead exposure and impairment of renal function. The Normative Aging Study. *The Journal of the American Medical Association, 275*(15), 1177–1181. PubMed PMID: 8609685.

96. Chung, H. K., Chang, Y. S., & Ahn, C. W. (2015). Effects of blood lead levels on airflow limitations in Korean adults: Findings from the 5th KNHNES 2011. *Environmental Research, 136,* 274–279. PubMed PMID: 25460646.

97. Leem, A. Y., Kim, S. K., Chang, J., Kang, Y. A., Kim, Y. S., Park, M. S., et al. (2015). Relationship between blood levels of heavy metals and lung function based on the Korean National Health and Nutrition Examination Survey IV-V. *International Journal of Chronic Obstructive Pulmonary Disease, 10,* 1559–1570. PubMed PMID: 26345298.

98. Rokadia, H., & Agarwal, S. (2013). Serum heavy metals and obstructive lung disease: Results from the National Health and Nutrition Examination Survey. *Chest, 143*(2), 388–397. PubMed PMID: 22911427.

99. Vigeh, M., Yokoyama, K., Seyedaghamiri, Z., Shinohara, A., Matsukawa, T., Chiba, M., et al. (2011). Blood lead at currently acceptable levels may cause preterm labour. *Occupational and Environmental Medicine, 68*(3), 231–234. PubMed PMID: 20798002.

100. Eum, K. D., Nie, L. H., Schwartz, J., Vokonas, P. S., Sparrow, D., Hu, H., et al. (2011). Prospective cohort study of lead exposure and electrocardiographic conduction disturbances in the Department of Veterans Affairs Normative Aging Study. *Environmental Health Perspectives, 119*(7), 940–944. PubMed PMID: 21414889.

101. Apostoli, P., Bellini, A., Porru, S., & Bisanti, L. (2000). The effect of lead on male fertility: A time to pregnancy (TTP) study. *American Journal of Industrial Medicine, 38*(3), 310–315. PubMed PMID: 10940969.

102. Buck Louis, G. M., Sundaram, R., Schisterman, E. F., Sweeney, A. M., Lynch, C. D., Gore-Langton, R. E., et al. (2012). Heavy metals and couple fecundity: the LIFE Study. *Chemosphere, 87*(11), 1201–1207. PubMed PMID: 22309709.

103. Benoff, S., Hurley, I. R., Millan, C., Napolitano, B., & Centola, G. M. (2003). Seminal lead concentrations negatively affect outcomes of artificial insemination. *Fertility and Sterility, 80*(3), 517–525. PubMed PMID: 12969691.

104. Benoff, S., Centola, G. M., Millan, C., Napolitano, B., Marmar, J. L., & Hurley, I. R. (2003). Increased seminal plasma lead levels adversely affect the fertility potential of sperm in IVF. *Human Reproduction, 18*(2), 374–383. PubMed PMID: 12571177.

105. Jackson, L. W., Cromer, B. A., & Panneerselvamm, A. (2010). Association between bone turnover, micronutrient intake, and blood lead levels in pre- and postmenopausal women, NHANES 1999-2002.

Environmental Health Perspectives, 118(11), 1590–1596. PubMed PMID: 20688594.

106. Thurtle, N., Greig, J., Cooney, L., Amitai, Y., Ariti, C., Brown, M. J., et al. (2014). Description of 3,180 Courses of chelation with dimercaptosuccinic acid in children ≤5 y with severe lead poisoning in Zamfara, Northern Nigeria: A retrospective analysis of programme data. *PLoS Medicine, 11*(10), e1001739. PubMed PMID: 25291378.

107. Flora, S. J., Pande, M., Kannan, G. M., & Mehta, A. (2004). Lead induced oxidative stress and its recovery following co-administration of melatonin or N-acetylcysteine during chelation with succimer in male rats. *Cellular and Molecular Biology (Noisy-Le-Grand, France), 50,* PubMed PMID: 15555419.

108. Weiss, B., Cory-Slechta, D. A., & Cox, C. (1990). Modification of lead distribution by diethyldithiocarbamate. *Fundamental and Applied Toxicology, 15*(4), 791–799. PubMed PMID: 1964918.

109. Chisolm, J. J., Jr. (2000). Safety and efficacy of meso-2,3-dimercaptosuccinic acid (DMSA) in children with elevated blood lead concentrations. *Journal of Toxicology. Clinical Toxicology, 38*(4), 365–375. PubMed PMID: 10930052.

110. Dietrich, K. N., Ware, J. H., Salganik, M., Radcliffe, J., Rogan, W. J., Rhoads, G. G., et al. (2004). Effect of chelation therapy on the neuropsychological and behavioral development of lead-exposed children after school entry. *Pediatrics, 114*(1), 19–26. PubMed PMID: 15231903.

111. Gulson, B., Mizon, K., Smith, H., Eisman, J., Palmer, J., Korsch, M., et al. (2002). Skeletal lead release during bone resorption: Effect of bisphosphonate treatment in a pilot study. *Environmental Health Perspectives, 110*(10), 1017–1023. PubMed PMID: 12361927.

112. Jin, Y., Yu, F., Liao, Y., Liu, S., Liu, M., Xu, J., et al. (2011). Therapeutic efficiency of succimer used with calcium and ascorbic acid in the treatment of mild lead-poisoning. *Environmental Toxicology and Pharmacology, 31*(1), 137–142. PubMed PMID: 21787678.

113. Flora, S. J., Pande, M., & Mehta, A. (2003). Beneficial effect of combined administration of some naturally occurring antioxidants (vitamins) and thiol chelators in the treatment of chronic lead intoxication. *Chemico-Biological Interactions, 145*(3), 267–280. PubMed PMID: 12732454.

114. Pande, M., & Flora, S. J. (2002). Lead induced oxidative damage and its response to combined administration of alpha-lipoic acid and succimers in rats. *Toxicology, 177*(2–3), 187–196. PubMed PMID: 12135622.

115. Sivaprasad, R., Nagaraj, M., & Varalakshmi, P. (2004). Combined efficacies of lipoic acid and 2,3-dimercaptosuccinic acid against lead-induced lipid peroxidation in rat liver. *The Journal of Nutritional Biochemistry, 15*(1), 18–23. PubMed PMID: 14711456.

116. Lin-Tan, D. T., Lin, J. L., Yen, T. H., Chen, K. H., & Huang, Y. L. (2007). Long-term outcome of repeated lead chelation therapy in progressive non-diabetic chronic kidney diseases. *Nephrology, Dialysis, Transplantation, 22*(10), 2924–2931. PubMed PMID: 17556414.

117. Čabarkapa, A., Borozan, S., Živković, L., Stojanović, S., Milanović-Čabarkapa, M., Bajić, V., et al. (2015). CaNa2EDTA chelation attenuates cell damage in workers exposed to lead—a pilot study. *Chemico-Biological Interactions, 242*, 171–178. PubMed PMID: 26460059.

118. Caylak, E., Aytekin, M., & Halifeoglu, I. (2008). Antioxidant effects of methionine, alpha-lipoic acid, N-acetylcysteine and homocysteine on lead-induced oxidative stress to erythrocytes in rats. *Experimental and Toxicologic Pathology, 60*((4–5), 289–294. PubMed PMID: 18407480.

119. Patrick, L. (2006). Lead toxicity part II: The role of free radical damage and the use of antioxidants in the pathology and treatment of lead toxicity. *Alternative Medicine Review: A Journal of Clinical Therapeutics, 11*(2), 114–127. PubMed PMID: 16813461.

120. Kasperczyk, S., Dobrakowski, M., Kasperczyk, A., Zalejska-Fiolka, J., Pawlas, N., Kapka-Skrzypczak, L., et al. (2014). Effect of treatment with N-acetylcysteine on non-enzymatic antioxidant reserves and lipid peroxidation in workers exposed to lead. *Annals of Agricultural and Environmental Medicine, 21*(2), 272–277. PubMed PMID: 24959775.

121. Kasperczyk, S., Dobrakowski, M., Kasperczyk, A., Ostałowska, A., & Birkner, E. (2013). The administration of N-acetylcysteine reduces oxidative stress and regulates glutathione metabolism in the blood cells of workers exposed to lead. *Clinical Toxicology (Philadelphia, Pa.), 51*(6), 480–486. PubMed PMID: 23731375.

122. Cao, X. J., Huang, S. H., Wang, M., Chen, J. T., & Ruan, D. Y. (2008). S-adenosyl-L-methionine improves impaired hippocampal long-term potentiation and water maze performance induced by developmental lead exposure in rats. *European Journal of Pharmacology, 595*(1–3), 30–34. PubMed PMID: 18713624.

123. Massadeh, A. M., Al-Safi, S. A., Momani, I. F., Alomary, A. A., Jaradat, Q. M., & AlKofahi, A. S. (2007). Garlic (Allium sativum L.) as a potential antidote for cadmium and lead intoxication: Cadmium and lead distribution and analysis in different mice organs. *Biological Trace Element Research, 120*(1–3), 227–234. PubMed PMID: 17916975.

124. Massadeh, A. M., Al-Safi, S. A., Momani, I. F., Al-Mahmoud, M., & Alkofahi, A. S. (2007). Analysis of cadmium and lead in mice organs: Effect of Nigella sativa L. (black cumin) on the distribution and immunosuppressive effect of cadmium-lead mixture in mice. *Biological Trace Element Research, 115*(2), 157–167. PubMed PMID: 17435259.

125. Gupta, S. C., Prasad, S., Kim, J. H., Patchva, S., Webb, L. J., et al. (2011). Multitargeting by curcumin as revealed by molecular interaction studies. *Natural Product Reports, 28*(12), 1937–1955. PubMed PMID: 21979811.

126. Shukla, P. K., Khanna, V. K., Khan, M. Y., & Srimal, R. C. (2003). Protective effect of curcumin against lead neurotoxicity in rat. *Human and Experimental Toxicology, 22*(12), 653–658. PubMed PMID: 14992327.

127. Flora, G., Gupta, D., & Tiwari, A. (2013). Preventive efficacy of bulk and nanocurcumin against lead-induced oxidative stress in mice, *Biological Trace Element Research, 152*(1), 31–40. PubMed PMID:23292317.

128. Dairam, A., Limson, J. L., Watkins, G. M., Antunes, E., & Daya, S. (2007). Curcuminoids, curcumin, and demethoxycurcumin reduce lead-induced memory deficits in male Wistar rats, *Journal of Agricultural and Food Chemistry, 55*(3), 1039–1044. PubMed PMID: 17263510.

129. Weiss, D., Tomasallo, C. D., Meiman, J. G., Alarcon, W., et al. Elevated Blood Lead Levels Associated with Retained Bullet Fragments—UnitedStates, 2003–2012. MMWR Morb Mortal Wkly Rep. 2017 Feb 10;66(5):130–133. PubMed PMID: 28182606.

14

Mercury

SUMMARY

- Presence in the population: Ubiquitous; at least 50% of the population has levels associated with physiological changes and health problems
- Major disease: Reduced central nervous system (CNS) function, cardiovascular diseases, hypothyroidism, blood sugar dysregulation, autoimmunity, nonalcoholic fatty liver disease (NAFLD)
- Primary sources: Fish, shellfish, dental amalgams; some areas of the country have elevated levels of mercury in air and water

- Best measure: Blood and urine mercury should be tested for current exposure, mercury mobilization test for body burden, and hair mercury for preconception care and cardiovascular risk
- Best intervention: Avoidance of mercury sources, then reduction of body burden with chelation and whole foods diet, N-acetyl cysteine (NAC), curcumin

DESCRIPTION

Mercury is present in three basic states: metallic/elemental, inorganic, and organic (methyl, ethyl, alkyl, and phenyl mercury). Each of these has its own sources, metabolism, half-life, and toxicological targets in humans.

Elemental or metallic mercury is primarily released as a vapor into the environment through combustion of mercury-containing compounds, such as mercury-contaminated coal, and is also found in older thermometers, thermostats, and dental fillings. Elemental mercury vapor is highly absorbed (70% to 80%) in the lungs and moved into the blood. Once in the body, elemental mercury is oxidized by catalase-hydrogen peroxide, forming divalent Hg^{2+}, a reactive species. This combines covalently with nearby sulfhydryl groups, including hemoglobin, reduced glutathione (GSH), cysteine, and cysteine-containing proteins such as albumin. Each molecule of mercury binds to two molecules of glutathione GSH,[1] thereby reducing GSH stores in the body.[2] Once in the circulation, it can easily cross both the blood-brain and placental barriers because of its fat-soluble nature and is fairly rapidly eliminated through the urine. Elemental mercury has a biphasic biological half-life ($t_{1/2}$), beginning with a rapid 1- to 3-day $t_{1/2}$, followed by a slower $t_{1/2}$ of 1 to 3 weeks.[3,4]

Metallic mercury in the environment is methylated by algae and bacteria in the soil and water. Fish absorb this methylmercury (MeHg) as water passes over their gills and from feeding on smaller fish. Because the $t_{1/2}$ of MeHg in fish is 2 years, large predator fish can accumulate substantial concentrations. MeHg binds tightly to muscle protein and is not reduced by any form of cooking.[5,6] Virtually all (95%–100%) of the MeHg in consumed fish is absorbed through the human gastrointestinal (GI) tract. MeHg blood levels peak between 4 and 14 hours after fish consumption, with a blood $t_{1/2}$ of 45 to 70 days.[7] Approximately two-thirds of MeHg is eliminated in the feces (complexed with GSH), and the remaining third is rendered inorganic and cleared through the urine. More than 70% of the MeHg dumped into the intestines is reabsorbed via enterohepatic recirculation, accounting for this long $t_{1/2}$.[8] Once MeHg is complexed with L-cysteine, it can be transported into the brain via methionine-uptake mechanisms.[9] Fortunately, uptake of MeHg into the brain by this mechanism can be blocked by the presence of L-methionine.[10] Once in the brain, it undergoes slow dealkylation to become inorganic mercury.[11]

Inorganic mercury, present as mercury salts, has been added to various "health-related" products, including facial creams.[12] This form of mercury is also conjugated with GSH in the liver and excreted into the bile for fecal release.

TOXICITY

Mercury is a powerful prooxidant promoting the formation of hydrogen peroxide, lipid peroxides, and hydroxyl radicals.[13] Mercury binds irreversibly with reduced GSH, causing the loss of up to two GSH molecules through the bile into the feces. Compounding this loss is the mercury-induced inhibition of GSH reductase, preventing the recycling of oxidized glutathione (GSSG) back to GSH.[14] At the same time, mercury also inhibits GSH synthetase, reducing the level of GSH production. Not only is mercury known to reduce the functioning of GSH transferases, it can also lead to the development of anti-glutathione transferase antibodies.[15] In addition, exposure to mercury reduces the activity of catalase, super oxide dismutase, GSH peroxidase, and paraoxonase 1, all of which are highly important for preventing oxidative stress.[16]

MeHg causes a dramatic dissolution of microtubules in platelets, red blood cells, neurons, and any other cell it is found in.[17] Mercury-induced dissolution of microtubules typically leads to apoptosis of those cells, whether they are neuronal or nonneuronal.[18,19] Mercury decreases the phagocytic activity of white blood cells and leads to apoptosis of both monocytes and lymphocytes.[20,21] Apoptosis of these and other cells appears to be secondary to the mercury-induced GSH depletion in the mitochondrial inner membrane. Regardless of the form of mercury, the percentage of cells undergoing apoptosis is dependent on the total mercury concentration. Mercury (as well as cadmium and lead) also causes a decrease in DNA content and an increase in collagenase-resistant protein formation in synovial joint tissue.[22]

Mercury is bound by selenium in the body, which can actually counteract mercuric chloride and MeHg toxicity.[23,24] Low selenium levels are found in persons with higher levels of mercury in the body.[25] Interestingly, persons complaining of mercury neurotoxicity symptoms

had significantly lower serum selenium levels than those who did not complain of symptoms.[26]

All forms of mercury have demonstrated toxic effects in humans and animals. MeHg is a potent neurotoxin via several mechanisms, including demyelination, oxidative stress, and autonomic dysfunction. MeHg also appears to lead to an increased risk for cardiovascular problems, including myocardial infarction. Metallic mercury is also neurotoxic, but to a lesser degree than MeHg. Metallic mercury interrupts the normal uptake and release of neurotransmitters and can result in excitability and irritability. All forms of mercury are renal toxins as well.

SOURCES

The primary sources of mercury for humans are the consumption of fish with high MeHg content in those who eat fish and dental amalgams in those who do not eat fish and have multiple amalgams.

Fish

Research has shown that women who consume at least nine fish meals per month have blood mercury levels seven times higher than women who do not eat fish.[27] Because of the increased production of coal-fired power plants in Asia releasing mercury into the air, the mercury level in the Pacific Ocean is expected to increase another 50% by 2050, with an equivalent MeHg increase in fish from those waters.[28] Almost the entire eastern seaboard, much of the Gulf of Mexico, well over 1.2 million miles of freshwater rivers, and more than 16 million acres of freshwater lakes in the United States have mercury advisories on them.[29] The US Environmental Protection Agency (EPA) places such warnings on waters containing fish with levels of mercury exceeding the limit of 1 parts per million (PPM) to warn consumers about the danger of eating the fish.

Nearly all fish contain trace amounts of MeHg, but fish living in areas of high pollution, like the Great Lakes, will have much higher levels of mercury and other pollutants.[30] MeHg levels for most fish range from 0.003 PPM to 1.5 PPM, with an average of approximately 0.3 PPM.[31] Usually only the large predator fish like shark and swordfish are found to have levels of MeHg reaching the US Food and Drug Administration (FDA) limit for human consumption of 1 PPM. The FDA lists commercially sold fish according to their average mercury content.[32] Restaurants often advertise "ahi tuna," which refers to either bigeye or yellowfin tuna. Both have quite high levels (Table 3.9), but bigeye averages almost twice the mercury content of yellowfin. Canned tuna is usually composed of smaller species of tuna such as skipjack and albacore and will typically have much lower levels, averaging about 0.17 PPM. However, tuna sold to schools for their lunch programs have been found to have levels of mercury higher than those found in grocery stores.[33]

Even though canned tuna has far lower levels of mercury than "high-mercury" fish such as swordfish and shark, it accounts for approximately 40% of the total MeHg intake because it is the most frequently consumed fish in the United States.[34] The next most frequently consumed fish in the United States is farmed salmon, which ranks among the lowest of mercury-containing fish, yet has also been associated with elevated blood mercury levels because of its regular consumption.[35] (Also see Chapter 3; farmed fish are very high in persistent organic pollutants.) Levels of mercury have been noted in Atlantic salmon that are quite close to levels found in canned tuna (Table 3.10).[36]

During pregnancy, MeHg easily crosses the placental barrier to reach the fetus and is present in the breast milk of lactating mothers who regularly consume seafood. The mercury concentration in the milk of these women has ranged from 2.45 µg/L in the Faroe Islands[37] to 3 µg/L in Sweden[38] and 7.6 µg/L in coastal Alaska.[39] The largest MeHg poisoning occurred between 1953 and 1960 in Minamata and Niigata, Japan, where industrial dumping of mercury into Minamata Bay led to chronic mercury toxicity in persons whose primary diet consisted of seafood from those waters.[40]

Industrial and Natural Sources

Mercury is ubiquitous in our environment, primarily because of its release into the atmosphere through the burning of coal and oil and from volcanic eruptions.

Incineration of medical waste and cremations also contribute to the environmental load of mercury.[41] Because dental amalgams are common in cadavers, a single crematorium facility releases an average of 5453 kg of mercury per year.[42] Older chlor-alkali plants still use mercury, resulting in end-product mercury contamination (including high-fructose corn syrup) along with higher mercury levels in those living proximal to the facilities.[43,44] Mercury in the air near coal-burning plants is discussed in Chapter 6.

Amalgams

One of the key reasons there has been controversy over the contribution of dental amalgams to the body load of mercury has been the design of many of the most influential studies. In general, when trying to determine the effect of amalgams (which are 55% mercury) on various measures of body load of mercury, using the number of teeth with fillings results in standard deviations that are so large that statistical significance is lost. However, when the surface area of fillings is used, the correlations with blood, urine, and brain mercury become statistically very strong. Counting the number of fillings is much better than simply the number of teeth with fillings, though not as significant as surface area. The reality is that studies using number of teeth have obfuscated a serious problem for more than a century.

Persons with amalgams on the occlusal surfaces of their teeth have demonstrated nine times higher nonstimulated levels of mercury vapor in their oral cavities than persons without amalgams. With chewing stimulation, an additional sixfold increase in elemental mercury levels occurs.[45] Mercury concentrations remain elevated during 30 minutes of continuous chewing and decline slowly over the following 90 minutes.[46] Similar increases in oral mercury levels have also been found in those with amalgams who have bruxism and during gum chewing, tooth brushing, or the consumption of hot drinks.[47,48] Blood mercury concentrations have been positively correlated with both the number and surface area of amalgam restorations and are significantly higher in those with amalgams than those without.[49] Individuals with 1 to 4 occlusal amalgams are estimated to have an average daily mercury exposure of 8 µg, whereas those with 12 or more occlusal amalgams may be exposed to 29 µg per day.[50] High copper amalgams can release up to 50 times more mercury vapor than standard amalgams.[51] Amalgams are also associated with higher urinary[52] and breast milk mercury levels but not with increased hair mercury.[53]

As shown in Fig. 14.1, research on cadavers has found a direct, statistically significant correlation between mercury in various parts of the brain and the number of amalgams in the mouth.[54]

Because this might be discounted as migration in dead tissue, the same correlation has also been shown in live tissues. A study of donated kidneys for transplant found that the number of amalgam surfaces had an R = 0.62 with amount of mercury in the kidneys.[55] Each additional

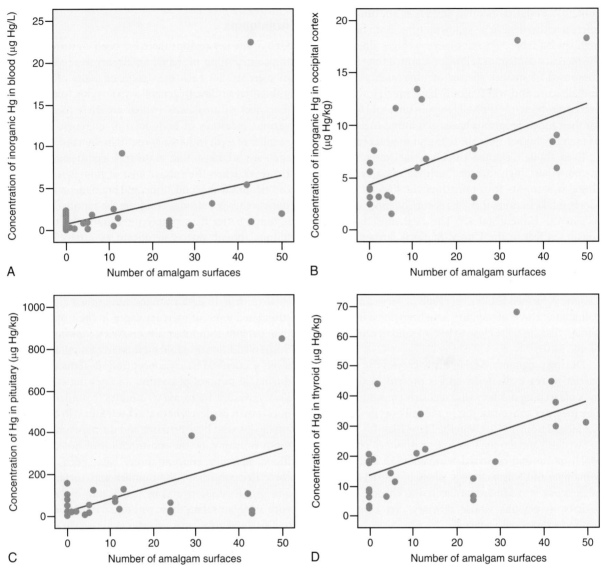

FIG. 14.1 Mercury in the brain correlates with the number of amalgam surfaces in the mouth. (From Guzzi, G., Grandi, M., Cattaneo, C., et al. [2006]. Dental amalgam and mercury levels in autopsy tissues. *The American Journal of Forensic Medicine and Pathology, 27*(1), 42–45.)

filling apparently caused a 6% increase in the amount of mercury in the kidney.

Other Mercury Exposure Sources

Mercury poisonings have occurred in individuals who lived or worked in buildings where mercury had formerly been used.[56,57,58] The improper cleaning of spilled mercury from broken thermometers has also resulted in mercury poisoning.[59] Mercury poisoning was found in persons living proximal to an inactive mercury mine in California and in individuals from several states who used mercury-containing face creams. Crema de Belleza-Manning facial cream was found to contain 6% to 10% mercury, and Nutrapeil Cremaning Plus was found to have 9.7% mercury.[61] Individuals living in older housing units have higher urinary mercury levels in addition to higher levels of cadmium, chlorophenoxy herbicides, and phthalates.[62]

BODY BURDEN

Mercury has been found in all populations that have been tested. Blood and urine mercury concentrations are commonly used as biomarkers of exposure to mercury, whereas hair is used to measure MeHg exposure. Recent exposure to mercury is reflected in both blood and urine, with urine giving a greater representation of metallic mercury, whereas blood favors MeHg.

The primary form of mercury in both hair and blood is MeHg, with more than 90% coming from the consumption of ocean fish and shellfish. Total blood mercury levels are directly associated with fish intake. Data from the 1999 to 2000 National Health and Nutritional Examination Survey (NHANES) revealed that women ages 16 to 49 years ingest a geometrical mean of 1.22 µg of mercury daily.[2] Those consuming fish twice weekly have a mean blood mercury level of 3.0 µg/L (Table 14.1).

The 2017 update to the Centers for Disease Control and Prevention (CDC) Fourth Report on Human Exposure provides data from the 2011 to 2014 NHANES, which measured total mercury, MeHg, ethyl mercury, and inorganic mercury (Table 14.2).[63] These US mercury ranges are closely reflected by those found in the populations of Canada, Mexico, Spain, Germany, the Czech Republic, and Italy.[64,65,66,67,68]

In the 2015 update to the Fourth Report, persons who identified themselves as Asian were included as a distinct ethnic group, in addition to Mexican Americans, non-Hispanic blacks, non-Hispanic whites, and all Hispanics. In previous years, Asian Americans were included with other populations under the general heading "Other." This group consistently had higher than normal mercury levels, which was ultimately found to correlate with the Asian Americans in the study. Because of higher fish intake in the Asian population, their mercury levels were higher across the board (Table 14.3).

The EPA reference value for blood mercury is less than 5.8 µg/L,[69] which more than 10% of the Asian ethnic group exceeded. The 95th percentile of blood mercury

TABLE 14.1 Blood Methylmercury (µg/L) in Women Ages 16 to 49, Years by Fish Intake, from NHANES 1999 to 2000

Fish Intake	Geo Mean	25th %	50th %	75th %	90th %	95th %
Never	0.43	ND	ND	0.60	1.4	2.1
<1 times/week	0.93	ND	0.82	1.80	4.4	6.4
≥1 times/week	2.04	0.83	2.56	5.54	8.8	11.6
≥2 times/week	2.70	1.12	3.02	6.68	12.0	13.4

From Mahaffey, K. R., Clickner, R. P., & Bodurow, C. C. (2004). Blood organic mercury and dietary mercury intake: National Health and Nutrition Examination Survey, 1999 and 2000. *Environmental Health Perspectives*, 112(5), 562–570.

TABLE 14.2 Blood and Urine Mercury Levels from NHANES 2011 to 2012

	Geo. Mean	50th %	75th %	90th %	95th %
Blood					
Total Hg (µg/L)	0.683	0.620	1.29	2.65	4.36
Methyl Hg (µg/L)	0.434	0.420	1.09	2.62	4.28
Ethyl Hg (µg/L)	<LOD	<LOD	<LOD	<LOD	<LOD
Inorganic Hg (µg/L)	<LOD	<LOD	<LOD	0.410	0.530
Urine					
Total Hg (µg/g creatinine)	0.246	0.200	0.470	1.07	1.64

From Harnly, M., Seidel, S., Rojas, P., Fornes, R., Flessel, P., Smith, D., et al. (1997). Biological monitoring for mercury within a community with soil and fish contamination. *Environmental Health Perspectives*, 105(4), 424–429.

TABLE 14.3   **Blood and Urine Mercury Levels Among Asians from NHANES 2011 to 2012**

	Geo. Mean	50th %	75th %	90th %	95th %
Blood					
Total Hg (µg/L)	1.86	2.30	4.32	7.71	10.3
Methyl Hg (µg/L)	1.58	2.16	4.35	7.57	10.5
Ethyl Hg (µg/L)	—	<LOD	<LOD	<LOD	0.160
Inorganic Hg (µg/L)	—	<LOD	0.350	0.550	0.700
Urine					
Total Hg (µg/g creatinine)	0.430	0.450	0.910	1.69	2.41

From Harnly, M., Seidel, S., Rojas, P., Fornes, R., Flessel, P., Smith, D., et al. (1997). Biological monitoring for mercury within a community with soil and fish contamination. *Environmental Health Perspectives*, *105*(4), 424–429.

TABLE 14.4   **Hair Mercury Levels (µg per Gram) in 16- to 49-Year-Old Women from NHANES 1999 to 2000**

Group	Geo. Mean	25th %	50th %	75th %	90th %	95th %
Total	0.20	0.09	0.19	0.42	1.11	1.73
No fish	0.11	0.05	0.10	0.20	0.40	0.55
Fish ≤2 times/month	0.20	0.10	0.19	0.39	0.79	1.26
Fish ≥3 times/month	0.38	0.17	0.34	0.81	1.75	2.75

From McDowell, M. A., Dillon, C. F., Osterloh, J., Bolger, P. M., Pellizzari, E., Fernando, R., et al. (2004). Hair mercury levels in U.S. children and women of childbearing age: reference range data from NHANES 1999 to 2000. *Environmental Health Perspectives*, *112*(11), 1165–1171.

in Asian Americans exceeds the blood level of mercury requiring emergency action to be taken (10 µg/L) set by the CDC.[70] Even though MeHg is reported to not clear well in the urine,[71] the increases in urinary mercury levels from one reported percentile to the next mirrored the increases seen for blood mercury.

MeHg present in the circulating blood during hair formation is incorporated into the follicles. Total blood mercury and blood MeHg levels are linearly related to total mercury in the hair. Because 80% of total hair mercury is MeHg, hair mercury levels are an excellent marker of MeHg exposure during the time of hair growth (typically 1–1.5 cm/month). Hair mercury levels have been significantly correlated with mercury levels in the cerebrum, cerebellum, heart, spleen, liver, and kidneys.[72] Levels of hair mercury were reported in the 1999 to 2000 NHANES, providing the first national ranges available for comparison with individual findings (Table 14.4).[73]

Because hair mercury is an excellent marker of ongoing MeHg exposure, this test has been recommended for women of reproductive age as a preconception tool to help prevent neurodevelopmental problems in their offspring.[74] The EPA reference dose for hair mercury is less than 1.0 µg/g.

However, both hair and urine mercury levels can be artificially reduced in persons with certain polymorphisms. GSH, GSH-conjugating enzymes, and selenium all play important roles in clearing mercury from the body. Individuals with genotypically reduced activity of three GSH transferase enzymes (GSTT1, GSTP1–105, GSTP1–114) are less able to clear mercury from the blood, resulting in lower urine and hair levels.[75] Similarly, those with a polymorphism in GSH synthase (GSS 5′) reducing the production of GSH also exhibit reduced hair and urine mercury levels. Reductions of both urinary and hair mercury levels are also found in persons with polymorphisms in selenoprotein processing.

In the body, mercury is also bound by thiol-rich metallothionein proteins. Of the four common isoforms of metallothionein, MT1M AA and MT2A CC both result in reduced urinary levels of mercury in dentists.[76] Those with either MT1A GA or GG and those with MT1M TT polymorphisms have less mercury in hair samples than should be present based on their blood MeHg levels.

These results suggest that individuals with such polymorphisms are less able to excrete mercury and are thus more susceptible to damage.

Detoxification/Excretion Processes

MeHg is primarily excreted through feces and hair, whereas inorganic and elemental mercury primarily exits through urine, with additional amounts leaving via breath, sweat, saliva, tears, and breast milk. Once in the body, mercury has a high affinity for sulfhydryl (thiol) groups and readily binds to available GSH and L-cysteine molecules. MeHg-L-cysteine is structurally similar to the amino acid methionine, and this molecular mimicry allows it to be a substrate for transport systems that carry methionine across cell membranes, including in the brain.

Once MeHg enters any cell in the body, some of it binds to GSH, forming a MeHg-GSH complex that can then be moved by membrane-bound efflux pumps. These pump transporters are members of the ATP-binding cassette (ABC) protein superfamily, including the multidrug-resistant proteins MRP1, 2, and 4, as well as the OATP3 transporters.[77] Mercury is moved from the blood into the urine through membrane-bound efflux pumps in the kidneys, primarily through the GSH-dependent multidrug-resistant protein 2 (MRP2).[78] Transport of both organic and inorganic mercury into the bile for excretion is also dependent on hepatic GSH stores. A depletion of GSH reduces the hepatic uptake of MeHg by 40% and reduces MeHg uptake by the kidney, thus inhibiting the two major pathways of mercury excretion.[79] Furthermore, any reduction of biliary mercury excretion results in increased body mercury levels and reduced renal uptake and excretion of mercury, because a large portion of the GSH-bound MeHg is reabsorbed from the intestines and then cleared through the kidneys.[80]

Clinical Significance

General Presentation. Beginning in the mid-20th century, mercury was released into the waters of Minamata Bay, Japan, affecting thousands of residents in the area. Minamata disease (MD) was the term used to describe the effects on those poisoned with MeHg; it presents with ataxia, speech impairment, constriction of visual field, hypoesthesia, dysarthria, hearing impairment, and sensory disturbances.[81] More than 1300 persons living in the Minamata Bay area, along with 446 controls, were assessed for subjective complaints 30 years after the spill

was discovered.[82] It was found that, in addition to the general symptoms, one of three major symptom groupings (sensory, arthritic, or muscular) would predominate the complaints in the affected individuals (Table 14.5).

A more recent study of persons with MeHg-related health problems (at levels lower than those found in Minamata) was done in a San Francisco, California, internal medicine practice.[83] Patients were selected for mercury blood testing based on either having a dietary history showing regular fish intake or having associated symptoms associated with excess mercury. This symptom picture consisted of fatigue, headache, decreased memory, decreased concentration, muscle or joint pain, hair loss and a metallic taste in the mouth. (Box 14.1).

A similar symptom list was used in a Canadian study of persons with amalgams to identify those needing amalgam removal and nutritional support.[84] Amalgam removal resulted in significant improvements in confusion, stomach problems, loss of sense of smell or taste, shakiness in hands, and coordination problems. Improvements in headaches and muscle weakness approached significance ($p \leq 0.1$). Supplementation, including N-acetyl cysteine and alpha lipoic acid, resulted in statistically significant

TABLE 14.5 Subjective Complaints Grouping Among Minamata Bay Residents with MeHg Exposure

Type	Complaint
General	Staggering
	Vertigo and dizziness
	Heart complaints
	Cramps
	Stiffness
	Dysesthesia
Sensory Dominant	Loss of touch sensation
	Loss of pain sensation
	Loss of thermal sensation
Arthritic Dominant	Arthredema
	Arthralgia
	Tinnitus and hearing difficulty
	Urinary complaints
Muscular Dominant	Muscular atrophy
	Muscular weakness

Modified from Fukuda, Y., Ushinjima, K., Kitano, T., Sakamoto, M., & Futatsuka, M. (1999). An analysis of subjective complaints in a population living in a methylmercury-polluted area. *Environmental Research, 81*, 100–107. PubMed PMID: 10433841.

BOX 14.1   Symptom Picture of Low-Level Mercury Burden

Symptoms Reflective of Mercury Burden in Fish Consumers[a]	Symptoms Improved After Amalgam Removal ($p < 0.05$)[b]
Fatigue	Headache
Headache	Memory loss
Decreased memory	Confusion
Decreased concentration	Coordination problems
Muscle pain	Hand tremors
Joint pain	Stomach problems
Hair loss	
Metallic taste	

[a]Hightower, J. M., & Moore, D. (2003). Mercury levels in high-end consumers of fish. *Environmental Health Perspectives, 111*(4), 604–608.
[b]Zwicker, J. D., Dutton, D. J., & Emery, J. C. (2014). Longitudinal analysis of the association between removal of dental amalgam, urine mercury and 14 self-reported health symptoms. *Environmental Health, 13,* 95.

TABLE 14.6   Mercury Toxicity Symptom Picture Used to Identify Mercury-Burdened Patients and the Most Commonly Improved Symptoms After Treatment

Symptom Type	Symptoms
Gross	Ataxia, intention tremor, incoordination, dysarthria
	Psychomotor retardation
Subtle	Fine tremor of tongue, lips, or outstretched fingers
	Hypersalivation with pooling of saliva
	Cold and erythematous hands and feet
	Labile mood
	Irritability, anxiety, depression, restlessness
	Cognitive problems (memory, concentration, cognition)
Symptoms most commonly improved after treatment	Fatigue
	Memory problems
	Depression

Modified from Wojcik, D. P., Godfrey, M. E., Christie, D., & Haley, B. E. (2006). Mercury toxicity presenting as chronic fatigue, memory impairment and depression: diagnosis, treatment, susceptibility, and outcomes in a New Zealand general practice setting (1994–2006). *Neuroendocrinology Letters, 27*(4), 415–423.

improvement in both memory loss and stomach problems.

A group in New Zealand used a set of mercury-related symptoms that appeared to be related to the Minamata disaster to identify persons with "chronic mercury toxicity" (Table 14.6).[85] Persons whose case fit into that symptom picture and who had a positive mercury mobilization test (discussed later) were then put on protocols for reducing their mercury load. Upon completion of the protocols, the most commonly improved symptoms were also those most commonly found in the cohort: memory problems, fatigue, and depression.

Cardiac Effects

- Hypertension
- Atherosclerosis and coronary vascular disease

Nonoccupational exposure to both elemental and methyl forms of mercury may predispose the individual to cardiovascular problems. Both short- and long-term increases in blood pressure have been documented among those poisoned in the Minamata Bay area in Japan.[86,87] Women who participated in the 1999 to 2000 NHANES trial exhibited a 1.83 mm Hg increase for each 1.3 µg/L increase in blood mercury.[88] Interestingly, this association was only significant for non–fish eaters. Two studies using hair mercury levels also found positive associations between mercury levels and blood pressure increases.[89,90]

Subjects in the Wisconsin Sleep Cohort study with the highest blood and hair mercury values were 1.9 and 4.0 times more likely to be hypertensive than those with lower mercury values.[91] Prenatal exposure to MeHg has been directly linked to elevated blood pressure and diminished heart rate variability when the children reached the age of 7 years.[92]

Hair mercury levels are associated with atherosclerotic disease, resulting in increased carotid intima-media thickness (CIMT).[93] Those with higher hair mercury levels were also found to be 56% more likely to have coronary heart disease (CHD), 60% more likely to have an acute myocardial infarction, and 68% more likely to have cardiovascular disease. In this study, the cardioprotective effects of docosahexaenoic and eicosapentaenoic acids were negated by the presence of MeHg. Heart tissue mercury levels in persons with cardiomyopathy were found to be 22,000 times higher than those in controls without CHD.[94] A study of Finnish and Swedish men revealed that hair mercury values were significantly associated with myocardial infarction, and that high hair mercury counteracted the benefit of fish oils in preventing heart disease.[95] Studies using toenail mercury as a measure of cumulative MeHg burden failed to find any increase in hypertension or cardiovascular disease risk related to this heavy metal,[96,97,98] making it apparent that toenail mercury is not a good method for identifying those with cardiovascular risk from mercury.

As mentioned earlier, paraoxonase 1, which quenches oxidized low-density lipoprotein and thereby provides cardioprotection, is inactivated by mercury.[16] This action of mercury alone would confer an increased risk for cardiovascular disease. A report from a group of mercury researchers assembled by the US EPA recently concluded that the weight of evidence indicates that MeHg is a contributing factor to acute myocardial infarction and that more research should be done to clarify this issue.[99]

Endocrine Effects
- Hypothyroidism
- Blood sugar dysregulation

Thyroid and blood sugar dysregulation are the two endocrine disorders attributed to nonoccupational mercury exposure. Mercury accumulates in the thyroid and reduces the uptake of iodine by binding to the sodium/iodide transporting molecule.[100] Mercury also inhibits deiodinase function in the peripheral tissues, preventing the production of triiodothyronine (T3) from thyroxine (T4).[101] Both adolescents and adults in the 2007 to 2008 NHANES had a negative association between blood mercury levels and total T3 and T4.[102] Adolescents also showed a higher risk for both antithyroglobulin and anti-thyroid peroxidase (TPO) antibodies. Women in the same NHANES cohort with blood mercury levels above 1.8 μg/L (approximately the 80th percentile) were more likely to have antithyroglobulin antibodies than those with blood mercury levels below 0.4 μg/L.[103]

Inorganic mercury causes pancreatic beta-cell dysfunction and apoptosis, which can fortunately be prevented with N-acetyl cysteine.[104] The association between blood mercury level and insulin resistance was assessed with data available from the 2008 to 2010 Korean NHANES (KNHANES).[105] This population consumes fish more frequently on average than the US population and thus has higher mean levels of blood mercury. This study used the homeostatic model Assessment for insulin resistance

(HOMA-IR) to assess insulin resistance. A significant correlation was found between blood mercury levels and fasting blood sugar, insulin, and insulin resistance. Data from the 2010 to 2012 KNHANES revealed that, compared with persons with the lowest quartile of mercury, those with the highest blood mercury were 62% more likely to have metabolic syndrome.[106] Adults in the Coronary Artery Risk Development in Young Adults (CARDIA) study with the highest toenail mercury levels were 65% more likely to develop type 2 diabetes than those with lower levels of mercury.[107]

Immune Effects
- Immune impairment
- Autoimmunity

Both inorganic and organic mercury exposure induces apoptosis of T cells through a combination of oxidative stress, reduction of GSH, and the release of cytochrome c from the mitochondria into the cytosol.[108,109] In addition, mercury reduces the release of T-helper 1 cytokines and increases those promoting T-helper 2 activity,[110] a phenomenon associated with depletion of GSH within the T cell.[111] Such an imbalance results in a reduction of cell-mediated immunity (leading to chronic infections) and an increase in allergic reactivity and autoimmunity.

In animal models, mercury has clearly been shown to promote autoimmunity.[112] People with systemic sclerosis and connective tissue disease often have elevated antifibrillarin antibodies. A group of individuals with high antifibrillarin antibodies had significantly higher urine mercury levels than did healthy controls.[113] Women participating in the 1999 to 2004 NHANES with higher levels of both blood and hair mercury were respectively 2.3 and 4.1 times more likely to have elevated antinuclear antibody (ANA) levels.[114] The mean levels of blood and hair mercury for the ANA-positive women were close to the CDC 75th percentile (Table 14.7). This association appears to be with MeHg, because urine mercury levels (primarily inorganic mercury) showed no association. When those with blood and hair values in the highest quartiles were compared with those with values in the lowest quartile, the odds ratios went to 11.41 for hair and 5.93 for blood.

The hair mercury levels associated with ANA in the previously discussed study were found in approximately 50% of NHANES participants, yet ANA-associated blood levels were found in 25%. For frequent fish consumers like Asian Americans, these levels were found in more

TABLE 14.7   Mercury Levels of ANA-Positive and ANA-Negative Women from NHANES 1999 to 2004

NHANES Year	ANA POSITIVE			ANA NEGATIVE		
	N	Blood Hg	Hair Hg	N	Blood Hg	Hair Hg
1999–2000	56	1.31 µg/L	0.27 PPM	396	1.01 µg/L	0.21 PPM
1999–2004	213	0.97 µg/L	NA	1139	0.91 µg/L	NA

Data from Somers, E. C., Ganser, M. A., Warren, J. S., Basu, N., Wang, L., Zick, S. M., et al. (2015). Mercury exposure and antinuclear antibodies among females of reproductive age in the United States: NHANES. *Environmental Health Perspectives, 123*(8), 792–798.

than 50%. Women from NHANES 2007 to 2008 with higher blood mercury levels were also more likely to have antithyroglobulin antibodies.[114] That group of women had a slightly higher blood mercury cutoff of 1.8 µg/L for having autoimmunity.

Neurological Effects

• Diminished CNS executive function

Mercury readily moves into the brain in both elemental and organic forms, as previously discussed. Blood MeHg levels are significantly correlated with mercury levels in the brain.[115] A blood MeHg level of 2.2 µg/L (CDC 50th percentile in Asians, <90th percentile in other ethnic groups) correlated with a 5 µg/kg mercury load in the cortex. In the brain, MeHg affects the mitochondria, endoplasmic reticulum, golgi complex, nuclear envelopes, and lysosomes. In nerve fibers, MeHg is localized primarily in myelin sheaths, where it leads to demyelination.[116] Fortunately, GSH, selenium, and cysteine have all demonstrated effectiveness at blocking mercury-induced neurotoxicity.[117]

Prenatal exposure to MeHg has resulted in ongoing neurobehavioral and neurocognitive defects in children.[118,119] Studies of children in the Faroe Islands whose mothers had a hair mercury value of more than 1 PPM have shown that these neurobehavioral defects persist at least through the age of 14 years.[120,121] Motor function, language skills, and memory were all diminished with prenatal MeHg exposure. Prenatal MeHg exposure also causes a reduction in children's IQ. Children with a cord blood mercury of 7.5 µg/L or higher were four times more likely to have an IQ below 80.[122] Children with higher cord blood mercury levels were also more likely to have attention deficit hyperactivity disorder (ADHD) in later years.[123] Maternal hair mercury levels within the NHANES values for fish eaters have also been associated with diminished visual memory, learning, and verbal memory in the offspring.[124]

Postnatal MeHg exposure is associated with diminished visuospatial processing and memory.[125] Amazonian children with hair mercury levels of more than 10 µg/g have poorer neuropsychological test results in motor function, attention, and visuospatial performance.[126] Dentists also perform significantly worse on neurobehavioral tests measuring motor speed (finger tapping), visual scanning (trail making), visuomotor coordination and concentration (digit symbol), verbal memory, visual memory, and visuomotor coordination speed.[127] Dentists with a mean blood mercury of 3.32 µg/L (versus 2.29 µg/L) and dental assistants with a mean blood mercury of 1.98 µg/L (versus 1.03 µg/L) exhibited statistically significant declines on multiple tests.[128] Those with a polymorphism in the coproporphyrinogen oxidase gene not only had worse performance on neurobehavioral testing, but also had greater depression, highlighted by feelings of worthlessness. Diminished complex information processing was found in fish-consuming corporate executives whose average blood mercury was 7.2 µg/L, falling within the 90th percentile for fish-consuming Asian Americans in the CDC Fourth Report.[129] Of particular interest, the authors of this study asserted that the benefits of higher omega-3s from fish consumption were not adequate to counter the effects of the mercury. These blood mercury levels were also found in the group of internal medicine patients in San Francisco.[81] The effect of blood mercury on neurobehavioral function was also assessed among participants of the Baltimore Memory Study.[130] The mean blood mercury level of this study group was 2.76 µg/L (CDC total 90th percentile, >50th percentile for Asian Americans). As blood mercury increased from that level, significant decrements in memory were found.

Hepatic Effects

- NAFLD
- Elevated alanine aminotransferase (ALT)

Elevations of serum ALT indicating NAFLD have been found to be associated with blood mercury levels. For men aged 18 to 20 years, ALT values of more than 37 IU/L are considered elevated, whereas the cutoff for men older than 21 years is a level above 48 IU/L. For women ages 18 to 20 years, an ALT level above 30 IU/L is considered elevated, and for those older than 21 years, an ALT level higher than 31 IU/L is considered elevated. In the NHANES 2003 to 2004 cohort, those with a blood mercury in the second quartile (25th to 50th percentile) were twice as likely to have elevated ALT.[131] Data collected from KNHANES showed that increasing blood mercury levels were associated with increases in AST and ALT and elevated gamma-glutamyltranspeptidase (GGTP) (>56 IU/L).[132,133]

ASSESSING BIOMARKERS

Mercury Levels

Current mercury exposure can be assessed with blood and urine, whereas hair gives an indication of exposure over the preceding 30 to 45 days.[124,134] As previously mentioned, both blood and hair provide the clearest indication of MeHg levels.[79,135] Urine mercury levels also reflect current exposure, but urine contains far more inorganic than organic mercury.[136] Blood, hair, and urine mercury values above the CDC 75th percentile would indicate the likelihood that current sources of mercury exposure are present for that individual. Cord blood mercury levels are an excellent indicator of fetal exposure to mercury, and measurement of those levels should become a standard part of birthing practices.[137] Table 14.8 illustrates the health markers associated with CDC percentiles for blood, urine, or hair mercury.

Both 2,3-dimercaptosuccinic acid (DMSA) and 2,3-dimercaptopropane-1-sulfonate (DMPS) have been used as mercury-mobilizing agents to assess body stores of inorganic mercury.[138,139] Urinary coproporphyrin levels were predictive of a positive mercury-mobilization test, indicating a high body burden of mercury in persons working in a dental office.[140] Mercury levels from mobilization tests have also been found to correlate with complex attention, perceptual motor tasks, and symptoms and mood scores on neuropsychological testing.[123] DMSA mobilization has resulted in a statistically significant 10-fold urinary mercury increase in fish eaters, whereas non–fish eaters experienced a fourfold increase. However, because of the low concentration of MeHg in urine, the mean levels of post-DMSA mercury for fish eaters were relatively low, even though the ranges went as high as 30 µg/g of creatinine.[135] DMPS mobilization resulted in a 10-fold increase in urinary mercury for mercury workers, a 5.9-fold increase for dentists, and a 3.8-fold increase in persons without amalgams.[141] Another study found 35- to 88-fold increases in urinary mercury in mercury workers after an oral challenge with 300 mg of DMPS.[142] When the total amounts of DMPS-mobilized urinary mercury were measured, workers dumped 1513 µg of mercury, dentists released 132.6 µg, and controls excreted only 3.78 µg over the following 48 hours.[143] With more than 90% of DMPS-bound mercury being released in the urine within the first 6 hours, the use of a 48-hour catch is unnecessary. After an intravenous DMPS dose of 3 mg/kg, a urine mercury dump of 50 µg or more has been considered a positive test.[83]

For DMSA and oral DMPS to be effective as mobilizing agents, unimpeded absorption and sufficient L-cysteine for proper conjugate must be in place. These issues are probable factors in the wide variance in the percentage increases in urinary mercury excretion. Individuals with positive antigliadin antibody levels, but without any of the celiac markers, have demonstrated very poor DMSA absorption.[144] When the mobilization test was repeated after a period of gluten abstinence sufficient to achieve negative antigliadin readings, excretion of lead

TABLE 14.8	**Health Markers Associated with CDC Percentiles for Blood, Urine, or Hair Mercury**		
50th %	**75th %**	**80th % (Approx)**	**95th %**
ALT increase	Antithyroglobulin ANA 8-OHdG	Neurocognitive defects	Cardiovascular disease Hypertension

and mercury dramatically increased to levels appropriate for their exposure histories. More than 90% of the urinary content of DMSA carrying heavy metals is conjugated with two molecules of L-cysteine.[136] Diminished L-cysteine or GSH has been shown to diminish mercury excretion, with repletion of those thiols leading to increased excretion.

The protocol for a mercury mobilization test is as follows:

1. Establish that the subject is not reactive to sulfur products (garlic, eggs, onions, etc.).
2. Collect the first morning urine for assessment of the baseline mercury level.
3. Mobilize with 30 mg/kg DMSA (up to 2250 mg), 10 mg/kg oral DMPS (300 mg), or 3 mg/kg intravenous (IV) DMPS (up to 250 mg).
4. Collect all urine over the next 4 hours for DMSA or 6 hours for DMPS for postmobilization measurement of toxic metals. The total amount of collected urine should be noted in milliliters and entered in the proper location on the laboratory requisition form so that total mercury release can be calculated.

Biomarkers of Biochemical and Physiological Damage

8-Hydroxy-2'-Deoxyguanosine. Mercury causes a great deal of oxidative damage throughout the body, including to the DNA. Hydroxyl radical damage to the DNA results in elevated levels of 8-hydroxy-2'-deoxyguanosine (8-OHdG) in the urine. Urinary 8-OHdG is both a general marker for oxidative stress and a fairly accurate predictor of chronic diseases (including cancer).[145] Persons without occupational exposure to mercury with mean blood and urine mercury levels of 0.91 μg/L and 0.95 μg/L had urinary 8-OHdG levels that averaged 2.08 ng/mg of creatinine (range 0.95–4.7).[146] Mercury workers with far higher blood and urine mercury levels had correspondingly higher urine 8-OHdG levels (mean 242.9 ng/mg of creatinine). Women exposed to both MeHg and inorganic mercury with urinary mercury levels of 5.3 μg/g of creatinine or more also had elevated 8-OHdG levels.[147] Elevated 8-OHdG levels have been documented in children whose urinary mercury was in the second to fourth quartiles.[148] Those children with a mean urinary mercury of 2.75 μg/g of creatinine had a mean 8-OHdG level of 17.7 μg/g of creatinine.

Porphyrins. Mercury is known to cause dysfunction in heme production, resulting in elevated levels of porphyrins.

Although urinary porphyrins are not a direct measure of the amount of mercury present in the body, they show that the mercury body burden is sufficient enough to disrupt the heme synthesis pathway. Mercury specifically inhibits the final steps in heme production by preventing the transitions of pentacarboxyporphyrinogen to coproporphyrinogen and coproporphyrinogen to protoporphyrinogen (Fig. 14.2).[149] Elevations of pentacarboxyporphyrin, precoproporphyrin, and coproporphyrin are the result of inhibiting these steps, and they have all been found to be elevated in children with mercury exposure from dental amalgams. Children with amalgam fillings present for the 8 years of the study had a statistically significant correlation between their mercury exposure and urinary levels of those three porphyrins. The porphyrin levels in the children with amalgams increased by 5% to 10% over the course of the study, whereas those without amalgams had no changes in their porphyrin counts. The levels of these porphyrins increase in a dose-dependent manner, and they can rise more than 300% in dental professionals.[150]

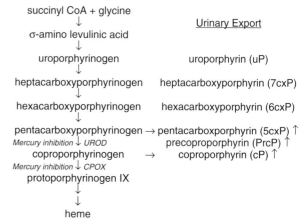

FIG. 14.2 A summary of the heme synthesis pathway and associated urinary porphyrins. Porphyrinogens appear in urine as porphyrin derivatives *(right)*. Mercury can cause increased urinary 5cxP, PrcP, and cP by inhibiting uroporphyrinogen decarboxylase *(UROD)* and/or coproporphyrinogen oxidase *(CPOX)*; urinary uP has not been reported to change with inhibition of these enzymatic steps. (From Geier, D. A., Carmody, T., Kern, J. K., King, P. G., & Geier, M. R. [2013]. A significant dose-dependent relationship between mercury exposure from dental amalgams and kidney integrity biomarkers: a further assessment of the Casa Pia children's dental amalgam trial. *Human & Experimental Toxicology, 32*(4), 434–440.)

Ferritin and Alanine Aminotransferase. As previously mentioned, blood levels of mercury in the NHANES second quartile and higher have been associated with elevated ALT values.[125] Data from the 2010 to 2012 KNHANES revealed that Korean men with blood mercury in the 75th percentile and higher were more than twice as likely to have elevated ferritin levels.[151]

Neurobehavioral Function. Although not specific for mercury, blood levels of mercury commonly found among the US population have been linked to several neurological functions that are easily assessed with in-office or web-based neurobehavioral/neurocognitive testing.

TREATMENT

Those individuals whose case presentation is in alignment with the common signs and symptoms of mercury-induced illness and whose onset of those problems coincides with known mercury exposure (Table 14.9) warrant further assessment.

Positive biomarker findings in persons fitting the previously described picture would indicate the need for intervention. Proper treatment for heavy metal exposure and overload follows the basic three-part environmental medicine approach of:
1. Avoiding further exposure
2. Reducing body burden
3. Reversing toxicant-induced damage

Avoidance

The first step in reducing mercury burden is to stop any ongoing exposure. Because fish intake is responsible for

the majority of mercury in humans, dietary changes can dramatically reduce mercury intake. For those without a clear dietary source of mercury, all the other sources of mercury previously listed must be examined. A follow-up blood or urine mercury measurement based on the known $t_{1/2}$ of the suspected form of mercury should be done to ensure that the true sources of mercury have been successfully eliminated. If such a reduction is not found, the probability of dietary non-compliance by the patient must be considered in cases of MeHg burden.

Reduction of Mercury Body Burden

Enhancing Normal Excretion. Because MeHg is primarily excreted through the bowel, it is not surprising that diet and the state of the microbiome can have a major effect on the excretion of mercury. One animal study reported that the $t_{1/2}$ of MeHg was reduced by 50% (doubling the rate of MeHg excretion) for those animals on a high-protein and low-fat diet, whereas animals on a milk diet (high fat) had a tripling of MeHg $t_{1/2}$.[152,153] Diets high in coconut oil and soy oil enhanced body retention of MeHg, whereas cod liver oil appeared to reduce it.[154] When diets enhanced with fish oil, soy oil, or lard were fed to animals exposed to MeHg, those with fish oil in their diets had the greatest fecal MeHg excretion levels, the highest liver MeHg levels (in preparation for biliary excretion), and the lowest brain MeHg levels (Table 14.10).[155]

Altering the microbiome with broad-spectrum antibiotics dramatically increased the $t_{1/2}$ of MeHg 10-fold.[170] Alternatively, consuming fiber that promotes a healthy microbiome appears to enhance biliary and fecal excretion of MeHg. Animals fed either 15% or 30% wheat bran diets had greater excretion of MeHg.[156] Not only was the $t_{1/2}$ of MeHg reduced by almost 50%, those animals were also found to have lower levels of MeHg in their brain tissue. Certain species of *Lactobacillus* have demonstrated the ability to sequester heavy metals and reduce their toxic effects *in vitro*.[157] Supplementation with *Lactobacillus rhamnosus*–containing yogurt was found to prevent an increase in blood mercury levels in pregnant fish eaters in Tanzania. A similar trend was seen in school children in the same study, but the results did not reach statistical significance.[158]

Weak acids, including GSH-complexed mercapturic acids, are readily recycled in the kidneys when the urine is acidic. Alkalinization has been used to reduce renal recycling and enhance urinary clearance of a number of

TABLE 14.9 Classic Signs and Symptoms of Low-Level Mercury Burden	
Classic Signs and Symptoms	**Classic Disease Presence**
Memory problems	Hypertension
Fatigue	Cardiovascular disease
Headache	Low thyroid
Cognitive difficulties	Autoimmune thyroiditis
Depression	Positive ANA
Musculoskeletal problems (diminished coordination, myalgia, tremors)	Blood sugar dysregulation (metabolic syndrome, insulin resistance, etc.)
Hair loss	NAFLD (elevated ALT)
Stomach issues	

TABLE 14.10   Effects of Different Fats on Tissue and Fecal MeHg Levels in ug/g

	MeHg dose (mg/kg/day)	Fish Oil	Soy Oil	Lard
Brain	0	0.04	0.30	0.07
MeHg	1	3.28	3.65	4.01
	3	14.7	15.3	16.1
Liver Hg	0	0.16	0.03	0.05
(for biliary	1	12.0	12.4	9.66
excretion)	3	54.0	45.2	45.7
Fecal Hg	0	0.20	0.26	0.23
	1	9.11	6.05	7.16
	3	31.4	27.1	24.5

From Jin, X., Lok, E., Bondy, G., Caldwell, D., Mueller, R., Kapal, K., et al. (2007) Modulating effects of dietary fats on methylmercury toxicity and distribution in rats. *Toxicology*, *230*(1), 22–44.

compounds.[159] The use of potassium citrate, typically used to alkalinize the urine, caused an increase in urinary mercury levels.[160] Other means of alkalinizing the urine may also be beneficial.

Utilizing Mercury-Mobilizing Agents. The thiol-containing compounds DMSA, DMPS, and NAC have all proven effective in effectively reducing the body burden of mercury. NAC is a nontoxic N-acetyl derivative of cysteine containing a thiol group. DMSA and DMPS contain two sulfhydryl groups each and possess the critical ability to bind mercury more tightly than it is bound to extracellular and intracellular thiols. When given to mercury-exposed pregnant animals, all three (DMSA, DMPS, and NAC) have exhibited the ability to reduce mercury levels in the fetal kidneys, brain, and liver.[161,162] Renal clearance of DMPS-, DMSA-, and NAC-mercury conjugates is mediated through MRP2 export proteins in the proximal tubules (see Fig. 14.3).[163,164] Proper MRP2 elimination of mercury is dependent upon adequate thiol stores and occurs daily even without DMSA or DMPS. By itself, NAC supplementation increases urinary MeHg excretion from 5- to 10-fold.[165] DMPS, DMSA, and NAC (30 mg/kg) are similar in their mercury-mobilizing effects.[164] When given separately, DMSA increased urinary mercury excretion by 163%, DMPS by 135%, and NAC by 131%. When given with potassium citrate to alkalinize

the urine, mercury excretion increased to 163% for both DMPS and NAC. Intravenous infusions of ascorbic acid have been recommended by some to clear mercury from the body; however, this therapy has demonstrated no such ability.[166]

DMPS was developed in 1951 and patented under the name Dimaval by Heyl Chem-Fabrik G (Berlin) for the treatment of mercury overload. DMPS increases urinary excretion of mercury and reduces mercury concentrations in the kidneys, blood, and brain.[135,136,140,167] Not only is DMPS safe and highly effective at body weight–adjusted doses in greatly increasing urinary mercury excretion,[168] it also has shown benefit in reversing mercury-associated symptoms.[169] A group of mercury-burdened individuals reported improvements in their complaints of tremors, memory loss, insomnia, and metallic taste in the mouth. They also demonstrated objective improvements in neurocognitive testing and rombergism.[170] Transdermal application of DMPS has shown no evidence of absorption into the blood or enhanced mercury excretion.[171]

DMSA (Succimer, or Chemet) is FDA approved for the treatment of lead but not mercury poisoning, although it has demonstrated a clear ability to reduce mercury levels.[172] The optimum body-weight dose of DMSA is 30 mg/kg/day given in three divided doses. Dividing the daily dose into thirds takes into account the DMSA peak in both blood and urine that occurs 4 hours postconsumption.[173] The use of body-weight doses of DMSA has been shown to be safe in children as young as 12 months of age.[174] Even with a DMSA overdose (185 mg/kg) in a 3-year-old child, no harm occurred.[175] With consecutive daily body-weight doses of DMSA, peak mercury excretion occurs on day 3.[172] DMSA primarily moves mercury from the kidneys, which contain the highest mercury concentration in the body,[176] but does not mobilize mercury from amalgams.[177]

It is generally recommended that DMSA or DMPS be given in several-day courses repeatedly with rest periods in between. Both DMSA and DMPS will increase the excretion of copper and zinc, although deficiencies of these minerals have not been noted.[178] The prescriber of Chemet (succimer) is cautioned to check for elevation of liver enzymes in the patient during the course of DMSA treatment.

Reversing Mercury-Induced Damage. N-acetyl cysteine was previously discussed with regard to its documented

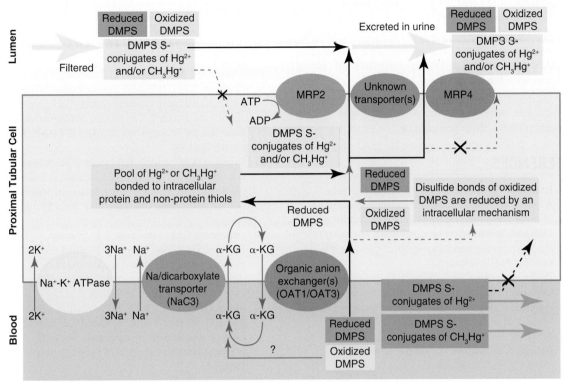

FIG. 14.3 Pathways for DMPS mobilization of mercury. (Reprinted with permission from Zalups, R. K., & Bridges, C. C. [2012]. Relationships between the renal handling of DMPS and DMSA and the renal handling of mercury. *Chemical Research in Toxicology, 25*(9), 1825–1838. Copyright 2012 American Chemical Society.)

ability to increase the excretion of MeHg and inorganic mercury from the body. It has also demonstrated both protection against and reversal of mercury-induced cellular and tissue damage throughout the body, especially when used in combination with selenium and zinc.[179,180] Both zinc[181] and selenium[182] have shown benefit by themselves in blocking mercury-induced hepatic and neurological damage, as has vitamin E.[183] The benefits of NAC include restoring GSH levels and antioxidant enzyme activities and reducing elevated levels of ALT. Both MeHg neurotoxicity via reduced DNA synthesis and apoptotic activity have been blocked and reversed by NAC supplementation.[184] It also offers protection to the neurons and astrocytes by depleting the GSH content in those cells.[185] NAC has demonstrated effectiveness at protecting the kidneys from mercury-induced oxidative damage[186,187] and protecting pancreatic beta cells.[104] NAC

appears to be a highly valuable supplement for mercury-exposed persons.

Curcumin has exhibited multiple benefits against mercury. At a dose of 80 mg/kg, it was shown to reduce peroxide levels, increase GSH, and restore the activity of catalase, GSH peroxidase, and superoxide dismutase.[188] Both premercury and postmercury consumption of curcumin reduced levels of mercury in the liver, kidneys, and brain, making this botanical a possible safe alternative for persons who cannot take the sulfhydryl-containing DMSA or DMPS.

Methionine has shown benefit in reducing MeHg transport into the brain,[10] and several studies have shown the benefit of selenium supplementation.[9,23–26] Alpha lipoic acid (ALA), which functions as an antioxidant, has been shown to ameliorate the neural oxidative damage caused by mercury.[189] However, controversy around the use of

ALA with mercury exists because of an animal study that used both intravenous MeHg and intravenous ALA.[190] In this study, the lowest dose of ALA (37.5 µmol/kg) doubled the excretion of MeHg, but each doubling of the ALA dose caused a marked reduction of MeHg excretion, with the highest dose (300 µmol/kg) effectively blocking MeHg release. Upon autopsy, the MeHg-exposed animals who were also given ALA had higher MeHg concentrations in their brain tissue.

REFERENCES

1. Fuhr, B. J., & Rabenstein, D. L. (1973). Nuclear magnetic resonance studies of the solution chemistry of metal complexes. IX. The binding of cadmium, zinc, lead, and mercury by glutathione. *Journal of the American Chemical Society*, 95(21), 6944–6950. PubMed PMID: 4784285.
2. De Souza Queiroz, M. L., Pena, S. C., Salles, T. S. I., de Capitani, E. M., & Olalla Saad, S. T. (1998). Abnormal antioxidant system in erythrocytes of mercury exposed workers. *Human & Experimental Toxicology*, 17, 225–230.
3. Barregård, L., Sällsten, G., Schütz, A., Attewell, R., Skerfving, S., & Järvholm, B. (1992). Kinetics of mercury in blood and urine after brief occupational exposure. *Archives of Environmental Health*, 47(3), 176–184. PubMed PMID: 1596100.
4. Sandborgh-Englund, G., Elinder, C. G., Johanson, G., Lind, B., Skare, I., & Ekstrand, J. (1998). The absorption, blood levels, and excretion of mercury after a single dose of mercury vapor in humans. *Toxicology and Applied Pharmacology*, 150(1), 146–153. PubMed PMID: 9630463.
5. Morgan, J. N., Berry, M. R., & Graves, R. L. (1997). Effects of commonly used cooking practices on total mercury concentration in fish and their impact on exposure assessments. *Journal of Exposure Analysis and Environmental Epidemiology*, 7(1), 119–133. PubMed PMID: 9076613.
6. Stopford, W., & Goldwater, L. J. (1975). Methylmercury in the environment: a review of current understanding. *Environmental Health Perspectives*, 12, 115–118.
7. Kershaw, T. G., Clarkson, T. W., & Dhahir, P. H. (1980). The relationship between blood levels and dose of methylmercury in man. *Archives of Environmental Health*, 35(1), 28–36. PubMed PMID: 7189107.
8. Miettinen, J. K. (1973). Absorption and elimination of dietary mercury(2+)ion and methylmercury in man. In M. W. Miller & T. W. Clarkson (Eds.), *Mercury, Mercurials, and Mercaptans*. New York: Plenum Press.
9. Kerper, L. E., Ballatori, N., & Clarkson, T. W. (1992). Methylmercury transport across the blood-brain barrier by an amino acid carrier. *The American Journal of Physiology*, 262(5 Pt. 2), R761–R765. PubMed PMID: 1590471.
10. Mokrzan, E. M., Kerper, L. E., Ballatori, N., & Clarkson, T. W. (1995). Methylmercury-thiol uptake into cultured brain capillary endothelial cells on amino acid system L. *The Journal of Pharmacology and Experimental Therapeutics*, 272(3), 1277–1284. PubMed PMID: 7891344.
11. Clarkson, T. W., Hursh, J. B., Sager, P. R., & Syversen, J. P. (1988). Mercury. In T. W. Clarkson, L. Friber, G. F. Nordberg, & P. R. Sager (Eds.), *Biological Monitoring of Toxic Metals* (pp. 199–246). New York: Plenum Press.
12. Dickenson, C. A., Woodruff, T. J., Stotland, N. E., Dobraca, D., & Das, R. (2013). Elevated mercury levels in pregnant woman linked to skin cream from Mexico. *American Journal of Obstetrics and Gynecology*, 209(2), e4–e5. PubMed PMID: 23685000.
13. Miller, O. M., Lund, B. O., & Woods, J. S. (1991). Reactivity of Hg(II) with superoxide: evidence for the catalytic dismutation of superoxide by Hg(II). *Journal of Biochemical Toxicology*, 6, 293–298. PubMed PMID: 1663557.
14. Zalups, R. K., & Lash, L. H. (1996). Interactions between glutathione and mercury in the kidney, liver and blood. In L. W. Chang (Ed.), *Toxicology of Metals* (pp. 145–163). Boca Raton, FL: CRC Press.
15. Motts, J. A., Shirley, D. L., Silbergeld, E. K., & Nyland, J. F. (2014). Novel biomarkers of mercury-induced autoimmune dysfunction: a cross-sectional study in Amazonian Brazil. *Environmental Research*, 132, 12–18. PubMed PMID: 24742722.
16. Pollack, A. Z., Sjaarda, L., Ahrens, K. A., Mumford, S. L., Browne, R. W., Wactawski-Wende, J., et al. (2014). Association of cadmium, lead and mercury with paraoxonase 1 activity in women. *PLoS ONE*, 9(3), e92152. PubMed PMID: 24682159.
17. Durham, H. D., Minotti, S., & Caporicci, E. (1997). Sensitivity of platelet microtubules to disassembly by methylmercury. *Journal of Toxicology and Environmental Health*, 48, 57–69. PubMed PMID: 8637058.
18. Falconer, M. M., Vaillant, A., Reuhl, K. R., Laferriere, N., & Brown, D. L. (1994). The molecular basis of microtubule stability in neurons. *Neurotoxicology*, 15, 109–122. PubMed PMID: 8090350.
19. Miura, K., Koide, N., Himeno, S., Hakagawa, I., & Imura, N. (1999). The involvement of microtubular disruption in methylmercury-induced apoptosis in

neuronal and nonneuronal cell lines. *Toxicology and Applied Pharmacology, 160*, 279–288. PubMed PMID: 10544062.

20. InSug, O., Datar, S., Koch, C. J., Shapiro, I. M., & Shenker, B. J. (1997). Mercuric compounds inhibit human monocyte function by inducing apoptosis: evidence for formation of reactive oxygen species, development of mitochondrial membrane permeability transition and loss of reductive reserve. *Toxicology, 124*, 211–224. PubMed PMID: 9482123.

21. Shenker, B. J., Guo, T. L., & Shapiro, I. M. (1998). Low-level methylmercury exposure causes human T-cells to undergo apoptosis: evidence of mitochondrial dysfunction. *Environmental Research, 77*, 149–159. PubMed PMID: 9600808.

22. Goldberg, R. L., Kaplan, S. R., & Fuller, G. C. (1983). Effect of heavy metals on human rheumatoid synovial cell proliferation and collagen synthesis. *Biochemical Pharmacology, 32*(18), 2763–2766. PubMed PMID: 6626246.

23. Ganther, H. E. (1978). Modification of methylmercury toxicity and metabolism by selenium and vitamin E: possible mechanisms. *Environmental Health Perspectives, 25*, 71–76. PubMed PMID: 720304.

24. Ganther, H. E. (1972). Selenium: relation to decreased toxicity of methylmercury in diets containing tuna. *Science, 175*, 1122. PubMed PMID: 5062150.

25. Drasch, G., Wanghofer, E., Roider, G., & Strobach, S. (1996). Correlation of mercury and selenium in the human kidney. *Journal of Trace Elements in Medicine and Biology, 10*(4), 251–254. PubMed PMID: 9021677.

26. Høl, P. J., Vamnes, J. S., Gjerdet, N. R., Eide, R., & Isrenn, R., (2001). Dental amalgam and selenium in blood. *Environmental Research, 87*(3), 141–146. PubMed PMID: 11771928.

27. Mahaffey, K. R., Clickner, R. P., & Bodurow, C. C. (2004). Blood organic mercury and dietary mercury intake: National Health and Nutrition Examination Survey, 1999 and 2000. *Environmental Health Perspectives, 112*(5), 562–570. PubMed PMID: 15064162.

28. Sunderland, E. M., Krabbenhoft, D. P., Moreau, J. W., Strode, S. A., & Landing, W. M. (2009). Mercury sources, distribution, and bioavailability in the North Pacific Ocean: insights from data and models. *Global Biogeochemical Cycles, 23*, GB2010.

29. U.S. Environmental Protection Agency. (2001). *National Listing of Fish Advisories (NLFA)*. Available at https://www.epa.gov/sites/production/files/2015-06/documents/maps-and-graphics-2011.pdf. (Accessed September 21, 2016.)

30. Tollefson, L., & Cordle, F. (1986). Methylmercury in fish: a review of residue levels, fish consumption and regulatory action in the United States. *Environmental Health Perspectives, 68*, 203–208.

31. U.S. Food and Drug Administration. (1994). Mercury in fish: cause for concern? *FDA Consumer*. Revised May 1995.

32. U.S. Food and Drug Administration. *Food: Mercury Levels in Commercial Fish and Shellfish (1990-2012)*. Available at http://www.fda.gov/food/foodborneillnesscontaminants/metals/ucm115644.htm. (Accessed September 26, 2016.)

33. Groth, E. *Tuna surprise: mercury in school lunches*. Available at http://mercurypolicy.org/wp-content/uploads/2012/09/mpp_tuna_surprise_final_final1.pdf. (Accessed September 21, 2016.)

34. Sunderland, E. M. (2007). Mercury exposure from domestic and imported estuarine and marine fish in the U.S. seafood market. *Environmental Health Perspectives, 115*(2), 235–242. [Epub 2006 Nov 20]. PubMed PMID: 17384771.

35. Nielsen, S. J., Kit, B. K., Aoki, Y., & Ogden, C. L. (2014). Seafood consumption and blood mercury concentrations in adults aged ≥20 y, 2007-2010. *The American Journal of Clinical Nutrition, 99*(5), 1066–1070. PubMed PMID: 24522443.

36. Sunderland, E. M. (2007). Mercury exposure from domestic and imported estuarine and marine fish in the U.S. seafood market. *Environmental Health Perspectives, 115*(2), 235–242. [Epub 2006 Nov 20]; PubMed PMID: 17384771.

37. Grandjean, P., Weihe, P., Needham, L. L., Burse, V. W., Patterson, D. G., Sampson, E. J., et al. (1995). Relation of a seafood diet to mercury, selenium, arsenic and polychlorinated biphenyl and other organochlorine concentrations in human milk. *Environmental Research, 71*, 29–38. PubMed PMID: 8757236.

38. Skerfving, S. (1988). Mercury in women exposed to methylmercury through fish consumption, and in their newborn babies and breast milk. *Bulletin of Environmental Contamination and Toxicology, 41*, 475–482. PubMed PMID: 3224165.

39. Galster, W. A. (1976). Mercury in Alaskan Eskimo mothers and infants. *Environmental Health Perspectives, 15*, 135–140. PubMed PMID: 1033830.

40. Watanabe, C., & Satho, H. (1996). Evolution of our understanding of methylmercury as health threat. *Environmental Health Perspectives, 104*, 367–378.

41. Agency for Toxic Substances and Disease Registry. *1999 toxicological profile for mercury*. http://www.atsdr.cdc.gov/substances/toxsubstance.asp?toxid=24 (Accessed September 26, 2016.)

42. Maloney, S. R., Phillips, C. A., & Mills, A. (1998). Mercury in the hair of crematoria workers. *Lancet, 352,* 1602.

43. Dufault, R., LeBlanc, B., Schnoll, R., Cornett, C., Schweitzer, L., Wallinga, D., et al. (2009). Mercury from chlor-alkali plants: measured concentrations in food product sugar. *Environmental Health: A Global Access Science Source, 8,* 2. PubMed PMID: 19171026.

44. Reis, A. T., Rodrigues, S. M., Araújo, C., Coelho, J. P., Pereira, E., & Duarte, A. C. (2009). Mercury contamination in the vicinity of a chlor-alkali plant and potential risks to local population. *The Science of the Total Environment, 407*(8), 2689–2700. PubMed PMID: 19211131.

45. Vimy, M. J. & Lorsheider, F. L. (1985). Intra-oral air mercury released from dental amalgams. *Journal of Dental Research, 64*(8), 1069–1071. PubMed PMID: 3860538.

46. Vimy, M. J., & Lorsheider, F. L. (1985). Serial measurements of intra-oral air mercury: estimation of daily dose from dental amalgams. *Journal of Dental Research, 64*(8), 1072–1075. PubMed PMID: 3860539.

47. Patterson, J. E., Weissberg, B., & Dennison, P. J. (1985). Mercury in human breath from dental amalgam. *Bulletin of Environmental Contamination and Toxicology, 34,* 459–468. PubMed PMID: 3986383.

48. Anthony, H., Birtwistle, S., Eaton, K., & Maberly, J. (Eds.). (1997). *Environmental Medicine in Clinical Practice* (pp. 204–208). Southampton, UK: BSAENM Publications.

49. Abraham, J. E., Svare, C. W., & Frank, C. W. (1984). The effect of dental amalgam restorations on blood mercury levels. *Journal of Dental Research, 63*(1), 71–73. PubMed PMID: 6582086.

50. Barregard, L., Sallsten, G., & Jarvholm, B. (1995). People with high mercury uptake from their own dental amalgam fillings. *Occupational and Environmental Medicine, 52,* 124–128. PubMed PMID: 7757165.

51. Brune, D., Gjerdet, N., & Paulsen, G. (1983). Gastrointestinal and in vitro release of copper, cadmium, indium, mercury and zinc from conventional and copper-rich amalgams. *Scandinavian Journal of Dental Research, 91,* 66–71. PubMed PMID: 6573763.

52. Trepka, M. J., Heinrich, J., Krause, C., Schulz, C., Wjst, M., Popescu, M., et al. (1997). Factors affecting internal mercury burdens among East German children. *Archives of Environmental Health, 52*(2), 134–138. PubMed PMID: 9124874.

53. Oskarsson, A., Schutz, A., Skerfving, S., Hallen, I. P., Ohlin, B., & Langerkvist, B. J. (1996). Total and inorganic mercury in breast milk and blood in relation to fish consumption and amalgam fillings in lactating women. *Archives of Environmental Health, 51*(3), 234–241. PubMed PMID: 8687245.

54. Guzzi, G., Grandi, M., Cattaneo, C., et al. (2006). Dental amalgam and mercury levels in autopsy tissues. *The American Journal of Forensic Medicine and Pathology, 27*(1), 42–45. PMID: 16501347.

55. Barregard, L., Fabricius-Lagging, E., Lundh, T., et al. (2010). Cadmium, mercury, and lead in kidney cortex of living kidney donors: Impact of different exposure sources. *Environmental Research, 110*(1), 47–54. PMID: 19931045.

56. Kissel, K. P. (1998). Teens fall ill after taking, playing with mercury. *The Seattle Times,* January 15.

57. Orloff, K. G., Ulirsch, G., Wilder, L., Block, A., Fagliano, J., & Pasqualo, J. (1997). Human exposure to elemental mercury in a contaminated residential building. *Archives of Environmental Health, 52*(3), 169–172. PubMed PMID: 9169625.

58. Fiedler, N., Udasin, I., Gochfeld, M., Buckler, G., Kelly-McNeil, K., & Kipen, H. (1999). Neuropsychological and stress evaluation of residential mercury exposure. *Environmental Health Perspectives, 107*(5), 343–347. PubMed PMID: 10210689.

59. Bonhomme, C., Gladyszaczak-Kohler, J., Cadou, A., Ilef, D., & Kadi, Z. (1996). Mercury poisoning by vacuum-cleaner aerosol. *Lancet, 347,* 115. PubMed PMID: 8538305.

60. Harnly, M., Seidel, S., Rojas, P., Fornes, R., Flessel, P., Smith, D., et al. (1997). Biological monitoring for mercury within a community with soil and fish contamination. *Environmental Health Perspectives, 105*(4), 424–429. PubMed PMID: 9189708.

61. Washington State Department of Health. (1996). Mercury poisoning cases traced to face cream. *EpiTRENDS, 1*(2), 4.

62. Shiue, I., & Bramley, G. (2015). Environmental chemicals mediated the effect of old housing on adult health problems: US NHANES, 2009-2010. *Environmental Science and Pollution Research International, 22*(2), 1299–1308. PubMed PMID: 25138559.

63. Centers for Disease Control and Prevention. *National Report on Human Exposure to Environmental Chemicals: Updated Tables, 2017.* Available at: www.cdc.gov/exposurereport (Accessed October 25, 2017.)

64. Adlard, B., Davis, K., Liang, C. L., S Curren, M., Rodríguez-Dozal, S., Riojas-Rodríguez, H., et al. (2014). Persistent organic pollutants (POPs) and metals in primiparous women: a comparison from Canada and Mexico. *The Science of the Total Environment, 500-501,* 302–313. PubMed PMID: 25233368.

65. Castaño, A., Sánchez-Rodríguez, J. E., Cañas, A., Esteban, M., Navarro, C., Rodríguez-García, A. C., et al. (2012). Mercury, lead and cadmium levels in the urine of 170 Spanish adults: a pilot human biomonitoring study. *International Journal of Hygiene and Environmental Health*, 215(2), 191–195. PubMed PMID: 21968334.

66. Becker, K., Schulz, C., Kaus, S., Seiwert, M., & Seifert, B. (2003). German Environmental Survey 1998 (GerES III): environmental pollutants in the urine of the German population. *International Journal of Hygiene and Environmental Health*, 206(1), 15–24. PubMed PMID: 12621899.

67. Benes, B., Spěváčková, V., Smíd, J., Cejchanová, M., Kaplanová, E., Cerná, M., et al. (2002). Determination of normal concentration levels of Cd, Pb, Hg, Cu, Zn and Se in urine of the population in the Czech Republic. *Central European Journal of Public Health*, 10(1–2), 3–5. PubMed PMID: 12096681.

68. Apostoli, P., Cortesi, I., Mangili, A., Elia, G., Drago, I., Gagliardi, T., et al. (2002). Assessment of reference values for mercury in urine: the results of an Italian polycentric study. *The Science of the Total Environment*, 289(1–3), 13–24. PubMed PMID: 12049389.

69. Mahaffey, K., Clickner, R., & Jeffries, R. (2009). *Adult women's blood mercury concentrations vary regionally in USA: association with patterns of fish consumption (NHANES 1999-2004) Environmental Health Perspective*, Jan;117(1), 47–53. PubMed PMID: 19165386.

70. Centers for Disease Control and Prevention. *Emergency Preparedness and Response: Mercury.* Available at https://emergency.cdc.gov/agent/mercury/mercelementalcasedef.asp. (Accessed September 21, 2016.)

71. Kingman, A., Albertini, T., & Brown, L. J. (1998). Mercury concentrations in urine and whole blood associated with amalgam exposure in a US military population. *Journal of Dental Research*, 77(3), 461–471. PubMed PMID: 9496919.

72. Suzuki, T., Hongo, T., Yoshinaga, J., Imai, H., Nakazawa, M., Matsuo, N., et al. (1993). The hair-organ relationship in mercury concentration in contemporary Japanese. *Archives of Environmental Health*, 48(4), 221–229. PubMed PMID: 8357270.

73. McDowell, M. A., Dillon, C. F., Osterloh, J., Bolger, P. M., Pellizzari, E., Fernando, R., et al. (2004). Hair mercury levels in U.S. children and women of childbearing age: reference range data from NHANES 1999-2000. *Environmental Health Perspectives*, 112(11), 1165–1171. PubMed PMID: 15289161.

74. Schoeman, K., Bend, J. R., & Koren, G. (2010). Hair methylmercury: a new indication for therapeutic monitoring. *Therapeutic Drug Monitoring*, 32(3), 289–293. PubMed PMID: 20445486.

75. Goodrich, J. M., Wang, Y., Gillespie, B., Werner, R., Franzblau, A., & Basu, N. (2011). Glutathione enzyme and selenoprotein polymorphisms associate with mercury biomarker levels in Michigan dental professionals. *Toxicology and Applied Pharmacology*, 257(2), 301–308. PubMed PMID: 21967774.

76. Wang, Y., Goodrich, J. M., Gillespie, B., Werner, R., Basu, N., & Franzblau, A. (2012). An investigation of modifying effects of metallothionein single-nucleotide polymorphisms on the association between mercury exposure and biomarker levels. *Environmental Health Perspectives*, 120(4), 530–534. PubMed PMID: 22233731. Erratum in: Environmental Health Perspectives. (2013). 121(1):A13.

77. Ballatori, N. (2002). Transport of toxic metals by molecular mimicry. *Environmental Health Perspectives*, 110(Suppl. 5), 689–694. PubMed PMID: 12426113. Review.

78. Bridges, C. C., Joshee, L., van den Heuvel, J. J., Russel, F. G., & Zalups, R. K. (2013). Glutathione status and the renal elimination of inorganic mercury in the Mrp2(-/-) mouse. *PLoS ONE*, 8(9), e73559. PubMed PMID: 24039982.

79. Alexander, J., & Aaseth, J. (1982). Organ distribution and cellular uptake of methyl mercury in the rat as influenced by the intra- and extracellular glutathione concentration. *Biochemical Pharmacology*, 31(5), 685–690. PubMed PMID: 7082336.

80. Zalups, R. K., Barfuss, D. W., & Lash, L. H. (1999). Relationships between alterations in glutathione metabolism and the disposition of inorganic mercury in rats: effects of biliary ligation and chemically induced modulation of glutathione status. *Chemico-Biological Interactions*, 123(3), 171–195. PubMed PMID: 10654838.

81. Ninomiya, T., Ohmori, H., Hashimoto, K., Tsuruta, K., & Ekino, S. (1995). Expansion of methylmercury poisoning outside of Minamata: and epidemiological study on chronic methylmercury poisoning outside Minamata. *Environmental Research*, 70, 47–50. PubMed PMID: 8603658.

82. Fukuda, Y., Ushinjima, K., Kitano, T., Sakamoto, M., & Futatsuka, M. (1999). An analysis of subjective complaints in a population living in a methylmercury-polluted area. *Environmental Research*, 81, 100–107. PubMed PMID: 10433841.

83. Hightower, J. M., & Moore, D. (2003). Mercury levels in high-end consumers of fish. *Environmental Health Perspectives*, 111(4), 604–608. PubMed PMID: 12676623.

84. Zwicker, J. D., Dutton, D. J., & Emery, J. C. (2014). Longitudinal analysis of the association between removal of dental amalgam, urine mercury and 14 self-reported health symptoms. *Environmental Health: A Global Access Science Source*, 13, 95. PubMed PMID: 25404430.

85. Wojcik, D. P., Godfrey, M. E., Christie, D., & Haley, B. E. (2006). Mercury toxicity presenting as chronic fatigue, memory impairment and depression: diagnosis, treatment, susceptibility, and outcomes in a New Zealand general practice setting (1994-2006). *Neuro Endocrinology Letters*, 27(4), 415–423. PubMed PMID: 16891999.

86. Inoue, S., Yorifuji, T., Tsuda, T., & Doi, H. (2012). Short-term effect of severe exposure to methylmercury on atherosclerotic heart disease and hypertension mortality in Minamata. *The Science of the Total Environment*, 417-418, 291–293. PubMed PMID: 22277149.

87. Yorifuji, T., Tsuda, T., Kashima, S., Takao, S., & Harada, M. (2010). Long-term exposure to methylmercury and its effects on hypertension in Minamata. *Environmental Research*, 110(1), 40–46. PubMed PMID: 19922910.

88. Vupputuri, S., Longnecker, M. P., Daniels, J. L., Guo, X., & Sandler, D. P. (2005). Blood mercury level and blood pressure among US women: results from the National Health and Nutrition Examination Survey 1999-2000. *Environmental Research*, 97(2), 195–200. PubMed PMID: 15533335.

89. Goodrich, J. M., Wang, Y., Gillespie, B., Werner, R., Franzblau, A., & Basu, N. (2013). Methylmercury and elemental mercury differentially associate with blood pressure among dental professionals. *International Journal of Hygiene and Environmental Health*, 216(2), 195–201. PubMed PMID: 22494934.

90. Hong, D., Cho, S. H., Park, S. J., Kim, S. Y., & Park, S. B. (2013). Hair mercury level in smokers and its influence on blood pressure and lipid metabolism. *Environmental Toxicology and Pharmacology*, 36(1), 103–107. PubMed PMID: 23603462.

91. Bautista, L. E., Stein, J. H., Morgan, B. J., Stanton, N., Young, T., & Nieto, F. J. (2009). Association of blood and hair mercury with blood pressure and vascular reactivity. *Wisconsin Medical Journal*, 108(5), 250–252. PubMed PMID: 19743756.

92. Sørensen, N., Murata, K., Budtz-Jørgensen, E., Weihe, P., & Grandjean, P. (1999). Prenatal methylmercury exposure as a cardiovascular risk factor at seven years of age. *Epidemiology (Cambridge, Mass.)*, 10(4), 370–375. PubMed PMID: 10401870.

93. Salonen, J. T., Seppänen, K., Lakka, T. A., Salonen, R., & Kaplan, G. A. (2000). Mercury accumulation and accelerated progression of carotid atherosclerosis: a population-based prospective 4-year follow-up study in men in eastern Finland. *Atherosclerosis*, 148(2), 265–273. PubMed PMID: 10657561.

94. Frustaci, A., Magnavita, N., Chimenti, C., Caldarulo, M., Sabbioni, E., Pietra, R., et al. (1999). Marked elevation of myocardial trace elements in idiopathic dilated cardiomyopathy compared with secondary cardiac dysfunction. *Journal of the American College of Cardiology*, 33(6), 1578–1583. PubMed PMID: 10334427.

95. Wennberg, M., Strömberg, U., Bergdahl, I. A., Jansson, J. H., Kauhanen, J., Norberg, M., et al. (2012). Myocardial infarction in relation to mercury and fatty acids from fish: a risk-benefit analysis based on pooled Finnish and Swedish data in men. *The American Journal of Clinical Nutrition*, 96(4), 706–713. PubMed PMID: 22894940.

96. Yoshizawa, K., Rimm, E. B., Morris, J. S., Spate, V. L., Hsieh, C. C., Spiegelman, D., et al. (2002). Mercury and the risk of coronary heart disease in men. *The New England Journal of Medicine*, 347(22), 1755–1760. PubMed PMID:12456851.

97. Mozaffarian, D., Shi, P., Morris, J. S., Spiegelman, D., Grandjean, P., Siscovick, D. S., et al. (2011). Mercury exposure and risk of cardiovascular disease in two U.S. cohorts. *The New England Journal of Medicine*, 364(12), 1116–1125. PubMed PMID: 21428767.

98. Mozaffarian, D., Shi, P., Morris, J. S., Grandjean, P., Siscovick, D. S., Spiegelman, D., et al. (2012). Mercury exposure and risk of hypertension in US men and women in 2 prospective cohorts. *Hypertension*, 60(3), 645–652. PubMed PMID: 22868395.

99. Roman, H. A., Walsh, T. L., Coull, B. A., Dewailly, É., Guallar, E., Hattis, D., et al. (2011). Evaluation of the cardiovascular effects of methylmercury exposures: current evidence supports development of a dose-response function for regulatory benefits analysis. *Environmental Health Perspectives*, 119(5), 607–614. PubMed PMID: 21220222.

100. Nishida, M., Yamamoto, T., Yoshimura, Y., & Kawada, J. (1986). Subacute toxicity of methylmercuric chloride and mercuric chloride on mouse thyroid. *Journal of Pharmacobio-Dynamics*, 9(4), 331–338. PubMed PMID: 3735055.

101. Tan, S. W., Meiller, J. C., & Mahaffey, K. R. (2009). The endocrine effects of mercury in humans and wildlife. *Critical Reviews in Toxicology*, 39(3), 228–269. PubMed PMID: 19280433.

102. Chen, A., Kim, S. S., Chung, E., & Dietrich, K. N. (2013). Thyroid hormones in relation to lead, mercury, and cadmium exposure in the National Health and Nutrition Examination Survey, 2007-2008.

Environmental Health Perspectives, 121(2), 181–186. PubMed PMID: 23164649.

103. Gallagher, C. M., & Meliker, J. R. (2012). Mercury and thyroid autoantibodies in U.S. women, NHANES 2007-2008. *Environment International, 40*, 39–43. PubMed PMID: 22280926.

104. Chen, Y. W., Huang, C. F., Yang, C. Y., Yen, C. C., Tsai, K. S., & Liu, S. H. (2010). Inorganic mercury causes pancreatic beta-cell death via the oxidative stress-induced apoptotic and necrotic pathways. *Toxicology and Applied Pharmacology, 243*(3), 323–331. PubMed PMID: 20006636.

105. Kim, K. N., Park, S. J., Choi, B., & Joo, N. S. (2015). Blood mercury and insulin resistance in nondiabetic Koreans (KNHANES 2008-2010). *Yonsei Medical Journal, 56*(4), 944–950. PubMed PMID: 26069115.

106. Chung, J. Y., Seo, M. S., Shim, J. Y., & Lee, Y. J. (2015). Sex differences in the relationship between blood mercury concentration and metabolic syndrome risk. *Journal of Endocrinological Investigation, 38*(1), 65–71. PubMed PMID: 25053396.

107. He, K., Xun, P., Liu, K., Morris, S., Reis, J., & Guallar, E. (2013). Mercury exposure in young adulthood and incidence of diabetes later in life: the CARDIA Trace Element Study. *Diabetes Care, 36*(6), 1584–1589. PubMed PMID: 23423697.

108. Guo, T. L., Miller, M. A., Shapiro, I. M., & Shenker, B. J. (1998). Mercuric chloride induces apoptosis in human T lymphocytes: evidence of mitochondrial dysfunction. *Toxicology and Applied Pharmacology, 153*(2), 250–257. PubMed PMID: 9878595.

109. Shenker, B. J., Guo, T. L., & Shapiro, I. M. (2000). Mercury-induced apoptosis in human lymphoid cells: evidence that the apoptotic pathway is mercurial species dependent. *Environmental Research, 84*(2), 89–99. PubMed PMID: 11068922.

110. de Vos, G., Abotaga, S., Liao, Z., Jerschow, E., & Rosenstreich, D. (2007). Selective effect of mercury on Th2-type cytokine production in humans. *Immunopharmacology and Immunotoxicology, 29*(3–4), 537–548. PubMed PMID: 18075863.

111. Peterson, J. D., Herzenberg, L. A., Vasquez, K., & Waltenbaugh, C. (1998). Glutathione levels in antigen-presenting cells modulate Th1 versus Th2 response patterns. *Proceedings of the National Academy of Sciences of the United States of America, 95*(6), 3071–3076. PubMed PMID: 9501217.

112. Vas, J., & Monestier, M. (2008). Immunology of mercury. *Annals of the New York Academy of Sciences, 1143*, 240–267. PubMed PMID: 19076354.

113. Arnett, F. C., Fritzler, M. J., & Holian, A. (2000). Urinary mercury levels in patients with autoantibodies to U3-RNP (fibrillarin). *The Journal of Rheumatology, 27*(2), 405–410. PubMed PMID: 10685806.

114. Somers, E. C., Ganser, M. A., Warren, J. S., Basu, N., Wang, L., Zick, S. M., et al. (2015). Mercury exposure and antinuclear antibodies among females of reproductive age in the United States: NHANES. *Environmental Health Perspectives, 123*(8), 792–798. PubMed PMID: 25665152.

115. Björkman, L., Lundekvam, B. F., Laegreid, T., Bertelsen, B. I., Morild, I., Lilleng, P., et al. (2007). Mercury in human brain, blood, muscle and toenails in relation to exposure: an autopsy study. *Environmental Health A Global Access Science Source, 6*, 30. PubMed PMID: 17931423.

116. Chang, L. W. (1977). Neurotoxic effects of mercury. A review. *Environmental Research, 14*, 329–373. PubMed PMID: 338298.

117. Park, S. T., Lim, K. T., Chung, Y. T., & Kim, S. U. (1996). Methylmercury-induced neurotoxicity in cerebral neuron culture is blocked by antioxidants and NMDA receptor antagonists. *Neurotoxicology, 17*(1), 37–45. PubMed PMID: 8784817.

118. Wu, J., Ying, T., Shen, Z., & Wang, H. (2014). Effect of low-level prenatal mercury exposure on neonate neurobehavioral development in China. *Pediatric Neurology, 51*(1), 93–99. PubMed PMID: 24938141.

119. Lam, H. S., Kwok, K. M., Chan, P. H., So, H. K., Li, A. M., Ng, P. C., et al. (2013). Long term neurocognitive impact of low dose prenatal methylmercury exposure in Hong Kong. *Environment International, 54*, 59–64. PubMed PMID: 23416249.

120. Budtz-Jorgensen, E., Grandjean, P., Keiding, N., White, R. F., & Weihe, P. (2000). Benchmark dose calculations of methylmercury-associated neurobehavioural deficits. *Toxicology Letters, 112-113*, 193–199. PubMed PMID: 10720731.

121. Debes, F., Budtz-Jørgensen, E., Weihe, P., White, R. F., & Grandjean, P. (2006). Impact of prenatal methylmercury exposure on neurobehavioral function at age 14 years. *Neurotoxicology and Teratology, 28*(5), 536–547. PubMed PMID: 17067778.

122. Jacobson, J. L., Muckle, G., Ayotte, P., Dewailly, É., & Jacobson, S. W. (2015). Relation of prenatal methylmercury exposure from environmental sources to childhood IQ. *Environmental Health Perspectives, 123*(8), 827–833. PubMed PMID: 25757069.

123. Boucher, O., Jacobson, S. W., Plusquellec, P., Dewailly, E., Ayotte, P., Forget-Dubois, N., et al. (2012). Prenatal methylmercury, postnatal lead exposure, and evidence of attention deficit/hyperactivity disorder among Inuit children in Arctic Québec. *Environmental Health Perspectives, 120*(10), 1456–1461. PubMed PMID: 23008274.

124. Orenstein, S. T., Thurston, S. W., Bellinger, D. C., Schwartz, J. D., Amarasiriwardena, C. J., Altshul, L. M., et al. (2014). Prenatal organochlorine and methylmercury exposure and memory and learning in school-age children in communities near the New Bedford Harbor Superfund site, Massachusetts. *Environmental Health Perspectives*, *122*(11), 1253–1259. PubMed PMID: 25062363.

125. Grandjean, P., Weihe, P., Debes, F., Choi, A. L., & Budtz-Jørgensen, E. (2014). Neurotoxicity from prenatal and postnatal exposure to methylmercury. *Neurotoxicology and Teratology*, *43*, 39–44. PubMed PMID: 24681285.

126. Grandjean, P., White, R. F., Nielsen, A., Cleary, D., & de Oliveira Santos, E. C. (1999). Methylmercury neurotoxicity in Amazonian children downstream from gold mining. *Environmental Health Perspectives*, *107*(7), 587–591. PubMed PMID: 10379006.

127. Ngim, C. H., Foo, S. C., Boey, K. W., & Jeyaratnam, J. (1992). Chronic neurobehavioural effects of elemental mercury in dentists. *British Journal of Industrial Medicine*, *49*, 782–790. PubMed PMID: 1463679.

128. Echeverria, D., Woods, J. S., Heyer, N. J., Rohlman, D., Farin, F. M., Li, T., et al. (2006). The association between a genetic polymorphism of coproporphyrinogen oxidase, dental mercury exposure and neurobehavioral response in humans. *NeurotoxicolTeratol*, *28*(1), 39–48. [Epub 2005 Dec 15]. PubMed PMID: 16343843.

129. Masley, S. C., Masley, L. V., & Gualtieri, C. T. (2012). Effect of mercury levels and seafood intake on cognitive function in middle-aged adults. *Integrative Medicine*, *11*(3), 32–39.

130. Weil, M., Bressler, J., Parsons, P., Bolla, K., Glass, T., & Schwartz, B. (2005). Blood mercury levels and neurobehavioral function. *The Journal of the American Medical Association*, *293*(15), 1875–1882. PubMed PMID: 15840862.

131. Lin, Y. S., Ginsberg, G., Caffrey, J. L., Xue, J., Vulimiri, S. V., Nath, R. G., et al. (2014). Association of body burden of mercury with liver function test status in the U.S. population. *Environment International*, *70*, 88–94. PubMed PMID: 24908642.

132. Lee, H., Kim, Y., Sim, C. S., Ham, J. O., Kim, N. S., & Lee, B. K. (2014). Associations between blood mercury levels and subclinical changes in liver enzymes among South Korean general adults: analysis of 2008-2012 Korean national health and nutrition examination survey data. *Environmental Research*, *130*, 14–19. PubMed PMID: 24525240.

133. Seo, M. S., Lee, H. R., Shim, J. Y., Kang, H. T., & Lee, Y. J. (2014). Relationship between blood mercury concentrations and serum γ-glutamyltranspeptidase level in Korean adults using data from the 2010 Korean National Health and Nutrition Examination Survey. *Clinica Chimica Acta*, *430*, 160–163. PubMed PMID: 24508988.

134. Harada, M., Nakanishi, J., Kunuma, S., Ohno, K., Kimura, T., Yamaguchi, H., et al. (1998). The present mercury contents of scalp hair and clinical symptoms in inhabitants of the Minamata area. *Environmental Research*, *77*, 160–164. PubMed PMID: 9600809.

135. Ruha, A. M., Curry, S. C., Gerkin, R. D., Caldwell, K. L., Osterloh, J. D., & Wax, P. M. (2009). Urine mercury excretion following meso-dimercaptosuccinic acid challenge in fish eaters. *Archives of Pathology & Laboratory Medicine*, *133*(1), 87–92. PubMed PMID: 19123743.

136. Halbach, S., Kremers, L., Willruth, H., Mehl, A., Welzl, G., Wack, F. X., et al. (1997). Compartmental transfer of mercury released from amalgam. *Human and Experimental Toxicology*, *16*, 667–672. PubMed PMID: 9426369.

137. Grandjean, P., Budtz-Jørgensen, E., Jørgensen, P. J., & Weihe, P. (2005). Umbilical cord mercury concentration as biomarker of prenatal exposure to methylmercury. *Environmental Health Perspectives*, *113*(7), 905–908. PubMed PMID: 16002381.

138. Aposhian, H. V., Maiorino, R. M., Gonzalez-Ramirez, D., Zuniga-Charles, M., Xu, Z., Hurlbut, K. M., et al. (1995). Mobilization of heavy metals by newer, therapeutically useful chelating agents. *Toxicology*, *97*(1–3), 23–38. PubMed PMID: 7716789.

139. Maiorino, R. M., Gonzalez-Ramirez, D., Zuniga-Charles, M., Xu, Z., Hurlbut, K. M., Aposhian, M. M., et al. (1996). Sodium 2,3-dimercaptopropane-1-sulfonate challenge test for mercury in humans. III. Urinary mercury after exposure to mercurous chloride. *The Journal of Pharmacology and Experimental Therapeutics*, *277*(2), 938–944. PubMed PMID: 8627576.

140. Gonzalez-Ramirez, D., Maiorino, R. M., Zuniga-Charles, M., Xu, Z., Hurlburt, K. M., Junco-Munoz, P., et al. (1995). Sodium 2,3-dimercaptopropane-1-sulfonate challenge test for mercury in humans: II. Urinary mercury, porphyrins and neurobehavioral changes of dental workers in Monterrey, Mexico. *The Journal of Pharmacology and Experimental Therapeutics*, *272*, 264–274. PubMed PMID: 7815341.

141. Molin, M., Schütz, A., Skerfving, S., & Sällsten, G. (1991). Mobilized mercury in subjects with varying exposure to elemental mercury vapour. *International Archives of Occupational and Environmental Health*, *63*(3), 187–192. PubMed PMID: 1917069.

142. Aposhian, H. V. (1998). Mobilization of mercury and arsenic in humans by sodium 2,3-dimercapto-1-propane sulfonate (DMPS). *Environmental Health Perspectives, 106*(Suppl. 4), 1017–1025. PubMed PMID: 9703487.

143. Nerudová, J., Cábelková, Z., Frantík, E., Lukás, E., Urban, P., Bláha, K., et al. (2000). Mobilization of mercury by DMPS in occupationally exposed workers and in model experiments on rats: evaluation of body burden. *International Journal of Occupational Medicine and Environmental Health, 13*(2), 131–146. PubMed PMID: 10967843.

144. Crinnion, W. J. (2009). The benefit of pre- and post-challenge urine heavy metal testing:part 2. *Alternative Medicine Review: A Journal of Clinical Therapeutics, 14*(2), 103–108. PubMed PMID: 19594221.

145. Valavanidis, A., Vlachogianni, T., & Fiotakis, C. (2009). 8-hydroxy-2' –deoxyguanosine (8-OHdG): A critical biomarker of oxidative stress and carcinogenesis. *Journal of Environmental Science and Health. Part C, Environmental Carcinogenesis & Ecotoxicology Reviews, 27*(2), 120–139. PubMed PMID: 19412858.

146. Chen, C., Qu, L., Li, B., Xing, L., Jia, G., Wang, T., et al. (2005). Increased oxidative DNA damage, as assessed by urinary 8-hydroxy-2'-deoxyguanosine concentrations, and serum redox status in persons exposed to mercury. *Clinical Chemistry, 51*(4), 759–767. PubMed PMID: 15695327.

147. Al-Saleh, I., Abduljabbar, M., Al-Rouqi, R., Elkhatib, R., Alshabbaheen, A., & Shinwari, N. (2013). Mercury (Hg) exposure in breast-fed infants and their mothers and the evidence of oxidative stress. *Biological Trace Element Research, 153*(1–3), 145–154. PubMed PMID: 23661328.

148. Al-Saleh, I., Al-Sedairi, A. A., & Elkhatib, R. (2012). Effect of mercury (Hg) dental amalgam fillings on renal and oxidative stress biomarkers in children. *The Science of the Total Environment, 431*, 188–196. PubMed PMID: 22683759.

149. Geier, D. A., Carmody, T., Kern, J. K., King, P. G., & Geier, M. R. (2013). A significant dose-dependent relationship between mercury exposure from dental amalgams and kidney integrity biomarkers: a further assessment of the Casa Pia children's dental amalgam trial. *Human and Experimental Toxicology, 32*(4), 434–440. PubMed PMID: 22893351.

150. Woods, J. S., Martin, M. D., Naleway, C. A., & Echeverria, D. (1993). Urinary porphyrin profiles as a biomarker of mercury exposure: studies on dentists with occupational exposure to mercury vapor. *Journal of Toxicology and Environmental Health, 40*(2–3), 235–246. PubMed PMID: 8230299.

151. Lee, Y. J., & Hwang, I. C. (2014). Relationship between serum ferritin level and blood mercury concentration using data from the Korean national health and nutrition examination survey (2010-2012). *Environmental Research, 135*, 271–275. PubMed PMID: 25462675.

152. Rowland, I. R., Robinson, R. D., & Doherty, R. A. (1984). Effects of diet on mercury metabolism and excretion in mice given methylmercury: role of gut flora. *Archives of Environmental Health, 39*(6), 401–408. PubMed PMID: 6524959.

153. Landry, T. D., Doherty, R. A., & Gates, A. H. (1979). Effects of three diets on mercury excretion after methylmercury administration. *Bulletin of Environmental Contamination and Toxicology, 22*(1–2), 151–158. PubMed PMID: 465772.

154. Højbjerg, S., Nielsen, J. B., & Andersen, O. (1992). Effects of dietary lipids on whole-body retention and organ distribution of organic and inorganic mercury in mice. *Food and Chemical Toxicology, 30*(8), 703–708. PubMed PMID: 1398351.

155. Jin, X., Lok, E., Bondy, G., Caldwell, D., Mueller, R., Kapal, K., et al. (2007). Modulating effects of dietary fats on methylmercury toxicity and distribution in rats. *Toxicology, 230*(1), 22–44. PubMed PMID: 17184894.

156. Rowland, I. R., Davies, M. J., & Evans, J. G. (1980). Tissue content of mercury in rats given methylmercuric chloride orally: influence of intestinal flora. *Archives of Environmental Health, 35*(3), 155–160. PubMed PMID: 7387196.

157. Monachese, M., Burton, J. P., & Reid, G. (2012). Bioremediation and tolerance of humans to heavy metals through microbial processes: a potential role for probiotics? *Applied and Environmental Microbiology, 78*(18), 6397–6404. PubMed PMID: 22798364.

158. Bisanz, J. E., Enos, M. K., Mwanga, J. R., Changalucha, J., Burton, J. P., Gloor, G. B., et al. (2014). Randomized open-label pilot study of the influence of probiotics and the gut microbiome on toxic metal levels in Tanzanian pregnant women and school children. *mBio, 5*(5), e01580–14. PubMed PMID: 25293764.

159. Proudfoot, A. T., Krenzelok, E. P., & Vale, J. A. (2004). Position paper on urine alkalinization. *Journal of Toxicology. Clinical Toxicology, 42*(1), 1–26. Review. PubMed PMID: 15083932.

160. Hibberd, A. R., Howard, M. A., & Hunnisett, A. G. (1998). Mercury from dental amalgam fillings: studies on oral chelating agents for assessing and reducing mercury burdens in humans. *Journal of Nutrition & Environmental Medicine, 8*, 219–231.

161. Bridges, C. C., Joshee, L., & Zalups, R. K. (2009). Effect of DMPS and DMSA on the placental and

fetal disposition of methylmercury. *Placenta*, *30*(9), 800–805. PubMed PMID: 19615742.

162. Aremu, D. A., Madejczyk, M. S., & Ballatori, N. (2008). N-acetylcysteine as a potential antidote and biomonitoring agent of methylmercury exposure. *Environmental Health Perspectives*, *116*(1), 26–31. PubMed PMID: 18197295.

163. Zalups, R. K., & Bridges, C. C. (2009). MRP2 involvement in renal proximal tubular elimination of methylmercury mediated by DMPS or DMSA. *Toxicology and Applied Pharmacology*, *235*(1), 10–17. PubMed PMID: 19063911.

164. Zalups, R. K., & Bridges, C. C. (2012). Relationships between the renal handling of DMPS and DMSA and the renal handling of mercury. *Chemical Research in Toxicology*, *25*(9), 1825–1838. PubMed PMID: 22667351.

165. Ballatori, N., Lieberman, M. W., & Wang, W. (1998). N-acetylcysteine as an antidote in methylmercury poisoning. *Environmental Health Perspectives*, *106*(5), 267–271. PubMed PMID: 9520359.

166. Dirks, M. J., Davis, D. R., Cheraskin, E., & Jackson, J. A. (1994). Mercury excretion and intravenous ascorbic acid. *Archives of Environmental Health*, *49*(1), 49–52.

167. Pingree, S. D., Simmonds, P. L., & Woods, J. S. (2001). Effects of 2,3-dimercapto-1-propanesulfonic acid (DMPS) on tissue and urine mercury levels following prolonged methylmercury exposure in rats. *Toxicological Sciences*, *61*(2), 224–233. PubMed PMID: 11353131.

168. Hurlburt, K. M., Maiorino, R. M., Mayersohn, M., Dart, R. C., Bruce, D. C., & Aposhian, H. V. (1994). Determination and metabolism of dithiol chelating agents XVI: pharmacokinetics of 2,3-dimercapto-1-propanesulfonate after intravenous administration to human volunteers. *Journal of Pharmacology and Experimental Therapeutics*, *268*(2), 662–668.

169. Bradberry, S. M., Sheehan, T. M., Barraclough, C. R., & Vale, J. A. (2009). DMPS can reverse the features of severe mercury vapor-induced neurological damage. *Clinical Toxicology (Philadelphia, Pa.)*, *47*(9), 894–898. PubMed PMID:19852623.

170. Böse-O'Reilly, S., Drasch, G., Beinhoff, C., Maydl, S., Vosko, M. R., Roider, G., et al. (2003). The Mt. Diwata study on the Philippines 2000: treatment of mercury intoxicated inhabitants of a gold mining area with DMPS (2,3-dimercapto-1-propane-sulfonic acid, Dimaval). *The Science of the Total Environment*, *307*(1–3), 71–82. PubMed PMID: 12711426.

171. Cohen, J. P., Ruha, A. M., Curry, S. C., Biswas, K., Westenberger, B., Ye, W., et al. (2013). Plasma and urine dimercaptopropanesulfonate concentrations after dermal application of transdermal DMPS (TD-DMPS). *Journal of Medical Toxicology*, *9*(1), 9–15. PubMed PMID:23143832.

172. Graziano, J. H. (1986). Role of 2,3-dimercaptosuccininc acid in the treatment of heavy metal poisoning. *Medical Toxicology*, *1*, 155–162. PubMed PMID:3023784.

173. Aposhian, H. V., Maiorino, R. M., Rivera, M., Bruce, D. C., Cart, R. C., Hurlburt, K. M., et al. (1992). Human studies with the chelating agents DMPS and DMSA. *Clinical Toxicology*, *30*(4), 505–528. PubMed PMID: 1331491.

174. Forman, J., Moline, J., Cernichiari, E., Sayegh, S., Torres, J. C., Landrigan, M. M., et al. (2000). A cluster of pediatric metallic mercury exposure cases treated with meso-2,3-dimercaptosuccinic acid (DMSA). *Environmental Health Perspectives*, *108*(6), 575–577. PubMed PMID: 10856034.

175. Sigg, T., Burda, A., Leikin, J. B., & Gossman, W. (1998). Umanos J. A report of pediatric succimer overdose. *Veterinary and Human Toxicology*, *40*(2), 90–91. PubMed PMID: 9554061.

176. Roels, H. A., Boeckx, M., Ceulemans, E., & Lauwerys, R. R. (1991). Urinary excretion of mercury after occupational exposure to mercury vapour and influence of the chelating agent meso-2,3-dimercaptosuccinic acid (DMSA). *British Journal of Industrial Medicine*, *48*(4), 247–253. PubMed PMID: 1851035.

177. Aposhian, H. V., Bruce, D. C., Alter, W., Dart, R. C., Hurlbut, K. M., & Aposhian, M. M. (1992). Urinary mercury after administration of 2,3-dimercaptopropane-1-sulfonic acid: correlation with dental amalgam score. *FASEB Journal*, *6*(7), 2472–2476. PubMed PMID: 1563599.

178. Aposhian, H. V. (1983). DMSA and DMPS-water soluble antidotes for heavy metal poisoning. *Annual Review of Pharmacology and Toxicology*, *23*, 193–215. PubMed PMID: 6307120.

179. Joshi, D., Mittal, D. K., Shukla, S., Srivastav, A. K., & Srivastav, S. K. (2014). N-acetyl cysteine and selenium protects mercuric chloride-induced oxidative stress and antioxidant defense system in liver and kidney of rats: a histopathological approach. *Journal of Trace Elements in Medicine and Biology*, *28*(2), 218–226. PubMed PMID: 24485406.

180. Joshi, D., Mittal, D., Shrivastav, S., Shukla, S., & Srivastav, A. K. (2011). Combined effect of N-acetyl cysteine, zinc, and selenium against chronic dimethylmercury-induced oxidative stress: a biochemical and histopathological approach. *Archives of Environmental Contamination and Toxicology*, *61*(4), 558–567. PubMed PMID: 21424224.

181. Afonne, O. J., Orisakwe, O. E., Ndubuka, G. I., Akumka, D. D., & Ilondu, N. (2000). Zinc protection of mercury-induced hepatic toxicity in mice. *Biological and Pharmaceutical Bulletin*, *23*(3), 305–308. PubMed PMID: 10726883.

182. Meinerz, D. F., de Paula, M. T., Comparsi, B., Silva, M. U., Schmitz, A. E., Braga, H. C., et al. (2011). Protective effects of organoselenium compounds against methylmercury-induced oxidative stress in mouse brain mitochondrial-enriched fractions. *Brazilian Journal of Medical and Biological Research*, *44*(11), 1156–1163. PubMed PMID: 22002094.

183. Kalender, S., Uzun, F. G., Demir, F., Uzunhisarcıklı, M., & Aslanturk, A. (2013). Aslanturk A. Mercuric chloride-induced testicular toxicity in rats and the protective role of sodium selenite and vitamin E. *Food and Chemical Toxicology*, *55*, 456–462. PubMed PMID: 23369933.

184. Falluel-Morel, A., Lin, L., Sokolowski, K., McCandlish, E., Buckley, B., & DiCicco-Bloom, E. (2012). N-acetyl cysteine treatment reduces mercury-induced neurotoxicity in the developing rat hippocampus. *Journal of Neuroscience Research*, *90*(4), 743–750. PubMed PMID: 22420031.

185. Kaur, P., Aschner, M., & Syversen, T. (2006). Glutathione modulation influences methyl mercury induced neurotoxicity in primary cell cultures of neurons and astrocytes. *Neurotoxicology*, *27*(4), 492–500. PubMed PMID: 16513172.

186. Ekor, M., Adesanoye, O. A., & Farombi, E. O. (2010). N-acetylcysteine pretreatment ameliorates mercuric chloride-induced oxidative renal damage in rats. *African Journal of Medicine and Medical Sciences*, *39*(Suppl.), 153–160. PubMed PMID: 22416658.

187. Girardi, G., & Elias, M. M. (1991). Effectiveness of N-acetylcysteine in protecting against mercuric chloride-induced nephrotoxicity. *Toxicology*, *67*(2), 155–164. PubMed PMID: 1674384.

188. Agarwal, R., Goel, S. K., & Behari, J. R. (2010). Detoxification and antioxidant effects of curcumin in rats experimentally exposed to mercury. *Journal of Applied Toxicology*, *30*(5), 457–468. PubMed PMID: 20229497.

189. Anuradha, B., & Varalakshmi, P. (1999). Protective role of DL-alpha-lipoic acid against mercury-induce neural lipid peroxidation. *Pharmacological Research*, *39*, 67–80.

190. Gregus, Z., Stein, A. F., Varga, F., & Klaasen, C. D. (1992). Effect of lipoic acid on biliary excretion of glutathione and metals. *Toxicology and Applied Pharmacology*, *114*, 88–96.

15

Other Metals
Gadolinium, Manganese, Thallium

SUMMARY

- Presence in population: Manganese (Mn) is an essential mineral and is required for proper health and development; gadolinium (Gd) and thallium (Tl) are nonessential and have no biological role; Gd is primarily present in individuals who have had imaging studies using contrast agents; Tl toxicity is rare
- Major diseases: The gastrointestinal, neurological, renal, and reproductive systems are particularly sensitive to toxic metal–induced impairment and dysfunction
- Primary sources: Diet (Mn, Tl), medical imaging contrast agent (Gd)
- Best measure: Hair analysis (Mn), urine and blood (Gd, Tl)
- Best intervention: Avoidance, antioxidants

DESCRIPTION

Toxic metals are used in a variety of industrial processes, and as a result, human exposure has dramatically increased during the last 50 years. Toxic metals are considered major environmental pollutants and are a common underlying factor in many cases of chemical overload. In some individuals, metals are the primary toxicants present.

The most prevalent toxic metals in humans are lead, mercury, cadmium, and arsenic. These metals are nonessential xenobiotics, and exposure is harmful to human health. Some metals, such as manganese and chromium, are essential for good health but may be toxic above certain levels.[1] Other metals have biological (e.g., vanadium), pharmacological (e.g., lithium), and medical (e.g., gadolinium) uses. Although exposure to several of these metals is prevalent, and sometimes therapeutically and/or medically necessary, the potential for toxic effects must be considered.

Gadolinium

Gadolinium is a rare earth metal with the atomic number 64. Gadolinium has no known biological role and is primarily used in medical imaging. Approximately 30% to 50% of all magnetic resonance imaging (MRI) scans use some kind of nonspecific gadolinium-based contrast agent (GBCA). The current US Food and Drug Adminstration (FDA)-approved GBCAs are gadobenate (Multi-Hance), gadobutrol (Gadavist), gadodiamide (Omniscan), gadopentetate (Magnevist), gadoterate (Dotarem), gadoteridol (ProHance), gadoversetamide (OptiMARK), gadoxetate (Eovist), and gadofosveset (Ablavar). Health Canada has recently published information cautioning practitioners on the use of these compounds because of renal and neurological concerns.[2]

Manganese

Manganese is the 12th most abundant element and constitutes about 0.1% of the Earth's crust. Manganese is an essential trace mineral and is involved in bone formation and brain development and in enzymes required for proper amino acid, cholesterol, and carbohydrate metabolism (e.g., arginase, glutamine synthetase, pyruvate carboxylase).[3] Manganese plays an important role in antioxidant defenses and forms part of the superoxide dismutase (MnSOD) enzyme system.

Thallium

Thallium is a rare but widely spread naturally occurring trace element with average concentrations of 0.3 to 0.5 µg/g in the continental crust. Thallium does not have any biological use and does not appear to be an essential element for life.

TOXICITY

Toxic metals cause damage in a variety of ways, including free radical production, enzyme poisoning, direct DNA damage, endocrine disruption, and mitochondrial or cell wall damage.[4]

Manganese

The exact mechanism of manganese toxicity is unknown. However, it has been hypothesized that it is associated with mitochondrial dysfunction, because manganese accumulates within mitochondria and adversely affects mitochondrial function by interfering with oxidative phosphorylation, inhibiting both NADPH dehydrogenase and NADH cytochrome c reductase, inhibiting cytochrome oxidase, and altering Leydig cell mitochondria.[5] Neurotoxic effects of manganese include disturbances in the dopaminergic system, gamma-aminobutyric acid (GABA) regulation, and glutamatergic-related excitotoxicity.[6] Manganese also causes oxidative damage, including autoxidation of dopamine, production of free radicals, depletion of cellular antioxidant defenses, and DNA fragmentation.[7,8]

Gadolinium

The trivalent free ion of gadolinium (Gd^{3+}) is extremely toxic and competes with a variety of cations, most notably Ca^{2+}. As a result, Gd^{3+} blocks many types of voltage-gated calcium channels, inhibiting those physiological processes and enzymes that depend on Ca^{2+} with an affinity for the reticuloendothelial system.[9] Chelation of gadolinium dramatically reduces its acute toxicity, with marked decline in LD_{50} of intravenous gadolinium-tetraazacyclododecanetetraacetic acid [Gd-DOTA (10.6 mmol/kg)] in mice compared with $GdCl_3$ (0.35 mmol/kg).[10] The amount of released gadolinium ions is the key determinant of toxic outcome, and the release is likely a consequence of Zn^{2+}, Cu^{2+}, and Ca^{2+} transmetallation in vivo.[11] Gadolinium may also induce toxicity through the release and stimulation of cytokines involved in tissue fibrosis, induction of fibronectin expression, apoptosis and necrosis in fibroblasts, mobilization of iron, and elevation of reactive oxygen species.[12]

Thallium

Thallium is highly toxic, and in the past, poisoning often resulted in death.[13] The toxicity of thallium-based compounds is mainly caused by the similarity between thallium ions and potassium ions. Toxic mechanisms of thallium may include disruption of sulfhydryl groups on the mitochondrial membrane interfering with the sodium-potassium ATPase, interference of riboflavin homeostasis, inhibition of cellular respiration, oxidative stress, and disruption of calcium homeostasis.[14] Common symptoms in nonfatal cases include fatigue, gastroenteritis, extremely painful sensory neuropathy, and alopecia.

SOURCES

The general population is exposed to metals at trace concentrations either voluntarily through supplementation or involuntarily through intake of contaminated food and water or contact with contaminated soil, dust, or air.

Manganese

For most individuals, manganese intake occurs primarily through food, with daily intake ranging from 2 to 9 mg. Ingestion from drinking water is assumed to represent a small portion of total intake, contributing less than 1%, although this can rise to 20% depending on manganese concentration in the water. Occupational exposure of manganese occurs in welding, dry cell battery manufacturing, automotive mechanics, mining, and agricultural application of manganese-containing pesticides (e.g., mancozeb). Airborne manganese from welding has been associated with "metal fume fever."[15] Manganese is also used as a contrast agent in nuclear magnetic resonance tomography and as a fuel additive (methylcyclopentandienyl manganese tricarbonyl).[16]

Gadolinium

Gadolinium has unusual ferromagnetic and superconductive properties and is used in microwave applications and in the production of phosphors in color televisions. The most common source of exposure occurs as a result of gadolinium-containing contrast agents used in diagnostic imaging (MRI).

Thallium

Thallium is used in the manufacturing of optical lenses, infrared optical instruments, imitation jewelry, scintillation counters, semiconductors, low-temperature thermometers, green-colored fireworks, and nuclear cardiography and as a chemical catalyst. Thallium was also included in rodenticides and insecticides, which, before its use was banned in these products, were the primary hazards to the general public. Atmospheric emissions from industrial facilities, such as metal mining, smelting, and cement plants using pyrite, have resulted in increased thallium concentrations. Most human exposure today is associated with contaminated food or drinking water. Reports indicate that high thallium concentrations may be found in green vegetables such as cabbage.[17]

BODY BURDEN AND ASSESSMENT

Manganese

The human body contains about 10 to 20 mg of manganese, half of which occurs in the bones and the remainder found in the liver, pancreas, pituitary gland, adrenal glands, and kidneys.[18] Ambient manganese can cross the blood-brain barrier, increasing the risk of neurotoxicity.[19] Although the brain takes up less manganese, it retains and accumulates manganese, primarily in the globus pallidus of basal ganglia. In cases of manganese intoxication, MRI can have diagnostic value, provided the scans are performed before cessation of exposure.[20] Common biological markers of manganese, such as blood or urine, have not proven to be practical.[21] However, hair manganese has shown promise as a biomarker, because it is not influenced by short-term variability of manganese exposure and has shown a significant linear association with 30-day time-weighted average manganese air exposure.[22]

Gadolinium

Despite normal renal function, there is increased evidence that gadolinium accumulates in tissues of patients exposed to gadolinium-based contrast agents during MRI. Gadolinium deposition has long been known to occur in bone tissue but can also be found in the skin,[23] kidneys, heart,[24]

liver,[25,26] spleen,[27] and brain.[28] Persistent high concentrations of gadolinium have been found in skin, some even 3 years after the last exposure, and if these residual gadolinium chelates dissociate into insoluble free Gd^{3+}, they can form complexes with tissue anions serving as potential sites for future harmful effects.[29]

Thallium

Thallium is absorbed through the skin and mucous membranes, is widely distributed throughout the body, and accumulates in bones, renal medulla, and the central nervous system.[30] Although it has been reported that thallium levels in normal humans is less than 1 parts per billion (PPB) in blood and urine and less than 10 PPB in tissues, its presence is abnormal in the human body and is considered lethal when it reaches 10 to 15 mg/kg of body weight.[31] Urine tests are considered to be the most accurate way to measure thallium, which can be detected in urine after 1 hour and up to 2 months after exposure.[32]

DETOXIFICATION/EXCRETION PROCESSES

Manganese

The amount of manganese absorbed orally from food by humans ranges between 1% and 5% depending on the amount and form of manganese.[33] Manganese is absorbed by the intestinal cells through its binding to transferrin, is transported into the cytosol by the divalent metal transporter-1 protein, and is eventually released from the cell into the circulation, where it binds to albumin and β-globulin for transport to peripheral tissues.[34] The half-life of slow-elimination manganese is about 37 to 39 days, less in people exposed to manganese.[35] Excretion is almost entirely fecal, and more than half is eliminated in the bile.[36] Inhaled manganese can bypass biliary excretion mechanisms and directly enter the systemic circulation. After intravenous contrast injection, normal regulation mechanisms are also bypassed. Because manganese can only be excreted slowly via the biliary system, decomplexation with release of free manganese prolongs elimination of the metal, increasing the danger of individual overdosing.[37]

Gadolinium

Gadolinium, in the form of the contrast agent gadodiamide, is almost exclusively excreted renally, and therefore has a markedly prolonged half-life in patients with renal failure.[38,39,40] In healthy humans, the half-life of gadolinium chelates is approximately 1.3 hours, whereas in patients with end-stage renal disease, it is prolonged to approximately 120 hours.[41]

Thallium

Thallium can enter the body through inhalation as a dust, ingestion from contaminated food and water, absorption through the skin, or intravenously as a contrast agent. Thallium spreads intravascularly within the first few hours of exposure and propagates through the central nervous system for several days.[42] The elimination half-life of thallium is between 1 and 30 days, depending on the route of exposure, dose, and time since and chronicity of ingestion, and it is excreted mainly in the urine.[43]

CLINICAL SIGNIFICANCE

The severity of signs and symptoms resulting from metal toxicity vary based on several factors, including the dose, route of exposure, and chemical species, as well as the age, gender, genetics, and nutritional status of exposed individuals. Early symptoms can include impaired ability to think or concentrate, fatigue, headache, indigestion, tremors, poor coordination, myalgia, anemia, asthma, allergies, "brain fog," infertility, and temperature dysregulation. The gastrointestinal, cardiovascular, neurological, renal, and reproductive systems are particularly sensitive to toxic metal–induced impairment and dysfunction. Chronic subacute exposure may lead to subtle or overt long-term problems in selected populations and is particularly concerning for children.

Cancer

A study examining the relationship between cancer and manganese concentration in drinking water in Huai'an, China, found that for every 1 µg/L increase in manganese concentration, there was a corresponding increase of $0.45/10^5$ new cancer cases and $0.35/10^5$ cancer deaths.[44] A large ecological study conducted in North Carolina also found that manganese concentration in groundwater correlates with cancer mortality.[45] For each log increase in groundwater manganese concentration, there was a corresponding county-level increase of 12.10 deaths/100,000 population in all-site cancer rates.

Thallium has been shown to decrease the activity of some drug-metabolizing enzymes dependent on cytochrome P-450 and therefore may interfere with the metabolism of organic carcinogens, increasing the risk of cancer.[46] Studies indicate that thallium compounds may have weak mutagenic effects, but no definitive effect on the induction of primary DNA damage or chromosomal damage has been shown.[47]

Gastrointestinal

Because manganese is absorbed and excreted by the liver, it is a target organ for toxicity, and manganese overload is common among patients with chronic liver disease.[48]

Case reports of acute pancreatitis have been reported after exposure to GBCAs, with one case requiring surgical intervention for acute necrotizing pancreatitis.[49,50]

Endocrine

A Korean study of welders exposed to manganese reported higher levels of thyroid-stimulating hormone (TSH), follicle-stimulating hormone (FSH), and luteinizing hormone (LH) among male welders compared with age-matched office workers, concluding that manganese suppresses the inhibitory feedback control of dopamine on the hypophyseal-pituitary axis.[51]

Neuropsychological

Manganese at levels found in some groundwater is associated with intellectual impairment in children. A cross-sectional study of 362 Canadian children examining the risk associated with drinking groundwater containing manganese on intellectual functioning found that a 10-fold increase in manganese values in water (MnW) was associated with a 2.4-point decrease in IQ score (95% confidence interval (CI): −3.9 to −0.9; $p < 0.01$).[52] Levels of manganese in tap water ranged between 1.0 and 2700 µg/L (median, 34 µg/L), and there was a 6.2-point difference in IQ between children in the lowest versus the highest MnW quintiles. In 11- to 13-year-old Chinese children, exposure to manganese-contaminated drinking water was associated with lower scores on tests of short-term memory, manual dexterity, and visual perceptual speed and lower mathematics and language scores.[53,54] A negative association was also determined between manganese levels in hair (0.472 µg/g) and verbal IQ scores in school-aged children.[55]

In children drinking home tap water, a 10-fold increment in manganese concentration in hair was associated with a 3.6- and 4.2-point reduction in memory and attention, respectively, and a 10-fold increase in manganese intake from water significantly decreased motor function by 1.3-fold.[56] Manganese exposure associated with drinking water was also significantly positively correlated with hyperactive and oppositional classroom behaviors in a study of 46 children in Quebec.[57]

Violent and aberrant behavior may be associated with manganese toxicity, because significantly elevated manganese levels were found in the hair of violent versus nonviolent prisoners.[58] Adults' scores on the Mini-Mental Status Examination, a dementia screening test, were inversely associated with blood manganese levels, showing a 12-fold increased risk of deficient cognitive performance.[59]

Neurological

Exposure to high levels of manganese results in a neurological disorder termed *manganism*. Manganese is a known neurotoxicant, with psychological and neurological disturbances producing symptoms similar to Parkinson's disease, including extrapyramidal motor system defects and altered behavior.[60] An overall prevalence estimate of parkinsonism of 15.6% has been observed in welders who had worked for 19 years compared with 0% in nonexposed controls.[61] Exposure to 0.22 mg Mn/m^3 air for a relatively short period (8.1–28 months) produced symptoms of manganism in 25.6% of welders, and blood concentrations of 5.85 μg/L to 14.6 μg/L in these welders were associated with a concomitant dose-dependent deterioration of neuropsychological function.[62] Adults who used methcathinone (i.e., ephedrone, a recreational stimulant) had greater urinary manganese than controls (8.68 μg/L vs. 4.27 μg/L, respectively) and developed impaired motor function, such as slurred speech and postural instability.[63] Animal studies suggest that iron deficiency or anemia may be a risk factor for manganese neurotoxicity.[64,65]

Renal

Animal studies have demonstrated that GBCA exposure causes nephrotoxicity, inducing necrosis and apoptosis in renal tubular cells.[66,67] The acute nephrotoxic effect of GBCA administration in humans was demonstrated in a case report of a 56-year-old woman with normal baseline renal function who developed acute renal failure after two consecutive vascular imaging procedures.[68]

Nephrogenic systemic fibrosis (NSF) is a systemic disease associated with exposure to gadolinium-based MRI contrast in patients with compromised renal function.[69] An odds ratio of 32.5 (95% CI, 1.9–549.2) has been observed for acquiring nephrogenic systemic fibrosis after gadolinium exposure.[70] Upon deposition in various tissues, gadolinium-based contrast agents are believed to play a role in NSF development by providing a target for fibrocyte recruitment and activation of the fibrotic process.[71] The principal manifestation is cutaneous, marked by plaque-like induration, thickening, and hyperpigmentation of the skin of the extremities and trunk, with facial sparing. Insoluble gadolinium-phosphate deposits have also been found in the liver, lungs, intestinal wall, kidneys, lymph nodes, skeletal muscle, dura matter, and cerebellum, primarily in vascular walls and fibrotic areas of patients with NSF.[72] Gadolinium deposition disease is a newly described entity that includes signs and symptoms that follow a pattern similar to, but not identical to, and also less severe than, those observed in NSF.[73]

Reproductive

The rate-limiting step in steroid hormone synthesis is the movement of cholesterol across the mitochondrial membrane, from the outer to the inner membrane, mediated by the steroidogenic acute regulatory (StAR) protein, with the conversion of cholesterol to pregnenolone by cytochrome P450 side-chain cleavage (CYPscc) initiating steroidogenesis.[74] Manganese is known to impede male reproductive function through a variety of mechanisms, including inhibition of StAR protein expression and/or function, mitochondrial dysfunction, and disturbance of calcium homeostasis, and at later stages, manganese may arrest the cell cycle and induce apoptosis of primary Leydig cells, leading to reduced steroidogenesis.[75] Ambient manganese exposure impairs male fertility, with high manganese levels associated with an increased risk of low sperm motility (OR = 5.5; 95% CI, 1.6–17.6) and low sperm concentration (OR = 2.4; 95% CI, 1.2–4.9).[76] Men with occupational exposure to manganese had decreased libido and increased sexual impotency.[77] In studies of the adult male rat, long-term ingestion of manganese sulfate suppressed sexual behavior, abolished territorial aggression, interfered with fertility, and caused anatomical changes in the reproductive system.[78] In female rats, manganese exposure induced abnormal development of reproductive tissues and altered gonadotropin secretion.[79]

Thallium crosses the placenta freely and produces abnormalities in animals as well as fetal demise, overt toxicity, and congenital abnormalities in humans.[80] Higher maternal urinary thallium levels are significantly associated with increased risk of low birth weight (OR = 1.52; 95% CI: 1.00–2.30 for the highest vs. lowest tertile), and the association was similarly elevated after adjustment for potential confounders (OR = 1.90; 95% CI: 1.01–3.58 for the highest vs. lowest tertile).[81]

INTERVENTION

Antioxidants are an essential component in the treatment and prevention of metal and chemical toxicity. Antioxidants protect the liver from damage and support detoxification processes. Antioxidants counteract oxidative stress by reducing the formation of free radicals. Dark-colored fruits and vegetables are rich sources of antioxidants. Several vitamins, minerals, and nutraceuticals also function as antioxidants.

Pretreatment with vitamin E has been shown to fully protect the manganese-induced increase in cerebral markers of oxidative damage, protects the cerebrum from neuronal oxidative damage, and protects neurons from dendritic degeneration.[82] In animal studies, melatonin attenuates manganese-induced motor dysfunction and neuronal loss and reverses manganese-induced oxidative injury.[83,84] Anthocyanins obtained from acai,[85] extracts of *Melissa officinalis*,[86] and silymarin[87] have also shown protective effects against manganese-induced oxidative stress.

N-acetylcysteine pretreatment inhibits gadolinium-induced cell death and endoplasmic reticulum stress and also protects against GBCA-induced nephrotoxicity in rats with chronic renal failure.[88]

Prussian blue has been used as a treatment for thallium toxicity, because the exchange of potassium ions in the crystal lattice with thallium ions leads to the binding of thallium in the intestine for extraction and elimination.[89]

REFERENCES

1. Trumbo, P., Yates, A. A., Schlicker, S., & Poos, M. (2001). Dietary reference intakes: vitamin A, vitamin K, arsenic, boron, chromium, copper, iodine, iron, manganese, molybdenum, nickel, silicon, vanadium, and zinc. *Journal of the American Dietetic Association, 101*(3), 294–301. PubMed PMID: 11269606.
2. Health Canada. (January 6, 2017). *Information Update - New safety information on injectable gadolinium-based contrast agents used in MRI scans.* Recalls and safety alerts. Available at http://healthycanadians.gc.ca/recall-alert-rappel-avis/hc-sc/2017/61676a-eng.php. (Accessed September 1, 2017).
3. Gunter, T. E., Gavin, C. E., Aschner, M., & Gunter, K. K. (2006). Speciation of manganese in cells and mitochondria: a search for the proximal cause of manganese neurotoxicity. *Neurotoxicology, 27*(5), 765–776. PubMed PMID: 16765446.
4. Flora, S. J., Mittal, M., & Mehta, A. (2008). Heavy metal induced oxidative stress & its possible reversal by chelation therapy. *The Indian Journal of Medical Research, 128*(4), 501–523. PubMed PMID: 19106443.
5. Cheng, J., Fu, J., & Zhou, Z. (2005). The mechanism of manganese-induced inhibition of steroidogenesis in rat primary Leydig cells. *Toxicology, 211*(1–2), 1–11. PubMed PMID: 15863243.
6. Fitsanakis, V. A., Au, C., Erikson, K. M., & Aschner, M. (2006). The effects of manganese on glutamate, dopamine and gamma-aminobutyric acid regulation. *Neurochemistry International, 48*(6–7), 426–433. PubMed PMID: 16513220.
7. Martinez-Finley, E. J., Gavin, C. E., Aschner, M., & Gunter, T. E. (2013). Manganese neurotoxicity and the role of reactive oxygen species. *Free Radical Biology & Medicine, 62*, 65–75. PubMed PMID: 23395780.
8. Latchoumycandane, C., Anantharam, V., Kitazawa, M., et al. (2005). Protein kinase Cdelta is a key downstream mediator of manganese-induced apoptosis in dopaminergic neuronal cells. *The Journal of Pharmacology and Experimental Therapeutics, 313*(1), 46–55. PubMed PMID: 15608081.
9. Abraham, J. L., & Thakral, C. (2008). Tissue distribution and kinetics of gadolinium and nephrogenic systemic fibrosis. *European Journal of Radiology, 66*(2), 200–207. PubMed PMID: 18374532.
10. Bousquet, J. C., Saini, S., Stark, D. D., et al. (1988). Gd-DOTA: characterization of a new paramagnetic complex. *Radiology, 166*(3), 693–698. PubMed PMID: 3340763.
11. Cacheris, W. P., Quay, S. C., & Rocklage, S. M. (1990). The relationship between thermodynamics and the toxicity of gadolinium complexes. *Magnetic Resonance Imaging, 8*(4), 467–481. PubMed PMID: 2118207.
12. Rogosnitzky, M., & Branch, S. (2016). Gadolinium-based contrast agent toxicity: a review of known and proposed mechanisms. *BioMetals, 29*(3), 365–376. PubMed PMID: 27053146.
13. No authors listed. (1972). Toxicity of thallium. *British Medical Journal, 3*(5829), 717. PubMed PMID: 5077906.
14. Mulkey, J. P., & Oehme, F. W. (1993). A review of thallium toxicity. *Veterinary and Human Toxicology, 35*(5), 445–453. PubMed PMID: 8249271.
15. Greenberg, M. I., & Vearrier, D. (2015). Metal fume fever and polymer fume fever. *Clinical Toxicology*

(Philadelphia, Pa.), 53(4), 195–203. PubMed PMID: 25706449.

16. Boudia, N., Halley, R., Kennedy, G., et al. (2006). Manganese concentrations in the air of the Montreal (Canada) subway in relation to surface automobile traffic density. *The Science of the Total Environment, 366*(1), 143–147. PubMed PMID: 16297437.

17. Ning, Z., He, L., Xiao, T., & Marton, L. (2015). High accumulation and subcellular distribution of thallium in green cabbage (Brassica oleracea L. Var. Capitata L.). *International Journal of Phytoremediation, 17*(11), 1097–1104. PubMed PMID: 26067081.

18. Gerber, G. B., Leonard, A., & Hantson, P. (2002). Carcinogenicity, mutagenicity and teratogenicity of manganese compounds. *Critical Reviews in Oncology/Hematology, 42*(1), 25–34. PubMed PMID: 11923066.

19. Elder, A., Gelein, R., Silva, V., Feikert, T., et al. (2006). Translocation of inhaled ultrafine manganese oxide particles to the central nervous system. *Environmental Health Perspectives, 114*(8), 1172–1178. PubMed PMID: 16882521.

20. Kim, Y. (2004). High signal intensities on T1-weighted MRI as a biomarker of exposure to manganese. *Industrial Health, 42*(2), 111–115. PubMed PMID: 15128159.

21. Laohaudomchok, W., Lin, X., Herrick, R. F., et al. (2011). Toenail, blood, and urine as biomarkers of manganese exposure. *Journal of Occupational and Environmental Medicine, 53*(5), 506–510. PubMed PMID: 21494156.

22. Reiss, B., Simpson, C. D., Baker, M. G., Stover, B., et al. (2016). Hair manganese as an exposure biomarker among welders. *The Annals of Occupational Hygiene, 60*(2), 139–149. PubMed PMID: 26409267.

23. Wang, Y. X., Schroeder, J., Siegmund, H., Idee, J. M., et al. (2015). Total gadolinium tissue deposition and skin structural finding following the administration of structurally different gadolinium chelates in healthy and ovariectomized female rats. *Quantitative Imaging in Medicine and Surgery [electronic resource], 5*(4), 534–545. PubMed PMID: 26435917.

24. Swaminathan, S., High, W. A., Ranville, J., et al. (2008). Cardiac and vascular metal deposition with high mortality in nephrogenic systemic fibrosis. *Kidney International, 73*(12), 1413–1418. PubMed PMID: 18401336.

25. Pascolo, L., Cupelli, F., Anelli, P. L., et al. (1999). Molecular mechanisms for the hepatic uptake of magnetic resonance imaging contrast agents. *Biochemical and Biophysical Research Communications, 257*(3), 746–752. PubMed PMID: 10208854.

26. Myrissa, A., Braeuer, S., Martinelli, E., et al. (2017). Gadolinium accumulation in organs of Sprague-Dawley rats after implantation of a biodegradable magnesium-gadolinium alloy. *Acto Biomater, 48,* 521–529. PubMed PMID: 27845277.

27. Barnhart, J. L., Kuhnert, N., Bakan, D. A., & Berk, R. N. (1987). Biodistribution of GdCl3 and Gd-DTPA and their influence on proton magnetic relaxation in rat tissues. *Magnetic Resonance Imaging, 5*(3), 221–231. PubMed PMID: 3626790.

28. Lohrke, J., Frisk, A. L., Frenzel, T., Schockel, L., et al. (2017). Histology and gadolinium distribution in the rodent brain after the administration of cumulative high doses of linear and macrocytic gadolinium-based contrast agents. *Investigative Radiology, 52*(6), 324–333. PubMed PMID: 28323657.

29. Thakral, C., Alhariri, J., & Abraham, J. L. (2007). Long-term retention of gadolinium in tissues from nephrogenic systemic fibrosis patient after multiple gadolinium-enhanced MRI scans: case report and implications. *Contrast Media and Molecular Imaging, 2*(4), 199–205. PubMed PMID: 17712863.

30. Peter, Al, & Viraraghavan, T. (2005). Thallium: a review of public health and environmental concerns. *Environment International, 31*(4), 493–501. PubMed PMID: 15788190.

31. Galvan-Arzate, S., & Santamaria, A. (1998). Thallium toxicity. *Toxicology Letters, 99*(1), 1–13. PubMed PMID: 9801025.

32. Krabowska, B. (2016). Presence of thallium in the environment: sources of contaminations, distribution and monitoring methods. *Environmental Monitoring and Assessment, 188*(11), 640. PubMed PMID: 27783348.

33. Johnson, P. E., Lykken, G. I., & Korynta, E. D. (1991). Absorption and biological half-life in humans of intrinsic and extrinsic 54Mn tracers from foods of plant origin. *The Journal of Nutrition, 121*(5), 711–717. PubMed PMID: 2019880.

34. Freeland-Graves, J. H., Mousa, T. Y., & Kim, S. (2016). International variability in diet and requirements of manganese: causes and consequences. *Journal of Trace Elements in Medicine and Biology, 38,* 24–32. PubMed PMID: 27264059.

35. Mahoney, J. P., & Small, W. J. (1968). Studies on manganese. 3. The biological half-life of radiomanganese in man and factors which affect this half-life. *The Journal of Clinical Investigation, 47*(3), 643–653. PubMed PMID: 5637148.

36. Maynard, L. S., & Fink, S. (1956). The influence of chelation on radiomanganese excretion in man and mouse. *The Journal of Clinical Investigation, 35*(8), 831–836. PubMed PMID: 13345885.

37. Misselwitz, B., Muhler, A., & Weinmann, H. J. (1995). A toxicologic risk for using manganese complexes?

A literature survey of existing data through several medical specialties. *Investigative Radiology, 30*(10), 611–620. PubMed PMID: 8557501.

38. Joffe, P., Thomsen, H. S., & Meusel, M. (1998). Pharmacokinetics of gadodiamide injection in patients with severe renal insufficiency and patients undergoing hemodialysis or continuous ambulatory peritoneal dialysis. *Academic Radiology, 5*(7), 491–502. PubMed PMID: 9653466.

39. Joffe, P., & Thomsen, H. S. (2011). The pharmacokinetics of gadodiamide in patients with severe renal insufficiency treated conservatively or undergoing hemodialysis or continuous ambulatory peritoneal dialysis. *Academic Radiology, 18*(8), 1060. PubMed PMID: 21718957.

40. Murata, N., Gonzalez-Cuyar, L. F., Murata, K., Fligner, C., et al. (2016). Macrocytic and other non-group 1 gadolinium contrast agents deposit low levels of gadolinium in brain and bone tissue: preliminary results from 9 patients with normal renal function. *Investigative Radiology, 51*(7), 447–453. PubMed PMID: 26863577.

41. Grobner, T., & Prischi, F. C. (2007). Gadolinium and nephrogenic systemic fibrosis. *Kidney International, 72*(3), 260–264. PubMed PMID: 17507905.

42. Ghaderi, A., Banafshe, H. R., Khodabandehlo, S., et al. (2017). Qualitative thallium urinary assays are almost as valuable as quantitative tests: implication for outpatient settings in low and middle income countries. *Electronic Physician [electronic resource], 9*(4), 4190–4194. PubMed PMID: 28607654.

43. Moore, D., House, I., & Dixon, A. (1993). Thallium poisoning: diagnosis may be elusive but alopecia is the clue. *British Medical Journal, 306*(6891), 1527–1529. PubMed PMID: 8518684.

44. Zhang, Q., Pan, E., Liu, L., Hu, W., et al. (2014). Study on the relationship between manganese concentrations in rural drinking water and incidence and mortality caused by cancer in Huai'an city. *BioMed Research International, 2014*, 645056. PubMed PMID: 25530966.

45. Spangler, J. G., & Reid, J. C. (2010). Environmental manganese and cancer mortality rates by county in North Carolina: an ecological study. *Biological Trace Element Research, 133*(2), 128–135. PubMed PMID: 19495573.

46. Fowler, B. A., Yamauchi, H., Conner, E. A., & Akkerman, M. (1993). Cancer risks for humans from exposure to the semiconductor metals. *Scandinavian Journal of Work, Environment and Health, 19*(Suppl. 1), 101–103. PubMed PMID: 8159952.

47. Rodriguez-Mercado, J. J., & Altamirano-Lozanzo, M. A. (2013). Genetic toxicology of thallium: a review. *Drug and Chemical Toxicology, 36*(3), 369–383. PubMed PMID: 22970858.

48. Rodriguez-Moreno, F., Gonzalez-Reimers, E., Santolaria-Fernandez, F., et al. (1997). Zinc, copper, manganese, and iron in chronic alcoholic liver disease. *Alcohol (Fayetteville, N.Y.), 14*(1), 39–44. PubMed PMID: 9014022.

49. Blasco-Perrin, H., Glaser, B., Pienkowski, M., Peron, J. M., & Payen, J. L. (2013). Gadolinium induced recurrent acute pancreatitis. *Pancreatology, 13*, 88–89. PubMed PMID: 23395575.

50. Erenoglu, C., Uluutku, A. H., Top, C., et al. (2007). Do MRI agents cause or worsen acute pancreatitis? *Ulusal Travma ve Acil Cerrahi Dergisi, 13*, 78–79. PubMed PMID: 17310418.

51. Kim, E. A., Cheong, H. K., Joo, K. D., Shin, J. H., et al. (2007). Effect of manganese exposure on the neuroendocrine system in welders. *Neurotoxicology, 28*(2), 263–269. PubMed PMID: 16950514.

52. Bouchard, M. F., Sauve, S., Barbeau, B., et al. (2011). Intellectual impairment in school-aged children exposed to manganese from drinking water. *Environmental Health Perspectives, 119*(1), 138–143. PubMed PMID: 20855239.

53. He, P., Liu, D. H., & Zhang, G. Q. (1994). Effects of high-level-manganese sewage irrigation on children's neurobehavior. *Zhonghua Yu Fang Yi Xue Za Zhi, 28*(4), 216–218. PubMed PMID: 7842882.

54. Zhang, G., Liu, D., & He, P. (1995). Effects of manganese on learning abilities in school children. *Zhonghua Yu Fang Yi Xue Za Zhi, 29*(3), 156–158. PubMed PMID: 7648952.

55. Wright, R. O., Amarasiriwardena, C., Woolf, A. D., Jim, R., & Bellinger, D. C. (2006). Neuropsychological correlates of hair arsenic, manganese, and cadmium levels in school-age children residing near a hazardous waste site. *Neurotoxicology, 27*(2), 210–216. PubMed PMID: 16310252.

56. Oulhote, Y., Mergler, D., Barbeau, B., et al. (2014). Neurobehavioral function in school-age children exposed to manganese in drinking water. *Environmental Health Perspectives, 122*(12), 1343–1350. PubMed PMID: 25260096.

57. Bouchard, M., Laforest, F., Vandelac, L., et al. (2007). Hair manganese and hyperactive behaviors: pilot study of school-age children exposed through tap water. *Environmental Health Perspectives, 115*(1), 122–127. PubMed PMID: 17366831.

58. Gottschalk, L. A., Rebello, T., Buchsbaum, M. S., et al. (1991). Abnormalities in hair trace elements as indicators of aberrant behavior. *Comprehensive Psychiatry, 32*(3), 229–237. PubMed PMID: 1884602.

59. Santos-Burgoa, C., Rios, C., Mercado, L. A., et al. (2001). Exposure to manganese: health effects on the general population, a pilot study in central Mexico. *Environmental Research*, 85(2), 90–104. PubMed PMID: 11161659.

60. Rodier, J. (1955). Manganese poisoning in Moroccan miners. *British Journal of Industrial Medicine*, 12(1), 21–35. PubMed PMID: 14351643.

61. Racette, B. A., Criswell, S. R., Lundin, J. I., et al. (2012). increased risk of parkinsonism associated with welding exposure. *Neurotoxicology*, 33(5), 1356–1361. PubMed PMID: 22975422.

62. Bowler, R. M., Nakagawa, S., Drezgic, M., Roels, H. A., et al. (2007). Sequelae of fume exposure in confined space welding: a neurological and neuropsychological case series. *Neurotoxicology*, 28(2), 298–311. PubMed PMID: 17169432.

63. Golasik, M., Wodowski, G., Gomolka, E., Herman, M., & Piekoszewski, W. (2014). Urine as a material for evaluation of exposure to manganese in methcathinone users. *Journal of Trace Elements in Medicine and Biology*, 28(3), 338–343. PubMed PMID: 24867657.

64. Erikson, K. M., Shihabi, Z. K., Aschner, J. L., & Aschner, M. (2002). Manganese accumulates in iron-deficient rat brain regions in a heterogeneous fahion and is associated with neurochemical alterations. *Biological Trace Element Research*, 87(1–3), 143–156. PubMed PMID: 12117224.

65. Garcia, S. J., Gellein, K., Syversen, T., & Aschner, M. (2007). Iron deficient and manganese supplemented diets alter metals and transporters in the developing rat brain. *Toxicological Sciences*, 95(1), 205–214. PubMed PMID: 17060373.

66. Elmstahl, B., Nyman, U., Leander, P., et al. (2006). Gadolinium contrast media are more nephrotoxic than iodine media. The importance of osmolality in direct renal artery injections. *European Radiology*, 16(12), 2712–2720. PubMed PMID: 16896701.

67. Heinrich, M. C., Kuhlmann, M. K., Kohlbacher, S., et al. (2007). Cytotoxicity of iodinated and gadolinium-based contrast agents in renal tubular cells at angiographic concentrations: in vitro study. *Radiology*, 242(2), 425–434. PubMed PMID: 17179401.

68. Akgun, H., Gonlusen, G., Cartwright, J., Jr., et al. (2006). Are gadolinium-based contrast media nephrotoxic? A renal biopsy study. *Archives of Pathology & Laboratory Medicine*, 130(9), 1354–1357. PubMed PMID: 16948524.

69. Cowper, S. E., Bucala, R., & Leboit, P. E. (2006). Nephrogenic fibrosing dermopathy/nephrogenic systemic fibrosis – setting the record straight. *Seminars in Arthritis and Rheumatism*, 35(4), 208–210. PubMed PMID: 16461067.

70. Marckmann, P., Skov, L., Rossen, K., Dupont, A., et al. (2006). Nephrogenic systemic fibrosis: suspected causative role of gadodiamide used for contrast-enhanced magnetic resonance imaging. *Journal of the American Society of Nephrology*, 17(9), 2359–2362. PubMed PMID: 16885403.

71. Mazhar, S. M., Shiehmorteza, M., Kohl, C. A., et al. (2009). Nephrogenic systemic fibrosis in liver disease: a systematic review. *Journal of Magnetic Resonance Imaging*, 30(6), 1313–1322. PubMed PMID: 19937937.

72. Sanyal, S., Marckmann, P., Scherer, S., & Abraham, J. L. (2011). Multiorgan gadolinium (Gd) deposition and fibrosis in a patient with nephrogenic systemic fibrosis – an autopsy-based review. *Nephrology, Dialysis, Transplantation*, 26(11), 3616–3626. PubMed PMID: 21441397.

73. Ramalho, M., Ramalho, J., Burke, L. M., & Semelka, R. C. (2017). Gadolinium retention and toxicity – an update. *Advances in Chronic Kidney Disease*, 24(3), 138–146. PubMed PMID: 28501075.

74. Shi, Z., Zhang, H., Ding, L., et al. (2009). The effect of perfluorododecanoic acid on endocrine status, sex hormones and expression of steroidogenic genes in pubertal female rats. *Reproductive Toxicology*, 27(3–4), 352–359. PubMed PMID: 19429406.

75. Cheng, J., Fu, J. L., & Zhou, Z. C. (2003). The inhibitory effects of manganese on steroidogenesis in rat primary Leydig cells by disrupting steroidogenic acute regulatory (StAR) protein expression. *Toxicology*, 187(2–3), 139–148. PubMed PMID: 12699903.

76. Wirth, J. J., Rossano, M. G., Daly, D. C., et al. (2007). Ambient manganese exposure is negatively associated with human sperm motility and concentration. *Epidemiolgy*, 18(2), 270–273. PubMed PMID: 17202870.

77. Emara, A. M., el-Ghawabi, S. H., Madkour, O. I., & el-Samra, G. H. (1971). Chronic manganese poisoning in the dry battery industry. *British Journal of Industrial Medicine*, 28(1), 78–82. PubMed PMID: 5101169.

78. Bataineh, H., Al-Hamood, M. H., & Elbetieha, A. M. (1998). Assessment of aggression, sexual behavior and fertility in adult male rat following long-term ingestion of four industrial metals salts. *Human and Experimental Toxicology*, 17(10), 570–576. PubMed PMID: 9821021.

79. Kim, S. I., Jang, Y. S., Han, S. H., Choi, M. J., et al. (2012). Effect of manganese exposure on the reproductive organs in immature female rats. *Development & Reproduction*, 16(4), 295–300. PubMed PMID: 25949103.

80. Hoffman, R. S. (2003). Thallium toxicity and the role of Prussian blue in therapy. *Toxicological Reviews*, 22(1), 29–40. PubMed PMID: 14579545.

81. Xia, W., Du, X., Zheng, T., et al. (2016). A case-control study of prenatal thallium exposure and low birth weight in China. *Environmental Health Perspectives, 124*(1), 164–169. PubMed PMID: 26009470.

82. Milatovic, D., Gupta, R. C., Yu, Y., et al. (2011). Protective effects of antioxidants and anti-inflammatory agents against manganese-induced oxidative damage and neuronal injury. *Toxicology and Applied Pharmacology, 256*(3), 219–226. PubMed PMID: 21684300.

83. Deng, Y., Jiao, C., Mi, C., Xu, B., et al. (2015). Melatonin inhibits manganese-induced motor dysfunction and neuronal los in mice: involvement of oxidative stress and dopaminergic neurodegeneration. *Molecular Neurobiology, 51*(1), 68–88. PubMed PMID: 24969583.

84. Deng, Y., Zhu, J., Mi, C., et al. (2015). Melatonin antagonizes Mn-induced oxidative injury through the activation of keap1-Nrf2-ARE signaling pathway in the striatum of mice. *Neurotoxicity Research, 27*(2), 156–171. PubMed PMID: 25288107.

85. De Silva Santos, V., Bisen-Hersh, E., Yu, Y., et al. (2014). Anthocyanin-rich acai (Euterpe oleracea Mart.) extract attenuates manganese-induced oxidative stress in rat primary astrocyte cultures. *Journal of Toxicology and Environmental Health. Part A, 77*(7), 390–404. PubMed PMID: 24617543.

86. Martins, E. N., Pessano, N. T., Leal, L., et al. (2012). Protective effect of Melissa officinalis aqueous extract against Mn-induced oxidative stress in chronically exposed mice. *Brain Research Bulletin, 87*(1), 74–79. PubMed PMID: 22020131.

87. Chtourou, Y., Fetoui, H., Sefi, M., et al. (2010). Silymarin, a natural antioxidant, protects cerebral cortex against manganese-induced neurotoxicity in adult rats. *Biometals: An International Journal on the Role of Metal Ions in Biology, Biochemistry, and Medicine, 23*(6), 985–996. PubMed PMID: 20503066.

88. Pereira, L. V., Shimizu, M. H., Rodrigues, L. P., et al. (2012). N-acetylcysteine protects rats with chronic renal failure from gadolinium-chelate nephrotoxicity. *PLoS ONE, 7,* e39528. PubMed PMID: 22815709.

89. Paton, W. D. (1972). Toxicity of thallium. *British Medical Journal, 4*(5831), 49. PubMed PMID: 5078424.

16

Fluoride

SUMMARY

- Presence in population: About 5% of the world's population (350 million people) consume artificially fluoridated water globally. In the United States, all residents are likely exposed to some degree of fluoride. It is estimated that 75% of a person's fluoride intake comes from their intake of water and processed beverages.[1]
- Major diseases: Dental fluorosis, fractures, bone pain, gastric irritation, thyroid dysfunction,

neurodevelopmental conditions, cardiovascular disease, death
- Primary sources: Water fluoridation, toothpaste (i.e., dentifrice), mouthwash, infant formula, seafood, tea, processed foods, pesticides
- Best measure: Urine, blood (serum)
- Best intervention: Avoidance, antioxidants

DESCRIPTION

Fluorine is the thirteenth most abundant element in the Earth's crust, leads all elements in electronegativity, is extremely reactive, and is rarely found in elemental form. Fluoride is the ionic form of the element fluorine.

The addition of fluoride to public drinking water supplies has been a topic of controversy since its introduction in the United States in 1950. Before this time, naturally occurring fluoride in ground water was the primary source. Several studies conducted during the 1930s and 1940s demonstrated an inverse relationship between the amount of dental caries and fluoride at concentrations of 1 part per million (PPM) or more in the water supply.[2,3,4] Because southern climates are warmer than northern regions, children living in high temperature areas consumed more water than children in the cooler northern regions.[5] As a result, fluoride recommendations by the Centers for Disease Control (CDC) and the American Dental Association (ADA) ranged from 0.7 PPM in warmer climates to 1.2 PPM in cooler climates. Over time, the amount of fluoride in the environment (also known as the *halo effect*) began to escalate from sources such as toothpaste, processed foods, processed beverages,

and pesticides, and the negative effects of excess fluoride started to increase. Because of this, in 2011, the CDC, ADA, and Environmental Protection Agency (EPA) proposed a modification to their recommendations for fluoride in drinking water to 0.7 PPM everywhere in the United States.[6]

Exposure to fluoride is now higher than ever (Fig. 16.1). Factors such as local environment, frequency of water consumption, duration of fluoride exposure, individual susceptibility, and use of fluoride-containing dentifrices all contribute to an individual's risk of fluoride toxicity.

TOXICITY

The lethal dose of soluble fluoride salts, such as sodium fluoride, is estimated to be between 5 and 10 g (equivalent to 32–64 mg/kg elemental fluoride/kg body weight).[7] The mechanism of toxicity involves combination of the fluoride anion with the calcium ions in the blood to form insoluble calcium fluoride, resulting in hypocalcemia. However, several studies indicate that sudden cardiac death after acute fluoride intoxication may be the result of hyperkalemia rather than hypocalcemia.[8,9,10]

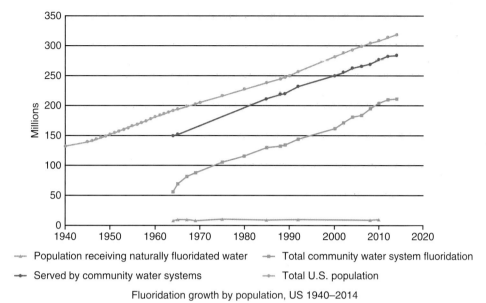

Fluoridation growth by population, US 1940–2014

FIG. 16.1 Amount of fluoridation in US water systems 1940 to 2014. (From Centers for Disease Control and Prevention. *Community water fluoridation.* Retrieved from https://www.cdc.gov/fluoridation/statistics/fsgrowth.htm

The most widespread examples of fluoride poisoning globally arise from consumption of ground water that is abnormally fluoride-rich. In the United States, cases of systemic toxicity and fatalities are rare. However, overexposures causing toxic signs and symptoms are not unusual, with dental products being the most common sources of acute overexposure.[11] Although fluorine is extremely reactive and toxic, fluoride has low electronegativity and associates with positive charged ions such as aluminum, calcium, and iron. Therefore the toxicity of fluoride depends on the environment in which it resides.[12] Fluoride has been associated with an increased risk of dental and skeletal fluorosis, joint pain, incomplete stress fractures, gastric irritation, impaired cognitive development, thyroid abnormalities, enzyme disruption, cardiovascular disease, and cancer.[13]

SOURCES

Fluoride is naturally present in low concentrations (0.01–0.3 PPM) when drinking water is sourced from surface water.

Most fluoride results from the production of cryolite, which is used in aluminum smelting. This process results in a significant amount of fluoride waste products, including two perfluorocarbons (PFCs); tetrafluoromethane (CF_4), hexafluoroethane (C_2F_6), hydrogen fluoride (HF) as gases; and sodium and aluminum fluorides as particulates.[14] HFs are toxic to vegetation, and PFCs are strong greenhouse gasses with long half-lives. Other industrial sources of fluoride include ceramics, aerosol propellants, pesticides, refrigerants, glassware, and Teflon cookware.

Sodium fluoride or sodium monofluorophosphate are often used in water fluoridation (Fig. 16.1) and in dental hygiene products as therapy in the prevention of tooth decay. Sources include community water, fluoride supplements, processed foods, beverages, toothpastes, mouth rinses, gels, foams, and varnishes.

Fluoride is also present in several foods in various concentrations. Table 16.1 lists some of the more common foods containing fluoride. Significant differences in fluoride content of foods exist as a result of variations in the fluoride content of groundwater as well as the use of fluoride-containing pesticides on crops.

BODY BURDEN

Saliva is a major carrier of topical fluoride. However, the concentration of fluoride in ductal saliva is only 0.016

TABLE 16.1   Examples of Fluoride Content in Foods

Food/Drink	Fluoride (mg per 100 g)
Alcoholic beverage, wine, table, white	0.202
Snacks, potato chips	0.105
Beverages, almond milk, ready to drink	0.069
Mollusks, oysters, eastern, wild	0.063
Beans, baked, canned, with pork	0.054
Bread, rye	0.051
Salami, Italian, pork	0.041
Cheese, cheddar	0.034

From U.S. Department of Agriculture. *USDA Food Composition Databases: Nutrient Lists.* Retrieved from https://ndb.nal.usda.gov/ndb/nutrients/report?nutrient1=313&nutrient2=&nutrient3=&&max=25&subset=1&offset=0&sort=c&totCount=82&measureby=g

PPM in areas where drinking water is fluoridated and 0.006 PPM in nonfluoridated areas.[15]

Total daily fluoride retention (TDFR) and daily urinary fluoride excretion (DUFE) can be used to indicate fluoride body burden; however, overnight fasting fluoride concentration may be a better indicator of chronic fluoride exposure or potential bone fluoride concentrations.[16] Fasting increases the rate of fluoride absorption to nearly 100%. After absorption from the gastrointestinal tract, fluoride is integrated into calcified tissues; 99% of all retained fluoride rests in the bone, and most is not exchangeable.[17]

Detoxification/Excretion Processes

About 25% of ingested fluoride is rapidly absorbed by the stomach, whereas much of the remainder is absorbed more slowly from the proximal small intestine.[18] Fluoride that is not absorbed is excreted in feces. Depending on the dose, plasma fluoride concentrations reach their peak 30 to 60 minutes after ingestion and return to preingestion levels within 8 hours.[19,20] Approximately 50% of ingested fluoride is excreted renally within a 24-hour period, whereas the other 50% is absorbed into the bones and teeth. The mechanisms of human renal fluoride excretion include glomerular filtration and tubular reabsorption.

Because tubular reabsorption of fluoride is pH-dependent, factors influencing acid-base status can affect urinary excretion and fluoride retention.[15,16] Factors that acidify the urine increase the retention of fluoride. There is no homeostatic mechanism to maintain circulating fluoride, and levels may increase and decrease rapidly depending on exposure, deposition in hard tissues, and excretion, especially in children.[21]

Clinical Significance

Dental Effects. For optimal dental health, the World Health Organization recommends a fluoride level from 0.5 to 1.0 mg/L of water, depending on climate. As of 2015, the US Health and Human Services Department recommends a maximum of 0.7 mg of fluoride per liter of water to maintain water fluoridation while reducing the occurrence of dental fluorosis. However, studies have shown that fluoridated levels exceeding 0.3 PPM have been associated with teeth mottling and discoloration.[22]

The prevalence of dental fluorosis in the United States has steadily increased since the introduction of fluoridated water in 1950 (Fig. 16.2). This trend has been seen both in communities with fluoridated water and in communities with nonfluoridated water.[23] Malnourishment contributes to an increased severity of dental fluorosis.[24]

Fluoride interferes with the cycles of mineralization and demineralization that occur throughout the life cycle of tooth enamel by interacting and competing with calcium and magnesium.[25,26] Research has shown that fluorosis is clearly more dependent on fluoride intake, whereas achieving a caries-free status has little to do with fluoride intake.[27] In a critical review, authors Stephen Peckham and Niyi Awofeso state, "While it might have been excusable in the 1950s to utilize an enzyme poison such as fluoride to undesirably alter dental architecture and to kill cariogenic bacteria, a better understanding of the pathogenesis of dental caries, coupled with development of antibiotics and probiotics with strong anticariogenic effects, diminishes any major future role for fluoride in caries prevention."[28] Several studies indicate that ingestion of fluoride, via any source, is an inefficient way of delivering fluoride to the teeth and contributes more to its adverse effects on human health.[7,29,30]

Neurological Effects. Fluoride causes oxidative stress in various organs, including the brain.[31] Fluoride can

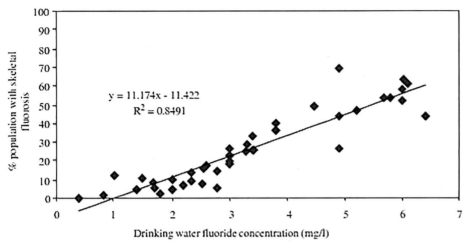

FIG. 16.2 Skeletal fluorosis and drinking water concentration. Fewtrell L, Smith S, Kay D, Bartram J. (2006). An attempt to estimate the global burden of disease due to fluoride in drinking water. *Journal of Water and Health*, 4(4), 533–542. Reproduced with permission from the copyright holders, IWA Publishing.

cross the blood-brain barrier and thus has been shown to have significant neurotoxic effects. Acute fluoride poisoning causes neurotoxicity in adults. In addition, animal models have demonstrated that fluoride affects learning and memory, perhaps by targeting hippocampal neurons.[32,33,34]

Fluoride has shown significant toxic affects on the neurodevelopment of children. Fluoride readily crosses the placenta,[35] and maternal exposure to high fluoride levels has been shown to have an adverse effect on fetal cerebral function and neurotransmitters. Several studies have shown a negative correlation between IQ levels and fluoridated water concentration (i.e., children who live in areas with high fluoride exposure have lower IQ scores than those who live in low exposure areas).[36,37,38]

Skeletal Effects. Skeletal fluorosis may occur when the daily dose of sodium fluoride is greater than 60 mg.[39] Increased osteoblastic activity occurs as a result of fluoride being trapped by the bone.[40] Fluoride demonstrates dose-response relationships being stimulatory to the precursors of osteoblasts at low doses and inhibitory to osteoclasts at high doses.[41] Individuals with skeletal

fluorosis develop progressive bone pain and stiffness of the entire body. Because fluoride is not a normal body component, once it is incorporated in bone, there are no normal mechanisms to mobilize it. Therefore fluoride is not removed from bone, and the accumulation can progress from bone weakening (approximately 3500 mg/kg) to arthritis-type bone pain (approximately 7000 mg/kg) to total immobility (approximately 10,000 mg/kg).[7] Complications of skeletal fluorosis include arthritis, radiculomyelopathy, quadriparesis, and pathological bone fractures.[42]

Kidney Effects. Impaired renal function appears to aggravate the harmful effects of fluoride and may increase fracture risk in individuals with even mild renal failure.[43] Urinary excretion of fluoride is reduced when creatinine clearance reaches values of about 25 mL/min.[44] A study of hemodialysis patients receiving more than 400 L of water per week showed that fluoride levels higher than 0.2 PPM cause significant morbidity and mortality.[45] An investigation of 210 children in China found that children drinking water with fluoride levels of 2 PPM had increased levels of N-acetyl glucosamine (NAG) and gamma-glutamyl transpeptidase (gamma-GT) in their urine, both of which are markers of renal tubular damage.[46] In addition, research has determined that fluoride levels in drinking water greater than 2.0 mg/L can cause renal damage in children, and the degree of damage increases with the fluoride content of drinking water.[47] Adults who have had renal damage because of fluoridated drinking water are vulnerable to chronic kidney disease (CKD) with continued consumption of water from the same source.[48]

Thyroid Effects.   Prolonged consumption of fluoridated water has the potential to suppress the function of the thyroid gland via several mechanisms.[49] Fluoride competes for thyroid-stimulating hormone (TSH) receptor sites on the thyroid gland, leading to a decrease in thyroid hormone production.[50] Fluoride has been shown to interfere with the activity of iodothyronine deiodinase, disrupting the conversion of T4 to T3.[51] Animal studies have shown a decrease in serum levels of T3 and T4 in fluorotic cows[52] and decreased serum T4 with increased serum TSH in fluoride-exposed pigs.[53] Thyroid hormone metabolism is disturbed in the peripheral tissues of children with dental fluorosis, resulting in thyroid hormone levels similar to those seen in iodine deficiency disorders.[54] In school-aged children with fluorosis, thyroid volume increases after puberty.[55] In addition, fluoride has been shown to induce cell apoptosis and increases reactive oxygen species in the thyroid gland.[56]

Gastrointestinal Effects.   Fluoridated drinking water can cause gastrointestinal distress because fluoride converts to HF in the stomach.[7] HF is a penetrating corrosive that can aggravate and prevent healing of ulcerative gastrointestinal tissue.[15] Acute exposure to HF causes gastrointestinal symptoms including nausea, vomiting, and abdominal pain secondary to bronchial ciliary action, which releases HF into the gastrointestinal tract.[57] Human studies have shown that abdominal discomfort can occur from drinking artificially fluoridated water at levels of 1 PPM.[58,59] Chronic atrophic gastritis with associated histological changes, including "cracked-clay" appearance, scanty microvilli, surface abrasions, and desquamated epithelium have been observed in individuals after consuming fluoride for long periods of time.[60] Chronic exposure to fluoride may also result in nonulcer dyspepsia.[61] Fluoride has been shown to be indirectly associated with a higher incidence of inflammatory bowel disease[62]

and may alter gastrointestinal motility via the cholinergic pathway.[63]

Cardiovascular Effects.   Fluoride accumulates in the aorta, and chronic ingestion is associated with changes in heart function, including decreased elastic properties of the aorta and left ventricular diastolic and global dysfunctions.[64,65] In addition, ECG abnormalities have been reported in areas with high natural fluoride levels.[66,67] An *in vitro* study of cultured myocardial cells showed that the heart cell beat rate slows with increasing fluoride levels in a concentration-dependent manner.[68] This is likely the result of fluoride binding with extracellular calcium, thus lowering the amount of calcium available for proper cardiac muscle contraction.

INTERVENTION

Treatment of fluoride toxicity should be based on minimizing risk factors and supporting the body's ability to abate the harmful effects of fluoride.

Curcumin

Curcumin has been shown to decrease lipid peroxidation and neurodegeneration associated with fluoride-induced neurotoxicity.[69] In addition, curcumin has shown protective effects on erythrocytes[70] and normalized serum creatinine, serum urea, and blood urea nitrogen in rats intoxicated with sodium fluoride.[71]

Gallic Acid

Gallic acid has been identified as an antioxidant from the plant *Peltiphyllum peltatum*. Gallic acid has been shown to suppress lipid peroxidation in erythrocytes in a dose-dependent manner.[72] Gallic acid has also been shown to inhibit toxicity and oxidative stress associated with sodium fluoride intoxication.[73] Epigallocatechin gallate (EGCG) has been shown to protect against fluoride-induced cardiotoxicity and dyslipidemia.[74]

Quercetin

Pretreatment with quercetin at 20 mg/kg for 1 week before sodium fluoride intoxication showed decreased thiobarbituric acid reactive substances (TBARS) levels, restoration of superoxide dismutase (SOD) and catalase activities, and modification of reduced glutathione.[75,76] Quercetin in combination with blackberry juice exhibits synergistic antioxidant effects in sodium fluoride intoxication,[77] and quercetin in combination with vitamin C has nephroprotective effects.[78]

Taurine

Taurine has neuroprotective and antioxidant properties. One study showed that taurine prevented fluoride-induced increases in hydrogen peroxide and lipid peroxidation levels while also increasing acetylcholinesterase and the antioxidant enzyme activities in the hypothalamus, cerebrum, and cerebellum.[79] Taurine has also been shown to protect against fluoride-induced renal toxicity by enhancing antioxidant enzyme activity, decreasing hydrogen peroxide and malondialdehyde levels, and increasing glutathione levels.[80] In addition, this same study showed that taurine restored the fluoride-mediated decrease in the circulatory concentrations of triiodothyronine and thyroxine.

Other

Several other antioxidants have shown benefit in fluoride-induced toxicity. Resveratrol was found to inhibit changes in metabolic activities, restoring antioxidant status, biogenic amine level, and structural organization of the brain in fluoride-intoxicated rats.[81] Oral supplementation with oleanolic acid, a plant triterpenoid, has been shown to ameliorate fluoride-induced alteration of brain metabolic functions.[82] Methionine has been shown to reduce the adverse effects of fluoride on soft tissue, whereas vitamin E prevents excessive accumulation of fluoride in bones and teeth.[83] Vitamin C and ginkgo have protective effects against the spatial learning and memory deficits that occur as a result of high levels of fluoride exposure.[84,85] Pomegranate juice,[86] rutin,[87] *Matricaria recutita L.* (German chamomile),[88] lycopene,[89] and silymarin[90] have all been shown to modify the levels of biochemical markers of oxidative stress associated with fluoride intoxication.

REFERENCES

1. Centers for Disease Control and Prevention. (2001). Recommendations for using fluoride to prevent and control dental carries in the United States. *MMWR. Recommendations and Reports: Morbidity and Mortality Weekly Report, 50*(RR–14), 1–42. PubMed PMID: 11521913.
2. Dean, H., & Elvove, E. (1937). Further studies on the minimum threshold of chronic endemic dental fluorosis. *Public Health Reports, 52*, 1249–1264.
3. Dean, H. T. (1943). Domestic water and dental caries: V. Additional studies of the relation of fluoride domestic waters to dental caries experience in 4,425 white children, aged 12 to 14 years, of 13 cities in 4 states. *Public Health Reports, 57*, 1155–1179.
4. Arnold, F. A., Likens, R. C., Russell, A. L., & Scott, D. B. (1962). Fifteenth year of the Grand Rapids fluoridation study. *Journal of the American Dental Association (1939), 65*, 780–785.
5. Richards, L. F., Westmoreland, W. W., Tashiro, M., McKay, C. H., & Morrison, J. T. (1967). Determining optimum fluoride levels for community water supplies in relation to temperature. *Journal of the American Dental Association (1939), 74*(3), 389–397. PubMed PMID: 4381074.
6. Carey, C. M. (2014). Focus on fluorides: update on the use of fluoride for the prevention of dental caries. *The Journal of Evidence-Based Dental Practice, 14*(Suppl.), 95–102. PubMed PMID: 24929594.
7. Centers for Disease Control and prevention. (2003). *Agency for Toxic Substances and Disease registry US. Fluorine, hydrogen fluoride and fluorides.* Washington, DC, USA: Dept of Health Services.
8. McIvor, M. E., Cummings, C. E., Mower, M. M., Wenk, R. E., et al. (1987). Sudden cardiac death from acute fluoride intoxication: the role of potassium. *Annals of Emergency Medicine, 16*(7), 777–781. PubMed PMID: 3592332.
9. Cummings, C. C., & McIvor, M. E. (1988). Fluoride-induced hyperkalemia: the role of Ca2+-dependent K+ channels. *The American Journal of Emergency Medicine, 6*(1), 1–3. PubMed PMID: 2446637.
10. McIvor, M. E., Cummings, C. C., Mower, M. M., Baltazar, R. F., Wenk, R. E., et al. (1985). The manipulation of potassium efflux during fluoride intoxication: implications for therapy. *Toxicology, 37*(3–4), 233–239. PubMed PMID: 3907018.
11. Whitford, Gm. (2011). Acute toxicity of ingested fluoride. *Monographs in Oral Science, 22*, 66–80. PubMed PMID: 21701192.
12. Sauerheber, R. (2013). Physiologic conditions affect toxicity of ingested industrial fluoride. *Journal of Environmental and Public Health, 2013*, 439490. PubMed PMID: 23840230.
13. National Research Council (NRC) (2006). *Fluoride in drinking water: a scientific review of EPA's standards.* Washington, DC: National Academies Press.
14. Marks, J., et al. *Perfluorocarbon (PFC) Generation during Primary Aluminum Production.* Available at https://www.epa.gov/sites/production/files/2016-02/documents/pfc_generation.pdf. (Accessed 17 April 2017).

15. Oliveby, A., Twetman, S., & Ekstrand, J. (1990). Diurnal fluoride concentration in whole saliva in children living in a high- and a low-fluoride area. *Caries Research, 24,* 44–47. PubMed PMID: 2293891.

16. Waterhouse, C., Taves, D., & Munzer, A. (1980). Serum inorganic fluoride: changes related to previous fluoride intake, renal function and bone resorption. *Clinical Science, 58*(2), 145–152. PubMed PMID: 7357834.

17. Whitford, G. M. (1994). Intake and metabolism of fluoride. *Advances in Dental Research, 8*(1), 5–14. PubMed PMID: 7993560.

18. Buzalaf, M., & Whitford, G. M. (2011). Fluoride metabolism. *Monographs in Oral Science, 22,* 20–36. PubMed PMID: 21701189.

19. Ekstrand, J., Fomon, S. J., Ziegler, E. E., & Nelson, S. E. (1994). Fluoride pharmacokinetics in infancy. *Pediatric Research, 35*(2), 157–163. PubMed PMID: 8165049.

20. Whitford, G. M. (1996). *Metabolism and toxicity of fluoride.* Karger.

21. Martins, C. C., Paiva, S. M., & Cury, J. A. (2011). Effect of discontinuation of fluoride intake from water and toothpaste on urinary excretion in young children. *Int J Environ Public Health, 8*(6), 2132–2141. PubMed PMID: 21776221.

22. European Commission. (2011). *Critical review of any new evidence on the hazard profile, health effects, and human exposure to fluoride and the fluoridating agents of drinking water.* Scientific Committee on Health and Environmental Risks (SCHER).

23. Fomon, S. J., Ekstrand, J., & Ziegler, E. E. (2000). Fluoride intake and prevalence of dental fluorosis: trends in fluoride intake with special attention to infants. *Journal of Public Health Dentistry, 60*(3), 131–139. PubMed PMID: 11109209.

24. Mahantesha, T., Dixit, U. B., Nayakar, R. P., Ashwin, D., Ramagoni, N. K., & Kamavaram Ellore, V. P. (2016). Prevalence of dental fluorosis and associated risk factors in Bangalkot District, Karnataka, India. *Int J Clin Pediatr Dent, 9*(3), 256–263. PubMed PMID: 27843259.

25. Powers, J. M., Craig, R. G., & Ludema, K. C. (1973). Wear of dental enamel. *Wear, 23*(2), 141–152.

26. White, D. J., & Nancollas, G. H. (1990). Physical and chemical considerations of the role of firmly and loosely bound fluoride in caries prevention. *Journal of Dental Research, 69*(Spec No), 587–594. PubMed PMID: 2179318.

27. Warren, J. J., Levy, S. M., Broffitt, B., Cavanaugh, J. E., Kanellis, M. J., & Weber-Gasparoni, K. (2009). Considerations on optimal fluoride intake using dental fluorosis and dental caries outcomes – a longitudinal study. *Journal of Public Health Dentistry, 69*(2), 111–115. PubMed PMID: 19054310.

28. Peckham, S., & Awofeso, N. (2014). Water fluoridation: a critical review of the physiological effects of ingested fluoride as a public health intervention. *Scientific World Journal, 2014,* 293019. Feb 26, PubMed PMID: 24719570.

29. Limeback, H. (1999). A re-examination of the pre-eruptive and post-eruptive mechanism of the anti-caries effects of fluoride: is there any anti-caries benefit from swallowing fluoride? *Community Dentistry and Oral Epidemiology, 27*(1), 62–71. PubMed PMID: 10086928.

30. Burt, B. A. (1999). The case for eliminating the use of dietary fluoride supplements for young children. *Journal of Public Health Dentistry, 59*(4), 269–274. PubMed PMID: 10682335.

31. Bharti, V. K., & Srivastava, R. S. (2009). Fluoride-induced oxidative stress in rat's brain and its amelioration by buffalo (Bubalus bubalis) pineal proteins and melatonin. *Biological Trace Element Research, 130*(2), 131–140. PubMed PMID: 19159082.

32. Mulleniz, P. J., Denbesten, P. K., Schunior, A., & Kernan, W. J. (1995r). Neurotoxicity of sodium fluoride in rats. *Neurotoxicology and Teratology, 17*(2), 169–177. PubMed PMID: 7760776.

33. Chioca, L. R., Raupp, Im, Da Cunha, C., Losso, E. M., & Andreatini, R. (2008). Subchronic fluoride intake induces impairment in habituation and active avoidance tasks in rats. *European Journal of Pharmacology, 579*(1–3), 196–201. PubMed PMID: 18001709.

34. Bhatnagar, M., Rao, P., Sushma, J., & Bhatnagar, R. (2002). Neurotoxicity of fluoride: neurodegeneration in hippocampus of female mice. *Indian Journal of Experimental Biology, 40*(5), 546–554. PubMed PMID: 12622200.

35. Agency for Toxic Substances and Disease Reistry. (2003). *Toxicological profile for fluorides, hydrogen fluoride, and fluorine (update).* Available: http://www.atsdr.cdc.gov/toxprofiles/tp11.pdf. (Accessed 13 March 2017).

36. Tang, Q. Q., Du, J., Ma, H. H., Jiang, S. J., & Zhou, X. J. (2008). Fluoride and children's intelligence: a meta-analysis. *Biological Trace Element Research, 126*(1–3), 115–120. PubMed PMID: 18695947.

37. Ding, Y., Gao, Yanhui, Sun, H., Han, H., Wang, W., Ji, X., et al. (2011). The relationships between low levels of urine fluoride on children's intelligence, dental fluorosis in endemic fluorosis areas in Hulunbuir, Inner Mongolia, China. *Journal of Hazardous Materials, 186*(2–3), 1942–1946. PubMed PMID: 21237562.

38. Choi, A. L., Sun, G., Zhang, Y., & Grandjean, P. (2012). Developmental fluoride neurotoxicity: a systemic review and meta-analysis. *Environmental Health Perspectives, 120*(10), 1362–1368. PubMed PMID: 22820538.

39. Cohen, P., & Gardner, F. H. (1966). Induction of skeletal fluorosis in two common demineralizing disorders. *JAMA: The Journal of the American Medical Association*, *195*, 962–963. PubMed PMID: 5952057.

40. Goodman, L., & Gilman, A. (1975). *Fluoride, the pharmacological basis of therapeutics* (5th ed.). New York: MacMillan.

41. Chachra, D., Turner, C., Dunipace, A., & Grynpas, M. (1999). The effect of fluoride treatment on bone minerals in rabbits. *Calcified Tissue International*, *64*(4), 345–351. PubMed PMID: 10089229.

42. Haimanot, R. T. (1990). Neurological complications of endemic skeletal fluorosis, with special emphasis on radiculo-myelopathy. *Paraplegia*, *28*(4), 244–251. PubMed PMID: 2172892.

43. Gerster, J. C., Charhon, S. A., Jaeger, P., et al. (1983). Bilateral fractures of femoral neck in patients with moderate renal failure receiving fluoride for spinal osteoporosis. *British Medical Journal (Clinical Research Ed.)*, *287*(6394), 723–725. PubMed PMID: 6311315.

44. Schiffl, H. H., & Biswanger, U. (1980). Human urinary fluoride excretion as influenced by renal function impairment. *Nephron*, *26*, 69–72. PubMed PMID: 7412962.

45. Ahmad, S. (2005). Essentials of water treatment in hemodialysis. *Hemodialysis International*, *9*(2), 127–134. PubMed PMID: 16191060.

46. Xiong, X., Liu, J., He, W., Xia, T., He, P., et al. (2007). Dose-effect relationship between drinking water fluoride levels and damage to liver and kidney functions in children. *Environmental Research*, *103*(1), 112–116. PubMed PMID: 16834990.

47. Liu, Jl, Xia, T., Yu, Y. Y., Sun, X. Z., Zhu, Q., He, W., et al. (2005). The dose-effect relationship of water fluoride levels and renal damage in children. *Wei Sheng Yan Jiu*, *34*(3), 287–288. PubMed PMID: 16111031.

48. Dharmaratne, R. W. (2015). Fluoride in drinking water and diet: the causative factor of chronic kidney diseases in the North Central Province of Sri Lanka. *Environmental Health and Preventive Medicine*, *20*(4), 237–242. PubMed PMID: 25916575.

49. Ge, Y., Ning, H., Wang, S., & Wang, J. (2005). DNA damage in thyroid gland cells of rats exposed to long-term intake of high fluoride and low iodine. *Fluoride*, *38*, 318–323.

50. Singh, N., Verma, K. G., Verma, P., Sidhu, G. K., & Sachdeva, S. (2014). A comparative study of fluoride ingestion levels, serum thyroid hormone and TSH level derangements, dental fluorosis status among school children from endemic and non-endemic fluorosis areas. *SpringerPlus*, *3*, 7. Jan 3, PubMed PMID: 24455464.

51. Clinch, C. (2009). Fluoride interactions with iodine and iodide: implications for breast health. *Fluoride*, *42*, 75–87.

52. Cinar, A., & Selcuk, M. (2005). Effect of chronic fluorosis in thyroxine, triiodothyronine and protein bound iodine in cows. *Fluoride*, *38*, 65–68.

53. Zhan, X. A., Li, J., Wang, M., & Xu, Z. R. (2006). Effects of fluoride on growth and thyroid function in young pigs. *Fluoride*, *39*, 95–100.

54. Susheela, A. K., Bhatnagar, M., Vig, K., & Mondal, N. K. (2005). Excess fluoride ingestion and thyroid hormone derangements in children living in Delhi, India. *Fluoride*, *38*, 98–108.

55. Kutlucan, A., Kale Koroglu, B., Numan Tamer, M., Aydin, Y., et al. (2013). The investigation of effects of fluorosis on thyroid volume in school-age children. *Med Glas (Zenica)*, *10*(1), 93–98. PubMed PMID: 23348169.

56. Zeng, Q., Cui, Y. S., Zhang, L., Fu, G., et al. (2012). Studies of fluoride on the thyroid cell apoptosis and mechanism. *Zhonghua Yu Fang Yi Xue Za Zhi*, *46*(3), 233–236. PubMed PMID: 22800594.

57. Na, J. Y., Woo, K. H., Yoon, S. Y., Cho, S. Y., Song, I. U., Kim, J. A., et al. (2013). Acute symptoms after a community hydrogen fluoride spill. *Ann Occup Environ Med*, *25*(1), 17. Sep 19, PubMed PMID: 24472561.

58. Waldbott, G. L. (1956). Incipient chronic fluoride intoxication from drinking water. II. Distinction between allergic reactions and drug intolerance. *International Archives of Allergy and Applied Immunology*, *9*(5), 241–249. PubMed PMID: 13428345.

59. Grimbergen, G. W. (1974). A double blind test for determination of intolerance to fluoridated water. *Fluoride*, *7*(3), 146–152.

60. Das, T. K., Susheela, A. K., Gupta, I. P., Dasarathy, S., & Tandon, R. K. (1994). Toxic effects of chronic fluoride ingestion on the upper gastrointestinal tract. *Journal of Clinical Gastroenterology*, *18*(3), 194–199. PubMed PMID: 8034913.

61. Gupta, I. P., Das, T. K., Susheela, A. K., Dasarathy, S., & Tandon, R. K. (1992). Fluoride as a possible aetiological factor in non-ulcer dyspepsia. *Journal of Gastroenterology and Hepatology*, *7*(4), 355–359. PubMed PMID: 1515558.

62. Follin-Arbelet, B., & Moum, B. (2016). Fluoride: a risk factor for inflammatory bowel disease. *Scandinavian Journal of Gastroenterology*, *51*(9), 1019–1024. PubMed PMID: 27199224.

63. Amira, S., Soufane, S., & Gharzouli, K. (2005). Effect of sodium fluoride on gastric emptying and intestinal transit in mice. *Experimental and Toxicologic Pathology*, *57*(1), 59–64. PubMed PMID: 16089320.

64. Varol, E., Akcay, S., Ersoy, I. H., Koroglu, B. K., & Varol, S. (2010). Impact of chronic fluorosis on left ventricular

diastolic and global functions. *The Science of the Total Environment, 408*(11), 2295–2298. PubMed PMID: 20206377.

65. Varol, E., Akcay, S., Ersoy, I. H., Ozaydin, M., Koroglu, B. K., & Varol, S. (2010). Aortic elasticity is impaired in patients with endemic fluorosis. *Biological Trace Element Research, 133*(2), 121–127. PubMed PMID: 20012382.

66. Xu, R. Y. (1997). Electrocardiogram analysis of patients with skeletal fluorosis. *Flouride, 303*(1), 16–18.

67. Takamori, T., Miyanaga, S., Kawahara, S., Okushi, H., Hirao, I., & Wakatsuki, H. (1956). EKG studies of inhabitants in high fluoride areas. *The Tokushima Journal of Experimental Medicine, 3*, 50.

68. Wang, F., Zhang, D., & Wang, R. (1998). Toxic effects of fluoride on beating myocardial cells cultured in vitro. *Fluoride, 31*(1), 26–32.

69. Sharma, C., Suhalka, P., Sukhwal, P., Jaiswal, N., & Bhatnagar, M. (2014). Curcumin attenuates neurotoxicity induced by fluoride: an in vivo evidence. *Pharmacogn Mag, 10*(37), 61–65. PubMed PMID: 24696547.

70. Nabavi, S. F., Nabavi, S. M., Abolhasani, F., Moghaddam, A. H., & Eslami, S. (2012). Cytoprotective effects of curcumin on sodium fluoride-induced intoxication in rat erythrocytes. *Bulletin of Environmental Contamination and Toxicology, 88*(3), 486–490. PubMed PMID: 22143374.

71. Nabavi, S. F., Moghaddam, A. H., Eslami, S., & Nabavi, S. M. (2012). Protective effects of curcumin against sodium fluoride-induced toxicity in rat kidneys. *Biological Trace Element Research, 145*(3), 369–374. PubMed PMID: 21901432.

72. Nabavi, S. F., Habtemariam, S., Sureda, A., Hajizedeh Moghaddam, A., Daglia, M., & Nabavi, S. M. (2013). In vivo protective effects of gallic acid isolated from Peltiphyllum peltatum against sodium fluoride-induced oxidative stress in rat erythrocytes. *Arhiv Za Higijenu Rada I Toksikologiju, 64*(4), 553–559. PubMed PMID: 24384762.

73. Nabavi, S. M., Habtemariam, S., Nabavi, S. F., Sureda, A., Daglia, M., Moghaddam, A. H., et al. (2013). Protective effect of gallic acid isolated from peltiphyllum peltatum against sodium fluoride-induced oxidatibe stress in rat's kidney. *Molecular and Cellular Biochemistry, 372*(1–2), 233–239. PubMed PMID: 23014933.

74. Miltonprabu, S., & Thangapandiyan, S. (2015). Epigallocatechin gallate potentially attenuates fluoride induced oxidative stress mediated cardiotoxicity and dyslipidemia in rats. *Journal of Trace Elements in Medicine and Biology: Organ of the Society for Minerals and Trace Elements (GMS)*, Jan, *29* 321=35. PubMed PMID: 25282272.

75. Nabavi, S. F., Nabavi, S. M., Latifi, A. M., Mirzaei, M., Habtemariam, S., & Moghaddam, A. H. (2012). Mitigating role or quescetin against sodium fluoride-induced oxidative stress in the rat brain. *Pharmaceutical Biology, 50*(11), 1380–1383. PubMed PMID: 22870923.

76. Nabavi, S. F., Nabavi, S. M., Mirzaei, M., & Moghaddam, A. H. (2012). Protective effect of quercetin against sodium fluoride induced oxidative stress in rat's heart. *Food Funct, 3*(4), 437–441. PubMed PMID: 22314573.

77. Hamza, R. Z., El-Shemawy, N. S., & Ismail, Ha. (2015). Protective effects of blackberry and quercetin on sodium fluoride-induced oxidative stress and histological changes in the hepatic, renal, testis, and brain tissue of male rats. *Journal of Basic and Clinical Physiology and Pharmacology, 26*(3), 237–251. PubMed PMID: 25918918.

78. Nabavi, S. M., Nabavi, S. F., Habtemariam, S., Moghaddam, A. H., & Latifi, A. M. (2012). Ameliorative effects of quercetin on sodium fluoride-induced oxidative stress in rat's kidney. *Renal Failure, 34*(7), 901–906. PubMed PMID: 22680615.

79. Adedara, I. A., Abolaji, A. O., Idris, U. F., Olabiyi, B. F., et al. (2017). Neuroprotective influence of taurine on fluoride-induced biochemical and behavioral deficits in rats. *Chemico-Biological Interactions, 261*, 1–10. PubMed PMID: 27840156.

80. Adedara, I. A., Ojuade, T. J., Olabiyi, B. F., Idris, U. F., Onibiyo, E. M., et al. (2017). Taurine ameliorates renal oxidative damage and thyroid dysfunction in rats chronically exposed to fluoride. *Biological Trace Element Research, 175*(2), 388–395. PubMed PMID: 27334436.

81. Pal, S., & Sarkar, C. (2014). Protective effect of resveratrol on fluoride induced alteration in protein and nucleic acid metabolism, DNA damage and biogenic amines in rat brain. *Environmental Toxicology and Pharmacology, 38*(2), 684–699. PubMed PMID: 25233527.

82. Sarkar, C., Pal, S., Das, N., & Dinda, B. (2014). Ameliorative effects of oleanolic acid on fluoride induced metabolic and oxidative dysfunctions in rat brain: experimental and biochemical studies. *Food Chen Toxicol, 66*, 224–236. PubMed PMID: 24468673.

83. Blaszczyk, I., Birkner, E., Gutowska, I., Romuk, E., & Chlubek, D. (2012). Influence of methionine and vitamin E on fluoride concentration in bones and teeth of rats exposed to sodium fluoride in drinking water. *Biological Trace Element Research, 146*(3), 335–339. PubMed PMID: 22068731.

84. Jetti, R., Raghuveer, C. V., & Malikarjuna, R. C. (2016). Protective effect of ascorbic acid and Ginkgo biloba against learning and memory deficits caused by fluoride.

Toxicology and Industrial Health, 32(1), 183–187. PubMed PMID: 24081631.

85. Raghu, J., Raghuveer, V. C., Rao, M. C., Somayaji, N. S., & Babu, P. B. (2013). The ameliorative effect of ascorbic acid and Ginkgo biloba on learning and memory deficits associated with fluoride exposure. *Interdiscip Toxicol, 6*(4), 217–221. PubMed PMID: 24678261.

86. Bouasla, A., Bouasla, I., Boumendjel, A., Abdennour, C., El Feki, A., & Messarah, M. (2016). Prophylactic effects of pomegranate (Punica granatum) juice on sodium fluoride induced oxidative damage in liver and erythrocytes of rats. *Canadian Journal of Physiology and Pharmacology, 94*(7), 709–718. PubMed PMID: 27124270.

87. Umarani, V., Muvvala, S., Ramesh, A., Lakshmi, B. V., & Sravanthi, N. (2015). Rutin potentially attenuates fluoride-induced oxidative stress-mediated cardiotoxicity, blood toxicity, and dyslipidemia in rats. *Toxicology Mechanisms and Methods, 25*(2), 143–149. PubMed PMID: 25560802.

88. Ranpariya, V. L., Parmar, S. K., Sheth, N. R., & Chandrashekhar, V. M. (2011). Neuroprotective activity of Matricaria recutita against fluoride-induced stress in rats. *Pharmaceutical Biology, 49*(7), 696–701. PubMed PMID: 21599496.

89. Mansour, H. H., & Tawfik, S. S. (2012). Efficacy of lycopene against fluoride toxicity in rats. *Pharmaceutical Biology, 50*(6), 707–711. PubMed PMID: 22133041.

90. Nabavi, S. M., Nabavi, S. F., Moghaddam, A. H., & Setzer, W. N. (2012). Mirzeai M. Effect of silymarin on sodium fluoride-induced toxicity and oxidative stress in rat cardiac tissues. *Anais Da Academia Brasileira de Ciencias, 84*(4), 1121–1126. PubMed PMID: 22964841.

17

Benzene, Toluene, Ethylbenzene, Xylenes (BTEX)

SUMMARY

- Presence in population: Ethylbenzene, and xylene are commonly found in blood and urine; benzene and toluene are slightly less common
- Major disease: Reduced fertility, respiratory problems, neurological
- Primary sources: Cigarette smoking, vehicular exhaust, nonconventional gas and oil exploration
- Best measure: Parent compounds in blood, metabolites in urine
- Best intervention: Avoidance, supplementation with amino acids and glutathione (GSH)

DESCRIPTION

Benzene, toluene, ethylbenzene, and the xylenes (BTEXs) are all volatile aromatic hydrocarbons produced commercially from coal and petroleum sources (Fig. 17.1). They are among the most commonly produced chemicals and are heavily used in industry. All are rapidly absorbed in the human body from dermal, oral, and inhalation exposures. All are rapidly distributed throughout the blood and fatty tissues of the body, including the brain, where they can dampen central nervous system (CNS) function.

TOXICITY

BTEXs all have the ability to suppress neuronal function, although this has only been documented in industrial exposure. Glues and paints that are high in toluene have been used as "drugs of abuse" to dampen brain function. Those who chronically use toluene for this effect are prone to permanent brain damage and dementia.[1] Benzene is listed by the International Agency for Research on Cancer (IARC) as a known human carcinogen, primarily associated with aplastic anemia.[2] Ethylbenzene is listed as a probable carcinogen, whereas toluene and xylene have

not been associated with cancers. BTEXs cause oxidative damage, and chronic exposures are associated with elevated 8-hydroxy-2′-deoxyquanosine (8-OHdG) levels and reduced GSH concentrations.[3,4]

SOURCES

Cigarette smoking is the single greatest source of BTEX exposure,[5] with urinary BTEX metabolites being significantly associated with cotinine.[6] For nonsmokers, vehicular exhaust is the primary exposure source. Individuals living close to busy roadways and industries have significantly higher levels of BTEXs.[7,8] In urban areas, ambient BTEX levels have been found to be higher during the summer and lower during the winter.[9] Higher personal exposure to BTEXs is also found in those who have an attached garage.[10] Benzene and toluene exposure occurs more when the windows are closed, and higher xylene exposure comes from using paint thinners or strippers. Up to 27.5% of high-octane gasoline is BTEX, and pumping gas increases personal exposure to toluene, ethylbenzene, and xylene. Commercial products with the highest levels of BTEXs include correction fluid (the use of which has declined significantly), marking pens, ballpoint pens, and glues.[11] Other commonly used commercial products found to

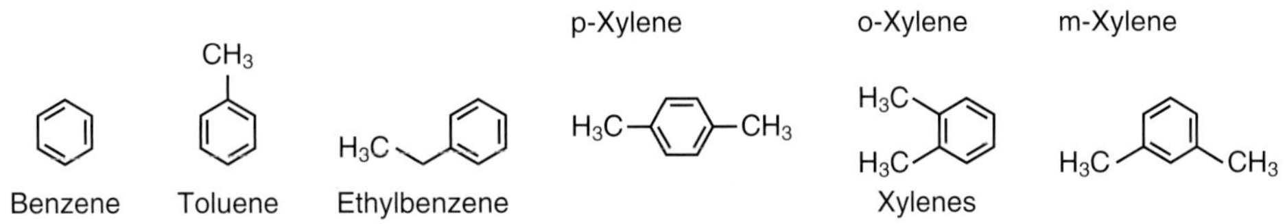

FIG. 17.1. BTEX structures.

TABLE 17.1	BTEX Blood Levels in NHANES 2001 to 2008 in ng/mL					
Solvent	NHANES	Geo Mean	50th %	75th %	90th %	95th %
Benzene	01/02	*	0.030	0.100	0.190	0.320
	03/04	*	0.027	0.064	0.170	0.260
	05/06	*	0.026	0.056	0.220	0.310
	07/08	*	<LOD	0.41	0.198	0.294
Toluene	01/02	0.156	0.160	0.340	0.670	1.06
	03/04	0.114	0.096	0.220	0.430	0.680
	05/06	0.137	0.120	0.230	0.550	0.814
	07/08	1.03	0.083	0.192	0.511	0.735
Ethylbenzene	01/02	0.034	0.030	0.050	0.090	0.140
	03/04	0.035	0.032	0.053	0.083	0.110
	05/06	0.038	0.035	0.059	0.100	0.140
	07/08	*	<LOD	0.038	0.038	0.122
m,p-Xylene	01/02	0.156	0.150	0.280	0.500	0.670
	03/04	0.136	0.130	0.200	0.280	0.340
	05/06	0.132	0.120	0.190	0.301	0.410
	07/08	0.079	0.072	0.130	0.231	0.343
o-Xylene	01/02	*	<LOD	0.070	0.100	0.130
	03/04	*	<LOD	0.051	0.072	0.090
	05/06	0.037	0.035	0.053	0.083	0.110
	07/08	*	<LOD	0.039	0.062	0.086

*No Geometric mean listed in NHANES, LOD—Level of detection.
Compiled from Centers for Disease Control and Prevention. (2017). *National Report on Human Exposure to Environmental Chemicals: Updated tables.* Available at www.cdc.gov/exposurereport/. (Accessed June 21, 2017).

contain these solvents include shoe polish and leather cleaner (toluene, ethylbenzene, and xylene) and air fresheners (toluene). Commercially available air fresheners containing toluene even have a carefully worded warning about the potential for drug abuse as part of the label. It was recently reported that individuals with detectable levels of blood benzene, typically around the Centers for Disease Control and Prevention (CDC) 75th percentile, reported sleeping on mattresses or pillows containing memory foam.[12] Most of these individuals also complained of various cognitive or mood problems, which ceased once the mattress or pillow was removed.

Unconventional gas and oil wells that use fracturing techniques, colloquially termed "fracking," have been linked with elevated levels of BTEXs, methane, and other air pollutants at residences in the area.[13,14] BTEXs are elevated during both the drilling of the well and the production of oil or gas from the well.[15] Workers at such sites also experience greater exposures.[16]

BODY BURDEN

BTEXs are rapidly cleared out of the body. Blood levels of these compounds reflect recent exposure to one of the sources previously mentioned. Chapter 53 discusses laboratory assessment and provides information on how to interpret blood solvent tests to identify likely exposure sources. The blood levels of BTEXs identified in four successive National Health and Nutritional Examination Survey (NHANES) trials are presented in Table 17.1.[17]

TABLE 17.2	BTEX Urinary Metabolites in NHANES 2011 to 2012 (µg/g creatinine)						
Metabolite	**Parent**	**Geo Mean**	**50th %**	**75th %**	**90th %**	**95th %**
N-acetyl-S-(phenyl)-L-cysteine	Benzene	*	<LOD	1.29	2.10	3.03
Phenylglyoxylic acid	Ethylbenzene + styrene	202	206	285	401	518
N-acetyl-S-(benzyl)-L-cysteine	Toluene	7.39	6.68	12.2	21.0	36.4
2-Methyl hippuric acid	Xylene	37.5	35.2	77.9	159	248
3- & 4-Methyl hippuric acid	Xylene	252	212	565	1050	1540

Although the data in Table 17.1 reveal that toluene and m,p-xylene are most common and occur in the highest amounts, this has not been shown in commercially available blood solvent testing. As discussed in Chapter 6, m,p-xylenes are commonly found markers of urban vehicular exhaust in those who have trouble eliminating solvents, but toluene has rarely been found. Table 17.2 shows the urinary metabolites of BTEXs, with phenylglyoxylic acid and 3,4-methylhippuric acid being present in the greatest amounts. The metabolite data indicate that ethylbenzene and styrene presence is high, along with m,p-xylene. The metabolite for toluene is present in the lowest levels in Table 17.2.

Detoxification/Excretion Processes

BTEXs are oxidized by cytochromes and then conjugated primarily with amino acids to make hippuric acids or with GSH to make N-acetyl cysteines, all of which are rapidly cleared through the kidneys. However, if the urine is acidic, these weak acids can be reabsorbed into the proximal tubules of the kidneys.

Clinical Significance
Respiratory Disorders

Individuals living within 1 km of oil and gas wells, where ambient BTEXs levels are higher, have more upper respiratory problems than those living more than 2 km away.[18] Exposure to ambient benzene, toluene, and ethylbenzene reduced lung function and caused lung inflammation in children, with wheezing.[19] Individuals in the 1999 to 2000 NHANES trial who were exposed to higher ambient levels of BTEXs were more than 60% more likely to have asthma.[20]

Reproductive Disorders

Women who are occupationally exposed to BTEXs are at greater risk of a variety of reproductive problems, including fertility and fetal health.[21] Ambient exposure to BTEX compounds has been associated with infertility and reduced fetal growth, as well as cardiovascular and allergic sensitization.[22]

INTERVENTION

Antioxidants, both dietary and supplemental, provide benefit in counteracting the oxidative stress caused by unavoidable BTEXs. Consumption of green tea has exhibited the ability to reverse oxidative stress in pump workers regularly exposed to high levels of BTEXs.[23] Supplementation with the primary conjugating agents glycine and taurine along with liposomal GSH are also prudent.

REFERENCES

1. Filley, C. M., Halliday, W., & Kleinschmidt-DeMasters, B. K. (2004). The effects of toluene on the central nervous system. *Journal of Neuropathology and Experimental Neurology*, 63(1), 1–12. PubMed PMID: 14748556.
2. World Health Organization, International Agency for Research on Cancer. *Benzene monograph*. Available at http://monographs.iarc.fr/ENG/Monographs/vol100F/mono100F-24.pdf. (Accessed 24 January 2018).
3. Xiong, F., Li, Q., Zhou, B., et al. (2016). Oxidative stress and genotoxicity of long-term occupational exposure to low levels of BTEX in gas station workers. *International Journal of Environmental Research and Public Health*, 13(12). pii: E1212. PubMed PMID: 27929445.
4. Lagorio, S., Tagesson, C., Forastiere, F., et al. (1994). Exposure to benzene and urinary concentrations of 8-hydroxydeoxyguanosine, a biological marker of oxidative damage to DNA. *Occupational and Environmental Medicine*, 51(11), 739–743. PubMed PMID: 7849850.
5. Symanski, E., Stock, T. H., Tee, P. G., & Chan, W. (2009). Demographic, residential, and behavioral determinants of elevated exposures to benzene, toluene, ethylbenzene, and xylenes among the U.S. population: Results from 1999-2000 NHANES. *Journal of Toxicology and*

Environmental Health. Part A, 72(14), 915–924. PubMed PMID: 19557620.

6. Brajenović, N., Karačonji, I. B., & Bulog, A. (2015). Evaluation of urinary BTEX, nicotine, and cotinine as biomarkers of airborne pollutants in nonsmokers and smokers. *Journal of Toxicology and Environmental Health. Part A*, 78(17), 1133–1136. PubMed PMID: 26460693.

7. Tsangari, X., Andrianou, X. D., Agapiou, A., et al. (2017). Spatial characteristics of urinary BTEX concentrations in the general population. *Chemosphere*, 173, 261–266. PubMed PMID: 28110016.

8. Lioy, P. J., Fan, Z., Zhang, J., et al. (2011). Personal and ambient exposures to air toxics in Camden, New Jersey. *Research Report (Health Effects Institute)*, 160, 3–127. PubMed PMID: 22097188.

9. Miri, M., Rostami Aghdam Shendi, M., Ghaffari, H. R., et al. (2016). Investigation of outdoor BTEX: Concentration, variations, sources, spatial distribution, and risk assessment. *Chemosphere*, 163, 601–609. PubMed PMID: 27589149.

10. Symanski, E., Stock, T. H., Tee, P. G., & Chan, W. (2009). Demographic, residential, and behavioral determinants of elevated exposures to benzene, toluene, ethylbenzene, and xylenes among the U.S. population: Results from 1999-2000 NHANES. *Journal of Toxicology and Environmental Health. Part A*, 72(14), 915–924. PubMed PMID:19557620.

11. Lim, S. K., Shin, H. S., Yoon, K. S., et al. (2014). Risk assessment of volatile organic compounds benzene, toluene, ethylbenzene, and xylene (BTEX) in consumer products. *Journal of Toxicology and Environmental Health. Part A*, 77(22–24), 1502–1521. PubMed PMID: 25343298.

12. Elgez, A. (2016). *Conditions Linked to Exposure in the Bedroom and How to Confirm Them*. Environmental Health Symposium, San Diego, CA. www.environmentalhealthsymposium.com.

13. Field, R. A., Soltis, J. J., Perez-Ballesta, P., et al. (2015). Distribution of air pollutants associated with oil and natural gas development measured in the Upper Green River Basin of Wyoming. *Elementa Science of the Anthropocene*, 3, 74.

14. Swarthout, R. F., Russo, R. S., Zhou, Y., et al. (2015). Impact of Marcellus Shale natural gas development in southwest Pennsylvania on volatile organic compound emissions and regional air quality. *Environmental Science & Technology*, 49(5), 3175–3184. PubMed PMID: 25594231.

15. Moore, C. W., Zielinska, B., Pétron, G., & Jackson, R. B. (2014). Air impacts of increased natural gas acquisition, processing, and use: A critical review. *Environmental Science & Technology*, 48(15), 8349–8359. PubMed PMID: 24588259.

16. Esswein, E. J., Snawder, J., King, B., Breitenstein, M., Alexander-Scott, M., & Kiefer, M. (2014). Evaluation of some potential chemical exposure risks during flowback operations in unconventional oil and gas extraction: Preliminary results. *Journal of Occupational and Environmental Hygiene*, 11(10), D174–D184. PubMed PMID: 25175286.

17. Centers for Disease Control and Prevention. (2017). *National Report on Human Exposure to Environmental Chemicals: Updated tables*. Available at www.cdc.gov/exposurereport/. (Accessed June 21, 2017).

18. Rabinowitz, P. M., Slizovskiy, I. B., Lamers, V., et al. (2015). Proximity to natural gas wells and reported health status: Results of a household survey in Washington County, Pennsylvania. *Environmental Health Perspectives*, 123(1), 21–26. PubMed PMID: 25204871.

19. Martins, P. C., Valente, J., Papoila, A. L., et al. (2012). Airways changes related to air pollution exposure in wheezing children. *The European Respiratory Journal*, 39(2), 246–253. PubMed PMID: 21719492.

20. Arif, A. A., & Shah, S. M. (2007). Association between personal exposure to volatile organic compounds and asthma among US adult population. *International Archives of Occupational and Environmental Health*, 80(8), 711–719. PubMed PMID: 17357796.

21. Sirotkin, A. V., & Harrath, A. H. (2017). Influence of oil-related environmental pollutants on female reproduction. *Reproductive Toxicology*, 71, 142–145. PubMed PMID: 28576684.

22. Bolden, A. L., Kwiatkowski, C. F., & Colborn, T. (2015). New look at BTEX: are ambient levels a problem? *Environmental Science & Technology*, 49(9), 5261–5276. PubMed PMID: 25873211.

23. Emara, A. M., & El-Bahrawy, H. (2008). Green tea attenuates benzene-induced oxidative stress in pump workers. *Journal of immunotoxicology*, 5(1), 69–80. PubMed PMID: 18382860.

18

Chlorinated Solvents
Trichloroethylene (TCE)/Perchloroethylene (PCE)/Tetrachloroethylene

SUMMARY

- Presence in population: Perchloroethylene (PCE) is present in indoor air; certain populations are exposed to trichloroethylene (TCE) in groundwater
- Major diseases: Diminished color vision; reduced reaction time; reproductive disorders and congenital anomalies; multiple cancers including kidney, lymphomas, multiple myelomas, breast, and liver

- Primary sources: Contaminated air and groundwater
- Best measure: 8-hydroxy-2′-deoxyquanosine (8-OHdG), water testing
- Best intervention: Water filtration, allowing dry-cleaned clothes to air out before bringing them into the home, whole food antioxidants, support for glutathione transferase activity

DESCRIPTION

TCE (Fig. 18.1A) is used as a solvent to remove grease from metal parts and as a substrate for other chemical compounds.[1] TCE has been used as an extraction solvent for greases, oils, fats, and waxes and has been used extensively in the dry-cleaning industry for fabrics. It has also been used in adhesives, lubricants, paints, varnishes, and paint strippers. Tetrachloroethylene, also known as PCE, has been one of the main dry-cleaning chemicals for decades and is used as an industrial degreaser. It is also used as a substrate for other compounds.[2]

TOXICITY

These chlorinated solvents adversely affect the central nervous system, liver, kidneys, and immune and reproductive systems. Fetal abnormalities are found in children born to parents with significant exposure to these solvents. Elevated levels of urinary trichloroacetic acid, the metabolite of TCE, have been positively correlated with urinary 8-OHdG levels, reflecting the oxidative stress that this compound causes.[3]

SOURCES

More than 2.4 million pounds of TCE were released into air, soil, and water by industrial waste in 2010.[4]

TCE has been found in more than 700 of the 1300 Superfund cleanup sites in the United States. Because it is so often found in the environment, most individuals will have some level of exposure to TCE in air, soil, or water. TCE breaks down quickly in air but slowly in soil and water, making those the most common vectors for exposure. PCE (Fig. 18.1B) is also found in drinking water, soil, and indoor environments and is commonly found at Superfund cleanup sites.[5] PCE is primarily released into the air, where it persists with an atmospheric half-life ($t_{1/2}$) of 100 days and can be carried long distances from the point of origin.[2] The median ambient indoor air concentration of PCE in the United States is 4.9 ug/m³, with an average concentration of 20.7 ug/m³.

The introduction of recently dry-cleaned clothing into homes increases levels of tetrachloroethylene, with concentrations reaching 300 μg/m³ and persisting for 48 hours.[6] Breath levels of tetrachloroethylene increased twofold to sixfold for those living in homes with dry-cleaned clothes. Tetrachloroethylene levels in the indoor air, personal air, and breath were directly correlated with the number of garments brought into the home. Elevated levels of tetrachloroethylene have also been found in the homes of those working in dry-cleaning establishments, related primarily to exhalation in the home.[7]

BODY BURDEN

These solvents have a very short $t_{1/2}$ and therefore are rarely found in the general population (Table 18.1).

Detoxification/Excretion Processes

TCE is oxidized by CYP450 into chloral hydrate (CH), trichloroacetic acid (TCA), and dichloroacetic acid (DCA). It can also be directly acted on by glutathione transferases to produce dichlorovinyl cysteine (DCVC)

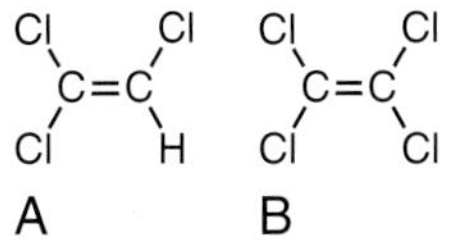

FIG. 18.1 (A) Chemical structure of trichloroethylene. (B) Chemical structure of tetrachloroethylene.

and dichlorovinyl glutathione (DCVG) (Fig. 18.2). All of these end products retain some degree of toxic action.

PCE is oxidized by cytochrome P450 (CYP) into trichloroacetyl chloride (TCAC), which can then be transformed into trichloracetic acid (TCA) or ethandioyl dichloride (EDD). It can be directly acted on by glutathione-s-transferase (GST), producing trichlorovinyl glutathione (TCVG), which can then be acted on by B-lyase, N-acetyl transferase (NAT), or more CYP450 to form other metabolites (Fig. 18.3).

Clinical Significance

Neurological. Both TCE and PCE are neurotoxic compounds that adversely affect color vision, visuospatial memory, and neuropsychological function (prolonged reaction time). Several studies have shown that the higher the PCE exposure, the greater the effect on color vision.

In a twin study, those with exposure to TCE had a risk of Parkinson's disease that was more than six times higher than their nonexposed sibling.[8]

Neoplasia. Parents of children from Camp Lejeune, North Carolina, where the water is contaminated with TCE, PCE, and benzene, had higher rates of preterm delivery and small for gestational age (SGA) babies.[9] Male marines stationed at Camp Lejeune also had a 40% to 270% greater risk of developing breast cancer.[10] Marines at Camp Lejeune were also more likely to die of a variety of cancers than marines stationed at Camp Pendleton, California (Table 18.2).[11] When exposure to TCE was singled out, the hazard ratio for dying from Hodgkin's lymphoma for those with the highest TCE exposure was 2.21.

Solvent	NHANES	Geo Mean	50th %	75th %	90th %	95th %
TCE	2001–2002	*	<LOD	<LOD	<LOD	<LOD
	2003–2004	*	<LOD	<LOD	<LOD	<LOD
	2005–2006	*	<LOD	<LOD	<LOD	<LOD
	2007–2008	*	<LOD	<LOD	<LOD	<LOD
PCE	2001–2002	*	<LOD	<LOD	0.100	0.190
	2003–2004	*	<LOD	<LOD	0.076	0.140
	2005–2006	*	<LOD	<LOD	0.070	0.126
	2007–2008	*	<LOD	<LOD	0.056	0.094

TABLE 18.1 Blood Levels of TCE and PCE in National Health and Nutritional Examination Survey (NHANES) 2001–2008 in ng/mL

Data from Centers for Disease Control and Prevention, National Report on Human Exposure to Environmental Chemicals. www.cdc.gov/exposurereport/.
*No geometric means were calculated, LOD—Level of detection.

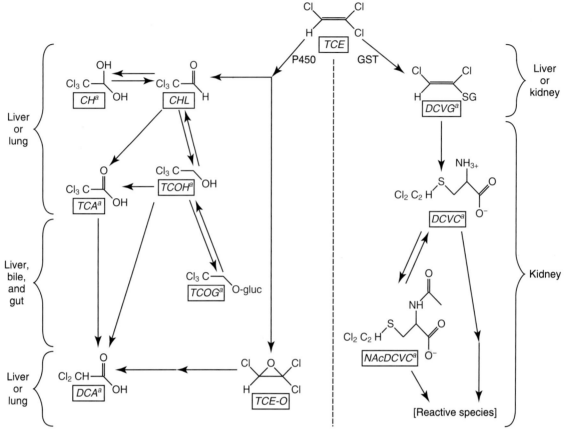

FIG. 18.2 CYP and GST biotransformation of TCE. (Chiu, W., Jinot, J., Scott, C. S., et al. (2013). Human health effects of trichloroethylene: Key findings and scientific issues. *Environmental Health Perspectives, 121*, 303–311.)

TABLE 18.2   Hazard Ratios for Marines Stationed at Camp Lejeune Compared with Those Stationed at Camp Pendleton

Cancer	Hazard Ratio
Multiple myeloma	1.68
Hodgkin's lymphoma	1.47
Esophageal	1.43
Liver	1.42
Kidney	1.35
Cervical	1.33
All cancers	1.10

Modified from Bove, F., Ruckart, P. Z., Maslia, M., & Larson, T. C. (2014). Evaluation of mortality among marines and navy personnel exposed to contaminated drinking water at USMC base Camp Lejeune: a retrospective cohort study. *Environmental Health, 13*(1), 10.

Data on cancer risk from PCE comes mostly from studies on persons working in the dry-cleaning industry, where PCE exposure is associated with bladder cancer, non-Hodgkin's lymphoma, and multiple myeloma.

Reproductive. Women exposed to tetrachloroethylene (also known as PCE) groundwater contamination were at more than three times greater risk for having a child with cleft palate or neural tube defects.[12] TCE is a more common contaminant in the soil and water than PCE. Wisconsin women living near an industry that emits TCE were more than three times more likely to give birth to a child with congenital heart defects.[13] Those living in an area in New York exposed to TCE through soil vapor intrusion also experienced higher rates of cardiac defects in their children as well as babies with lower birth weight.[14]

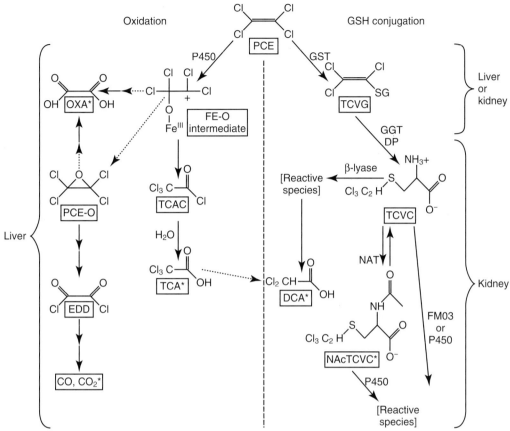

FIG. 18.3 CYP and GST biotransformation of PCE. (From Chiu, W., Jinot, J., Scott, C. S., et al. [2013]. Human health effects of trichloroethylene: Key findings and scientific issues. *Environmental Health Perspectives, 121*, 303–311.)

Immunological Effects. Because TCE has contaminated so many groundwater sites in the United States, the National Exposure Registry has been tracking adverse health effects in persons exposed to TCE. When Wistar rats were given water with TCE levels similar to what homeowners in those areas were getting, the animals produced increased levels of the Th2 cytokine, IL-4, and developed type 1 allergic reactivity.[15] Currently more than 4000 individuals living in homes supplied with TCE-contaminated well water, all near Superfund sites, are being monitored for health outcomes. As the cumulative exposure level increases, these homeowners exhibit significantly more problems with respiratory allergies, asthma, emphysema, stroke, and hearing impairment.[16]

Persons exposed to TCE from contaminated municipal drinking water have higher rates of systematic lupus erythematosus (SLE).[17] Exposure to TCE via drinking water can also increase the risk of developing scleroderma by 2.5-fold in men.[18]

INTERVENTION

The easiest way to prevent exposure to PCE in the home is to not have recently dry-cleaned clothing in the home. If dry-cleaning is necessary, it is recommended that the dry-cleaned clothes (or other materials) are aired out on a porch or in a garage or left in the car trunk for at least 48 hours. The use of a high-quality indoor air purifier will also help to reduce the level of ambient solvents in indoor air. Reverse osmosis filtration would be a prudent choice if the water supply has TCE in it, although a whole-house water filter would be the best choice, because

TCE is released into the air with showers, washing dishes, and similar activities.

Because both compounds are conjugated with glutathione, supplementation with N-acetyl cysteine (NAC) or liposomal glutathione and a diet rich in members of the brassica family as well as curcumin and green tea (all of which enhance glutathione transferase function) are indicated.

Oxidative stress from these compounds can be best addressed with botanical and whole food antioxidants.

REFERENCES

1. *Agency for Toxic Substances and Disease Registry. Toxicological Profile for Trichloroethylene.* (2014). https://www.atsdr.cdc.gov/toxprofiles/tp19.pdf. (Accessed June 23, 2017).
2. *Agency for Toxic Substances and Disease Registry. Toxicological Profile for Tetrachloroethylene.* (2014). https://www.atsdr.cdc.gov/toxprofiles/tp18.pdf. (Accessed June 23, 2017).
3. Abusoglu, S., Celik, H. T., Tutkun, E., et al. (2014). 8-Hydroxydeoxyguanosine as a useful marker for determining the severity of trichloroethylene exposure. *Archives of Environmental and Occupational Health, 69,* 180–186. PubMed PMID: 24325749.
4. U.S. Environmental Protection Agency. *TRI explorer. Release Trends Report.* https://iaspub.epa.gov/triexplorer/tri_release.chemical. (Accessed July 11, 2017).
5. U.S. Environmental Protection Agency. *National Priorities List (NPL).* http://www.epa.gov/superfund. (Accessed July 11, 2017).
6. Thomas, K. W., Pellizzari, E. D., Perritt, R. L., & Nelson, W. C. (1991). Effect of dry-cleaned clothes on tetrachloroethylene levels in indoor air, personal air and breath for residents of several New Jersey homes. *Journal of Exposure Analysis and Environmental Epidemiology, 1*(4), 475–490. PubMed PMID: 1824329.
7. Aggazzotti, G., Fantuzzi, G., Righi, E., et al. (1994). Occupational and environmental exposure to perchloroethylene in dry cleaners and their family members. *Archives of Environmental Health, 49*(6), 487–493. PubMed PMID: 7818292.
8. Goldman, S. M., Quinlan, P. J., Ross, G. W., et al. (2012). Solvent exposures and Parkinson disease risk in twins. *Annals of Neurology, 71*(6), 776–784. PubMed PMID: 22083847.
9. Ruckart, P. Z., Bove, F. J., & Maslia, M. (2014). Evaluation of contaminated drinking water and preterm birth, small for gestational age, and birth weight at Marine Corps Base Camp Lejeune, North Carolina: A cross-sectional study. *Environmental Health: A Global Access Science Source, 13,* 99. PubMed PMID: 25413571.
10. Ruckart, P. Z., Bove, F. J., Shanley, E., 3rd, & Maslia, M. (2015). Evaluation of contaminated drinking water and male breast cancer at Marine Corps Base Camp Lejeune, North Carolina: A case control study. *Environmental Health: A Global Access Science Source, 14,* 74. PubMed PMID: 26376727.
11. Bove, F., Ruckart, P. Z., Maslia, M., & Larson, T. C. (2014). Evaluation of mortality among marines and navy personnel exposed to contaminated drinking water at USMC base Camp Lejeune: A retrospective cohort study. *Environmental Health: A Global Access Science Source, 13*(1), 10. PubMed PMID: 24552493.
12. Aschengrau, A., Weinberg, J. M., Janulewicz, P. A., et al. (2009). Prenatal exposure to tetrachloroethylene-contaminated drinking water and the risk of congenital anomalies: A retrospective cohort study. *Environmental Health: A Global Access Science Source, 8,* 44. PubMed PMID: 19778411.
13. Yauck, J. S., Malloy, M. E., Blair, K., Simpson, P. M., & McCarver, D. G. (2004). Proximity of residence to trichloroethylene-emitting sites and increased risk of offspring congenital heart defects among older women. *Birth Defects Research. Part A, Clinical and Molecular Teratology, 70*(10), 808–814. PubMed PMID: 15390315.
14. Forand, S. P., Lewis-Michl, E. L., & Gomez, M. I. (2012). Adverse birth outcomes and maternal exposure to trichloroethylene and tetrachloroethylene through soil vapor intrusion in New York State. *Environmental Health Perspectives, 120*(4), 616–621. PubMed PMID: 22142966.
15. Seo, M., Yamagiwa, T., Kobayashi, R., et al. (2008). Augmentation of antigen-stimulated allergic responses by a small amount of trichloroethylene ingestion from drinking water. *Regulatory Toxicology and Pharmacology, 52*(2), 140–146. PubMed PMID: 18721841.
16. Burg, J. R., & Gist, G. L. (1999). Health effects of environmental contaminant exposure: An intrafile comparison of the trichloroethylene subregistry. *Archives of Environmental Health, 54*(4), 231–241. PubMed PMID: 10433181.
17. Kilburn, K. H., & Warshaw, R. H. (1992). Prevalence of symptoms of systemic lupus erythematosus (SLE) and of fluorescent antinuclear antibodies associated with chronic exposure to trichloroethylene and other chemicals in well water. *Environmental Research, 57*(1), 1–9. PubMed PMID: 1740091.
18. Cooper, G. S., Makris, S. L., Nietert, P. J., & Jinot, J. (2009). Evidence of autoimmune-related effects of trichloroethylene exposure from studies in mice and humans. *Environmental Health Perspectives, 117*(5), 696–702. PubMed PMID: 19479009.

19

Styrene

SUMMARY

- Presence in population: Blood levels are only found in about 25% of the population, but urinary metabolites are found in all persons tested
- Major disease: Autism spectrum disorder (ASD) risk, reductions in vision and hearing, genotoxicity, increased cancer risk

- Primary sources: Smoking, vehicular exhaust, foods, memory foam mattresses
- Best measure: Urinary metabolites or blood styrene levels
- Best intervention: Avoidance, antioxidants, N-acetyl cysteine (NAC), garlic

DESCRIPTION

Styrene (Fig. 19.1) is produced from ethylbenzene and is then used in numerous manufacturing processes as polystyrene (PS), acrylonitrile-butadiene-styrene (ABS), styrene-acrylonitrile (SAN), styrene-butadiene rubber (SBR), styrene-butadiene latex (SBL), or unsaturated polyester resins (UPR) used in fiberglass. All told, the worldwide production of styrene-containing products generates $60 billion in annual revenue (Fig. 19.2).[1]

TOXICITY

Styrene causes oxidative damage, leading to elevated malondialdehyde levels and depleted glutathione (GSH) levels.[2] This oxidative damage is accompanied by DNA adducts and elevated 8-hydroxy-2'-deoxyquanosine (8-OHdG) levels.[3]

SOURCES

In addition to the millions of individuals who work in or live near styrene manufacturing facilities, smoking is probably the biggest source of styrene exposure.[4,5] Blood styrene levels can be up to four times higher in smokers than nonsmokers. Styrene is commonly found in urban air, both from industry and in areas of higher motor vehicle traffic. In addition to cigarette smoke, styrene can be introduced into the home air by photocopiers and laser printers.[6] It was recently reported that individuals with detectable levels of blood styrene, typically above the United States Centers for Disease Control (CDC) 95th percentile, reported sleeping on mattresses or pillows containing memory foam.[7] Most of these individuals also complained of various cognitive or mood problems, which ceased once the mattress or pillow was removed. On commercially available styrene blood tests, styrene is otherwise quite rarely found.

Styrene and ethylbenzene are found in foodstuffs as a result of migration from polystyrene food containers.[8,9] Styrene migration is dependent on fat content in the food and storage temperature as well as length of exposure.[10,11] Greater migration of styrene will therefore occur in foods like cheese and hamburger, hotdogs, or steaks, all of which are commonly wrapped in plastic. Heating leftover meals in Styrofoam containers in a microwave would undoubtedly increase styrene content in the food. Cooking pork in thermoset polyester dishes (microwave safe) for 1.5 hours resulted in a styrene migration range of 6 to 2400 µg/kg and 6 to 34 µg/kg for ethylbenzene.[12] Consuming hot liquids in Styrofoam or high-impact polystyrene cups also increases styrene consumption.[13] Hot drinks with higher fat content (cream in coffee) have greater styrene transfer to the beverage. Total daily exposure for styrene for persons in the United States is estimated at 3 parts per billion (PPB) (9 µg/day), and it is estimated at 1 to 4 µg/day for residents of the United Kingdom.[14]

BODY BURDEN

Table 19.1 presents the data from four successive National Health and Nutritional Examination Survey (NHANES) cohorts on blood styrene levels. Styrene was not found

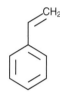

FIG. 19.1 Styrene structure.

in the blood frequently enough to calculate either a geometrical mean (GM) or a 50th percentile. Blood styrene levels could only be calculated for 25% of the measured population.

In contrast to the data presented in Table 19.1, the 2011–2012 NHANES measured the primary urinary metabolites of styrene and found the two main metabolites to be present throughout the study cohort. It is evident from the data in Table 19.2 that amino acid conjugation is the primary route of phase 2 biotransformation for styrene and that GSH conjugation only occurs in individuals with the highest styrene exposure.

Detoxification/Excretion Processes

Styrene is oxidized by CYP2B6, 1A2, or 2E1 into styrene oxide, which is then hydrolyzed by epoxide hydrolase into styrene glycol. This compound is then conjugated primarily with amino acids to form mandelic acid (MA),

6 major styrene resin families (20 million tons, more than 40 billion pounds)

PS - polystyrene
cups, plates, toys, packaging, dairy containers, building constr., cassettes

ABS - acrylonitrile-butadiene styrene
appliances, transportation, business machines

SAN - styrene-acrylonitrile
appliances, battery castings, packaging, automotive materials, housewares

SBR - styrene-butadiene rubber
tires, automotive applications

SBL - styrene-butadiene latex
carpet and upholstery backing, coatings

UPR - unsaturated polyester resins
boats, bath tubs, shower stalls, spas, hot tubs, cultured marble

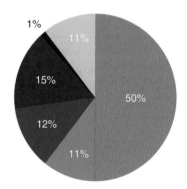

Industry estimates

FIG. 19.2 Six major styrene resin families (20 million tons, more than 40 billion pounds). (From The Styrene Forum, Information on the Styrene Industry Worldwide. http://www.styreneforum. org/industry_index.html)

TABLE 19.1	Blood Styrene Levels (ng/mL) in NHANES Participants					
	Year	GM	50th %	75th %	90th %	95th %
Styrene	2001–2002	*	<LOD	0.080	0.130	0.200
	2003–2004	*	<LOD	0.050	0.089	0.120
	2005–2006	*	<LOD	0.047	0.099	0.130
	2007–2008	*	<LOD	0.045	0.096	0.130

*no geometric mean was given LOD—Level of detection.
Data from Centers for Disease Control and Prevention, National Report on Human Exposure to Environmental Chemicals. www.cdc.gov/exposurereport/.

TABLE 19.2 Urinary Metabolites of Styrene Found in NHANES 2011 to 2012 (µg/g Creatinine)

Metabolite	Parent	GM	50th %	75th %	90th %	95th %
Phenylglyoxylic acid	Ethylbenzene/styrene	202	206	285	401	518
N-acetyl-S-(phenyl-2-hydroxyethyl)-L-cysteine	Styrene	*	<LOD	1.34	2.28	3.34
Mandelic acid	Styrene	167	158	232	363	513

*no geometric mean given LOD—level of detection.
Data from Centers for Disease Control and Prevention, National Report on Human Exposure to Environmental Chemicals. www.cdc.gov/exposurereport/.

phenylglyoxylic acid (PGA), or hippuric acids, although it can also be conjugated with GSH to make phenyl-2-hydroxyethyl mecapturic acid.[15] As reflected in Table 19.2, the majority of inhaled or ingested styrene is metabolized into MA and PGA. A very small amount (<7.5%) of styrene is also excreted into the urine unchanged. Styrene exhibits a biphasic half-life, beginning with rapid clearance ($t_{1/2}$ of 0.58 hours) followed by more prolonged clearance ($t_{1/2}$ of 13.0 hours).

Clinical Significance

Virtually all of the published health data on styrene exposure comes from workplace exposures, where it has been causally linked to immunological, neurological, reproductive, and developmental problems along with genotoxicity and neoplasia.[15] DNA adducts and single-strand DNA breaks are commonly found in styrene workers.[16] In 2011, styrene was listed by the Department of Health and Humans Services as "reasonably anticipated to be a human carcinogen."[17]

Neurological problems including hearing loss, vestibular dysfunction, and reduced color vision occur with styrene exposure.[18,19,20] It was noted that color discrimination worsened as levels of MA increased, but color vision loss was not associated with length of time working with styrene.

Living in an area with high ambient levels of styrene can increase the risk of having a child with ASD by 80%.[21]

INTERVENTION

Antioxidants, both dietary and supplemental, provide benefit in counteracting the oxidative stress and potential DNA damage caused by unavoidable styrene. NAC supplementation in rats was able to reduce the levels of hearing loss from styrene exposure.[22] The main sulfur compounds in garlic were shown to limit the genotoxicity of styrene.[23] Supplementation with the primary conjugating agents glycine and taurine along with liposomal GSH is also prudent.

REFERENCES

1. The Styrene Forum. *Information on the styrene industry worldwide.* Available at http://www.styreneforum.org/industry_index.html. (Accessed June 22, 2017.)
2. Sati, P. C., Khaliq, F., Vaney, N., et al. (2011). Pulmonary function and oxidative stress in workers exposed to styrene in plastic factory: Occupational hazards in styrene-exposed plastic factory workers. *Human and Experimental Toxicology, 30*(11), 1743–1750. PubMed PMID: 21382913.
3. Wongvijitsuk, S., Navasumrit, P., Vattanasit, U., et al. (2011). Low level occupational exposure to styrene: Its effects on DNA damage and DNA repair. *International Journal of Hygiene and Environmental Health, 214*(2), 127–137. PubMed PMID: 21030303.
4. Chambers, D. M., Ocariz, J. M., et al. (2011). Impact of cigarette smoking on volatile organic compound (VOC) blood levels in the U.S. population: NHANES 2003-2004. *Environment International, 37*(8), 1321–1328. PubMed PMID: 21703688.
5. Boyle, E. B., Viet, S. M., Wright, D. J., et al. (2016). Assessment of exposure to VOCs among pregnant women in the National Children's Study. *International Journal of Environmental Research and Public Health, 13*(4), 376. PubMed PMID: 27043585.
6. Wallace, L. A., Pellizzari, E. D., Hartwell, T. D., et al. (1987). The TEAM (Total Exposure Assessment Methodology) Study: personal exposures to toxic substances in air, drinking water, and breath of 400 residents of New Jersey, North Carolina, and North Dakota. *Environmental Research, 43*(2), 290–307. PubMed PMID: 3608934.
7. Elgez, A. *Conditions Linked to Exposure in the Bedroom and How to Confirm Them.* (2016). Environmental Health Symposium, San Diego, CA. www.environmentalhealthsymposium.com.
8. Tang, W., Hemm, I., & Eisenbrand, G. (2000). Estimation of human exposure to styrene and ethylbenzene. *Toxicology, 144*, 39–50. PubMed PMID:10781869.
9. Genualdi, S., Nyman, P., & Begley, T. (2014). Updated evaluation of the migration of styrene monomer and oligomers from polystyrene food contact materials

to foods and food simulants. *Food Additives & Contaminants. Part A, Chemistry, Analysis, Control, Exposure & Risk Assessment, 31*(4), 723–733. PubMed PMID: 24383702.

10. Tawfik, M. S., & Huyghebaert, A. (1998). Polystyrene cups and containers: Styrene migration. *Food Additives and Contaminants, 15*(5), 592–599. PubMed PMID: 9829045.

11. Lickly, T. D., Lehr, K. M., & Welsh, G. C. (1995). Migration of styrene from polystyrene foam food contact articles. *Food and Chemical Toxicology, 33*(6), 475–481.

12. Gramshaw, J. W., & Vandenburg, H. J. (1995). Compositional analysis of samples of thermoset polyester and migration of ethylbenzene and styrene from thermoset polyester into pork during cooking. *Food Additives and Contaminants, 12*(2), 223–234.

13. Khaksar, M. R., & Ghazi-Khansari, M. (2009). Determination of migration monomer styrene from GPPS (general purpose polystyrene) and HIPS (high impact polystyrene) cups to hot drinks. *Toxicology Mechanisms and Methods, 19*(3), 257–261. PubMed PMID: 19750020.

14. Lickly, T. D., Breder, C. V., & Rainey, M. L. (1995). A model for estimating the daily dietary intake of a substance from food contact articles: Styrene from polystyrene food contact polymers. *Regulatory Toxicology and Pharmacology, 21*(3), 406–417.

15. Agency for Toxic Substances and Disease Registry. Toxic Substances Portal: Styrene. Available at: https://www.atsdr.cdc.gov/toxprofiles/tp.asp?id=421&tid=74. (Accessed June 22, 2017.)

16. Henderson, L. M., & Speit, G. (2005). Review of the genotoxicity of styrene in humans. *Mutation Research, 589*(3), 158–191. PubMed PMID: 15878141.

17. National Institute of Health National Institute of Environmental Sciences National Toxicology Program. *14th Report on Carcinogens.* Available at https://ntp.niehs.nih.gov/pubhealth/roc/index-1.html. (Accessed June 22, 2017.)

18. Fetoni, A. R., Rolesi, R., Paciello, F., et al. (2016). Styrene enhances the noise induced oxidative stress in the cochlea and affects differently mechanosensory and supporting cells. *Free Radical Biology & Medicine, 101,* 211–225. PubMed PMID: 27769922.

19. Pleban, F., Oketope, O., & Shrestha, L. (2017). Occupational styrene exposure on auditory function among adults: a systematic review of selected workers. *Safety and Health at Work, 8*(4), 329–336. www.e-shaw.org

20. Kishi, R., Eguchi, T., Yuasa, J., et al. (2001). Effects of low-level occupational exposure to styrene on color vision: Dose relation with a urinary metabolite. *Environmental Research, 85*(1), 25–30. PubMed PMID: 11161648.

21. Kalkbrenner, A. E., Daniels, J. L., Chen, J. C., Poole, C., Emch, M., & Morrissey, J. (2010). Perinatal exposure to hazardous air pollutants and autism spectrum disorders at age 8. *Epidemiology (Cambridge, Mass.), 21*(5), 631–641. PubMed PMID: 20562626.

22. Yang, W. P., Hu, B. H., Chen, G. D., et al. (2009). Protective effect of N-acetyl-L-cysteine (L-NAC) against styrene-induced cochlear injuries. *Acta Oto-Laryngologica, 129*(10), 1036–1043. PubMed PMID: 19051069.

23. Guyonnet, D., Belloir, C., Suschetet, M., et al. (2001). Antimutagenic activity of organosulfur compounds from Allium is associated with phase II enzyme induction. *Mutation Research, 495*(1–2), 135–145. PubMed PMID: 11448651.

20

Organochlorine Pesticides

SUMMARY

- Presence in population: Because of their persistence and high use, these toxicants are present in the adipose tissues of virtually everyone
- Major diseases: Immune, neurological, cardiovascular, and endocrine disorders as well as several neoplasms
- Primary sources: Maternal-fetal transfer; lactation; consumption of beef, dairy products, and fish
- Best measure: Blood testing that reports both ng/mL in blood and ng/g in lipid (lipid adjusted)
- Best intervention: Sauna, enhancement of fecal fat excretion (using pancreatic lipase inhibitors)

DESCRIPTION

The organochlorine pesticides (OCPs) are a family of biologically persistent, bioaccumulating compounds composed of ringed structures to which any number of chlorine molecules are attached (Fig. 20.1). These compounds are highly lipophilic, which leads to their bioaccumulation, as does the new-to-nature character of their high level of halogenation, which makes them extremely difficult to break down by biological processes. This is why pharmaceutical scientists add halogens to drugs to lengthen their half-lives (J. Bland, personal communication, July 29, 2017).

The pesticide abilities of dichlorodiphenyl-trichloro-ethane (DDT) were discovered in 1939, and it was used during World War II to control typhus and malaria. It was then used agriculturally beginning in 1945, until it was banned for this purpose in 1972.

TOXICITY

The chlorinated pesticides as a class kill pests primarily through disruption of axonal ion flux, which inhibits impulse transmission along the axon. The acute toxicity (poisoning) signs and symptoms of these chlorinated compounds, including headache, nausea, vomiting, hyperesthesias, irritability, confusion, convulsions, respira-tory depression, cardiac arrhythmias, aplastic anemias, and porphyria cutanea tardas, are rarely seen, because these compounds have mostly been banned for use in the United States. Long-term effects of low levels of these fat-soluble and bioaccumulative pesticides in animals and humans are less clear. The effects of these compounds are most often seen secondary to mitochondrial toxicity in the neurological, immunological, and endocrinological systems, although they can also affect the cardiovascular, respiratory, gastrointestinal, and other systems in the body.

All of these organochlorine compounds, with the exception of dieldrin, have been shown to induce the functioning of 1A and 2B cytochromes (which will increase the production of free radicals) and deplete glutathione levels. So, not only do they possess prooxidant action themselves, they increase free radical production via phase one and reduce available cellular antioxidant levels.

SOURCES

The primary source of exposure to OCPs comes from consumption of foods contaminated with them. Because of their fat-soluble and bioaccumulative nature, they are mostly found in animal products, including breast milk,

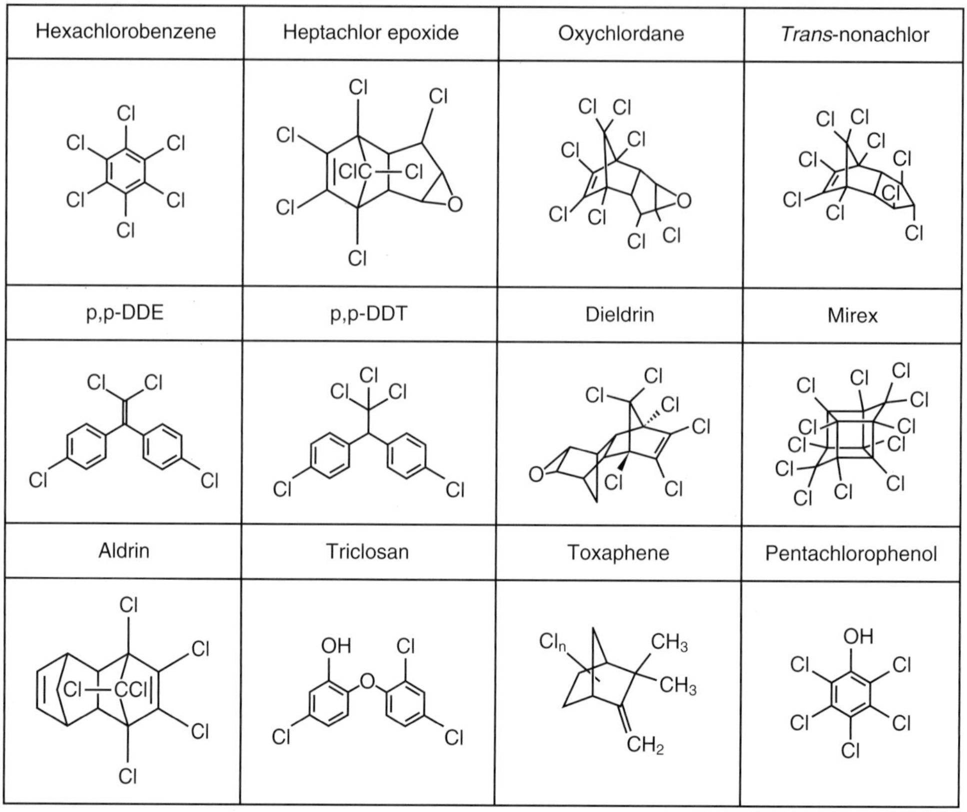

FIG. 20.1 Organochlorine pesticides.

TABLE 20.1	**OCP Exposures in the Western Diet**							
POP	Cantaloupe	Carrot	Cheese	Cucumber	Peanuts	Radish	Farmed Salmon	Summer Squash
Chlordane				X		X		X
DDE	X	X	X	X	X	X	X	X
DDT		X				X	X	X
Dieldrin	X	X	X	X	X	X	X	X
Endrin	X			X		X		X
Heptachlor	X		X	X	X	X	X	X
HCB			X				X	X
Toxaphene	X			X	X	X		X

dairy, meats, and fish. Data on 12 persistent organic pollutants (POPs) in foods assayed in the US Food and Drug Administration (FDA) Total Diet Survey (TDS) and the U.S. Department of Agriculture (USDA) Pesticide Data Program (PDP) were used to determine the toxicant content of typical meals consumed in the Northeast, Southeast, West, and Midwest United States.[1] Southeastern

daily meal plans would provide 70 POP exposures daily, western would have 66, northeastern 64, and midwestern 63, whereas a typical holiday dinner alone would provide 38 POP exposures. Table 20.1 shows the OCP exposures from a typical daily US diet.[1]

POP residues were found in meat, poultry, and dairy products as well as baked goods, fruits, and vegetables.

TABLE 20.2   OCP Compounds in NHANES 2001 to 2002, in PPB, in Serum and Adjusted for Circulating Lipids

Compounds	CDC 50th % PPB	CDC 50th % ng/g Lipid	CDC 75th % PPB	CDC 75th % ng/g Lipid	CDC 90th % PPB	CDC 90th % ng/g Lipid	CDC 95th % PPB	CDC 95th % ng/g Lipid
HCB	<LOD	<LOD	<LOD	<LOD	<LOD	<LOD	<LOD	<LOD
Heptachlor epoxide	<LOD	<LOD	<LOD	<LOD	0.102	14.8	0.153	21.6
Oxychlordane	0.69	11.1	0.143	21.7	0.248	36.3	0.352	49.7
Trans nonachlor	0.1112	17.9	0.217	33.7	0.389	56.3	0.589	78.2
DDE (p-p)	1.57	250	3.97	597	8.81	1400	15.4	2320
DDT (p-p)	<LOD	<LOD	<LOD	<LOD	<LOD	<LOD	0.184	26.5
Dieldrin	<LOD	<LOD	<LOD	<LOD	0.109	15.2	0.146	20.3
Mirex	<LOD	<LOD	<LOD	<LOD	0.101	15.8	0.414	57.1

LOD—Level of detection.

The total daily amount of DDT that could possibly be ingested by one individual consuming foods contaminated by DDT/dichlorodiphenyl-dichloroethylene (DDE) was 3154 µg/d (Chapter 3, Table 3.2).

Spanish butter has been shown to have elevated levels of hexachorobenzene (HCB), beta-hexachlorocyclohexane (HCH), and lindane.[2] Mexican butter was found to contain lindane in 91% of samples, HCB in 90%, p,p-DDE in 88%, alpha-HCH in 63%, p,p-DDT in 42%, beta-HCH in 38%, and o,p-DDT in 17%.[3] Lactation remains the primary method of reducing body burden of POPs in mammals and, as such, provides a level of exposure to all breastfed infants.[4-6]

BODY BURDEN

The Centers for Disease Control and Prevention (CDC) measured the levels of several organochlorine pesticides (OCP) compounds in the National Health and Nutritional Examination Survey (NHANES) 1999 to 2000, 2001 to 2002, and 2003 to 2004 (Table 20.2).

DDE is found regularly in the population, along with two of the chlordane compounds that were used as termiticides in North America for several decades.

Detoxification/Excretion Processes

In humans, OCPs are stored in tissues based on their fat content, with higher OCP levels found in omental fat (Fig. 20.2).[7] Once in the body, they can undergo slow dechlorination, along with some oxidation and hydrolysis action. Some of these compounds are also conjugated with glutathione, but it fails to dramatically enhance the excretion of these very lipophilic, difficult to detoxify substances.

Clinical Significance

Hexachlorobenzene. HCB is a byproduct in the manufacturing of chemical solvents, other chlorine-containing compounds, and pesticides. Small amounts of HCB can be produced by combustion of waste and other compounds. It is also an industrial byproduct of the chlor-alkali and wood preservative industries. HCB was widely used as a pesticide until 1965 but is no longer used commercially in the United States. HCB was also used as a fungicide for control of mold and fungi in cereal grains, primarily wheat. The CDC study did not find enough HCB to establish any standards, so the presence of any level of HCB is abnormal and should be considered actionable.

Exposure sources. The CDC estimates that the average exposure to HCB from foods is 1 µg/kg of body weight. The foods that HCB was found most commonly in as a part of the FDA TDS were mostly from cows, with 25% of ground beef samples having HCB, 66% of all nonorganic butter, and 18% of all American cheese samples.[8] It was also found in 41% of all lamb chops and 50% of all Atlantic salmon (farmed) steaks. Of these, the highest levels were found in nonorganic butter. Higher levels in the blood may also be from industrial exposure or from living close to a waste facility. The Environmental Protection Agency (EPA) toxic release inventory database found at www.scorecard.org or https://www.epa.gov/toxics-release-inventory-tri-program can be used to help assess these exposure sources.

Adverse health effects
- Diabetes risk is increased to an odds ratio of 4.5 with the presence of HCB.[9]
- Childhood obesity is increased to an odds ratio of 2.5 to 3.0 with maternal serum levels of HCB.[10]

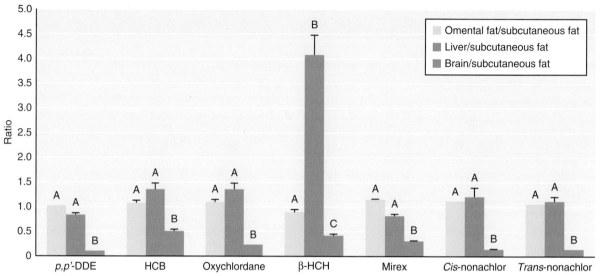

FIG. 20.2 Organochlorine concentrations in various tissues relative to subcutaneous fat samples. (From Dewailly, E., Mulvad, G., Pedersen, H. S., Ayotte, P., Demers, A., Weber, J. P., Hansen, J. (1999). Concentration of organochlorines in human brain, liver, and adipose tissue autopsy samples from Greenland. *Environmental Health Perspectives, 107*(10), 823–828.)

- Testicular cancer rates are higher in men (odds ratio (OR) 4.4) whose mothers had high serum HCB levels.[11]
- Reduction of total T4 occurs with increased levels of HCB (T4 dropped 0.32 μg/dL per each unit increase [in ng/mL] of HCB).[12]
- Rates of soft-tissue sarcomas and thyroid cancers are increased in persons living close to industries that emit HCBs.[13]
- There is an increased risk of porphyria with neurological manifestations.[14]
- Risk of childhood otitis media is increased to an OR of 2.38 when present with DDE.[15]
- Risk of positive Epstein Barr early antigen and of non-Hodgkin's lymphoma is increased (OR 5.3 with "above median" levels of HCB).[16]
- HCB exposure may be related to increased risk of autoimmunity.[17]
- Patients with cronic fatigue syndrome have higher levels of HCB and/or DDE.[18]
- HCB suppresses gamma-interferon production.[19]

Heptachlor Epoxide. Heptachlor and its metabolite heptachlor epoxide (HCE) are chlordanes, a group of chlorinated compounds that were used agriculturally until 1974 and as termiticides commonly throughout

North America until 1988. Bacteria in the soil and in the livers of humans and animals will transform heptachlor through cytochrome 1A1 to the much more toxic and biologically persistent epoxide form. Once a house has been treated with chlordane, it can be found in dust for the life of the home, contaminating anyone living in the home who breathes the dust. Heptachlor is still approved for the treatment of fire ants in underground transformers.

Exposure sources. A major source of exposure is living in a home (built before 1988) in which the chlordane was applied in the crawlspace where the furnace or air conditioning ducts now run. If those ducts have leaking connections (common in older ductwork), chlordane-contaminated dust will be sucked into the intake ducts and distributed throughout the house. Because heptachlor and HCE stick to soil and dust, another source comes from tracking in dirt from outdoors. In many areas of the country, places that were formerly orchards or farmland have now been turned into housing developments. Those areas in which heptachlor was used before 1974 can have soil contaminated with HCE that will make it into the dirt and dust of homes. This is especially true in homes where shoes are worn indoors and that have carpeting for the HCE to stick to.

The next greatest source of exposure is through foods, typically seafood, dairy, meats, and poultry. In the TDS,[8] the foods that were highest in HCE were very similar to those in which HCB was found. Fifty percent of the butter samples (nonorganic) had HCE. It was also found in 34% of all samples of cream cheese and salmon steaks (farmed Atlantic salmon), 32% of all samples of ground beef, and 30% of all samples of Swiss and cheddar cheeses. Interestingly, 25% of all samples of Hubbard squash also had HCE in them.

Chlordanes have been found in all studies of breast milk in North America. Thus these children had transplacental transfer of chlordanes and many had breast milk exposure as well.

Adverse health effects
- HCE, as the epoxide form, is a powerful prooxidant and difficult to clear through normal phase two conjugation.
- High maternal levels of HCE lead to increased rates of cryptorchidism in male offspring.[20]
- HCE has demonstrated the ability to be an initiator, promoter, and progressor of breast cancer.[21,22]
- Higher HCE blood levels increase the risk of non-Hodgkin's lymphoma (third quartile levels have an OR of 1.82, fourth quartile levels have an OR of 3.41).[23]
- HCE is neurotoxic to the dopaminergic system and may lead to an increased risk for parkinsonism.[24]
- HCE presence, along with other chlorinated compounds, can lead to increased atherosclerosis.[25]

Oxychlordane. Oxychlordane is the major metabolite of the various chlordane and nonachlor compounds that were used agriculturally until 1974 and residentially until 1988. It is one that is found commonly in all persons living in North America who have been measured for levels of persistent pollutants in their blood. As a human metabolite, it has not been found in food, because it is produced by the liver after the individual is exposed through air, water, or food to chlordanes and nonachlors. This metabolite is, unfortunately, about eight times more toxic than its parent compounds and is more bioaccumulative.[26]

Exposure sources. Oxychlordane is present in the same sources as listed above for HCE.
Adverse health effects
- There is a greatly increased risk of diabetes (OR 14.7) associated with high levels of oxychlordane.[27]

- Oxychlordane exposure increases the risk of non-Hodgkin's lymphoma (OR 2.68).[28]
- Oxychlordane introduces an increased risk (OR 1.63) of seminoma (testicular germ cell tumor).[29]
- It increases the increased risk of prostate cancer.[30]
- Immunosuppression of cell-mediated immune response to pathogens occurs.[31]
- Natural killer cell ability to lyse tumor cells is decreased.[32]
- The likelihood of developing erectile dysfunction is increased.[33]

Transnonachlor. Transnonachlor is another of the major chlordane compounds that was used agriculturally from 1953 to 1974 and as a termiticide until 1988.

Exposure sources. The same exposure sources listed for the other chlordanes also apply here. The most likely source is exposure to dirt or dust that is already contaminated with it. Homes built before 1988 that have the original ductwork still intact offer particular risk. Unfortunately, a number of individual homeowners chose to apply the chlordane themselves, and in these cases, the chlordane may be inside the home itself.

Dietary sources of transnonachlor were surprisingly few in the TDS, with the most frequent finding being in sweet cucumber pickles (around 25% of all samples) rather than dairy and beef like the other chlordanes.

Transnonachlor is found in most persons tested for it.
Adverse health effects
- The adverse effects of the chlordanes are very similar. Many of the cancer and other health associations are found with transnonachlor as well, just in differing levels.
- There is increased obesity and risk of diabetes, with the highest odds ratio of all organochlorine compounds for diabetes, at 37.7.[27]

Dichlorodiphenyl-Dichloroethylene (DDE). This metabolite of dichloro-diphenyl-trichloroethane (DDT) is the most ubiquitous and abundant of all the chlorinated pesticides. When DDT is produced, it consists of a combination of DDT and DDE. The rate of breakdown in the environment (in temperate climates, the soil half-life is 20–30 years) is measured by the changing ratios of DDE to DDT. Once in the human body, DDT is broken down to DDE within about 6 months. Many published research articles will use the term DDT or total DDT to include DDT, DDE, and dichlorodiphenyldichloroethane (DDD). Because DDE is the most commonly found DDT compound, the main aspects of all the DDTs are reviewed under DDE.

DDT was first synthesized in 1874; its pesticide abilities were discovered in 1939, and it was used in wartime to control typhus and malaria. It was put into agricultural use in the United States in 1945 and was banned for use in 1972. Production in this country was not banned, so it was still manufactured and sent to other countries, often as part of U.S. agricultural aid. The DDTs are found throughout the globe, including the Arctic and Antarctic, because they have been carried by wind across the planet.

The DDTs are highly lipid soluble and are stored in all lipid-rich tissues of the body, including adipose tissue, the liver, and the brain. It has been estimated that 1 part per billion (PPB) DDT in serum would mean 5 to 10 PPB in the brain, 47 PPB in the liver, and 100 to 300 PPB in fat cells. DDE has been found in all samples of breast milk across the globe. Unfortunately, the levels of DDE in some of these human samples exceeded what would have been allowed to be sold commercially in any other milk product.

Exposure sources. The major source of exposure is through diet. In the years 1986 to 1991, the average adult in the United States consumed an average of 0.8 μg of DDT a day. The largest fraction of DDT in a person's diet comes from meat, poultry, dairy products, and fish, including sport fish. A number of freshwater fish advisories in certain lakes and rivers in the U.S. have been posted because of DDT contamination of trout and other fish. Leafy vegetables will often contain more DDT than other vegetables, possibly because DDT in the air is deposited on the leaves, and infants may be exposed by drinking breast milk.

The most recent TDS assessment of DDE in food reveals that DDE is present in many of the most commonly consumed food items in the western diet (Table 20.3). The following chart shows those foods in which it was found commonly in this FDA survey. In each percentage grouping, the foods are given with the most contaminated foods first.

The other main sources are from the dust or dirt in a home contaminated with DDE. This could occur in an older dwelling where DDT was used or in newer housing projects that were built on or around previously contaminated soil. These levels can also come from airborne contamination of DDE/DDT when it is used agriculturally

TABLE 20.3 **Foods with the Highest DDE Content According to the TDS**		
Food	Percentage of Samples Positive for DDE (%)	Mean Concentration of DDE in PPM
Catfish (farm raised)	100	0.032
Butter (nonorganic)	100	0.02
Spinach (nonorganic)	100	0.01
Salmon steaks (farmed Atlantic)	100	0.008
American cheese, processed	100	0.006
Cream cheese	100	0.004
Candy bar, chocolate, nougat, nuts	100	0.001
Quarter-pound cheeseburger	98	0.004
Meatloaf (homemade)	98	0.002
Quarter-pound burger	98	0.002
Lamb chops	95	0.005
Sour cream	93	0.0028
Fast food egg, ham, biscuit breakfast	93	0.0024
Pizza, pepperoni	93	0.0012
Ground beef	91	0.002
Pizza, cheese	90	0.0015
Collard greens, nonorganic	89	0.0045
Hotdogs	89	0.002
Half and half	82	0.002
Vanilla ice cream	80	0.0012
Lasagna, beef	80	0.0008
Cheddar cheese	77	0.003
Peanut butter, creamy	75	0.0016
Baked potato, with skin (nonorganic)	73	0.0013

in other parts of the world before making its way across the globe via wind.

Sport fishing is another potential source of DDT exposure for those persons who consume their catch. The Department of Fish and Game for the state the fish is caught in offers advisories for any toxic presence in their waterways. Anyone planning on fishing in any state, including coastal waterways, should obtain this information before consuming their catch.

All children are exposed in utero, and through breast milk if they are breastfed.

Adverse health effects. In general, DDE causes ongoing neurological problems (including cognitive difficulties, headaches, and depression) along with immune and endocrinological problems. Various cancers are also associated with DDE presence. Breast cancer is not listed, because there have been and continue to be articles published that both do and do not show a correlation. One intriguing study reported that higher rates of breast cancer were related to DDT exposure occurring before the age of 14 years.[34]

- Prenatal exposure to DDE led to increased findings of hyporeflexia[35] and attention problems[36] in infants, and caused a delay in mental and psychomotor development identifiable at the age of 13 months.[37] It also led to decreased cognitive skills for these children that was still evident when they became preschoolers.[38]
- Prenatal exposure to DDE, HCB, and dieldrin increases the risk of otitis media, and higher levels led to the otitis becoming recurrent.[39]
- Prenatal DDE exposure also increases the rate of asthma in children (with the highest levels of DDE having a relative risk of 2.6).[40]
- DDE increases the rate of mast cell degranulation and increases the risk of allergy and asthma.[41-43]
- Elevated serum DDE significantly reduces mitogen-induced lymphocyte proliferation response,[44] resulting in cell-mediated immune deficiency, and may increase the incidence of herpes zoster.[45]
- DDE and other chlorinated pesticides are found in higher levels of the substantia nigra in persons with parkinsonism.[46] It also disrupts the transport of dopamine in the brain.[47]
- DDE and HCB are associated with chronic fatigue syndrome.[18]
- DDE is also associated with higher rates of type 2 diabetes.[9,48]
- DDE levels are associated with a 71% increased risk of developing testicular germ cell tumors.[29]
- Above median levels of DDE (and other chlorinated compounds) may lead to increased risk of developing pancreatic cancer[49] and will lead to tremendously shorter survival times in persons with pancreatic cancer.[50]

- DDE levels below medial levels were associated with a greatly elevated risk factor (OR 3.2) for liver cancer.[51]
- DDE levels almost doubled the risk (OR 1.9) for endometrial cancer.[52]
- DDE and other environmental endocrine disruptors have also been associated with increased rates of precocious puberty.[53]
- DDE showed a clear correlation with both preterm births and small-for-gestational-age babies.[54]
- DDE was the most frequently found chlorinated compound in a study of infertile women and their male partners,[55] with the highest residue levels being negatively associated with fertilization.
- DDE levels are also associated with multiple abnormalities in semen indices and sperm amount, motility, and quality.[56]
- DDE can also lead to early menopause.[57]
- DDE levels are associated with greater risk of endometriosis and reduced functioning of natural killer cells.[58]
- DDE can lead to altered levels of thyroid hormones.[59]

Dichlorodiphenyl-Trichloroethane. See the earlier section on DDE. The sources are similar, except that DDT is present in much smaller quantities. The health problems are virtually the same.

The main difference is the frequency with which DDE and DDT are found and their respective levels. Although a small amount of DDT can be found in the adipose tissues of almost everybody, it is rarely found in the serum. Because of the time it takes for DDT to be metabolized to DDE in the body, if DDT is found in the serum, it typically indicates current exposure (probably by foods) within the preceding 6 months.

In the TDS,[8] the greatest source of DDT was nonorganic spinach.

Dieldrin. From the 1950s until 1970, dieldrin and a similar compound, Aldrin, were used extensively as insecticides on crops such as corn and cotton. They were both approved by the EPA in 1972 for killing termites and were used as termiticides until 1987. Aldrin is metabolized into dieldrin after entering the body or the environment (where sunlight and bacteria bring about the production of dieldrin). Dieldrin does not break down in water and is not easily volatilized for release into the air. It sticks very strongly to soil, sediment, and dust particles. It can be taken up by plants and stored in their leaves and roots. Fish or animals that eat dieldrin-contaminated materials store a large amount of the dieldrin in their fat. Animals or fish that eat other animals have levels of dieldrin in their fat many times higher because of bioaccumulation. Humans, who are at the top of the food chain, will then be the final repository of dieldrin.

Exposure sources. The most common exposures to aldrin and dieldrin occur from contaminated foods that include fish or shellfish from contaminated lakes or streams, root crops, dairy products, and meats. Exposure to aldrin and dieldrin also occurs when water or air comes into contact with contaminated soil at hazardous waste sites (listed at www.epa.gov). People with the greatest potential for exposure include those who live in homes that were once treated for termites with aldrin or dieldrin, because exposure to these toxins can still occur years after they were applied in a home.

Squash, cucumber, and zucchini plants have the ability to clean aldrin and dieldrin from the soil and accumulate it in their fruits, which we typically eat.[60] This is reflected in the 10 foods listed in the TDS as having the highest levels of dieldrin. If aldrin and dieldrin are still in the soil from decades earlier, even if these vegetables are grown organically, they will still have high levels of these toxins in them. Of course, these plants can also be used to clean the soil of these pesticides; it is just not recommended to either eat their fruits or compost them.

Foods with the highest levels of dieldrin in the FDA TDS

1. Summer squash (0.007 parts per million [PPM])
2. Hubbard squash (0.005 PPM)
3. Dill cucumber pickles (0.004 PPM)
4. Sweet cucumber pickles (0.003 PPM)
5. Raw peeled cucumbers (0.003 PPM)
6. Pumpkin pie (0.0024 PPM)
7. Atlantic salmon (0.002 PPM)
8. Cream cheese (0.0008 PPM)
9. Creamy peanut butter (0.00076 PPM)
10. Cheddar cheese (0.0007 PPM)

Adverse health effects

- Dieldin disrupts dopamine transport in the brain.[47]
- Dieldrin increases oxidative damage in the brain (nigrostriatal pathway)[61] and may lead to increased rates of parkinsonism.[62] It is also significantly associated with existing diagnoses of parkinsonism.[63]
- Dieldrin is associated with increased rates of hypothyroidism.[64]

- Dieldrin adversely affects the Leydig cells, reducing their production of testosterone, and could contribute to infertility.[65]
- Dieldrin is associated with increased rates of lung cancer,[66] breast cancer,[67] and non-Hodgkin's lymphoma.[21]
- Dieldrin may also increase pancreatic cancer mortality.[68]
- Dieldrin increases superoxide production and causes neutrophil inflammation.[69]

Mirex. Mirex was used as a pesticide to control fire ants mostly in the southeastern part of the United States until 1978. It was also used as a flame retardant additive under the trade name Dechlorane in plastics, rubber, paint, paper, and electrical goods from 1959 to 1972. Mirex is found attached to soil and dust, like many of these other compounds.

Once in the bloodstream, Mirex is carried to many parts of the body, where it is stored, mainly in fat. Mirex is not broken down in the body by the biotransformation processes.

Exposure sources. The most likely way for people in the general population to be exposed to Mirex is by eating food, particularly fish, taken from contaminated areas. Currently, three states (Ohio, New York, and Pennsylvania) have issued warnings to the public that fish (primarily fish caught in Lake Ontario) may contain Mirex. The FDA TDS has not measured other foods for Mirex, so exposure sources are not clearly delineated.

Adverse health effects. In rodents, Mirex causes liver, adrenal, and blood cancer. In humans, it causes trembling, tiredness, weakness, increased oxidative damage, and neurological and immunological problems. Most of the published studies that looked for adverse health effects of Mirex were done while looking at a number of chlorinated compounds. As a single agent, it has not been well studied, so there are no specific articles on its effects.

Intervention

The first step in intervention is to identify exposure sources and remediate them. Cleansing protocols can also be prescribed to enhance the clearance of these persistent toxins from the body. Sauna therapy has demonstrated the ability to mobilize OCPs in sweat. DDT, DDE, methoxychlor, endrin, and endosulfan sulfate were all mobilized in sweat in the blood, urine, and sweat (BUS) study.[70] In these individuals, the chlorinated pesticides were found more often in sweat than in urine or serum, with some compounds only found in sweat. Saunas and colonic irrigations have been used to reduce the blood concentration of PCBs and chlorinated pesticides as well.[71]

Various dietary measures have been shown to increase the normal bowel excretion of these fat-soluble toxins. Daily use of rice bran fiber (RBF) has been documented in several studies in Japan to be able to increase the clearance of POPs and should work for all OCPs.[72-74] Chlorophyll and all chlorophyll-containing foods are also tremendous at increasing the excretion of these persistent fat-soluble toxins in feces.[75-77] Increasing these in the diet or through daily supplementation will slowly increase excretion of these compounds from the body. The polyphenols found highest in white and green teas have also been shown to increase excretion of fat-soluble toxicants.[78]

There is intriguing, but very inconsistent, research on the use of bile sequestrants to increase excretion of OCPs. See Chapter 26, for discussion.

In addition to increasing excretion of these compounds from the body, high amounts of a combination of nutrient and botanical antioxidants to protect the tissues and cells that are under assault from the toxic compounds should be used.

REFERENCES

1. Schafer, K. S., & Kegley, S. E. (2002). Persistent toxic chemicals in the US food supply. *Journal of Epidemiology and Community Health*, *56*(11), 813–817. PubMed PMID: 12388566.
2. Badia-Vila, M., Ociepa, M., Mateo, R., & Guitart, R. (2000). Comparison of residue levels of persistent organochlorine compounds in butter from Spain and from other European countries. *Journal of Environmental Science and Health. Part. B, Pesticides, Food Contaminants, and Agricultural Wastes*, *35*(2), 201–210. PubMed PMID: 10736769.
3. Waliszewski, S. M., Villalobos-Pietrini, R., Gómez-Arroyo, S., & Infanzón, R. M. (2003). Persistent organochlorine pesticides in Mexican butter. *Food Additives and Contaminants*, *20*(4), 361–367. PubMed PMID: 12775478.
4. Chávez-Almazán, L. A., Diaz-Ortiz, J., Alarcón-Romero, M., et al. (2016). Influence of breastfeeding time on levels of organochlorine pesticides in human milk of a Mexican population. *Bulletin of Environmental Contamination and Toxicology*, *96*(2), 168–172. PubMed PMID: 26602567.
5. Lignell, S., Winkvist, A., Bertz, F., et al. (2016). Environmental organic pollutants in human milk before and after weight loss. *Chemosphere*, *159*, 96–102. PubMed PMID: 27281542.
6. Müller, M. H., Polder, A., Brynildsrud, O. B., et al. (2017). Organochlorine pesticides (OCPs) and polychlorinated biphenyls (PCBs) in human breast milk and associated health risks to nursing infants in Northern Tanzania. *Environmental Research*, *154*, 425–434. PubMed PMID: 28196346.
7. Dewailly, E., Mulvad, G., Pedersen, H. S., et al. (1999). Concentration of organochlorines in human brain, liver, and adipose tissue autopsy samples from Greenland. *Environmental Health Perspectives*, *107*(10), 823–828. PubMed PMID: 10504150.
8. U.S. Food and Drug Administration. *Total Diet Study. Analytical Results*. Available at https://www.fda.gov/food/foodscienceresearch/totaldietstudy/ucm184293.htm. (Accessed July 11, 2017.)
9. Codru, N., Schymura, M. J., Negoita, S., et al. (2007). Diabetes in relation to serum levels of polychlorinated biphenyls and chlorinated pesticides in adult Native Americans. *Environmental Health Perspectives*, *115*(10), 1442–1447. PubMed PMID: 17938733.
10. Smiths, A., Ribas-Fito, N., Garcia, R., et al. (2008). Exposure to hexachlorobenzene during pregnancy increases the risk of overweight in children aged 6 years. *Acta Paediatrica (Oslo, Norway)*, *97*, 1465–1469. PubMed PMID: 18665907.
11. Hardell, L., van Bavel, B., Lindstrom, G., et al. (2003). Increased concentrations of polychlorinated biphenyls, hexachlorbenzene, and chlordanes in mothers of men with testicular cancer. *Environmental Health Perspectives*, *111*, 930–934. PubMed PMID: 12782494.
12. Sala, M., Sunyer, J., Herrero, C., To-Figueras, J., & Grimalt, J. (2001). Association between serum concentrations of hexachlorobenzene and polychlorinated biphenyls with thyroid hormone and liver enzymes in a sample of the general population. *Occupational and Environmental Medicine*, *58*, 172–177. PubMed PMID: 11171930.
13. Grimalt, J. O., Sunyer, J., Moreno, V., et al. (1994). Risk excess of soft-tissue sarcoma and thyroid cancer in a community exposed to airborne organochlorinated compound mixtures with a high hexachlorobenzene content. *International Journal of Cancer*, *56*, 200–203. PubMed PMID: 8314301.
14. Peters, H. A., Cripps, D. J., Gocmen, A., et al. (1986). Neurotoxicity of hexachlorobenzene-induced porphyria turcica. In: Hexachlorobenzene: Proceedings of an International Symposium. *IARC Scientific Publications*, (77), 575–579. PubMed PMID: 3036698.
15. Karmaus, W., Kuehr, J., & Kruse, H. (2001). Infections and atopic disorders in children and organochlorine

exposure. *Archives of Environmental Health*, 56, 485–492. PubMed PMID: 11958547.

16. Hardell, E., Eriksson, M., Lindstrom, G., et al. (2001). Case-control study on concentrations of organohalogen compounds and titers of antibodies to Epstein-Barr virus antigens in the etiology of non-Hodgkin lymphoma. *Leukemia & Lymphoma*, 42, 619–629. PubMed PMID: 11697490.

17. Michielsen, C. C., van Loveren, H., & Vos, J. G. (1999). The role of the immune system in hexachlorobenzene-induced toxicity. *Environmental Health Perspectives*, 107(Suppl. 5), 783–792. PubMed PMID: 10502545.

18. Dunstan, R. H., Donohoe, M., Taylor, W., et al. (1995). A preliminary investigation of chlorinated hydrocarbons and chronic fatigue syndrome. *The Medical Journal of Australia*, 163, 294–297. PubMed PMID: 7565234.

19. Daniel, V., Huber, W., Bauer, K., et al. (2001). Associations of blood levels of PCB, HCHS, and HCB with numbers of lymphocyte subpopulations, in vitro lymphocyte response, plasma cytokine levels, and immunoglobulin autoantibodies. *Environmental Health Perspectives*, 109, 173–178. PubMed PMID: 11266339.

20. Pierik, F. H., Klebanoff, M. A., Brock, J. W., & Longnecker, M. P. (2007). Maternal pregnancy serum levels of heptachlor epoxide, hexachlorobenzene, and beta hexachlorocyclohexane and risk of cryptorchidism in offspring. *Environmental Research*, 105, 364–369. PubMed PMID: 17532317.

21. Cassidy, R. A., Natarajan, S., & Vaughan, G. M. (2005). The link between the insecticide heptachlor epoxide, estradiol and breast cancer. *Breast Cancer Research and Treatment*, 90, 55–64. PubMed PMID: 15770527.

22. Khanjani, N., English, D. R., & Sim, M. R. (2006). An ecological study of organochlorine pesticides and breast cancer in rural Victoria, Australia. *Archives of Environmental Contamination and Toxicology*, 50, 452–461. PubMed PMID: 16489419.

23. Quintana, P. J., Delfino, R. J., Korrick, S., et al. (2004). Adipose tissue levels of organochlorine pesticides and polychlorinated biphenyls and risk of non-Hodgkins lymphoma. *Environmental Health Perspectives*, 112, 854–861. PubMed PMID: 15175172.

24. Richardson, J. R., Caudle, W. M., Wang, M. Z., et al. (2008). Developmental heptachlor exposure increases susceptibility of dopamine neurons to N-methyl-4-phenyl-1,2,3,6-tetrahydropyridine (MPTP) in a gender-specific manner. *Neurotoxicology*, 29, 855–863. PubMed PMID: 18577399.

25. Pines, A., Cucos, S., Ever-Hadani, P., et al. (1986). Levels of some organochlorine residues in blood of patients with arteriosclerotic disease. *The Science of*

the Total Environment, 54, 135–155. PubMed PMID: 3101173.

26. Bondy, G., Armstrong, C., Coady, L., et al. (2003). Toxicity of the chlordane metabolite oxychlordane in female rats: Clinical and histopathological changes. *Food and Chemical Toxicology*, 41, 291–301. PubMed PMID: 12480304.

27. Lee, D. H., Lee, I. K., Song, K., et al. (2006). A strong dose-response relationship between serum concentrations of persistent organic pollutants and diabetes: Results from the National Health and Examination Survey 1999-2002. *Diabetes Care*, 29, 1638–1644. PubMed PMID: 16801591.

28. Spinelli, J. J., Ng, C. H., Weber, H. P., et al. (2007). Organochlorines and risk of non-Hodgkin's lymphoma. *International Journal of Cancer*, 1212, 2767–2775. PubMed PMID: 17722095.

29. McGlynn, K. A., Quraishi, S. M., Graubard, B. I., et al. (2008). Persistent organochlorine pesticides and risk of testicular germ cell tumors. *Journal of the National Cancer Institute*, 100, 663–671. PubMed PMID: 18445826.

30. Ritchie, J. M., Vial, S. L., Fuortes, L. J., et al. (2003). Organochlorines and risk of prostate cancer. *Journal of Occupational and Environmental Medicine*, 45, 692–702. PubMed PMID: 12855910.

31. Johnson, K. W., Kaminski, N. E., & Munson, A. E. (1987). Direct suppression of cultured spleen cell responses by chlordane and the basis for differential effects on in vivo and in vitro immunocompetence. *Journal of Toxicology and Environmental Health*, 22, 497–515. PubMed PMID: 3694709.

32. Beach, T. M., & Whalen, M. M. (2006). Effects of organochlorine pesticides on interleukin secretion from lymphocytes. *Human and Experimental Toxicology*, 25, 651–659. PubMed PMID: 17211983.

33. Polsky, J. Y., Aronson, K. J., Heaton, J. P., & Adams, M. A. (2007). Pesticides and polychlorinated biphenyls as potential risk factors for erectile dysfunction. *Journal of Andrology*, 28, 28–37. PubMed PMID: 16899811.

34. Cohn, B. A., Wolff, M. S., Cirillo, P. M., & Sholtz, R. I. (2007). DDT and breast cancer in young women: New data on the significance of age at exposure. *Environmental Health Perspectives*, 115, 1406–1414. PubMed PMID: 17938728.

35. Rogan, W. J., Gladen, B. C., McKinney, J. D., Carreras, N., et al. (1986). Neonatal effects of transplacental exposures to PCBs and DDE. *The Journal of Pediatrics*, 109, 335–341.

36. Saqiv, S. K., Nugent, J. K., Brazelton, T. B., Choi, A. L., et al. (2008). Prenatal organochlorine exposure and

measures of behavior in infancy using the neonatal behavioral assessment scale. *Environmental Health Perspectives, 116,* 666–673.

37. Ribas-Fito, N., Cardo, E., Sala, M., Eulalia de Muga, M., et al. (2003). Breastfeeding, exposure to organochlorine compounds, and neurodevelopment in infants. *Pediatrics, 115,* e580–e585.

38. Ribas-Fito, N., Torrent, M., Carrizo, D., Munoz-Ortiz, L., et al. (2006). In utero exposure to background concentrations of DDT and cognitive functioning among preschoolers. *American Journal of Epidemiology, 164,* 955–962.

39. Dewailly, E., Ayotte, P., Burneau, S., Gingras, S., Belles-Isles, M., & Roy, R. (2000). Susceptibility to infections and immune status in Inuit infants exposed to organochlorines. *Environmental Health Perspectives, 108,* 205–211.

40. Sunyer, J., Torrent, M., Garcia-Esteban, R., Ribas-Fito, N., et al. (2006). Early exposure to dichlorodiphenyldichloroethylene, breastfeeding and asthma at age six. *Clinical and Experimental Allergy, 36,* 1236–1241.

41. Narita, S., Goldblum, R. M., Watson, C. S., Brooks, E. G., et al. (2007). Environmental estrogens induce mast cell degranulation and enhance IgE-mediated release of allergic mediators. *Environmental Health Perspectives, 115,* 48–52.

42. Sunyer, J., Torrent, M., Munoz-Ortiz, L., Ribas-Fito, N., et al. (2005). Prenatal dichlordiphenyldichloroethylene (DDE) and asthma in children. *Environmental Health Perspectives, 113,* 1787–1790.

43. Karmaus, W., Kuehr, J., & Kruse, H. (2001). Infections and atopic disorders in children and organochlorine exposure. *Archives of Environmental Health, 56,* 485–492.

44. Vine, M. F., Stein, L., Weigle, K., Schroeder, J., Degnan, D., Tse, C. K. E., et al. (2000). Effects on the immune system associated with living near a pesticide dumpsite. *Environmental Health Perspectives, 108,* 1113–1124.

45. Arndt, V., Vine, M. F., & Weigle, K. (1999). Environmental chemical exposures and risk of herpes zoster. *Environmental Health Perspectives, 107*(10), 835–841.

46. Corrigan, F. M., Wienburg, C. L., Shore, R. F., Daniel, S. E., & Mann, D. (2000). Organochlorine insecticides in substantia nigra in Parkinson's disease. *Journal of Toxicology and Environmental Health. Part A, 59,* 229–234.

47. Hatcher, J. M., Delea, K. C., Richardson, J. R., Pennell, K. D., & Miller, G. W. (2008). Disruption of dopamine transport by DDT and its metabolites. *Neurotoxicology, 29,* 682–690.

48. Rignell-Hydbom, A., Rylander, L., & Hagmar, L. (2007). Exposure to persistent organochlorine pollutants and type 2 diabetes mellitus. *Human and Experimental Toxicology, 26,* 447–452.

49. Porta, M., de Basea, M. B., Benavides, F. G., Lopez, T., et al. (2008). Differences in serum concentrations of organochlorine compounds by occupational social class in pancreatic cancer. *Environmental Research, 108,* 370–379.

50. Hardell, L., Carlberg, M., Hardell, K., Bjornfoth, H., et al. (2007). Decreased survival in pancreatic cancer patients with high concentrations of organochlorine in adipose tissue. *Biomedicine & Pharmacotherapy, 61,* 659–664.

51. McGlynn, K. A., Abnet, C. C., Zhang, M., Sun, X. D., et al. (2006). Serum concentrations of 1,1,1-trichlor-2,2-bis(p-chlorophenyl)ethane (DDT) and 1,1-dichloro-2,2-bis(p-chlorophenyl)ethylene (DDE) and risk of primary liver cancer. *Journal of the National Cancer Institute, 98,* 1005–1010.

52. Hardell, L., van Bavel, B., Linstrom, G., Bjornfoth, H., et al. (2004). Adipose tissue concentrations of p,p-DDE and the risk for endometrial cancer. *Gynecologic Oncology, 95,* 706–711.

53. Lu, J. P., Zheng, L. X., & Cai, D. P. (2006). Study on the level of environmental endocrine disruptors in serum of precocious puberty patients. *Zhonghua Yu Fang Xue Za Zhi [Chinese Journal of Preventive Medicine], 40,* 88–92.

54. Longnecker, M. P., Klebanoff, M. A., Zhou, H., & Brock, J. W. (2001). Association between maternal serum concentration of the DDT metabolite DDE and preterm and small-for-gestational-age babies at birth. *Lancet, 358,* 110–114.

55. Younglai, W. V., Foster, W. G., Hughes, E. G., Trim, H. K., & Jarrell, J. F. (2002). Levels of environmental contaminants in human follicular fluid, serum, and seminal plasma of couples undergoing in vitro fertilization. *Archives of Environmental Contamination and Toxicology, 43,* 121–126.

56. Aneck-Hahn, N. H., Schulenburg, G. W., Bornman, M. S., Farias, P., & de Jager, C. (2007). Impaired semen quality associated with environmental DDT exposure in young men living in a malaria area in the Limpopo Province, South Africa. *Journal of Andrology, 28,* 423–434.

57. Akkina, J., Reif, J., Keefe, T., & Bachand, A. (2004). Age at natural menopause and exposure to organochlorine pesticides in Hispanic women. *Journal of Toxicology and Environmental Health. Part A, 67,* 1407–1422.

58. Quaranta, M. G., Porpora, M. G., Mattioli, B., Giordani, L., et al. (2006). Impaired NK cell-mediated cytotoxic activity and cytokine production in patients with endometriosis: A possible role for PCBs and DDE. *Life Sciences, 79,* 491–498.

59. Asawasinsopon, R., Prapamontol, T., Prakobvitayakit, O., et al. (2006). The association between organochlorine and thyroid hormone levels in cord serum: A study from northern Thailand. *Environment International, 32,* 554–559.

60. Donnarumma, L., Pompi, V., Faraci, A., & Conte, E. (2008). Uptake of organochlorine pesticides by zucchini cultivars grown in polluted soils. *Communications in Agricultural and Applied Biological Sciences, 73,* 853–859.

61. Hatcher, J. M., Richardson, J. R., Guillot, T. S., McCormack, A. L., et al. (2007). Dieldrin exposure induces oxidative damage in the mouse nigrostriatal dopamine system. *Experimental Neurology, 204,* 619–630.

62. Richardson, J. R., Caudle, W. M., Wang, M., Dean, E. D., Pennell, K. D., & Miller, G. W. (2006). Developmental exposure to the pesticide dieldrin alters the dopamine system and increases neurotoxicity in an animal model of Parkinson's disease. *FASEB Journal, 20,* 1695–1697.

63. Fleming, L., Mann, J. B., Bean, J., Briggle, T., & Sanchez-Ramos, J. R. (1994). Parkinson's disease and brain levels of organochlorine pesticides. *Annals of Neurology, 36,* 100–103.

64. Rathore, M., Bhatnagar, P., Mathur, D., & Saxena, G. N. (2002). Burden of organochlorine pesticides in blood and its effect on thyroid hormones in women. *The Science of the Total Environment, 295,* 207–215.

65. Fowler, P. A., Abramovich, D. R., Haites, N. E., Cash, P., et al. (2007). Human fetal testis Leydig cell disruption by exposure to the pesticide dieldrin at low concentrations. *Human Reproduction, 22,* 2919–2927.

66. Purdue, M. P., Hoppin, J. A., Blair, A., Dosemeci, M., & Alavanja, M. C. (2007). Occupational exposure to organochlorine insecticides and cancer incidence in the Agricultural Health Study. *International Journal of Cancer, 120,* 642–649.

67. Hoyer, A. P., Grandjean, P., Jorgensen, T., Brock, J. W., & Hartvig, H. B. (1998). Organochlorine exposure and risk of breast cancer. *Lancet, 352,* 1816–1820.

68. Clary, T., & Ritz, B. (2003). Pancreatic cancer mortality and organochlorine pesticide exposure in California, 1989-1996. *American Journal of Industrial Medicine, 43,* 306–313.

69. Pelletier, M., & Girard, D. (2002). Dieldrin induces human neutrophil superoxide production via protein kinase C and tyrosine kinases. *Human and Experimental Toxicology, 21,* 415–420.

70. Genuis, S. J., Lane, K., & Birkholz, D. (2016). Human elimination of organochlorine pesticides: blood, urine, and sweat study. *BioMed Research International, 2016,* 1624643. PubMed PMID: 27800487.

71. Crinnion, W. Unpublished research. Southwest College of Naturopathic Medicine. 2010.

72. Morita, K., Hamamura, K., & Iida, T. (1995). Binding of PCB by several types of dietary fiber in vivo and in vitro. *Fukuoka Igaku Zasshi, 86,* 212–217.

73. Morita, K., Hirakawa, H., Matsueda, T., et al. (1993). Stimulating effect of dietary fiber on fecal excretion of polychlorinated dibenzofuans (PCDF) and polychlorinated dibenzo-p-dioxins (PCDD) in rats. *Fukuoka Igaku Zasshi, 84,* 273–281.

74. Nagayama, J., Takasuga, T., Tsuji, H., et al. (2003). Active elimination of causative PCDFs/DDs congeners of Yusho by one year intake of FEBRA in Japanese people. *Fukuoka Igaku Zasshi, 94,* 118–125.

75. Morita, K., Ogata, M., & Hasegawa, T. (2001). Chlorophyll derived from chlorella inhibits dioxin absorption from the gastrointestinal tract and accelerates dioxin excretion in rats. *Environmental Health Perspectives, 109,* 289–294.

76. Morita, K., Matsueda, T., & Iida, T. (1999). Effect of green vegetables on digestive tract absorption of polychlorinated dibenzo-p-dioxins and polychlorinated dibenzofurans in rats. *Fukuoka Igaku Zaashi, 90,* 171–183.

77. Morita, K., Matsueda, T., Iida, T., & Hasegawa, T. (1999). Chlorella accelerates dioxin excretion in rats. *The Journal of Nutrition, 129,* 1731–1736.

78. Hsu, T. F., Kusumoto, A., Abe, K., et al. (2006). Oolong tea increased fecal fat. *European Journal of Clinical Nutrition, 60*(11), 1330–1336.

21

Organophosphate Pesticides

SUMMARY

- Presence in population: Organophosphate pesticides (OPs) represent approximately 50% of all the insecticide use worldwide, and, with the exception of individuals consuming all organic foods, their metabolites are found ubiquitously
- Major diseases: Suicide, neurotoxicity, cancer, cardiovascular disease, neurodevelopmental issues, decreased IQ in children, increased incidence attention deficit hyperactivity disorder (ADHD)

- Primary sources: Conventionally grown foods, agricultural pesticides
- Best measure: Red blood cell cholinesterase, urinary metabolites
- Best intervention: Atropine plus pralidoxime, antioxidants, organically grown diet

DESCRIPTION

OPs (Fig. 21.1) were first recognized in the early 19th century. After the discovery of the cholinergic effects of OPs, they were developed into nerve gas warfare agents in the 1930s and were first used agriculturally in 1940. When organochlorine insecticides, such as dichlorodiphenyl-trichloroethane (DDT), were banned in the 1970s, organophosphate insecticides became the most commonly used form of insect control.

OPs are some of the most commonly used insecticides around the world in a variety of agricultural and domestic settings. There are approximately 100 known OPs, of which 36 are still registered for use in the United States (Table 21.1). All of them are toxic.

TOXICITY

OPs are acutely neurotoxic at high doses. The type of pesticide, the duration and route of exposure, and the individual's health status are determining factors in the degree of toxicity. Toxicity is usually rated according to the LD_{50} in rats, which roughly differentiates between very toxic (e.g., parathion LD_{50} 13 mg/kg; World Health Organization [WHO]: Class IA) and generally safe (e.g., temephos LD_{50} 8600 mg/kg; WHO: unlikely to cause acute hazard) pesticides.[1] All OPs share a common mechanism of action functioning as acetylcholinesterase (AChE) inhibitors through phosphorylation of the AChE enzyme. By attaching to the serine hydroxyl group on AChE, OPs prevent acetylcholine (ACh) from interacting with the cholinesterase enzyme and being broken down. This leads to accumulation of ACh at the synapses of parasympathetic and myoneural junctions and in the autonomic nervous ganglia, causing muscarinic, nicotinic, and central nervous system (CNS) effects.[2] Because of the elevated concentration of ACh, the brain is initially overstimulated, leading to sensory and behavioral disturbances, incoordination, and depressed motor function. Later, as the end plates depolarize, there is paralysis of neural transmission that eventually impairs the diaphragm and causes respiratory paralysis.

The AChE-phosphate bond is strengthened after the initial exposure in a process known as *aging*. The aging reaction involves the loss of an alkyl group from the phosphoryl adduct bound to the enzyme. Depending on

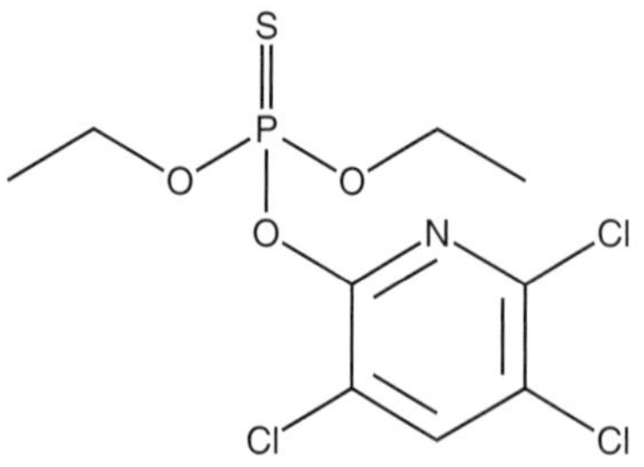

FIG. 21.1 Chlorpyrifos.

the time of aging of the agent, reactivation of the enzyme through dephosphorylation is possible using a compound known as an *oxime.* 2-pyridine aldoxime methyl chloride (2-PAM), or pralidoxime, is currently the only Food and Drug Administration (FDA)-approved oxime in the United States.[3] If pralidoxime is not given within 24 to 48 hours, the antidote may be ineffective, and the AChE-phosphate bond can become strong enough that physiological recovery depends on new synthesis of AChE.[4] Red blood cell AChE levels show 15% to 24% inhibition after a 2-hour organophosphate exposure, with a recovery rate of 4% to 9% per hour.[5] AChE is restored in about 2 weeks, and the whole body can take up to 3 months to fully recover.

In some cases, the onset of toxicity and aging can be delayed. Fenthion and chlorfenthion are fat-soluble organophosphorus compounds that can redistribute from fat stores over time, continuing to inhibit cholinesterase for days.[6] Others, such as parathion and malathion, must first be metabolically converted by CYP450 3A4 into the neurotoxic oxon form. Oxons are more toxic but break down more readily. Dermal exposure may also cause a delay in absorption and onset of cholinesterase inhibition for up to 18 hours.[7]

At low doses, OPs may have a variety of toxic actions, including disruption of nuclear transcription factors that control cell replication, differentiation, and apoptosis[8]; interference with neural cell development and neurotransmitter systems (serotonin and dopamine)[9]; and alteration of synaptic formation.[10,11] Free radical–mediated damage related to pesticide exposure has also been evidenced by an increase of malondialdehyde, protein carbonyl groups, advanced oxidation protein products, glutathione peroxidase, superoxide dismutase, and a decrease in glutathione, Na^+/K^+-ATPase, and vitamin C levels.[12,13]

Toxicity of organophosphates is heightened by the presence of solvents (e.g., toluene, xylene, cyclohexanone) that are common in commercial preparations as "inert ingredients." Neurotoxicity resulting from the combination of solvents and organophosphates can cause axonal and myelin degeneration in distal fibers. For example, human poisoning with dimethoate EC40 (a formula containing cyclohexanone, xylene, a surfactant, and dimethoate) is characterized by respiratory failure, distributive shock, cardiovascular collapse, and neuromuscular dysfunction.[14] The addition of the cyclohexanone solvent is required for toxicity, and when it is absent no neuromuscular toxicity or markedly attenuated cardiotoxicity occur.[15] In addition, cumulative toxicity has demonstrated additive or potentiation effects when two or more organophosphates are absorbed together or when they are combined with other pesticides, including herbicides, carbamates, and pyrethroids.[16,17,18,19]

Carbamate insecticides have similar cholinesterase-inhibiting toxicity; however, they involve reversible carbamylation, not phosphorylation. Carbamate toxicity impairs CNS function and affects muscarinic and nicotinic receptors where the carbamate-cholinesterase bonds spontaneously hydrolyze. Because of this, the half-life is relatively short, inactivating the poison in 1 to 2 hours, with clinical recovery in several hours. Studies have shown that mixed poisonings with organophosphate compounds and carbamates are common, with approximately 35% of poisonings involving mixed exposures.[20]

SOURCES

OPs are mainly used in agriculture. However, organophosphates (triaryl phosphates) are also found in solvents, plasticizers, flame retardants, and extreme pressure additives (e.g., lubricants). The chemical warfare agent sarin gas is also an organophosphate.[21] Occupational exposures primarily occur among agricultural workers, industrial workers, and pest control exterminators. Residential sources include pesticide use by exterminators around homes, individual house and yard use of pesticides, ingestion of conventionally grown fruits and vegetables, accidental exposure, and public areas close to farms.[22] OPs are not as persistent in the environment as organochlorine pesticides; however, OPs cause adverse human health effects. It has been estimated that 80% to 90% of American households use pesticides.[23] One study demonstrated that all children tested in one elementary school in the United States excreted organophosphate metabolites without knowingly having been exposed to OP

TABLE 21.1 Organophosphates, Commercial Products

Highly Toxic[a]	Moderately Toxic[a]	Highly Toxic[a]	Moderately Toxic[a]
Azinphos-methyl (Guthion, Gusathion)	Acephate (Orthene)	Mevinphos (Phosdrin, Duraphos)	Malathion (Cython)
Bomyl (Swat)[b]	Bensulide (Betasan, Prefar)	Mipafox (Isopestox, Pestox, XV)[b]	Merphos (Folex, Easy Off-D)
Carbophenothion (Trithion)	Bromophos-ethyl (Nexagan)[b]	Monocrotophos (Azodrin)	Methyl trithion, dimethoate (Cygon, DeFend)[b]
Chlorfenvinphos (Apachlor, Birlane)	Bromophos (Nexion)[b]	Phorate (Thimet, Rampart, AASTAR)	Naled (Dibrom)
Chlormephos (Dotan)[b]	Chlorphoxim (Baythion-C)[b]	Phosfolan (Cyolane, Cylan)[b]	Oxydemeton-methyl (Metasystox-R)[b]
Chlorthiophos (Celathion)[b]	Chlorpyrifos (Dursban, Lorsban, Brodan)	Phosphamidon (Dimecron)	Oxydeprofos (Metasystox-S)[b,c]
Coumaphos (Co-Ral, Asuntol)	Crotoxyphos (Ciodrin, Cypon)	Prothoate (Fac)[b,c]	Phenkapton (G 28029)[b]
Cyanofenphos (Surecide)	Crufomate (Ruelene)[b]	Schradan (OMPA)[b]	Phenthoate (dimephenthoate)[b]
Demeton (Syntox)[c]	Cyanophos (Cyanox)[b]	Sulfotep (Thiotepp, Bladafum, Dithione)	Phosalone (Zolone)
Dialifor (Torak)	Cythioate (Proban, Cyflee)[b]	Terbufos (Counter, Contraven)	Phosmet (Imidan, Prolate)
Dicrotophos (Bidrin)	DEF (De-Green, E-Z-Off D)	Tetraethyl pyrophosphate (TEPP)[b]	Phoxim (Baythion)[b]
Dimefos (Hanane, Pestox, XIV)[b]	Demetron-S-methyl (Duratox, Metasystox-R)[b]		Primiphos-ethyl (Primicid)[b]
Dioxathion (Delnav)	Diazinon (Spectracide)		Primiphos-methyl (Actellic)
Disulfoton (Disyston)[c]	Dichlofenthion (VC-13, Nemacide)		Profenofos (Curacron)
			Propetamphos (Safrotin)
Endothion[b]	Dichlorvos (DDVP,Vapona)		Propyl thiopyrophosphate (Aspon)[b]
EPN	Edifenphos[b]		Pyrazophos (Afugan, Curamil)[b]
Ethyl parathion (E605, parathion, thiophos)	EPBP (S-Seven)[b]		Pyridaphenthion (Ofunack)[b]
Famphur (Famfos, Bo-Ana, Bash)	Ethion (Ethanox)		Quinalphos (Bayrusil)[b]
Fenamiphos (Nemacur)	Ethoprop (Mocap)		Ronnel (Fenchlorphos, Korlan)
Fenophosphon (trichloronate, Agritox)[b]	Etrimfos (Ekamet)[b]		Sulprofos (Bolstar, Helothion)[b]
Fensulfothion (Dasanit)	Fenitrothion (Accothion, Agrothion, Sumithion)		Temephos (Abate, Abathion)
Fonofos (Dyfonate, N-2790)	Fenthion (mercaptophos, Entex, Baytex, Tiguvon)		Tetrachlorvinphos (Gardona, Apex, Stirofos)
Fosthietan (Nem-A-Tak)	Formothion (Anthio)[b]		Thiometon (Ekatin)[b]
Isofenphos (Amaze, Oftanol)	Heptenophos (Hostaquick)[b]		Triazophos (Hostathion)[b]
Mephosfolan (Cytrolane)[b,c]	IBP (Kitazin)		Trichlorfon (Dylox, Dipterex, Proxol, Neguvon)
Methamidophos (Monitor)	Iodofenphos (Nuvanol-N)[b]		
Methidathion (Supracide, Ultracide)	Isoxathion (E-48, Karphos)[b]		
Methyl parathion (E601, Penncap-M)	Leptophos (Phosvel)[b]		

[a]"Highly toxic" organophosphates have listed oral LD_{50} values (rat) less than 50 mg/kg; "moderately toxic" agents have LD_{50} values in excess of 50 mg/kg and less than 500 mg/kg.

[b]Products no longer registered in the United States.

[c]These organophosphates are systemic; they are taken up by the plant and translocated into foliage and sometimes into the fruit.

compounds.[24] As can be seen in Fig. 21.2, children who eat primarily conventionally grown foods have urine levels of OPs nine times higher than those of children who eat primarily organically grown foods.

BODY BURDEN

Exposure to OPs can be through contact with the skin, ingestion, or inhalation. Systemic absorption varies with the specific agents as well as the route of exposure. The primary route of OP exposure for the general population is through the diet.[25,26] Blood samples can measure red blood cell AChE and plasma butyrylcholinesterase (pseudocholinesterase) levels to determine exposure of

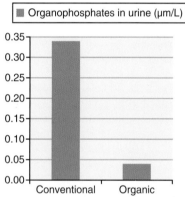

FIG. 21.2 Children who eat conventionally grown foods have nine-times higher body load of organophosphate pesticides. (From Curl, C. L., Fenske, R. A., Elgethun, K. [2003]. Organophosphorus pesticide exposure of urban and suburban preschool children with organic and conventional diets. *Environmental Health Perspectives, 111*, 377–382.)

OPs.[27] Studies have shown that red cell cholinesterase activity is better correlated with the severity of exposure than plasma cholinesterase activity.[28,29]

Levels of the various OP compounds in residents of the United States have been studied as part of the ongoing National Health and Nutritional Examination Survey (NHANES) trial and published by the Centers for Disease Control and Prevention (CDC) in their Exposure Report.[30] Table 21.2 summarizes the organophosphate metabolites findings published in the January 2017 updated tables to the Fourth Report.

Detoxification/Excretion Processes

Breakdown of organophosphates occurs primarily by hydrolysis in the liver. The human paraoxonase gene family has three members, PON1, PON2, and PON3, that function as lactonases/lactonizing enzymes.[31,32] Many organothiophosphates are converted from thions to oxons (arylesters) by cytochrome P-450 systems. Although oxons are more toxic than thions, they break down more readily than thions. PON1 hydrolyzes the toxic oxon metabolites of several OPs, including parathion, diazinon, and chlorpyrifos, producing dialkyl phosphates (DAPs) and phenols.[33] Children younger than 2 years have lower levels of PON1 and are therefore more susceptible to the adverse effects of organophosphates.[34] PON1 is prone to polymorphic changes at positions 55 and 192, which can alter its function dramatically.[35]

Individuals with reduced PON1 function are at increased risk for neurotoxic damage from OPs and can develop neurological disorders that are strongly associated with neuroinflammation.[36] Individuals with either the PON1-192 G/A or G/G polymorphisms (both of which result in reduced activity) were more prone to

TABLE 21.2 **Dialkyl Phosphate Metabolites of Urinary Organophosphate Pesticides (ug/g creatinine)**

Toxicant	Mean	75th %	90th %	95th %
Diethylphosphate (DEP)	*	3.20	8.86	15.7
Dimethylphosphate (DMP)	*	9.10	20.0	33.6
Diethylthiophosphate (DETP)	*	1.24	2.46	3.92
Dimethylthiophosphate (DMTP)	2.34	5.91	17.5	33.7
Diethyldithiophosphate (DEDTP)	*	< LOD	< LOD	< LOD
Dimethyldithiophosphate (DMDTP)	*	< LOD	2.63	6.12

LOD: limit of detection.
* : Not calculated; proportion of results below limit of detection was too high to provide a valid result.
From Centers for Disease Control and Prevention. National Report on Human Exposure to Environmental Chemicals. Retrieved from www.cdc.gov/exposurereport/.

neurotoxic effects of organophosphates than were those with the same exposure who had suffered a traumatic brain injury.[37] Children with low PON1 activity who are residentially exposed to OPs are up to three times more likely to develop brain tumors.[38,39] Although B-cell malignancies are already linked with environmental toxicants, individuals with the PON1-192 G/G (lowest activity) can have a fourfold increased risk of developing lymphoma.[40] Those with the PON1-55 M/M variant who were exposed to organophosphates were more than twice as likely to develop Parkinson's disease.[41] Reduced PON1 activity has also been linked to the development of dementia and Alzheimer's disease.[42,43] In fact, Mini Mental Status Examination results show a positive correlation with paraoxonase activity. Low paraoxonase activity has also been associated with depression and bipolar disorders.[44]

Alkyl phosphates and phenols can often be detected in the urine after pesticide absorption and may be used to identify and quantify the actual pesticide involved in poisonings.[45] Diethyldithiophosphate (DEDTP), diethylthiophosphate (DETP), diethyldiphosphate (DEDP), dimethyldithiophosphate (DMDTP), dimethylthiophosphate (DMTP), and dimethylphosphate (DMP) are the six known DAPs and have longer *in vivo* half-lives and clearance periods than their parent compounds. The excretion of metabolites demonstrates a biphasic reaction and varies based on the compound and level of exposure. One study evaluated the urinary excretion of DAPs in individuals poisoned by quinalphos or chlorpyrifos and found that the urinary metabolite half-life in the fast excretion phase was 5.5 to 53.6 hours for quinalphos and 3.5 to 5.5 hours for chlorpyrifos, and in the slow excretion phase, half-life for both compounds was between 66.5 and 127.9 hours.[46]

Clinical Significance

The typical symptoms associated with acute organophosphate poisoning include salivation, lacrimation, urination, defecation, gastrointestinal upset (e.g., cramps, diarrhea, vomiting), and emesis (SLUDGE). Acute symptoms occur within minutes to hours. Chronic exposure has been linked to several common neurological conditions (see Chapter 42).

Cancer. Non-Hodgkin's lymphoma (NHL) risk is higher in people occupationally exposed to OP compounds.[47] A study of farmers in Nebraska showed organophosphate exposure was significantly associated with NHL risk (OR

= 1.9), and risk increased with days per year of use to OR = 3.1 for 21 or more days.[48] Significantly elevated risks for leukemia have been observed with exposure to specific animal insecticides, including crotoxyphos (OR = 11.1), dichlorvos (OR = 2.0), and famphur (OR = 2.2).[49] There has also been research associating agricultural pesticide use (chlorpyrifos and coumaphos) with an increased risk of glioma.[50] Another study found that pesticide applicators in the highest quartile of chlorpyrifos lifetime exposure days (>56 days) had a relative risk of lung cancer 2.18 times (95% CI, 1.31–3.64) that of those with no exposure.[51]

Cardiovascular System. Cardiac toxicity from acute OP poisoning involves three phases: 1) a period of increased sympathetic tone; 2) a prolonged parasympathetic phase; and 3) Q-T interval prolongation with malignant ventricular arrhythmias of the "torsade de pointes" type and ventricular fibrillation.[52,53] Some possible mechanisms of cardiotoxicity include sympathetic and parasympathetic overactivity, hypoxemia, acidosis, electrolyte derangements, and a direct toxic effect of the compounds on the myocardium.[54,55] Hypertension and sinus tachycardia are nicotinic effects, whereas hypotension and sinus bradycardia are cholinergic manifestations.[56] The incidence of cardiovascular diseases, such as coronary artery disease and congestive heart failure, in cases of OP poisoning has been estimated to be 1.3 times higher than those of non-OP poisoning.[57] Death from cardiovascular effects often occurs as a result of arrhythmias or severe and refractory hypotension.[58,59]

Endocrine Disruption. Evidence is increasing regarding the metabolic effects of organophosphates and their potential effect on obesity and diabetes. Organophosphate-induced interference with the pathway synthesizing cyclic adenosine monophosphate (AMP) during critical developmental periods permanently alters the cellular responses to multiple neurotransmitters, hormones, cytokines, and trophic signals that operate through cyclic (AMP).[60,61] As a result, OPs produce lasting effects on metabolism in a manner consistent with prediabetes-like dysfunction.[62] Although OPs produce diabetes-like effects, each agent may have unique characteristics surrounding circulating insulin, glucose, and lipids. For example, chlorpyrifos impairs glucose homeostasis through increased circulating insulin levels and attendant hyperlipidemia,[63] whereas parathion induces a deficiency in the uptake and utilization of glucose by the cell.[64] Animal studies have shown that subchronic organophosphate exposure, similar to human exposure, can lead to enhanced weight gain and diabetes-like changes in hepatic energy metabolism.[65,66]

Developmental Neurotoxicity. Data in laboratory animals suggests that exposures to OPs during pregnancy or early life can impair fetal growth and neurocognitive development in the offspring.[67] CNS damage may be aggravated through noncholinergic mechanisms that involve alterations in the expression and function of nuclear transcription factors that control cell replication, differentiation, and apoptosis.[68] Chlorpyrifos administered to developing rats, in doses that do not evoke signs of overt toxicity, decreases DNA synthesis and elicits damage from early stages of neural cell replication through late stages of axonogenesis and terminal differentiation.[69] OP exposure has been negatively associated with several cognitive and behavioral conditions in human children, including lowered IQ,[70,71] ADHD,[72,73] impaired social functioning,[74] and pervasive developmental disorder.[75] Children born to mothers in the top 20% of organophosphate levels have a 7.0 lower IQ compared with children born to mothers in the lowest 20% of body load, even after correcting for psychosocial factors.[76]

Neuropathy. Neurological symptoms of OP poisoning are several and occur at various times postexposure. Weakness, fasciculations, cramps, and twitching occur acutely. Once the cholinergic phase has settled down, paralysis of limb muscles, neck flexors, motor cranial nerves, and respiratory muscles occurs 24 to 96 hours after poisoning and lasts up to 18 days.[77] Symptoms of delayed polyneuropathy typically occur 1 to 4 weeks after acute organophosphate exposure and are characterized by distal degeneration of axons of both the peripheral and central nervous systems.[78] Early signs are paresthesias, which then progress to weakness, ataxia, gait changes, or flaccid paralysis. An etiological attribute of delayed polyneuropathy is believed to be the inhibition of neuropathy target esterase (NTE), which can be inhibited by phosphates, phosphonates, and phosphoramidates when more than 70% of the enzyme is inhibited.[79] A study of pesticide applicators working with chlorpyrifos found that they did not perform as well with pegboard and postural sway tests and reported significantly more problems with memory, emotional states, fatigue, and loss of muscle strength.[80] Weakness of specific muscle groups at sites of dermal exposure, cranial nerve palsies,[81]

supranuclear gaze palsy,[82] laryngeal paralysis,[83] and diaphragmatic paralysis have all been reported after OP exposure.[84] Box 21.1 provides a complete list of neurological manifestations of OP poisoning.

Suicide. Pesticide self-poisoning is a major health problem, accounting for approximately one-third of the world's suicides.[85] Self-poisoning with organophosphate insecticides is responsible for more than two-thirds of the 250,000 to 370,000 pesticide-related deaths per year.[86,87] A World Health Organization (WHO) task group estimated that there may be one million serious unintentional poisonings each year and an additional two million people hospitalized for suicide attempts with pesticides.[88]

INTERVENTION

Acute exposure is typically treated using a combination of pralidoxime chloride and atropine. Atropine is an anticholinergic medication and, more specifically, an antimuscarinic agent. The therapeutic action of atropine results from its binding with the synaptic receptor replacing ACh, and therefore blocking synaptic transmission.[89] Atropine antagonizes the muscarinic-like actions of ACh on structures innervated by postganglionic cholinergic nerves and on smooth muscles that respond to endogenous ACh (e.g., exocrine glands, cardiac muscle). 2-PAM or pralidoxime is attracted to the anionic site of AChE where it reacts with and removes the cholinesterase inhibitor. Atropine and 2-PAM are synergistic in their effects, and the effectiveness of atropine plus 2-PAM is 35 times greater than with atropine alone.[90]

Considering that the main route of OP exposure for the general population is through the diet, direct action can be taken to reduce exposure by consuming organic foods. In a study of adults consuming a mostly organic diet for 7 days, urinary DAP levels decreased by nearly 90%, suggesting that not only is there greater dietary exposure to OP pesticides from conventionally produced foods, but that the majority of ingested OP pesticides are metabolized and excreted within a week of ingestion.[91] Studies in children have demonstrated significant and immediate reductions in OP exposure after consuming an organic diet for as little as 5 days.[25,92,93] Consumption of organic fruits, vegetables, and juice can reduce children's exposure levels from above to below the US Environmental Protection Agency's current guidelines into a range of negligible risk.[94]

BOX 21.1   Neurological Manifestations of Organophosphate Poisoning

Paralysis
- Acute paralysis
- Intermediate paralysis syndrome
- Organophosphate induced delayed polyneuropathy
- Localized permanent paralysis
- Diaphragmatic paralysis
- Laryngeal paralysis
- Cranial nerve palsy
- Supranuclear gaze palsy

Impaired Consciousness
- Unconsciousness
- Coma
- Delayed onset organophosphate induced encephalopathy

Neuropsychiatric
- Impaired memory
- Confusion
- Irritability
- Lethargy
- Psychoses

Extra-Pyramidal
- Dystonia
- Resting tremor

- Cog-wheel rigidity
- Chorea
- Bradykinesia

Ocular
- Supranuclear gaze palsy
- Optic neuropathy
- Retinal degeneration
- Myopia
- Cortical visual loss

Ataxia
- Early onset, self-limiting
- Delayed neurotoxic ataxia

Other
- Fasciculations
- Convulsions
- Delirium
- Guillain-Barre syndrome
- Sphincter involvement
- Ototoxicity

Data from Peter, J. V., Sudarsan, T. I., Moran, J. L. (2014). Clinical features of organophosphate poisoning: a review of different classification systems and approaches. *Indian Journal of Critical Care Medicine*, 18(11), 735–745. PubMed PMID: 25425841.

Studies have shown many benefits in using nutraceuticals for the treatment of OP poisoning. In chlorpyrifos-treated rats, zinc protected hepatocytes from the disruptions in the membranous organelles and narrowing and blocking of biliary channels that typically occurs as a result of chlorpyrifos exposure.[95] Zinc treatment also improved total leukocyte, neutrophil, and lymphocyte counts in OP-poisoned animals[96] and increased levels of glutathione, catalase, and glutathione-S-transferase.[97]

Organophosphates increase free radical production. Several natural antioxidants have proven to be effective in mitigating the damage from OP poisoning. Lycopene has shown a protective effect by neutralizing the decreased antioxidant enzyme activity and increased reactive oxygen species formation caused by organophosphate toxicity.[98,99] Ellagic acid,[100] propolis,[101,102] boron,[103] vitamin C,[104,105] vitamin E/selenium,[106] and vitamin E/curcumin[107] have also shown protective effects against OP-induced oxidative stress.

REFERENCES

1. WHO. (2001). *WHO recommended classification of pesticides by hazard and guidelines to classification 2000-2001*. WHO/PCS/01.4. World Health Organization; Geneva.
2. Wadia, R. S., Sadagopan, C., Amin, R. B., & Sardesai, H. V. (1974). Neurological manifestations of organophophorous insecticide poisoning. *Journal of Neurology, Neurosurgery, and Psychiatry, 37*(7), 841–847. PubMed PMID: 4853328.
3. Agency for Toxic Substances and Disease Registry. (2007 Oct 16). *Cholinesterase inhibitors: including insecticides and chemical warfare nerve agents Part 4- Section 11 Management strategy3: medications 2-PAM (2-pyridine aldoxime methylchloride)*

(pralidoxime). https://www.atsdr.cdc.gov/csem/
csem.asp?csem=11&po=23. (Accessed 30 March 2017).

4. Taylor, P. (1985). Anticholinesterase agents. In A. G.
Gilman & L. S. Goodman (Eds.), *The pharmacological
basis of therapeutics* (pp. 110–128). New York:
Macmillian Publishing Co, Inc.

5. He, F., Chen, S., Tang, X., Gan, W., Tao, B., & Wen, B.
(2002). Biological monitoring of combined exposure
to organophosphates and pyrethroids. *Toxicology
Letters*, *134*, 119–124.

6. Howland, M. S. (2002). Antidotes in depth:
pralidoxime. In L. R. Glodfrank, N. E. Flomenbaum,
N. A. Leni, et al. (Eds.), *Glodfrank's toxicological
emergencies* (pp. 1361–1365). New York: McGraw Hill.

7. Sidell, F. R. (1997). Nerve ahents. In F. R. Sidell, E.
T. Takafuji, & D. R. Franz (Eds.), *Medical aspects of
chemical and biological wrfare* (pp. 129–179). Falls
Church, Virginia: Office of the Surgeon General,
United States Army.

8. Dam, K., Seidler, F. J., & Slotkin, T. A. (2003).
Transcriptional biomarkers distinguish between
vulnerable periods for developmental neurotoxicity of
chlorpyrifos: implications for toxicogenomics. *Brain
Research Bulletin*, *59*(4), 261–265. PubMed PMID:
12464398.

9. Aldridge, J. E., Meyer, A., Seidler, F. J., & Slotkin,
T. A. (2005). Alterations in central nervous system
serotonergic and dopaminergic synaptic activity in
adulthood after prenatal or neonatal chlorpyrifos
exposure. *Environmental Health Perspectives*, *113*(8),
1027–1031. PubMed PMID: 16079074.

10. Slotkin, T. A., Cousins, M. M., Tate, C. A., & Seidler,
F. J. (2001). Persistent cholinergic presynaptic deficits
after neonatal chlorpyrifos exposure. *Brain Research*,
902(2), 229–243. PubMed PMID: 11384617.

11. Qiao, D., Seidler, F. J., Tate, C. A., Cousins, M.
M., & Slotkin, T. A. (2003). Fetal chlorpyrifos
exposure: adverse effects on brain cell development
and cholinergic biomarkers emerge postnatally
and continue into adolescence and adulthood.
Environmental Health Perspectives, *111*(4), 536–544.
PubMed PMID: 12676612.

12. Amara, I. B., Soudani, N., Troudi, A., Hakim, A.,
et al. (2012). Dimethoate induced oxidative damage
and histopathological changes in lung of adult rats:
modulatory effects of selenium and/or vitamin E.
Biomedical and Environmental Sciences, *25*(3), 340–351.
PubMed PMID: 22840586.

13. Ben Amara, I., Soudani, N., Hakim, A., Bouaziz,
H., Troudi, A., Zeghal, K. M., et al. (2012).
Dimethoate-induced oxidative damage in erythrocytes
of female adult rats: possible protective effect of

vitamin E and selenium supplemented to diet.
Toxicology and Industrial Health, *28*(3), 222–237.
PubMed PMID: 21976143.

14. Eddleston, M., Eyer, P., Worek, F., Mohamed, F.,
Senarathna, L., et al. (2005). Differences between
organophosphorous insecticides, in human
self-poisoning: a prospective cohort study. *Lancet*,
366(9495), 1452–1459. PubMed PMID: 16243090.

15. Eddleston, M., Street, J. M., Self, I., Thompson, A.,
King, T., et al. (2012). A role for solvents in the
toxicity of agricultural organophosphorous pesticides.
Toxicology, *294*(2–3), 94–103. PubMed PMID:
22365945.

16. Scholz, N. L., Truelove, N. K., Labenia, J. S., Baldwin,
D. H., & Collier, T. K. (2006). Dose-additive inhibition
of chinook salmon acetylcholinesterase activity
by mixtures of organophosphate and carbamate
insecticides. *Environmental Toxicology and Chemistry*,
25(5), 1200–1207. PubMed PMID: 16704049.

17. Axelrad, J. C., Howard, C. V., & McLean, W. G. (2002).
Interactions between pesticides and components of
pesticide formulations in an in vitro neurotoxicity test.
Toxicology, *173*(3), 259–269. PubMed PMID: 11960678.

18. Ahmad, M. (2007). Potentiation/antagonism of
pyrethroids with organophosphate insecticides in
Bemisia tabaci (Homoptera: Aleyrodidae). *Journal
of Economic Entomology*, *100*(3), 886–893. PubMed
PMID: 17598552.

19. Costa, L. G., & Murphy, S. D. (1983). Unidirectional
cross-tolerance between the carbamate insecticide
propoxur and the organophosphate disulfoton in mice.
Fundamental and Applied Toxicology, *3*(5), 483–488.
PubMed PMID: 6642106.

20. Carlton, F. B., Simpson, W. M., et al. (1998). Pesticides.
In L. M. Haddad, M. W. Shannon, & J. F. Winchester
(Eds.), *Clinical management of poisoning and drug
overdose* (pp. 836–845). Philadelphia: WB Saunders
Company.

21. Wikipedia. *Sarin*. Available at https://en.wikipedia.org/
wiki/Sarin. (Accessed 20 April 2017).

22. Jaga, K., & Dharmani, C. (2003). Sources of exposure
to and public health implications of organophosphate
pesticides. *Revista Panamericana de Salud Publica*,
14(3), 171–185. PubMed PMID: 14653904.

23. Landrigan, P. J., Claudio, L., Markowitz, S. B.,
Berkowitz, G. S., et al. (1999). Pesticides and
inner-city children: exposures, risks, and prevention.
Environmental Health Perspectives, *107*(Suppl. 3),
431–437. PubMed PMID: 10346991.

24. Duggan, A., Charnley, G., Chen, W., Chukwudebe,
A., Hawk, R., Krieger, R. I., et al. (2003). Di-alkyl
phosphate biomonitoring data: assessing cumulative

exposure to organophosphate pesticides. *Regulatory Toxicology and Pharmacology*, 37(3), 382–395. PubMed PMID: 12758218.

25. Wilson, N. K., Chuang, J. C., Lyu, C., Menton, R., & Morgan, M. K. (2003). Aggregate exposures of nine preschool children to persistent organic pollutants at day care and at home. *Journal of Exposure Analysis and Environmental Epidemiology*, 13(3), 187–202. PubMed PMID: 12743613.

26. Lu, C., Barr, D. B., Pearson, M. A., & Waller, L. A. (2008). Dietary intake and its contribution to longitudinal organophosphorous pesticide exposure in urban/suburban children. *Environmental Health Perspectives*, 116(4), 537–542. PubMed PMID: 18414640.

27. Eddleston, M., Buckley, N. A., Eyer, P., & Dawson, A. H. (2008). Management of acute organophosphorous pesticide poisoning. *Lancet*, 371(9612), 597–607. PubMed PMID: 17706760.

28. Bobba, R., Venkataraman, B. V., Pais, P., & Joseph, T. (1996). Correlation between the severity of symptoms in prganophosphorous poisoning and cholinesterase activity (RBC and plasma) in humans. *Indian Journal of Physiology and Pharmacology*, 40(3), 249–252. PubMed PMID: 8950142.

29. Brahmi, N., Mokline, A., Kouraichi, N., Ghorbel, H., et al. (2006). Prognostic value of human erythrocyte acetylcholinesterase in acute organophosphate poisoning. *The American Journal of Emergency Medicine*, 24(7), 822–827. PubMed PMID: 17098105.

30. Centers for Disease Control and Prevention. (2017). *National Report on Human Exposure to Environmental Chemicals: Updated tables*. Available at www.cdc.gov/exposurereport/. (Accessed 30 April 2017).

31. Primo-Parmo, S. L., Sorenson, R. C., Teiber, J., & La Du, B. N. (1996). The human serum paraoxonase/arylesterase gene (PON1) in one member of a multigene family. *Genomics*, 33, 498–507. PubMed PMID: 8661009.

32. Draganov, D. I. (2010). Lactonases with organophosphatase activity: structural and evolutionary perspectives. *Chemico-Biological Interactions*, 187(1–3), 370–372. PubMed PMID: 20122908.

33. Davies, H. G., Richter, R. J., Keifer, M., Broomfield, C. A., Sowalla, J., & Furlong, C. E. (1996). The effect of the human serum paraoxonase polymorphism is reversed with diazoxon, soman and sarin. *Nature Genetics*, 14(3), 334–336. PubMed PMID: 8896566.

34. Echobichon, J. D., & Stephens, D. S. (1973). Perinatal development of human blood esterases. *Clinical Pharmacology and Therapeutics*, 14(10), 41–47. PubMed PMID: 4734200.

35. Searles Nielsen, S., Mueller, B. A., De Roos, A. J., Viernes, H. M., Farin, F. M., & Checkoway, H. (2005). Risk of brain tumors in children and susceptibility to organophosphorus insecticides: the potential role of paraoxonase (PON1). *Environmental Health Perspectives*, 113(7), 909–913. PubMed PMID: 16002382.

36. Costa, L. G., Giordano, G., Cole, T. B., Marsillach, J., & Furlong, C. E. (2013). Paraoxonase 1 (PON1) as a genetic determinant of susceptibility to organophosphate toxicity. *Toxicology*, 307, 115–122. PubMed PMID: 22884923.

37. Lee, B. W., London, L., Paulauskis, J., Myers, J., & Christiani, D. C. (2003). Association between human paraoxonase gene polymorphism and chronic symptoms in pesticide-exposed workers. *Journal of Occupational and Environmental Medicine*, 45(2), 118–122. PubMed PMID: 12625227.

38. Searles Nielsen, S., Mueller, B. A., De Roos, A. J., Viernes, H. M., Farin, F. M., & Checkoway, H. (2005). Risk of brain tumors in children and susceptibility to organophosphorus insecticides: the potential role of paraoxonase (PON1). *Environmental Health Perspectives*, 113(7), 909–913. PubMed PMID: 16002382.

39. Searles Nielsen, S., McKean-Cowdin, R., Farin, F. M., Holly, E. A., Preston-Martin, S., & Mueller, B. A. (2010). Childhood brain tumors, residential insecticide exposure, and pesticide metabolism genes. *Environmental Health Perspectives*, 118(1), 144–149. PubMed PMID: 20056567.

40. Conesa-Zamora, P., Ruiz-Cosano, J., Torres-Moreno, D., Español, I., Gutiérrez-Meca, M. D., Trujillo-Santos, J., et al. (2013). Polymorphisms in xenobiotic metabolizing genes (EPHX1, NQO1 and PON1) in lymphoma susceptibility: a case control study. *BMC Cancer*, 13, 228. PubMed PMID: 23651475.

41. Manthripragada, A. D., Costello, S., Cockburn, M. G., Bronstein, J. M., & Ritz, B. (2010). Paraoxonase 1, agricultural organophosphate exposure, and Parkinson disease. *Epidemiology (Cambridge, Mass.)*, 21(1), 87–94. PubMed PMID: 19907334.

42. Wehr, H., Bednarska-Makaruk, M., Graban, A., Lipczyńska-Łojkowska, W., Rodo, M., Bochyńska, A., et al. (2009). Paraoxonase activity and dementia. *Journal of the Neurological Sciences*, 283(1–2), 107–108. PubMed PMID: 19268306.

43. Bednarska-Makaruk, M. E., Krzywkowski, T., Graban, A., Lipczyńska-Łojkowska, W., Bochyńska, A., Rodo, M., et al. (2013). Paraoxonase 1 (PON1) gene-108C>T and p.Q192R polymorphisms and arylesterase activity of the enzyme in patients with dementia. *Folia*

Neuropathologica, 51(2), 111–119. PubMed PMID: 23821382.

44. Bortolasci, C. C., Vargas, H. O., Souza-Nogueira, A., Barbosa, D. S., Moreira, E. G., Nunes, S. O., et al. (2014). Lowered plasma paraoxonase (PON)1 activity is a trait marker of major depression and PON1 Q192R gene polymorphism-smoking interactions differentially predict the odds of major depression and bipolar disorder. *Journal of Affective Disorders, 159*, 23–30. PubMed PMID: 24679385.

45. Davies, J. E., & Peterson, J. C. (1997). Surveillance of occupational, accidental, and incidental exposure to organophosphate pesticides using urine alkyl phosphate and phenolic metabolite measurements. *Annals of the New York Academy of Scien, 837*, 257–268. PubMed PMID: 9472345.

46. Vasilic, Z., Drevenkar, V., Rumenjak, V., Stengl, B., & Frobe, Z. (1992). Urinary excretion of diethylphosphorous metabolites in persons poisoned by quinalphos or chlorpyrifos. *Archives of Environmental Contamination and Toxicology, 22*, 351–357. PubMed PMID: 1375016.

47. Waddell, B. L., Zahm, S. H., Baris, D., Weisenburger, D. D., Holmes, F., Burmeister, L. F., et al. (2001). Agricultural use of organophosphate pesticides and the risk of non-Hodgkin's lymphoma among male farmers (United States). *Cancer Causes and Control, 12*(6), 509–517. PubMed PMID: 11519759.

48. Zahm, S. H., Weisenburger, D. D., Babbitt, R. C., Saal, R. C., Cantor, K. P., & Blair, A. (1988). A case-control study of non-Hodgkin's lymphoma and agricultural factors in Eastern Nebraska. *American Journal of Epidemiology, 128*, 901.

49. Brown, L. M., Blair, A., Gibson, R., Everett, G. D., Cantor, K. P., Schuman, L. M., et al. (1990). Pesticide exposure and other agricultural risk factors for leukemia among men in Iowa and Minnesota. *Cancer Research, 50*(20), 6585–6591. PubMed PMID: 2208120.

50. Lee, W. J., Colt, J. S., Heineman, E. F., McComb, R., Weisenburger, D. D., Lijinsky, W., et al. (2005). Agricultural pesticide use and risk of glioma in Nebraska, United States. *Occupational and Environmental Medicine, 62*(11), 786–792. PubMed PMID: 16234405.

51. Lee, W. J., Blair, A., Hoppin, J. A., Lubin, J. H., Rusiecki, J. A., Sandler, D. P., et al. (2004). Cancer incidence among pesticide applicators exposed to chlorpyrifos in the Agricultural Health Study. *Journal of the National Cancer Institute, 96*(23), 1781–1789. PubMed PMID: 15572760.

52. Karki, P., Ansari, J. A., Bhandary, S., & Koirala, S. (2004). Cardiac and electrocardiographical manifestations of acute organoposphate poisoning. *Singapore Medical Journal, 45*(8), 385–389. PubMed PMID: 15284933.

53. Ludomirsky, A., Klein, H. O., Sarelli, P., Becker, B., Hoffman, S., et al. (1982). Q-T prolongation and polymorphous ("torsade de pointes") ventricular arrhythmias associated with organophosphorous insecticide poisoning. *American Journal of Cardiology, 49*(7), 1654–1658. PubMed PMID: 7081053.

54. Velmurugan, G., Venkatesh Babu, D. D., & Ramasamy, S. (2013). Prolonged monocrotophos intake induces cardiac oxidative stress and myocardial damage in rats. *Toxicology, 307*, 103–108. PubMed PMID: 23228476.

55. Lyzhnikov, E. A., Savina, A. S., & Shepelev, V. M. (1975). Pathogenesis of disorders of cardiac rhythm and conductivity in acute organophosphate insecticide poisoning. *Kardiologiia, 15*(9), 126–129. PubMed PMID: 1230517.

56. Lovejoy, F. H., & Linden, C. (1991). Acute poison and drug over dosage. In *Harrison's priniciples of internal medicine* (12th ed., p. 2178). New York: McGraw-Hill.

57. Hung, D. Z., Yang, H. J., Li, Y. F., Lin, C. L., et al. (2015). The long-term effects of organophosphates poisoning as a risk factor of CVDs: a nationwide population-based cohort study. *PLoS ONE, 10*(9), e0137632. PubMed PMID: 26339906.

58. Davies, J., Roberts, D., Eyer, P., Buckley, N., & Eddleston, M. (2008). Hypotension in severe dimethoate self-poisoning. *Clinical Toxicology (Philadelphia, Pa.), 46*(9), 880–884. PubMed PMID: 19003596.

59. Chacko, J., & Elangovan, A. (2010). Late onset, prolonged asystole following organophosphate poisoning: a case report. *Journal of Medical Toxicology, 6*(3), 311–314. PubMed PMID: 20532843.

60. Adigun, A. A., Seidler, F. J., & Slotkin, T. A. (2010). Disparate developmental neurotoxicants converge on the cyclic AMP signaling cascade, revealed by transcriptional profiles in vitro and in vivo. *Brain Research, 1316*, 1–16. PubMed PMID: 20026089.

61. Adigun, A. A., Ryde, I. T., Seidler, F. J., & Slotkin, T. A. (2010). Organophosphate exposure during a critical developmental stage reprograms adenylyl cyclase signaling in PC12 cells. *Brain Research, 1329*, 36–44. PubMed PMID: 20298678.

62. Adigun, A. A., Wrench, N., Seidler, F. J., & Slotkin, T. A. (2010). Neonatal organophosphorous pesticide exposure alters the developmental trajectory of cell-signaling cascades controlling metabolism: differential effects of diazinon and parathion. *Environmental Health Perspectives, 118*(2), 210–215. PubMed PMID: 20123610.

63. Slotkin, T. A., Brown, K. K., & Seidler, F. J. (2005). Developmental exposure of rats to chlorpyrifos elicits sex-selective hyperlipidemia and hyperinsulinemia in adulthood. *Environmental Health Perspectives*, *113*(10), 1291–1294. PubMed PMID: 16203236.

64. Lassiter, T. L., Ryde, I. T., Mackillop, E. A., Brown, K. K., Levin, E. D., Seidler, F. J., et al. (2008). Exposure of neonatal rats to parathion elicits sex-selective reprogramming of metabolism and alters the response to a high-fat diet in adulthood. *Environmental Health Perspectives*, *116*(11), 1456–1462. PubMed PMID: 19057696.

65. Meggs, W. J., & Brewer, K. L. (2007). Weight gain associated with chronic exposure to chlorpyrifos in rats. *Journal of Medical Toxicology*, *3*(3), 89–93. PubMed PMID: 18072142.

66. Abdollahi, M., Donyavi, M., Pourmourmohammadi, S., & Saadat, M. (2004). Hyperglycemia associated with increased hepatic glycogen phosphorylase and phosphoenolpyruvate carboxykinase in rats following subchronic exposure to malathion. *Comparative Biochemistry and Physiology. Toxicology and Pharmacology*, *137*(4), 343–347. PubMed PMID: 15228952.

67. Eskenazi, B., Bradman, A., & Castorina, R. (1999). Exposures of children to organophosphate pesticides and their potential adverse health effects. *Environmental Health Perspectives*, *107*(Suppl. 3), 409–419. PubMed PMID: 10346990.

68. Dam, K., Seidler, F. J., & Slotkin, T. A. (2005). Transcriptional biomarkers distinguish between vulnerable periods for developmental neurotoxicity of chlorpyrifos: implications for toxicogenomics. *Brain Research Bulletin*, *59*(4), 261–265. PubMed PMID: 12464398.

69. Slotkin, T. A. (1999). Developmental cholinotoxicants: nicotine and chlorpyrifos. *Environmental Health Perspectives*, *107*(Suppl. 1), 71–80. PubMed PMID: 10229709.

70. Rauh, V., Arunajadai, S., Horton, M., Perera, F., Hoepner, L., Barr, D. B., et al. (2011). Seven-year neurodevelopmental scores and prenatal exposure to chlorpyrifos, a common agricultural pesticide. *Environmental Health Perspectives*, *119*(8), 1196–1201. PubMed PMID: 21507777.

71. Bouchard, M. F., Chevrier, J., Harley, K. G., Kogut, K., et al. (2011). Prenatal exposure to organophosphate pesticides and IQ in 7-year-old children. *Environmental Health Perspectives*, *119*(8), 1189–1195. PubMed PMID: 21507776.

72. Marks, A. R., Harley, K., Bradman, A., Kogut, K., et al. (2010). Organophosphate pesticide exposure and attention in young Mexican-American children: the CHAMACOS study. *Environmental Health Perspectives*, *118*(12), 1768–1774. PubMed PMID: 21126939.

73. Rauh, V. A., Garfinkel, R., Perera, F. P., Andrews, H. F., et al. (2006). Impact of prenatal chlorpyrifos exposure on neurodevelopment in the first 3 years of life among inner-city children. *Pediatrics*, *118*(6), e1845–e1859. PubMed PMID:17116700.

74. Furlong, M. A., Engel, S. M., Barr, D. B., & Wolff, M. S. (2014). Prenatal exposure to organophosphate pesticides and reciprocal social behavior in childhood. *Environment International*, *70*, 125–131. PubMed PMID: 24934853.

75. Eskenazi, B., Marks, A. R., Bradman, A., Harley, K., et al. (2007). Organophosphate pesticide exposure and neurodevelopment in young Mexican-American children. *Environmental Health Perspectives*, *115*(5), 792–798. PubMed PMID: 17520070.

76. Bouchard, M. F., Chevrier, J., Harley, K. G., et al. (2011). Prenatal Exposure to Organophosphate Pesticides and IQ in 7-Year Old Children. *Environmental Health Perspectives*, *119*(8), 1189–1195.

77. Senanayake, N., & Karalliedde, L. (1987). Neurotoxic effects of organophosphorous insecticides. An intermediate syndrome. *The New England Journal of Medicine*, *316*(13), 761–763. PubMed PMID: 3029588.

78. Lotti, M., & Moretto, A. (2005). Organophosphate-induced delayed polyneuropathy. *Toxicological Reviews*, *24*(1), 37–49. PubMed PMID: 16042503.

79. Jokanovic, M., Stukalov, P. V., & Kosanovic, M. (2002). Organophosphate induced delayed polyneuropathy. *Current Drug Targets. CNS and Neurological Disorders*, *1*(6), 593–602. PubMed PMID: 12769600.

80. Steenland, K., Dick, R. B., Howell, R. J., Chrislip, D. W., Hines, C. J., Reid, T., et al. (2000). Neurologic function among termiticide applicators exposed to chlorpyriphos. *Environmental Health Perspectives*, *108*(4), 293–300. PubMed PMID: 10753086.

81. Narendra, J., Chethankmar, J. G., & Rao, B. B. (1989). Cranial nerve palsies in organophosphorous poisoning. *The Journal of the Association of Physicians of India*, *37*(11), 732–733. PubMed PMID: 2632551.

82. Liang, T. W., Balcer, L. J., Solomon, D., Messe, S. R., & Galetta, S. L. (2003). Supranuclear gaze palsy and opsoclonus after Diazinon poisoning. *Journal of Neurology, Neurosurgery, and Psychiatry*, *74*(5), 677–679. PubMed PMID: 12700320.

83. Indudharan, R., Win, M. N., & Noor, A. R. (1998). Laryngeal paralysis in organophosphorous poisoning. *The Journal of Laryngology and Otology*, *112*(1), 81–82. PubMed PMID: 9538454.

84. Rivett, K., & Potgieter, P. D. (1987). Diaphragmatic paralysis after organophosphate poisoning. A case report. *South African Medical Journal, 72*(12), 881–882. PubMed PMID: 3424038.

85. Eddleston, M., & Phillips, M. R. (2004). Self-poisoning with pesticides. *BMJ (Clinical Research Ed.), 328*(7430), 42–44. PubMed PMID: 14703547.

86. Gunnell, D., Eddleston, M., Phillips, M. R., & Konradsen, F. (2007). The global distribution of fatal pesticide self-poisoning: systematic review. *BMC Public Health, 7*, 357. PubMed PMID: 18154668.

87. Eddleston, M. (2000). Patterns and problems of deliberate self-poisoning in the developing world. *QJM: Monthly Journal of the Association of Physicians, 93*(11), 715–731. PubMed PMID: 11077028.

88. Jeyaratnam, J. (1990). Acute pesticide poisoning: a major global health problem. *World Health Statistics Quarterly, 43*(3), 139–144. PubMed PMID: 2238694.

89. Namba, T. (1971). Cholinesterase inhibition by organophosphorus compunds and its clinical effects. *Bulletin of the World Health Organization, 44*(1-2-3), 289–307. PubMed PMID: 4941660.

90. O-Leary, J. F., Kunkel, A. M., et al. (1996). Efficacy and limitations of oxime-atropine treatment of arganophosphorous anticholinesterase poisoning. *The Journal of Pharmacology and Experimental Therapeutics, 132*, 50–57.

91. Oates, L., Cohen, M., Braun, L., Schembri, A., & Taskova, R. (2014). Reduction in urinary organophosphate pesticide metabolites in adults after a week-long organic diet. *Environmental Research, 132*, 105–111. PubMed PMID: 24769399.

92. Lu, C., Toepel, K., Irish, R., Fenske, R. A., Barr, D. B., & Bravo, R. (2006). Organic diets significantly lower children's dietary exposure to organophosphorous pesticides. *Environmental Health Perspectives, 114*(2), 260–263. PubMed PMID: 16451864.

93. Bradman, A., Quiros-Alcala, L., Castorina, R., et al. (2015). Effect of organic diet intervention on pesticide exposures in young children living in low-income urban and agricultural communities. *Environmental Health Perspectives, 123*(10), 1086–1093. PubMed PMID: 25861095.

94. Curl, C. L., Fenske, R. A., & Elgethun, K. (2003). Organophosphorous pesticide exposure of urban and suburban preschool children with organic and conventional diets. *Environmental Health Perspectives, 111*(3), 377–382. PubMed PMID: 12611667.

95. Goel, A., & Dhawan, D. K. (2001). Zinc supplementation prevents liver injury in chlorpyrifos-treated rats. *Biological Trace Element Research, 82*(1–3), 185–200. PubMed PMID: 11697766.

96. Goel, A., Dani, V., & Dhawan, D. K. (2006). Role of zinc in mitigating the toxic effects of chlorpyrifos on hematological alterations and electron microscopic observations in rat blood. *Biometals: An International Journal on the Role of Metal Ions in Biology, Biochemistry, and Medicine, 19*(5), 483–492. PubMed PMID: 16937254.

97. Goel, A., Dani, V., & Dhawan, D. K. (2005). Protective effects of zinc on lipid peroxidation, antioxidant enzymes and hepatic histoarchitecture in chlopyrifos-induced toxicity. *Chemico-Biological Interactions, 156*(2–3), 131–140. PubMed PMID: 16169541.

98. Ural, M. S. (2013). Chlopyrifos-induced changes in oxidant/antioxidant status and haematological parameters of Cyprinus carpio carpio: ameliorative effect of lycopene. *Chemosphere, 90*(7), 2059–2064. PubMed PMID: 23312461.

99. Yonar, S. M. (2013). Toxic effects of malathion in carp, Cyprinus carpio carpio: protective role of lycopene. *Ecotoxicology and Environmental Safety, 97*, 223–229. PubMed PMID: 23932509.

100. Ural, M. S., Yonar, M. E., & Mise Yonar, S. (2015). Protective effect of ellagic acid on oxidative stress and antioxidant status in Cyprinus carpio carpio during malathion exposure. *Cellular and Molecular Biology (Noisy-Le-Grand, France), 61*(5), 58–63. PubMed PMID: 26516111.

101. Enis Yonar, M., Yonar, S. M., Ural, M. S., Silici, S., & Dusukcan, M. (2012). Protective role of propolis in chlorpyrifos-induced changes in the haematological parameters and the oxidative/antioxidative status of Cyprinus carpio carpio. *Food and Chemical Toxicology : An International Journal Published for the British Industrial Biological Research Association, 50*(8), 2703–2708. PubMed PMID: 22634289.

102. Yonar, S. M., Ural, M. S., Silici, S., & Yonar, M. E. (2014). Malathion-induced changes in the haematological profile, the immune response, and the oxidative/antioxidant status of Cyprinus carpio carpio: protective role of propolis. *Ecotoxicology and Environmental Safety, 102*, 202–209. PubMed PMID: 24480596.

103. Coban, F. K., Ince, S., Kucukkurt, I., Demirel, H. H., & Hazman, O. (2015). Boron attenuates malathion-induced oxidative stress and acethycholinesterase inhibition in rats. *Drug and Chemical Toxicology, 38*(4), 391–399. PubMed PMID: 25342379.

104. Eroglu, S., Pandir, D., Uzun, F. G., & Bas, H. (2013). Protective role of vitamins C and E in dichlorvos-induced oxidative stress in human erythrocytes in vitro. *Biological Research*, *46*(1), 33–38. PubMed PMID: 23760412.

105. Ozkan, F., Gunduz, S. G., Berkoz, M., Hunt, A. O., & Yalin, S. (2012). The protective role of ascorbic acid (vitamin C) against chlorpyrifos-induced oxidative stress in Oreochromis niloticus. *Fish Physiology and Biochemistry*, *38*(3), 635–643. PubMed PMID: 21818541.

106. Aboul-Soud, M. A., Al-Othman, A. M., El-Desoky, G. E., Al-Othman, Z. A., Yusuf, K., Ahmad, J., et al. (2011). Hepatoprotective effects of vitamin E/selenium against malathion-induced injuries on the antioxidant status and apoptosis-related gene expression in rats. *The Journal of Toxicological Sciences*, *36*(3), 285–296. PubMed PMID: 21628957.

107. Hassani, S., Sepand, M. R., Jafari, A., Jaafari, J., et al. (2015). Protective effects of curcumin and vitamin E against chlorpyrifos-induced lung oxidative damage. *Human and Experimental Toxicology*, *34*(6), 668–676. PubMed PMID: 25233897.

22

Pyrethroid Pesticides

SUMMARY

- Presence in population: Most common commercial household insecticide; significant contamination in diet; average daily intake of permethrin is about 3.2 μg per day
- Major diseases: Neurotoxicity, endocrine disruption, gastrointestinal symptoms, cardiovascular symptoms
- Primary sources: Contaminated food and water, home pesticide use
- Best measure: Urine metabolites
- Best intervention: Avoidance, antioxidants

DESCRIPTION

Pyrethrum is one of the oldest known insecticides and is derived from the flowerheads of two species of asters: *Chrysanthemum cinerariifolium* and *C. coccineum*. Pyrethrins are purified pyrethrum and refer to the original plant-derived mixture from the chrysanthemum flowers. Pyrethroid pesticides are artificial pyrethrin-like insecticides synthesized in a laboratory based on the structure of the six insecticidal constituents of the natural product pyrethrum. By 2002, their use had grown to represent 18% of the United States' dollar value of the insecticide market,[1] and pyrethroids now constitute most commercial household insecticides.

Pyrethroids consist of two groups and are organized by their chemical structure. Type I pyrethroids are devoid of a cyano moiety at the α-position [e.g., allethrin (See Fig. 22.1)] and type II pyrethroids have an α-cyano moiety (e.g., cypermethrin).[2] Permethrin is the most commonly used synthetic type I pyrethroid insecticide and is widely used in agricultural and domestic applications. Box 22.1 lists most of the synthetic pyrethroid insecticides registered for use in the United States.

TOXICITY

Pyrethroids are excitatory neurotoxins that function primarily by preventing the closure of voltage-gated sodium channels in the axonal membranes, thus preventing repolarization of the nerves and paralyzing the organism.[3] Some pyrethroids may also act on voltage-gated calcium and chloride channels, which contribute to their toxicity.[4,5] Type I pyrethroids cause hyperexcitation, ataxia, tremor, and paralysis ("T syndrome"), whereas type II pyrethroids cause hypersensitivity, salivation, and choreoathetosis ("CS syndrome").[6] Although this system is widely recognized, the categories are not absolute or mutually exclusive, because some compounds exhibit elements of both syndromes. For example, both type I and type II pyrethroids can act as preconvulsants via gamma-amino butyric acid (GABA)-ergic and glutamatergic systems.[7,8] Other signs and symptoms of toxicity include abnormal facial sensation; dizziness; headache; fatigue; vomiting; diarrhea; irritability to sound and touch; and, in severe cases, pulmonary edema, muscle fasciculations, seizures, and coma.

Toxicity of pyrethroids to humans has been reported to be at least three orders of magnitude lower than that

BOX 22.1   Pyrethroid Pesticides Registered for Use in the United States

Type I Pyrethroids	Type II Pyrethroids
Allethrin (Fig 22.1)	Cyfluthrin
Bifenthrin	Cyhalothrin
Bioresmethrin	Cypermethrin
Permethrin	Cyphenothrin
Phenothrin	Deltamethrin
Prallethrin	Esfenvalerate
Resmethrin	Fenvalerate
Tefluthrin	Fenpropathrin
Tetramethrin	Flucythrinate
	Flumethrin
	Fluvalinate
	Tralomethrin

to insects.[9] In rats, most pyrethroids have acute oral lethal dose, 50% (LD_{50}) values after administration in vegetable oils between 50 and 500 mg/kg and are considered moderately toxic by Environmental Protection Agency (EPA) standards.[4] Almost all reported human poisonings relate to type II pyrethroids, which generally cause more severe symptoms than type I.[10]

Toxicity of pyrethroids may be increased because of interactions with other pesticides. For example, when organophosphate insecticides were administered to mice *in vivo* before dosing with transpermethrin, the organophosphate pesticide (OP) compounds strongly inhibited liver microsomal esterase activity, thus increasing the *in vivo* toxicity of the pyrethroid.[11] Organophosphates and carbamates are carboxylesterase (CE) inhibitors and therefore have synergistic effects on pyrethroid toxicity.[12]

Oxidative stress may play a critical role in the toxic effect of pyrethroids. Permethrin has been shown to increase superoxide anion production and the activity of the hydrogen peroxide–myeloperoxidase system in rat polymorphonuclear neutrophils.[13] Pyrethroid exposure induces lipid peroxide and protein oxidation and depletes reduced glutathione.[14]

SOURCES

Relatively hydrophobic with significant aquatic toxicity, pyrethroids bind tightly to soil and have a soil half-life of 12 days.[15] Pyrethroids are registered for numerous uses on a wide variety of crops, on golf courses, in homes and gardens, for landscaping, in nurseries, and at structural sites and for treatment of ectoparasitic disease.[16] Over the last decade, pyrethroid insecticides have been at the forefront of malaria control using insecticide-treated nets and residual spraying.[17] The main route of exposure to pyrethroids for the general public is through dietary intake.[18]

BODY BURDEN

Absorption varies significantly depending on the route of exposure. Inefficient absorption and rapid metabolic detoxification result in very low levels of systemic toxicity after dermal exposure.[19] The lipophilicity of pyrethroids favors absorption in the gastrointestinal and respiratory tracts.[20] One study evaluated absorption of cypermethrin after administration orally or dermally and found much greater absorption by the oral route (27%–57% of the administered dose) compared with the dermal route (0.85%–1.8% of the administered dose).[21] Once absorbed, pyrethroids are typically internally distributed between liver, kidney, muscle, brain, and fat, with an estimated half-life of 12 days.[22,23,24]

Levels of the various pyrethroid compounds in residents of the United States have been studied as part of the ongoing National Health and Nutritional Examination Survey (NHANES) trial and published by the Centers for Disease Control and Prevention (CDC) in their Exposure Report.[25] Table 22.1 summarizes the pyrethroid metabolite findings published in the January 2017 updated tables to the Fourth Report.

Detoxification/Excretion Processes

One of the major catabolic pathways involved in the clearance of pyrethroids from the body is hydrolysis. CEs are hepatic enzymes that metabolize ester-containing xenobiotics such as pyrethroids.[26] CEs for hydrolysis and CYP450 enzymes for oxidation play critical roles in the metabolism of pyrethroids.[27] In some cases, human alcohol and aldehyde dehydrogenases are the enzymes involved in oxidation.[28] Not all pyrethroids are metabolized in the same way, indicating the presence of isozymes, resulting in interindividual variability in CE activity.[29]

The blood half-life of pyrethroids is on the order of tens of hours[30] but can vary significantly based upon the agent involved, dose, exposure time, route of exposure, and the individual's rate of metabolism.[31] For example, the type II pyrethroid cyfluthrin is metabolized very

TABLE 22.1 CDC Fourth Report January 2017 Update: Urinary Pyrethroid Pesticides (µg/g Creatinine)

Toxicant	Mean	75th %	90th %	95th %
Trans-3-(2,2-dichlorovinyl)-2,2-dimethylcyclopropane carboxylic acid	Not calculated	< LOD	2.10	4.37
Cis-2-(2,2-dibromovinyl)-2,2-dimethylcyclopropane carboxylic acid	Not calculated	< LOD	< LOD	< LOD
4-fluoro-3-phenoxybenzoic acid	Not calculated	< LOD	< LOD	< LOD
3-phenoxybenzoic acid	0.438	1.01	2.88	5.44

< LOD, less than the limit of detection.
Modified from Centers for Disease Control and Prevention. National Report on Human Exposure to Environmental Chemicals: Updated Tables, January 2017. Available atwww.cdc.gov/exposurereport/.

quickly (19–86 minutes), with an elimination half-life for its metabolites of about 6 hours,[32] whereas the elimination half-life for permethrin is 8.67 hours.[33] Most pyrethroids and their metabolites are rapidly excreted in urine and feces, with more than 90% excreted within 1 week after exposure.[34]

Pyrethroid metabolites can be measured in urine, with the following detected in occupationally exposed workers up to 3.5 days after exposure: cis- and trans-3-(2,2-dichlorovinyl)-2,2-dimethylcyclopropanecarboxylic acid, cis-3-(2,2-dibromovinyl)-2,2-dimethylcyclopropanecarboxylic acid, 3-phenoxybenzoic acid, and 4-fluoro-3-phenoxybenzoic acid.[35]

Clinical Significance

The risk of exposure and adverse effects in the general population are increased by the abundance and variety of pyrethroid uses as well as by higher body loads of other environmental toxicants that affect detoxification and act via similar toxic mechanisms. Pyrethroids have shown a variety of clinical effects including neurotoxicity; immunotoxicity; cardiotoxicity; hepatotoxicity; reproductive, genotoxic, and hematotoxic effects; digestive system toxicity; and cytotoxicity.[36]

Cardiovascular. *In vitro* studies on animal hearts show prolonged action potentials and altered spontaneous rhythmic contractions affecting both the amplitude and frequency of contractions after exposure to pyrethroid insecticides.[37] Action potential prolongation has been attributed to the direct effects of pyrethroids on cardiac sodium channels.[38] Early life exposure to pyrethroids may lead to long-term consequences such as cardiac hypotrophy and increased intracellular calcium influx in the heart.[39]

Endocrine. Type I and type II pyrethroids cause adrenal activation in rats, with an increase in blood adrenaline and noradrenaline accompanying motor signs.[40] Subacute doses of permethrin have been shown to cause reproductive toxicity, leading to a deregulation of spermatogenesis, strong deformations in the microstructure of the epididymis, and disruption in testosterone concentrations.[41] Occupational exposure to fenvalerate has been shown to decrease sperm motion parameters and increase the abnormality of viscidity and coagulation of semen,[42] as well as increase sperm DNA damage.[43] Enantiomers of bifenthrin induced cell proliferation through the estrogen response pathway via the estrogen receptor.[44]

Gastrointestinal. Evaluation of 48 patients with oral poisoning from insecticides containing permethrin showed the most common signs and symptoms involve the gastrointestinal system, including sore throat, mouth ulceration, dysphagia, epigastric pain, vomiting, and melena.[45] Vomiting, diarrhea, and a burning sensation in the oral cavity have been reported after oral intoxication with permethrin.[46]

Hepatic. Exposure to bifenthrin can induce liver injury through caspase-mediated mitochondrial-dependent cell death, a process associated with oxidative stress.[47] Animal studies have shown that exposure to the pyrethroid metofluthrin produced hepatocellular tumors through CYP2B induction, increased hepatocellular DNA replication, and increased hepatocyte proliferation.[48] However, further evaluation concluded that metofluthrin would not have any hepatocarcinogenic activity in humans.[49]

Neuropathic. The most commonly reported symptom associated with dermal exposure is paresthesia,

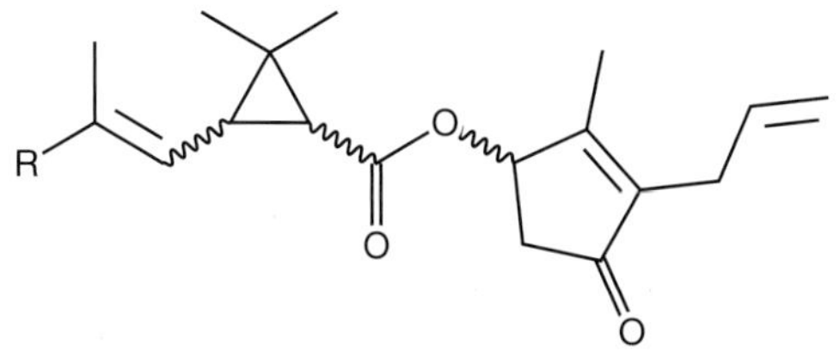

FIG. 22.1 Allethrin. (CC BY-SA 3.0 [http://creativecommons.org/licenses/by-sa/3.0] / User: CYL / Wikimedia Commons / https://commons.wikimedia.org/w/index.php?curid = 17998563.)

characterized by numbness, itching, burning, or tingling.[50] A study evaluating the effects of pyrethroids applied to human earlobes demonstrated transient paresthesia as the only symptom, developing within 30 minutes of exposure, peaking by 8 hours, and resolving by 24 to 32 hours after exposure.[51]

Residual effects after acute pyrethroid intoxication include cerebroorganic disorders (reduced intellectual performance, with 20%–30% reduction of endurance during mental work, and personality disorders), visual disturbances, dysacousia, sensomotor-polyneuropathy in the lower legs, and vegetative nervous disorders (paroxysmal tachycardia, increased heat sensitivity, orthostatic hypotonia, and reduced exercise tolerance).[52] Cases of multiple chemical sensitivities developing after high-dose exposure to pyrethroid insecticides have been reported.[53] Pyrethroids have also shown negative effects on neurobehavior, including impairment of schedule-controlled operant response, decreased grip strength, incoordination, and an increase in acoustic-evoked startle response amplitude.[54]

INTERVENTION

As with most toxicants, avoidance is primary. No specific conventional medication exists for pyrethroid toxicity, and treatment is primarily based on symptom relief. Decontamination of the skin with soap and water and flushing of the eyes with water or saline may be helpful. The use of natural antioxidants does appear to provide benefit. Vitamin E has shown to be effective in the treatment of parasthesias resulting from dermal contact with pyrethroids. One study showed dermal application of vitamin E applied from 29 hours before to 15 minutes after pyrethroid exposure reduced skin sensations, with protection lasting more than 5 hours.[55] Several

studies have evaluated the benefits of antioxidants after exposure of rats to permethrin. Treatment with 200 mg/kg of vitamins E and C protected erythrocytes against plasma membrane lipid peroxidation and maintained the activity of glutathione peroxidase.[56] Vitamin E plus coenzyme Q10 reversed the negative effect of permethrin on the central nervous system, restoring plasma membrane fluidity and preserving glutathione levels.[57] After permethrin exposure, olive leaf extract has shown genoprotective effects via inhibition of oxidative stress and scavenging of free radicals.[58,59] Resveratrol has also shown a genoprotective effect, diminishing indices on chromosome aberrations and sister chromatid exchange tests.[60]

REFERENCES

1. Pickett, J. A. (2004). New opportunities in neuroscience, but a great danger that some may be lost. In D. J. Beadle, I. R. Mellor, & P. N. R. Usherwood (Eds.), *Neurotox '03: Neurotoxicological Targets from Functional Genomics and Proteomics* (pp. 1–10). London: Society of Chemical Industry.
2. Nasuti, C., Cantalamessa, F., Falcioni, G., & Gabbianelli, R. (2003). Different effects of type I and type II pyrethroids on erythrocyte plasma membrane properties and enzymatic activity in rats. *Toxicology, 191*(2–3), 233–244. PubMed PMID: 12965126.
3. Soderlund, D. M. (2012). Molecular mechanisms of pyrethroid insecticide neurotoxicity: Recent advances. *Archives of Toxicology, 86*(2), 165–181. PubMed PMID: 21710279.
4. Soderlund, D. M., Clark, J. M., Sheets, L. P., Mullin, L. S., et al. (2002). Mechanisms of pyrethroid neurotoxicity: Implications for cumulative risk assessment. *Toxicology, 171*(1), 3–59. PubMed PMID: 11812616.
5. Breckenridge, C. B., Holden, L., Sturgess, N., Weiner, M., et al. (2009). Evidence for a separate mechanism of toxicity for the type I and the type II pyrethroid insecticides. *Neurotoxicology, 30*(Suppl. 1), S17–S31. PubMed PMID: 19766671.
6. Ray, D. E., & Fry, J. R. (2006). A reassessment of the neurotoxicity of pyrethroid insecticides. *Pharmacology & Therapeutics, 111*(1), 174–193. PubMed PMID: 16324748.
7. Devaud, L. L., Szot, P., & Murray, T. F. (1986). PK 11195 antagonism of pyrethroid-induced proconvulsant activity. *European Journal of Pharmacology, 121*(2), 269–273. PubMed PMID: 3699096.
8. Pham Huu Chanh, A., Navarro-Delmasure, C., et al. (1984). Pharmacological effects of delmethrin on the

central nervous system. *Arzneimittel-Forschung, 34*(2), 175–181. PubMed PMID: 6539110.

9. Schettgen, T., Heudorf, U., Drexler, H., & Angerer, J. (2002). Pyrethroid exposure of the general population: is this due to diet. *Toxicology Letters, 134*(1–3), 141–145. PubMed PMID: 12191872.

10. Ray, D. E., & Forshaw, P. J. (2000). Pyrethroid insecticides: Poisoning syndromes, synergies, and therapy. *Journal of Toxicology. Clinical Toxicology, 38*(2), 95–101. PubMed PMID: 10778904.

11. Gaughan, L. C., Engel, J. L., & Casida, J. E. (1980). Pesticide interactions: Effects of organophosphorous pesticides on the metabolism, toxicity, and persistence of selected pyrethroid insecticides. *Pesticide Biochemistry and Physiology, 14*, 81–85.

12. Sogorb, M. A., & Vilanova, E. (2002). Enzymes involved in the detoxification of organophosphorous, carbamate and pyrethroid insecticides through hydrolysis. *Toxicology Letters, 128*(1–3), 215–228. PubMed PMID: 11869832.

13. Gabbianelli, R., Falcioni, M. L., Nasuti, C., Cantalamessa, F., Imada, I., & Inoue, M. (2009). Effect of permethrin insecticide on rat polymorphonuclear neutrophils. *Chemico-Biological Interactions, 182*(2–3), 245–252. PubMed PMID: 19772857.

14. Vontas, J. G., Small, G. J., & Hemingway, J. (2001). Glutathione S-transferases as antioxidant defence agents confer pyrethroid resistance in Nilaparvata lugens. *The Biochemical Journal, 357*(Pt. 1), 65–72. PubMed PMID: 11415437.

15. Hladik, M. L., & Kuivila, K. M. (2009). Assessing the occurrence and distribution of pyrethroids in water and suspended sediments. *Journal of Agricultural and Food Chemistry, 57*(19), 9079–9085. PubMed PMID: 19754147.

16. Spurlock, F., & Lee, M. (2008). Synthetic pyrethroid use patterns, properties, and environmental effects. In J. Gan, F. Spurlock, P. Hendley, & D. Weston (Eds.), *Synthetic Pyrethroids: Occurrence and Behavior in Aquatic Environments* (pp. 3–25). Washington, DC: American Chemical Society.

17. Ranson, H., N'guessan, R., Lines, J., Moiroux, N., Nkuni, Z., & Corbel, V. (2011). Pyrethroid resistance in African anopheline mosquitos: What are the implications for malaria control? *Trends in Parasitology, 27*(2), 91–98. PubMed PMID: 20843745.

18. Agency for Toxic Substances and Disease Registry. (2007). *Toxicological profile for pyrethrins and pyrethroids.* Available at https://www.atsdr.cdc.gov/ToxProfiles/tp155-c1.pdf. (Accessed April 9, 2017.)

19. Clark, J. M. (1995). Effects and mechanisms of action of pyrethrin and pyrethroid insecticides. In L. W. Chang & R. S. Dyer (Eds.), *Handbook of Neurotoxicology* (pp. 511–546). New York: Marcel Dekker.

20. Kavlock, R., Chernoff, N., Baron, R., Linder, R., et al. (1979). Toxicity studies with decamethrin, a synthetic pyrethroid insecticide. *Journal of Environmental Pathology and Toxicology, 2*(3), 751–765. PubMed PMID: 370325.

21. Woollen, B. H., Marsh, J. R., Laird, W. J., & Lesser, J. E. (1992). The metabolism of cypermethrin in man: Differences in urinary metabolite profiles following oral and dermal administration. *Xenobiotica, 22*(8), 983–991. PubMed PMID: 1413886.

22. Crawford, M. J., Croucher, A., & Hutson, D. H. (1981). Metabolism of cis- and trans-cypermethrin in rats. Balance and tissue retention study. *Journal of Agricultural and Food Chemistry, 29*(1), 130–135. PubMed PMID: 7204747.

23. Ueda, K., Gaughan, L. C., & Casida, J. E. (1975). Metabolism of (+)-trans- and (+)-cis-resmethrin in rats. *Journal of Agricultural and Food Chemistry, 23*(1), 106–115. PubMed PMID: 1133269.

24. Cole, L. M., Ruzo, L. O., Wood, E. J., & Casida, J. E. (1982). Pyrethroid metabolism: Comparative fate in rats of tralomethrin, tralocythrin, deltamethrin, and (1R, alpha S)-cis-cypermethrin. *Journal of Agricultural and Food Chemistry, 30*(4), 631–636. PubMed PMID: 6811643.

25. Centers for Disease Control and Prevention. *National Report on Human Exposure to Environmental Chemicals: Updated Tables, January 2017.* Available at www.cdc.gov/exposurereport/. (Accessed October 25, 2017.)

26. Satoh, T., & Hosokawa, M. (1998). The mammalian carboxylesterases: From molecules to functions. *Annual Review of Pharmacology and Toxicology, 38*, 257–288. PubMed PMID: 9597156.

27. Casida, J. E., Gammon, D. W., Glickman, A. H., & Lawrence, L. J. (1983). Mechanisms of selective action of pyrethroid insecticides. *Annual Review of Pharmacology and Toxicology, 23*, 413–438. PubMed PMID: 6347050.

28. Choi, J., Rose, R. L., & Hodgson, E. (2002). In vitro human metabolism of permethrin: The role of human alcohol and aldehyde dehydrogenases. *Pesticide Biochemistry and Physiology, 73*, 117–128.

29. Wheelock, C. E., Wheelock, A. M., Zhang, R., Stok, J. E., Morisseau, C., et al. (2003). Evaluation of alpha-cyanoesters as fluorescent substrates for examining interindividual variation in general and pyrethroid-selective esterases in human liver microsomes. *Analytical Biochemistry, 315*(2), 208–222. PubMed PMID: 12689831.

30. Anadon, A., Martinez-Larranaga, M. R., Fernandez-Cruz, M. L., Diaz, M. J., Fernandez, M. C., & Martinez,

M. A. (1996). Toxicokinetics of deltamethrin and its 4'-HO-metabolite in the rat. *Toxicology and Applied Pharmacology*, *141*(1), 8–16. PubMed PMID: 8917670.

31. Leng, G., & Lewalter, J. (1999). Role of individual susceptibility in risk assessment of pesticides. *Occupational and Environmental Medicine*, *56*(7), 449–453. PubMed PMID: 10472315.

32. Leng, G., Leng, A., Kuhn, K. H., et al. (1997). Human dose-excretion studies with the pyrethroid insecticide cyfluthrin: Urinary metabolite profile following inhalation. *Xenobiotica*, *27*, 1272–1283. PubMed PMID: 9460232.

33. Anadon, A., Martinez-Larranaga, M. R., Diaz, M. J., & Bringas, P. (1991). Toxicokinetics of permethrin in the rat. *Toxicology and Applied Pharmacology*, *110*(1), 1–8. PubMed PMID: 1871768.

34. Roberts, T. R., & Hutson, D. H. (1999). *Metabolic Pathways of Agrochemicals. Part 2: Insecticides and Fungicides*. Cambridge: Royal Society of Chemistry.

35. Leng, G., Kuhn, K. H., & Idel, H. (1996). Biological monitoring of pyrethroid metabolites in urine of pest control operators. *Toxicology Letters*, *88*(1–3), 215–220. PubMed PMID: 8920739.

36. Wang, X., Martinez, M. A., Dai, M., Chen, D., Ares, I., et al. (2016). Permethrin-induced oxidative stress and toxicity and metabolism. A review. *Environmental Research*, *149*, 86–104. PubMed PMID: 27183507.

37. Spencer, C. I., Yuill, K. H., Borg, J. J., Hancox, J. C., & Kozlowski, R. Z. (2001). Actions of pyrethroid insecticides on sodium currents, action potentials, and contractile rhythm in isolated mammalian ventricular myocytes and perfused hearts. *The Journal of Pharmacology and Experimental Therapeutics*, *298*(3), 1067–1082. PubMed PMID: 11504804.

38. Spencer, C. I., & Sham, J. S. (2005). Mechanisms underlying the effects of the pyrethroid tefluthrin on action potential duration in isolated rat ventricular myocytes. *The Journal of Pharmacology and Experimental Therapeutics*, *315*(1), 16–23. PubMed PMID: 15980056.

39. Vadhana, M. S. D., Arumugam, A. A., Carloni, M., Nasuti, C., & Gabbianelli, R. (2013). Early life permethrin treatment leads to long-term cardiotoxicity. *Chemosphere*, *93*(6), 1029–1034. PubMed PMID: 23806482.

40. Cremer, J. E., & Seville, M. P. (1985). Changes in regional cerebral blood flow and glucose metabolism associated with sympoms of pyrethroid toxicity. *Neurotoxicology*, *6*(3), 1–12. PubMed PMID: 4047507.

41. Issam, C., Zohra, H., Monia, Z., & Hassen, B. C. (2011). Effects of dermal sub-chronic exposure of pubescent male rats to permethrin (PRMT) on the histological structures of the genital tract, testosterone, and lipoperoxidation. *Experimental and Toxicologic Pathology*, *63*(4), 393–400. PubMed PMID: 20381324.

42. Lifeng, T., Shoulin, W., Junmin, J., Xuezhao, S., et al. (2006). Effects of fenvalerate exposure on semen quality among occupational workers. *Contraception*, *73*(1), 92–96. PubMed PMID: 16371303.

43. Bian, Q., Xu, L. C., Wang, S. L., Xia, Y. K., et al. (2004). Study on the relation between occupational fenvalerate exposure and spermatozoa DNA damage of pesticide factory workers. *Occupational and Environmental Medicine*, *61*(12), 999–1005. PubMed PMID: 15550606.

44. Wang, L., Liu, W., Yang, C., Pan, Z., et al. (2007). Enantioselectivity in estrogenic potential and uptake of bifenthrin. *Environmental Science & Technology*, *41*(17), 6124–6128. PubMed PMID: 17937291.

45. Yang, P. Y., Lin, J. L., Hall, A. H., Tsao, T. C., & Chern, M. S. (2002). Acute ingestion poisoning with insecticide formulations containing the pyrethroid permethrin, xylene, and surfactant: A review of 48 cases. *Journal of Toxicology. Clinical Toxicology*, *40*(2), 107–113. PubMed PMID: 12126181.

46. Gotoh, Y., Kawakami, M., Matsumoto, N., & Okada, Y. (1998). Permethrin emulsion ingestion: Clinical manifestations and clearance of isomers. *Journal of Toxicology. Clinical Toxicology*, *36*(1–2), 57–61. PubMed PMID: 9541045.

47. Zhang, Y., Lu, M., Zhou, P., et al. (2015). Multilevel evaluations of potential liver injury of bifenthrin. *Pesticide Biochemistry and Physiology*, *122*, 29–37. PubMed PMID: 26071804.

48. Deguchi, Y., Yamada, T., Hirose, Y., Nagahori, H., et al. (2009). Mode of action analysis for the synthetic pyrethroid metofluthrin-induced rat liver tumors: Evidence for hepatic CYP2B induction and hepatocyte proliferation. *Toxicological Sciences*, *108*(1), 69–80. PubMed PMID: 19176366.

49. Yamada, T., Uwagawa, S., Okuno, Y., et al. (2009). Case study: An evaluation of the human relevance of the synthetic pyrethroid metofluthrin-induced liver tumors in rats based on mode of action. *Toxicological Sciences*, *108*(1), 59–68. PubMed PMID: 19176367.

50. Vijverberg, H. P., & van den Bercken, J. (1990). Neurotoxicological effects and the mode of action of pyrethroid insecticides. *Critical Reviews in Toxicology*, *21*(2), 105–126. PubMed PMID: 1964560.

51. Flannigan, S. A., & Tucker, S. B. (1985). Variation in cutaneous sensation between synthetic pyrethroid insecticides. *Contact Dermatitis*, *13*(3), 140–147. PubMed PMID: 4053596.

52. Muller-Mohnssen, H. (1999). Chronic sequelae and irreversible injuries following acute pyrethroid intoxication. *Toxicology Letters, 107*(1–3), 161–176. PubMed PMID: 10414793.

53. Muller-Mohnssen, H. (1996). Multiple chemical sensitivity (MCS) syndrome. *Gesundheitswesen, 58*(7), 415–416. PubMed PMID: 8963109.

54. Wolansky, M. J., & Harill, J. A. (2008). Neurobehavioral toxicology of pyrethroid insecticides in adult animals: A critical review. *Neurotoxicology and Teratology, 30*(2), 55–78. PubMed PMID: 18206347.

55. Malley, L. A., Cagen, S. Z., Parker, C. M., et al. (1985). Effect of vitamin E and other amelioratory agents on the fenvalerate-mediated skin sensation. *Toxicology Letters, 29*(1), 51–58. PubMed PMID: 2867622.

56. Gabbianelli, R., Nasuti, C., Falcioni, G., & Cantalamessa, F. (2004). Lymphocyte DNA damage in rats exposed to pyrethroids: Effect of supplementation with vitamins E and C. *Toxicology, 203*(1–3), 17–26. PubMed PMID: 15363578.

57. Nasuti, C., Falcioni, M. L., Nwankwo, I. E., Cantalamessa, F., & Gabbianelli, R. (2008). Effect of permethrin plus antioxidants on locomotor activity and striatum in adolescent rats. *Toxicology, 251*(1–3), 45–50. PubMed PMID: 18692543.

58. Turkez, H., & Togar, B. (2011). Olive (Olea europaea L.) leaf extract counteracts genotoxicity and oxidative stress of permethrin in human lymphocytes. *The Journal of Toxicological Sciences, 36*(5), 531–537. PubMed PMID: 22008529.

59. Turkez, H., Togar, B., & Polat, E. (2012). Olive leaf extract modulates permethrin induced genetic and oxidative damage in rats. *Cytotechnology, 64*(4), 459–464. PubMed PMID: 22262123.

60. Turkez, H., & Aydin, E. (2013). The genoprotective activity of resveratrol on permethrin-induced genotoxic damage in cultured human lymphocytes. *Brazilian Archives of Biology and Technology, 56*, 405–411.

23

Glyphosate and Petroleum Distillates

SUMMARY

- Presence in population: Ubiquitous
- Major diseases: Endocrine disruption, cancer, renal failure
- Primary sources: Conventional foods, water contamination, agricultural and home use herbicides
- Best measure: Urine glyphosate or glyphosate metabolite concentration
- Best intervention: Avoidance, consumption of organic non-GMO foods

DESCRIPTION

Different combinations of glyphosate (N-[phospho-nomethyl] glycine) and petroleum distillates are used in conventional agriculture and around the home and are marketed under names such as Roundup Rodeo, and Accord. Glyphosate was registered in the United States in 1974 as a broad-spectrum contact herbicide to kill weeds in fields before the planting of crops and for weed control in a variety of noncrop settings. Glyphosate kills plants by inhibiting the shikimic acid pathway via the direct inhibition of 5-enolpyruvylshikimate 3-phosphate synthase, resulting in a decrease in aromatic amino acid production.[1] Considering that all higher animals, including humans, lack the shikimic acid pathway, it has been presumed that glyphosate is safe and has limited toxicity.

Glyphosate-based formulations range from agricultural concentrates requiring dilution before use (containing 30% to 50% or more glyphosate) to ready-to-use formulations (1% to 5% glyphosate) marketed for domestic use. Glyphosate-based herbicides (GBHs) are the most commonly used pesticides in the United States, and coinciding with the introduction of genetically engineered, herbicide-tolerant (GE-HT) crops in 1996, a rapid increase in use has occurred over the last two decades. It is estimated that 90% of the transgenic crops grown worldwide are glyphosate resistant,[2] with the major agricultural uses in the production of soybeans, corn, cotton, wheat, hay, and pasture and fallow land.[3] As can be seen in Table 23.1, glyphosate use in the agricultural sector rose 300-fold from 1974 to 2014, and although it has been on the market for 42 years, two-thirds of the total volume of glyphosate applied has occurred in just the last 10 years.[4]

This chapter includes assessments of glyphosate, its Roundup formulations, and the "inert" adjuvants used in Roundup formulations worldwide.

TOXICITY

It can be difficult to assess the toxicity of any given substance because many studies assume, albeit incorrectly, that no one is exposed to more than one toxicant at a time, and that the subjects involved are completely free from any toxicants before the exposure being considered. Cumulative exposure certainly poses greater risk. Complex mixtures, dose additivity, and synergism between and among hormones and chemicals complicate toxicity studies. For example, glyphosate alone does not show the same toxicity characteristics as Roundup, and the differences in toxicity may be attributed to the other chemicals contained in Roundup or a synergistic effect of glyphosate and the "inert" ingredients.[5]

TABLE 23.1   Glyphosate Use in the United States: 1974 to 2014 (Data in Thousands of Pounds)

	1974	1982	1990	1995	2000	2005	2010	2012	2014
Glyphosate use	1400	7800	12,700	40,000	98,500	179,690	260,804	261,807	276,425
Agricultural	800	5000	7400	27,500	78,750	157,500	235,814	236,318	249,906
Nonagricultural	600	2800	5300	12,500	19,750	22,190	24,989	25,489	26,519

Modified from Benbrook, C. M. (2016). Trends in glyphosate herbicide use in the United States and globally. *Environmental Sciences Europe, 28*(1), 3.

Most pesticides are formulated commercial mixtures containing multiple constituents, which are often kept confidential and are labeled as inert, plus a declared active ingredient (DAI), which is commonly the only ingredient tested in toxicological studies. The lack of transparency regarding ingredients, along with the multitude of chemicals included in Roundup, not only makes it difficult for consumers to make educated choices but also hinders research on the true toxic effects of GBHs. In cases of toxicity, source identification can be hampered by a lack of information regarding product ingredients, including those listed as inert—the solvents, preservatives, surfactants, and other coformulants added to pesticides by the manufacturer—as well as chemicals that may be present as byproducts, residual starting materials, processing aids, and contaminants. It can be difficult to separate the toxicity of glyphosate from that of the formulation as a whole or to determine the direct contribution of coformulants to overall toxicity.[6]

Roundup contains glyphosate (i.e., the DAI), which can be used as five different salts, and "inert" constituents, such as the surfactant polyethoxylated tallow amine (POEA), which vary in nature and concentration. "Inert" ingredients are added to make the product easier to use and/or more effective. For example, surfactants are nearly universally present in herbicides to aid uniform spreading of droplets on leaves as well as to improve penetration of the herbicide into the plants.[7] They also appear to significantly contribute to the toxicity profile of glyphosate-containing herbicides.[8] Surfactants have been identified as the chemicals primarily responsible for the toxicity of GBHs to nontarget species.[9] Research has demonstrated that Roundup formulations and coformulants alone are up to 1000 times more toxic to human cells then the DAI, glyphosate, at 24-hour exposure.[10] Federal law classifies all pesticide ingredients that do not harm pests as "inert." The inert ingredients contained in GBHs are clearly not harmless; they simply do not kill insects or weeds. Table 23.2 lists a variety of inert ingredients that have been found in glyphosate-based herbicides as well as symptoms that result from exposure to these specific chemicals.[11]

Compared with glyphosate alone, which supposedly produces no effects, dilution levels far below agricultural recommendations of glyphosate formulation exposure—the products actually used—have been shown to produce increases in reactive oxygen species (ROS), nitrotyrosine formation, superoxide dismutase (SOD) activity, and glutathione (GSH) activity and induce apoptosis.[12] The addition of surfactants to glyphosate formulations enhances the toxicity of the mixture, causing an increase in ROS production and antioxidant defenses in cell cultures.[13] Oxidative stress after exposure to glyphosate formulations has a cytotoxic effect on several organisms, including maize and rice leaves, bullfrog tadpoles, earthworms (*Lumbriculus variegatus*), and microalgae (*Chlorella kessleri*).[14] In humans, the volume of surfactant ingested, and not necessarily the type, is more significant in GBH intoxication. Ingestion of 8 mL caused (in rank order) hypotension (47.1%), mental deterioration (38.6%), respiratory failure (30.0%), acute kidney injury (17.1%), and arrhythmia (10.0%) in humans.[15]

Glyphosate and Roundup

Glyphosate has an oral acute LD_{50} (the dose that causes death in 50% of a population of test animals) of >4200 mg/kg in rats, and an acute dermal LD_{50} of >2000 mg/kg of body weight in rabbits.[16] The toxicity of glyphosate may vary based on the glyphosate salt formulation. For example, isopropylamine (IPA) salt showed increased cardiovascular effects (e.g., QTc prolongation and PR prolongation) and increased fatalities compared with the glyphosate ammonium salt.[17] GBHs present DNA-damaging and endocrine-disrupting effects on human

TABLE 23.2   **Inert Ingredients in GBHs and Their Related Symptoms**

Ingredient	Symptoms	Ingredient	Symptoms
• Ammonium sulfate	• Eye irritation • Nausea • Diarrhea • Allergic respiratory reactions • Prolonged exposure causes permanent eye damage	• Methyl pyrrolidinone	• Eye irritation • Fetal loss and reduced fetal weight in laboratory animals
• Benzisothiazolone	• Eczema • Skin irritation • Light-induced allergic reaction	• Pelargonic acid	• Eye irritation • Skin irritation • Respiratory tract irritation
• 1,4-Dioxane	• Mammary cancer • Liver cancer • Nasal cancer • Genotoxic effects	• Polyethoxylated tallow amine (POEA)	• Eye burns • Skin erythema, swelling, and blistering • Nausea • Diarrhea
• Formaldehyde	• Eye irritation • Nose irritation • Throat irritation • Increased incidence of lung and nasopharyngeal cancer	• Potassium hydroxide	• Irreversible eye injury • Deep skin ulcers • Severe digestive tract burns • Severe respiratory irritation
• 3-Iodo-2-propynyl butylcarbamate (IPBC)	• Eye irritation • Increased incidence of miscarriage in laboratory tests • Allergic skin reactions	• Sodium sulfite	• Eye irritation • Skin irritation • Vomiting • Diarrhea • Skin allergies • Severe allergic reactions
• Isopropylamine	• Destroys tissue of the mucous membranes and upper respiratory tract • Wheezing • Laryngitis • Headache • Nausea	• Sorbic acid	• Severe skin irritation • Nausea • Vomiting • Chemical pneumonitis • Sore throat • Allergic reactions

Data from Cox, C. (2000). Glyphosate factsheet. *Journal of Pesticide Reform, 108,* 3. Retrieved from www.eastbaypesticidealert.org/Glyphosate%20Factsheet%201.htm

cells at levels 800 times lower than the level authorized in some food or feed, with the nature of the adjuvants changing the toxicity more than glyphosate itself.[18]

The use of GBHs is ubiquitous, and human exposure to known or suspected endocrine-disrupting chemicals (EDCs) has been documented in the United States and worldwide.[19] Mechanisms by which EDCs act in the body include direct and indirect action on estrogen receptors; antiandrogenic effects; thyroid effects; disruption of enzymes and nuclear and membrane receptors involved in steroidogenesis, steroid metabolism, and protein/peptide synthesis; and molecular epigenetic changes.[20,21,22] Roundup formulations have various mechanisms of toxicity, including inhibition of steroidogenesis and expression of the steroidogenic acute regulatory protein (StAR—the rate-limiting step in steroid hormone synthesis),[23] effects on apoptosis and necrosis in various cells,[24] disruption of cellular membranes, partial inhibition of mitochondrial complexes, and uncoupling of oxidative phosphorylation, which all may be interrelated.[25] Glyphosate alone alters estrogen receptors, with rapid activation of estrogen receptor-β (ERβ) and slower but prolonged activation of ERα, and has shown a synergistic additive estrogenic effect with genistein, a phytoestrogen in soybeans.[26] Glyphosate demonstrates toxicity to several human enzymes, including acetylcholinesterase (AChE), lactate dehydrogenase (LDH), aspartate aminotransferase (AST), alanine aminotransferase (ALT), and alkaline phosphatase (ALP), with IC50 values (the concentration of compound that inhibits 50% of the enzyme activity in 1 hour at 37°C) of 714.5, 750, 54.2, 270.8, and 71.4 mM, respectively.[27]

Glyphosate decreases the hepatic level of cytochrome P450 and monooxygenase activities and the intestinal activity of aryl hydrocarbon hydroxylase,[28] which may explain the gastrointestinal effects associated with glyphosate toxicity. In high concentrations, Roundup produces significant sister-chromatid exchanges in human lymphocytes correlating with the swelling experienced by persons poisoned by Roundup.[29] Significant DNA damage to erythrocytes has been shown to occur after exposure to Roundup.[30] These effects significantly impair tissue perfusion and can aggravate symptoms such as chest pain and dyspnea. Cytotoxicity of Roundup is significantly higher than glyphosate alone: the equivalent LC_{50} of 56.4 µg/mL of glyphosate in the form of Roundup and 1640 µg/mL for technical grade glyphosate.[31]

Aminomethylphosphonic acid (AMPA) and polyoxyethylene tallow amine (POEA) independently and synergistically damage cell membranes at different concentrations; their mixtures are more harmful than glyphosate; and through apoptosis and necrosis, they change human cell permeability and amplify toxicity already induced by glyphosate.[32] Generally, the order of toxicity for these chemicals is POEA, Roundup, > glyphosate acid, IPA salt of glyphosate.[33] However, with the recent introduction of petroleum distillate to the formulas, the hierarchy is likely to change, because it appears petroleum distillate is even more toxic than POEA.

Aminomethylphosphonic Acid

AMPA is the primary metabolite of glyphosate. AMPA is also more persistent than glyphosate, with a half-life in soil of 25 to 240 days.[34,35] Although the LD_{50} is 8300 mg/kg of body weight in rats, subchronic tests show AMPA causes an increase in LDH, a decrease in liver weight, and excessive cell division in the lining of the urinary bladder. AMPA has been shown to be clastogenic on human cells *in vitro* and genotoxic both *in vitro* and *in vivo*.[36] At quantities starting at 0.05 mM, AMPA induces hemolysis, and at 0.25 mM, AMPA is able to create on *in vitro* human erythrocytes.[37]

Polyoxyethylene Tallow Amine

The surfactant POEA appears to be the most toxic against human cells when tested in hepatic, embryonic, and placental cell lines and is considered to be responsible for glyphosate toxicity.[38] Far below toxicity thresholds, POEA inhibits aromatase (the enzyme responsible for the conversion of androgens to estrogen), disrupts mitochondrial function, and is 1200 to 2000 times more cytotoxic than glyphosate.[39] Even at the lowest concentrations tested, inhalation of POEA and preparations containing POEA caused gasping, congested eyes, reduced activity, weight loss, and lung irritation. POEA in low doses produces biphasic muscle relaxation in the motoric activity of rat intestine, and high doses induce an irreversible myorelaxant response exceeding the toxicity of commercial Roundup formulations.[40] In addition to disrupting cellular metabolic activity, mitochondrial activity, and cell proliferation, POEA has been shown to be the most toxic surfactant to cell membrane integrity ($p < 0.01$).[41] Toxic effects of POEA are likely the result of tissue erosion of the mucous membranes and linings of the gastrointestinal and respiratory tracts.[42] In piglets, POEA affected hemodynamics, reducing the cardiac index and left-ventricular stroke work index, resulting in death, whereas glyphosate (NaOH) had no similar effects.[43]

Petroleum Distillate

Naphtha is a highly used solvent with excellent lipid-soluble properties, which accounts for most of its cellular toxicity, in that it solubilizes membrane lipids, leading to their instability and dysfunction.[44] Intentional injection produces erythema, swelling, and necrosis at the injection site, and after accidental exposure, symptoms may include chest pain, dyspnea, hemorrhagic pneumonitis, seizures, and respiratory collapse.[45] Myoglobulinuria has been noted after naphtha ingestion, and it may cause direct myocardial toxicity.[46]

A study of coformulants of GBHs on human cell toxicity, including formulations containing POEA, showed R WeatherMAX, a product developed to bypass the problem of POEA toxicity, was the most toxic GBH among those tested.[39] The formulation provided limited information other than the presence of the light aromatic petroleum distillate naphtha as a differentiating factor. Unfortunately, the lack of transparency surrounding the exact nature of inert ingredients contained in GBHs have resulted in limited toxicity studies evaluating the potential harm of these chemicals.

SOURCES

Glyphosate is primarily used in agriculture in concentrated doses. Glyphosate use has tripled since 1997, largely related to the increasing popularity of Roundup Ready crops (e.g., corn and soybeans).[47] These foods are genetically modified specifically to be resistant to glyphosate, leading to an increase in the amount sprayed around them. The dramatic increases in volume applied have led to significant increases in the levels of glyphosate and its primary metabolite, AMPA, being detected in air,[48] soil,[49] and water.[50] Primary routes of human exposure to glyphosate include ingestion of contaminated food, occupational/workplace exposure, contact with contaminated soil, drinking or bathing in contaminated water, and off-target drift after application to crops.[51]

A 2014 study commissioned by Moms Across America tested 21 drinking water samples with no apparent methodology for ensuring a representative distribution. Nonetheless, the results were alarming. Thirteen of the samples had glyphosate levels ranging from 85 to 330 parts per billion (PPB), and more worrisome was that 76 to 166 PPB of glyphosate was found in breast milk samples that were tested.[52]

BODY BURDEN

Mean concentrations of glyphosate of 73.6 ± 28.2 µg/L of blood have been found in people whose only known exposure was from ingesting genetically modified foods.[53] In cases of intoxication, blood glyphosate concentrations ranged from 0.6 to 150 mg/L (mean 61 mg/L) in mild to moderate cases and 690 to 7480 mg/L (mean 4146 mg/L) in severe cases.[54] In fatal cases in which greater than 190 mL of GBH was consumed (36% w/v glyphosate), a glyphosate blood level higher than 734 mg/L was the best predictor of death.[55]

The US Centers for Disease Control and Prevention (CDC) provides extensive information regarding exposure to 250 exogenous chemicals and metals found in US residents, but it does not include glyphosate. It is estimated that glyphosate is regularly found in urine at levels corresponding to a dietary daily intake of around 0.1 to 3.3 µg/kg of body weight per day, and studies show only 30% to 50% of glyphosate and AMPA concentrations in urine reach or exceed the limit of quantification of 0.1 µg/L.[56] Both glyphosate and AMPA can be measured in the urine, but until the CDC includes them in its ongoing study, no national reference values are available to aid interpretation.

Detoxification/Excretion Processes

Glyphosate is rapidly absorbed, with a peak concentration generally within 4 to 6 hours, followed by an apparent half-life of 10 to 14 hours.[57] Animal studies demonstrate that approximately 35% to 40% of orally administered glyphosate is absorbed from the gastrointestinal tract, and 1% of glyphosate persists after 7 days, mainly in the colon and bone.[58] Around 98% to 99% of administered glyphosate is recovered as the parent compound in urine and feces within 48 hours, with limited metabolism of glyphosate to AMPA attributed to gut microflora metabolism.[59] One case showed that glyphosate was still present in serum 5 days postingestion in a patient with renal failure treated with hemodialysis.[60]

Clinical Significance

Accidental ingestion of domestic glyphosate formulations is generally associated with mild, transient gastrointestinal symptoms. The concentrated formula Roundup (41% glyphosate as the IPA salt and 15% POEA) can cause gastrointestinal corrosive effects, including mouth, throat, and epigastric pain; dysphagia; renal and hepatic impairment; respiratory distress; impaired consciousness; pulmonary edema; shock; arrhythmias; metabolic acidosis; hyperkalemia; and death.[61,62,63] Acute pancreatitis has also been reported after glyphosate-surfactant oral intoxication.[64] Inhalation may cause oral or nasal discomfort, tingling, or throat irritation. Eye exposure may lead to mild conjunctivitis, and dermal exposure to ready-to-use glyphosate formulations can cause irritation and photo-contact dermatitis,[65] but this may be related to the preservative Proxel (benzisothiazolin-3-one).

Cancer. In animal studies, Roundup is associated with increased DNA adducts,[66] mutagenic effects, and chromosomal aberrations.[67] Genetically modified (GM) Roundup-Ready corn and soy fed to rats led to an increased risk of mammary tumors in females, which occurred in response to both Roundup and the GM food alone.[68]

Non-Hodgkin's lymphoma (NHL) has increased rapidly since the early 1970s, and exposure to herbicides, including glyphosate, decades before diagnosis increases the risk of developing NHL.[69] In male farmers, exposure to glyphosate is associated with a twofold increased risk of developing NHL (OR = 2.1; 95% CI, 1.1–4.0).[70] A Canadian multicenter population-based study of men in a variety of occupations also showed an OR of 2.1 (95% CI, 1.2–3.7) for developing NHL with increased frequency of exposure to Roundup.[71] A pooled analysis of NHL and hairy cell leukemia (HCL) showed a relationship between glyphosate exposure and increased risk of disease (OR = 3.04; 95% CI, 1.08–8.52).[72] A case-control study of 121 males with HCL showed similar association between disease and GBH exposure (OR = 2.9; CI 95%, 1.4–5.9).[73] A metaanalysis of nearly 3 decades' worth of epidemiological research on the relationship between NHL and exposure to occupational pesticides demonstrated a strong significant association between B cell lymphoma, a subtype of NHL, and glyphosate exposure (OR = 2.0; 95% CI, 1.1–3.6).[74] Using data from the Agricultural Health Study, there was a 60% to 80% increased risk of melanoma associated with glyphosate use and a more than twofold increased risk of multiple myeloma.[75]

Neurological. An epidemiological study conducted in the Red River Valley of Minnesota showed an increase in attention deficit disorder (ADD) and attention deficit hyperactivity disorder (ADHD) in children of male farmers who applied GBHs (OR = 3.6; 95% CI, 1.3–9.6).[76] In single-pesticide models, neural tube defects have been associated with mothers' exposure to GBHs (OR = 1.5; 95% CI, 1.0–2.4).[77]

Renal. Epidemiological research has found a strong correlation between glyphosate use and the kidney failure epidemic. Of course, association does not prove causation. Animal research shows that chronic exposure at very low dosages causes kidney damage. A 2-year study of drinking water for rats showed that just 0.1 PPB of glyphosate resulted in cellular kidney abnormalities and significant chronic kidney deficiencies.[68] Several unpublished research projects conducted by Monsanto, some performed nearly 4 decades ago, demonstrated urinary abnormalities, hyperplasia of the urinary bladder, and significant reproductive and developmental toxicity after glyphosate exposure at various levels.[78,79,80,81]

Research conducted in Sri Lanka found that those who drank well water contaminated with glyphosate had a higher incidence of kidney failure in proportion to concentrations starting at 0.7 PPB, and farmers spraying glyphosates in the fields had a 5.4-fold increased incidence of kidney disease.[82] The European standard for water contamination is 0.1 PPB, while the US Environmental Protection Agency (EPA) standard is an inexplicable 700 PPB.[83] Case reports after intentional ingestion of Roundup have demonstrated acute renal failure, with oliguria,[84] electrolyte abnormalities, acidosis, cardiovascular collapse, and death.[85]

Reproductive Effects. At low nontoxic concentrations, Roundup damages testicular cells, leading to a 35% decrease in testosterone levels.[86] In addition, low doses of Roundup (36 PPM) have also been shown to induce oxidative stress, leading to Sertoli cell death in prepubertal rat testes, likely as a result of Ca^{2+} overload and cell signaling misregulation.[87] The Ontario Farm Family Health Study reported a reduction of fertility in women exposed to GBH.[88] Preconception exposure to glyphosate increases the risk of early abortion (Odds ratio (OR) = 1.4; 95% confidence interval (CI), 1.1–1.9) as well as late spontaneous abortion (OR = 1.7; 95% CI, 1.0–2.9).[89] Miscarriage (OR = 1.5; 95% CI, 0.8–2.7) and preterm delivery (OR = 2.4; 95% CI, 0.8–7.9) have also been associated with glyphosate exposure.[90]

INTERVENTION

Treatment of glyphosate poisoning is primarily of a supportive nature. Early use of hemodialysis may improve the prognosis of patients despite the vigorous supportive treatment for GBH intoxication.[91]

Considering the main route of GBH exposure for the general population is through the diet, direct action can be taken to reduce exposure by consuming organic foods. The median glyphosate concentration in urine (around 1 PPB) of people consuming predominantly organic food was significantly lower than that of people consuming conventional food.[92] Indeed, several studies have confirmed that an organic diet significantly reduces exposure to numerous pesticides.[93,94,95] Fig. 23.1 clearly shows that eating an organically grown diet results in significantly lower glyphosate levels and that sicker people have higher glyphosate levels.

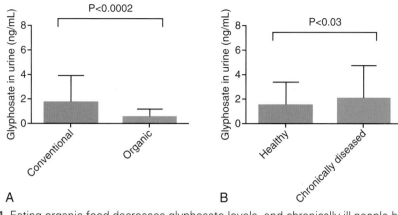

FIG. 23.1 Eating organic food decreases glyphosate levels, and chronically ill people have higher glyphosate levels. (A) Comparison of glyphosate excretion in urine of humans with conventional (N = 99) and predominantly organic (N = 41) foods. (B) Glyphosate in healthy (N = 102) and chronically diseased (N = 199) humans. (From Goen, T., Schmidt, L., Lichtensteiger, W., & Schlumpf, M. [2017]. Efficiency control of dietary pesticide intake reduction by human biomonitoring. *International Journal of Hygiene and Environmental Health, 220*(2 Pt A), 254–260.)

REFERENCES

1. Schonbrunn, E., Eschenburg, S., Shuttleworth, W. A., et al. (2001). Interaction of the herbicide glyphosate with its target enzyme 5-enolpyruvylshikimate 3-phosphate synthase in atomic detail. *Proceedings of the National Academy of Sciences of the United States of America, 98*(4), 1376–1380. PubMed PMID: 11171958.

2. Duke, S. O., & Powles, S. B. (2008). Glyphosate: a once-in-a-century herbicide. *Pest Management Science, 64*(4), 319–325. PubMed PMID: 18273882.

3. Fernandez-Cornejo, J., Nehring, R., Osteen, C., et al.; U.S. Department of Agriculture. Economic Research Service. (2014 May). *Pesticide use in US agriculture: 21 selected crops 1960-2008.* Economic Information bulletin Number 124. https://www.ers.usda.gov/webdocs/publications/43854/46734_eib124.pdf?v=41830. (Last accessed July 26, 2017.)

4. Benbrook, C. M. (2016). Trends in glyphosate herbicide use in the United States and globally. *Environmental Sciences Europe, 28*(1), 3. PubMed PMID: 27752438.

5. Moore, L. J., Fuentes, L., et al. (2012). Relative toxicity of the components of the original formulation of Roundup to five North American anurans. *Ecotoxicology and Environmental Safety, 78*, 128–133. PubMed PMID: 22137360.

6. Bradberry, S. M., Proudfoot, A. T., & Vale, J. A. (2004). Glyphosate poisoning. *Toxicological Reviews, 23*(3), 159–167. PubMed PMID: 15862083.

7. Haefs, R., Schmitz-Eiberger, M., Mainx, H., et al. (2002). Studies on a new group of biodegradable surfactants for glyphosate. *Pest Management Science, 58*(8), 825–833. PubMed PMID: 12192908.

8. Lee, H. L., Kan, C. D., Tsai, C. L., Liou, M. J., & Guo, H. R. (2009). Comparative effects of the formulation of glyphosate-surfactant herbicides on hemodynamics in swine. *Clinical Toxicology (Philadelphia, Pa.), 47*(7), 651–658. PubMed PMID: 19663613.

9. Annett, R., Habibi, H. R., & Hontela, A. (2014). Impact of glyphosate and glyphosate-based herbicides on the freshwater environment. *Journal of Applied Toxicology, 34*(5), 458–479. PubMed PMID: 24615870.

10. Mesnage, R., Defarge, N., Spiroux de Vendômois, J., et al. (2014). Major pesticides are more toxic to human cells than their declared active principles. *BioMed Research International, 2014*, 179691. PubMed PMID: 24719846.

11. Cox, C. (2000). Glyphosate factsheet. *Journal of Pesticide Reform, 108*, 3. At www.eastbaypesticidealert.org/Glyphosate%20Factsheet%201.htm. (Accessed July 25, 2017.)

12. Chaufan, G., Coalova, I., & Rios de Molina Mdel, C. (2014). Glyphosate commercial formulation causes cytotoxicity, oxidative effects, and apoptosis on human cells: differences with its active ingredient. *International Journal of Toxicology, 33*(1), 29–38. PubMed PMID: 24434723.

13. Coalova, I., Rios de Molina Mdel, C., & Chaufan, G. (2014). Influence of the spray adjuvant on the toxicity

effects of a glyphosate formulation. *Toxicology in Vitro*, *28*(7), 1306–1311. PubMed PMID: 24999230.

14. Romero, D. M., Rios de Molina, M. C., & Juarez, A. B. (2011). Oxidative stress induced by a commercial glyphosate formulation in a tolerant strain of Chlorella kessleri. *Ecotoxicology and Environmental Safety*, *74*(4), 741–747. PubMed PMID: 21074853.

15. Seok, S. J., Park, J. S., Hong, J. R., et al. (2011). Surfactant volume is an essential element in human toxicity in acute glyphosate herbicide intoxication. *Clinical Toxicology (Philadelphia, Pa.)*, *49*(10), 892–899. PubMed PMID: 22077202.

16. Williams, G. M., Kroes, R., & Munro, I. C. (2000). Safety evaluation and risk assessment of the herbicide Roundup and its active ingredient, glyphosate, for humans. *Regulatory Toxicology and Pharmacology*, *31*(2 Pt. 1), 117–165. PubMed PMID: 10854122.

17. Moon, J. M., Chun, B. J., Cho, Y. S., et al. (2017 Jun 13). Cardiovascular effects and fatality may differ according to the formulation of glyphosate salt herbicide. *Cardiovascular Toxicology*, [Epub ahead of print]. PubMed PMID: 28612304.

18. Gasnier, C., Dumont, C., Benachour, N., et al. (2009). Glyphosate-based herbicides are toxic and endocrine disruptors in human cell lines. *Toxicology*, *262*(3), 184–191. PubMed PMID: 19539684.

19. Gore, A. C., Chappell, V. A., Fenton, S. E., et al. (2015). Executive summary to EDC-2: The Endocrine Society's second scientific statement on endocrine-disrupting chemicals. *Endocrine Reviews*, *36*(6), 593–602. PubMed PMID: 26414233.

20. Waring, R. H., & Harris, R. M. (2005). Endocrine disruptors: a human risk? *Molecular and Cellular Endocrinology*, *244*(1–2), 2–9. PubMed PMID: 16271281.

21. Buck Louis, G. M., Gray, L. E., Jr., et al. (2008). Environmental factors and puberty timing: expert panel research needs. *Pediatrics*, *121*(Suppl. 3), S192–S207. PubMed PMID: 18245512.

22. Anway, M. D., & Skinner, M. K. (2006). Epigenetic transgenerational actions of endocrine disruptors. *Endocrinology*, *147*(6 Suppl.), S43–S49. PubMed PMID: 16690803.

23. Walsh, L. P., McCormick, C., Martin, C., & Stocco, D. M. (2000). Roundup inhibits steroidogenesis by disrupting steroidogenic acute regulatory (StAR) protein expression. *Environmental Health Perspectives*, *108*(8), 769–776. PubMed PMID: 10964798.

24. Kwiatkowski, M., Pawel, J., & Bukowska, B. (2013). Glyphosate and its formulations – toxicity, occupational and environmental exposure. *Medycyna Pracy*, *64*(5), 717–729. PubMed PMID: 24502134.

25. Peixoto, F. (2005). Comparative effects of the Roundup and glyphosate on mitochondrial oxidative phosphorylation. *Chemosphere*, *61*(8), 1115–1122. PubMed PMID: 16263381.

26. Thongpraisang, S., Thiantanawat, A., Rangkadilok, N., et al. (2013). Glyphosate induces human breast cancer cells growth via estrogen receptors. *Food and Chemical Toxicology*, *59*, 129–136. PubMed PMID: 23756170.

27. El-Demerdash, F. M., Yousef, M. I., & Elegamy, E. I. (2001). Influence of paraquat, glyphosate, and cadmium on the activity of some serum enzymes and protein electrophoretic behavior (in vitro). *Journal of Environmental Science and Health. Part. B, Pesticides, Food Contaminants, and Agricultural Wastes*, *36*(1), 29–42. PubMed PMID: 11281253.

28. Hietanen, E., Linnainmaa, K., & Vainio, H. (1983). Effects of phenoxyherbicides and glyphosate on the hepatic and intestinal biotransformation activities in the rat. *Acta Pharmacologica et Toxicologica*, *53*(2), 103–112. PubMed PMID: 6624478.

29. Vigfusson, N. V., & Vyse, E. R. (1980). The effect of the pesticides Dexon, Captan, and Roundup on sister-chromatid exchanges in human lymphocytes in vitro. *Mutation Research*, *79*(1), 53–57. PubMed PMID: 7432366.

30. Clements, C., Ralph, S., & Petras, M. (1997). Genotoxicity of select herbicides in Rana catesbeiana tadpoles using the alkaline single-cell gel DNA electrophoresis (comet) assay. *Environmental and Molecular Mutagenesis*, *29*(3), 277–288. PubMed PMID: 9142171.

31. Martinez, A., Reyes, I., & Reyes, N. (2007). Cytotoxicity of the herbicide glyphosate in human peripheral blood mononuclear cells. *Biomedica: Revista Del Instituto Nacional de Salud*, *27*(4), 594–604. PubMed PMID: 18320126.

32. Benachour, N., & Seralini, G. E. (2009). Glyphosate formulations induce apoptosis and necrosis in human umbilical, embryonic, and placental cells. *Chemical Research in Toxicology*, *22*(1), 97–105. PubMed PMID: 19105591.

33. Tsui, M. T., & Chu, L. M. (2003). Aquatic toxicity of glyphosate-based formulations: comparisons between different organisms and the effects of environmental factors. *Chemosphere*, *52*(7), 1189–1197. PubMed PMID: 12821000.

34. Grandcoin, A., Piel, S., & Baures, E. (2017). Aminomethylphosphonic acid (AMPA) in natural waters: its sources, behavior and environmental fate. *Water Research*, *117*, 187–197. PubMed PMID: 28391123.

35. Battaglin, W., Kolpin, D., Scribner, E., et al. (2005). Glyphosate, other herbicides, and transformation

products in Midwestern streams. *Journal of the American Water Resources Association*, 41, 323–332.

36. Manas, F., Peralta, L., Raviolo, J., et al. (2009). Genotoxicity of AMPA, the environmental metabolite of glyphosate, assessed by the Comet assay and cytogenetic tests. *Ecotoxicology and Environmental Safety*, 72(3), 834–837. PubMed PMID: 19013644.

37. Kwiatkowska, M., Huras, B., & Bukowska, B. (2014). The effect of metabolites and impurities of glyphosate on human erythrocytes (in vitro). *Pesticide Biochemistry and Physiology*, 109, 34–43. PubMed PMID: 24581382.

38. Mesnage, R., Bernay, B., & Seralini, G. E. (2013). Ethoxylated adjuvants of glyphosate-based herbicides are active principles of human cell toxicity. *Toxicology*, 313(2–3), 122–128. PubMed PMID: 23000283.

39. Defarge, N., Takacs, E., Lozano, V. L., et al. (2016). Co-formulants in glyphosate-based herbicides disrupt aromatase activity in human cells below toxic levels. *International Journal of Environmental Research and Public Health*, 13(3), Pii:E264. PubMed PMID: 26927151.

40. Chlopecka, M., Mendel, M., Dziekan, N., & Karlik, W. (2017). The effect of glyphosate-based herbicide Roundup and its co-formulant, POEA, on the motoric activity of rat intestine – in vitro study. *Environmental Toxicology and Pharmacology*, 49, 156–162. PubMed PMID: 28049099.

41. Song, H. Y., Kim, Y. H., Seok, S. J., et al. (2012). Cellular toxicity of surfactants used as herbicide additives. *Journal of Korean Medical Science*, 27(1), 3–9. PubMed PMID: 22219606.

42. Sribanditmongkol, P., Jutavijittum, P., Pongraveevongsa, P., et al. (2012). Pathological and toxicological findings in glyphosate-surfactant herbicide fatality: a case report. *The American Journal of Forensic Medicine and Pathology*, 33(3), 234–237. PubMed PMID: 22835958.

43. Lee, H. L., Kan, C. D., Tsai, C. L., et al. (2009). Comparative effects of the formulation of glyphosate-surfactant herbicides on hemodynamics in swine. *Clinical Toxicology (Philadelphia, Pa.)*, 47(7), 651–658. PubMed PMID: 19663613.

44. Rush, M. D., Schoenfeld, C. N., & Watson, W. A. (1998). Skin necrosis and venous thrombosis from subcutaneous injection of charcoal lighter fluid (naphtha). *The American Journal of Emergency Medicine*, 16(5), 508–511. PubMed PMID: 9725968.

45. Shusterman, E. M., Williams, S. R., & Childers, B. J. (1999). Soft tissue injection of hydrocarbons: a case-report and review of the literature. *The Journal of Emergency Medicine*, 17(1), 63–65. PubMed PMID: 9950390.

46. Roberge, R. J., Crippen, D. R., Jayadevappa, D., & Kosek, T. L. (2001). Acute myocardial infarction and renal failure following naphtha ingestion. *The Journal of Emergency Medicine*, 21(3), 243–247. PubMed PMID: 11604278.

47. Battaglin, W. A., Thurman, E. M., Kolpin, D. W., et al. (2003). *Work plan for determining the occurrence of glyphosate, its transformation product AMPA, other herbicide compounds, and antibiotics in Midwestern United States streams, 2002: U.S. Geological Survey Open-File Report 03-69.*

48. Chang, F. C., Simcik, M. F., & Capel, P. D. (2011). Occurrence and fate of the herbicide glyphosate and its degredate aminomethylphosphonic acid in the atmosphere. *Environmental Toxicology and Chemistry*, 30(3), 548–555. PubMed PMID: 21128261.

49. Borggaard, O. K., & Gimsing, A. L. (2008). Fate of glyphosate in soil and the possibility of leaching to ground and surface waters: a review. *Pest Management Science*, 64(4), 441–456. PubMed PMID: 18161065.

50. Coupe, R. H., Kalkhoff, S. J., Capel, P. D., & Gregoire, C. (2012). Fate and transport of glyphosate and aminomethylphosphonic acid in surface waters of agricultural basins. *Pest Management Science*, 68(1), 16–30. PubMed PMID: 21681915.

51. McQueen, H., Callan, A. C., & Hinwood, A. L. (2012). Estimating maternal and prenatal exposure to glyphosate in the community setting. *International Journal of Hygiene and Environmental Health*, 215(6), 570–576. PubMed PMID: 22261298.

52. Honeycutt, Z., & Rowlands, H. *Glyphosate Testing Report: Findings in American Mothers' Breast Milk, Urine and Water.* Moms Across America. Available at http://www.momsacrossamerica.com/glyphosate_testing_results. (Accessed November 18, 2015.)

53. Aris, A., & Leblanc, S. (2011). Maternal and fetal exposure to pesticides associated to genetically modified foods in Eastern Townships of Quebec, Canada. *Reproductive Toxicology*, 31(4), 528–533. PubMed PMID: 21338670.

54. Zouaoui, K., Dulaurent, S., Gaulier, J. M., et al. (2013). Determination of glyphosate and AMPA in blood and urine from humans: about 13 cases of acute intoxication. *Forensic Science International*, 226(1–3), e20–e25. PubMed PMID: 23291146.

55. Roberts, D. M., Buckley, N. A., Mohamed, F., et al. (2010). A prospective observational study of the clinical toxicology of glyphosate-containing herbicides in adults with acute self-poisoning. *Clinical Toxicology (Philadelphia, Pa.)*, 48(2), 129–136. PubMed PMID: 20136481.

56. Conrad, A., Schroter-Kermani, C., Hoppe, H. W., et al. (2017). Glyphosate in German adults – time trend (2001-2015) of human exposure to a widely

used herbicide. *International Journal of Hygiene and Environmental Health*, *220*(1), 8–16. PubMed PMID: 27838355.

57. Anadon, A., Martinez-Larranaga, M. R., Martinez, M. A., et al. (2009). Toxicokinetics of glyphosate and its metabolite aminomethyl phosphonic acid in rats. *Toxicology Letters*, *190*(1), 91–95. PubMed PMID: 19607892.

58. Brewster, D. W., Warren, J., & Hopkins, W. E., 2nd. (1991). Metabolism of glyphosate in Sprague-Dawley rats: tissue distribution, identification, and quantitation of glyphosate-derived materials following a single oral dose. *Fundamental and Applied Toxicology*, *17*(1), 43–51. PubMed PMID: 1916078.

59. Bus, J. S. (2015). Analysis of Moms Across America report suggesting bioaccumulation of glyphosate in U.S. mother's breast milk: implausibility based on inconsistency with available body of glyphosate animal toxicokinetic, human biomonitoring, and physico-chemical data. *Regulatory Toxicology and Pharmacology*, *73*(3), 758–764. PubMed PMID: 26520181.

60. Cartigny, B., Azaroual, N., Imbenotte, M., et al. (2008). Quantitative determination of glyphosate in human serum by 1H NMR spectroscopy. *Talanta*, *74*(4), 1075–1078. PubMed PMID: 18371753.

61. Tominack, R. L., Yang, G. Y., Tsai, W. J., et al. (1991). Taiwan National Poison Center survey of glyphosate-surfactant herbicide ingestions. *Journal of Toxicology. Clinical Toxicology*, *29*(1), 91–109. PubMed PMID: 2005670.

62. Lee, H. L., Chen, K. W., Chi, C. H., et al. (2000). Clinical presentations and prognostic factors of a glyphosate-surfactant herbicide intoxication: a review of 131 cases. *Academic Emergency Medicine*, *7*(8), 906–910. PubMed PMID: 10958131.

63. Stella, J., & Ryan, M. (2004). Glyphosate herbicide formulation: a potentially lethal ingestion. *Emergency Medicine Australasia*, *16*(3), 235–239. PubMed PMID: 15228468.

64. Hsiao, C. T., Lin, L. J., Hsiao, K. Y., et al. (2008). Acute pancreatitis caused by severe glyphosate-surfactant oral intoxication. *The American Journal of Emergency Medicine*, *26*(3), 384.e3–384.e5. PubMed PMID: 18358975.

65. Penagos, H., Ruepert, C., Partanen, T., et al. (2004). Pesticide patch test series for the assessment of allergic contact dermatitis among banana plantation workers in Panama. *Dermatitis: Contact, Atopic, Occupational, Drug*, *15*(3), 137–145. PubMed PMID: 15724348.

66. Peluso, M., Munnia, A., Bolognesi, C., & Parodi, S. (1998). 32P-postlabeling detection of DNA adducts in mice treated with the herbicide Roundup. *Environmental and Molecular Mutagenesis*, *31*(1), 55–59. PubMed PMID: 9464316.

67. Rank, J., Jensen, A. G., Skov, B., et al. (1993). Genotoxicity testing of the herbicide Roundup and its active ingredient glyphosate isopropylamine using the mouse bone marrow micronucleus test, Salmonalls mutagenicity test, and Allium anaphase-telophase test. *Mutation Research*, *300*(1), 29–36. PubMed PMID: 7683765.

68. Seralini, G. E., Clair, E., Mesnage, R., et al. (2014). Republished study: long-term toxicity of a Roundup herbicide and a Roundup-tolerant genetically modified maize. *Environmental Sciences Europe*, *26*(1), 14. PubMed PMID: 27752412.

69. Hardell, L., & Eriksson, M. (1999). A case-control syudy of non-Hodgkin's lymphoma and exposure to pesticides. *Cancer*, *85*(6), 1353–1360. PubMed PMID: 10189142.

70. De Roos, A. J., Zahm, S. H., Cantor, K. P., et al. (2003). Integrative assessment of multiple pesticides as risk factors for non-Hodgkin's lymphoma among men. *Occupational and Environmental Medicine*, *60*(9), E11. PubMed PMID: 12937207.

71. McDuffie, H. H., Pahwa, P., McLaughlin, J. R., et al. (2001). Non-Hodgkin's lymphoma and specific pesticide exposures in men: cross-Canada study of pesticides and health. *Cancer Epidemiology, Biomarkers and Prevention*, *10*(11), 1155–1163. PubMed PMID: 11700263.

72. Hardell, L., Eriksson, M., & Nordstrum, M. (2002). Exposure to pesticides as risk factor for non-Hodgkin's lymphoma and hairy cell leukemia: pooled analysis of two Swedish case-control studies. *Leukemia and Lymphoma*, *43*(5), 1043–1049. PubMed PMID: 12148884.

73. Nordstrum, M., Hardell, L., Magnuson, A., et al. (1998). Occupational exposures, animal exposure and smoking as risk factors for hairy cell leukemia evaluated in a case-control study. *British Journal of Cancer*, *77*(11), 2048–2052. PubMed PMID: 9667691.

74. Schinasi, L., & Leon, M. E. (2014). Non-Hodgkin lymphoma and occupational exposure to agricultural pesticide chemical groups and active ingredients: a systematic review and meta-analysis. *International Journal of Environmental Research and Public Health*, *11*(4), 4449–4527. PubMed PMID: 24762670.

75. De Roos, A. J., Blair, A., Rusiecki, J. A., et al. (2005). Cancer incidence among glyphosate-exposed pesticide applicators in the Agricultural Health Study. *Environmental Health Perspectives*, *113*(1), 49–54. PubMed PMID: 15626647.

76. Garry, V. F., Harkins, M. E., Erickson, L. L., et al. (2002). Birth defects, season of conception, and sex of

children born to pesticide applicators living in the Red River Valley of Minnesota, USA. *Environmental Health Perspectives*, 110(Suppl. 3), 441–449. PubMed PMID: 12060842.

77. Rull, R. P., Ritz, B., & Shaw, G. M. (2006). Neural tube defects and maternal residential proximity to agricultural pesticide applications. *American Journal of Epidemiology*, 163(8), 743–753. PubMed PMID: 16495467.

78. IRDC. (1980a). *Test article – technical glyphosate: teratology study in rats. Unpublished report prepared by International Research and Development Corporation, Mattawan, MI*. Submitted to WHO by Monsanto Ltd. (Study No. 401-054; Reference No. IR-79-018).

79. Bio/Dynamics Inc. (1981b). *A three-generation reproduction study in rats with glyphosate*. Final Report. Unpublished report prepared by Bio/Dynamics Inc., Division of Biology and Safety Evaluation, East Millstone, NJ. Submitted to WHO by Monsanto Ltd. (Project No. 77-2063; BDN-77-147).

80. Bio/Dynamics Inc. (1983). *A chronic feeding study of glyphosate (Roundup technical) in mice*. Unpublished report prepared by Bio/Dynamics Inc., Division of Biology and Safety Evaluation, East Millstone, NJ. Submitted to WHO by Monsanto Ltd. (Project No. 77-2061; BDN-77-420).

81. Monsanto. (1990a). *Chronic study of glyphosate administered in feed to albino rats*. Unpublished report prepared and submitted to WHO by Monsanto Ltd., Monsanto Environmental Health Laboratory, St. Louis, MO (Project No. MSL-10495).

82. Jayasumana, C., Paranagama, P., Agampodi, S., et al. (2015). Drinking well water and occupational exposure to Herbicides is associated with chronic kidney disease, in Padavi-Sripura, Sri Lanka. *Environmental Health: A Global Access Science Source*, 14, 6.

83. U.S. Environmental Protection Agency. *Glyphosate & Ground Water & Drinking Water*. Available at https://safewater.zendesk.com/hc/en-us/article s/212076457-4-What-are-EPA-s-drinking-water-regul ations-for-glyphosate-. (Accessed November 15, 2017.)

84. Sampoogna, R. V., & Cunard, R. (2007). Roundup intoxication and a rationale for treatment. *Clinical Nephrology*, 68(3), 190–196. PubMed PMID: 17915625.

85. Garlich, F. M., Goldman, M., Pepe, J., et al. (2014). Hemodialysis clearance of glyphosate following a life-threatening ingestion of glyphosate-surfactant herbicide. *Clinical Toxicology (Philadelphia, Pa.)*, 52(1), 66–71. PubMed PMID: 24400933.

86. Clair, E., Mesnage, R., Travert, C., & Seralini, G. E. (2012). A glyphosate-based herbicide induces necrosis and apoptosis in mature rat testicular cells in vitro, and testosterone decrease at lower levels. *Toxicology in Vitro*, 26(2), 269–279. PubMed PMID: 22200534.

87. de Liz Oliveira Cavalli, V. L., Cattani, D., Heinz Rieg, C. E., et al. (2013). Roundup disrupts male reproductive functions by triggering calcium-mediated cell death in rat testis and Sertoli cells. *Free Radical Biology & Medicine*, 65, 335–346. PubMed PMID: 23820267.

88. Curtis, K. M., Savitz, D. A., Weinberg, C. R., & Arbuckle, T. E. (1999). The effect of pesticide exposure on time to pregnancy. *Epidemiology (Cambridge, Mass.)*, 10(2), 112–117. PubMed PMID: 10069244.

89. Arbuckle, T. E., Lin, Z., & Mery, L. S. (2001). An exporatory analysis of the effect of pesticide exposure on the risk of spontaneous abortion in an Ontario farm population. *Environmental Health Perspectives*, 109(8), 851–857. PubMed PMID: 11564623.

90. Savitz, D. A., Arbuckle, T., Kaczor, D., & Curtis, K. M. (1997). Male pesticide exposure and pregnancy outcome. *American Journal of Epidemiology*, 146(12), 1025–1036. PubMed PMID: 9420527.

91. Moon, J. M., Min, Y. I., & Chun, B. J. (2006). Can early hemodialysis affect the outcome of the ingestion of glyphosate herbicide? *Clinical Toxicology (Philadelphia, Pa.)*, 44(3), 329–332. PubMed PMID: 16749554.

92. Kruger, M., Schledorn, P., Wieland, S., et al. (2014). Detection of glyphosate residues in animals and humans. *Journal of Environmental & Analytical Toxicology*, 4, 2.

93. Goen, T., Schmidt, L., Lichtensteiger, W., & Schlumpf, M. (2017). Efficiency control of dietary pesticide intake reduction by human biomonitoring. *International Journal of Hygiene and Environmental Health*, 220(2 Pt. A), 254–260. PubMed PMID: 27939065.

94. Lu, C., Toepel, K., Irish, R., et al. (2006). Organic diets significantly lower children's dietary exposure to organophosphorous pesticides. *Environmental Health Perspectives*, 114(2), 260–263. PubMed PMID: 16451864.

95. Bradman, A., Quiros-Alcala, L., Castorina, R., et al. (2015). Effect of organic diet intervention on pesticide exposures in young children living in low-income urban and agricultural communities. *Environmental Health Perspectives*, 123(10), 1086–1093. PubMed PMID: 25861095.

24

Chlorophenoxy Herbicides

SUMMARY

- Presence in population: 2,4-D is found ubiquitously
- Major disease: Monoclonal gammopathy of undetermined significance (MGUS), non-Hodgkin's lymphoma (NHL), prostate and gastric cancers, Alzheimer's disease, parkinsonism, light chain autoimmune amyloidosis, thyroiditis, heart disease, and diabetes

- Primary sources: Carpet dust, wheat products
- Best measure: No testing is currently available for 2,4-D
- Best intervention: Control indoor dust, removing carpeting and not wearing shoes indoors, avoiding nonorganic wheat products.

DESCRIPTION

Chlorophenoxy herbicides (Fig. 24.1) have been used for decades to control broadleaf weeds in agriculture, on roadways, along railroads, in parks and golf courses, and on commercial and residential lawns. These compounds are chemical analogs of auxins and cause uncontrolled and lethal growth in broadleaf plants. The US military used a combination of 2,4-D and 2,4,5-T, commonly known as Agent Orange, for deforestation of more than 3.6 million acres in Southeast Asia during the Vietnam War.

The most commonly used chlorophenoxy herbicide is 2,4-di-chlorophenoxy acetic acid (2,4-D), with more than 40 million pounds applied annually in the United States. Others in this class include 2-(2,4-dichlorophenoxy) propionic acid (2,4-DP); 2,4,5-trichlorophenoxy acetic acid (2,4,5-T); 3,6-dichloro-o-anisic acid (Dicamba); 4-chloro-2-methyl-phenoxy acetic acid (MCPA); 2-(4-chloro-2-methylphenoxy) butyric acid (MCPB); and 2-(4-chloro-2-methylphenoxy) proprionic acid (Mecoprop).

TOXICITY

Chlorophenoxy herbicides are prooxidants that cause cellular damage, mitochondrial dysfunction, and disrup

tion of acetylcoenzyme A metabolism.[1] Long-term toxicity comes from their contamination with dioxins, a byproduct of some types of hydrocarbon chlorination. Although several dioxins are present in these herbicides, the combination of 2,4-D and 2,4,5-T (Agent Orange) contains 2,3,7,8-tetrachlorodibenzo[p]dioxin (TCDD), widely regarded as the most toxic dioxin.

SOURCES

Millions of pounds of chlorophenoxy herbicides have been used agriculturally since they were first produced in the 1940s. Recently, glyphosate-based herbicides have somewhat eclipsed chlorophenoxy herbicides as the primary agricultural herbicide class, but they are still high-use agricultural chemicals.[2] The half-life of 2,4-D in the air is 19 hours, in soil 6 days, and in water 15 days under aerobic conditions and up to 333 days in anaerobic conditions. Contact can come during application or when swimming in water containing runoff. It has been found in 83% of homes studied in North Carolina and 98% in Ohio, with urinary levels found in 87% and 97% of the participants in each location. Carpet dust samples in both North Carolina and Ohio had the highest concentrations of 2,4-D in the home, followed by hand wipes (dermal levels of 2,4-D) and solid food.[3] When source

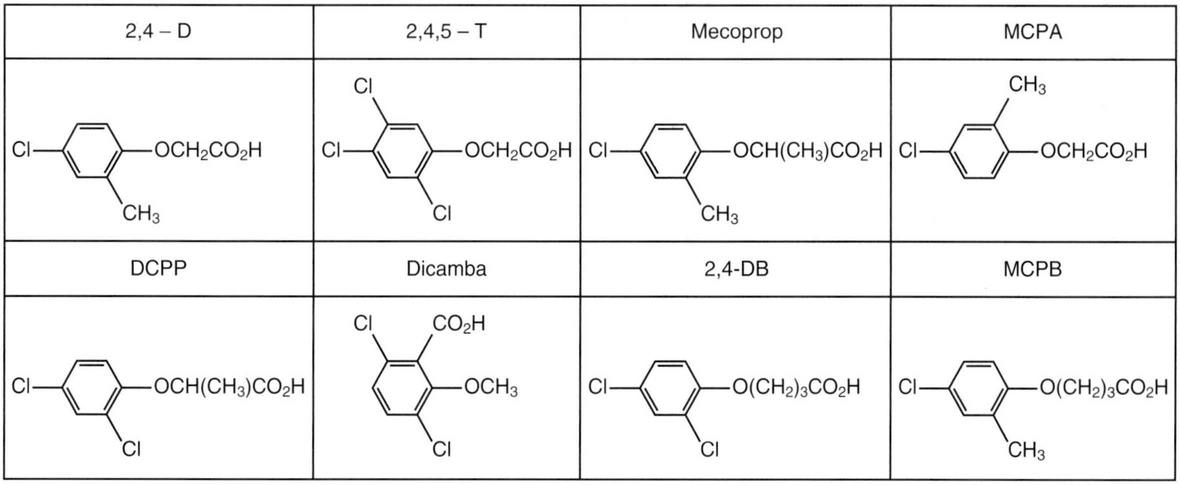

FIG. 24.1 Chemical structure of chlorophenoxy herbicides.

TABLE 24.1 Food with 2,4-D Residue Out of Eight Samples		
Food	Number Found	Mean PPM
Whole wheat bread	7	0.00169
Cracked wheat bread	6	0.00098
White bread	6	0.00060
Raisin bran cereal	6	0.00035
Fried rice, meatless	3	0.00015
Enriched white rice	1	0.00025

From Food and Drug Administration. (2017). *Total Diet Study*. Retrieved from www.fda.gov/food/foodscienceresearch/totaldietstudy/default.htm

exposure was correlated with average urine 2,4-D levels (found positive in more than 95% of those tested), the only source with a significant positive correlation was diet. The Food and Drug Administration Total Diet Study (FDA TDS) found 2,4-D in a small percentage of the cereals and breads tested. If applied to the lawn, it is then tracked into the home by pets or humans and transferred to carpets, fabrics, and home dust.[4] In a contaminated home, children are estimated to have up to 10-fold greater exposure to this herbicide. Table 24.1 shows 2,4-D residue from eight samples of several foods.

BODY BURDEN

2,4-D is found throughout the North American population assessed in the National Health and Nutritional Examination Survey (NHANES) trial (Table 24.2). However, the North Carolina/Ohio study revealed that it would require three to four urine samples in children and two to nine samples in adults to get a reliable measurement of daily exposure. This is related to the short half-life of 2,4-D in humans, which varies between 10 and 33 hours. Furthermore, because 2,4-D is ubiquitously found, this implies that constant ongoing exposure is occurring.

Detoxification/Excretion Processes

2,4-D is rapidly eliminated through urine intact.

Clinical Significance

Between 1998 and 2002, the US Poison Control Centers reported more than 11,000 cases of chlorophenoxy herbicide poisoning.[1] The literature contains case reports of individuals drinking these compounds as a means of committing suicide.[5]

An increased risk for NHL has repeatedly been found for farmers working with 2,4-D.[6,7,8,9] Air Force personnel who participated in Operation Ranch Hand, the spraying of Agent Orange during the Vietnam War have a 2.4-fold increased risk for MGUS and a 2.19-fold risk for prostate cancer.[10,11] They also have increased risk for amyloidosis,

TABLE 24.2 Urinary 2,4-D Levels in NHANES 2009 to 2010 (µg/g Creatinine)					
	GM	50th %	75th %	90th %	95th %
2,4-dichlorophenoxyacetic acid	.321	.301	.500	.983	1.55

From Centers for Disease Control and Prevention. (2017). *National Report on Human Exposure to Environmental Chemicals.* Retrieved from www.cdc.gov/exposurereport

have a 32% increased risk for hypertension, are 50% more likely to have diabetes, are 52% more likely to have heart disease, and are 62% more likely to have chronic respiratory problems.[12,13] They are also more than twice as likely to have elevated liver enzymes.[14]

Compared with those without exposure, the Vietnam veterans from Korea who were exposed to Agent Orange were more likely to have amyloidosis (odds ratio (OR) 3.20), autoimmune thyroiditis (OR 1.93), Alzheimer's disease (OR 1.64), and endocrinopathies (OR 1.43).[15]

Hypothyroidism is also more likely to be found in pesticide applicators who have "ever used" 2,4-D, 2,4,5-T or Dicamba.[16] Use of 2,4-D has also been associated with a 2.59-fold increased risk for parkinsonism and an 85% increased risk for gastric cancer.[17,18]

INTERVENTION

Avoidance remains the main intervention for this herbicide. If it is being used for lawn care, pets should not be allowed to run on the lawn after application, and shoes should not be worn in the home. Removal of indoor carpeting would eliminate the major source of indoor chlorophenoxy herbicides. Indoor dust control would also be critical. Urinary alkalinization is considered to be one of the best treatments for acute chlorophenoxy poisoning.[1,19]

REFERENCES

1. Bradberry, S. M., Proudfoot, A. T., & Vale, J. A. (2004). Poisoning due to chlorophenoxy herbicides. *Toxicological Reviews, 23*(2), 65–73. Review. PubMed PMID: 15578861.
2. EPA *Pesticides industry sales and usage 2008-2012 market estimates.* https://www.epa.gov/sites/production/files/2017-01/documents/pesticides-industry-sales-usage-2016_0.pdf. (Accessed July 21, 2017.)
3. Morgan, M., Sheldon, L., Thomas, K., et al. (2008). Adult and children's exposure to 2,4-D from multiple sources and pathways. *Journal of Exposure Science & Environmental Epidemiology, 18,* 486–494. PubMed PMID: 18167507.
4. Nishioka, M. G., Lewis, R. G., Brinkman, M. C., et al. (2001). Distribution of 2,4-D in air and on surfaces inside residences after lawn applications: comparing exposure estimates from various media for young children. *Environmental Health Perspectives, 109*(11), 1185–1191. PubMed PMID: 11713005.
5. Roberts, D. M., Seneviratne, R., Mohammed, F., et al. (2005). Intentional self-poisoning with the chlorophenoxy herbicide 4-chloro-2-methylphenoxyacetic acid (MCPA). *Annals of Emergency Medicine, 46*(3), 275–284. PubMed PMID: 16126140.
6. Hoar, S. K., Blair, A., Holmes, F. F., et al. (1986). Agricultural herbicide use and risk of lymphoma and soft-tissue sarcoma. *The Journal of the American Medical Association, 256*(9), 1141–1147. Erratum in: *The Journal of the American Medical Association.* (1986). *256*(24):3351. PubMed PMID: 3801091.
7. Woods, J. S., Polissar, L., Severson, R. K., et al. (1987). Soft tissue sarcoma and non-Hodgkin's lymphoma in relation to phenoxyherbicide and chlorinated phenol exposure in western Washington. *Journal of the National Cancer Institute, 78*(5), 899–910. PubMed PMID: 3471999.
8. Zahm, S. H., Weisenburger, D. D., Babbitt, P. A., et al. (1990). A case-control study of non-Hodgkin's lymphoma and the herbicide 2,4-dichlorophenoxyacetic acid (2,4-D) in eastern Nebraska. *Epidemiology (Cambridge, Mass.), 1*(5), 349–356. PubMed PMID: 2078610.
9. Smith, A. M., Smith, M. T., La Merrill, M. A., et al. (2017). 2,4-dichlorophenoxyacetic acid (2,4-D) and risk of non-Hodgkin lymphoma: a meta-analysis accounting for exposure levels. *Annals of Epidemiology, 27*(4), 281–289, e4. PubMed PMID: 28476329.
10. Landgren, O., Shim, Y. K., Michalek, J., et al. (2015). Agent Orange exposure and monoclonal gammopathy of undetermined significance: An Operation Ranch Hand veteran cohort study. *JAMA Oncology, 1*(8), 1061–1068. PubMed PMID: 26335650.
11. Chamie, K., DeVere White, R. W., Lee, D., Ok, J. H., & Ellison, L. M. (2008). Agent Orange exposure, Vietnam War veterans, and the risk of prostate cancer. *Cancer, 113*(9), 2464–2470. PubMed PMID: 18666213.

12. Department of Veterans Affairs. (2009). Presumptive service connection for disease associated with exposure to certain herbicide agents: AL amyloidosis. Final rule. *Federal Register, 74*(87), 21258–21260. PubMed PMID: 19507326.

13. Kang, H. K., Dalager, N. A., Needham, L. L., et al. (2006). Health status of Army Chemical Corps Vietnam veterans who sprayed defoliant in Vietnam. *American Journal of Industrial Medicine, 49*(11), 875–884. PubMed PMID: 17006952.

14. Michalek, J. E., Ketchum, N. S., & Longnecker, M. P. (2001). Serum dioxin and hepatic abnormalities in veterans of Operation Ranch Hand. *Annals of Epidemiology, 11*(5), 304–311. PubMed PMID: 11399444.

15. Yi, S. W., Hong, J. S., Ohrr, H., & Yi, J. J. (2014). Agent Orange exposure and disease prevalence in Korean Vietnam veterans: the Korean veteran's health study. *Environmental Research, 133*, 56–65. PubMed PMID: 24906069.

16. Goldner, W. S., Sandler, D. P., Yu, F., et al. (2013). Hypothyroidism and pesticide use among male private pesticide applicators in the agricultural health study. *Journal of Occupational and Environmental Medicine, 55*(10), 1171–1178. PubMed PMID: 2406477.

17. Tanner, C. M., Ross, G. W., Jewell, S. A., et al. (2009). Occupation and risk of parkinsonism: a multicenter case-control study. *Archives of Neurology, 66*(9), 1106–1113. PubMed PMID: 19752299.

18. Mills, P. K., & Yang, R. C. (2007). Agricultural exposures and gastric cancer risk in Hispanic farm workers in California. *Environmental Research, 104*(2), 282–289. PubMed PMID: 17196584.

19. Flanagan, R. J., Meredith, T. J., Ruprah, M., et al. (1990). Alkaline diuresis for acute poisoning with chlorophenoxy herbicides and ioxynil. *Lancet, 335*(8687), 454–458. PubMed PMID: 1968179.

25

Bisphenol A
[4,4'-dihydroxy-2,2-diphenylpropane]

SUMMARY

- Presence in population: It is estimated that in 2008, the total world production of bisphenol A (BPA) was approximately 5.2 million metric tons;[1] BPA is found in a wide variety of applications and is ubiquitous

- Major diseases: Endocrine-related disorders
- Primary sources: Food packaging, thermal paper, toys, healthcare equipment, dental materials
- Best measure: Urine BPA concentration
- Best intervention: Avoidance, antioxidants

DESCRIPTION

BPA (Fig. 25.1) is an industrial chemical that was first synthesized in 1891 by condensing two phenol groups and one acetone molecule. BPA has since been used as a monomer in the manufacturing of polymers such as polycarbonate, epoxy resins, polysulfone, and polyacrylate; a component in the processing of polyvinyl chloride (PVC) plastics; and a precursor for the synthesis of the flame retardant tetrabromobisphenol-A.[2] End-use applications include plastic food and drink packaging, kitchenware, inner coatings of cans and jar lids, water bottles, electrical and electronic goods, electronic storage media, and marine and car coatings.

In 2008, the total world production of BPA was approximately 5.2 million metric tons.[1] Safety and side effects profiles of BPA emerged in the late 1990s when it was found to leach out of plastics and into experimental animals, resulting in chromosomal anomalies in their offspring.[3] The presence of BPA in the environment and consumer products has since garnered a lot of attention regarding the potential for human harm from exposure and bioaccumulation.

TOXICITY

Free forms of BPA display estrogenic activity through the classical nuclear estrogen receptors. BPA has been shown to bind to a membrane-associated estrogen receptor, producing nongenomic steroid action and stimulate rapid cellular response at concentrations lower than expected.[4] BPA is also associated with progesterone deficiency.[5] Increasing concentrations of BPA reduce the effect of an androgen receptor agonist in a dose-dependent manner.[6] BPA binds to the thyroid hormone receptor, antagonizing its activation,[7] and exerts a direct effect on thyroid follicular cells, altering expression of the genes involved in thyroid hormone synthesis.[8] Animal studies indicate that BPA causes oxidative stress, generating highly reactive toxic intermediates in the liver, kidney, testes, and brain.[9,10]

SOURCES

There are various routes of human exposure to BPA, including ingestion, inhalation, and transdermal absorption. The main sources of BPA exposure include food

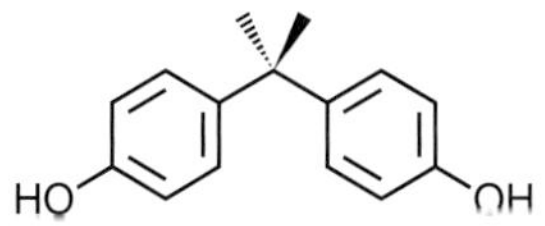

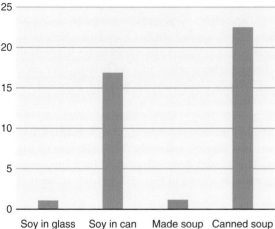

FIG. 25.1 Bisphenol A.

HO—⟨ ⟩—⟨ ⟩—OH

BPA (µg/L urine)

FIG. 25.2 Canned foods have high levels of BPA.

TABLE 25.1 Urinary BPA Concentrations in the 2011 to 2012 NHANES (ug/g creatinine)

	Mean	50th %	75th %	90th %	95th %
BPA	1.72	1.58	2.86	4.62	8.24

BPA, Bisphenol A.
From Centers for Disease Control and Prevention, National Report on Human Exposure to Environmental Chemicals. www.cdc.gov/exposurereport.

because of the electronic equipment used in those settings.[21] As a result of more frequent hand-to-mouth contact, toddlers have a larger intake of house dust compared with adults and therefore have higher exposure to toxicants via ingestion.[22] Thermal paper commonly used in cash registers and credit card terminals and recycled paper contain up to 2.3% BPA.[23,24] The average amount of BPA transferred to the skin after holding thermal paper for 5 seconds is 1.1 µg per finger, and about 10 times higher if the fingers are wet or greasy.[25] BPA may be present as an impurity in dental composite resins and is likely more relevant for patients with multiple or large dental restorations.[26]

BODY BURDEN

The Centers for Disease Control and Prevention estimates that 93% of Americans 6 years of age or older have detectable urine levels of BPA.[27] The current tolerable daily intake (TDI) value derived by the European Food Safety Authority is set at 50 µg/kg body weight per day.[28] Urinary data suggests that estimated median exposure to BPA is in the range of 0.01 to 0.05 µg/kg body weight per day for adults and 0.02 to 0.12 µg/kg body weight per day for children, with a 95th percentile exposure estimate of 0.27 µg/kg body weight per day for the general population.[29] Table 25.1 lists the urinary BPA concentrations from the 2011 to 2012 National Health and Nutritional Examination Survey (NHANES).

A review of more than 80 biomonitoring studies measuring BPA concentrations in human tissues and fluids indicated that adults, adolescents, and children are overwhelmingly exposed to BPA, and unconjugated BPA in blood poses significant risk from internal exposure.[30] BPA is lipophilic and may accumulate in fat. Rodents chronically exposed to BPA had levels 8 to 10 times higher in brown fat than in serum.[31] A small study of 20 women

packaging, dust, dental materials,[11] healthcare equipment,[12] thermal paper,[13,14] toys, and products for children and infants. Although BPA is not persistent in the environment, exposure appears to be continuous.

Exposure from food is primary, with greater than 90% of BPA exposure being dietary based.[15,16] This results from BPA leaching into food from either the release of unpolymerized monomers or the slow decay of polymer bonds in polycarbonates, leading to monomer release into proximal foods and liquids.[17] Research has shown significant increases (up to 1200%) in urinary BPA levels after consumption of canned foods.[18] Studies show 80% to 100% of free BPA migrates into food during sterilization,[19] and heating temperature has more influence on migration than heating time.[20] Fig. 25.2 shows a comparison between urinary BPA after consumption of two servings of canned soy milk versus soy milk in glass, and one daily 12-ounce serving of fresh soup versus canned soup.

Nonfood sources of BPA contribute approximately 1% to 5% of exposure and vary significantly among subsets of the population. Higher concentrations of BPA can be found in indoor dust in laboratories and offices measured BPA in adipose tissue and found a mean of 3.2 ng BPA/g fat and 8.2 ng chlorinated BPA/g fat.[32]

Detoxification/Excretion Processes

Unconjugated BPA is the biologically active form of BPA. It is metabolized in the liver and gut wall to form BPA glucuronide, which is delivered to the blood and then the kidneys to be excreted in the urine.[33] BPA conjugates have an estimated half-life in the human body of 5.4 hours.[34] However, many tissues, including the intestines, lungs, liver, kidneys, and placentas of animals and humans, have been shown to contain β-glucuronidase, an enzyme that is able to deconjugate BPA and release its active form, thus delaying the elimination process.[35]

Clinical Significance

BPA may play a role in the pathogenesis of several endocrine disorders, including female and male infertility, precocious puberty, hormone-dependent tumors such as breast and prostate cancer, hyperplasia of the endometrium, and several metabolic disorders including polycystic ovary syndrome (PCOS), insensitivity to insulin, and diabetes.[36,37] Higher seminal BPA levels are associated with decreased sperm concentration, decreased motility, abnormal sperm morphology, and decreased total sperm count.[38]

Higher urinary BPA concentrations have been associated with chronic obstructive pulmonary disease,[39] cardiovascular disease, diabetes, and elevated blood levels of the liver enzymes gamma-glutamyltransferase and alkaline phosphatase.[40] A follow-up study confirmed an association between higher urinary concentrations of total BPA and an increased prevalence of coronary heart disease.[41] Animal studies found chronic exposure to BPA reduces successful cardiac remodeling after myocardial infarction[42] and increases ventricular arrhythmias after ischemia-reperfusion injury.[43]

Exposure to BPA during early development may contribute to genital tract abnormalities, obesity, and attention deficit hyperactivity disorder (ADHD).[44] Although ADHD is more common in males, prenatal BPA exposure has been found to be associated with increased externalizing behaviors (i.e., aggression, hyperactivity) in female toddlers.[45] Mean prenatal BPA is associated with increased odds of wheeze at 6 months of age (adjusted odds ratio [AOR] = 2.3; 95% confidence interval [CI]: 1.3, 4.1), but not at 3 years of age (AOR = 1.2; 95% CI, 1.0–1.5).[46] A 2015 Taiwanese study of 453 children from the Childhood Environment and Allergic Diseases Study

cohort found urinary BPA glucuronide levels to be significantly associated with asthma at ages 3 and 6 years, with approximately 70% of the total effect of BPA exposure on asthma mediated by immunoglobulin E (IgE) levels.[47]

In women, elevated BPA levels are associated with recurrent miscarriages,[48] fetuses with an abnormal karyotype,[49] decreased number of oocytes retrieved in *in vitro* fertilization (IVF) treatment,[50] and chromosomal abnormalities.[51]

Independent of potential confounders (e.g., body mass index, alcohol intake, blood pressure, or serum cholesterol levels), a positive association has been shown between higher levels of urinary BPA and prediabetes.[52] BPA directly blocks insulin receptor sites and distributes to adipose tissue, where it is slowly released into the bloodstream, causing insulin resistance.[53,54] This not only increases the incidence of diabetes, but also increases obesity, especially accumulation of visceral fat. This is well demonstrated by increasing waist-to-hip ratio, as shown in Fig. 25.3. Urinary concentrations

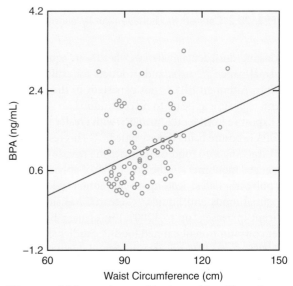

FIG. 25.3 BPA correlates with visceral fat. (From Savastano, S., Tarantino, G., D'Esposito, V., Passaretti, F., Cabaro, S., Liotti, A., Liguoro, D., Perruolo, G., Ariemma, F., Finelli, C., Beguinot, F., Formisano, P., Valentino, R. [2015]. Bisphenol-A plasma levels are related to inflammatory markers, visceral obesity and insulin-resistance: A cross-sectional study on adult male population. *Journal of Translational Medicine, 13,*169.) Licensed under a Creative Commons Attribution-ShareAlike 4.0 International License (http://creativecommons.org/licenses/by/4.0/).

of total BPA are associated with oxidative stress, which may also lead to increased fasting glucose levels.[55] The threshold for doubling the risk for diabetes is 5.0 μg/L urine.

INTERVENTION

As with most toxicants, avoidance is the most effective intervention. Because of the ubiquitous presence of BPA, total avoidance is virtually impossible, but with 90% of exposure coming from foods, the majority can easily be avoided. Induced sweating may be a clinically useful tool to facilitate the release of BPA through the skin to increase elimination.[17] Because BPA has been shown to induce oxidative stress, the use of antioxidants is critical.

BPA exposure is associated with PCOS and reduced progesterone levels. N-acetylcysteine (NAC) was found to improve ovulation rates and increase progesterone levels in PCOS when given at 1200 mg/day for 5 days, starting on the third day of the cycle.[56] Coadministration of NAC (100 mg/kg orally) antagonized the effect of BPA-induced cognitive dysfunction and attenuated the BPA-induced increase in malondialdehyde (MDA) levels and decreased glutathione (GSH) levels in the brains of rats.[57]

Research has shown that curcumin effectively attenuates the spectrum of effects of BPA-triggered insulin resistance.[58] *In vitro* and *in vivo* studies of the developing rat brain showed that curcumin protects against BPA-induced hippocampal neurotoxicity.[59]

Melatonin significantly attenuated brain oxidative stress, modulated apoptotic-regulating proteins, and protected against apoptosis in BPA-treated rats.[60] Melatonin has been shown to modulate the levels of GSH, superoxide dismutase, and catalase as well as the MDA and hydrogen peroxide concentrations in the testes and sperm, suggesting a protective effect against the reproductive toxicity of BPA.[61] Melatonin may also prevent the potential genotoxicity of BPA.[62]

In young women, treatment with wheat sprout (*Triticum aestivum*) juice reduced urinary BPA levels, suggesting possible reduction of BPA absorption or metabolism and excretion.[63] Selenium treatment mitigated BPA-induced inflammation and oxidative stress in lung tissue.[64] Alpha-lipoic acid and alpha-tocopherol were both shown to prevent oxidative damage in liver and ovarian tissues caused by BPA exposure.[65]

BISPHENOL ANALOGS

As a result of concerns regarding the use of BPA, manufacturers have shifted to using bisphenol analogs. Bisphenol S (BPS) and bisphenol F (BPF) are the two most common analogs used in BPA-free products. BPS and BPF have been found in many everyday products, such as personal care products (e.g., body lotions, face creams, liquid foundations),[66] paper products (e.g., thermal receipts, flyers, magazines, newspapers, paper towels, toilet paper),[67] and food (e.g., condiments, dairy products, cereals, meat).[68] Several animal studies have shown endocrine-disrupting effects of BPS and BPF similar to those associated with BPA exposure. BPS exposure in rats caused an induction of uterine growth,[69] and in zebrafish, BPS exposure caused decreases in gonad weight, alterations in plasma estrogen and testosterone,[70] and reproductive disruption (e.g., decreased egg production, increased time to hatch, decreased sperm count).[71] BPF has shown estrogenic (e.g., uterine growth),[72] androgenic (e.g., increased weight of testes), and thyroidogenic (e.g., increased thyroid weight, altered thyroid hormone concentrations) effects.[73] The estrogenic potency of BPS and BPF is on the same order of magnitude as the potency of BPA.[74] Although human studies are not yet available, there is little reason to think these substitutions are any less toxic.

REFERENCES

1. Arnold, S. M., Clark, K. E., Staples, C. A., Klecka, G. M., et al. (2013). Relevance of drinking water as a source of human exposure to bisphenol A. *Journal of Exposure Science and Environmental Epidemiology*, 23(2), 137–144. PubMed PMID: 22805988.
2. Geens, T., Goeyens, L., & Covaci, A. (2011). Are potential sources for human exposure to bisphenol-A overlooked? *International Journal of Hygiene and Environmental Health*, 214(5), 339–347. PubMed PMID: 21570349.
3. Hunt, P. A., Koehler, K. E., Susiarjo, M., Hodges, C. A., Ilagan, A., et al. (2003). Bisphenol A exposure causes meiotic aneuploidy in the female mouse. *Current Biology*, 13(7), 546–553. PubMed PMID: 12676084.
4. Welshons, W. V., Nagel, S. C., & vom Saal, F. S. (2006). Large effects from small exposures. III. Endocrine mechanisms mediating effects of bisphenol A at levels of human exposure. *Endocrinology*, 147(6 Suppl.), S56–S69. PubMed PMID: 16690810.

5. Windham, G. C., Lee, D., Mitchell, P., et al. (2005). Exposure to organochlorine compounds and effects on ovarian function. *Epidemiology (Cambridge, Mass.)*, 16(2), 182–190.

6. Bonefield-Jorgensen, E. C., Long, M., Hofmeister, M. V., et al. (2007). Endocrine-disrupting potential of bisphenol A, bisphenol A dimethacrylate, 4-n-nonylphenol, and 4-n-octylphenol, in vitro: New data and a brief review. *Environmental Health Perspectives*, 115(Suppl. 1), 69–76.

7. Pearce, E. N., & Braverman, L. E. (2009). Environmental pollutants and the thyroid. *Best Practice and Research. Clinical Endocrinology and Metabolism*, 23(6), 801–813.

8. Gentilcore, D., Porreca, I., Rizzo, F., et al. (2013). Bisphenol A interferes with thyroid specific gene expression. *Toxicology*, 304, 21–31. PubMed PMID: 23238275.

9. Kabuto, H., Amakawa, M., & Shishibori, T. (2004). Exposure to bisphenol A during embryonic/fetal life and infancy increases oxidative injury and causes underdevelopment of the brain and testis in mice. *Life Sciences*, 74(24), 2931–2940. PubMed PMID: 15051418.

10. Obata, T., & Kubota, S. (2000). Formation of hydroxy radicals by environmental estrogen-like chemicals in rat striatum. *Neuroscience Letters*, 296(1), 41–44. PubMed PMID: 11099829.

11. Fleisch, A. F., Sheffield, P. E., Chinn, C., Edelstein, B. L., & Landrigan, P. J. (2010). Bisphenol A and related compounds in dental materials. *Pediatrics*, 126(4), 760–768. PubMed PMID: 20819896.

12. Haishima, Y., Hayashi, Y., Yagami, T., & Nakamura, A. (2001). Elution of bisphenol-A from hemodialyzers consisting of polycarbonate and polysulfone resins. *Journal of Biomedical Materials Research*, 58(2), 209–215. PubMed PMID: 11241341.

13. Ozaki, A., Yamaguchi, Y., Fujita, T., Kuroda, K., & Endo, G. (2004). Chemical analysis and genotoxicological safety assessment of paper and paperboard used for food packaging. *Food and Chemical Toxicology*, 42(8), 1323–1337. PubMed PMID: 15207384.

14. Geens, T., Goeyens, L., Kannan, K., Neels, H., & Covaci, A. (2012). Levels of bisphenol-A in thermal paper receipts from Belgium and estimation of human exposure. *The Science of the Total Environment*, 435-436, 30–33. PubMed PMID: 22846760.

15. Wilson, N. K., Chuang, J. C., Morgan, M. K., Lordo, R. A., & Sheldon, L. S. (2007). An observational study of the potential exposures of preschool children to pentachlorophenol, bisphenol-A, and nonylphenol at home and daycare. *Environmental Research*, 103(1), 9–20. PubMed PMID: 16750524.

16. Miyamoto, K., & Kotake, M. (2006). Estimation of daily bisphenol A intake of Japanese individuals with emphasis on uncertainty and variability. *Environmental Sciences: An International Journal of Environmental Physiology and Toxicology*, 13(1), 15–29. PubMed PMID: 16685249.

17. Genuis, S. J., Beesoon, S., Birkholz, D., & Lobo, R. A. (2012). Human excretion of bisphenol A: Blood, urine, and sweat (BUS) study. *Journal of Environmental and Public Health*, 2012, 185731. PubMed PMID: 22253637.

18. Carwile, J. L., Ye, X., Zhou, X., et al. (2011). Canned soup consumption and urinary bisphenol A: A randomized crossover trial. *The Journal of the American Medical Association*, 306(20), 2218–2220.

19. Goodson, A., Robin, H., Summerfield, W., & Cooper, I. (2004). Migration of bisphenol A from can coatings – effects of damage, storage conditions and heating. *Food Additives and Contaminants*, 21(10), 1015–1026. PubMed PMID: 15712526.

20. Kang, J. H., & Kondo, F. (2003). Determination of bisphenol A in milk and dairy products by high-performance liquid chromatography with fluorescence detection. *Journal of Food Protection*, 66(8), 1439–1443. PubMed PMID: 12929832.

21. Loganathan, S. N., & Kannan, K. (2011). Occurrence of bisphenol A in indoor dust from two locations in the eastern United States and implications for human exposures. *Archives of Environmental Contamination and Toxicology*, 61(1), 68–73. PubMed PMID: 21221962.

22. Jones-Otazo, H. A., Clarke, J. P., Diamond, M. L., Archbold, J. A., et al. (2005). Is house dust the missing exposure pathway for PBDEs? An analysis of the urban fate and human exposure to PBDEs. *Environmental Science & Technology*, 39(14), 5121–5130. PubMed PMID: 16082939.

23. Liao, C., & Kannan, K. (2011). Widespread occurrence of bisphenol A in paper and paper products: Implications for human exposure. *Environmental Science & Technology*, 45(21), 9372–9379. PubMed PMID: 21939283.

24. Mendum, T., Stoler, E., Van Benschoten, H., & Warner, J. C. (2011). Concentration of bisphenol A in thermal paper. *Green Chemistry Letters and Reviews*, 4, 81–86.

25. Biedermann, S., Tschudin, P., & Grob, K. (2010). Transfer of bisphenol A from thermal printer paper to the skin. *Analytical and Bioanalytical Chemistry*, 398(1), 571–576. PubMed PMID: 20623271.

26. Van Landuyt, K. L., Nawrot, T., Geebelen, B., De Munck, J., et al. (2011). How much do resin-based dental materials release? A meta-analytical approach. *Dental Materials*, 27(8), 723–747. PubMed PMID: 21664675.

27. Calafat, A. M., Ye, X., Wong, L. Y., Reidy, J. A., & Needham, L. L. (2008). Exposure of the U.S. population to bisphenol A and 4-tertiary-octylphenol: 2003-2004. *Environmental Health Perspectives, 116*(1), 39–44. PubMed PMID: 18197297.

28. European Food Safety Authority. (2006). Opinion of the scientific panel on food additives, flavourings, processing aids and materials in contact with food on a request from the commission related to 2,2-bis(4-hydroxyphenyl) propane (Bisphenol A). Question number EFSA-Q-2005-100. *EFSA Journal, 426,* 1–75.

29. Lakind, J. S., & Naiman, D. Q. (2008). Bisphenol A (BPA) daily intakes in the United States: Estimates from the 2003-2004 NHANES urinary BPA data. *Journal of Exposure Science and Environmental Epidemiology, 18*(6), 608–615. PubMed PMID: 18414515.

30. Vandenberg, L. N., Chahoud, I., Heindel, J. J., et al. (2012). Urinary, circulating, and tissue biomonitoring studies indicate widespread exposure to bisphenol A. *Ciencia & Saude Coletiva, 17*(2), 407–434.

31. Nunez, A. A., Kannan, K., Giesy, J. P., Fang, J., & Clemens, L. G. (2001). Effects of bisphenol A on energy balance and accumulation in brown adipose tissue in rats. *Chemosphere, 42*(8), 917–922. PubMed PMID: 11272914.

32. Fernandez, M. F., Arrebola, J. P., Taoufiki, J., et al. (2007). Bisphenol-A and chlorinated derivatives in adipose tissue of women. *Reproductive Toxicology, 24*(2), 259–264. PubMed PMID: 17689919.

33. Volkel, W., Bittner, N., & Dekant, W. (2005). Quantitation of bisphenol A and bisphenol A glucuronide in biological samples by high performance liquid chromatography-tandem mass spectrometry. *Drug Metabolism and Disposition: The Biological Fate of Chemicals, 33*(11), 1748–1757. PubMed PMID: 16103135.

34. Volkel, W., Colnot, T., Csanady, G. A., Filser, J. G., & Dekant, W. (2002). Metabolism and kinetics of bisphenol A in humans at low doses following oral administration. *Chemical Research in Toxicology, 15*(10), 1281–1287. PubMed PMID: 12387626.

35. Ginsberg, G., & Rice, D. C. (2009). Does rapid metabolism ensure negligible risk from bisphenol A? *Environmental Health Perspectives, 117*(11), 1639–1643. PubMed PMID: 20049111.

36. Anses, French Agency for Food, Environmental and Occupational Health and Safety. (2011). Effects sanitaires du Bisphenol A: Saisines No. 2009-SA-0331 et No. 2010-SA-0197. Rapport d'expertise collective. http://www.anses.fr/documents/CHIM-Ra-BisphenolA.pdf. (Accessed April 14, 2017.)

37. Soto, A. M., Vandenberg, L. N., Maffini, M. V., & Sonnenschein, C. (2008). Does breast cancer start in the womb? *Basic and Clinical Pharmacology and Toxicology, 102*(2), 125–133. PubMed PMID: 18226065.

38. Vitku, J., Sosvorova, L., Chlupacova, T., et al. (2015). Differences in bisphenol A and estrogen levels in the plasma and seminal plasma of men with different degrees of infertility. *Physiological Research, 64*(Suppl. 2), S303–S311. PubMed PMID: 26680493.

39. Erden, E. S., Motor, S., Ustun, I., Demirkose, M., et al. (2014). Investigation of bisphenol A as an endocrine disruptor, total thiol, malondialdehyde, and C-reactive protein levels in chronic obstructive pulmonary disease. *European Review for Medical and Pharmacological Sciences, 18*(22), 3477–3483. PubMed PMID: 25491624.

40. Lang, I. A., Galloway, T. S., Scarlett, A., Henley, W. E., Depledge, M., Wallace, R. B., et al. (2008). Association of urinary bisphenol A concentrations with medical disorders and laboratory abnormalities in adults. *The Journal of the American Medical Association, 300*(11), 1303–1310. PubMed PMID: 18799442.

41. Melzer, D., Rice, N. E., Lewis, C., Henley, W. E., & Galloway, T. S. (2010). Association of urinary bisphenol A concentration with heart disease: Evidence from NHANES 2003/06. *PLoS ONE, 5*(1), e8673. PubMed PMID: 20084273.

42. Patel, B. B., Kasneci, A., Bolt, A. M., et al. (2015). Chronic exposure to bisphenol A reduces successful cardiac remodeling after an experimental myocardial infarction in male C57bl/6n mice. *Toxicological Sciences, 146*(1), 101–115. PubMed PMID: 25862758.

43. Yan, S., Song, W., Chen, Y., Hong, K., et al. (2013). Low-dose bisphenol A and estrogen increase ventricular arrhythmias following ischemia-reperfusion in female rat hearts. *Food and Chemical Toxicology, 56,* 75–80. PubMed PMID: 23429042.

44. Sharpe, R. M., & Skakkebaek, N. E. (1993). Are oestrogens involved in falling sperm counts and disorders of the male reproductive tract? *Lancet, 341*(8857), 1392–1395. PubMed PMID: 8098802.

45. Braun, J. M., Yolton, K., Dietrich, K. N., Hornung, R., et al. (2009). Prenatal bisphenol A exposure and early childhood behavior. *Environmental Health Perspectives, 117*(12), 1945–1952. PubMed PMID: 20049216.

46. Spanier, A. J., Kahn, R. S., Kunselman, A. R., et al. (2012). Prenatal exposure to bisphenol A and child wheeze from birth to 3 years of age. *Environmental Health Perspectives, 120*(6), 916–920. PubMed PMID: 22334053.

47. Wang, I. J., Chen, C. Y., & Bornehag, C. G. (2016). Bisphenol A exposure may increase the risk of development af atopic disorders in children.

International Journal of Hygiene and Environmental Health, 219(3), 311–316. PubMed PMID: 26765087.

48. Sugiura-Ogasawara, M., Ozaki, Y., Sonta, S., Makino, T., & Suzumori, K. (2005). Exposure to bisphenol A is associated with recurrent miscarriage. *Human Reproduction, 200*(8), 2325–2329. PubMed PMID: 15947000.

49. Yamada, H., Furuta, I., Kato, E. H., Kataoka, S., et al. (2002). Maternal serum and amniotic fluid bisphenol A concentrations in the early second trimester. *Reproductive Toxicology, 16*(6), 735–739. PubMed PMID: 12401500.

50. Mok-Lin, E., Ehrlich, S., Williams, P. L., Petrozza, J., et al. (2010). Urinary bisphenol A concentrations and ovarian response among women undergoing IVF. *International Journal of Andrology, 33*(2), 385–393. PubMed PMID: 20002217.

51. Yang, M., Kim, S. Y., Chang, S. S., Lee, I. S., & Kawamoto, T. (2006). Urinary concentrations of bisphenol A in relation to biomarkers of sensitivity and effect and endocrine-related health effects. *Environmental and Molecular Mutagenesis, 47*(8), 571–578. PubMed PMID: 16795089.

52. Sabanayagam, C., Teppala, S., & Shankar, A. (2013). Relationship between urinary bisphenol A levels and prediabetes among subjects free of diabetes. *Acta Diabetologica, 50*(4), 625–631. PubMed PMID: 23636267.

53. Wang, T., Li, M., Chen, B., et al. (2012). Urinary bisphenol A (BPA) concentration associates with obesity and insulin resistance. *The Journal of Clinical Endocrinology and Metabolism, 97*(2), E223–E227.

54. Calafat, A. M., Ye, X., Wong, L. Y., Reidy, J. A., & Needham, L. L. (2008). Exposure of the U.S. population to bisphenol A and 4-tertiary-octylphenol: 2003-2004. *Environmental Health Perspectives, 116*(1), 39–44. PubMed PMID: 18197297.

55. Hong, Y. C., Park, E. Y., Park, M. S., Ko, J. A., Oh, S. Y., et al. (2009). Community level exposure to chemicals and oxidative stress in adult population. *Toxicology Letters, 184*(2), 139–144. PubMed PMID: 19049859.

56. Badawy, A., State, O., & Abdelgawad, S. (2007). N-acetylcysteine and clomiphene citrate for induction of ovulation in polycystic ovary syndrome: A cross-over trial. *Acta Obstetricia et Gynecologica Scandinavica, 86*(2), 218–222.

57. Jain, S., Kumar, C. H., Suranagi, U. D., & Mediratta, P. K. (2011). Protective effect of N-acetylcysteine on bisphenol A-induced cognitive dysfunction and oxidative stress in rats. *Food and Chemical Toxicology, 49*(6), 1404–1409. PubMed PMID: 21440025.

58. Geng, S., Wang, S., Zhu, W., Xie, C., et al. (2017). Curcumin attenuates BPA-induced insulin resistance in HepG2 cells through suppression of JNK/p38 pathways. *Toxicology Letters, 272*, 75–83. PubMed PMID: 28300666.

59. Tiwari, S. K., Agarwal, S., Tripathi, A., & Chaturvedi, R. K. (2016). Bisphenol-A mediated inhibition of hippocampal neurogenesis attenuated by curcumin via canonical Wnt pathway. *Molecular Neurobiology, 53*(5), 3010–3029. PubMed PMID: 25963729.

60. El-Missiry, M. A., Othman, A. I., Al-Abdan, M. A., & El-Sayed, A. A. (2014). Melatonin ameliorates oxidative stress, modulates death receptor pathway proteins, and protects the rat cerebrum against bisphenol-A-induced apoptosis. *Journal of the Neurological Sciences, 347*(1–2), 251–256. PubMed PMID: 25454643.

61. Othman, A. I., Edrees, G. M., El-Missiri, M. A., et al. (2016). Melatonin controlled apoptosis and protected the testes and sperm quality against bisphenol A-induced oxidative toxicity. *Toxicology and Industrial Health, 32*(9), 1537–1549. PubMed PMID: 25537623.

62. Wu, H. J., Liu, C., Duan, W. X., et al. (2013). Melatonin ameliorates bisphenol A-induced DNA damage in the germ cells of adult male rats. *Mutation Research, 752*(1–2), 57–67. PubMed PMID: 23402883.

63. Yi, B., Kasai, H., Lee, H. S., et al. (2011). Inhibition by wheat sprout (Triticum aestivum) juice of bisphenol A-induced oxidative stress in young women. *Mutation Research, 724*(1–2), 64–68. PubMed PMID: 21736952.

64. Abedellhaffez, A. S., El-Aziz, E. A., Aziz, M. A., & Ahmed, A. M. (2017). Lung injury induced by bisphenol A: A food contaminant, is ameliorated by selenium supplementation. *Pathophysiology*, pii:S0928-4680(17), 30006–30008. [Epub ahead of print]; PubMed PMID: 28285737.

65. Avci, B., Bahadir, A., Tuncel, O. K., & Bilgici, B. (2016). Influence of alpha-tocopherol and alpha-lipoic acid on bisphenol-A-induced oxidative damage in liver and ovarian tissue of rats. *Toxicology and Industrial Health, 32*(8), 1381–1390. PubMed PMID: 25548375.

66. Liao, C., & Kannan, K. (2014). A survey of alkylphenols, bisphenols, and triclosan in personal care products from China and the United Sates. *Archives of Environmental Contamination and Toxicology, 67*(1), 50–59. PubMed PMID: 24639116.

67. Liao, C., Liu, F., & Kannan, K. (2012). Bisphenol S, a new bisphenol analogue, in paper products and currency bills and its association with bisphenol A residues. *Environmental Science & Technology, 46*(12), 6515–6522. PubMed PMID: 22591511.

68. Liao, C., & Kannan, K. (2013). Concentrations and profiles of bisphenol A and other bisphenol analogues in foodstuffs from the United States and their implications

for human exposure. *Journal of Agricultural and Food Chemistry*, *61*(19), 4655–4662. PubMed PMID: 23614805.

69. Yamasaki, K., Noda, S., Imatanaka, N., & Yakabe, Y. (2004). Comparative study of the uterotrophic potency of 14 chemicals in a uterotrophic assay and their receptor-binding affinity. *Toxicology Letters*, *146*(2), 111–120. PubMed PMID: 14643963.

70. Ji, K., Hong, S., Kho, Y., & Choi, K. (2013). Effects of bisphenol S exposure on endocrine functions and reproduction of zebrafish. *Environmental Science & Technology*, *47*(15), 8793–8800. PubMed PMID: 23806087.

71. Naderi, M., Wong, M. Y., & Gholami, F. (2014). Developmental exposure of zebrafish (Danio rerio) to bisphenol-S impairs subsequent reproduction potential and hormonal balance in adults. *Aquatic Toxicology (Amsterdam, Netherlands)*, *148*, 195–203. PubMed PMID: 24508763.

72. Stroheker, T., Chagnon, M. C., Pinnert, M. F., et al. (2003). Estrogenic effects of food wrap packaging xenoestrogens and flavonoids in female Wistar rats: A comparative study. *Reproductive Toxicology*, *17*(4), 421–432. PubMed PMID: 12849853.

73. Higashihara, N., Shiraishi, K., Miyata, K., et al. (2007). Subacute oral toxicity study of bisphenol F based on the draft protocol for the "Enhanced OECD Test Guideline no. 407." *Archives of Toxicology*, *81*(12), 825–832. PubMed PMID: 17628788.

74. Rochester, J. R., & Bolden, A. L. (2015). Bisphenol S and F: A systematic review and comparison of the hormonal activity of bisphenol A substitutes. *Environmental Health Perspectives*, *123*(7), 643–650. PubMed PMID: 25775505.

26

Phthalates

SUMMARY

- Presence in population: Phthalates are found in the dust of all homes and commercial buildings, with multiple phthalate metabolites detectable in the urine of all persons tested
- Major disease: Infertility, low testosterone, obesity, diabetes, allergies, asthma, autism, mood disorder, reduced cognition

- Primary sources: Solid plastic products in the home, plastic-covered foods, personal care products, house dust
- Best measure: Review of home for phthalate-containing products and urinary phthalate metabolites
- Best intervention: Avoidance

DESCRIPTION

Phthalates are worldwide high-production chemicals that can be used in many ways, such as to make plastics more flexible and resilient and to solubilize fragrances in health and beauty aids. They are weakly bound to the plastics and are therefore easily released into the surrounding environment. Phthalates are often roughly grouped into two categories based on molecular weight: high-molecular-weight (HMW) or low-molecular-weight (LMW) compounds. The structures shown in Fig. 26.1 give an indication of where these compounds fall on that scale. Diethyl phthalate (DEP) and diisononyl phthalate (DiNP) are LMW, while diethylhexyl phthalate (DEHP) and dibenzyl phthalate (DBzP) are HMW. HMW phthalates are typically solid at room temperature, whereas LMW phthalates are liquid.

SOURCES

Consumer Products

Phthalates are found in many kinds of consumer goods (Box 26.1). HMW phthalates are found in shower curtains, raincoats, toys, polyvinyl chloride flooring, furniture polishes, plastic food wrap, etc. Phthalates are released from these products into the environment, where they contaminate the dust throughout the home or office.[1,2] LMW phthalates are typically found in liquid personal care products such as fragrances, body lotion, shower gel, shampoos, nail polish, and other products, which are then inhaled, with some minimal dermal exposure as well.

Food

Plastics can contaminate food by simple contact with plastic food wrap (see Table 3.7). A total phthalate level of 42.50 µg/g was found in the top tortilla of a package of tortillas that was tested in the US Food and Drug Administration Total Diet Study (FDA TDS). That level of phthalate had migrated from the ink on the packaging into the tortilla, whereas the tortillas below it and further from the ink had very little phthalate. Numerous articles have documented the transfer of plasticizers from various food wraps into food.[3,4] Plastic migrates into food based on fat content, the length of time the wrap is in contact, and heat exposure.[5]

DEHP is found in plastic bottled beverages[6] and in meals prepared by food service workers wearing disposable polyvinyl chloride (PVC) gloves.[7,8] DEHP levels in lunches packed with the use of PVC gloves ranged from 0.80 to 11.8 mg/kg, whereas levels of only 0.012 to 0.30 mg were found in lunches made without gloves. Fast food

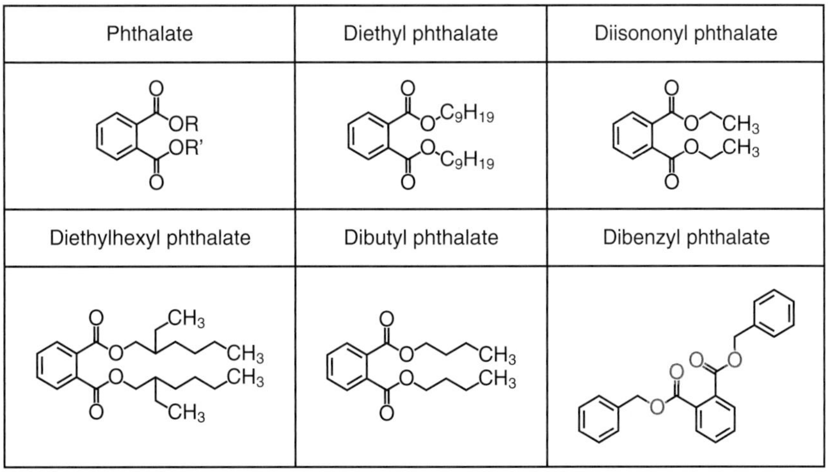

FIG. 26.1. Structures of some common phthalates.

BOX 26.1 Phthalate-Containing Consumer Products

Adhesives
Automotive parts
Detergents
Flooring (vinyl)
Raincoats
Cleaning products
Food packaging
Household furnishings
Garden hoses
Cosmetics
Shampoos
Lotions
Fragrances
Plastic bags
Children's toys
Pharmaceuticals

consumption is also positively associated with increased levels of urinary phthalates.[9]

Air

DEP is used in the production of fragrances and is found in air fresheners.[10] Phthalates are commonly found in the dust of homes, schools, and workplaces.[11] HMW phthalates such as DEHP are higher in homes with polyvinyl flooring, foam mattresses, shower curtains, and other plastic materials.[12,13] Plastic-coated wallpaper, often found in bathrooms, releases more DEHP when the ambient moisture content increases (as it would during showering).[14]

Personal Care Products

LMW phthalates like DEP and dimethyl phthalate (DMP) are found together in all perfumes,[15] as well as liquid soaps, shower gel, body lotion, hair products, nail polish, and other products.[16] Persons using those products have correspondingly higher levels of phthalate metabolites in their urine.

BODY BURDEN

Thirteen of the fifteen different phthalates that are measured in the ongoing National Health and Nutritional Examination Survey (NHANES) trials are routinely found in North American residents (Table 26.1).

Detoxification/Excretion Processes

All phthalates used in industry are in the di- form, but with biotransformation are excreted in the mono- form. Hence, DEHP becomes mono ethylhexyl phthalate (MEHP), etc. Phthalates are conjugated with glucuronates and are rapidly cleared from the body.[17] Fig. 26.2 shows the biotransformation of phthalates.

DEHP is metabolized to one of four compounds: mono-ethyl-hexyl phthalate (MEHP), mono-(2-ethyl-5-hydroxyhexyl) phthalate (MEHHP), mono-(2-ethyl-5-oxohexyl) phthalate (MEOHP), or mono-(2-ethyl-5-carboxypentyl) phthalate (MECPP). The half-life of

TABLE 26.1   **CDC Fourth Report 2017 Update (NHANES 2011–2014)**

Compound	Parent Compound	Mean[a]	50th %	75th %	90th %	95th %
MEHP	DEHP	1.55	1.46	2.73	4.91	8.47
MEHHP	"	8.99	8.46	14.1	25.3	37.7
MEOHP	"	5.78	5.51	8.99	15.6	23.4
MECCP	"	14.7	14.1	22.7	38.9	59.8
MCNP	DiNP	2.83	2.50	4.59	9.36	14.6
MCOP	"	22.4	20.4	54.1	118	194
MiNP	"	*	1.08	2.69	7.88	17.6
MMP	"	*	1.32	2.84	6.13	11.0
MCPP	DMP	3.42	2.86	6.00	15.8	36.6
MBzP	BzBP	5.15	4.96	9.49	17.4	26.7
MiBP	DiBP	6.83	6.77	11.6	19.4	27.5
MnBP	DBP, BzBP	8.66	9.04	15.8	27.9	41.2
MEP	DEP	43.2	34.4	94.2	263	541

BzBP, Benzylbutyl phthalate; *DBP*, di-n-butyl-phthalate; *DEHP*, diethylhexyl phthalate; *DEP*, diethyl phthalate; *DiBP*, Di-isobutyl phthalate; *DiNP*, diisononyl phthalates; *DMP*,; *MBzP*, monobenzyl phthalate; *MCNP*, Mono-(carboxynonyl) phthalate; *MCOP*, Mono-(carboxyoctyl) phthalate; *MCPP*, Mono-(3-carboxypropyl) phthalate; *MECCP*,; *MEHHP*,; *MEHP*, mono-ethyl-hexyl phthalate; *MEOHP*, Mono-(2-ethyl-5-oxohexyl) phthalate; *MEP*, Mono-ethyl phthalate; *MiBP*, Mono-isobutyl phthalate; *MiNP*, Mono-isononyl phthalate; *MMP*, Mono-methyl phthalate; *MnBP*, Mono-n-butyl phthalate.
[a]Urinary phthalates in µg/g creatinine.
*no geometric mean calculated

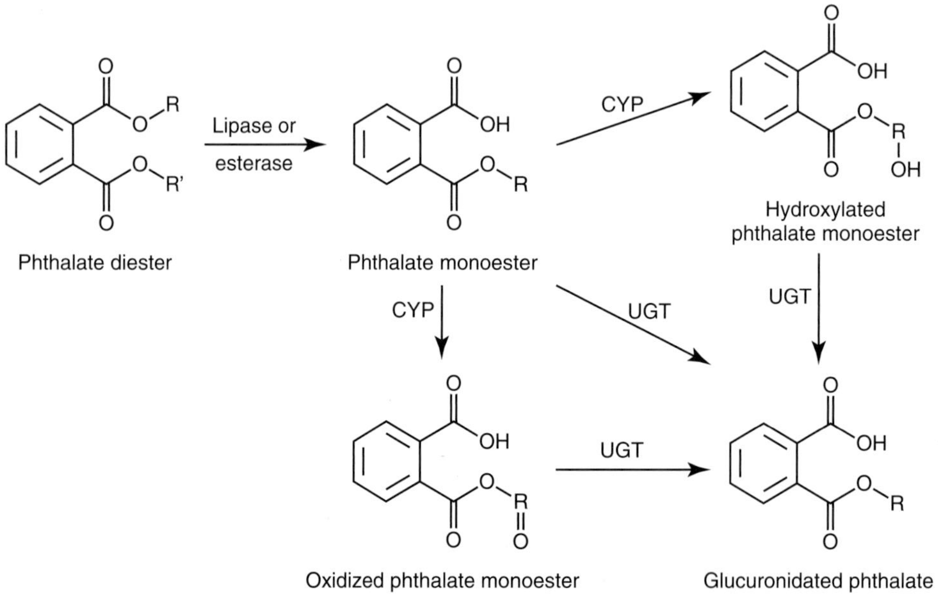

FIG. 26.2 Basic biotransformation of phthalates. (From North, M. L., Takaro, T. K., Diamond, M. L., & Ellis, A. K. [2014]. Effects of phthalates on the development and expression of allergic disease and asthma. *Annals of Allergy, Asthma & Immunology, 112*(6), 496–502.)

MEHP is 12 hours, whereas the other metabolites have a half-life of 24 hours.[18] However, the half-life of DEHP in water is thought to be 100 years. The half-life of DEP is listed as 2.2 days.[19]

Clinical Significance

Mitochondrial Disruption. Phthalates, specifically HMW MEHP, have been shown to reduce mitochondrial succinate dehydrogenase activity and to reduce cellular adenosine triphosphate (ATP) by 20%.[20] MEHP was the most potent inhibitor of mitochondrial activity, followed by di-n-butyl phthalate (DBT) and di-mono-n-butyl phthalate (DMBT).[21] MEHP also demonstrates an ability to inhibit beta-oxidation of certain fatty acids in the mitochondria by about 50% to 60%.[22] This undoubtedly plays a role in phthalates increasing the rates of obesity and diabetes.[23] Inhibition of mitochondrial function is responsible for phthalates' adverse effect on Sertoli cells, leading to male infertility. Phthalates have been found in significantly higher levels in infertile men, where they are linked with mitochondrial depolarization along with increased levels of reactive oxygen species and lipid peroxidases.[24]

Endocrine Disruption

Diabetes. A substantial amount of animal research shows that phthalates block insulin receptor sites, impair glucose transporter 4, and induce epigenetic changes that disrupt blood sugar regulation and the oxidation of glucose for energy.[25] These effects begin *in utero,* increase during lactation in a phthalate-contaminated mother, and accumulate throughout an exposed life.[26,27]

An increased risk of developing metabolic syndrome (MetS) has been associated with higher concentrations of certain phthalate metabolites.[28] Phthalates such as di-2-ethyl-hexl phthalate, DEP, dibutyl phthalate, dimethyl phthalate, DBzP, and DiNP are associated with the development of type 2 diabetes and obesity by interfering with various cell-signaling pathways involved in weight and glucose homeostasis.[29] A PubMed search with the terms "diabetes" and "phthalates" and the limit "humans" yielded 78 hits (July 2017), half of which were published in the previous 5 years. This is an emerging area of research that will likely show progressively worse results as the body load in the population continues to increase.

Reproductive effects. In utero exposure to phthalates appears to alter progesterone and follicle-stimulating hormone (FSH) levels in the offspring.[30] Phthalate

presence in young girls has been associated with both delayed menarche[31] and premature breast development (thelarche).[32] Young Puerto Rican girls with thelarche had serum DEHP levels averaging 450 parts per billion, whereas those without thelarche averaged only 70 PPB.

Women presenting at a German fertility clinic with endometriosis had significantly higher levels of DEHP than were found in controls.[33] Women with leiomyomas also had higher urinary phthalate levels than those without fibroids.[34]

Maternal levels of phthalates during pregnancy have been associated with long-term hormonal imbalance in male children when they reached the age of 14 years.[35] Maternal urinary levels of MEHP were positively associated with sex hormone binding globulin (SHBG) and inversely associated with total testosterone levels. Maternal levels of the LMW Mono-isobutyl phthalate (MiBP) (often found in fingernail polish) were also inversely associated with testosterone levels. Boys exposed to higher levels of phthalates *in utero* also experienced delayed puberty. Data from the 2011 to 2012 NHANES trial revealed that in boys aged 6–12 years, adult men, and adult women, urinary levels of MEHP were associated with lower testosterone levels.[36] The clear inverse relationship between phthalates and testosterone levels has been repeatedly established across the globe.[37,38]

A correlation was found in men attending an infertility clinic between urinary levels of Mono-ethyl phthalate MEP and DNA damage in their sperm.[39] Another group of infertile men showed inverse associations between Mono-isononyl phthalate MiNP and MEHP levels, testosterone levels, and sperm viability.[40] Elevated urinary levels of LMW phthalates were significantly associated with a 20% reduction in male fertility.[41]

Obesity. Male participants in the 1999 to 2002 NHANES trial had a significant positive correlation between urinary levels of monobenzyl phthalate (MBzP), MEHHP, MEOHP, and MEP, and both increasing waist circumference and insulin resistance.[42] The correlation was strongest in 20- to 59-year-old men, with MBzP causing increased belt size in all quartiles. MEP was also found to be positively associated with waist circumference in adolescent girls.[43] In 70-year-old Swedish women, Mono-isobutyl phthalate MiBP and Mono-methyl phthalate MMP were positively related to waist circumference and truncal fat mass.[44] LMW phthalates Mono-n-butyl phthalate MnBP, MEP, and MiBP were significantly associated with obesity in boys and adolescents in the 2007 to 2010 NHANES trial.[45] HMW phthalate metabolites, especially metabolites of DEHP (MEHP, MEHHP, MEOHP), were significantly associated with increased rates of obesity in all adults from the same cohort. Data from both the 1999 to 2004 and 2003 to 2008 NHANES confirmed these findings among adult women.[46,47]

Thyroid. Phthalates have various mechanisms of action on thyroid homeostasis, including interfering with the activity of the sodium/iodine symporter,[48] inhibiting T3 uptake in cells,[49] and competitively binding to transthyretin (TTR).[50] Significant mild negative correlations were found between TT4 and FT4 and urinary phthalate monoesters in pregnant women exposed to di-n-butyl-phthalate (DBP).[51] In adult men, there was an inverse association between urinary concentration of MEHP and serum levels of FT4 and T3.[52]

Immune. Three different HMW phthalates have been associated with higher rates of allergic and respiratory problems. The presence of butyl benzyl phthalate (BBzP) in house dust is associated with rhinitis and eczema, whereas DEHP is associated with asthma.[53] Another HMW phthalate metabolite, MBzP, is also associated with higher levels of asthma in adults but not in children.[54] DEHP is in all vinyl chloride products, and BBzP is in both vinyl and carpet tiles and some artificial leather products. Phthalates have been shown to induce Th2 immune response, with increased Th2 cytokine production, as well as increased immunoglobulin E (IgE) and immunoglobulin G (IgG).[55]

Neurological. Maternal exposure to mono-n-butyl, monoisobutyl, and monobenzyl phthalates resulted in reduced scores on both the Mental Development Index and Psychomotor Index for their daughters by age 2 years.[56] Maternal levels of these phthalates were also associated with a 6.7- to 7.6-point drop in IQ in their offspring by age 7 years.[57] Prenatal exposure to HMW phthalates was associated with delinquent and aggressive behavior in 8-year-old Taiwanese children, with the strongest associations with maternal MEHP and MEOHP levels.[58]

Autism. In a Swedish study following families over a 5-year period, a connection between vinyl flooring and a diagnosis of autism, Asperger's, or Tourette's syndrome was noted.[59] In addition to increased rates of these diagnoses in children whose parents had vinyl flooring in the bedroom, risk was also associated with parental smoking, condensation on the windows, and reduced ventilation in the home.

Mood. US residents older than 60 years who participated in the 2006 to 2012 NHANES trial who had higher urine levels of two common phthalates (mono-carboxypropylphthalates and mono-n-butyl phthalate) were more than twice as likely to be depressed as those with lower phthalate levels.[60]

INTERVENTION

Avoidance of phthalates has been documented to result in a reduction of these compounds in the urine.[61,62] Lifestyle choices have clearly demonstrated the ability to rapidly reduce exposure to phthalates.[63] Individuals who participated in a 5-day Buddhist retreat that included a vegetarian diet (primarily grown at the monastery) experienced a reduction in both LMW and HMW phthalates and antibiotic metabolites in their urine. They also had a reduction in their malondialdehyde levels, indicating a reduction in oxidative stress.[64] Significant reductions in urinary phthalate levels have been found in young girls when they reduced their frequency of handwashing, ceased drinking from plastic cups, and used less shower gel and shampoo.[65] The greatest reduction of phthalates is attainable by avoiding the use of body lotion, deodorant, perfume and colognes, antiaging facial creams, and bottled water.[66,67] The authors of *Slow Death by Rubber Duck* did a 2-day avoidance of all personal care products followed by 2 days of using normally applied products.[68] After the 2-day avoidance, the level of the LMW MEP was 64 ng/L. After liberal use of personal care products for 2 days, the MEP urine level increased to 1410 ng/L.

REFERENCES

1. Larsson, K., Lindh, C. H., Jönsson, B. A., et al. (2017). Phthalates, non-phthalate plasticizers and bisphenols in Swedish preschool dust in relation to children's exposure. *Environment International, 102*, 114–124. PubMed PMID: 28274486.
2. Ait Bamai, Y., Araki, A., Kawai, T., et al. (2016). Exposure to phthalates in house dust and associated allergies in children aged 6-12years. *Environment International, 96*, 16–23. PubMed PMID: 27588698.
3. Castle, L., Mayo, A., & Gilbert, J. (1989). Migration of plasticizers from printing inks into foods. *Food Additives*

and Contaminants, 6(4), 437–443. PubMed PMID: 2792462.

4. Castle, L., Mercer, A. J., Startin, J. R., & Gilbert, J. (1988). Migration from plasticized films into foods. 3. Migration of phthalate, sebacate, citrate and phosphate esters from films used for retail food packaging. *Food Additives and Contaminants*, 5(1), 9–20. PubMed PMID: 3356285.

5. Page, B. D., & Lacroix, G. M. (1995). The occurrence of phthalate ester and di-2-ethylhexyl adipate plasticizers in Canadian packaging and food sampled in 1985-1989: A survey. *Food Additives and Contaminants*, 12(1), 129–151.

6. Yang, J. F., Yang, L. M., Zheng, L. Y., et al. (2017). Phthalates in plastic bottled non-alcoholic beverages from China and estimated dietary exposure in adults. *Food Additives & Contaminants. Part B, Surveillance*, 10(1), 44–50. PubMed PMID: 27719622.

7. Tsumura, Y., Ishimitsu, S., Saito, I., et al. (2003). Estimated daily intake of plasticizers in 1-week duplicate diet samples following regulation of DEHP-containing PVC gloves in Japan. *Food Additives and Contaminants*, 20(4), 317–324. PubMed PMID: 12775472.

8. Tsumura, Y., Ishimitsu, S., Kaihara, A., et al. (2001). Di(2-thylhexyl) phthalate contamination of retail packed lunches caused by PVC gloves used in the preparation of foods. *Food Additives and Contaminants*, 18(6), 569–579. PubMed PMID: 11407756.

9. Zota, A. R., Phillips, C. A., & Mitro, S. D. (2016). Recent fast food consumption and bisphenol A and phthalates exposures among the U.S. population in NHANES, 2003-2010. *Environmental Health Perspectives*, 124(10), 1521–1528. PMID: 27072648.

10. Kim, S., Hong, S. H., Bong, C. K., & Cho, M. H. (2015). Characterization of air freshener emission: The potential health effects. *The Journal of Toxicological Sciences*, 40(5), 535–550. PubMed PMID: 26354370.

11. Larsson, K., Lindh, C. H., Jönsson, B. A., et al. (2017). Phthalates, non-phthalate plasticizers and bisphenols in Swedish preschool dust in relation to children's exposure. *Environment International*, 102, 114–124. PubMed PMID: 28274486.

12. Jeon, S., Kim, K. T., & Choi, K. (2016). Migration of DEHP and DINP into dust from PVC flooring products at different surface temperature. *The Science of the Total Environment*, 547, 441–446. PubMed PMID: 26824397.

13. Sukiene, V., Gerecke, A. C., Park, Y. M., et al. (2016). Tracking SVOCs' transfer from products to indoor air and settled dust with deuterium-labeled substances. *Environmental Science & Technology*, 50(8), 4296–4303. PubMed PMID: 27019300.

14. Hsu, N. Y., Liu, Y. C., Lee, C. W., et al. (2017). Higher moisture content is associated with greater emissions of DEHP from PVC wallpaper. *Environmental Research*, 152, 1–6. PubMed PMID: 27736685.

15. Al-Saleh, I., & Elkhatib, R. (2016). Screening of phthalate esters in 47 branded perfumes. *Environmental Science and Pollution Research International*, 23(1), 455–468. PubMed PMID: 26310707.

16. Philippat, C., Bennett, D., Calafat, A. M., & Picciotto, I. H. (2015). Exposure to select phthalates and phenols through use of personal care products among Californian adults and their children. *Environmental Research*, 140, 369–376. PubMed PMID: 25929801.

17. Hanioka, N., Kinashi, Y., Tanaka-Kagawa, T., Isobe, T., & Jinno, H. (2017). Glucuronidation of mono(2-ethylhexyl) phthalate in humans: Roles of hepatic and intestinal UDP-glucuronosyltransferases. *Archives of Toxicology*, 91(2), 689–698. PubMed PMID: 27071666.

18. Agency for Toxic Substances & Disease Registry. *Diethylhexyl phthalate toxicological profile*. https://www.atsdr.cdc.gov/toxprofiles/tp.asp?id=684&tid=65. (Accessed July 18, 2017.)

19. Agency for Toxic Substances & Disease Registry. *Diethyl phthalate toxicological profile*. https://www.atsdr.cdc.gov/toxprofiles/tp.asp?id=603&tid=112. (Accessed July 18, 2017.)

20. Chapin, R. E., Gray, T. J., Phelps, J. L., & Dutton, S. L. (1988). The effects of mono-(2-ethylhexyl)-phthalate on rat Sertoli cell enriched primary cultures. *Toxicology and Applied Pharmacology*, 92(3), 467–479. Pubmed PMID: 3353991.

21. Melnick, R. L., & Schiller, C. M. (1982). Mitochondrial toxicity of phthalate esters. *Environmental Health Perspectives*, 45, 51–56. Pubmed PMID: 7140696.

22. Winberg, L. D., & Badr, M. Z. (1995). Mechanism of phthalate-induced inhibition of hepatic mitochondrial beta-oxidation. *Toxicology Letters*, 76(1), 63–69. Pubmed PMID: 7701518.

23. Stahlhut, R. W., van Wijngaarden, E., Dye, T. D., Cook, S., & Swan, S. H. (2007). Concentrations of urinary phthalate metabolites are associated with increased waist circumference and insulin resistance in adult US males. *Environmental Health Perspectives*, 115, 876–882. Pubmed PMID: 17589594.

24. Pant, N., Shukla, M., Kumar Patel, D., et al. (2008). Correlation of phthalate exposures with semen quality. *Toxicology and Applied Pharmacology*, 231(1), 112–116. PubMed PMID: 18513777.

25. Rajesh, P., & Balasubramanian, K. (2014). Di(2-ethylhexyl)phthalate exposure impairs insulin receptor and glucose transporter 4 gene expression in L6

myotubes. *Human and Experimental Toxicology, 33*(7), 685–700. PMID: 24130215.

26. Rajesh, P., & Balasubramanian, K. (2014). Phthalate exposure in utero causes epigenetic changes and impairs insulin signalling. *The Journal of Endocrinology, 223*(1), 47–66. PMID: 25232145.

27. Mangala Priya, V., Mayilvanan, C., Akilavalli, N., et al. (2014). Lactational exposure of phthalate impairs insulin signaling in the cardiac muscle of F1 female albino rats. *Cardiovascular Toxicology, 14*(1), 10–20. PMID: 24297258.

28. James-Todd, T. M., Huang, T., Seely, E. W., & Saxena, A. R. (2016). The association between phthalates and metabolic syndrome: The National Health and Nutrition Examination Survey 2001-2010. *Environmental Health: A Global Access Science Source, 15*, 52. PubMed PMID: 27079661.

29. Stojanoska, M. M., Milosevic, N., Milic, N., & Abenavoli, L. (2016). The influence of phthalates and bisphenol A on the obesity development and glucose metabolism disorders. *Endocrine*, [Epub ahead of print]. PubMed PMID: 27822670.

30. Su, P. H., Chen, J. Y., Lin, C. Y., et al. (2014). Sex steroid hormone levels and reproductive development of eight-year-old children following in utero and environmental exposure to phthalates. *PLoS ONE, 9*(9), e102788. PubMed PMID: 25207995.

31. Wolff, M. S., Pajak, A., Pinney, S. M., et al.; Breast Cancer and Environment Research Program. (2017). Associations of urinary phthalate and phenol biomarkers with menarche in a multiethnic cohort of young girls. *Reproductive Toxicology, 67*, 56–64. PubMed PMID: 27851993.

32. Colon, I., Caro, D., Bourdony, C. J., & Rosario, O. (2000). Identification of phthalate esters in the serum of young Puerto Rican girls with premature breast development. *Environmental Health Perspectives, 108*, 895–900. PubMed PMID: 11017896.

33. Cobellis, L., Latini, G., De Felice, C., et al. (2003). High plasma concentrations of di-(2-ethylhexyl)-phthalate in women with endometriosis. *Human Reproduction, 18*(7), 1512–1515. PubMed PMID: 12832380.

34. Kim, J. H., Kim, S. H., Oh, Y. S., et al. (2017). In vitro effects of phthalate esters in human myometrial and leiomyoma cells and increased urinary level of phthalate metabolite in women with uterine leiomyoma. *Fertility and Sterility, 107*(4), 1061–1069.e1. PubMed PMID: 28292620.

35. Ferguson, K. K., Peterson, K. E., Lee, J. M., et al. (2014). Prenatal and peripubertal phthalates and bisphenol A in relation to sex hormones and puberty in boys. *Reproductive Toxicology, 47*, 70–76. PubMed PMID: 24945889.

36. Meeker, J. D., & Ferguson, K. K. (2014). Urinary phthalate metabolites are associated with decreased serum testosterone in men, women, and children from NHANES 2011-2012. *The Journal of Clinical Endocrinology and Metabolism, 99*(11), 4346–4352. PubMed PMID: 25121464.

37. Joensen, U. N., Frederiksen, H., Blomberg Jensen, M., et al. (2012). Phthalate excretion pattern and testicular function: A study of 881 healthy Danish men. *Environmental Health Perspectives, 120*(10), 1397–1403. PubMed PMID: 22832070.

38. Meeker, J. D., Calafat, A. M., & Hauser, R. (2009). Urinary metabolites of di(2-ethylhexyl) phthalate are associated with decreased steroid hormone levels in adult men. *Journal of Andrology, 30*(3), 287–297. PubMed PMID: 19059903.

39. Duty, S. M., Singh, N. P., Silva, M. J., et al. (2003). The relationship between environmental exposures to phthalates and DNA damage in human sperm using the neutral comet assay. *Environmental Health Perspectives, 111*(9), 1164–1169. PubMed PMID: 12842768.

40. Jurewicz, J., Radwan, M., Sobala, W., et al. (2013). Human urinary phthalate metabolites level and main semen parameters, sperm chromatin structure, sperm aneuploidy and reproductive hormones. *Reproductive Toxicology, 42*, 232–241. PubMed PMID: 24140385.

41. Buck Louis, G. M., Sundaram, R., Sweeney, A. M., et al. (2014). Urinary bisphenol A, phthalates, and couple fecundity: The Longitudinal Investigation of Fertility and the Environment (LIFE) Study. *Fertility and Sterility, 101*(5), 1359–1366. PubMed PMID: 24534276.

42. Stahlhut, R. W., van Wijngaarden, E., Dye, T. D., Cook, S., & Swan, S. H. (2007). Concentrations of urinary phthalate metabolites are associated with increased waist circumference and insulin resistance in adult U.S. males. *Environmental Health Perspectives, 115*(6), 876–882. PubMed PMID: 17589594.

43. Hatch, E. E., Nelson, J. W., Qureshi, M. M., et al. (2008). Association of urinary phthalate metabolite concentrations with body mass index and waist circumference: A cross-sectional study of NHANES data, 1999-2002. *Environmental Health: A Global Access Science Source, 7*, 27. PubMed PMID: 18522739.

44. Lind, P. M., Roos, V., Rönn, M., et al. (2012). Serum concentrations of phthalate metabolites are related to abdominal fat distribution two years later in elderly women. *Environmental Health: A Global Access Science Source, 11*, 21. PubMed PMID: 22472124.

45. Buser, M. C., Murray, H. E., & Scinicariello, F. (2014). Age and sex differences in childhood and adulthood

obesity association with phthalates: Analyses of NHANES 2007-2010. *International Journal of Hygiene and Environmental Health*, *217*(6), 687–694. PubMed PMID: 24657244.

46. Yaghjyan, L., Sites, S., Ruan, Y., & Chang, S. H. (2015). Associations of urinary phthalates with body mass index, waist circumference and serum lipids among females: National Health and Nutrition Examination Survey 1999-2004. *International Journal of Obesity (2005)*, *39*(6), 994–1000. PubMed PMID: 25644057.

47. Trasande, L., Attina, T. M., Sathyanarayana, S., et al. (2013). Race/ethnicity-specific associations of urinary phthalates with childhood body mass in a nationally representative sample. *Environmental Health Perspectives*, *121*(4), 501–506. PubMed PMID: 23428635.

48. Breous, E., Wenzel, A., & Loos, U. (2005). The promotor of the human sodium/iodide symporter responds to certain phthalate plasticisers. *Molecular and Cellular Endocrinology*, *244*(1–2), 75–78. PubMed PMID: 16257484.

49. Shimada, N., & Yamauchi, K. (2004). Characteristics of 3,5,3'-triiodothyronine (T3)-uptake system of tadpole red blood cells: Effect of endocrine-disrupting chemicals on cellular T3 response. *The Journal of Endocrinology*, *183*(3), 627–637. PubMed PMID: 15590988.

50. Ishihara, A., Nishiyama, N., Sugiyama, S., & Yamauchi, K. (2003). The effect of endocrine disrupting chemicals on thyroid hormone binding to Japanese quail thransthyretin and thyroid hormone receptor. *General and Comparative Endocrinology*, *134*(1), 36–43. PubMed PMID: 13129501.

51. Huang, P. C., Kuo, P. L., Guo, Y. L., Liao, P. C., & Lee, C. C. (2007). Associations between urinary phthalate monoesters and thyroid hormones in pregnant women. *Human Reproduction*, *22*(10), 2715–2722. PubMed PMID: 17704099.

52. Meeker, J. D., Calafat, A. M., & Hauser, R. (2007). Di(2-ethylhexyl) phthalate metabolites may alter thyroid hormone levels in men. *Environmental Health Perspectives*, *115*(7), 1029–1034. PubMed PMID: 17637918.

53. Bornehag, C. G., Sundell, J., Weschler, C. J., et al. (2004). The association between asthma and allergic symptoms in children and phthalates in house dust: A nested case-control study. *Environmental Health Perspectives*, *112*, 1393–1397. PubMed PMID: 15471731.

54. Hoppin, J. A., Jaramillo, R., London, S. J., et al. (2013). Phthalate exposure and allergy in the U.S. population: Results from NHANES 2005-2006. *Environmental Health Perspectives*, *121*(10), 1129–1134. PubMed PMID: 23799650.

55. Bornehag, C. G., & Nanberg, E. (2009). Phthalate exposure and asthma in chidren. *International Journal of Andrology*, *33*, 1–13. PubMed PMID: 20059582.

56. Doherty, B. T., Engel, S. M., Buckley, J. P., et al. (2016). Prenatal phthalate biomarker concentrations and performance on the Bayley Scales of Infant Development-II in a population of young urban children. *Environmental Research*, *152*, 51–58. PubMed PMID: 27741448.

57. Factor-Litvak, P., Insel, B., Calafat, A. M., et al. (2014). Persistent associations between maternal prenatal exposure to phthalates on child IQ at age 7 years. *PLoS ONE*, *9*(12), e114003. PubMed PMID: 25493564.

58. Lien, Y. J., Ku, H. Y., Su, P. H., et al. (2015). Prenatal exposure to phthalate esters and behavioral syndromes in children at 8 years of age: Taiwan Maternal and Infant Cohort Study. *Environmental Health Perspectives*, *123*(1), 95–100. PubMed PMID: 25280125.

59. Larsson, M., Weiss, B., Janson, S., et al. (2009). Associations between indoor environmental factors and parental-reported autistic spectrum disorders in children 6-8 years of age. *Neurotoxicology*, *30*(5), 822–831. PubMed PMID: 19822263.

60. Kim, K. N., Choi, Y. H., Lim, Y. H., & Hong, Y. C. (2016). Urinary phthalate metabolites and depression in an elderly population: National Health and Nutrition Examination Survey 2005-2012. *Environmental Research*, *145*, 61–67. PubMed PMID: 26624239.

61. Koch, H. M., Lorber, M., Christensen, K. L., et al. (2013). Identifying sources of phthalate exposure with human biomonitoring: Results of a 48h fasting study with urine collection and personal activity patterns. *International Journal of Hygiene and Environmental Health*, *216*(6), 672–681. PubMed PMID: 23333758.

62. Harley, K. G., Kogut, K., Madrigal, D. S., et al. (2016). Reducing phthalate, paraben, and phenol exposure from personal care products in adolescent girls: Findings from the HERMOSA Intervention Study. *Environmental Health Perspectives*, *124*(10), 1600–1607. PubMed PMID: 26947464.

63. Sathyanarayana, S., Alcedo, G., Saelens, B. E., et al. (2013). Unexpected results in a randomized dietary trial to reduce phthalate and bisphenol A exposures. *Journal of Exposure Science and Environmental Epidemiology*, *23*(4), 378–384. PubMed PMID: 23443238.

64. Ji, K., Lim Kho, Y., Park, Y., & Choi, K. (2010). Influence of a five-day vegetarian diet on urinary levels of antibiotics and phthalate metabolites: A pilot study with "Temple Stay" participants. *Environmental Research*, *110*(4), 375–382. PubMed PMID: 20227070.

65. Chen, C. Y., Chou, Y. Y., Lin, S. J., & Lee, C. C. (2015). Developing an intervention strategy to reduce phthalate exposure in Taiwanese girls. *The Science of the Total Environment, 517*, 125–131. PubMed PMID: 25725197.

66. Romero-Franco, M., Hernández-Ramírez, R. U., Calafat, A. M., Cebrián, M. E., Needham, L. L., Teitelbaum, S., et al. (2011). Personal care product use and urinary levels of phthalate metabolites in Mexican women. *Environment International, 37*(5), 867–871. PubMed PMID: 21429583.

67. Lewis, R. C., Meeker, J. D., Peterson, K. E., Lee, J. M., Pace, G. G., Cantoral, A., et al. (2013). Predictors of urinary bisphenol A and phthalate metabolite concentrations in Mexican children. *Chemosphere, 93*(10), 2390–2398. PubMed PMID: 24041567.

68. Smith, R., & Lourie, B. (2011). *Slow Death by Rubber Duck: The Secret Danger of Everyday Things.* New York: Counterpoint Press.

27

Polybrominated Diphenyl Ethers

SUMMARY

- Presence in population: Polybrominated diphenyl ethers (PBDEs) are found in 100% of residential dust samples and ubiquitously in human serum, with levels rising over the last two decades
- Major diseases: Lower testosterone levels, hypothyroidism, neurodevelopment disorders
- Primary sources: House dust, fish, maternal-fetal transfer
- Best measure: Currently no laboratory assessments are available for PBDEs
- Best intervention: Avoidance, sauna, enhancement of fecal fat release

DESCRIPTION

PBDEs (Fig. 27.1) have been used since the 1970s as flame retardants added to foam padding, textiles, and plastics. Hexabromobiphenyl 153 was removed from the market after a mislabeling accident resulted in this polybrominated biphenyl (PBB) being sold as animal feed in Michigan in the early 1970s, yet it is still found in virtually all North American residents (Table 27.1).[1] PBDEs typically contain three or more bromines, with those containing five or fewer being the most bioaccumulative. The most commonly used PBDE is decabromodiphenyl ether (deca-BDE) (not measured in the National Health and Nutritional Examination Survey [NHANES]), which was added to polystyrene, nylon, polypropylene, other polymers, adhesives, wire insulation, textiles, and cases for computers and televisions.[2] Antimony trioxide was also added to some PBDEs to enhance their flame retardant ability. Beginning in 2003, several states, including California, Washington, and Maine, banned the sale of certain PBDEs. In 2009, PBDEs were listed as persistent organic pollutants (POPs) by the Stockholm Convention for Persistent Organic Pollutants.[3]

TOXICITY

PBDEs do not bind aryl hydrocarbon receptors (AhRs), so they do not cause dioxin-like toxicity, but they are often contaminated with polybrominated dibenzodioxins (PBDDs) and dibenzofurans (PBDFs), which can induce cytochromes P450 (CYPs), leading to increased oxidative stress. PBDEs cause oxidative damage to DNA and are genotoxic as well as mitochondrial poisons.[2,4,5] PBDEs have also been officially listed as endocrine disrupting chemicals by the Endocrine Society.[6,7]

SOURCES

With the exception of the brominated flame retardant BDE-209, household dust is the primary source of PDBEs found in human serum (Fig. 27.2).[8] PBDEs are highest in fish, meats, and dairy products, with fish having the highest levels (mean of 1120 pg/g) (Table 27.2).[9,10] Sardines topped the charts with an average PBDE content of 3726 pg/g, again making them the most POP-contaminated fish. Farmed salmon were the next most contaminated, with levels of 1999, 3082, and 1732 pg/g. Wild Alaskan salmon had far lower levels of 141 and 605 pg/g. The mean level of PDBEs in all the meats tested was 383 pg/g, with levels varying widely from sample to sample in the same food category. For example, three samples of bacon had 39 pg/g, whereas two others contained 105 and 165 pg/g. One pork sausage sample had a whopping 1426 pg/g, yet another only contained 195 pg/g, and some hotdogs had 1348 pg/g. In addition to dust and fish intake,

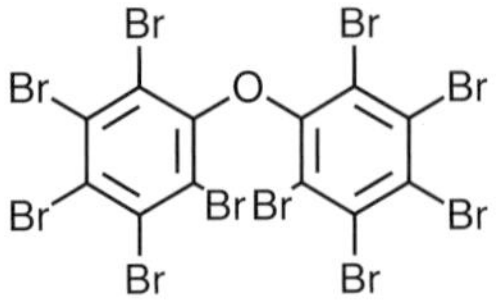

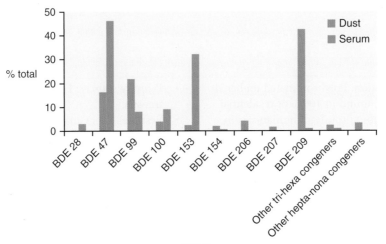

FIG. 27.1. Basic structure of polybrominated diphenyl ether with 10 bromine molecules.

FIG. 27.2. Polybrominated diphenyl ethers in dust and serum. (Reprinted with permission from Johnson, P. I., Stapleton, H. M., Sjodin, A., & Meeker, J. D. [2010]. Relationships between polybrominated diphenyl ether concentrations in house dust and serum. *Environmental Science & Technology, 44*(14), 5627–5632. Copyright 2010 American Chemical Society.

TABLE 27.1	**Polybrominated Diphenyl Ethers and Polybrominated Biphenyl Hexabromobiphenyl (BB153) in the National Health and Nutritional Examination Survey 2003 to 2004 in ng/g Lipid (Lipid Adjusted)**					
Polybrominated Diphenyl Ether	**Number of bromine molecules**	**Geometric Mean**	**50th percentile**	**75th percentile**	**90th percentile**	**95th percentile**
BDE-17	3	*	<LOD	<LOD	<LOD	<LOD
BDE-28	3	1.19	1.10	2.20	4.80	8.00
BDE-47	4	20.5	19.2	41.1	85.1	163
BDE-66	4	*	<LOD	<LOD	<LOD	1.30
BDE-85	5	*	<LOD	<LOD	<LOD	4.10
BDE-99	5	*	<LOD	9.20	21.7	42.2
BDE-100	5	3.93	3.60	7.80	18.4	36.5
BDE-153	6	5.69	4.80	11.3	32.6	65.7
BDE-154	6	*	<LOD	0.900	2.10	4.20
BDE-183	7	*	<LOD	<LOD	<LOD	<LOD
BB-153	6	2.29	2.20	4.40	12.8	27.2

From Centers for Disease Control and Prevention. National Report on Human Exposure to Environmental Chemicals: Updated tables, 2017. Retrieved from https://www.cdc.gov/exposurereport/pdf/fourthreport.pdf
*no geometric mean calculated LOD—level of detection.

TABLE 27.2	Polybrominated Diphenyl Ether Content in Fish and Hamburger (pg/g)				
	Wild Salmon	**Farmed Salmon**	**Sardines**	**Catfish/Tuna/Tilapia/Cod**	**Hamburger**
PBDE	373 pg/g	2253 pg/g	3726 pg/g	228.6 pg/g	168.5 pg/g

Data from Schecter, A., Colacino, J., Haffner, D., Patel K., Opel M., Päpke O., et al. (2010). Perfluorinated compounds, polychlorinated biphenyls, and organochlorine pesticide contamination in composite food samples from Dallas, Texas, USA. *Environmental Health Perspectives, 118*(6), 796–802; Hayward, D., Wong, J., & Krynitsky, A. J. (2007). Polybrominated diphenyl ethers and polychlorinated biphenyls in commercially wild caught and farm-raised fish fillets in the United States. *Environmental Research, 103*(1), 46–54; van Leeuwen, S. P., van Velzen, M. J., Swart, C. P., van der Veen I., Traag W. A., et al. (2009). Halogenated contaminants in farmed salmon, trout, tilapia, pangasius, and shrimp. *Environmental Science & Technology, 43*(11), 4009–4015.

maternal-fetal transfer is another source of PBDE contamination.[11]

BODY BURDEN

In the 2003 to 2004 NHANES, 10 PBDEs were assessed (Table 27.1), with 4 of the 10 being found ubiquitously. Subsequently, mean levels of PBDE-47 were found to have doubled by 2008 to 2009 in a group of pregnant Californians, indicating a potential rise in PBDE burden.[12] PBDE levels have also increased in Chinese women in the last decade.[13] Canadian fetal PBDE levels have shown the biggest increase: a fivefold rise between 1998 and 2006.[14]

Detoxification/Excretion Processes

The research on PBDE detoxification in humans is very incomplete. PBDEs are metabolized by both phase I and phase II, including oxidative and reductive debromination, cytochrome P450 (CYP) biotransformation, and/or phase II conjugation (glucuronidation and sulfation).[15] Oxidative hydroxylation by CYP450 2B6 to become hydroxylated PBDEs appears to have greater toxic action against cells and tissues.[16]

PBDEs with 8 to 10 bromines have a blood half-life in humans ranging from 15 to 91 days but can be persistent in adipose tissue.[17] The half-lives of the various PBDEs in humans appear to be highly variable according to type and exposure source. Although the previously discussed study found a serum half-life of 15 to 91 days in those industrially exposed, several studies of an environmentally exposed population found 4.5 or more years.[18] Rate of excretion slows in proportion to body mass index (BMI). Some PBDEs bioaccumulate in the human placenta as well.[19]

Clinical Significance

Endocrine Disruption. As penta-BDE levels increase in men, levels of follicle-stimulating hormone (FSH) decrease, whereas sex hormone-binding globulin (SHBG) and estradiol increase, and a rise in deca-BDE blood levels corresponds with a reduction in testosterone levels.[20]

PBDEs, pentabromophenol (PBP), and tetrabromobisphenol A (TBBPA) have structural resemblance to thyroxine (T4) and are potent competitors for T4 binding to transthyretin (TTR).[21] PBDEs suppress TH-regulated gene expression in humans and interfere with TH signaling.[22] Several animal studies indicate that PBDEs decrease the levels of circulating thyroid hormones,[23,24,25] and perinatal maternal exposure reduces thyroid hormones prenatally and postnatally.[26,27,28] Elevated levels of PBDE in children are associated with higher thyroid stimulating hormone (TSH) levels and a tendency for lower T4 and higher FT3.[29] High serum levels of BDE-47 and BDE-100, along with total BDEs, can increase the risk for hypothyroidism by 70%.[30]

Neurodevelopment. Prenatal exposure to elevated maternal serum PBDE is inversely associated with reading skills and positively associated with externalizing behavior by age 8 years.[31] A 10-fold increase in maternal BDE-153 increased the likelihood of the child having behavioral problems by age 8 years by almost fourfold, along with a 2.34-fold risk for decreased executive functioning.[32] Postnatal PBDE exposure was also associated with reduced attention and executive functioning in 9-year-old girls.[33] Six-year-old children living in homes with high levels of PBDE in the dust are up to 80% more likely to have diminished verbal comprehension and working memory.[34]

INTERVENTION

The primary source of PBDE exposure can be mitigated by following the dust-control and indoor air purification recommendations listed in Chapter 60. Ceasing consumption of sardines and farmed salmon also reduces exposure. Body burden of existing PBDE should be reduced by following the protocols in Chapter 62.

The only apparent direct human study of enhancing PBDE excretion was recently published by Genuis et al. They found induced sweating to be effective at excreting multiple PBDEs.[35] Of particular interest is that many of the subjects had no apparent PBDEs in the serum even though they were symptomatic and their sweat levels were high.

REFERENCES

1. Fries, G. F. (1985). The PBB episode in Michigan: An overall appraisal. *Critical Reviews in Toxicology*, *16*(2), 105–156. Review. PubMed PMID: 3002722.
2. Agency for Toxic Substances & Disease Registry. (2017). *Toxicological Profile for Polybrominated Diphenyl Ethers (PBDEs)*. https://www.atsdr.cdc.gov/toxprofiles/tp207.pdf. (Accessed July 31, 2017.)
3. Stockholm Convention. The BRS blog. Available at http://chm.pops.int. (Accessed July 30, 2017.)
4. Souza, A. O., Tasso, M. J., Oliveira, A. M., et al. (2016). Evaluation of polybrominated diphenyl ether toxicity on HepG2 cells: Hexabrominated congener (BDE-154) is less toxic than tetrabrominated congener (BDE-47). *Basic and Clinical Pharmacology and Toxicology*, *119*(5), 485–497. PubMed PMID: 27060917.
5. Yeh, A., Kruse, S. E., Marcinek, D. J., & Gallagher, E. P. (2015). Effect of omega-3 fatty acid oxidation products on the cellular and mitochondrial toxicity of BDE 47. *Toxicology in Vitro*, *29*(4), 672–680. PubMed PMID: 25659769.
6. Diamanti-Kandarakis, E., Bourguignon, J. P., Giudice, L. C., Hauser, R., Prins, G. S., Soto, A. M., et al. (2009). Endocrine-disrupting chemicals: An Endocrine Society scientific statement. *Endocrine Reviews*, *30*(4), 293–342. PubMed PMID: 19502515.
7. Gore, A. C., Chappell, V. A., Fenton, S. E., Flaws, J. A., Nadal, A., Prins, G. S., et al. (2015). EDC-2: The Endocrine Society's Second Scientific Statement on Endocrine-Disrupting Chemicals. *Endocrine Reviews*, *36*(6), E1–E150. PubMed PMID: 26544531.
8. Johnson, P. I., Stapleton, H. M., Sjodin, A., & Meeker, J. D. (2010). Relationships between polybrominated diphenyl ether concentrations in house dust and serum. *Environmental Science & Technology*, *44*(14), 5627–5632. PubMed PMID: 20521814.
9. Schecter, A., Päpke, O., Harris, T. R., et al. (2006). Polybrominated diphenyl ether (PBDE) levels in an expanded market basket survey of U.S. food and estimated PBDE dietary intake by age and sex. *Environmental Health Perspectives*, *114*(10), 1515–1520. PubMed PMID: 17035135.
10. Wang, H. S., Jiang, G. M., Chen, Z. J., et al. (2013). Concentrations and congener profiles of polybrominated diphenyl ethers (PBDEs) in blood plasma from Hong Kong: Implications for sources and exposure route. *Journal of Hazardous Materials*, *261*, 253–259. PubMed PMID: 23939206.
11. Chen, Z. J., Liu, H. Y., Ho, K. L., et al. (2016). Hydroxylated polybrominated diphenyl ethers (OH-PBDEs) in paired maternal and neonatal samples from South China: Placental transfer and potential risks. *Environmental Research*, *148*, 72–78. PubMed PMID: 27035923.
12. Zota, A. R., Park, J. S., Wang, Y., et al. (2011). Polybrominated diphenyl ethers, hydroxylated polybrominated diphenyl ethers, and measures of thyroid function in second trimester pregnant women in California. *Environmental Science & Technology*, *45*(18), 7896–7905. PubMed PMID: 21830753.
13. Chen, Z. J., Liu, H. Y., Cheng, Z., et al. (2014). Polybrominated diphenyl ethers (PBDEs) in human samples of mother-newborn pairs in South China and their placental transfer characteristics. *Environment International*, *73*, 77–84. PubMed PMID: 25090577.
14. Doucet, J., Tague, B., Arnold, D. L., et al. (2009). Persistent organic pollutant residues in human fetal liver and placenta from Greater Montreal, Quebec: A longitudinal study from 1998 through 2006. *Environmental Health Perspectives*, *117*(4), 605–610. PubMed PMID: 19440500.
15. Hakk, H., & Letcher, R. J. (2003). Metabolism in the toxicokinetics and fate of brominated flame retardants—a review. *Environment International*, *29*(6), 801–828.
16. Stapleton, H. M., Kelly, S. M., Pei, R., et al. (2009). Metabolism of polybrominated diphenyl ethers (PBDEs) by human hepatocytes in vitro. *Environmental Health Perspectives*, *117*(2), 197–202. PubMed PMID: 19270788.
17. Thuresson, K., Höglund, P., Hagmar, L., et al. (2006). Apparent half-lives of hepta- to decabrominated diphenyl ethers in human serum as determined in occupationally exposed workers. *Environmental Health Perspectives*, *114*(2), 176–181. PubMed PMID: 16451851.

18. Blanck, H. M., Marcus, M., Hertzberg, V., et al. (2000). Determinants of polybrominated biphenyl serum decay among women in the Michigan PBB cohort. *Environmental Health Perspectives, 108*(2), 147–152.

19. Leonetti, C., Butt, C. M., Hoffman, K., et al. (2016). Concentrations of polybrominated diphenyl ethers (PBDEs) and 2,4,6-tribromophenol in human placental tissues. *Environment International, 88,* 23–29. PubMed PMID: 26700418.

20. Johnson, P. I., Stapleton, H. M., Mukherjee, B., Hauser, R., & Meeker, J. D. (2013). Associations between brominated flame retardants in house dust and hormone levels in men. *The Science of the Total Environment, 445-446,* 177–184. PubMed PMID: 23333513.

21. Meerts, I. A., van Zanden, J. J., Luijks, E. A., et al. (2000). Potent competitive interactions of some brominated flame retardants and related compounds with human transthyretin in vitro. *Toxicological Sciences, 56*(1), 95–104. PubMed PMID: 10869457.

22. Zheng, J., He, C. T., Chen, S. J., Yan, X., et al. (2017). Disruption of thyroid hormone (TH) levels and TH-regulated gene expression be polybrominated diphenyl ethers (PBDEs), polychlorinated biphenyls (PCBs), and hydroxylated PCBs in e-waste recycling workers. *Environment International, 102,* 138–144. PubMed PMID: 28245931.

23. Fowles, J. R., Fairbrother, A., Beacher-Steppan, L., & Kerkvliet, N. I. (1994). Immunologic and endocrine effects of the flame-retardant pentabromodiphenyl ether (DE-71) in C57BL/6J mice. *Toxicology, 86*(1–2), 49–61. PubMed PMID: 8134923.

24. Zhou, T., Ross, D. G., DeVito, M. J., & Crofton, K. M. (2001). Effects of short-term in vivo exposure to polybrominated diphenyl ethers on thyroid hormones and hepatic enzyme activities in weanling rats. *Toxicological Sciences, 61*(1), 76–82. PubMed PMID: 11294977.

25. Stoker, T. E., Laws, S. C., Crofton, K. M., Hedge, J. M., et al. (2004). Assessment of DE-71, a commercial polybrominated diphenyl ether (PBDE) mixture, in the EDSP male and female pubertal protocols. *Toxicological Sciences, 78*(1), 144–155. PubMed PMID: 14999130.

26. Kim, T. H., Lee, Y. J., Lee, E., Kim, M. S., et al. (2009). Effects of gestational exposure to decabromodiphenyl ether on reproductive parameters, thyroid hormone levels, and neuronal development in Sprague-Dawley rats offspring. *Journal of Toxicology and Environmental Health. Part A, 72*(21–22), 1296–1303. PubMed PMID: 20077200.

27. Kodavanti, P. R., Coburn, C. G., Moser, V. C., MacPhail, R. C., et al. (2010). Developmental exposure to a commercial PBDE mixture, DE-71: Neurobehavioral, hormonal, and reproductive effects. *Toxicological Sciences, 116*(1), 297–312. PubMed PMID: 20375078.

28. Lema, S. C., Dickey, J. T., Scholtz, I. R., & Swanson, P. (2008). Dietary exposure to 2,2',4,4'-tetrabromodiphenyl ether (PBDE-47) alters thyroid status and thyroid hormone-regulated gene transcription in the pituitary and brain. *Environmental Health Perspectives, 116*(12), 1694–1699. PubMed PMID: 19079722.

29. Jacobson, M. H., Barr, D. B., Marcus, M., et al. (2016). Serum polybrominated diphenyl ether concentrations and thyroid function in young children. *Environmental Research, 149,* 222–230. PubMed PMID: 27228485.

30. Oulhote, Y., Chevrier, J., & Bouchard, M. F. (2016). Exposure to polybrominated diphenyl ethers (PBDEs) and hypothyroidism in Canadian women. *The Journal of Clinical Endocrinology and Metabolism, 101*(2), 590–598. PubMed PMID:26606679.

31. Zhang, H., Yolton, K., Webster, G. M., et al. (2017). Prenatal PBDE and PCB exposures and reading, cognition, and externalizing behavior in children. *Environmental Health Perspectives, 125*(4), 746–752. PubMed PMID: 27385187.

32. Vuong, A. M., Yolton, K., Webster, G. M., et al. (2016). Prenatal polybrominated diphenyl ether and perfluoroalkyl substance exposures and executive function in school-age children. *Environmental Research, 147,* 556–564. PubMed PMID: 26832761.

33. Sagiv, S. K., Kogut, K., Gaspar, F. W., et al. (2015). Prenatal and childhood polybrominated diphenyl ether (PBDE) exposure and attention and executive function at 9-12 years of age. *Neurotoxicology and Teratology, 52*(Pt. B), 151–161. PubMed PMID: 26271888.

34. Chevrier, C., Warembourg, C., Le Maner-Idrissi, G., et al. (2016). Childhood exposure to polybrominated diphenyl ethers and neurodevelopment at six years of age. *Neurotoxicology, 54,* 81–88. PubMed PMID: 26955917.

35. Genuis, S. K., Birkholz, D., & Genuis, S. J. (2017). Human excretion of polybrominated diphenyl ether flame retardants: blood, urine, and sweat study. *BioMed Research International, 2017,* 3676089. PMID: 28373979.

28

Polychlorinated Biphenyls

SUMMARY

- Presence in population: 36 polychlorinated biphenyls (PCBs) are found ubiquitously in the North American population
- Major diseases: Recurrent infections, allergies, asthma, autoimmunity, autism spectrum disorder (ASD), lower IQ, attention deficit hyperactivity disorder (ADHD), hypothyroid, infertility, miscarriage, diabetes, breast cancer

- Primary sources: Consuming foods contaminated with polychlorinated biphenyls (PCBs) including Atlantic salmon and sardines
- Best measure: Serum testing for a small number of commonly found PCBs is available
- Best intervention: Avoidance, chlorophyll, rice bran fiber, green tea, sauna

DESCRIPTION

PCBs (Fig. 28.1) were used extensively as heat exchangers for electrical transformers and hydraulic fluids, and were added to paints, oils, joint caulking, and floor tiles. The production of PCBs in the United States ceased in 1979 because of the findings that these compounds were highly persistent, bioaccumulated, and associated with severe health problems.[1] More than 1.5 billion pounds of 200 different PCBs were made in the United States, so products made before 1977 may still contain PCBs, including old fluorescent lighting fixtures, electrical devices or appliances containing PCB capacitors, and electrical transformers, as well as old microscope oil and hydraulic fluids. Since the signing of the Stockholm Convention[2] in 2001, there has been a worldwide ban on the production and use of PCBs. Unfortunately, production of PCBs recently began anew in the People's Republic of North Korea.

TOXICITY

PCBs are generally divided into two classifications, those with dioxin-like activity (the ability to bind to the aryl hydrocarbon [AhR] receptor) and those without.

Dioxin-like PCBs have either a coplanar or mono-ortho substitute. Dioxin-like PCBs are often rated using the toxic equivalency factor (TEF), which relates their dioxin-like toxic effect. In addition to the structure dictating toxic effect, the total number of chlorine molecules can affect the degree of water- and fat-solubility and toxicity as well. Both groups of PCBs have demonstrated toxic effects.

SOURCES

Because of PCBs' fat solubility and biological persistence, they are found mostly in fatty foods, which remain the main source of PCB exposure in the general population. The highest content of PCBs in one dietary study was found in dairy products, meat, and fish.[3] The estimated dietary intake of PCBs for an average adult was 0.027 μg/kg/day in 1978 and had declined to less than 0.001 μg/kg/day by 1991.[4] In the 2004 to 2005 Food and Drug Administration Total Diet Study (FDA TDS), 100% of the salmon samples were found to contain PCBs and dichlorodiphenyldichloroethylene (DDE). Currently 50% of world fish consumption comes from aquaculture,[5] and two-thirds of all salmon consumed in North America

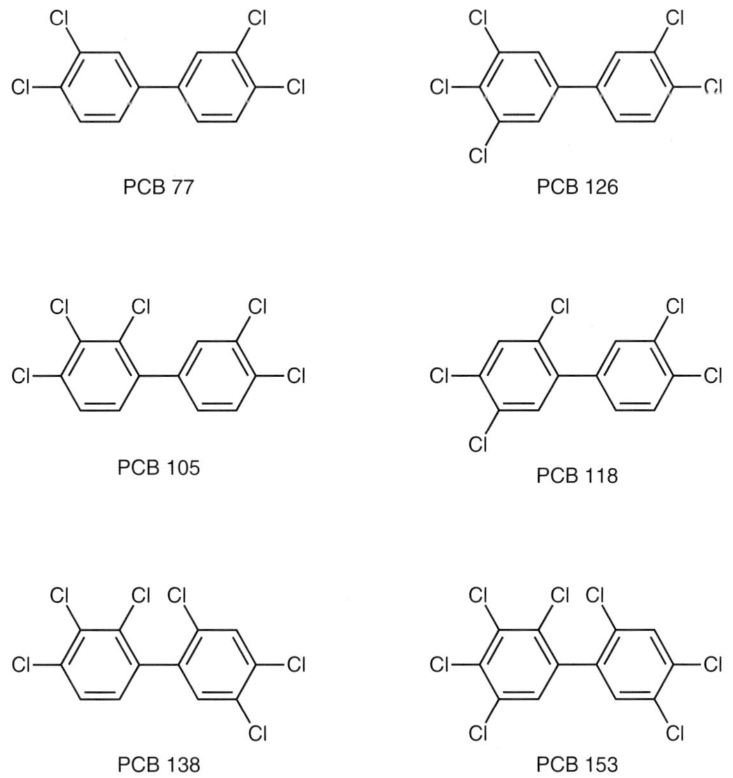

FIG. 28.1. Chemical structure of some of the most commonly found PCBs. (From Gauger, K. J., Giera, S., Sharlin, D. S., Bansal, R., Iannacone, E., & Zoeller RT. [2007]. Polychlorinated biphenyls 105 and 118 form thyroid hormone receptor agonists after cytochrome P4501A1 activation in rat pituitary GH3 cells. *Environmental Health Perspectives. 115*(11),1623–1630.)

is farmed.[6] It has been estimated that farmed salmon is responsible for 97% of dietary persistent organic pollutant (POP) exposure.[7] POP levels were assessed in 700+ salmon (totaling approximately 2 metric tons of farmed and wild salmon) from around the globe.[8] Fourteen persistent chlorinated compounds were found in significantly higher levels in farmed salmon than in wild salmon. The only compound that did not reach statistical significance was lindane, which was still higher in farmed than wild salmon. The four compounds with the greatest differences were PCBs, dioxins, toxaphene, and dieldrin. The PCB content in farmed salmon averaged 42.5 ng/g, whereas the wild Alaskan salmon averaged only 3.2 ng/g. Fish samples from farms off the coast of Washington State and Chile had lower PCB concentrations than salmon farmed near Scotland and the Faroe Islands. POP levels

in the fish samples paralleled the POP levels in the fish pellets used in those areas.[9] Another study revealed the average PCB content in farm-raised Atlantic salmon to be 28 to 38 ng/g, whereas PCB content in wild Alaskan salmon averaged 2.8 to 13.7 ng/g.[10] The PCBs found in Atlantic salmon, dominated by highly toxic PCB 138, 153, and 180, are different from those in Alaskan salmon, which have fewer chlorine molecules and greater water solubility and are far less toxic to humans. Some changes have been made to the fish pellets fed to farmed salmon, resulting in a decrease in some of the POPs present in the fish.[11] Unfortunately, the levels of PCBs 135, 153, and 180 have remained about the same. Farmed shrimp and tilapia, along with cod, are relatively free of the POPs found in farmed salmon, providing less-toxic fish alternatives.[7]

Sport fishing in the Great Lakes and other areas of the country remains another exposure source of POPs for those who eat their catch.[12,13,14] Table 3.3 (Chapter 3—Food Pollution) compares PCB content among sardines, wild Alaskan salmon, farmed Atlantic salmon, and hamburger. Sardines had the highest concentration of the highly toxic PCBs 138, 153, and 180, followed closely by farmed salmon and hamburger.[15,16]

BODY BURDEN

Serum values of chlorinated pesticides and PCBs are typically reported both as parts per billion (PPB) present in serum and as lipid-adjusted values (ng/g lipid). Adjusting the fat-soluble persistent toxicants to the amount of lipid in the blood provides a good representation for the level of those compounds in adipose storage (total body burden).[17] The Centers for Disease Control and Prevention (CDC) exposure report provides both PPB and ng/g lipid values for chlorinated pesticides and PCBs, and lists them according to the mean and 50th, 75th, 90th, and 95th percentiles found in the US population.[1] These levels provide an excellent reference point to determine which ones have higher than normal amounts. It must be kept in mind that higher POP levels can sometimes be found in persons undergoing weight loss.[18] The lipid-adjusted values provide a means of assessing the effectiveness of depuration protocol when done before and after treatment. The CDC Fourth Report contained 36 PCBs that were present ubiquitously in the 2003 to 2004 National Health and Nutritional Examination Survey (NHANES), with another (PCB 169) found in only 25% of the population (Table 28.1).

Detoxification/Excretion Processes

PCBs are initially acted upon by CYP450, primarily the 1A and the 3A series, to arene oxides, which are then either hydroxylated or conjugated with glutathione. Depending on the number and position of chlorine molecules, one or more arene oxide intermediates may be formed from each PCB congener. However, certain PCBs like 153 appear to be resistant to biotransformation. The half-lives of the various PCBs in humans are of great concern, ranging from 1 to 47 years.[19] PCBs also act as inducers for CYPs 1A, 2B, and 3A.

Clinical Significance

Immune System Effects. PCBs increase the likelihood of having recurrent infections.[20,21,22] They also increase type 1 allergic reactivity and incidence of asthma.[23,24] However, of perhaps greatest concern is the increased risk of multiple presentations of autoimmunity.[25,26,27,28,29] This may help explain the increasing incidence of virtually all autoimmune diseases.

Neurological Effects. *In utero* exposure to PCB affects intellectual functioning in children[30] and increases the risk for ASD.[31] Children exposed to PCBs *in utero* have increased cognitive defects, poorer gross motor function, and decreased visual recognition memory.[32] Exposed children also have lower IQ levels and increased rates of hyperactivity, both of which persist throughout childhood.[33,34,35] Adults consuming PCB-contaminated fish experienced increased problems with memory and learning.[36] Persons exposed to PCB gas had chronic neurological problems, including slower reaction time (for both simple and choice reactions), faster sway speed, diminished color discrimination and visual performance, and constricted visual field. They also had diminished scores on digit symbols, vocabulary, and verbal recall and embedded memory.[37] The potential role of PCB exposure in the dementia epidemic must be seriously considered.

Endocrine Effects. PCBs adversely affect thyroid hormone levels, including elevated antithyroid antibodies.[38,39,40] As PCB serum levels increase, T3 and T4 decrease.[41] Women exposed to PCBs report higher incidence of stillbirth, more abnormal menstrual bleeding, and greater incidence of endometriosis than nonexposed women.[42] High PCB levels can cause increased rates of miscarriage.[43] PCB serum levels have been linked to infertility in both men and women and to failed *in vitro* fertilization (IVF).[44,45] *In utero* PCB exposure reduced estradiol levels in 8-year-old children and caused shorter fundal and uterine length in girls.[46] PCBs and other chlorinated compounds led to increased risk for type 2 diabetes.[47]

Adverse Health Effects of Specific PCBs

- Together, PCBs 118, 138, 153, and 180 exhibit adverse immune effects on children.[48]

TABLE 28.1 Levels of PCBs in NHANES 2003 to 2004

Compound	CDC 50th %		CDC 75th %		CDC 90th %		CDC 95th %	
	PPB	ng/g lipid	PPB	ng/g lipid	PPB	ng/g lipid	PPB	ng/g lipid
Nondioxin-like								
PCB 28	0.030	4.96	0.041	6.79	0.057	9.39	0.067	11.3
PCB 44	0.013	2.05	0.018	3.03	0.026	4.40	0.032	5.70
PCB 49	0.008	1.35	0.012	1.90	0.016	2.80	0.019	3.53
PCB 52	0.017	2.74	0.024	4.17	0.035	5.91	0.043	7.60
PCB 66	0.008	1.37	0.012	1.97	0.019	3.10	0.025	4.10
PCB 74	0.027	4.36	0.058	8.72	0.104	15.8	0.153	22.3
PCB 87	0.005	0.900	0.008	1.32	0.012	2.02	0.017	2.70
PCB 99	0.024	3.79	0.042	6.53	0.082	13.0	0.119	18.0
PCB 101	0.010	1.70	0.016	2.70	0.027	4.40	0.033	5.83
PCB 110	0.007	1.20	0.012	1.96	0.019	3.40	0.026	4.42
PCB 138, 158	0.095	15.1	0.206	30.5	0.359	55.4	0.477	75.3
PCB 146	0.014	2.21	0.032	4.80	0.054	8.27	0.077	11.7
PCB 149	0.004	0.600	0.006	0.900	0.009	1.45	0.011	1.90
PCB 151	<LOD	<LOD	0.003	0.420	0.004	0.700	0.006	1.00
PCB 153	0.135	20.8	0.283	43.3	0.477	71.8	0.624	97.1
PCB 170	0.041	6.30	0.087	12.9	0.144	21.7	0.188	28.2
PCB 172	0.006	0.900	0.012	1.80	0.021	2.98	0.027	4.16
PCB 177	0.008	1.30	0.018	2.77	0.034	5.30	0.047	7.20
PCB 178	0.008	1.20	0.016	2.50	0.029	5.24	0.041	6.10
PCB 180	0.114	18.0	0.246	37.1	0.409	63.7	0.534	81.5
PCB 183	0.010	1.60	0.021	3.29	0.039	5.86	0.054	7.90
PCB 187	0.029	4.60	0.065	10.1	0.115	17.2	0.167	24.3
PCB 194	0.026	4.19	0.056	8.47	0.096	14.3	0.129	19.1
PCB 195	0.005	0.900	0.012	1.98	0.022	3.40	0.031	4.51
PCB 196, 203	0.022	3.40	0.044	6.70	0.082	11.8	0.101	15.0
PCB 199	0.023	3.80	0.056	8.30	0.100	14.9	0.127	18.9
PCB 206	0.015	2.34	0.034	5.00	0.060	9.20	0.086	13.7
PCB 209	0.008	1.18	0.021	3.20	0.049	7.58	0.073	11.1
Dioxin-like								
	Fg/g	Pg/g lipid	Fg/g	Pg/g lipid	Fg/g	Pg/g lipid	Fg/g	Pg/g lipid
PCB 126	89.8	14.7	159	24.8	308	46.7	475	68.7
PCB 169	<LOD	<LOD	133	19.5	203	31.0	269	40.6
	PPB	Ng/g lipid	PPB	Ng/g lipid	PPB	Ng/g lipid	PPB	Ng/g lipid
PCB 105	0.007	1.09	0.012	1.90	0.027	4.04	0.043	8.24
PCB 118	0.032	5.19	0.066	10.4	0.143	21.8	0.216	31.3
PCB 156	0.021	3.29	0.048	7.00	0.075	11.4	0.103	15.3
PCB 157	0.005	0.800	0.011	1.73	0.018	2.80	0.024	3.80
PCB 167	0.004	0.700	0.010	1.60	0.020	2.99	0.026	4.10

- PCB 153 was shown to have a significant association with diabetes risk.[49,50]
- Together, PCBs 28, 52, 101, 118, 138, 153, and 180 are associated with low T4 and elevated γ-glutamy transferase.[51]
- PCB 118 mimics T3 action.[52]
- PCBs 153 and 126 can target the nervous system and thyroid.[53]
- PCB 126 is associated with estrogenic[54] and adrenal effects[55] and is immunotoxic.[56]

- PCBs 118, 138, 153, and 180 were higher in breast adipose tissue from breast cancer patients than from women who were free of breast cancer.[57,58]
- PCBs 138/158 and 153 increase ASD risk up to 80%.[31]

INTERVENTION

Various dietary measures have demonstrated the ability to increase normal bowel excretion of these persistent pollutants (see Chapter 62—Gastrointestinal and Renal Elimination), resulting in reduction of the half-lives of PCBs. Daily use of rice bran fiber (RBF) has been documented in several studies in Japan to be able to increase the clearance of PCBs.[59,60,61] Chlorophyll and all chlorophyll-containing foods also facilitate the excretion of PCBs through the stool.[62,63,64] Increasing these in the diet or with supplementation on a daily basis will slowly increase excretion of these compounds from the body. In addition to chlorophyll-containing agents, polyphenols found in white and green teas have also been shown to increase excretion of fat-soluble toxins.[65]

A small number of intriguing studies have shown that bile sequestrants are very effective at decreasing body load of PCBs, likely by increasing fecal excretion. One study found that colestimide (dosage not disclosed) decreased blood PCB levels by 23% after 6 months.[66] Another controlled study had participants eat potato chips made with either olestra or vegetable oil. The olestra group experienced an 8% drop in PCBs compared with 4% in the controls. However, the high dosage of 15 g/d of olestra (22 fat-free Pringles [no longer commercially available]) resulted in 25% experiencing the typical loose stool adverse reaction associated with such agents.[67] Olestra was also used on an overweight diabetic male in Australia who was severely poisoned with PCBs. He suffered from chloracne, a common symptom of PCB overload, along with headaches and numbness in his lower body that got worse with any weight loss. He consumed seven potato chips containing only 16 grams of Olestra daily for two years without any adverse bowel effects. At the end of those 24 months he was 40 pounds lighter, had normal cholesterol, was no longer diabetic and had a dramatic drop in his adipose PCB stores from 1254 mg/kg to 56. He was able to do all this without other dietary changes and without experiencing any chloracne.

Sauna therapy protocols (see Chapter 61—Sauna) have also demonstrated effectiveness at reducing body burden of PCBs.[68,69,70]

REFERENCES

1. U.S. Environmental Protection Agency. *EPA Bans PCB Manufacture; Phases Out Uses.* [EPA press releas, April 19, 1979] Available at https://archive.epa.gov/epa/aboutepa/epa-bans-pcb-manufacture-phases-out-uses.html. (Accessed July 21, 2017.)
2. Stockholm Convention. The BRS blog. Available at http://chm.pops.int. (Accessed July 21, 2017.)
3. Zuccato, E., Clavarese, S., Mariani, G., Mangiapan, S., Grasso, P., Guzzi, A., et al. (1999). Level, sources and toxicity of polychlorinated biphenyls in the Italian diet. *Chemosphere, 38*(12), 2753–2765.
4. Gunderson, E. L. (1995). FDA Total Diet Study, July 1986-April 1991, dietary intakes of pesticides, selected elements, and other chemicals. *Journal of AOAC International, 78*(6), 1353–1363.
5. National Oceanic and Atmospheric Administration Fisheries Service. *Basic Questions about Aquaculture.* January 12, 2012. Available at http://www.nmfs.noaa.gov/aquaculture/faqs/faq_aq_101.html#4howmuch. (Accessed April 29, 2017.)
6. Knapp, G., et al. *The Great Salmon Run: Competition Between Wild and Farmed Salmon.* Available from http://www.iser.uaa.alaska.edu/Publications/2007_01-GreatSalmonRun.pdf. (Accessed April 29, 2017.)
7. van Leeuwen, S. P., van Velzen, M. J., Swart, C. P., et al. (2009). Halogenated contaminants in farmed salmon, trout, tilapia, pangasius, and shrimp. *Environmental Science & Technology, 43*(11), 4009–4015. PubMed PMID: 19569323.
8. Hites, R. A., Foran, J. A., Carpenter, D. O., et al. (2004). Global assessment of organic contaminant in farmed salmon. *Science, 303*, 226–229. PubMed PMID: 14716013.
9. Carlson, D. L., & Hites, R. A. (2005). Polychlorinated biphenyls in salmon and salmon feed: global differences and bioaccumulation. *Environmental Science & Technology, 39*(19), 7389–7395. PubMed PMID: 16245806.
10. Ikonomou, M. G., Higgs, D. A., Gibbs, M., et al. (2007). Flesh quality of market-size farmed and wild British Columbia salmon. *Environmental Science & Technology, 41*(2), 437–443. PubMed PMID:17310704.
11. Nøstbakken, O. J., Hove, H. T., Duinker, A., et al. (2015). Contaminant levels in Norwegian farmed Atlantic salmon (Salmo salar) in the 13-year period from 1999 to 2011. *Environment International, 74*, 274–280. PubMed PMID: 25454244.
12. Hanrahan, L. P., Falk, C., Anderson, H. A., et al. (1999). Serum PCB and DDE levels of frequent Great Lakes sport fish consumers: a first look. The Great Lakes

Consortium. *Environmental Research*, *80*(2 Pt. 2), S26–S37. PubMed PMID: 10092417.

13. Newsome, W. H., & Andrews, P. (1993). Organochlorine pesticides and polychlorinated biphenyl cogeners in commercial fish from the Great Lakes. *Journal of AOAC International*, *76*(4), 707–710. PubMed PMID: 8374320.

14. He, J. P., Stein, A. D., Humphrey, H. E., et al. (2001). Time trends in sport-caught Great Lakes fish consumption and serum polychlorinated biphenyl levels among Michigan anglers, 1973-1993. *Environmental Science & Technology*, *35*(3), 435–440. PubMed PMID: 11351711.

15. Schecter, A., Colacino, J., Haffner, D., et al. (2010). Perfluorinated compounds, polychlorinated biphenyls, and organochlorine pesticide contamination in composite food samples from Dallas, Texas, USA. *Environmental Health Perspectives*, *118*(6), 796–802. PubMed PMID: 20146964.

16. Hayward, D., Wong, J., & Krynitsky, A. J. (2007). Polybrominated diphenyl ethers and polychlorinated biphenyls in commercially wild caught and farm-raised fish fillets in the United States. *Environmental Research*, *103*(1), 46–54. PubMed PMID: 16769049.

17. Patterson, D. G., Jr., Needham, L. L., Pirkle, J. L., Roberts, D. W., Bagby, J., Garrett, W. A., et al. (1988). Correlation between serum and adipose tissue levels of 2,3,7,8-tetrachlorodibenzo-p-dioxin in 50 persons from Missouri. *Archives of Environmental Contamination and Toxicology*, *17*(2), 139–143. PubMed PMID: 3355228.

18. Lim, J. S., Son, H. K., Park, S. K., Jacobs, D. R., Jr., & Lee, D. H. (2011). Inverse associations between long-term weight change and serum concentrations of persistent organic pollutants. *International Journal of Obesity (2005)*, *35*(5), 744–747. PubMed PMID: 20820170.

19. Agency for Toxic Substances & Disease Registry. Polychlorinated Biphenyls (PCBs). https://www.atsdr.cdc.gov/substances/toxsubstance.asp?toxid=26. (Accessed July 23, 2017.)

20. Weisglas-Kuperus, N., Patadin, S., Berbers, G. A. M., Sas, T. C. J., Mulder, P. G. H., Sauer, P. J. J., et al. (2000). Immunologic effects of background exposure to polychlorinated biphenyls and dioxins in Dutch preschool children. *Environmental Health Perspectives*, *108*, 1203–1207.

21. Dewailly, E., Ayotte, P., Burneau, S., Gingras, S., Belles-Isles, M., & Roy, R. (2000). Susceptibility to infections and immune status in Inuit infants exposed to organochlorines. *Environmental Health Perspectives*, *108*, 205–211.

22. Heilmann, C., Budtz-Jørgensen, E., Nielsen, F., Heinzow, B., Weihe, P., & Grandjean, P. (2010). Serum concentrations of antibodies against vaccine toxoids in children exposed perinatally to immunotoxicants.

Environmental Health Perspectives, *118*(10), 1434–1438. PubMed PMID: 20562056.

23. Grandjean, P., Poulsen, L. K., Heilmann, C., Steuerwald, U., & Weihe, P. (2010). Allergy and sensitization during childhood associated with prenatal and lactational exposure to marine pollutants. *Environmental Health Perspectives*, *118*(10), 1429–1433. PubMed PMID: 20562055.

24. Stølevik, S. B., Nygaard, U. C., Namork, E., Haugen, M., Kvalem, H. E., Meltzer, H. M., et al. (2011). Prenatal exposure to polychlorinated biphenyls and dioxins is associated with increased risk of wheeze and infections in infants. *Food and Chemical Toxicology*, *49*(8), 1843–1848. PubMed PMID: 21571030.

25. Gallagher, C. M., McElroy, A. E., Smith, D. M., Golightly, M. G., & Meliker, J. R. (2013). Polychlorinated biphenyls, mercury, and antinuclear antibody positivity, NHANES 2003-2004. *International Journal of Hygiene and Environmental Health*, *216*(6), 721–727. PubMed PMID: 23419585.

26. Tsai, P. C., Ko, Y. C., Huang, W., Liu, H. S., & Guo, Y. L. (2007). Increased liver and lupus mortalities in 24-year follow-up of the Taiwanese people highly exposed to polychlorinated biphenyls and dibenzofurans. *The Science of the Total Environment*, *374*(2–3), 216–222. PubMed PMID: 17257654.

27. Lee, D. H., Steffes, M., & Jacobs, D. R. (2007). Positive associations of serum concentration of polychlorinated biphenyls or organochlorine pesticides with self-reported arthritis, especially rheumatoid type, in women. *Environmental Health Perspectives*, *115*(6), 883–888. PubMed PMID: 17589595.

28. Cebecauer, L., Radikova, Z., Rovensky, J., Koska, Imrich, R., Ksinantova, L., et al. (2009). Increased prevalence and coincidence of antinuclear and antithyroid antibodies in the population exposed to high levels of polychlorinated pollutants cocktail. *Endocrine Regulations*, *43*(2), 75–81. PubMed PMID: 19856712.

29. Schell, L. M., Gallo, M. V., Ravenscroft, J., & DeCaprio, A. P. (2009). Persistent organic pollutants and anti-thyroid peroxidase levels in Akwesasne Mohawk young adults. *Environmental Research*, *109*(1), 86–92. PubMed PMID: 18995849.

30. Jacobson, S., Fein, G., Jacobson, J., Schwartz, P., & Dowler, J. (1985). The effect of intrauterine PCB exposure on visual recognition memory. *Child Development*, *56*, 853–860.

31. Lyall, K., Croen, L. A., Sjödin, A., et al. (2017). Polychlorinated biphenyl and organochlorine pesticide concentrations in maternal mid-pregnancy serum samples: association with autism spectrum disorder and intellectual disability. *Environmental Health Perspectives*, *125*(3), 474–480. PubMed PMID: 27548254.

32. Jacobson, J. L., & Jacobson, S. W. (1997). Evidence for PCBs as neurodevelopmental toxicant in humans. *Neurotoxicol*, *18*(2), 415–424.

33. Chen, Y.-C. J., Guo, Y.-L., Hsu, C.-C., & Rogan, W. J. (1992). Cognitive development of Yu-Cheng ('Oil disease') children prenatally exposed to heat-degraded PCBs. *The Journal of the American Medical Association*, *268*(22), 3213–3218.

34. Chen, Y.-C. J., Yu, M.-L. M., Rogan, W. J., Gladden, B. C., & Hsu, C.-C. (1994). A 6-year follow-up of behavior and activity disorders in the Taiwan Yu-Cheng children. *American Journal of Public Health*, *84*(3), 415–421.

35. Lai, T.-J., Liu, X., Guo, Y. L., et al. (2002). A cohort study of behavior problems and intelligence in children with high prenatal polychlorinated biphenyl exposure. *Archives of General Psychiatry*, *59*(11), 1061–1066.

36. Schantz, S., Gasior, D., Polverejan, E., et al. (2001). Impairments of memory and learning in older adults exposed to polychlorinated biphenyls via consumption of Great Lakes fish. *Environmental Health Perspectives*, *109*(6), 605–611.

37. Kilburn, K. H. (2000). Visual and neurobehavioral impairment associated with polychlorinated biphenyls. *NeuroToxicology*, *21*(4), 489–500. PMID: 11022858.

38. Gerhard, I., Mongo, B., Krahe, J., & Runnebaum, B. (1999). Chlorinated hydrocarbons in infertile women. *Environmental Research*, *80*, 299–310.

39. Langer, P., Tajtakova, M., Fodor, G., et al. (1998). Increased thyroid volume and prevalence of thyroid disorders in an area heavily polluted by polychlorinated biphenyls. *European Journal of Endocrinology*, *139*, 402–409.

40. Li, M.-H., & Hansen, L. G. (1996). Enzyme induction and acute endocrine effects in prepubertal female rats receiving environmental PCB/PCDF/PCDD mixtures. *Environmental Health Perspectives*, *104*(7), 712–722.

41. Hagmar, L., Rylander, L., Dyremark, E., et al. (2001). Plasma concentrations of persistent organochlorines in relation to thyrotropin and thyroid hormone levels in women. *International Archives of Occupational and Environmental Health*, *74*, 184–188.

42. Yu, M. L., Guo, Y. L., Hsu, C.-C., & Rogan, W. J. (2000). Menstruation and reproduction in women with polychlorinated biphenyl (PCB) poisoning: long-term follow-up interviews of the women from the Taiwan Yucheng cohort. *International Journal of Epidemiology*, *29*, 672–677.

43. Leoni, V., Fabiani, L., Marinelli, G., et al. (1989). PCB and other organochlorine compounds in blood of women with or without miscarriage: a hypothesis of correlation. *Ecotoxicology and Environmental Safety*, *17*, 1–11.

44. Younglai, W. V., Foster, W. G., Hughes, E. G., Trim, H. K., & Jarrell, J. F. (2002). Levels of environmental contaminants in human follicular fluid, serum, and seminal plasma of couples undergoing in vitro fertilization. *Archives of Environmental Contamination and Toxicology*, *43*, 121–126. PubMed PMID: 12045882.

45. Meeker, J. D., Maity, A., Missmer, S. A., Williams, P. L., Mahalingaiah, S., Ehrlich, S., et al. (2011). Serum concentrations of polychlorinated biphenyls in relation to in vitro fertilization outcomes. *Environmental Health Perspectives*, *119*(7), 1010–1016. PubMed PMID:21345762.

46. Su, P. H., Huang, P. C., Lin, C. Y., Ying, T. H., Chen, J. Y., & Wang, S. L. (2012). The effect of in utero exposure to dioxins and polychlorinated biphenyls on reproductive development in eight year-old children. *Environment International*, *39*(1), 181–187. PubMed PMID: 22208758.

47. Lee, D. H., Lee, I. K., Jin, S. H., Steffes, M., & Jacobs, D. R., Jr. (2007). Association between serum concentrations of persistent organic pollutants and insulin resistance among nondiabetic adults: results from the National Health and Nutrition Examination Survey 1999-2002. *Diabetes Care*, *30*(3), 622–628.

48. Weisglas-Kuperus, N., Patandin, S., Berbers, G. A. M., et al. (2000). Immunologic effects of background exposure to polychlorinated biphenyls and dioxins in Dutch preschool children. *Environmental Health Perspectives*, *108*, 1203–1207.

49. Lee, D. H., Toscano, W., Lee, I. K., et al. (2006). A strong dose-response relation between serum concentrations of persistent organic pollutants and diabetes. *Diabetes Care*, *29*, 1638–1644.

50. Rylander, L., Rignell-Hydbom, A., & Hagmar, L. (2005). A cross-sectional study of the association between persistent organochlorine pollutants and diabetes. *Environmental Health*, *4*, 28.

51. Sala, M., Sunyer, J., Herrero, C., To Figueras, J., & Grimalt, J. (2001). Association between serum concentrations of hexachlorobenzene and polychlorinated biphenyls with thyroid hormone and liver enzymes in a sample of the general population. *Occupational and Environmental Medicine*, *58*, 172–177.

52. Fritsche, E., Cline, J. E., Nguyen, N. H., et al. (2005). Polychlorinated biphenyls disturb differentiation of normal human neural progenitor cells: clue for involvement of thyroid hormone receptors. *Environmental Health Perspectives*, *113*, 871–876.

53. Costa, L. G., Fattori, V., Giordano, G., & Vitalone, A. (2007). An in vitro approach to assess the toxicity of certain food contaminants: methylmercury and polychlorinated biphenyls. *Toxicology*, *237*, 65–76.

54. Matthews, J., Wihlen, B., Heldring, N., et al. (2007). Co-planar 3,3',4,4',5-pentachlorinated biphenyl and

non-co-planar 2,2',4,6,6'-pentachlorinated biphenyl differentially induce recruitment of estrogen receptor alpha to aryl hydrocarbon receptor target genes. *The Biochemical Journal, 406*, 343–345.

55. Li, L. A., & Wang, P. W. (2005). PCB 126 induces differential changes in androgen, cortisol and aldosterone biosynthesis in human adrenocortical H295R cells. *Toxicological Sciences, 85*, 530–540.

56. Riecke, K., Schmidt, A., & Stahlmann, R. (2003). Effects of 2,3,7,8-TCDD and PCB126 on human thymic epithelial cells in vitro. *Archives of Toxicology, 77*(6), 358–364.

57. Guttes, S., Failing, G., Neumann, K., Kleinstein, J., et al. (1998). Chloroganic pesticides and polychlorinated biphenyls in breast tissue of women with benign and malignant breast diseases. *Archives of Environmental Contamination and Toxicology, 35*, 140–147.

58. Stallman, S. C., Djordjevic, M. V., Muscat, J. E., Gong, L., Bernstein, D., et al. (2000). Breast cancer risk in relation to adipose concentrations of organochlorine pesticides and polychlorinated biphenyls in Long Island, New York. *Cancer Epidemiology, Biomarkers & Prevention, 9*, 1241–1249.

59. Morita, K., Hamamura, K., & Iida, T. (1995). Binding of PCB by several types of dietary fiber in vivo and in vitro. *Fukuoka Igaku Zasshi, 86*, 212–217.

60. Morita, K., Hirakawa, H., Matsueda, T., et al. (1993). Stimulating effect of dietary fiber on fecal excretion of polychlorinated dibenzofuans (PCDF) and polychlorinated dibenzo-p-dioxins (PCDD) in rats. *Fukuoka Igaku Zasshi, 84*, 273–281.

61. Nagayama, J., Takasuga, T., Tsuji, H., et al. (2003). Active elimination of causative PCDFs/DDs congeners of Yusho by one year intake of FEBRA in Japanese people. *Fukuoka Igaku Zasshi, 94*, 118–125.

62. Morita, K., Ogata, M., & Hasegawa, T. (2001). Chlorophyll derived from chlorella inhibits dioxin absorption from the gastrointestinal tract and accelerates dioxin excretion in rats. *Environmental Health Perspectives, 109*, 289–294.

63. Morita, K., Matsueda, T., & Iida, T. (1999). Effect of green vegetables on digestive tract absorption of polychlorinated dibenzo-p-dioxins and polychlorinated dibenzofurans in rats. *Fukuoka Igaku Zaashi, 90*, 171–183.

64. Morita, K., Matsueda, T., Iida, T., & Hasegawa, T. (1999). Chlorella accelerates dioxin excretion in rats. *The Journal of Nutrition, 129*, 1731–1736.

65. Hsu, T. F., Kusumoto, A., Abe, K., et al. (2006). Oolong tea increased fecal fat. *European Journal of Clinical Nutrition, 60*(11), 1330–1336.

66. Sakurai, K., Fukata, H., Todaka, E., et al. (2006). Colestimide reduces blood polychlorinated biphenyl (PCB) levels. *Internal Medicine (Tokyo, Japan), 45*(5), 327–328. PMID: 16596004.

67. Jandacek, R. J., Heubi, J. E., Buckley, D. B., et al. (2014). Reduction of the body burden of PCBs and DDE by dietary intervention in a randomized trial. *The Journal of Nutritional Biochemistry, 25*, 483–488. PMID: 24629911.

68. Tretjak, Z., Root, D. E., Tretjak, A., Slivnik, R., et al. (1990). Xenobiotic reduction and clinical improvements in capacitor workers: a feasible method. *Journal of Environmental Science and Health, A25*(7), 731–751.

69. Dahlgren, J., Cecchini, M., Takhar, H., & Paepke, O. (2007). Persistent organic pollutants in 9/11 World Trade Center rescue workers: reduction following detoxification. *Chemosphere, 69*(8), 1320–1325. [Epub 2007 Jan 17]; PubMed PMID: 17234251.

70. Kilburn, K. H., Warsaw, R. H., & Shields, M. G. (1989). Neurobehavioral dysfunction in firemen exposed to polycholorinated biphenyls (PCBs): possible improvement after detoxification. *Archives of Environmental Health, 44*(6), 345–350. PubMed PMID: 2514627.

29

Perfluorocarbons
Perfluoroalkyl Substances

SUMMARY

- Presence in population: 12 perfluoroalkyl substances (PFASs) were measured in the US National Health and Nutrition Examination Survey (NHANES) from 1999 to 2008; of these, 4 were found in 95% of participants: perfluorooctanoic acid (PFOA), perfluorooctane sulfonic acid (PFOS), perfluorohexane sulfonic acid (PFHxS), and perfluorononanoic acid (PFNA)
- Major diseases: PFOA is listed as a possible carcinogen in humans and an immune system hazard; lower bone mineral density and osteoporosis among women has also been observed, as well as an association with non-high-density lipoprotein (HDL) cholesterol; PFASs also adversely affect thyroid function, blood sugar regulation, and fertility
- Primary sources: Food is generally the primary source, in part via protective water- and stain-resistant coatings on clothing, furnishings, and nonstick housewares; breast milk is the primary source of exposure for infants; groundwater, locally caught fish, and indoor air (household dust) are also potential exposure points
- Best measure: Serum perfluorinated compound (PFC) levels
- Best intervention: Bile acid sequestrants, antioxidants

DESCRIPTION

PFCs comprise a wide range of chemicals consisting of an alkyl chain (4–14 carbons), which is partially or fully fluorinated, with different functional groups attached. PFCs include perfluoroalkyl carboxylic acids (e.g., PFOA, PFDA), perfluoroalkyl sulfonic acids (e.g., PFOS, PFBS), perfluoroalkyl sulfonamides (e.g., PFOS), and other PFCs, such as fluorotelomer alcohols (e.g., fluorotelomer). PFCs have been produced since at least the 1950s and are used in many industrial and manufacturing applications, including production of nonstick cookware, waterproof and breathable textiles, and protective coatings for paper, food packing materials, leather conditioner, sealants, and carpets.[1] Because they represent a high proportion of environmental PFCs, PFOA and PFOS are often the primary contaminants measured (Fig. 29.1). Despite a voluntary phase-out in the production of PFOS in 2002 and PFOA in 2015, both compounds are extremely persistent, resulting in widespread exposure. For example, in surface water, the half-lives of PFOS and PFOA are 41 and 92 years, respectively, and in the human body range from 2 to 8 years.[2]

Given that perfluorinated chemicals are found in nearly 100% of people sampled in national studies, are extremely persistent in the environment and human tissues, and are linked to a number of chronic and diverse conditions, clinicians must improve their recognition of these synthetic toxins. Additionally, most of the PFCs in humans exist in mixtures both with each other and with other contaminants, with very little known about the toxicity of such complex mixtures. Much more research is needed to better understand PFC toxicity, as well as optimal strategies for avoidance, detoxification, and elimination.

perfluorooctanoic acid (PFOA; CAS# 335-67-1)   perfluorooctane sulfonate (PFOS; CAS# 1763-23-1)

FIG. 29.1 Structure of perfluorooctanoic acid and perfluorooctane sulfonic acid.

Toxicity

The US National Toxicology Program has concluded that both PFOA and PFOS are "presumed to be immune hazards to humans based on a high level of evidence." Both compounds have been shown to suppress antibody responses, leading to greater susceptibility to infectious disease, and to increase hypersensitivity reactions, suggesting multiple mechanisms of immune modulation. In human leukocytes, PFOS and PFOA decreased natural killer cell activity and impaired the release of tumor necrosis factor (TNF)-α following lipopolysaccharide (LPS) stimulation.[3] PFOA-induced immunotoxicity appears to be mediated via peroxisome proliferator–activated receptor alpha (PPAR-α), a ligand-activated transcription factor involved in the regulation of gene expression, lipid metabolism, glucose homeostasis, cell proliferation, and inflammation. PFOS inhibited LPS-induced I-κB degradation, preventing a necessary step for normal cellular inflammatory response.[4]

PFCs have also been shown to induce mitochondrial dysfunction and oxidative stress; when exposed to PFOA, osteoblasts had collapse of the mitochondrial membrane potential (MMP), cardiolipin peroxidation, and cytochrome c release, and decreased adenosine triphosphate (ATP) levels, with overall loss of cell viability.[5] In liver and brain mitochondria, PFOA was shown to increase reactive oxygen species production, collapse the MMP, and arrest the activity of mitochondrial complexes I, II (liver only), and III.[6]

PFCs may also act as endocrine disruptors, at least in part by altering the regulation of genes associated with steroidogenesis.[7] The net effect appears to be a reduction of testosterone synthesis and an induction of estrogen effects.[8-10] Thyroid function may also be disrupted; some PFASs compete with thyroxine for binding to the thyroid hormone transport protein transthyretin (TTR), lowering thyroid hormone levels, whereas others (including PFOA and PFHxS) increase T4 and T3 levels, though there appears to be a gender-dependent effect.[11,12]

Associations have also been found between PFCs and both cardiovascular and metabolic abnormalities. PFCs have been linked to accumulation of hepatic lipids, hepatic insulin resistance, and hepatic steatosis, likely due to upregulation of fatty acid accumulation.[13,14] Unfortunately, PFCs appear to cross the placental barrier and pass through breast milk, with early exposure associated with a number of adverse outcomes, including dyslipidemia.[15,16]

PFCs have also been shown to be carcinogenic in animal studies and linked to an increase in cancer mortality among exposed humans, including breast, prostate, and bladder cancer.[17,18]

SOURCES

PFCs have widespread usage, including industrial applications such as coatings on fabrics, carpets, and paper, as well as in insecticides, paints, cosmetics, and firefighting foams. They have also made their way into public water drinking systems, drinking water wells, and soil, and because they do not evaporate easily, the air surrounding industrial sources. The diverse exposure sources have made it difficult to determine the relative contribution from different pathways, which may also be influenced by age and geographical location.

Diet is an important source of PFC exposure, perhaps the most significant. A Norwegian study found that consumption of fish and shrimp, age, breastfeeding history, and area of residence were all significantly associated with blood levels of PFCs; indeed, seafood contributed 38% of the dietary intake of PFOA and 81% of PFOS, and was a major determinant of serum concentration.[19] A study based in Singapore supported the link with fish and shellfish, and also found both a positive association with red meat and poultry intake and an inverse association with grain and soy intake.[20] An analysis of US foods also found the largest contributors in dietary intake to be meat and fish (likely from bioaccumulation), with lesser amounts coming from vegetables, dairy, and eggs.[21] However, an analysis of NHANES data from 2003 to 2008 found that dietary factors accounted for only 10.4% to 21.2% of the explained variation in serum levels.[22]

Although dietary exposure appears to be the primary determinant of serum level for some groups, inhalation of indoor air may also be significant (particularly inhalation of office air), yet ingestion of dust by infants/toddlers may be the most relevant, as they are more likely to lie, crawl, or play on treated carpets.[23-25] Repeated Scotchgard™ treatment of indoor carpets resulted in highly elevated levels of PFHxS and moderately high levels of PFOA and PFOS in a Canadian family.[26]

In areas where PFCs are produced or used, drinking water is often a significant source of ongoing exposure. As one of the most extreme examples, individuals near a fluorochemical facility in Washington, West Virginia, where PFOA was used in fluoropolymer production, had PFOA concentrations 190-fold higher than the lifetime health advisory recommended by the US Environmental Protection Agency (EPA) and serum levels of PFOA 20 times higher than the US general population.[27] An analysis of US drinking water sources found that 16.5 million residents were at or above minimum reporting levels, positively associated with proximity to industrial sites, military fire training areas, airports, and wastewater treatment plants (Fig. 29.2).[28] Supporting this finding, firefighters have been found to have serum concentrations of some PFCs (perfluorodecanoic acid) three times higher than the general population.[29]

As previously mentioned, placental and breast milk transfer can be a significant source of exposure. Duration of exclusive breastfeeding, for example, was associated with an increase in most PFCs by up to 30% per month, with decreases following cessation of breastfeeding.[30] PFOS, PFOA, perfluorononanoic acid (PFNA), perfluoroundecanoic acid (PFUnDa), and perfluorodecanoic acid (PFDA) have all been detected in fetal organs, with cord blood values ranging between 30% and 79% of maternal concentrations.[31,32]

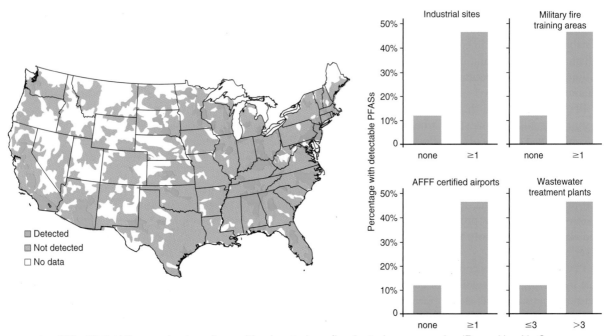

FIG. 29.2 U.S.groundwater sites with elevated perfluorinated compounds. (From Hu, X. C., Andrews, D. Q., Lindstrom, A. B., Burton, T. A., Schaider, L. A., Grandjean, P., Lohmann, R., Carignan, C. C., Blum, A., Balan, S. A., Higgins, C. P., Sunderland, E. M. [2016]. Detection of poly and perfluoroalkyl substances (PFASs) in U.S. drinking water linked to industrial sites, military fire training areas, and wastewater treatment plants. *Environmental Science & Technology Letters*, 3(10), 344–350.)

BODY BURDEN

PFCs typically do not accumulate in lipids, and exposure levels are usually monitored with serum levels. The two most abundant PFCs in human serum samples are PFOA and PFOS, with half-lives estimated to be 3.8 years and 5.4 years, respectively.[33] PFOS is now listed by the Stockholm Convention as a persistent organic pollutant (POP).[34] As previously mentioned, exposure is primarily via ingestion and inhalation among adults, though prenatal and breast milk exposure have been linked to a body burden in 6-month-old infants similar to adults.[35]

Detoxification/Excretion Processes

Although persistent, PFCs are thought to be mostly excreted by biliary excretion from the liver, with a lesser role played by the kidneys. They may be reabsorbed and transported back to the liver via enterohepatic circulation, and then reexcreted in the bile.[36] PFCs are often converted into perfluorinated acids (PFAs), which bind to serum proteins, are not further metabolized, are eliminated slowly, and are distributed primarily to the serum, liver, and kidneys.[37] Animal studies suggest hepatic levels of some PFCs (PFOS specifically) may be as much as 12-fold higher than serum levels.[38] Additionally, PFAs tend to persist in serum and are shunted back and forth between the liver and serum, resulting in elevated blood levels long after initial exposure. The strength of the carbon-fluorine bond is thought to explain the stability of these compounds and lack of metabolism.

Very little has been published on specific pathways of detoxification, although in mothers with the null genotype for glutathione S-transferase M1 (GSTM1), the concentrations of several PFCs were linked to low birth weight, suggesting a role for glutathione detoxification.[39] Animal studies have shown glutathione depletion with PFOS exposure, supporting this association.[40]

Clinical Significance

Immune Toxicity. Exposure to PFCs has been associated with impaired antibody response, including a diminished vaccine response. A prospective birth cohort study following approximately 600 children found that serum levels of PFCs showed "uniformly negative associations with antibody levels, especially at age 7 years, except the tetanus antibody level following PFOS exposure was not statistically significant." Overall antibody concentration was roughly half in children who had twice the serum level of PFCs, who also had a 2.38- and 4.2-fold increased likelihood for falling below protective tetanus and diphtheria levels, respectively, by age 7.[41] A recent report on this longitudinal study identified continued reduction of antibody protection through age 13.[42] This supports the finding that infectious disease risk increases with PFC exposure; in an analysis of more than 1500 mother–child pairs, maternal plasma levels of PFOS increased the odds of total infectious disease in children by 60%, when comparing the highest and the lowest quartile.[43]

A systematic review of 64 studies examining childhood exposure to PFC and health outcomes found evidence for positive associations between exposure and asthma (as well as dyslipidemia, renal function, and age at menarche).[15] This was in part based upon NHANES data that found a nearly 20% increase in asthma diagnoses among children with higher PFOA exposure.[44] In addition to asthma, other immune-mediated inflammatory conditions may also be notable; eczema risk was found to be 40% to 50% lower among children 12 to 24 months old who had low prenatal exposure.[45]

Cancer. As previously mentioned, an increase in cancer risk and/or mortality with PFC exposure has been documented, including breast, prostate, and bladder cancer.[17,18] Breast cancer risk appears to be modified by both the BRCA1 founder mutation and polymorphisms in estrogen detoxification pathways, including single nucleotide polymorphisms (SNPs) in CYP1A1 and CYP17.[46] Among individuals with high PFOA exposure (living near a chemical plant), an increase in the risk for kidney and testicular cancer has also been cited.[47]

Cardiovascular/Metabolic. A nested cohort study that enrolled more than 750 participants found statistically significant positive associations between PFOA and PFOS with total cholesterol.[48] Similarly, in a study with more than 800 women, both PFOS and PFOA were found to have a positive association with cholesterol levels, even after adjusting for dietary intake, at a similar magnitude to that found with saturated fat intake.[49] A significant positive association between low-density lipoprotein cholesterol and triglycerides among children has also been documented, particularly for PFOS and perfluorotetradecanoic acid (PFTA).[50]

A positive association between PFOA and PFOS concentrations and serum alanine transaminase (ALT) levels has also been found, indicating hepatocellular damage with exposure.[51] The accumulation of hepatic lipids may also play a role in hepatic insulin resistance. Indeed, in a study with more than 500 adult participants, the risk for impaired glucose homeostasis and diabetes was elevated in those with higher PFOS exposure (diabetes odds ratio [OR] = 3.37 [95% confidence interval (CI) 1.18–9.65]).[52]

Bone Health. Data from more than 2000 adults participating in 2005 to 2008 NHANES found lower lumbar spine bone mineral density (BMD) in nonmenopausal women with higher serum PFOS levels.[53] Though the effect was considered marginal/subclinical, it may be relevant when combined with other sources of bone loss. Analysis of 2009 to 2010 NHANES data had a more robust finding: Although both men and women had an inverse association with femoral neck BMD, in women, the prevalence of osteoporosis was significantly higher in the highest versus lowest quartiles of PFOA, PFHxS, and PFNA, with adjusted ORs of 2.59, 13.20, and 3.23, respectively.[54]

Endocrine Disruption. NHANES data between 1999 and 2006 found that women in the higher quartile of PFOA serum levels (≥ 5.7 ng/mL) had a 2.24 OR for thyroid disease compared with quartiles 1 and 2, yet men had a near significant trend (OR = 2.12). For PFOS exposure, men in the highest quartile (≥ 36.8 ng/mL) had an OR of 2.68 for treated thyroid disease, yet the association with PFOS among women was not significant.[55]

In Swedish seniors, urinary levels of PFNA showed a significant nonlinear relationship with diabetes presence (OR 1.96).[56] Levels of PFOA were also significantly related to the proinsulin/insulin ratio, which is a measure of insulin secretion.

In a cohort study of more than 2000 Canadian women, for each standard deviation increase in PFOA and PFHxS, the odds of infertility increased by 31% and 27%, respectively, with no significant association observed for PFOS.[57] A negative effect of PFCs on sperm parameters, including spermatozoa DNA fragmentation, was observed in men with exposure.[58] Analysis of the male offspring (age 19–21) of a pregnancy cohort also found that *in utero* exposure to PFOA was associated with lower adjusted sperm concentration and total sperm count, as well as higher luteinizing hormone (LH) and follicle-stimulating hormone (FSH) levels.[59] As previously mentioned, PFOS has been associated with reduced testosterone levels in men,[10] and PFCs have been positively associated with earlier age of menopause, as well as the rate of hysterectomy. Women in the third tertile for PFHxS had a nearly 70% higher likelihood of early menopause compared with those in the first tertile.[60]

INTERVENTION

Very little data has been published on interventions that limit PFC toxicity, emphasizing the importance of reducing exposure. Because PFCs/PFAs are secreted into bile, the use of bile acid sequestrants has been suggested to help reduce body burden. The use of cholestyramine in rats increased PFC excretion approximately 10-fold and reduced both serum and hepatic levels.[61] In an anecdotal report, cholestyramine appeared to be of benefit for a patient with elevated PFCs, particularly PFHxS, whereas sauna depuration, zeolites, and saponin compounds did not.[37] With the failure of sauna to enhance PFC excretion, phlebotomy was successfully used to reduce elevated PFC levels in six individuals.[62]

Other therapies of potential value include choline, vitamin C, and anthocyanin supplementation, as well as glutathione precursors. In mice, choline supplementation prevented both the oxidative damage and alterations in hepatic lipid metabolism observed with PFOS exposure.[63] In a double-blind controlled trial, vitamin C was shown to eliminate the effects on insulin resistance observed with PFC exposure.[64] Similarly, several mitochondrial deficits induced by PFOA toxicity were attenuated with anthocyanin usage, likely due to its antioxidant effects.[65] As previously mentioned, PFCs may have greater toxicity among those with impaired glutathione synthesis. Additionally, altered methylation of glutathione-S-transferase Pi (GSTP) gene promoter by PFOA may partly account for its mechanism of toxicity (i.e., by inhibiting glutathione production).[66] Supplementation with glutathione precursors such as N-acetylcysteine may help to counter this deficit in those with a genotype capable of producing sufficient glutathione.

REFERENCES

1. Corsini, E., Luebke, R. W., Germolec, D. R., et al. (2014). Perfluorinated compounds: emerging POPs with potential immunotoxicity. *Toxicology Letters*, 230(2), 263–270. PubMed PMID: 24503008.

2. National Toxicology Program. (2016). *Monograph on Immunotoxicity Associated with Exposure to Perfluorooctanoic Acid (PFOA) or Perfluorooctane Sulfate (PFOS)*. Research Triangle Park, NC; National Toxicology Program.

3. Brieger, A., Bienefeld, N., Hasan, R., et al. (2011). Impact of perfluorooctanesulfonate and perfluorooctanoic acid on human peripheral leukocytes. *Toxicology in Vitro*, 25(4), 960–968. PubMed PMID: 21397682.

4. Corsini, E., Avogadro, A., Galbiati, V., et al. (2011). In vitro evaluation of the immunotoxic potential of perfluorinated compounds (PFCs). *Toxicology and Applied Pharmacology*, 250(2), 108–116. PubMed PMID: 21075133.

5. Choi, E. M., Suh, K. S., Rhee, S. Y., et al. (2017). Perfluorooctanoic acid induces mitochondrial dysfunction in MC3T3-E1 osteoblast cells. *Journal of Environmental Science and Health. Part A, Toxic/Hazardous Substances & Environmental Engineering*, 52(3), 281–289. PubMed PMID: 27901621.

6. Mashayekhi, V., Tehrani, K. H., Hashemzaei, M., et al. (2015). Mechanistic approach for the toxic effects of perfluorooctanoic acid on isolated rat liver and brain mitochondria. *Human and Experimental Toxicology*, 34(10), 985–996. PubMed PMID: 25586001.

7. Shi, Z., Ding, L., Zhang, H., et al. (2009). Chronic exposure to perfluorododecanoic acid disrupts testicular steroidogenesis and the expression of related genes in male rats. *Toxicology Letters*, 188(3), 192–200. PubMed PMID: 19397962.

8. Bjerregaard-Olesen, C., Ghisari, M., et al. (2016). Activation of the estrogen receptor by human serum extracts containing mixtures of perfluorinated alkyl acids from pregnant women. *Environmental Research*, 151, 71–79. PubMed PMID: 27451001.

9. Sonthithai, P., Suriyo, T., Thiantanawat, A., et al. (2016). Perfluorinated chemicals, PFOS and PFOA, enhance the estrogenic effects of 17β-estradiol in T47D human breast cancer cells. *Journal of Applied Toxicology*, 36(6), 790–801. PubMed PMID: 26234195.

10. Joensen, U. N., Veyrand, B., Antignac, J. P., et al. (2013). PFOS (perfluorooctanesulfonate) in serum is negatively associated with testosterone levels, but not with semen quality, in healthy men. *Human Reproduction*, 28(3), 599–608. PubMed PMID: 23250927.

11. Shah-Kulkarni, S., Kim, B. M., Hong, Y. C., et al. (2016). Prenatal exposure to perfluorinated compounds affects thyroid hormone levels in newborn girls. *Environment International*, 94, 607–613. PubMed PMID: 27395336.

12. Wen, L. L., Lin, L. Y., Su, T. C., et al. (2013). Association between serum perfluorinated chemicals and thyroid function in U.S. adults: the National Health and Nutrition Examination Survey 2007-2010. *The Journal of Clinical Endocrinology and Metabolism*, 98(9), E1456–E1464. PubMed PMID: 23864701.

13. Das, K. P., Wood, C. R., Lin, M. T., et al. (2017). Perfluoroalkyl acids-induced liver steatosis: Effects on genes controlling lipid homeostasis. *Toxicology*, 378, 37–52. PubMed PMID: 28049043.

14. Qiu, T., Chen, M., Sun, X., et al. (2016). Perfluorooctane sulfonate-induced insulin resistance is mediated by protein kinase B pathway. *Biochemical and Biophysical Research Communications*, 477(4), 781–785. PubMed PMID: 27363333.

15. Rappazzo, K. M., Coffman, E., & Hines, E. P. (2017). Exposure to perfluorinated alkyl substances and health outcomes in children: a systematic review of the epidemiologic literature. *International Journal of Environmental Research and Public Health*, 14(7), pii: E691. PubMed PMID: 28654008.

16. Lv, Z., Li, G., Li, Y., Ying, C., et al. (2013). Glucose and lipid homeostasis in adult rat is impaired by early-life exposure to perfluorooctane sulfonate. *Environmental Toxicology*, 28(9), 532–542. PubMed PMID: 23983163.

17. Nakayama, S., Harada, K., Inoue, K., et al. (2005). Distributions of perfluorooctanoic acid (PFOA) and perfluorooctane sulfonate (PFOS) in Japan and their toxicities. *Environmental Sciences*, 12(6), 293–313. PubMed PMID: 16609670.

18. Wielsøe, M., Kern, P., & Bonefeld-Jørgensen, E. C. (2017). Serum levels of environmental pollutants is a risk factor for breast cancer in Inuit: a case control study. *Environmental Health: A Global Access Science Source*, 16(1), 56. PubMed PMID: 28610584.

19. Haug, L. S., Thomsen, C., Brantsaeter, A. L., et al. (2010). Diet and particularly seafood are major sources of perfluorinated compounds in humans. *Environment International*, 36(7), 772–778. PubMed PMID: 20579735.

20. Liu, Y., Su, J., van Dam, R. M., et al. (2017). Dietary predictors and plasma concentrations of perfluorinated alkyl acids in a Singapore population. *Chemosphere*, 171, 617–624. PubMed PMID: 28056448.

21. Schecter, A., Colacino, J., Haffner, D., et al. (2010). Perfluorinated compounds, polychlorinated biphenyls, and organochlorine pesticide contamination in composite food samples from Dallas, Texas, USA. *Environmental Health Perspectives*, 118(6), 796–802. PubMed PMID: 20146964.

22. Jain, R. B. (2014). Contribution of diet and other factors to the levels of selected polyfluorinated compounds: data from NHANES 2003-2008. *International Journal*

of Hygiene and Environmental Health, 217(1), 52–61. PubMed PMID: 23601780.

23. Shoeib, M., Harner, T., M Webster, G., & Lee, S. C. (2011). Indoor sources of poly- and perfluorinated compounds (PFCS) in Vancouver, Canada: implications for human exposure. *Environmental Science & Technology, 45*(19), 7999–8005. PubMed PMID: 21332198.

24. Fraser, A. J., Webster, T. F., Watkins, D. J., et al. (2013). Polyfluorinated compounds in dust from homes, offices, and vehicles as predictors of concentrations in office workers' serum. *Environment International, 60*, 128–136. PubMed PMID: 24041736.

25. Egeghy, P. P., & Lorber, M. (2011). An assessment of the exposure of Americans to perfluorooctane sulfonate: a comparison of estimated intake with values inferred from NHANES data. *Journal of Exposure Science and Environmental Epidemiology, 21*(2), 150–168. PubMed PMID: 20145679.

26. Beesoon, S., Genuis, S. J., Benskin, J. P., & Martin, J. W. (2012). Exceptionally high serum concentrations of perfluorohexanesulfonate in a Canadian family are linked to home carpet treatment applications. *Environmental Science & Technology, 46*(23), 12960–12967. PubMed PMID:23102093.

27. Hoffman, K., Webster, T. F., Bartell, S., et al. (2011). Private drinking water wells as a source of exposure to perfluorooctanoic acid (PFOA) in communities surrounding a fluoropolymer production facility. *Environmental Health Perspectives, 119*, 92–97. PubMed PMID: 20920951.

28. Hu, X. C., Andrews, D. Q., Lindstrom, A. B., et al. (2016). Detection of poly- and perfluoroalkyl substances (PFASs) in U.S. drinking water linked to industrial sites, military fire training areas, and wastewater treatment plants. *Environment Science & Technology Letters, 3*(10), 344–350. PubMed PMID: 27752509.

29. Dobraca, D., Israel, L., McNeel, S., et al. (2015). Biomonitoring in California firefighters: metals and perfluorinated chemicals. *Journal of Occupational and Environmental Medicine, 57*(1), 88–97. PubMed PMID: 25563545.

30. Mogensen, U. B., Grandjean, P., Nielsen, F., et al. (2015). Breastfeeding as an exposure pathway for perfluorinated alkylates. *Environmental Science & Technology, 49*(17), 10466–10473. PubMed PMID: 26291735.

31. Mamsen, L. S., Jönsson, B. A. G., et al. (2017). Concentration of perfluorinated compounds and cotinine in human foetal organs, placenta, and maternal plasma. *The Science of the Total Environment, 596-597*, 97–105. PubMed PMID: 28426990.

32. Gützkow, K. B., Haug, L. S., Thomsen, C., et al. (2012). Placental transfer of perfluorinated compounds is selective—a Norwegian mother and child sub-cohort study. *International Journal of Hygiene and Environmental Health, 215*(2), 216–219. PubMed PMID: 21937271.

33. Olsen, G. W., Burris, J. M., Ehresman, D. J., Froehlich, J. W., Seacat, A. M., Butenhoff, J. L., et al. (2007). Half-life of serum elimination of perfluorooctanesulfonate, perfluorohexanesulfonate, and perfluorooctanoate in retired fluorochemical production workers. *Environmental Health Perspectives, 115*, 1298–1305. PubMed PMID: 17805419.

34. Stockholm Convention. *The BRS blog. The new POPs under the Stockholm Convention*. Available at http://chm.pops.int/TheConvention/ThePOPs/TheNewPOPs/tabid/2511/Default.aspx. (Accessed September 1, 2017.)

35. Fromme, H., Mosch, C., Morovitz, M., et al. (2010). Pre- and postnatal exposure to perfluorinated compounds (PFCs). *Environmental Science & Technology, 44*(18), 7123–7129. PubMed PMID: 20722423.

36. Lau, C., Anitole, K., Hodes, C., Lai, D., et al. (2007). Perfluoroalkyl acids: a review of monitoring and toxicological findings. *Toxicological Sciences, 99*, 366–394. PubMed PMID: 17519394.

37. Genuis, S. J., Birkholz, D., Ralitsch, M., et al. (2010). Human detoxification of perfluorinated compounds. *Public Health, 124*(7), 367–375. PubMed PMID: 20621793.

38. Seacat, A. M., Thomford, P. J., et al. (2003). Sub-chronic dietary toxicity of potassium perfluorooctanesulfonate in rats. *Toxicology, 183*(1–3), 117–131. PubMed PMID: 12504346.

39. Kwon, E. J., Shin, J. S., Kim, B. M., et al. (2016). Prenatal exposure to perfluorinated compounds affects birth weight through GSTM1 polymorphism. *Journal of Occupational and Environmental Medicine, 58*(6), e198–e205. PubMed PMID: 27206125.

40. Khansari, M. R., Yousefsani, B. S., Kobarfard, F., et al. (2017). In vitro toxity of perfluorooctane sulfonate on rat liver hepatocytes: probability of destructive binding to CYP 2E1 and involvement of cellular proteolysis. *Environmental Science and Pollution Research International*, PubMed PMID: 28842823.

41. Grandjean, P., Andersen, E. W., Budtz-Jørgensen, E., et al. (2012). Serum vaccine antibody concentrations in children exposed to perfluorinated compounds. *The Journal of the American Medical Association, 307*(4), 391–397. PubMed PMID: 22274686.

42. Grandjean, P., Heilmann, C., Weihe, P., et al. (2017). Serum vaccine antibody concentrations in adolescents

exposed to perfluorinated compounds. *Environmental Health Perspectives*, *125*(7), 077018. PMID: 28749778.

43. Goudarzi, H., Miyashita, C., Okada, E., et al. (2017). Prenatal exposure to perfluoroalkyl acids and prevalence of infectious diseases up to 4 years of age. *Environment International*, *104*, 132–138. PubMed PMID: 28392064.

44. Humblet, O., Diaz-Ramirez, L. G., Balmes, J. R., et al. (2014). Perfluoroalkyl chemicals and asthma among children 12-19 years of age: NHANES (1999-2008). *Environmental Health Perspectives*, *122*(10), 1129–1133. PubMed PMID: 24905661.

45. Okada, E., Sasaki, S., Kashino, I., et al. (2014). Prenatal exposure to perfluoroalkyl acids and allergic diseases in early childhood. *Environment International*, *65*, 127–134. PubMed PMID: 24486970.

46. Ghisari, M., Eiberg, H., Long, M., et al. (2014). Polymorphisms in phase I and phase II genes and breast cancer risk and relations to persistent organic pollutant exposure: a case-control study in Inuit women. *Environmental Health: A Global Access Science Source*, *13*(1), 19. PubMed PMID: 24629213.

47. Barry, V., Winquist, A., & Steenland, K. (2013). Perfluorooctanoic acid (PFOA) exposures and incident cancers among adults living near a chemical plant. *Environmental Health Perspectives*, *121*(11–12), 1313–1318. PubMed PMID: 24007715.

48. Eriksen, K. T., Raaschou-Nielsen, O., McLaughlin, J. K., et al. (2013). Association between plasma PFOA and PFOS levels and total cholesterol in a middle-aged Danish population. *PLoS ONE*, *8*(2), e56969. PubMed PMID: 23441227.

49. Skuladottir, M., Ramel, A., Rytter, D., et al. (2015). Examining confounding by diet in the association between perfluoroalkyl acids and serum cholesterol in pregnancy. *Environmental Research*, *143*(Pt A), 33–38. PubMed PMID: 26432473.

50. Zeng, X. W., Qian, Z., Emo, B., et al. (2015). Association of polyfluoroalkyl chemical exposure with serum lipids in children. *The Science of the Total Environment*, *512-513*, 364–370. PubMed PMID: 25638651.

51. Gallo, V., Leonardi, G., Genser, B., et al. (2012). Serum perfluorooctanoate (PFOA) and perfluorooctane sulfonate (PFOS) concentrations and liver function biomarkers in a population with elevated PFOA exposure. *Environmental Health Perspectives*, *120*(5), 655–660. PubMed PMID: 22289616.

52. Su, T. C., Kuo, C. C., Hwang, J. J., et al. (2016). Serum perfluorinated chemicals, glucose homeostasis and the risk of diabetes in working-aged Taiwanese adults. *Environment International*, *88*, 15–22. PubMed PMID: 26700417.

53. Lin, L. Y., Wen, L. L., Su, T. C., et al. (2014). Negative association between serum perfluorooctane sulfate concentration and bone mineral density in US premenopausal women: NHANES, 2005-2008. *The Journal of Clinical Endocrinology and Metabolism*, *99*(6), 2173–2180. PubMed PMID: 24606077.

54. Khalil, N., Chen, A., Lee, M., et al. (2016). Association of perfluoroalkyl substances, bone mineral density, and osteoporosis in the U.S. population in NHANES 2009-2010. *Environmental Health Perspectives*, *124*(1), 81–87. PubMed PMID: 26058082.

55. Melzer, D., Rice, N., Depledge, M. H., et al. (2010). Association between serum perfluorooctanoic acid (PFOA) and thyroid disease in the U.S. National Health and Nutrition Examination Survey. *Environmental Health Perspectives*, *118*(5), 686–692. PubMed PMID: 20089479.

56. Lind, L., Zethelius, B., Salihovic, S., et al. (2014). Circulating levels of perfluoroalkyl substances and prevalent diabetes in the elderly. *Diabetologia*, *57*(3), 473–479. PubMed PMID: 24337155.

57. Vélez, M. P., Arbuckle, T. E., & Fraser, W. D. (2015). Maternal exposure to perfluorinated chemicals and reduced fecundity: the MIREC study. *Human Reproduction*, *30*(3), 701–709. PubMed PMID: 25567616.

58. Governini, L., Guerranti, C., De Leo, V., et al. (2015). Chromosomal aneuploidies and DNA fragmentation of human spermatozoa from patients exposed to perfluorinated compounds. *Andrologia*, *47*(9), 1012–1019. PubMed PMID: 25382683.

59. Vested, A., Ramlau-Hansen, C. H., et al. (2013). Associations of in utero exposure to perfluorinated alkyl acids with human semen quality and reproductive hormones in adult men. *Environmental Health Perspectives*, *121*(4), 453–458. PubMed PMID: 23360585.

60. Taylor, K. W., Hoffman, K., Thayer, K. A., et al. (2014). Polyfluoroalkyl chemicals and menopause among women 20-65 years of age (NHANES). *Environmental Health Perspectives*, *122*(2), 145–150. PubMed PMID: 24280566.

61. Johnson, J. D., Gibson, A. J., & Ober, R. E. (1984). Cholestyramine-enhanced fecal elimination of carbon-14 in rats after administration of ammonium perfluorooctanoate or potassium perfluorooctanesulfonate. *Fundamental and Applied Toxicology*, *4*, 972–976. PubMed PMID: 6519377.

62. Genuis, S. J., Liu, Y., Genuis, Q. I., & Martin, J. W. (2014). Phlebotomy treatment for elimination of perfluoroalkyl acids in a highly exposed family: a retrospective case-series. *PLoS ONE*, *9*(12), e114295. PubMed PMID: 25504057.

63. Zhang, L., Krishnan, P., Ehresman, D. J., et al. (2016). Editor's Highlight: Perfluorooctane sulfonate-choline ion pair formation: a potential mechanism modulating hepatic steatosis and oxidative stress in mice. *Toxicological Sciences, 153*(1), 186–197. PubMed PMID: 27413108.

64. Kim, J. H., Park, H. Y., Jeon, J. D., et al. (2016). The modifying effect of vitamin C on the association between perfluorinated compounds and insulin resistance in the Korean elderly: a double-blind, randomized, placebo-controlled crossover trial. *European Journal of Nutrition, 55*(3), 1011–1020. PubMed PMID: 25939797.

65. Yuan, Z., Zhang, J., Tu, C., et al. (2016). The protective effect of blueberry anthocyanins against perfluorooctanoic acid-induced disturbance in planarian (Dugesia japonica). *Ecotoxicology and Environmental Safety, 127*, 170–174. PubMed PMID: 26836138.

66. Tian, M., Peng, S., Martin, F. L., et al. (2012). Perfluorooctanoic acid induces gene promoter hypermethylation of glutathione-S-transferase Pi in human liver L02 cells. *Toxicology, 296*(1–3), 48–55. PubMed PMID: 22425687.

30

Parabens

SUMMARY

- Presence in population: Exposure is ubiquitous
- Major diseases: Endocrine and reproductive disruption
- Best measure: Urinary metabolites
- Best intervention: Avoidance

DESCRIPTION

Methyl-, ethyl-, propyl-, butyl-, and benzylparabens, all esters of p-hydroxybenzoic acid (Fig. 30.1), are widely used in cosmetics, pharmaceuticals, foods, and beverages as antimicrobial agents and preservatives. Because of their low cost, inertness, broad spectrum of activity, and low toxicity, parabens are commonly used throughout the world. Paraben exposure comes mainly from the use of personal care products containing propylparaben and/or methylparaben.[1] After water, parabens are the second most common ingredient in cosmetics and are present in approximately 80% of personal care products (PCPs; also known as *health and beauty aids [HABAs]*). Products that often contain parabens include hand soap, body lotion, shampoo, conditioner, face lotion, facial cleanser, foundation, lipstick, mascara, hair spray, mousse, hair gel, toothpaste, and sunscreen.[2] Therefore, when consumers use these products, parabens can come into contact with the skin, hair, scalp, lips, mucosae (oral, ocular, and vaginal), axillae, and nails. PCPs may be used occasionally or on a daily basis, and their use may extend over a period of years, leading to nearly continuous exposure. A 1995 study showed that nearly all (99%) leave-on cosmetics and more than 75% of rinse-off cosmetics contained parabens.[3]

TOXICITY

Because of their potential estrogenicity, the presence of parabens in tissue is a concern regarding breast cancer.

Although the exact health effects of parabens are currently unknown, they do possess some estrogenic activity, can adversely affect the breakdown of endogenous estrogens, and cause mitochondrial dysfunction. An *in vitro* yeast-based estrogen assay found that the four most widely used parabens (methyl-, ethyl-, propyl-, and butylparabens) were all weakly estrogenic, and the magnitude of the body's estrogenic response increased relative to alkyl group size.[4] Specifically, methylparaben produced the weakest response (2,500,000-time less potent than 17β-estradiol), followed by ethylparaben (150,000-times less potent), propylparaben (30,000-times less potent), and butylparaben (10,000-times less potent).

In addition, parabens and their common metabolite, p-hydroxybenzoic acid, have been shown to possess androgen antagonist activity, to act as inhibitors of sulfotransferase enzymes, and to possess genotoxic activity.[5] Parabens can indirectly affect estrogen levels via inhibition of sulfotransferase activity inside the cytosol of human skin cells, causing estrogen levels to remain higher than normal.[6] Methyl- and propylparabens are also potent inhibitors of mitochondrial function.[7,8] This effect on mitochondrial function has been proposed as a mechanism for parabens possible role in male infertility.[9]

BODY BURDEN

The Centers for Disease Control and Prevention (CDC) has been monitoring the level of butyl-, ethyl-, methyl-, and propylparabens since 2005. Butyl- and ethylparabens

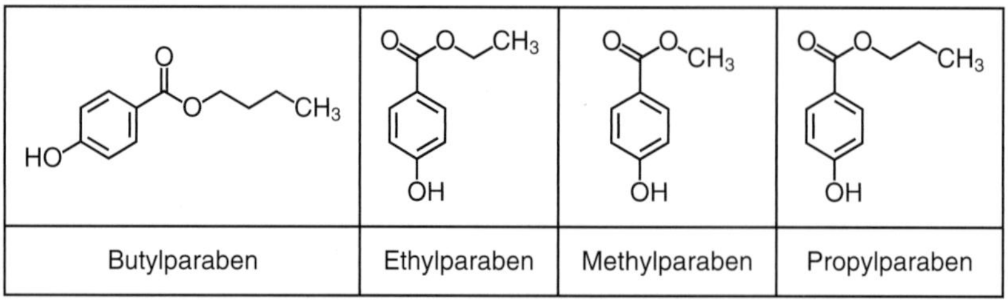

FIG. 30.1 Paraben structure.

TABLE 30.1   **Urinary Parabens—CDC Fourth Report from National Health and Nutritional Examination Survey 2011 to 2014**

Compound	Mean (ug/g creatinine)	50th %	75th %	90th %	95th %
Butylparaben	*	<LOD	0.250	3.50	10.0
Ethylparaben	*	<LOD	5.41	36.6	99.3
Methylparaben	48.2	41.8	180.0	410.0	653.0
Propylparaben	5.74	4.75	36.7	124.0	222.0

Data from Centers for Disease Control and Prevention. (2017). National Report on Human Exposure to Environmental Chemicals: Updated tables. (www.cdc.gov/exposurereport)
*No mean calculated LOD—Level of detection.

have only been found in about 25% of the population, and methyl- and propylparabens are found ubiquitously throughout North America (Table 30.1).

DETOXIFICATION/EXCRETION PROCESSES

Animal studies have shown that parabens are quickly absorbed from the gastrointestinal tract and metabolized. Parabens are lipophilic, can be absorbed through the skin, and are found intact in tissue. In fact, these compounds have been found in breast cancer tissue at levels ranging from 20 to 100 ng/g tissue.[10] Once in the bloodstream, parabens are conjugated in the liver with glycine, sulfate, or glucuronate for excretion in the urine. About 80% to 85% of parabens are excreted in urine, predominantly in their conjugated forms, within the first 24 hours of administration,[11] and p-hydroxyhippuric acid has been identified as the major but nonspecific metabolite.[12]

Clinical Significance

Endocrine. Parabens have weak estrogenic activity and have been shown to induce the growth of MCF-7 human breast cancer cells *in vitro,*[13] leading some researchers to suggest their potential as initiators or promoters of breast cancer. Part of the concern arises from an increasing number of breast cancers that occur in the upper outer quadrant, where paraben-containing antiperspirant is applied.[14] Parabens demonstrate multiple cancer hallmarks and characteristics, including the following: 1) they have been measured as present in 99% of human breast tissue samples; 2) they possess estrogenic activity and can stimulate sustained proliferation of human breast cancer cells at concentrations measurable in the breast; 3) they can inhibit the suppression of breast cancer cell growth by hydroxytamoxifen; 4) long-term exposure (> 20 weeks) to parabens leads to increased migratory and invasive activity in human breast cancer cells; 5) methylparaben increases the mechanistic target of rapamycin (mTOR), a key regulator of energy metabolism; and 6) parabens can cause DNA damage at high concentrations in a short term.[15]

Butylparaben has been reported to affect reproductive tract development in rats, causing significant decreases in sperm count and sperm motility in the epididymis.[16] The addition of parabens to the diet of postweaning male rats resulted in decreased daily sperm production and sperm efficiency in the testis, and the exposure level at which this disruption was observed was the same as the upper-limit acceptable daily intake of parabens (10 mg/kg body weight/day).[17] Male partners in infertile couples with above average levels of methylparaben were 81% more likely to experience failure of *in vitro* fertilization (IVF) with their partners.[18]

INTERVENTION

Choosing PCPs that are labeled as free of parabens and other unwanted endocrine disruptors can significantly reduce personal exposure to these harmful toxicants. A study of female Latina teens showed that after only 3 days of avoidance, urinary concentrations of methyl- and propylparaben decreased by 43.9% and 45.4%, respectively.[19] Use reduction targeted at endocrine disrupting chemicals (EDCs) in consumer products has the potential to significantly decrease occupational and residential exposures. However, the lack of transparency regarding ingredients, along with the multitude of chemicals included in PCPs, not only makes it difficult for consumers to make educated choices, but also hinders research on the true toxic effects of PCPs. Apps like ThinkDirty are now available to quickly assess the level of toxic constituents in PCPs. A number of websites are good resources to help navigate product labels and reduce exposure to toxicants contained in PCPs:

- Good Guide™—http://www.goodguide.com
- Green Seal™—http://www.greenseal.org/
- Environmental Protection Agencys Design for the Environment program—https://www.epa.gov/safer choice/design-environment-programs-initiatives-and-projects
- Environmental Working Group—http://www.ewg.org/skindeep

REFERENCES

1. Msagati, T. A., Barri, T., et al. (2008). Analysis and quantification of parabens in cosmetic products by utilizing hollow fibre-supported liquid membrane and high performance liquid chromatography with ultraviolet detection. *International Journal of Cosmetic Science*, 30(4), 297–307. PubMed PMID: 18713076.
2. Kirchhof, M. G., & de Gannes, G. C. (2013). The health controversies of parabens. *Skin Therapy Letter*, 18(2), 5–7. PubMed PMID: 23508773.
3. Rastogi, S. C., Schouten, A., et al. (1995). Contents of methyl-, ethyl-, propyl-, butyl-, and benzylparaben in cosmetic products. *Contact Dermatitis*, 32(1), 28–30. PubMed PMID: 7720367.
4. Routledge, E. J., Parker, J., et al. (1998). Some alkyl hydroxyl benzoate preservatives (parabens) are estrogenic. *Toxicology and Applied Pharmacology*, 153(1), 12–19. PubMed PMID: 9875295.
5. Darbre, P. D., & Harvey, P. W. (2008). Paraben esters: Review of recent studies of endocrine toxicity, absorption, esterase and human exposure, and discussion of potential human health risks. *Journal of Applied Toxicology*, 28(5), 561–578. PubMed PMID: 18484575.
6. Prusakiewicz, J. J., Harville, H. M., Zhang, Y., et al. (2007). Parabens inhibit human skin estrogen sulfotransferase activity: Possible link to paraben estrogenic effects. *Toxicology*, 232, 248–256.
7. Soni, M. G., Taylor, S. L., Greenberg, N. A., & Burdock, G. A. (2002). Evaluation of the health aspects of methyl paraben: A review of the published literature. *Food and Chemical Toxicology*, 40, 1335–1373.
8. Soni, M. G., Burdock, G. A., Taylor, S. L., & Greenberg, N. A. (2001). Safety assessment of propyl paraben: A review of the published literature. *Food and Chemical Toxicology*, 39, 513–532.
9. Tavares, R. S., Martins, F. C., Oliveira, P. J., et al. (2009). Parabens in male infertility – is there a mitochondrial connection? *Reproductive Toxicology*, 27, 1–7.
10. Darbre, P. D., Aljarrah, A., Miller, W. R., et al. (2004). Concentrations of parabens in human breast tumours. *Journal of Applied Toxicology*, 24, 5–13.
11. Ye, X., Bishop, A. M., et al. (2006). Parabens as urinary biomarkers of exposure in humans. *Environmental Health Perspectives*, 114(12), 1843–1846. PubMed PMID: 17185273.
12. Moos, R. K., Angerer, J., et al. (2016). Metabolism and elimination of methyl-, iso-, and n-butyl paraben in human urine after single oral dosage. *Archives of Toxicology*, 90(11), 2699–2709. PubMed PMID: 26608183.
13. Byford, J. R., Shaw, L. E., Drew, M. G., et al. (2002). Oestrogenic activity of parabens in MCF7 human breast cancer cells. *The Journal of Steroid Biochemistry and Molecular Biology*, 80, 49–60.
14. Darbre, P. D., & Harvey, P. W. (2008). Paraben esters: Review of recent studies on endocrine toxicity, absorption, esterase and human exposure, and discussion of potential human health risks. *Journal of Applied Toxicology : JAT*, 28, 561–578.
15. Darbre, P. D., & Harvey, P. W. (2014). Parabens can enable hallmarks and characteristics of cancer in human breast epithelial cells: A review of the literature with reference to new exposure data and regulatory status. *Journal of Applied Toxicology*, 34(9), 925–938. PubMed PMID: 25047802.

16. Kang, K. S., Che, J. H., Ryu, D. Y., et al. (2002). Decreased sperm number and motile activity on the F1 offspring maternally exposed to butyl p-hydroxybenzoic acid (butyl paraben). *The Journal of Veterinary Medical Science / The Japanese Society of Veterinary Science, 64*(3), 227–235. PubMed PMID: 11999442.

17. Oishi, S. (2002). Effects of propyl paraben on the male reproductive system. *Food and Chemical Toxicology, 40*(12), 1807–1813. PubMed PMID: 12419695.

18. Dodge, L. E., Williams, P. L., Williams, M. A., Missmer, S. A., Toth, T. L., Calafat, A. M., et al. (2015). Paternal urinary concentrations of parabens and other phenols in relation to reproductive outcomes among couples from a fertility clinic. *Environmental Health Perspectives, 123*(7), 665–671. PubMed PMID: 25767892.

19. Harley, K. G., Kogut, K., et al. (2016). Reducing phthalate, paraben, and phenol exposure from personal care products in adolescent girls: Findings from the HERMOSA intervention study. *Environmental Health Perspectives, 124*(10), 1600–1607. PubMed PMID: 26947464.

31

Mold and Water-Damaged Building Toxicity

SUMMARY

- Presence in population: Ubiquitous
- Major diseases: Respiratory, neurological (cognition, executive function, and vision), reduced immune function, fatigue
- Primary sources: Water-damaged buildings

- Best measure: Mold spore count, Environmental Relative Moldiness Index (ERMI), urinary mycotoxins
- Best intervention: Avoidance, complete remediation of damaged area, antioxidant support

INTRODUCTION

Molds are fungi that grow best in warm, damp, and humid conditions. In general, any area with a relative humidity greater than 80% in the presence of organic materials supports mold growth. A relative humidity over 90% is ideal for proliferation. There are tens of thousands of species that spread and reproduce by making spores, which can survive harsh environmental conditions. According to the Centers for Disease Control and Prevention (CDC), the most common indoor molds are of the *Cladosporium, Penicillium, Alternaria,* and *Aspergillus* families.[1] *Stachybotrys chartarum,* also known as "black mold," is also found indoors where there is a constant moisture source.

The concept of mold toxicity as an unrecognized cause of chronic disease has been around the integrative medicine community for quite some time. This is especially true for cases of adult-onset asthma, two-thirds of which appear to be caused by toxins released from water-damaged buildings. Research shows that as many as 50% of residential and work environments have water damage, and 10% to 50% of indoor environments in Europe, North America, Australia, India, and Japan have clinically significant mold problems.[2] The percentages are higher in river valleys and coastal areas.

Mold toxicity should be considered in all patients with any chronic respiratory condition and whose illness history is clearly linked to their residence. This chapter addresses the research evaluating this concept for respiratory conditions, the incidence in the population, diagnosis, intervention, and the far more complicated and controversial nonrespiratory mold-related conditions.

TOXINS PRODUCED IN WATER-DAMAGED BUILDINGS

The research is unequivocal that water-damaged buildings expose their occupants to a diverse range of toxins, with many physiologically damaging effects. They are produced by chemical, microbial, and physical processes that break down building materials. Box 31.1 lists the World Health Organization's (WHO's) primary indicators of dampness and microbial growth.

Indoor environments contain a complex mixture of live and dead microorganisms, fragments of dead organisms, toxins, allergens, volatile microbial organic compounds, and other chemicals. Damp building materials contribute to the production of undesirable organisms and toxins, including 1) molds, which release biological agents, toxic chemicals, and spores; 2) bacteria, which release biological agents, toxic chemicals, and spores; 3) protozoa; 4) viruses; 5) dust mites (i.e., arachnids of many different species); 6) rodents and cockroaches, which can carry infectious agents;

and 7) the release of chemicals and particles from building materials.

Box 31.2 lists some of the biological and chemical toxins that have been found. These data are by no means complete; rather, this is a list of toxic agents that are most harmful and/or most prevalent.

HEALTH EFFECTS

Since about 2005, a broad international consensus has been reached that mold and dampness in buildings significantly increases disease risk and is a public health hazard. The primary manifestations of damp building toxicity are immunological (e.g., stimulation, suppression, autoimmunity), toxic (e.g., neurotoxicity, genotoxicity, reproductive damage), and inflammatory. A clear majority of the peer-reviewed published research on damp building toxicity focuses on respiratory conditions, and various government reports, such as one that was commissioned by the CDC and released by the Institute of Medicine in 2004, concluded that only for respiratory conditions is there sufficient evidence of causation by mold or damp buildings.[3] The primary clinical indications in the WHO and CDC reports, listed in Box 31.3, have been shown

---

BOX 31.1 Primary Indicators of Dampness and Microbial Growth

- Condensation on surfaces or in structures such as windows
- Visible mold, especially black mold
- Perceived moldy odor
- Poorly maintained air conditioning systems
- A history of water damage (exterior leaks, wet basement, leaking plumbing)

From Pizzorno J. Is Mold Toxicity Really a Problem for Our Patients? Part I—Respiratory Conditions. Integrative Medicine: A Clinician's Journal. 2016;15(2):6-10.

BOX 31.3 Clinical Conditions Indicative of Dampness and Mold

Common Conditions	Common Symptoms	Rare Conditions
• Allergic rhinitis • Exacerbation of asthma • Respiratory infections	• Cough • Upper respiratory tract (nose and throat) symptoms • Wheeze	• Allergic alveolitis • Allergic fungal sinusitis • Chronic rhinosinusitis • Hypersensitivity pneumonitis

From Pizzorno J. Is Mold Toxicity Really a Problem for Our Patients? Part I—Respiratory Conditions. Integrative Medicine: A Clinician's Journal. 2016;15(2):6-10.

BOX 31.2 Partial List of Toxic Agents Found in Dust and Air of Damp Buildings

Allergens

- Dust mite allergens—Dust mites produce the predominant inhalation allergens in most of the world. Most common are proteases from *Dermatophagoides pteronyssinus* and *Dermatophagoides farinae.*
- Fungal allergens—These allergens have the strongest correlations with asthma. They are typically glycopeptides with enzymatic properties and are usually found in spores, hyphae, and fungal fragments.

Biologicals

- Beta-glucans—These are proinflammatory, nonallergenic, water-insoluble, structural cell wall components found in most fungi, some bacteria, most higher plants, and many lower plants.
- Multiple organic molecules—These include endotoxins, ergosterol (vitamin D_2), and penicillin G (which may

further aggravate symptoms in patients allergic to this class of antibiotics).
- Mycotoxins—These are metabolites produced by fungi, which can cause a toxic response in animals and humans, often at very low concentrations.
- Methane VOC (MVOC)—Several fungi produce volatile metabolites depending on species and substrate.

Toxic Chemicals

- Phthalates
- Formaldehyde
- Volatile organic compounds (VOCs)—Examples include alcohols, aldehydes, ketones, terpenes, esters, aromatic compounds, amines, and sulfur-containing compounds.

From Pizzorno J. Is Mold Toxicity Really a Problem for Our Patients? Part I—Respiratory Conditions. Integrative Medicine: A Clinician's Journal. 2016;15(2):6-10.

to improve with remediation of dampness and eradication of microbial overgrowth in buildings. The increased risk has been found throughout the population and is not limited to those with atopy as was originally alleged. Research supports that exposure to mold and dampness increases the risk of allergy to other allergens such as house dust mites and pollen, not just fungi, and causes epigenetic modulation that upregulates many inflammatory genes.[4] This may help explain the nonrespiratory conditions considered mold-related by the integrative medicine (IM) community.

A diverse range of physiological dysfunctions can be caused by toxins released in water-damaged buildings, and many have associated diseases. The term *sick building syndrome (SBS)* is often used to describe this phenomenon. Tables 31.1 and 31.2 list toxins, organisms, physiological dysfunctions, and diseases associated with water-damaged buildings. As can be seen in these tables, toxic metabolites have very diverse physiological effects, including disrupting mitochondrial function, misbalancing nitric oxide synthesis, and increasing inflammatory mediators, neurotoxicity, cytotoxicity, immune suppression, carcinogenesis, and mutagenesis. When adding in biochemical individuality, almost any chronic clinical condition could be caused or aggravated by these toxins. A significant challenge is that statistical and generic research make documenting such effects in specific patients difficult to prove. In addition, the differences between human and animal physiology, dramatically varying dosages, sensitization, and genetic polymorphisms further complicate the clinical situation.

Note that the "Disease" columns in Tables 31.1 and 31.2 are full of unknowns, as the research simply has not been done or is inconclusive when considering population groups.

Mold: Asthma, Asthma-Related, and Respiratory Conditions

The research is clear that mold and damp building exposure is a major factor in the asthma epidemic. Studies have shown that dampness or mold in houses causes 21% of asthma in the U.S. and a 30% to 50% increase in asthma and asthma-related health problems.[5,6] The incidence may be much higher, as one study found that 67% of adult-onset asthma started after working in a water-damaged office building.[7] The rare condition allergic alveolitis (also known as *extrinsic allergic alveolitis* or *hypersensitivity pneumonitis*) is likely primarily due to mold reactivity and has a strong correlation with the use of contaminated air humidifiers. Inhalation fever (also known as *toxic pneumonitis, humidifier fever,* or *organic dust toxic syndrome*) also results from contaminated humidifiers.

The research is clear: every patient suffering any kind of chronic respiratory condition—especially those of adult onset—must be fully evaluated for mold/damp building exposure. Symptoms such as dyspnea, wheeze, cough, respiratory infections, bronchitis, allergic rhinitis, eczema, vocal cord dysfunction, and upper respiratory tract difficulties should also be included. Once an individual has become sensitized, he or she becomes much more reactive to even low to modest mold exposure as

TABLE 31.1 Toxic Metabolites Produced by Bacteria Isolated from Water-Damaged Materials and Indoor Air

Metabolites	Organisms	Physiological Effects	Diseases
Valinomycin	*Streptomyces griseus*	Mitochondrial poison	Unknown
Leptomycin B	*Streptomyces* species	Inhibition of inducible nitric oxide synthetase	Unknown
Toxic peptide	*Bacillus amyloliquefaciens*	Depolarized transmembrane, decreased adenosine triphosphate (ATP), and nicotinamide adenine dinucleotide (NADH) cell death	Unknown
Mitochondrial toxin	*Bacillus pumilus*	Disruption of mitochondrial membrane	Unknown
Mitochondrial toxin	*Nocardiopsis* species	Disruption of mitochondrial membrane	Unknown
Cytostatic compounds	Coculture of *S. chartarum* and *S. californicus*	Cytotoxic compounds that are just as toxic as doxorubicin and actinomycin D	Unknown

Modified from Pizzorno J. Is Mold Toxicity Really a Problem for Our Patients? Part I—Respiratory Conditions. Integrative Medicine: A Clinician's Journal. 2016;15(2):6-10.

TABLE 31.2   Mycotoxins Produced by Toxic Molds

Metabolites	Organisms	Physiological Effects	Diseases
Gliotoxin	Aspergillus fumigatus, A. terreus, A. flavus, A. niger, Trichoderma virens, Penicillium species Candida albicans	Immune toxicity, immunosuppression, neurotoxicity	Invasive aspergillosis
Aflatoxin B1, kojic acid, aspergillic acid, nitropropionic acid	Aspergillus flavus	Liver pathology and cancer, immune toxicity, neurotoxicity	Carcinogenesis
Fumigaclavines, fumitoxins, fumitremorgins, verruculogen, gliotoxin	Aspergillus fumigatus	Lung disease, neurotoxicity, tremors, immune toxicity	Aspergillosis
Ochratoxin A		Immunosuppression	Balkan endemic nephropathy (BEN)
Urinary tract tumors	Aspergillus niger		BEN
Aspergillosis	Penicillium verrucosom	Lung disease	
Ochratoxin A	Aspergillus ochraceus	Nephropathology	Urinary tract damage
Xanthomegnin, Viomellein, Violaxanthin			Tumors
Penicillic acid	Aspergillus westerdijkiae, A. steynii, Penicillium aurantiogriseum	Nephropathy, carcinogenesis	
Sterigmatocystin, 5-methoxysterigmato cystin	Aspergillus versicolor	Liver pathology and cancer	Carcinogenesis
Chaetomiums	Chaetomium globosum	Cytotoxicity	Unknown
Chaetoglobosin A and C		Cell division	Unknown
Griseofulvin	Memnoniella echinata	Carcinogenesis	Unknown
Dechlorogriseofulvins			Reproductive toxin
Trichodermin			Hypersensitivity
Trichoderma		Protein synthesis inhibition	
Mycophenolic acid	Penicillium brevicompactum	Cytotoxic, mutagenic	Unknown
Botryodiplodin	Penicillium expansum	Immune toxicity, cytotoxic	Unknown
Patulin, Chaetoglobosin, Roquefortine C			Tremors
Citrinin	Penicillium citrinum	Nephrotoxicity, potentially genotoxic	
Verrucosidins	Penicillium plonicium	Cytotoxicity	Tremors
Nephrotoxic glyco-peptides			Nephropathology
Trichothecenes	Trichoderma species	Trichothecene toxicity	Unknown
Trichodermol, Trichodermin, Gliotoxin, Viridin		Immunotoxicity	Immune impairment
Fumonisins	Fusarium verticillioides (also known as F. moniliforme)	Neural tube defects in animals and humans	Central nervous system birth defects
Spirocyclic	Stachybotrys chartarum	Respiratory bleeding	Pulmonary bleeding
Drimanes, roridin		Protein synthesis inhibition	
Satratoxins (F, G, H)		Neurotoxicity	
Hydroxyroridin E		Cytotoxicity	
Verrucarin J, Trichodermin, Dolabellanes, Altrones B, C; Stachybotryslactams		Immune toxicity	

From Pizzorno J. Is Mold Toxicity Really a Problem for Our Patients? Part I—Respiratory Conditions. Integrative Medicine: A Clinician's Journal. 2016;15(2):6-10.

well as to other allergens. The symptom and disease associations are far stronger when dust levels rather than air levels of mold products are measured. This seems logical, as air levels are much more likely to vary dramatically, whereas dust levels show average exposure over time.

Mold: Nonrespiratory Conditions

The role of indoor mold exposure in water-damaged buildings and its relationship to nonrespiratory conditions are not as clear. The WHO does not provide any support for the nonrespiratory conditions considered important indicators of mold problems, but reports, "Microbial growth may result in greater numbers of spores, cell fragments, allergens, mycotoxins, endotoxins, β-glucans, and volatile organic compounds in indoor air. *The causative agents of adverse health effects have not been identified conclusively* [emphasis added], but an excess level of any of these agents in the indoor environment is a potential health hazard." The italicized phrase highlights why this has been such a challenging issue to address quantitatively, as the causative agents can be so diverse, and clinical effects appear to be highly dependent on individual susceptibility and sensitivity.

Although damage from mold/damp buildings can affect all systems of the body, the two nonrespiratory systems primarily affected are the neurological and immunological systems. According to the WHO, "Although mycotoxins can induce a wide range of adverse health effects in both animals and human beings, the evidence that they play a role in health problems related to indoor air is extremely weak."[2] The CDC issued a report in 2004 that asserts there is no conclusive evidence of nonrespiratory conditions being caused by mold or damp buildings. Review of the current recommendations shows no apparent change in the CDC's position.[8] Although these statements appear highly conclusive, they are based on a limited body of published research and are likely outdated, and we respectfully disagree.

Research in this area has been limited, as it has been very difficult to build cohorts of individuals exposed to mycotoxins and unexposed controls and then create a study to evaluate them. This is primarily due to the significant limitations of the testing technology used to determine the presence of hidden indoor mold. There are various testing approaches, and each one has unique limitations and many false negatives. Additionally, human testing for toxin load of mold via sampling tissue and body fluids is significantly limited. At the time of this publication, only 4 mycotoxin groups with 15 individual toxins could be tested. There are probably hundreds of mycotoxins, possibly even an order of magnitude more. Another challenge with standard research is that statistical results in population groups inherently obfuscate individual susceptibility. This, of course, is important for suffering patients who are outside the statistical norms. Clearly, toxins affect individuals in different ways depending on their genetics, synergistic toxins present, and nutritional status. Studies that evaluate the most important variables of genetics, toxin exposure, and nutritional status and their complex effects on health need to be conducted.

Mycotoxins

A tremendous amount of research has been published on the clinical effects of mycotoxins. Although this is the area of most interest in the IM community, aside from the respiratory effects of mycotoxins, the research is disappointingly limited.

A comprehensive review published in 2004 evaluated the research on the physiological effects of mold toxins.[9] The research included the symptoms of people living or working in water-damaged buildings. Particularly important is that the researchers compared the symptoms of those people with an "unexposed" control population. This is critical, as too often ignoring false positives overstates the significance of symptoms. This is a conservative view, as the "controls" may have included individuals being exposed to hidden active mold, which is estimated to be as high as 50%. Table 31.3 shows which symptoms have the best predictive value for suspicion of mold exposure. As can be seen, neurological symptoms are predominant.

Studies comparing mycotoxins with pesticides have concluded that mycotoxins are more toxic to humans than are pesticides.[10] In addition, fungal metabolites have synergistic genotoxic and other harmful effects.[11]

Microbial Volatile Organic Compounds

In addition to mycotoxins, active molds produce microbial volatile organic compounds (mVOCs). mVOCs are low molecular weight compounds that include numerous alcohols, esters, ethers, ketones, aldehydes, terpenoids, thiols, and derivatives of these compounds. Because these compounds are small and volatile, they can diffuse into the air and enter the body through the lungs and skin.

TABLE 31.3   Symptoms Caused by Mold Toxicity/Water-Damaged Buildings

Symptom	% In Exposed Population	% In Controls	P Value
Memory problems	5.1	3.3	0.0002
Spaciness	4.8	3.2	0.0007
Excessive fatigue	5.8	4.3	0.0001
Coughing	4.6	3.2	0.001
Slurred speech	4.5	3.1	0.002
Weak voice	4.1	2.8	0.003
Watery eyes	4.6	3.4	0.004
Lightheadedness	4.4	3.2	0.006
Dizziness	4.3	3.1	0.005
Weakness	4.2	3.0	0.008
Headache	5.2	4.1	0.005
Throat discomfort	4.5	3.4	0.008
Sinus discomfort	4.7	3.6	
Coordination problems	4.0	2.9	
Nasal symptoms	5.1	4.1	
Bloating	4.2	3.2	
Visual changes	3.9	2.9	
Rash	3.9	2.9	

From Pizzorno J. Is Mold Toxicity Really a Problem for Our Patients? Part I—Respiratory Conditions. Integrative Medicine: A Clinician's Journal. 2016;15(2):6-10.

Some researchers have suggested that mVOCs function as mycotoxins and have proposed the term *volatoxin*.[12] Research has also shown that mVOCs may be more toxic to humans than are the chemicals traditionally recognized as industrial toxins. For example, I-octen-3-ol has been shown to be more toxic to human embryonic stems cells than toluene.[13] Another study reported that fungal VOCs had a greater toxic effect than formaldehyde, xylene, benzene, and toluene.[14] mVOCs increase inflammation biomarkers such as myeloperoxidase, lysozyme, and eosinophil cationic protein, which causes headache, nausea, and mucosal irritation.[15] One study reported that "the impact of fungal VOCs, 2-octenal and oct-1-en-3-ol, on bone marrow stromal cells that are vital for the appropriate development and activation of the immune system showed increased membrane fluidity."[16] The same study also stated that "these vast changes in membranes are known to contribute to the breakdown of normal cellular function and possibly lead to death." mVOCs induce neurotoxicity in the drosophila model even at very low concentrations, inducing locomotor defects and changes in antigen-labeled dopaminergic neurons.[17] Another drosophila study showed that the mVOC 1-octen3-ol induces nitric oxide–mediated inflammatory response.[18]

Neurotoxicity

Neurotoxicity is associated with mycotoxins and other chemicals produced by mold. One study examined neurobehavioral and pulmonary impairment in 105 adults with indoor exposure to molds and 100 adults exposed to chemicals and, although it is nearly impossible to find a control group without toxin exposure, compared them with 202 "unexposed" community referents.[19] Researchers examined several respiratory measures and found 6.1% abnormalities in mold-exposed individuals and 7.1% in chemical-exposed individuals compared with 1.2% abnormalities in controls. This is consistent with the clearly demonstrable respiratory effects previously mentioned. Neurologically, they found statistically significant problems in both exposed groups: decreased balance, longer reaction times, increased blink reflex latency, increased color discrimination errors, decreased visual field, and reduced grip strength. They also found several measures of cognitive and memory performance were abnormal in both exposed groups. Interestingly, little difference was found in virtually all measures between the mold- and chemical-exposed populations.

A study of 100 individuals exposed to mold in their homes found multiple neurological deficits in 70% and abnormalities in T and B cells in more than 80% of the patients.[20] A study of 95 employees working in a well-documented water-damaged school building compared with 110 "unexposed" controls found statistically significant loss of visual contrast sensitivity (VCS), an apparently sensitive measure of neurodysfunction, in addition to the usual respiratory problems.[21]

Individuals exposed to satratoxin (SH), a trichothecene, and microbial organisms showed a chronic immune response (inflammation and oxidative stress), leading to neural damage.[22] According to the researchers, their results demonstrate that "regardless of whether the neurons were exposed to SH alone or under additive effects, sensitivity of the neurons to these compounds is high and neurological system cell damage can occur from SH exposure." In addition, data demonstrate that constant activation of inflammatory and apoptotic pathways at low levels amplifies the devastation and leads to neurological cell damage from indirect events triggered by the presence of a trichothecene mycotoxin. They concluded that "from this study and others, we show that neurological system cell damage from exposure to mycotoxins is a potential public health threat for occupants of water-damaged buildings."

Immunotoxicity

Several studies have clearly shown mold-induced immunotoxicity. The research in humans convincingly shows chronic mold/damp building exposure increases production of multiple inflammatory measures and alters immune function mediators. The immune systems of those working in damp buildings reacting to exposure showed a 2- to 1000-fold increase in production of a wide variety of inflammatory/immune mediators.[23]

Researchers who have shown an association between multiple sclerosis (MS) and fungal toxins have proposed that MS is primarily a mold toxin disease.[24] Gliotoxin, a heat-stable secondary metabolite produced by various species of *Aspergillus* and *Candida,* suppresses immune function, increases blood–brain barrier permeability, and is highly neurotoxic. As is well known, incidence of MS increases with distance from the equator, which also correlates with mold exposure and decreased vitamin D—a critical nutrient for immune system modulation. It is possible that MS is primarily due to the combination of mold exposure and vitamin D deficiency.

Another study examining chronic fatigue syndrome (CFS) patients showed a high correlation between CFS diagnosis and the presence of mycotoxins in the patient's urine. Of the 102 CFS patients studied, 93% had one mycotoxin present, and almost 30% had two or more mycotoxins present.[25] Further research is warranted to better understand this association.

Foodborne Mycotoxins

Foodborne mycotoxins are abiotic metabolites produced by certain fungi that grow on a variety of food crops. The clinical significance of foodborne mycotoxins depends on frequency of occurrence and/or severity of the disease(s) they produce. The most concerning mycotoxins include aflatoxins-AF (B_1, B_2, G_1, G_2), fumonisins (FB_1, FB_2), zearalenone (ZEA), trichothecenes (T-2 toxin, deoxynivalenol DON, HT-2), ochratoxin A (OTA), citrinin (CIT), penicillic acid (PA), and certain ergot alkaloids.[26] These toxic secondary metabolites are produced by fungi primarily in the genera *Aspergillus, Penicillium,* and *Fusarium.*[27]

Single mycotoxins produce a wide range of physiological effects. For example, OTA possesses teratogenic, embryotoxic, genotoxic, neurotoxic, immunosuppressive, carcinogenic, and nephrotoxic properties.[28,29] The carcinogenic effects of foodborne mold contamination are well documented (e.g., aflatoxins, fumonisins, OTA).[30,31,32] In addition, foodborne mycotoxins have been shown to cause impaired child growth (aflatoxins), neural tube defects (fumonisins), immunotoxicity (DON), gastroenteritis (DON), and renal disease (OTA).[33] Most of these conditions occur after ingestion of mycotoxin-contaminated food products (most often grains or products made from grains), but other routes of exposure exist.

Further exacerbating the deleterious effects of mycotoxins are the additive or synergistic effects that occur because of the co-occurrence of foodborne mycotoxins. The combined toxicity of mycotoxins is hard to predict based on the toxic effect of a single mycotoxin. Many studies show that OTA-CIT,[34,35] OTA-PA,[36,37] OTA-FB_1,[38,39,40] and OTA-AF[41] combinations have additive or synergistic actions.[42]

DIAGNOSIS/ASSESSMENT

A detailed medical history and comprehensive physical examination continue to be foundational in the diagnosis of toxicant exposure. A thorough history should include questions regarding the patient's work and home environments (does he or she spend time in a home or office building with dampness problems?), chronic respiratory symptoms (e.g., coughing, sinusitis, rhinitis), adult-onset allergic or respiratory symptoms, and whether mold is obviously present in the environment according to visibility or odor.

The level of humidity in the various parts of the building can be easily measured by a variety of readily available and inexpensive monitors. A more sophisticated and clinically validated method is to directly measure the contaminants in the air, on surfaces, or in dust. There are four primary methods: culture, nonculture, chemical assay for key toxic molecules, and immunoassay. The advantage of culturing is being able to definitively determine the organisms involved. The disadvantages include delay, cost, difficulty in culturing itself, and poor reproducibility between the several different collection and culturing protocols.

The nonculture protocols count the number of particles and organisms caught by the collection tools, such as air filtration or liquid capturing. The advantage with nonculture protocols is quantification. The primary disadvantage is poor differentiation, but this can be improved with various staining methods (e.g., lactophenol blue for fungal spores).

The chemical assay depends on the toxins to be evaluated. Typical assessment methodologies include polymerase chain reaction (PCR), immunoassays, gas chromatography, high-pressure liquid chromatography, and mass spectrometry. In general, immunoassays are used to determine allergen types.

Regardless of the methodology used, dust samples are generally more sensitive and accurate measures than air samples and have better clinical correlation.

An on-site inspection for the presence of mold includes visual inspection of typical locations for water damage, mold growth, and available sample collection. ERMI is a well-documented assessment for the likelihood of mold contamination in a building utilizing dust samples.[43] High ERMI ratings in a building are directly associated with increased asthma risk for persons in the structure.[44,45] Other methods include mold spore collection inside (usually in two areas) and outside the home. This method identifies any mold that is present inside the building but not outside the building. It can also identify which molds are present indoors at a higher level than they would be found outdoors. Either of these methods can identify a mold-infested home. Although these assessments are not inexpensive, if the core cause of an unresolved clinical problem can be identified and treated, it is well worth the investment. Box 31.4 shows several national associations, individuals, and companies and their certifications that can be used to test for the presence of mold.

Clinical Evaluation

Table 31.4 alphabetically lists the conditions and symptoms that should alert clinicians to a mold/damp building problem. These can be simply summed up as any chronic, unexplained respiratory tract problem.

A number of laboratories run a wide range of tests that can help with diagnosis. For example, LabCorp offers 58 tests for the search term "mold." These tests include mold identification through DNA and culturing, checking antibodies to specific molds, and measuring various inflammatory markers.

For individual patients, enzyme-linked immunosorbent assay (ELISA) testing can be used to detect 15 mycotoxins both in the patient and in the environment and assess the relationship between the two. Additionally, qualitative polymerase chain reaction (QPCR) can detect and quantify the presence of 36 molds in human tissue and the environment. Genetic testing is available to help identify those individuals most susceptible to mold toxins and other environmental toxins. Genetic single-nucleotide polymorphisms (SNPs), proteomics, and other markers of cellular function of the immune, detoxification, mitochondrial, and methylation systems may help identify those most susceptible, those most affected, and potential treatment options. In addition, assessing potential nutritional deficiencies and levels of other environmental toxins may help identify those with increased individual susceptibility. As additional research is completed, it will be imperative to improve and expand these technologies. Given the complex nature of the interaction between the human genome and environmental toxins, this seems a problem likely to be solved, at least in part, by applying the science of bioinformatics. Such an approach will help us understand more fully the relationship (i.e., severity and magnitude) of indoor mold exposure to human health.

BOX 31.4   Certifications and Certification Organizations

- ACAC—American Council of Accredited Certifications
- AIHA—American Industrial Hygiene Association
- CMC—Certified Mold Consultant
- CIEC—Certified Indoor Environmental Consultant
- CIH—Certified Industrial Hygienist w/mold experience

TABLE 31.4   Diseases and Symptoms Caused or Aggravated by Mold/Damp Buildings

Diseases	Symptoms
Allergic rhinitis	Bronchitis
Allergic alveolitis (hypersensitivity pneumonitis)	Cough
Asthma	Dyspnea
Chronic respiratory infections	Hoarseness
Eczema	Vocal cord dysfunction
Inhalation fever (toxic pneumonitis, humidifier fever, or organic dust toxic syndrome)	Wheeze

INTERVENTION

Decrease Exposure

Intervention begins by addressing the cause, which in the case of mold primarily involves avoidance of further exposure. There is no substitute for fixing the foundational causes: excessive building humidity from poor design or water damage, inadequate ventilation, and contaminated air conditioning vents. Specifically addressing these causes is beyond the scope of this chapter and requires professional assistance. Nonetheless, unless these causes are corrected, focusing treatment solely on the patient may not be sufficient when the problem is almost entirely due to the environment. In many ways, this is a problem of civilization.

Several studies in both children and adults have objectively assessed the clinical effects of addressing building moisture. An excellent review paper evaluated eight studies (total of 6538 participants) for the effects of building remediation. Researchers found moderate-quality evidence in adults that repairing houses decreased asthma-related symptoms (Odds ratio (OR) 0.64) and respiratory infections (OR 0.57). For children, they reported moderate-quality evidence for a reduction in the number of acute care visits (mean difference −0.45).[46]

Complete care requires more than building remediation. However, it is necessary to begin there. Dealing with building moisture will facilitate the efficacy of allergen control as well as dietary, nutritional, and herbal medicine treatments for asthma and other chronic respiratory conditions.

REFERENCES

1. Centers for Disease Control and Prevention. *Basic Facts about Mold*. Available at https://www.cdc.gov/mold/faqs.htm#indoor. (Accessed February 1, 2016.)
2. WHO Regional Office for Europe. (2009). *WHO guidelines for indoor air quality: dampness and mould*. World Health Organization Germany: Druckpartner Moser. Available at http://www.who.int/indoorair/publications/7989289041683/en/. (Accessed November 15, 2017.)
3. Institute of Medicine. Committee on Damp Indoor Spaces and Health, Board on Health Promotion and Disease Prevention of the National Academies (2004). *Damp indoor spaces and health*. Washington, DC: National Academies Press.
4. Miller, J. D., & McMullin, D. R. (2014). Fungal secondary metabolites as harmful indoor air contaminants: 10 years on. *Applied Microbiology and Biotechnology*, 98(24), 9953–9966.
5. Mudarri, D., & Fisk, W. J. (2007). Public health and economic impact of dampness and mold. *Indoor Air*, 17(3), 226–235.
6. Fisk, W. J., Lei-Gomez, Q., & Mendell, M. J. (2007). Meta-analyses of the associations of respiratory health effects with dampness and mold in homes. *Indoor Air*, 17(4), 284–296.
7. Cox-Ganser, J. M., White, S. K., Jones, R., et al. (2005). Respiratory morbidity in office workers in a water-damaged building. *Environmental Health Perspectives*, 113, 485–490.
8. Centers for Disease Control and Prevention. Basic Facts about Mold. *Mold: basic facts*. Available at http://www.cdc.gov/mold/faqs.htm#affect. (Accessed February 15, 2016.)
9. Campbell, A. W., Thrasher, J. D., Gray, M. R., & Vojdani, A. (2004). Mold and mycotoxins: effects on the neurological and immune systems in humans. *Advances in Applied Microbiology*, 55, 375–406.
10. Paterson, R. R., & Lima, N. (2010). Toxicology of mycotoxins. *Experientia Supplementum*, 100, 31–63.
11. Juil, K., Seong-Hwan, P., Hun Do, K., Kim, D., Moon, Y. (2016). Interference with mutagenic aflatoxin B1-induced checkpoints through antagonistic action of ochratoxin A in intestinal cancer cells: a molecular explanation on potential risk of crosstalk between carcinogens. *Oncotarget*, 7(26):39627–39639.
12. Bennett, J. W., & Inamdar, A. A. (2015). Are some fungal volatile organic compounds (VOCs) mycotoxins? *Toxins*, 7, 3785–3804.
13. Inamdar, A. A., Moore, J. C., Cohen, R. I., & Bennett, J. W. (2012). A model to evaluate the cytotoxicity of the fungal volatile organic compound 1-octen-3-ol in human embryonic stem cells. *Mycopathologia*, 173, 13–20.
14. Inamdar, A. A., Zaman, T., Morath, S. U., Pu, D. C., & Bennett, J. W. (2014). Drosophila melanogaster as a model to characterize fungal volatile organic compounds. *Environmental Toxicology*, 29(7), 829–836.
15. Wålindera, R., Ernstgårdb, L., Norbäcka, D., et al. (2008). Acute effects of 1-octen-3-ol, a microbial volatile organic compound (MVOC)—An experimental study. *Toxicology Letters*, 181, 141–147.
16. Hokeness, K., Kratch, J., Nadolny, C., et al. (2014). The effects of fungal volatile organic compounds on bone marrow stromal cells. *Canadian Journal of Microbiology*, 60(1), 1–4.

17. Inamdar, A. A., Masurekar, P., & Bennett, J. W. (2010). Neurotoxicity of fungal volatile organic compounds in Drosophila melanogaster. *Toxicological Sciences, 117*(2), 418–426.

18. Inamdar, A. A., & Bennett, J. W. (2014). A common fungal volatile organic compound induces a nitric oxide mediated inflammatory response in Drosophila melanogaster. *Scientific Reports* 4, Article number:3833.

19. Kilburn, K. H. (2009). Neurobehavioral and pulmonary impairment in 105 adults with indoor exposure to molds compared to 100 exposed to chemicals. *Toxicology and Industrial Health, 25*(9–10), 681–692.

20. Rea, W. J., Didriksen, N., Simon, T. R., et al. (2003). Effects of toxic exposure to molds and mycotoxins in building-related illnesses. *Archives of Environmental Health, 58*(7), 399–405.

21. Thomas, G., Burton, N. C., Mueller, C., et al. (2012). Comparison of work-related symptoms and visual contrast sensitivity between employees at a severely water-damaged school and a school without significant water damage. *American Journal of Industrial Medicine, 55*(9), 844–854.

22. Karunasena, E., Larranaga, M. D., Simoni, J. S., et al. (2010). Building-associated neurological damage modeled in human cells: A mechanism of neurotoxic effects by exposure to mycotoxins in the indoor environment. *Mycopathologia, 170*(6):377–390.

23. Rosenblum Lichtenstein, J. H., Hsu, Y. H., Gavin, I. M., et al. (2015). Environmental mold and mycotoxin exposures elicit specific cytokine and chemokine responses. *PLoS ONE, 10*(5), e0126926.

24. Purzycki, C. B., & Shain, D. H. (2010). Fungal toxins and multiple sclerosis: a compelling connection. *Brain Research Bulletin, 82*(1–2), 4–6.

25. Brewer, J. H., Thrasher, J. D., Straus, D. C., et al. (2013). Detection of mycotoxins in patients with chronic fatigue syndrome. *Toxins, 5*(4), 605–617.

26. Richard, J. L. (2007). Some major mycotoxins and their mycotoxicoses – an overview. *International Journal of Food Microbiology, 119*(1–2), 3–10.

27. Lee, H. J., & Ryu, D. (2015). Advances in mycotoxin research: public health perspectives. *Journal of Food Science, 80*(12), T2970–T2983.

28. O'Brien, E., Heussner, A. H., & Dietrich, D. R. (2001). Species-, sex-, and cell type-specific effects of ochratoxin A and B. *Toxicological Sciences, 63*, 256–264.

29. International Agency for Research on Cancer. (1993). Ochratoxin A in some naturally occurring substances: food items and constituents, heterocyclic aromatic amines and mycotoxins. *IARC Monographs on the Evaluation of Carcinogenic Risks to Humans, 56*, 489–521.

30. Pfohl-Leszkowicz, A., Petkova-Bocharova, T., Chernozemsky, I. N., & Castegnaro, M. (2002). Balkan endemic nephropathy and associated urinary tract tumors: a review on aetiological causes and the potential role of mycotoxins. *Food Additives and Contaminants, 19*, 282–302.

31. Pfohl-Leszkowicz, A., & Manderville, R. A. (2007). Ochratoxin A: an overview on toxicity and carcinogenicity in animals and humans. *Molecular Nutrition & Food Research, 51*, 61–99.

32. IARC. (2002). Some traditional herbal medicines, some mycotoxins, naphthalene, and styrene. *IARC Monographs on the Evaluation of Carcinogenic Risks to Humans, 82*, 301–366.

33. Wu, F., Groopman, J. D., & Pestka, J. J. (2014). Public health impacts of foodborne mycotoxins. *Annual Review of Food Science and Technology, 5*, 351–372.

34. Kumar, M., Dwivedi, P., Sharma, A. K., Singh, N. D., & Patil, R. D. (2007). Patil Ochratoxin A and citrinin nephrotoxicity in New Zealand white rabbits: an ultrastructural assessment. *Mycopathologia, 163*, 21–30.

35. Kitchen, D. N., Carlton, W. W., & Tuite, J. (1997). Ochratoxin A and citrinin induced nephrosis in beagle dogs I. II. Pathology. *Veterinary Pathology 14*, 261–272.

36. Parker, R., Phillips, T., Kubena, L., Russell, L. H., & Heidelbaugh, N. D. (1982). Inhibition of pancreatic carboxypeptidase A: a possible mechanism of interaction between penicillic acid and ochratoxin A. *Journal of Environmental Science and Health, B17*, 77–91.

37. Stoev, S. D., Vitanov, S., Anguelov, G., Petkova-Bocharova, T., & Creppy, E. E. (2001). Experimental mycotoxic nephropathy in pigs provoked by a mouldy diet containing ochratoxin A and penicillic acid. *Veterinary Research Communications, 25*, 205–223.

38. Segvic Klaric, M. (2012). Adverse effects of combined mycotoxins. *Arhiv Za Higijenu Rada I Toksikologiju, 63*, 519–530.

39. Creppy, E. E., Chirappa, P., Baudrimont, I., Borracci, P., Moukha, S., & Carratu, M. R. (2004). Synergistic effects of fumonisin B1 and ochratoxin A: are in vitro cytotoxicity data predictive of in vivo acute toxicity? *Toxicology, 201*, 115–123.

40. Domijan, A. M., Peraica, M., Vrdoljak, A. L., Radic, B., Zlender, V., & Fuchs, R. (2007). The involvement of oxidative stress in ochratoxin A and fumonisin B1 toxicity in rats. *Molecular Nutrition & Food Research, 51*, 1147–1151.

41. Grenier, B., & Oswald, I. P. (2011). Mycotoxin co-contamination of food and feed: meta-analysis of publications describing toxicological interactions. *World Mycotoxin Journal, 4*, 285–313.

42. Hadjeba-Medjdoub, K., Faucet-Marquis, V., Tozlovanu, M., et al. (2011). Synergistic effect of three nephrotoxic and carcinogenic mycotoxins (citrinin, fumonisin, ochratoxin A) on human kidney cells viability and genotoxicity. In R. Antolovic & T. Milicevic (Eds.), *Power of Fungi and Mycotoxins in Health and Disease; Primosten, Croatia* (p. 57). Zagreb, Croatia: Croatian Mycrobiological Society.

43. Täubel, M., Karvonen, A. M., Reponen, T., et al. (2015). Application of the Environmental Relative Moldiness Index in Finland. *Applied and Environmental Microbiology*, 82(2), 578–584. PubMed PMID: 26546428.

44. Vesper, S., & Wymer, L. (2016). The relationship between environmental relative moldiness index values and asthma. *International Journal of Hygiene and Environmental Health*, 219(3), 233–238. PubMed PMID: 26861576.

45. McSharry, C., Vesper, S., Wymer, L., et al. (2015). Decreased FEV1 % in asthmatic adults in Scottish homes with high Environmental Relative Moldiness Index values. *Clinical and Experimental Allergy*, 45(5), 902–907. PubMed PMID: 25580663.

46. Sauni, R., Uitti, J., Jauhiainen, M., et al. (2013). Remediating buildings damaged by dampness and mould for preventing or reducing respiratory tract symptoms, infections and asthma (Review). *Evidence-Based Child Health*, 8(3), 944–1000.

32

Ozone

SUMMARY

- Presence in population: All individuals inhale ozone (O_3) every day
- Major diseases: Asthma, reduced lung function, cardiovascular disease, and diabetes
- Primary sources: Combustion byproducts and volatile organic compounds (VOCs) reacting with sunlight

- Best measure: Government-sponsored O_3 monitoring stations, which are available in certain areas, can provide average levels of O_3 concentration
- Best intervention: Remove sources of indoor O_3 generation, use activated charcoal filters to reduce indoor O_3 levels, supplement antioxidants to ameliorate oxidative damage

DESCRIPTION

O_3 is a colorless gas, a powerful oxidizing agent, and a normal constituent of the atmosphere. Stratospheric O_3 forms a layers between 10 and 30 miles above the Earth's surface that protects it from the harmful ultraviolet rays of the sun. In contrast, ground level (tropospheric) O_3 causes damage to mammalian respiratory tracts, and crops and other plants. In the United States, O_3 is responsible for $500 million dollars of crop damage per year.[1] Ground level O_3 is produced from the interaction of sunlight with solvents (VOCs) or nitrogen dioxide. Sunlight and hot weather combine with vehicular and industrial emissions to form high levels of O_3, one of the primary constituents of smog. Ground level O_3 concentrations change seasonally, with the highest levels in the summer. Daily levels also vary with the amount of sunlight present and anthropogenic activities, including traffic congestion (Fig. 32.1).

The current Environmental Protection Agency (EPA) standard for an 8-hour average "primary" exposure to O_3 of 0.075 PPM was established in 2008. A new standard of 0.070 PPM was set in 2015, which will be implemented from 2019 through 2023.[2] O_3 from East Asia has increased overall springtime levels of O_3 in Washington State and other areas since 1985.[3] Levels of O_3 in China increased 7% between 2005 and 2010, and are responsible for a considerable amount of tropospheric O_3 in the western United States.[4] The European Union set a maximum daily 8-hour average of 120 µg/m^3 (0.06 PPM) that should not be exceeded more than 25 days each year.[5] The World Health Organization (WHO) has set 100 µg/m^3 as the daily maximum 8-hour average.

TOXICITY

O_3 is a powerful prooxidant that interacts with a wide range of cellular components and tissues.[6] O_3 also reduces levels of antioxidants in the body. Ascorbic acid levels in bronchial lavages of nine persons exposed to 0.2 PPM of O_3 for 2 hours were found to drop.[7] O_3 exposure has been repeatedly linked to triggering and worsening of respiratory problems.

SOURCES

Some tropospheric O_3 comes from the stratosphere, whereas the majority comes from anthropogenic sources of vehicular exhaust and VOCs interacting with sunlight. Forest fires are also a major source of O_3.[8]

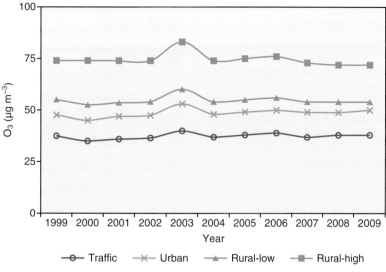

FIG. 32.1 Annual pattern of O_3 for traffic, industrial, and rural sites in Europe from 1999 to 2009. (From Sousa S. I., Alvim-Ferraz M. C., & Martins F. G. [2013]. Health effects of ozone focusing on childhood asthma: What is now known—a review from an epidemiological point of view. *Chemosphere, 90*[7], 2051–2058.)

Indoor levels of O_3 initially come from intake of outdoor air through heating, ventilation, and air conditioning (HVAC) systems; doorways; windows; and airflow under doors and through unsealed building envelopes. Indoor sources of O_3 include laser printers, photocopiers, ion generators, and electrostatic precipitators for air cleaning.[9,10,11] Some companies sell O_3 generators for "air purification." Unfortunately, controlled studies in laboratories and residential settings show that these systems actually increase particulate matter, particularly when there is a terpene source such as a pine oil–based cleaner.[12]

Clinical Significance
- Respiratory disease
- Cardiovascular disease
- Type 2 diabetes mellitus (T2DM)

Respiratory. The following are the most common respiratory problems related to O_3 exposure:
- Airway irritation and inflammation
- Aggravation of asthma and coughing
- Wheezing and breathing difficulties during exercise or outdoor activities
- Increased susceptibility to respiratory illnesses like pneumonia and bronchitis

Urban joggers exposed to O_3 exhibited increased markers of chronic respiratory inflammation.[13] Adverse respiratory function with O_3 exposure was also found in hikers ages 18 to 64 in New Hampshire. With each 50 parts per billion (PPB) (not parts per million (PPM)) incremental increase in ambient O_3 levels, the hikers experienced a 2.6% decline in forced expiratory volume in 1 second (FEV_1) and a 2.2% decline in forced vital capacity (FVC).[14] Those hikers with a history of asthma or wheezing had a fourfold greater response to O_3 than the others. Children exposed to higher levels of ground level O_3 have greater rates of asthma and rhinitis than children in areas with less O_3.[15] College students exposed to high ambient O_3 had statistically significantly poorer lung function, as shown by lower FEV_1 and FEV_{25-75} (between 25–75%).[16] They also exhibited more respiratory symptoms of cough, phlegm, and wheezing that were not due to colds. Acute ambient exposure in children resulted in marked reduction in FVC and FEV_1 the day after exposure to elevated O_3 (< 80 PPB).[17] Hospital admissions for pneumonia are higher when ambient O_3 levels increase.[18] A large study of 36 US cities showed that a 5 PPB increase in ground level O_3 led to an increase in hospital admissions for pneumonia.[19]

Cardiovascular. Health damage from O_3 goes beyond the respiratory tract, and to the cardiovascular system as well. Animals exposed to 0.5 PPM of O_3 for 8 hours a day exhibited altered blood pressure, heart rate, and endothelial-dependent vascular function, oxidative stress, mitochondrial damage, and the development of athero-sclerotic plaque.[20] O_3 exposure is also associated with increased mortality for city dwellers.[21]

Diabetes. Very small increases in ground level O_3 can also increase the risk for developing T2DM.[22]

ASSESSMENT

The level of O_3 (and other pollutants) in a specific area can be found at www.airnow.gov/.

Some counties may have active O_3 monitoring sites that can be accessed via their official websites (typically www.countyname.gov), then search for "ozone" or "ozone map." O_3 advisories for US national parks are available at https://nature.nps.gov/air/data/current/advisory/advisory.cfm.

INTERVENTION
Avoidance

Removing of indoor sources of O_3 generation is the first step in reducing exposure. This includes removing indoor ion or O_3 generators. If printers or copiers need to be used, they should be put in a room that has an exhaust fan constantly moving the air outside the building. Clean HVAC filters can remove a small amount of O_3 from home air.[23] Reductions of up to 20% of indoor O_3 levels can be obtained with commercially available charcoal air filters.[24] Activated charcoal filters can remove at least 60% of indoor O_3 and possibly up to 90%.[25,26]

Passive reduction of indoor O_3 levels can also be obtained by the use of passive removal materials (PRMs), the most effective of which is clay paint.[27]

Supplementation

Antioxidant repletion can help to mitigate damage from O_3.[28] Cyclists who supplemented with 15 mg beta carotene, 75 mg vitamin E, and 650 mg vitamin C experienced none of the adverse effects of O_3 in any of the respiratory parameters tested, whereas all of those without supplementation did.[29]

REFERENCES

1. U.S. Environmental Protection Agency. *Ozone Pollution.* Available at https://www.epa.gov/ozone-pollution. (Accessed April 23, 2017.)
2. U.S. Environmental Protection Agency. *Ozone Pollution: Setting and Reviewing Standards to Control Ozone Pollution.* Available at https://www.epa.gov/ozone-pollution/setting-and-reviewing-standards-control-ozone-pollution. (Accessed August 3, 2017.)
3. Cooper, O. R., Parrish, D. D., Stohl, A., et al. (2010). Increasing springtime ozone mixing ratios in the free troposphere over western North America. *Nature, 463*(7279), 344–348. PubMed PMID: 20090751.
4. Verstraeten, W. W., Neu, J. L., Williams, J. E., et al. (2015). Rapid increases in tropospheric ozone production and export from China. *Nature Geoscience, 8,* 690–695.
5. European Environment Agency. *Air Quality in Europe – 2016 report.* https://www.eea.europa.eu/publications/air-quality-in-europe-2016. (Accessed August 2, 2017.)
6. Servais, S., Boussouar, A., Molnar, A., et al. (2005). Age-related sensitivity to lung oxidative stress during ozone exposure. *Free Radical Research, 39*(3), 305–316. PubMed PMID: 15788235.
7. Mudway, I., Krishna, M., Frew, A., et al. (1999). Compromised concentrations of ascorbate in fluid lining the respiratory tract in human subjects after exposure to ozone. *Occupational and Environmental Medicine, 56,* 473–481. PubMed PMID: 10472319.
8. Jaffe, D., Chand, D., Hafner, W., et al. (2008). Influence of fires on O_3 concentrations in the western U.S. *Environmental Science & Technology, 42*(16), 5885–5891. PubMed PMID: 18767640.
9. Singh, B. P., Kumar, A., Singh, D., et al. (2014). An assessment of ozone levels, UV radiation and their occupational health hazard estimation during photocopying operation. *Journal of Hazardous Materials, 275,* 55–62. PubMed PMID: 24857892.
10. Kim, K. H., Szulejko, J. E., Kumar, P., et al. (2017). Air ionization as a control technology for off-gas emissions of volatile organic compounds. *Environmental Pollution, 225,* 729–743. PubMed PMID: 28347612.
11. Destaillats, H., Maddalena, R. L., Singer, B. C., et al. (2008). Indoor pollutants emitted by office equipment: A review of reported data and information needs. *Atmospheric Environment, 42,* 1371–1388.
12. Hubbard, H. F., Coleman, B. K., Sarwar, G., & Corsi, R. L. (2005). Effects of an ozone-generating air purifier on

indoor secondary particles in three residential dwellings. *Indoor Air*, 15(6), 432–444.

13. Kinney, P. L., Nilsen, D. M., Lippmann, M., et al. (1996). Biomarkers of lung inflammation in recreational joggers exposed to ozone. *American Journal of Respiratory and Critical Care Medicine*, 154(5), 1430–1435. PubMed PMID: 8912760.

14. Korrick, S., Neas, L., Dockery, D., et al. (1998). Effects of ozone and other pollutants on the pulmonary function of adult hikers. *Environmental Health Perspectives*, 106(2), 93–99. PubMed PMID: 9435151.

15. Kim, B. J., Kwon, J. W., Seo, J. H., et al. (2011). Association of ozone exposure with asthma, allergic rhinitis, and allergic sensitization. *Annals of Allergy, Asthma and Immunology*, 107(3), 214–219, e1. PubMed PMID: 21875539.

16. Glizia, A., & Kinney, P. L. (1999). Long-term residence in areas of high ozone: associations with respiratory health in a nationwide sample of nonsmoking young adults. *Environmental Health Perspectives*, 107(8), 675–679. PubMed PMID: 10417367.

17. Chen, P. C., Lai, Y. M., Chan, C. C., et al. (1999). Short-term effect of ozone on the pulmonary function of children in primary school. *Environmental Health Perspectives*, 107(11), 921–925. PubMed PMID: 10544161.

18. Tsai, S. S., & Yang, C. Y. (2014). Fine particulate air pollution and hospital admissions for pneumonia in a subtropical city: Taipei, Taiwan. *Journal of Toxicology and Environmental Health. Part A*, 77(4), 192–201. PubMed PMID: 24555678.

19. Medina-Ramon, M., Zanobetti, A., & Schwartz, J. (2006). The effect of ozone and PM10 on hospital admissions for pneumonia and chronic obstructive pulmonary disease: a national multicity study. *American Journal of Epidemiology*, 163(6), 579–588. PubMed PMID: 16443803.

20. Chuang, G. C., Yang, Z., Westbrook, D. G., et al. (2009). Pulmonary ozone exposure induces vascular dysfunction, mitochondrial damage, and atherogenesis. *American Journal of Physiology. Lung Cellular and Molecular Physiology*, 297(2), L209–L216. PubMed PMID: 19395667.

21. Chen, C., Zhao, B., & Weschler, C. J. (2012). Assessing the influence of indoor exposure to "outdoor ozone" on the relationship between ozone and short-term mortality in U.S. communities. *Environmental Health Perspectives*, 120(2), 235–240. PubMed PMID: 22100611.

22. Jerrett, M., Brook, R., White, L. F., et al. (2017). Ambient ozone and incident diabetes: A prospective analysis in a large cohort of African American women. *Environment International*, 102, 42–47. PubMed PMID: 28153529.

23. Zhao, P., Siegel, J., & Corsi, R. (2007). Ozone removal by HVAC filters. *Atmospheric Environment*, 41, 3151–3160.

24. Aldred, J. R., Darling, E., Morrison, G., et al. (2016). Benefit-cost analysis of commercially available activated carbon filters for indoor ozone removal in single-family homes. *Indoor Air*, 26(3), 501–512. PubMed PMID: 25952610.

25. Lin, C.-C., & Chen, H.-Y. (2014). Impact of HVAV filter on indoor air quality in terms of ozone removal and carbonyls generation. *Atmospheric Environment*, 89, 29–34.

26. Lee, P., & Davidson, J. (1999). Evaluation of activated carbon filters for removal of ozone at the PPB level. *American Industrial Hygiene Association Journal*, 60(5), 589–600. PubMed PMID: 10529990.

27. Darling, E., Morrison, G., & Corsi, R. L. (2016). Passive removal materials for indoor ozone control. *Building and Environment*, 106, 33–44.

28. Romieu, I., Meneses, F., Ramirez, M., et al. (1998). Antioxidant supplementation and respiratory functions among workers exposed to high levels of ozone. *American Journal of Respiratory and Critical Care Medicine*, 158(1), 226–232. PubMed PMID: 9655734.

29. Grievink, L., Jansen, S., van't Veer, P., & Brunekreef, B. (1998). Acute effects of ozone on pulmonary function of cyclists receiving antioxidant supplements. *Occupational and Environmental Medicine*, 55, 13–17. PubMed PMID: 9536157.

33

Particulate Matter and Polycyclic Aromatic Hydrocarbons

SUMMARY

- Presence in population: Ubiquitous
- Major diseases: Neoplasia, cardiovascular, respiratory, allergic reactivity
- Primary sources: Vehicular exhaust: diesel exhaust produces the most damaging emissions
- Best measure: Currently no laboratory measurement is available other than oxidative stress (8-OHdG)
- Best interventions: Air purifiers in the home, antioxidants from whole foods, botanicals agents and supplements, fish oil

DESCRIPTION

Particulate Matter

Particulate matter (PM; also referred to as *particulate pollution*) is a combination of liquid droplets (aerosols) and solid particles like dust, soot, smoke, and dirt. PM carries a number of chemicals, including multiple polycyclic aromatic hydrocarbons and volatile organic compounds, which account for some of their toxic health effects.[1]

PM is differentiated according to particle size, with "coarse" particles that are less than 10 micrometers but larger than 2.5 micrometers designated PM_{10}. PM_{10} is often encountered near dusty roadways and industries. Fine particles are between 2.5 and 0.1 micrometers in diameter and are designated $PM_{2.5}$. Ultrafine particles, also called *nanoparticles,* are less than 0.1 micrometer in size and are more soluble than their larger counterparts. These are referred to as ultrafine particles (UFP) or $PM_{0.1}$.

Any PM less than 10 micrometers is readily absorbed in the lungs and then distributed throughout the body. Ultrafine PM levels in the livers of rats 18 to 24 hours after exposure were found to be five times higher than the PM levels in their lungs.[2] PM has also shown the ability to travel from the nose into the brain via the olfactory nerve.[3] PM of iron oxide, India ink, and titanium dioxide initially identified in alveolar macrophages was found a day later not only in the lung (highest concentration) but also in the liver, kidney, heart, tracheobronchial and mediastinal lymph nodes, anterior and posterior nasal cavities, brain, and blood. At 7 days postexposure, it was still found in the lungs, liver, and blood.[4] Rats exposed once to UFP and then sacrificed after 3 weeks, 2 months, or 6 months showed that PM concentrations in the brain, heart, spleen, liver, and lungs from the single exposure slowly reduced over time, with the lungs retaining the most.[5] Individuals with constant daily exposure would be expected to have these particles, with their adsorbed toxicants, throughout their bodies.

Polyaromatic Hydrocarbons

Numerous chemical compounds are adsorbed to PM, including polycyclic aromatic hydrocarbons (PAHs) (Fig. 33.1).[6] PAHs are highly lipophilic. They are found naturally in oil, coal, and tar deposits and are also formed during incomplete burning of coal, oil, and gas for fuels; incineration of garbage; smoking of tobacco; and charbroiling of meat. In short, burning anything will produce PAHs.

TOXICITY

PM causes significant oxidative damage in the tissues and organs it is distributed to[7,8,9] and has been associated with

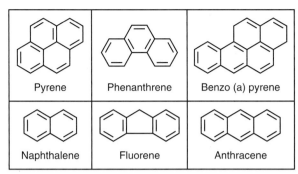

FIG. 33.1 Chemical structure of common PAHs.

TABLE 33.1 Major PAH Compounds in the Air, Along with Their Status as Carcinogens and Presence in Diesel Exhaust

Most Common PAHs	EPA-Listed Probable Carcinogens	Present in Diesel Exhaust
Acenaphthene		
Acenaphthylene		X
Anthracene		X
Benz-anthracene	X	X
Benzo-a-pyrene [BaP]	X	X
Benzo-e-pyrene		X
Benzo-b-fluoranthene	X	X
Benzo-j-fluoranthene		X
Benzo-k-fluoranthene	X	X
Benzo-g,h,i-perylene		X
Chrysene	X	X
Dibenzo-anthracene	X	
Fluoranthene		X
Fluorene		X
Indenol-pyrene	X	X
Phenanthrene		X
Pyrene		X

increased 8-hydroxy-2-deoxyguanosine (8-OHdG) levels and mortality, primarily from cardiovascular,[10,11] respiratory,[12] and neoplastic diseases.[13,14] Diesel exhaust particles (DEPs), high in benzo[a]pyrene (BaP) levels, reduce intracellular glutathione (GSH) levels, as well as the function of GSH transferase and other antioxidant enzymes.[15] PM$_{2.5}$ from vehicular exhaust gives higher risk of all diseases than PM$_{2.5}$ from nonvehicular sources.

SOURCES

Humans are exposed to PAHs from consuming foods cooked over open flames, especially meats.[16] Vehicular exhaust comprises the single greatest source of health-damaging air pollutants. Among vehicle types, diesel exhaust is the largest single source of PM, contributing up to 100 times more than gasoline engines and responsible for up to 90% of the total outdoor PM.[17] Diesel engines (both stationary and vehicular) also produce significant levels of carbon monoxide (CO), sulfur and nitrogen oxides, and other ozone-forming compounds. Diesel exhaust is a combination of gaseous compounds and DEPs. DEPs are built around a carbon core with a large surface area to which hundreds of chemicals and metals are attached. DEPs are either PM$_{2.5}$ "fine particles" or PM$_{0.1}$.

Both PM and PAHs are known to damage mitochondria and suppress their proper functioning.[9,18,19] The Environmental Protection Agency (EPA) has determined that the PAHs BaP, benz[a]anthracene, benzo[b]fluoranthene, benzo[k]fluoranthene, chrysene, dibenz[a,h]anthracene, and indeno[1,2,3- c,d]pyrene are probable human carcinogens.[20] BaP is the main lung carcinogen in cigarette smoke[21] and vehicular exhaust.[22] The 17 most common PAHs as well as their carcinogenic ratings by the EPA and their presence in diesel exhaust are presented in Table 33.1.

As shown, diesel exhaust is the major source of the most common PAHs, including those that are absolute (BaP) or probable carcinogens.

The digging of unconventional natural gas (UNG) wells, often referred to as "fracking," is a relatively new and alarming source of air and water emissions. There are more than 1 million active gas and oil wells, compressors, and processing stations in the United States.[23] Tens of thousands of those are fracking wells that emit tons of PAHs and volatile organic compounds (VOCs) daily into the air.[24]

Fig. 6.3 (Chapter 6, Outdoor Air Pollution, pg 9) shows the concentrations of total PAHs along with phenanthrene and the carcinogenic BaP that are produced by UNG wells. Both total PAHs and phenanthrene concentrations are still elevated over a mile away from each site. Areas that contain UNG sites typically have a high number within each county, making the levels of these toxic pollutants quite high. This will result in rural dwellers being exposed to PAH levels that would more typically be experienced by their urban counterparts.[25]

TABLE 33.2   Urinary PAH Metabolites in 2017 CDC Fourth Report (ng/g)

PAH	Parent Compound	Mean	50th %	75th %	90th %	95th %
2-OH fluorene	Fluorene	273	211	439	1340	2110
3-OH fluorene	"	107	80.6	185	753	1170
9-OH fluorene	"	279	248	490	934	1370
1-OH phenanthrene	Phenanthrene	143	134	218	357	519
2-OH phenanthrene	"	69.2	62.2	106	182	248
3-OH phenanthrene	"	70.5	62.6	118	226	325
4-OH phenanthrene	"	23.3	22.0	36.9	65.0	106
1–OH pyrene	Pyrene	127	119	215	395	542
1-OH naphthalene	Naphthalene	1.90	1.51	4.15	13.4	20.4
2-OH naphthalene	"	4.72	4.32	9.30	17.6	23.4

BODY BURDEN

All 10 of the PAHs tested for in the Centers for Disease Control and Prevention (CDC) Fourth Report were found ubiquitously throughout the North American population (Table 33.2).[26]

Detoxification/Excretion Processes

The fat solubility allows PAHs to easily penetrate cell membranes and remain in tissues. However, metabolism of PAHs occurs in all tissues of the body, resulting in more water-soluble and excretable compounds. The CYP1A series oxidizes PAHs into a more toxic epoxide form that can then be conjugated with GSH, glucuronides, or sulfate esters. Phase one biotransformation of PAHs can also result in dihydrodiols, phenols, and quinones. The half-life of PAHs in humans ranges from 2.5 to 6.1 hours.[27] Clearly, humans are good at detoxifying PAHs. Unfortunately, a substantial portion of the population is constantly exposed.

Clinical Significance

Mortality. Increased mortality has been associated with elevated levels of PM_{10}. Persons living in larger cities are 15% to 17% more likely to die prematurely than people living in cities with cleaner air. In Phoenix, Arizona, cardiovascular mortality was significantly associated with $PM_{2.5}$, PM_{10}, and elemental carbon.[28]

Cardiovascular. PM_{10} was found to lead to increased levels of platelets and fibrinogen[29] and C reactive protein.[30] PM exposure has been associated with indicators of autonomic function of the heart, including increased heart rate, decreased heart rate variability, and increased cardiac arrhythmias. Several markers of increased risk for sudden cardiac death have also been associated with PM exposure.[31] In older (>65 years of age) residents of Tokyo, ambient levels of PM_{10} were positively associated with hospital admissions for angina, cardiac insufficiency, hypertension, myocardial infarction, asthma, chronic bronchitis, and pneumonia.[32]

Living close to a major roadway alone confers increased risk of dying from a myocardial infarction (MI). By collecting data on home location from 3886 persons presenting to hospitals with acute MI, it was found that those living between 200 and 1000 meters from a major roadway were 13% more likely to have a fatal MI than were those living more than 1000 meters away. If they lived 100 to 200 meters from a major roadway, they were 19% more likely to die from an MI. Those who lived closest to high traffic (within 100 meters) had the highest risk of dying from an MI, with an odds ratio (OR) of 1.27.[33] And, although PM from vehicular exhaust is clearly associated with cardiovascular disease, PM from cooking fires is thought to be a main factor in cardiovascular disease (CVD) evident in ancient mummies.[34]

Neoplasia. Lung cancer risk for persons occupationally exposed to diesel exhaust, the greatest source of $PM_{0.1}$, was 19% to 68% higher than for those who were non-exposed, whereas gasoline exhaust had only a weakly positive and nonsignificant association with lung cancer.[35] Squamous cell and large cell carcinomas were higher in those exposed to diesel exhaust. Similar risk values were found in Canadians; moderate exposure to diesel exhaust showed a 20% increased risk for lung cancer, while those with greater diesel exposure showed a 60% increased risk.[36] Various components of air pollution have also been closely linked to increased rates of mortality from lung cancer.[37,38,39] Both men and women had higher rates of lung cancer with increasing levels of PM_{10} (Odd ratio (OR) 5.21 for men and OR 1.21 for women).

Respiratory. Children in the Netherlands living within 100 m of a freeway (with high truck traffic) had significantly more cough, wheeze, rhinitis, and diagnosed asthma than those living farther away.[40] Italian researchers found that the amount of truck traffic on the streets where the children resided was significantly associated with increased risk of bronchitis (OR 1.69), bronchiolitis (OR 1.74), and pneumonia (OR 1.84) as well as persistent phlegm (OR 1.68) and wheezing (OR 1.86) that was severe enough to limit speech.[41] Another Netherlands study of families living on busy roadways found that girls had a significantly higher risk for wheezing and using respiratory medication.[42] In the same study, adults living on busy streets were 80% more likely to have dyspnea (95% confidence interval (CI) 1.1–3.0). Exposure to higher levels of PM_{10} in Marseilles, France, was associated with higher rates of bronchial hyperreactivity and symptoms of asthma.[43]

Immunological

Direct exposure to diesel exhaust has been linked to the development of asthma, which persists even after exposure ceases.[44] Animal models have revealed that exposure to diesel emission particles increases immunoglobulin E (IgE) responsiveness to ovalbumin.[45] Japanese individuals living along main roads lined with older cedar trees (heavier pollen count) and heavy traffic (heavier DEP exposure) had higher rates of cedar pollen allergy (13.2%) than those living in cedar forest areas with low traffic (5.1%).[46]

Neurological. Exposure to $PM_{2.5}$ has a clear negative association with cognitive development.[47] Children in Mexico City with no clear risk factors for cognitive deficits living in highly $PM_{2.5}$-polluted areas exhibited clear cognitive deficiencies.[48] In older men (average age of 71), increased PM exposure resulted in reduced cognitive functioning; those with the highest level of exposure experienced a mental decline equivalent to 1.9 years of aging.[49] Women between the ages of 70 and 81 with higher long-term exposure to $PM_{2.5}$ and $PM_{2.5-10}$ exhibited a cognitive decline equivalent to 2 years of aging.[50]

INTERVENTION

Avoidance

Home air purifiers—stand-alone electrical units containing pleated electrostatic HVAC filters for individual rooms—have been studied for their effectiveness. A minimum efficiency rating value (MERV) 12–containing unit rated for 150 square feet reduced $PM_{2.5}$ levels by 57%, and the residents experienced a drop in inflammatory markers and both systolic and diastolic blood pressure (Table 33.3).[51] Similar units in homes of smokers produced a significant ($>30 \ \mu g/m^3$) reduction in mean levels of $PM_{0.1}$, $PM_{2.5}$, and PM_{10}.[52] In addition, the average FEV_1 of the occupants increased by 217 mL, systolic blood pressure dropped by 7.9 mm Hg, and diastolic dropped by 4.5 mm Hg.

Introducing HEPA units with only 60% effectiveness at clearing PM into homes in an area with high levels of wood smoke reduced indoor levels of $PM_{2.5}$.[53] After only 7 days of using the units, the residents of those homes had a 9.4% improvement in endothelial function and a 32.6% average drop in their high-sensitivity C-reactive protein (hs-CRP) levels.[54] Other commercially available HEPA units have reduced indoor $PM_{2.5}$ levels between 40% and 50%.[55,56] Such units have roughly the same effectiveness at clearing $PM_{2.5}$ as the units containing replaceable high-MERV furnace filters, which are far less expensive to replace.

TABLE 33.3 Reduction in Blood Pressure and Inflammatory Markers After 48 Hours of Residence in a Room with a MERV 12 Filter Unit

Cardiovascular	Biomarkers
Systolic pressure – avg. 2.7 mm Hg drop Diastolic pressure – avg. 4.8% mm Hg drop Exhaled nitrous oxide – 17% drop	IL-1B – 58% reduction Soluble CD40 ligand – 55% reduction Myeloperoxidase – 33% reduction Monocyte chemoattractant protein 1–17.5% reduction

Data from Chen, R., Zhao, A., Chen, H., Zhao, Z., Cai, J., Wang, C., et al. (2015). Cardiopulmonary benefits of reducing indoor particles of outdoor origin: a randomized, double-blind crossover trial of air purifiers. *Journal of the American College of Cardiology, 65*(21), 2279–2287.

Antioxidants

Because these pollutants cause so much oxidative damage, dietary antioxidants, supplements, botanical agents, and fish oil have been used to alleviate their toxic effects. Women who consume more fruits and vegetables in their diets have lower levels of DNA adducts and are less likely to have low-birth-weight babies even though they have high PAH exposure.[57] Broccoli intake reduces DNA damage in smokers by 41%[58] and is also associated with a reduction of lung cancer incidence of up to 22%.[59]

Persons with higher serum levels of vitamins C and E are not as likely to have increased asthma or chronic obstructive pulmonary disease (COPD) events when the ambient level of $PM_{2.5}$ increases.[60] Female smokers taking only 500 mg of vitamin C and 400 IU of vitamin E daily had a 31% drop in BaP DNA adducts.[61] Those smokers who had intact GSTM1 genes and took antioxidant vitamins had a 43% reduction in DNA adducts.

Curcumin can prevent the powerful prooxidant effects of BaP and enhance levels of GSH and the activity of GSH peroxidase, GSH reductase, GSH transferase, superoxide dismutase, and catalase.[62] These actions resulted in lower BaP-DNA adducts in animals given curcumin. The application of green or black tea to ground meat before cooking prevented the production of mutagenic PAH compounds that normally occur with cooking.[63] Heavy smokers who consumed 4 cups of decaffeinated green tea daily had significant drops in their urinary 8-OHdG levels, while all the other groups had an increase in DNA oxidative damage.[64]

When fish oil capsules were given to elderly nursing home residents in Mexico City, the typical PAH-induced depletion of GSH levels and superoxide dismutase activity was greatly diminished.[65] A dose of 3 grams of fish oil daily was also found to block the adverse cardiac effects of PAHs in a group of middle-aged adults.[66] Although even small fluctuations in $PM_{2.5}$ levels can affect heart-rate variability, 2 grams of fish oil daily were able to attenuate that effect in elderly individuals.[67]

REFERENCES

1. Yu, J. Z., Huang, X. H., Ho, S. S., & Bian, Q. (2011). Nonpolar organic compounds in fine particles: Quantification by thermal desorption-GC/MS and evidence for their significant oxidation in ambient aerosols in Hong Kong. *Analytical and Bioanalytical Chemistry*, *401*(10), 3125–3139. PubMed PMID: 21983947.
2. Oberdorster, G., Sharp, Z., Atudorel, V., et al. (2002). Extrapulmonary translocation of ultrafine carbon particles following whole-body inhalation exposure of rats. *Journal of Toxicology and Environmental Health. Part A*, *65*(20), 1531–1543. PubMed PMID: 12396867.
3. Oberdorster, G., Sharp, Z., Atudorel, V., et al. (2004). Translocation of inhaled ultrafine particles to the brain. *Inhalation Toxicology*, *16*(607), 437–445. PubMed PMID: 15204759.
4. Takenaka, S., Karg, E., Roth, C., et al. (2001). Pulmonary and systemic distribution of inhaled ultrafine silver particles in rats. *Environmental Health Perspectives*, *109*(Suppl. 4), 547–551. PubMed PMID: 11544161.
5. Semmler, M., Seitz, J., Erbe, R., et al. (2004). Long-term clearance kinetics of inhaled ultrafine insoluble iridium particles from the rat lung, including transient translocation into secondary organs. *Inhalation Toxicology*, *16*(6–7), 453–459. PubMed PMID: 15204761.
6. Yu, J. Z., Huang, X. H., Ho, S. S., & Bian, Q. (2011). Nonpolar organic compounds in fine particles: Quantification by thermal desorption-GC/MS and evidence for their significant oxidation in ambient aerosols in Hong Kong. *Analytical and Bioanalytical Chemistry*, *401*(10), 3125–3139. PubMed PMID: 21983947.
7. Oh, S. M., Kim, H. R., Park, Y. J., et al. (2011). Organic extracts of urban air pollution particulate matter (PM2.5)-induced genotoxicity and oxidative stress in human lung bronchial epithelial cells (BEAS-2B cells). *Mutation Research*, *723*(2), 142–151. PubMed PMID: 21524716.
8. Frikke-Schmidt, H., Roursgaard, M., Lykkesfeldt, J., et al. (2011). Effect of vitamin C and iron chelation on diesel exhaust particle and carbon black induced oxidative damage and cell adhesion molecule expression in human endothelial cells. *Toxicology Letters*, *203*(3), 181–189. PubMed PMID: 21421028.
9. Harrison, C. M., Pompilius, M., Pinkerton, K. E., & Ballinger, S. W. (2011). Mitochondrial oxidative stress significantly influences atherogenic risk and cytokine-induced oxidant production. *Environmental Health Perspectives*, *119*(5), 676–681. PubMed PMID: 21169125.
10. Zhang, P., Dong, G., Sun, B., et al. (2011). Long-term exposure to ambient air pollution and mortality due to cardiovascular disease and cerebrovascular disease in Shenyang, China. *PLoS ONE*, *6*(6), e20827. PubMed PMID: 21695220.

11. Ito, K., Mathes, R., Ross, Z., et al. (2011). Fine particulate matter constituents associated with cardiovascular hospitalizations and mortality in New York City. *Environmental Health Perspectives, 119*, 467–473. PubMed PMID: 21463978.

12. Guaita, R., Pichiule, M., Maté, T., Linares, C., & Díaz, J. (2011). Short-term impact of particulate matter (PM(2.5)) on respiratory mortality in Madrid. *International Journal of Environmental Health Research, 21*(4), 260–274. PubMed PMID: 21644129.

13. Katanoda, K., Sobue, T., Satoh, H., et al. (2011). An association between long-term exposure to ambient air pollution and mortality from lung cancer and respiratory diseases in Japan. *Journal of Epidemiology, 21*(2), 132–143. PubMed PMID: 21325732.

14. Shah, P. P., Singh, A. P., Singh, M., et al. (2008). Interaction of cytochrome P4501A1 genotypes with other risk factors and susceptibility to lung cancer. *Mutation Research, 639*(1–2), 1–10. PubMed PMID: 18082227.

15. Al-Humadi, N. H., Siegel, P. D., Lewis, D. M., et al. (2002). Alteration of intracellular cysteine and glutathione levels in alveolar macrophages and lymphocytes by diesel exhaust particle exposure. *Environmental Health Perspectives, 110*(4), 349–353. PubMed PMID: 11940452.

16. Oz, F., & Yuzer, M. O. (2016). The effects of cooking on wire and stone barbecue at different cooking levels on the formation of heterocyclic aromatic amines and polycyclic aromatic hydrocarbons in beef steak. *Food Chemistry, 203*, 59–66. PubMed PMID: 26948589.

17. Air Quality Expert Group. (2005). *Particulate matter in the United Kingdom*. London; Defra. http://webarchive.nationalarchives.gov.uk/20130402151656/http://archive.defra.gov.uk/environment/quality/air/airquality/publications/particulate-matter/index.htm. (Accessed April 23, 2017.)

18. Xia, T., Kovochich, M., & Nel, A. E. (2007). Impairment of mitochondrial function by particulate matter (PM) and their toxic components: Implications for PM-induced cardiovascular and lung disease. *Frontiers in Bioscience, 12*, 1238–1246. PubMed PMID: 17127377.

19. Jiang, Y., Zhou, X., Chen, X., et al. (2011). Benzo(a)pyrene-induced mitochondrial dysfunction and cell death in p53-null Hep3B cells. *Mutation Research, 726*(1), 75–83. PubMed PMID: 21911080.

20. Centers for Disease Control and Prevention, Agency for Toxic Substances & Disease Registry. *Toxic Substances Portal: Polycyclic Aromatic Hydrocarbons (PAHs)*. Public Health Statement for Polycyclic Aromatic Hydrocarbons (PAHs). Available at http://www.atsdr.cdc.gov/PHS/PHS.asp?id=120&tid=25. (Accessed April 23, 2017.)

21. Alexandrov, K., Rojas, M., & Satarug, S. (2010). The critical DNA damage by benzo(a)pyrene in lung tissues of smokers and approaches to preventing its formation. *Toxicology Letters, 198*(1), 63–68. PubMed PMID: 20399842.

22. Armstrong, B., Hutchinson, E., Unwin, J., & Fletcher, T. (2004). Lung cancer risk after exposure to polycyclic aromatic hydrocarbons: A review and meta-analysis. *Environmental Health Perspectives, 112*(9), 970–978. PubMed PMID: 15198916.

23. Fracktracker alliance. Oil and Gas Information by location. https://www.fracktracker.org/map/. (Accessed January 29, 2017.)

24. Swarthout, R. F., Russo, R. S., Zhou, Y., et al. (2015). Impact of Marcellus Shale natural gas development in southwest Pennsylvania on volatile organic compound emissions and regional air quality. *Environmental Science & Technology, 49*(5), 3175–3184. PubMed PMID: 25594231.

25. Field, R., Soltis, J., McCarthy, M., Murphy, S., & Montague, D. (2015). Influence of oil and gas field operations on spatial and temporal distributions of atmospheric non-methane hydrocarbons and their effect on ozone formation in winter. *Atmospheric Chemistry and Physics, 15*, 3527–3542.

26. Centers for Disease Control and Prevention. (January 2017). *National Report on Human Exposure to Environmental Chemicals: Updated Tables*. Available at www.cdc.gov/exposurereport/. (Accessed October 25, 2017.)

27. Li, Z., Romanoff, L., Bartell, S., et al. (2012). Excretion profiles and half-lives of ten urinary polycyclic aromatic hydrocarbon metabolites after dietary exposure. *Chemical Research in Toxicology, 25*(7), 1452–1461. PubMed PMID: 22663094.

28. Mar, T. F., Norris, G. A., Koenig, J. Q., & Larson, T. V. (2000). Associations between air pollution and mortality in Phoenix, 1995-1997. *Environmental Health Perspectives, 108*(4), 347–353. PubMed PMID: 10753094.

29. Schwartz, J. (2001). Air pollution and blood markers of cardiovascular risk. *Environmental Health Perspectives, 109*(Suppl. 3), 405–409. PubMed PMID: 11427390.

30. Donaldson, K., Stone, V., Seaton, A., & MacNee, W. (2001). Ambient particle inhalation and cardiovascular system: Potential mechanisms. *Environmental Health Perspectives, 109*(Suppl. 40), 523–527. PubMed PMID: 11544157.

31. Dockery, D. W. (2001). Epidemiologic evidence of cardiovascular effects of particulate air pollution. *Environmental Health Perspectives, 109*(Suppl. 4), 483–486. PubMed PMID: 11544151.

32. Ye, F., Piver, W. T., Ando, M., & Portier, C. J. (2001). Effects of temperature and air pollutants on cardiovascular and respiratory diseases for males and females older than 65 years of age in Tokyo, July and August 1980-1995. *Environmental Health Perspectives*, *109*(4), 355–359. PubMed PMID: 11335183.

33. Rosenbloom, J. I., Wilker, E. H., Mukamal, K. J., Schwartz, J., & Mittleman, M. A. (2012). Residential proximity to major roadway and 10-year all-cause mortality after myocardial infarction. *Circulation*, *125*(18), 2197–2203. PubMed PMID: 22566348.

34. Thompson, R. C., Allam, A. H., Lombardi, G. P., et al. (2013). Atherosclerosis across 4000 years of human history: The Horus study of four ancient populations. *Lancet*, *381*(9873), 1211–1222. PubMed PMID: 23489753.

35. Velleneuve, P. J., Parent, M. E., Sahni, V., Johnson, K. C., & Canadian Cancer Registries Epidemiology Research Group. (2011). Occupational exposure to diesel and gasoline exhaust emissions and lung cancer in Canadian men. *Environmental Research*, *111*(5), 727–735. PubMed PMID: 2156265.

36. Parent, M. E., Rousseau, M. C., Boffetta, P., Cohen, A., & Siemiatycki, J. (2007). Exposure to diesel and gasoline engine emissions and the risk of lung cancer. *American Journal of Epidemiology*, *165*(1), 53–62. PubMed PMID: 17062632.

37. Reymão, M. S., Cury, P. M., Lichtenfels, A. J., et al. (1997). Urban air pollution enhances the formation of urethane-induced lung tumors in mice. *Environmental Research*, *74*(2), 150–158. PubMed PMID: 9339228.

38. Tokiwa, H., Nakanishi, Y., Sera, N., Hara, N., & Inuzuka, S. (1998). Analysis of environmental carcinogens associated with the incidence of lung cancer. *Toxicology Letters*, *99*, 33–41. PubMed PMID: 9801028.

39. Biggeri, A., Barbone, F., Lagazio, C., Bovenzi, M., & Stanta, G. (1996). Air pollution and lung cancer in Trieste, Italy: Spatial analysis of risk as a function of distance from sources. *Environmental Health Perspectives*, *104*, 750–754. PubMed PMID: 8841761.

40. Van Vliet, P., Knape, M., de Hartog, J., et al. (1977). Motor vehicle exhaust and chronic respiratory symptoms in children living near freeways. *Environmental Research*, *74*, 122–132. PubMed PMID: 9339225.

41. Ciccone, G., Forastiere, F., Agabiti, N., et al. (1998). Road traffic and adverse respiratory effects in children. SIDRIA Collaborative Group. *Occupational and Environmental Medicine*, *55*(11), 771–778. PubMed PMID: 9924455.

42. Oosterlee, A., Drijver, M., Lebret, E., & Brunekreef, B. (1966). Chronic respiratory symptoms in children and adults living along streets with high traffic density. *Occupational and Environmental Medicine*, *53*, 241–247. PubMed PMID: 8664961.

43. Jammes, Y., Delpierre, S., Delvolgo, M. J., Humbert-Tena, C., & Burnet, H. (1998). Long-term exposure of adults to outdoor air pollution is associated with increased airway obstruction and higher prevalence of bronchial hyper responsiveness. *Archives of Environmental Health*, *53*(6), 372–377. PubMed PMID: 9886154.

44. Wade, J. F., & Newman, L. S. (1993). Diesel asthma, reactive airway disease following overexposure to locomotive exhaust. *Journal of Occupational Medicine*, *35*(2), 149–154. PubMed PMID: 8433186.

45. Takafuji, S., Suzuki, S., Koizumi, K., et al. (1987). Diesel-exhaust particulates inoculated by the intranasal route have and adjuvant activity for IgE production in mice. *The Journal of Allergy and Clinical Immunology*, *79*, 639–645. PubMed PMID 2435776.

46. Ishizaki, T., Koizumi, K., Ikemori, R., et al. (1987). Studies of prevalence of Japanese cedar pollinosis among residents in a densely cultivated area. *Annals of Allergy*, *58*, 265–270. PubMed PMID: 3565861.

47. Basagaña, X., Esnaola, M., Rivas, I., et al. (2016). Neurodevelopmental deceleration by urban fine particles from different emission sources: a longitudinal observational study. *Environmental Health Perspectives*, *124*(10), 1630–1636. PubMed PMID: 27128166.

48. Calderón-Garcidueñas, L., Mora-Tiscareño, A., Ontiveros, E., Gómez-Garza, G., et al. (2008). Air pollution, cognitive deficits and brain abnormalities: A pilot study with children and dogs. *Brain and Cognition*, *68*(2), 117–127. PubMed PMID: 18550243.

49. Power, M. C., Weisskopf, M. G., Alexeeff, S. E., Coull, B. A., Spiro, A., 3rd, & Schwartz, J. (2011). Traffic-related air pollution and cognitive function in a cohort of older men. *Environmental Health Perspectives*, *119*(5), 682–687. PubMed PMID: 21172758.

50. Weuve, J., Puett, R. C., Schwartz, J., Yanosky, J. D., Laden, F., & Grodstein, F. (2012). Exposure to particulate air pollution and cognitive decline in older women. *Archives of Internal Medicine*, *172*(3), 219–227. PubMed PMID: 22332151.

51. Chen, R., Zhao, A., Chen, H., Zhao, Z., Cai, J., Wang, C., et al. (2015). Cardiopulmonary benefits of reducing indoor particles of outdoor origin: A randomized, double-blind crossover trial of air purifiers. *Journal of the American College of Cardiology*, *65*(21), 2279–2287. PubMed PMID: 26022815.

52. Weichenthal, S., Mallach, G., Kulka, R., Black, A., Wheeler, A., You, H., et al. (2013). A randomized double-blind crossover study of indoor air filtration and acute changes in cardiorespiratory health in a First

Nations community. *Indoor Air*, *23*(3), 175–184. PubMed PMID: 23210563.

53. McNamara, M. L., Thornburg, J., Semmens, E. O., Ward, T. J., & Noonan, C. W. (2017). Reducing indoor air pollutants with air filtration units in wood stove homes. *The Science of the Total Environment*, *592*, 488–494. PubMed PMID: 28320525.

54. Allen, R. W., Carlsten, C., Karlen, B., Leckie, S., van Eeden, S., Vedal, S., et al. (2011). An air filter intervention study of endothelial function among healthy adults in a woodsmoke-impacted community. *American Journal of Respiratory and Critical Care Medicine*, *183*(9), 1222–1230. PubMed PMID: 21257787.

55. Kajbafzadeh, M., Brauer, M., Karlen, B., Carlsten, C., van Eeden, S., & Allen, R. W. (2015). The impacts of traffic-related and woodsmoke particulate matter on measures of cardiovascular health: A HEPA filter intervention study. *Occupational and Environmental Medicine*, *72*(6), 394–400. PubMed PMID: 25896330.

56. Karottki, D. G., Spilak, M., Frederiksen, M., Gunnarsen, L., Brauner, E. V., Kolarik, B., et al. (2013). An indoor air filtration study in homes of elderly: Cardiovascular and respiratory effects of exposure to particulate matter. *Environmental Health: A Global Access Science Source*, *12*, 116. PubMed PMID: 24373585.

57. Pedersen, M., Schoket, B., Godschalk, R. W., et al. (2013). Bulky DNA adducts in cord blood, maternal fruit-and-vegetable consumption, and birth weight in a European mother-child study (NewGeneris). *Environmental Health Perspectives*, *121*(10), 1200–1206. PubMed PMID: 23906905.

58. Riso, P., Martini, D., Møller, P., et al. (2010). DNA damage and repair activity after broccoli intake in young healthy smokers. *Mutagenesis*, *25*(6), 595–602. PubMed PMID: 20713433.

59. Lam, T. K., Gallicchio, L., Lindsley, K., et al. (2009). Cruciferous vegetable consumption and lung cancer risk: A systematic review. *Cancer Epidemiology, Biomarkers and Prevention*, *18*(1), 184–195. PubMed PMID: 19124497.

60. Canova, C., Dunster, C., Kelly, F. J., et al. (2012). PM10-induced hospital admissions for asthma and chronic obstructive pulmonary disease: The modifying effect of individual characteristics. *Epidemiology*, *23*(4), 607–615. PubMed PMID: 22531667.

61. Mooney, L. A., Madsen, A. M., Tang, D., et al. (2005). Antioxidant vitamin supplementation reduces benzo(a) pyrene-DNA adducts and potential cancer risk in female smokers. *Cancer Epidemiology, Biomarkers and Prevention*, *14*(1), 237–242. PubMed PMID: 15668500.

62. Sehgal, A., Kumar, M., Jain, M., & Dhawan, D. K. (2013). Modulatory effects of curcumin in conjunction with piperine on benzo(a)pyrene-mediated DNA adducts and biotransformation enzymes. *Nutrition and Cancer*, *65*(6), 885–890. PubMed PMID: 23909733.

63. Weisburger, J. H., Veliath, E., Larios, E., et al. (2002). polyphenols inhibit the formation of mutagens during the cooking of meat. *Mutation Research*, *516*(1–2), 19–22. PubMed PMID: 11943606.

64. Hakim, I. A., Harris, R. B., Chow, H. H., et al. (2004). Effect of a 4-month tea intervention on oxidative DNA damage among heavy smokers: Role of glutathione S-transferase genotypes. *Cancer Epidemiology, Biomarkers and Prevention*, *13*(2), 242–249. PubMed PMID: 14973088.

65. Romieu, I., Garcia-Esteban, R., Sunyer, J., et al. (2008). The effect of supplementation with omega-3 polyunsaturated fatty acids on markers of oxidative stress in elderly exposed to PM(2.5). *Environmental Health Perspectives*, *116*(9), 1237–1242. PubMed PMID: 18795169.

66. Tong, H., Rappold, A. G., Diaz-Sanchez, D., et al. (2012). Omega-3 fatty acid supplementation appears to attenuate particulate air pollution-induced cardiac effects and lipid changes in healthy middle-aged adults. *Environmental Health Perspectives*, *120*(7), 952–957. PubMed PMID: 22514211.

67. Romieu, I., Téllez-Rojo, M. M., Lazo, M., et al. (2005). Omega-3 fatty acid prevents heart rate variability reductions associated with particulate matter. *American Journal of Respiratory and Critical Care Medicine*, *172*(12), 1533–1540. PubMed PMID: 16210665.

34

Sulfur and Nitrogen Oxides

SUMMARY

- Presence in population: Ubiquitous
- Major disease: Lung cancer, reduced cell-mediated immunity, allergies, asthma, chronic obstructive pulmonary disease (COPD), hypertension, acute myocardial infarction (MI)

- Primary sources: Vehicular exhaust, coal fired power plants, volcanoes, smoking
- Best measure: Currently no measure for these ubiquitous air pollutants exists
- Best intervention: Indoor air purification

DESCRIPTION

Sulfur and nitrogen oxides are two of the six most common and most damaging pollutants that the US Environmental Protection Agency (EPA) has listed as Criteria Air Pollutants criteria air pollutants (CAPs). The other four major pollutants are particle pollution (see Chapter 6, Outdoor Air Pollution), ground level ozone, carbon monoxide, and lead. These six are called "criteria" air pollutants because their permissible levels are derived from either human health–based or environment-based criteria (i.e., science-based guidelines; Box 34.1). These criteria are referred to as "primary" when they are based on human health outcomes and "secondary" when they are associated with environmental or property damage.[1]

TOXICITY

Sulfur Oxides

If contaminated with sulfur, combustion of fossil fuels produces a number of sulfur oxide gasses, the most common of which is sulfur dioxide (SO_2), shown in Fig. 34.1. Seventy-three percent of all SO_2 emissions come from coal-fired power plants with another 20% from industrial facilities. Volcanoes are the only natural source for SO_2. The EPA first set a 24-hour standard of 140 parts per billion (PPB) for SO_2 in 1971. The 3-hour average

was set at 500 PPB, and an annual average was set at 30 PPB.[2] Sulfur oxides in the atmosphere can be transformed to H_2SO_4, the primary component in acid rain.

Nitrogen Oxides

There are two major nitrogen oxide air pollutants, nitrogen dioxide (NO_2) and nitric oxide (NO), both of which are produced by combustion from vehicles, stationary sources, appliances, and smoking (Fig. 34.2). Nitrogen oxides can react other airborne chemicals in with sunlight resulting in the production of acid rain or smog.

SOURCES

Burning fossil fuels releases sulfur and nitrogen oxide, and using gas stoves or smoking releases other nitrogen oxides.

BODY BURDEN

Oxides of sulfur and nitrogen have not yet been assessed by the Centers for Disease Control and Prevention (CDC).

Detoxification/Excretion Processes

Sulfur oxides rapidly change into sulfites, bisulfites, and hydrogen ions in the body. Sulfite oxidase can then act on these sulfites to produce sulfates that are rapidly

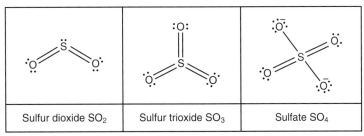

FIG. 34.1 Common sulfur oxide structures.

Sulfur dioxide SO$_2$	Sulfur trioxide SO$_3$	Sulfate SO$_4$

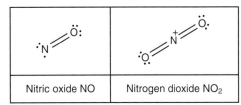

FIG. 34.2 Common nitrogen oxide structures.

Nitric oxide NO	Nitrogen dioxide NO$_2$

BOX 34.1   The Six Environmental Protection Agency Criteria Air Pollutants

- Particulate Matter
- Ozone
- Carbon monoxide
- Sulfur oxides
- Nitrogen oxides
- Lead

excreted in urine. SO_2 can also be conjugated with glutathione, the metabolites of which will also be cleared through urine.

Clinical Significance

Outdoor air levels of SO_2 have been associated with increased rates of asthma in French children,[3] and industrial exposure to SO_2 was associated with bronchial hyperresponsiveness and a reduced forced expiratory volume in 1 second (FEV_1)/forced vital capacity (FVC) ratio.[4] In Taiwanese children, SO_2 levels were associated with increased incidence of asthma and of contracting the flu.[5] Maternal exposure to SO_2 has also been associated with a greater risk of a preterm delivery[6] and of having a low-birth-weight baby.[7]

Nitrogen dioxide is a powerful respiratory irritant that can lead to asthma, decreased lung function, pulmonary edema, and diffuse lung injury.[8] Emergency room visits for asthma are increased 1 to 5 days after outdoor levels of NO_2 spike.[9,10] Nitrogen dioxide exposure in individuals with allergenic tendencies increases their reactivity to airborne pollens.[11,12] These individuals will then react allergically to levels of pollen that previously did not induce a reaction. At least part of this allergic sensitization occurs because NO_2 increases eosinophil activation.[13] Low levels of nitrogen oxides in the air can cause eye, nose, throat, and lung irritation and inflammation. Clinical

presentations can include cough, shortness of breath, fatigue, and nausea.[14] Exposure to low levels can also result in fluid build-up in the lungs 1 or 2 days after exposure.

Mortality. Increased mortality has been associated with elevated levels of particulate matter >10 microns in diameter (PM_{10}). Persons living in larger cities are 15% to 17% more likely to die a prematurely than are people who live in cities with cleaner air. In Phoenix, Arizona, total a study showed that mortality was significantly associated with ambient SO_2 and NO_2 levels. Cardiovascular mortality was significantly associated with CO, NO_2, SO_2, particulate matter >2.5 microns in diameter $PM_{2.5}$, PM_{10}, and elemental carbon.[15] In Sao Paulo, Brazil, 15% of the deaths were attributable to CO, 13% to SO_2, and 7% to PM_{10}.[16] In Sydney, Australia, increased mortality has been found with exposures to PM, ozone, and NO_2.[17]

Neoplasia. Ambient air pollution has also been linked to increased risk of lung cancer in nonsmoking adults in California. Both men and women had higher rates of lung cancer with increasing levels SO_2 (odds ratio (OR) 2.66 for men and OR 2.14 for women).[18]

Immune. Children living in areas with high SO_2 and NO_2 were found to have higher rates of asthma, rhinitis, eczema, and conjunctivitis.[19] Exposing mice to a mixture of ozone and NO_2 reduced cell-mediated immune response (CMI). Daily 3-hour exposure to 0.5 parts per million (PPM) of NO_2 and 0.1 PPM of ozone resulted in the highest drop in CMI, as evidenced by increased mortality rates and shortened survival time after exposure to streptococcal pneumonia.[20]

Respiratory. Men living in downtown Marseilles, France had higher rates of bronchial hyperreactivity and symptoms of asthma that were significantly associated with the NO_2 and PM_{10} levels.[21] NO_2 peaks are clearly associated with increased asthmatic prevalence.[22] Expectant mothers with asthma are also more likely to experience a preterm delivery when NO levels are high.[23] In asthmatics, exposure to SO_2 after ozone exposure (0.120 PPM for 45 min) resulted in a significant decrease in FEV and maximal flow at 50% of FVC (Vmax50) (compared with FEV and Vmax50 without ozone preexposure).[24] Spikes in SO_2 increase the risk for hospitalization with COPD, upper respiratory tract infections, and acute MI.[25,26]

Cardiovascular. Elevated levels of SO_2 are significantly associated with both hypertension and acute MIs.[23,27]

INTERVENTION

The best intervention is the use of high quality air purifiers in indoor spaces.

REFERENCES

1. U.S. Environmental Protection Agency. *Criteria Air Pollutants*. Available at https://www.epa.gov/criteria-air-pollutants (Accessed 24 April 2017).
2. U.S. Environmental Protection Agency. *Reviewing National Ambient Air Quality Standards (NAAQS): Scientific and Technical Information*. Available at https://www.epa.gov/naaqs (Accessed 23 April 2017).
3. Penard-Morand, C., Charpin, D., Raherison, C., et al. (2005). Long-term exposure to background air pollution related to respiratory and allergic health in schoolchildren. *Clinical and Experimental Allergy: Journal of the British Society for Allergy and Clinical Immunology, 35*(10), 1279–1287. PubMed PMID: 16238786.
4. Abramson, M. J., Benke, G. P., Cui, J., et al. (2010). Is potroom asthma due more to sulphur dioxide than fluoride? An inception cohort study in the Australian aluminium industry. *Occupational and Environmental Medicine, 67*(10), 679–685. PubMed PMID: 20798006.
5. Liao, C. M., Hsieh, N. H., & Chio, C. P. (2011). Fluctuation analysis-based risk assessment for respiratory virus activity and air pollution associated asthma incidence. *The Science of the Total Environment, 409*(18), 3325–3333. PubMed PMID: 21663946.
6. Sagiv, S. K., Mendola, P., Loomis, D., et al. (2005). A time-series analysis of air pollution and preterm birth in Pennsylvania, 1997-2001. *Environmental Health Perspectives, 113*(5), 602–606. PubMed PMID: 15866770.
7. Dugandzic, R., Dodds, L., Steib, D., & Smith-Doiron, M. (2006). The association between low level exposures to ambient air pollution and term low birth weight: a retrospective cohort study. *Environmental Health: A Global Access Science Source, 5*, 3. (PubMed PMID: 16503975).
8. U.S. Environmental Protection Agency. *Indoor Air Quality (IAQ): Nitrogen Dioxide's Impact on Indoor Air Quality*. Available at https://www.epa.gov/indoor-air-quality-iaq/nitrogen-dioxides-impact-indoor-air-quality (Accessed 15 November 2017).
9. Pereira, G., Cook, A., De Vos, A. J., & Holman, C. D. (2010). A case-crossover analysis of traffic-related air pollution and emergency department presentations for asthma in Perth, Western Australia. *The Medical Journal of Australia, 193*(9), 511–514. PubMed PMID: 21034384.
10. Krmpoti, D., Luzar-Stiffler, V., Rakusic, N., et al. (2011). Effects of traffic air pollution and hornbeam pollen on adult asthma hospitalizations in Zagreb. *International Archives of Allergy and Immunology, 156*(1), 62–68. PubMed PMID: 21447960.
11. Strand, V., Svartengren, M., Rak, S., Barck, C., & Bylin, G. (1998). Repeated exposure to an ambient level of NO2 enhances asthmatic response to a nonsymptomatic allergen dose. *The European respiratory journal, 12*(1), 6–12. PubMed PMID: 9701406.
12. Wang, J. H., Devalia, J. L., Duddle, J. M., et al. (1995). Effects of six-hour exposure to nitrogen dioxide on early phase nasal response to allergen challenge in patients with a history of seasonal allergic rhinitis. *The Journal of Allergy and Clinical Immunology, 96*(5 Pt. 1), 669–676. PubMed PMID: 7599684.
13. Wang, J. H., Duddle, J., Devalia, J. L., & Davies, R. J. (1995). Nitrogen dioxide increases eosinophil activation in the early-phase response to nasal allergen provocation. *International Archives of Allergy and Immunology, 107*(1–3), 103–105. PubMed PMID: 7613114.
14. Agency for Toxic Substances and Disease Registry. *Nitrogen oxide toxicological fact sheets*. https://

www.atsdr.cdc.gov/toxfaqs/tf.asp?id=396&tid=69 (Accessed 30 July 2017).

15. Mar, T. F., Norris, G. A., Koenig, J. Q., & Larson, T. V. (2000). Associations between air pollution and mortality in Phoenix, 1995-1997. *Environmental Health Perspectives*, 108(4), 347–353. PubMed PMID: 10753094.

16. Coneicao, G. M. S., Miraglia, S. G. E. K., Kishi, H. S., et al. (2001). Air pollution and child mortality: a time-series study in Sao Paulo, Brazil. *Environmental Health Perspectives*, 109(Suppl. 3), 347–350. PubMed PMID: 11427383.

17. Morgan, G., Corbett, S., Wlodarczyk, J., & Lewis, P. (1998). Air pollution and daily mortality in Sydney, Australia, 1989 through 1993. *American journal of public health*, 88, 759–764. PubMed PMID: 9585741.

18. Beeson, W. L., Abbey, D. E., & Knutsen, S. F. (1998). Long-term concentrations of ambient air pollutants and incident lung cancer in California adults: results from the AHSMOG study. Adventist Health Study on Smog. *Environmental Health Perspectives*, 106(12), 813–822. PubMed PMID: 9831542.

19. Kim, Y. K., Baek, D., Koh, Y. I., et al. (2001). Outdoor air pollutants derived from industrial processes may be causally related to the development of asthma in children. *Annals of Allergy, Asthma and Immunology*, 86(4), 456–460. PubMed PMID: 11345292.

20. Ehrlich, R., & Findlay, J. C. (1979). Effects of repeated exposures to peak concentrations of nitrogen dioxide and ozone on resistance to streptococcal pneumonia. *Journal of Toxicology and Environmental Health*, 5, 621–642. PubMed PMID: 385895.

21. Jammes, Y., Delpierre, S., Delvolgo, M. J., et al. (1998). Long-term exposure of adults to outdoor air pollution in associated with increased airway obstruction and higher prevalence of bronchial hyper responsiveness. *Archives of Environmental Health*, 53(6), 372–377. PubMed PMID: 9886154.

22. Greenberg, N., Carel, R. S., Derazne, E., et al. (2017). Modeling long-term effects attributed to nitrogen dioxide (NO_2) and sulfur dioxide (SO_2) exposure on asthma morbidity in a nationwide cohort in Israel. *Journal of Toxicology and Environmental Health. Part A*, 80(6), 326–337. PubMed PMID: 28644724.

23. Mendola, P., Wallace, M., Hwang, B. S., et al. (2016). Preterm birth and air pollution: Critical windows of exposure for women with asthma. *The Journal of Allergy and Clinical Immunology*, 138(2), 432–440, e5. PubMed PMID: 26944405.

24. Koenig, J. Q., Covert, D. S., Hanley, W. S., et al. (1990). Prior exposure to ozone potentiates subsequent response to sulfur dioxide in adolescent asthmatic subjects. *The American Review of Respiratory Disease*, 141, 377–380. PubMed PMID: 2301855.

25. Khaniabadi, Y. O., Daryanoosh, S. M., Hopke, P. K., et al. (2017). Acute myocardial infarction and COPD attributed to ambient SO2 in Iran. *Environmental Research*, 156, 683–687. PubMed PMID: 28477578.

26. Li, R., Jiang, N., Liu, Q., et al. (2017). Impact of Air Pollutants on Outpatient Visits for Acute Respiratory Outcomes. *International Journal of Environmental Research and Public Health*, 14(1), PubMed PMID: 28067786.

27. Cai, Y., Zhang, B., Ke, W., et al. (2016). Associations of Short-Term and Long-Term Exposure to Ambient Air Pollutants With Hypertension: A Systematic Review and Meta-Analysis. *Hypertension*, 68(1), 62–70. PubMed PMID: 27245182.

35

Endotoxicity

SUMMARY

- Presence in population: Common
- Major disease: Disruption of xenobiotic biotransformation, endothelial dysfunction, chronic fatigue syndrome, diabetes, nonalcoholic fatty liver disease (NAFLD) and nonalcoholic steatohepatitis (NASH), neuroinflammation, metabolic syndrome, obesity
- Primary sources: Bioaerosols, gram-negative infections, gram negative bowel flora overgrowth
- Best measure: Signs and symptoms, diet diary
- Best intervention: Whole foods or Mediterranean diet, whole food fibers, probiotics, antioxidants, polyphenols

DESCRIPTION

Endotoxins are lipopolysaccharides (LPSs) from the cell walls of gram-negative bacteria such as *Enterobacteriaceae, Neisseriaceae,* and *Pseudomonadaceae.* This term is used to differentiate LPSs from toxic compounds secreted by living organisms called exotoxins. LPSs are composed of two main regions, the oligosaccharide outer shell called O-antigen and the toxic inner phospholipid membrane called lipid-A. The actual carbohydrate and lipid makeup of endotoxins varies between bacterial strains and species with varying degrees of toxicity of the lipid A component. One bacterial cell contains approximately 3.5 million LPS molecules. Upon bacterial cell death, cell wall lysis occurs, releasing LPS to interact with intestinal cell membranes and surface proteins. The outer portion of the O component is typically made up of between four to six hexoses, primarily glucose, galactose, and N-acetyl-glucosamine. The toxic lipid A portion is made up of fatty acids attached to disaccharides (Fig. 35.1).

SOURCES

- Bioaerosols
  - Water-damaged buildings
- Gram-negative bacterial infections
- Gram-negative intestinal bacteria
  - Higher in people with high-fat diets (e.g., the typical Western diet)

Endotoxins are widely present in the external environment, including dust, animal waste, food, and other material exposed to gram-negative bacteria. Airborne endotoxin levels, also called bioaerosols, are often quite high in water-damaged buildings.[1] Inhalation of high levels of endotoxins can cause inflammation in the respiratory tract, resulting in asthma, bronchiectasis, and pneumonia.

Internal sources of endotoxins include gram-negative bacterial infections and gram-negative bowel flora. LPSs are elevated with any gram-negative infection and cause of much of the morbidity in people with sepsis.

LPS levels can increase from meals, depending on what food is consumed. When 12 healthy men consumed three slices of toast with 50 grams of butter (900 kcal), their median plasma LPS concentration increased by 50%.[2] Another group of volunteers consumed either a high-fat breakfast sandwich and hash browns or an American Heart Association (AHA)–approved meal of oatmeal, milk, orange juice, raisins, peanut butter, and an English muffin.[3] The high-fat, high-carbohydrate breakfast of sandwich and hash browns increased LPS

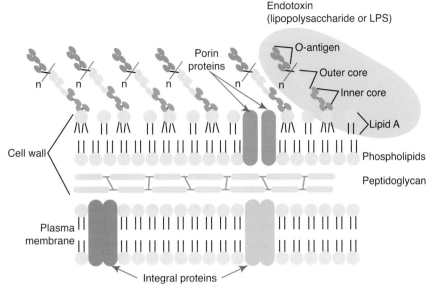

FIG. 35.1 Schematic representation of endotoxin (lipopolysaccharide [LPS]) structure and localization in gram-negative bacteria. (From Laurent, G. J., & Shapiro, S. D. [2006]. In P. J. Bertics, M. L. Gavala, & L. C. Denlinger [Eds.], *Encyclopedia of respiratory medicine*. s.v. "endotoxins" [pp. 80–85]. Cambridge, MA: Academic Press.)

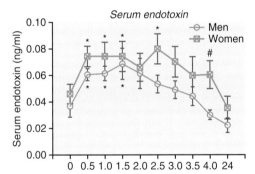

FIG. 35.2 Serum endotoxin levels in binge-drinking men and women after alcohol consumption. (From Bala, S., Marcos, M., Gattu, A., Catalano, D., & Szabo, G. [2014]. Acute binge drinking increases serum endotoxin and bacterial DNA levels in healthy individuals. *PLoS One, 9*[5], e96864.)

levels significantly, whereas the AHA-approved meal did not. Serum endotoxin levels increased in healthy volunteers who consumed saturated fats with a meal, whereas those who consumed a meal with omega-3 fats had a reduction in circulating endotoxins.[4] Binge drinking dramatically increased circulating LPS levels (Fig. 35.2),[5]

but moderate drinkers (< 20 grams/week) had endotoxin levels lower than nondrinkers.[6] Eight individuals with similar endotoxin levels went on either a Western diet or a "prudent" diet for a month. At the end of the month, those on the prudent diet had an average drop in endotoxin levels by 31% whereas those on the Western diet averaged a 71% increase.[7]

Intestinal LPS appears to have two avenues of transport from the intestinal lumen to portal circulation. Lipids in the intestines can carry LPS through enterocytes to circulation, which is the most likely reason that high-fat meals increase the circulating endotoxin concentration. However, if the tight junctions are compromised with any inflammatory condition, even from food allergy–induced histamine release, LPS will move paracellularly into portal circulation. After entry into portal circulation, LPS is picked up by Kupffer cells. Once in the liver, LPS can be bound by lipopolysaccharide binding protein (LBP) that carries it through the bloodstream. Hepatic production of LBP increases as the level of LPS entering the liver goes up.[8] LBP-bound LPS is more readily picked up by lipoproteins, including chylomicrons, high density lipoproteins (HDL), and low density lipoproteins (LDL), and carried throughout the body.

TOXICITY

Inflammation

LBP-bound LPS activates CD14 binding sites on monocytes more than nonbound LPS.[9] LPS binding to CD14 receptors activates toll-like receptor 4 (TLR4) via the lipid A portion, which in turn activates nuclear factor kappa-light-chain-enhancer of activated B cells (NF-κβ), IL-1β, and IL-6, initiating the inflammatory process. Although TLR4 can be activated by other bacterial compounds, it appears to be the specific binding site for LPS. Human cells that express TLR4, and are therefore prone to inflammation from LPS binding, are listed on Box 35.1. LPS activation also results in higher levels of IL-17, which is associated with serious neuroinflammation and debilitating autoimmunity.[10] LPS leaves the liver in higher amounts when the blood lipid content is elevated, as it will be readily carried by the chylomicrons. Fatty liver conditions, both alcohol and non–alcohol related, are associated with higher levels of circulating endotoxins.[11] Of course, a high-fat diet alters the *Firmicutes* to *Bacteroidetes* ratio of the intestinal microbiota with a result of more LPS being produced to be carried by the lipids. *Bifidobacteria* counts, reduced by high-fat diets, are inversely correlated with LPS counts in portal circulation. High-fat diets also increase the activation of mast cells and the release of tumor necrosis factor-α (TNF-α), all of which increase gut permeability and LPS movement into the bloodstream.[12] The ability of high-fat diets to increase endotoxemia is a major mechanism by which high-fat diets are associated with inflammation. This was reflected by the study in which either a fast food or AHA-approved breakfast was consumed.[3] Along with the increase in LPS in those consuming egg or sausage muffins,

---

BOX 35.1   Human Cells That Express TLR4

- Monocytes
- Macrophages
- Granulocytes
- Adipocytes
- Microglia
- Astrocytes
- Oligodendrocytes
- Vessel endothelium
- Brain endothelium
- Heart
- Small intestine
- Colon
- Lung

From Vaure, C., & Liu, Y. (2014). A comparative review of toll-like receptor 4 expression and functionality in different animal species. *Frontiers in Immunology, 5,* 316.

---

levels of reactive oxygen species increased along with thiobarbituric acid reactive substances (TBARS), as did NF-κβ and the expression of TLR4.

DETOXIFICATION/EXCRETION PROCESSES

The liver and spleen play primary roles in clearing LPS from the blood.[13]

CLINICAL SIGNIFICANCE

Effects on Biotransformation, Excretion, and Glutathione Production

LPS presence adversely affects the biotransformation (phases 1 and 2) of xenobiotic compounds in the body. LPS suppress cytochrome P450 (CYP450) messenger RNA and reduce levels of both NADPH-cytochrome c-reductase and cytochrome b5, two of the three critical components needed for all phase 1 oxidation.[14] LPS reduce sex-specific cytochrome activity in women by 17% and in men by 35%. LPS exposure results in a general reduction of all cytochromes levels and has been specifically linked to reduced activity of the 1A, 2B, 2E, 3A, and 4A families.[15,16] High circulating levels of maternal LPS had also been linked to reduced hepatic CYP3A4 levels in fetal livers.[17] LPS downregulates glutamyl-cysteine ligase, one of the two critical enzymes for glutathione synthesis resulting in lower levels of available glutathione.[18] LPS also reduces the effectiveness of phase 2 glutathione transferase activity, preventing the rapid clearance of xenobiotics from circulation. In addition, LPS reduces the production of S-adenosylmethionine necessary for proper methylation.[19]

Cardiovascular and Chronic Fatigue

Elevated levels of TNF-α, interleukin-6 (IL-6), and IL-17 (from LPS activation of TLR4) move through the bloodstream and affect all parts of the body. Not surprisingly, LPS has been found to cause endothelial inflammation, a precursor to atherosclerotic plaque formation.[20] Among a group of atrial fibrillation patients, the higher the level of circulating LPS, the more likely they were to have a major cardiac event.[21]

Patients with diagnosed chronic fatigue syndrome (CFS), now called myalgic encephalomyelitis, have significantly higher circulating LPS levels than healthy controls (119.43 pg/mL versus 74.74 pg/mL).[22] They also have higher levels of LBP (49 μg/mL versus 37 μg/mL in controls), higher CD14 (49 μg/mL versus 39 μg/mL in controls), and high-sensitivity C-reactive protein (hsCRP; 46 mg/L versus 34 mg/L in controls). Interestingly, the CFS patients also had lower intestinal microbiome diversity with clearly diminished Firmicutes populations.

Diabetes, Obesity, and Metabolic Syndrome

Obese individuals have almost three times the amount of LBP in their blood than nonobese, and their inflammatory markers match the rise in LBP and may be one of the mechanisms for obesity, increasing diabetes risk.[23,24] Elevated blood levels of LBP are associated with obesity, metabolic syndrome, and type 2 diabetes (T2DM).[12] Elevated levels of LPS and their concomitant proinflammatory markers appear to impair pancreatic beta cell function.[25] Healthy volunteers who received an infusion of endotoxin developed insulin resistance and an increased production of proin-flammatory cytokines.[26] A review of 30 studies on endotoxemia and diabetes mellitus revealed that, on average, type 1 diabetes (T1DM) cases have 235.7% higher LPS blood levels and T2DM cases have 66.4% higher LPS blood levels than persons without diabetes.[27]

A very interesting Russian study showed that LPS levels were higher in T1DM patients at the onset of the disease than they were after having diabetes for 2 years.[28] Those just diagnosed with T1DM averaged 882% higher LPS levels than healthy controls whereas those who had the disease at least 2 years averaged 492% higher. This may indicate that endotoxicity is a factor in the development of T1DM.

Individuals with T2DM have a greater increase in circulating endotoxin levels after a high-fat meal compared with healthy controls, indicating an exaggerated response.[29] The increase in plasma LPS concentration can last for close to 4 hours, which would result in a constant elevation of endotoxin, and the resulting inflammation and oxida-tive damage through the majority of each day. This is undoubtedly due in part to the increased gut permeability found in diabetics.[30]

Persons with metabolic syndrome have greater expres-sion of TLR4 on their monocytes than healthy controls.[31] They also have enhanced production of NF-κβ binding and release of IL-1β upon exposure to LPS. Another study found that persons with metabolic syndrome had higher blood endotoxin levels, and that those endotoxin levels correlated with increased monocyte polarization to the M1 proinflammatory phenotype.[32]

Fatty Liver

Endotoxin levels are significantly higher in persons with NAFLD than healthy controls (10.6 EU/mL versus 3.9 EU/mL).[33] The average level of endotoxins in NAFLD patients was virtually identical to those with T2DM, and a significant association between endotoxin and insulin resistance was noted. NAFLD patients are more likely to have small intestinal bowel overgrowth and increased intestinal permeability, both of which will increase the amount of circulating endotoxins.[34,35] Circulating levels of endotoxin, LBP, and an endotoxin-specific IgG (EndoCab IgG) were measured in 920 individuals, 263 of whom had diagnosed NAFLD.[36] All of those with NAFLD had higher LBP but lower circulating endotoxins or EndoCab IgG than the controls, which included 78 individuals who later developed NAFLD. Once those individuals were identified, it was noted that they had higher baseline LBP levels than the other controls, indicating that high LBP could be causative for fatty liver. LBP was also correlated with fasting glucose, insulin resistance, and triglycerides. EndoCab IgG was positively associated with intrahepatic triglyceride content. Persons with NASH have even higher levels of LBP than those with NAFLD.[37] In these subjects, LBP also correlated with steatosis and ballooning scores but did not correlate with fibrosis. In addition, EndoCab IgG showed no difference between those with NASH and NAFLD and has no correlation with histological changes in the liver.

Neuroinflammation

In an animal model of sepsis, LPS administration caused microglial activation and a release of proinflammatory cytokines leading to neuroinflammation and cognitive decline.[38] The microglial activation and cognitive decline were still present in the animals 2 months after the LPS exposure. Not only are TNF-α and IL-6 elevated post-LPS exposure, but IL-17 is as well.[10] TLR4 activation contrib-utes to neuronal degeneration in animal models of Alzheimer's disease.[39] LPS neuroinflammation causes defects in memory and learning, and it also significantly reduces levels of brain-derived neurotrophic factor (BDNF).[40] Depression, another common manifestation of neuroinflammation, is also noted with LPS-induced microglial activation.[41] Healthy adults who were given a bolus of LPS experienced increased depression and anxiety along with elevations of TNF-α, IL-6, and IL-10.[42] Pain thresholds were also seen to be reduced in adults given LPS,[43] as was long-term memory.[44]

INTERVENTION

Dietary

Intermittent fasting was shown to be helpful in reducing LPS-induced neuroinflammation in an animal model.[45] Rats in the intermittent fasting group did not experience the same cognitive decline post-LPS injection as those fed regularly. Intermittent fasting also prevented elevation of inflammatory cytokines typically seen after LPS exposure, as well as a reduction in BDNF.

In a study of atrial fibrillation patients, it was noted that those who had higher scores for adherence to the Mediterranean diet had lower LPS levels, along with fewer major adverse cardiovascular events.[21] When individual foods were assessed for their relation to LPS levels, fruits and legumes held the strongest inverse correlation, with both of those being foods high in indigestible fiber that stimulates increased production of Firmicutes bacteria. Walnuts, another common component of the Mediterranean diet, have the ability to reduce LPS-induced neuroinflammation.[46] Adults who consumed polyphenol-rich bilberry juice daily for 4 weeks had significantly lower levels of C-reactive protein (CRP), IL-6, and LPS-induced NF-κβ activation than those taking placebo.[47]

Omega-3 Fatty Acids. Diets high in omega-3 fatty acids have already demonstrated the ability to reduce postprandial levels of endotoxins,[4] as have diets high in carotenoids.[48] Consumption of an almond-based beverage enriched with docosahexaenoic acid (DHA) successfully reduced inflammatory cytokine production from LPS in young male athletes.[49] Supplementation with 3600 mg of EPA/DHA daily reduced LPS-generated fever and inflammatory biomarkers, whereas dosing with only 900 mg/daily had no effect.[50] Fish oil supplementation in septic patients improved their inflammatory cytokine levels and diminished their length of hospital stay.[51]

Fiber and Probiotics. Because of the association with intestinal microbial balance and endotoxicity, it is not surprising that whole-food fibers and probiotics would have a beneficial effect on LPS levels. Overweight adults, who normally have higher circulating postprandial LPS levels,[52] had a dose-dependent drop in LPS when they

consumed diets supplemented with soluble fiber from legumes.[53] Along with a reduction in LPS came a reduction in their CRP levels. Healthy young athletes who took a combination of *Lactobacillus* and *Bifidobacteria* species experienced a significant reduction in endotoxin levels.[54] Almost 60% of the HIV patients who took a *Saccharomyces boulardii* supplement daily for 12 weeks had a reduction of LBP and IL-6, whereas only 6% of the placebo group showed reductions.[55] The use of a purgative agent made from rhubarb, buckthorn, and Chinese knotweed reduced circulating LPS and NF-κβ in animals.[56]

Antioxidants

Eight weeks of N-acetyl cysteine (NAC) supplementation in sarcoid patients resulted in reduced TNF-α output from their bronchial tissue post-LPS stimulation.[57] Intravenous NAC attenuated LPS-induced inflammation and elevation of blood pressure in adult volunteers.[58] Intravenous ascorbic acid reversed the LPS-induced depletion of vitamin C and impairment of endothelial-derived nitric oxide activity.[59] Oral vitamin E supplementation in nonasthmatic adults attenuated the respiratory effect of endotoxin inhalation.[60]

Botanicals

Prophylactic treatment with glycyrrhizin before LPS injection dramatically reduced inflammatory markers in animals after receiving LPS.[61] Licorice also reduced the memory deficit normally present in LPS-induced neuroinflammation. Licorice extract has also demonstrated the ability to protect the lungs from LPS damage.[62] Ginseng extract reduced microglial activation in LPS-exposed animals and prevented the normal increase in inflammatory cytokines in those mice.[63] Epigallocatechin-3-gallate, the primary polyphenol in green tea, prevented LPS neuroinflammation, neuronal cell death, memory impairment, and deposition of amyloid protein in animals.[64] LPS inhibition of CYP3A2 can be prevented by the supplementation of either curcumin or melatonin.[65,66]

REFERENCES

1. Salonen, H., Duchaine, C., Létourneau, V., Mazaheri, M., Clifford, S., & Morawska, L. (2013). Endotoxins in indoor air and settled dust in primary schools in a subtropical climate. *Environmental Science & Technology*, *47*(17), 9882–9890. PubMed PMID: 23927534.

2. Erridge, C., Attina, T., Spickett, C. M., & Webb, D. J. (2007). A high-fat meal induces low-grade endotoxemia: Evidence of a novel mechanism of postprandial inflammation. *The American Journal of Clinical Nutrition*, 86(5), 1286–1292. PubMed PMID: 17991637.

3. Ghanim, H., Abuaysheh, S., Sia, C. L., et al. (2009). Increase in plasma endotoxin concentrations and the expression of Toll-like receptors and suppressor of cytokine signaling-3 in mononuclear cells after a high-fat, high-carbohydrate meal: Implications for insulin resistance. *Diabetes Care*, 32(12), 2281–2287. PubMed PMID: 19755625.

4. Lyte, J. M., Gabler, N. K., & Hollis, J. H. (2016). Postprandial serum endotoxin in healthy humans is modulated by dietary fat in a randomized, controlled, cross-over study. *Lipids in Health and Disease*, 15(1), 186. PubMed PMID: 27816052.

5. Bala, S., Marcos, M., Gattu, A., et al. (2014). Acute binge drinking increases serum endotoxin and bacterial DNA levels in healthy individuals. *PLoS ONE*, 9(5), e96864. PubMed PMID: 24828436.

6. Wong, V. W., Wong, G. L., Chan, H. Y., et al. (2015). Bacterial endotoxin and non-alcoholic fatty liver disease in the general population: A prospective cohort study. *Alimentary Pharmacology and Therapeutics*, 42(6), 731–740. PubMed PMID:26202818.

7. Pendyala, S., Walker, J. M., & Holt, P. R. (2012). A high-fat diet is associated with Endotoxemia that originates from the gut. *Gastroenterology*, 142(5), 1100–1101.e2. PubMed PMID: 22326433.

8. Van Amersfoort, E. S., Van Berkel, T. J., & Kuiper, J. (2003). Receptors, mediators, and mechanisms involved in bacterial sepsis and septic shock. *Clinical Microbiology Reviews*, 16(3), 379–414. PubMed PMID: 12857774.

9. Schumann, R. R., Leong, S. R., Flaggs, G. W., et al. (1990). Structure and function of lipopolysaccharide binding protein. *Science*, 249(4975), 1429–1431. PubMed PMID: 2402637.

10. Sun, J., Zhang, S., Zhang, X., et al. (2015). IL-17A is implicated in lipopolysaccharide-induced neuroinflammation and cognitive impairment in aged rats via microglial activation. *Journal of Neuroinflammation*, 12, 165. PubMed PMID: 26373740.

11. Kitabatake, H., Tanaka, N., Fujimori, N., et al. (2017). Association between endotoxemia and histological features of nonalcoholic fatty liver disease. *World Journal of Gastroenterology*, 23(4), 712–722. PubMed PMID: 28216979.

12. Piya, M. K., Harte, A. L., & McTernan, P. G. (2013). Metabolic endotoxaemia: Is it more than just a gut feeling? *Current Opinion in Lipidology*, 24(1), 78–85. PubMed PMID: 23298961.

13. Shao, B., Lu, M., Katz, S. C., et al. (2007). A host lipase detoxifies bacterial lipopolysaccharides in the liver and spleen. *The Journal of Biological Chemistry*, 282(18), 13726–13735. PMID: 17322564.

14. Morgan, E. T. (1989). Suppression of constitutive cytochrome P-450 gene expression in livers of rats undergoing an acute phase response to endotoxin. *Molecular Pharmacology*, 36(5), 699–707. PubMed PMID: 2511427.

15. Tajima, M., Ikarashi, N., Okaniwa, T., et al. (2013). Consumption of a high-fat diet during pregnancy changes the expression of cytochrome P450 in the livers of infant male mice. *Biological and Pharmaceutical Bulletin*, 36(4), 649–657. PubMed PMID: 23358370.

16. Warren, G. W., Poloyac, S. M., Gary, D. S., et al. (1999). Hepatic cytochrome P-450 expression in tumor necrosis factor-alpha receptor (p55/p75) knockout mice after endotoxin administration. *The Journal of Pharmacology and Experimental Therapeutics*, 288(3), 945–950. PubMed PMID: 10027830.

17. Li, X. Y., Zhang, C., Wang, H., et al. (2008). Tumor necrosis factor alpha partially contributes to lipopolysaccharide-induced downregulation of CYP3A in fetal liver: Its repression by a low dose LPS pretreatment. *Toxicology Letters*, 179(2), 71–77. PubMed PMID: 18501536.

18. van der Crabben, S. N., Stegenga, M. E., Blümer, R. M., et al. (2011). Erythrocyte glutathione concentration and production during hyperinsulinemia, hyperglycemia, and endotoxemia in healthy humans. *Metabolism: Clinical and Experimental*, 60(1), 99–106. PubMed PMID: 20850847.

19. Ko, K., Yang, H., Noureddin, M., et al. (2008). Changes in S adenosylmethionine and GSH homeostasis during endotoxemia in mice. *Laboratory Investigation; a Journal of Technical Methods and Pathology*, 88(10), 1121–1129. PubMed PMID: 18695670.

20. Li, Y. Y., Zhang, G. Y., He, J. P., et al. (2017). Ufm1 inhibits LPS-induced endothelial cell inflammatory responses through the NF-κB signaling pathway. *International Journal of Molecular Medicine*, 39(5), 1119–1126. PubMed PMID: 28393202.

21. Pastori, D., Carnevale, R., Nocella, C., et al. (2017). Gut-derived serum lipopolysaccharide is associated with enhanced risk of major adverse cardiovascular events in atrial fibrillation: Effect of adherence to Mediterranean diet. *Journal of the American Heart Association*, 6(6), PubMed PMID: 28584074.

22. Giloteaux, L., Goodrich, J. K., Walters, W. A., et al. (2016). Reduced diversity and altered composition of the gut microbiome in individuals with myalgic

encephalomyelitis/chronic fatigue syndrome. *Microbiome, 4*(1), 30. PubMed PMID: 27338587.

23. Sun, L., Yu, Z., Ye, X., et al. (2010). A marker of endotoxemia is associated with obesity and related metabolic disorders in apparently healthy Chinese. *Diabetes Care, 33*(9), 1925–1932. PubMed PMID: 20530747.

24. Boutagy, N. E., McMillan, R. P., Frisard, M. I., & Hulver, M. W. (2016). Metabolic endotoxemia with obesity: Is it real and is it relevant? *Biochimie, 124*, 11–20. PubMed PMID: 26133659.

25. Monte, S. V., Caruana, J. A., Ghanim, H., et al. (2012). Reduction in endotoxemia, oxidative and inflammatory stress, and insulin resistance after Roux-en-Y gastric bypass surgery in patients with morbid obesity and type 2 diabetes mellitus. *Surgery, 151*(4), 587–593. PubMed PMID: 22088821.

26. Mehta, N. N., McGillicuddy, F. C., Anderson, P. D., et al. (2010). Experimental Endotoxemia induces adipose inflammation and insulin resistance in humans. *Diabetes, 59*(1), 172–181. PubMed PMID: 19794059.

27. Gomes, J. M., Costa, J. A., & Alfenas, R. C. (2017). Metabolic endotoxemia and diabetes mellitus: A systematic review. *Metabolism: Clinical and Experimental, 68*, 133–144. PubMed PMID: 28183445.

28. Okorokov, P. L., Anikhovskaia, I. A., Volkov, I. E., & Iakovlev, MIu. (2011). [Intestinal endotoxin in induction of type 1 diabetes]. *Fiziologiia Cheloveka, 37*(2), 138–141, (Russian). PubMed PMID: 21542330.

29. Harte, A. L., Varma, M. C., Tripathi, G., et al. (2012). High fat intake leads to acute postprandial exposure to circulating endotoxin in type 2 diabetic subjects. *Diabetes Care, 35*(2), 375–382. PubMed PMID: 22210577.

30. Allin, K. H., Nielsen, T., & Pedersen, O. (2015). Mechanisms in endocrinology: Gut microbiota in patients with type 2 diabetes mellitus. *European Journal of Endocrinology, 172*(4), R167–R177. PubMed PMID: 25416725.

31. Jialal, I., Huet, B. A., Kaur, H., et al. (2012). Increased toll-like receptor activity in patients with metabolic syndrome. *Diabetes Care, 35*(4), 900–904. PubMed PMID: 22357188.

32. Chen, X., & Devaraj, S. (2014). Monocytes from metabolic syndrome subjects exhibit a proinflammatory M1 phenotype. *Metabolic Syndrome and Related Disorders, 12*(7), 362–366. PubMed PMID: 24847781.

33. Harte, A. L., da Silva, N. F., Creely, S. J., et al. (2010). Elevated endotoxin levels in non-alcoholic fatty liver disease. *Journal of Inflammation (London, England), 7*, 15. PubMed PMID: 20353583.

34. Farhadi, A., Gundlapalli, S., Shaikh, M., et al. (2008). Susceptibility to gut leakiness: A possible mechanism for endotoxaemia in non-alcoholic steatohepatitis. *Liver International, 28*(7), 1026–1033. PubMed PMID: 18397235.

35. Miele, L., Valenza, V., La Torre, G., et al. (2009). Increased intestinal permeability and tight junction alterations in nonalcoholic fatty liver disease. *Hepatology, 49*(6), 1877–1887. PubMed PMID: 19291785.

36. Wong, V. W., Wong, G. L., Chan, H. Y., et al. (2015). Bacterial endotoxin and non-alcoholic fatty liver disease in the general population: A prospective cohort study. *Alimentary Pharmacology and Therapeutics, 42*(6), 731–740. PubMed PMID: 26202818.

37. Kitabatake, H., Tanaka, N., Fujimori, N., et al. (2017). Association between endotoxemia and histological features of nonalcoholic fatty liver disease. *World Journal of Gastroenterology, 23*(4), 712–722. PubMed PMID: 28216979.

38. Weberpals, M., Hermes, M., Hermann, S., et al. (2009). NOS2 gene deficiency protects from sepsis-induced long-term cognitive deficits. *The Journal of Neuroscience, 29*(45), 14177–14184. PubMed PMID: 19906966.

39. Walter, S., Letiembre, M., Liu, Y., et al. (2007). Role of the toll-like receptor 4 in neuroinflammation in Alzheimer's disease. *Cellular Physiology and Biochemistry: International Journal of Experimental Cellular Physiology, Biochemistry, and Pharmacology, 20*(6), 947–956. PubMed PMID: 17982277.

40. Schnydrig, S., Korner, L., Landweer, S., et al. (2007). Peripheral lipopolysaccharide administration transiently affects expression of brain-derived neurotrophic factor, corticotropin and proopiomelanocortin in mouse brain. *Neuroscience Letters, 429*(1), 69–73. PubMed PMID: 17976910.

41. Shi, Z., Ren, H., Huang, Z., et al. (2016). Fish oil prevents lipopolysaccharide-induced depressive-like behavior by inhibiting neuroinflammation. *Molecular Neurobiology*, PubMed PMID: 27815837.

42. Kullmann, J. S., Grigoleit, J. S., Lichte, P., et al. (2013). Neural response to emotional stimuli during experimental human endotoxemia. *Human Brain Mapping, 34*(9), 2217–2227. PubMed PMID: 22461242.

43. Benson, S., Kattoor, J., Wegner, A., et al. (2012). Acute experimental endotoxemia induces visceral hypersensitivity and altered pain evaluation in healthy humans. *Pain, 153*(4), 794–799. PubMed PMID: 22264996.

44. Grigoleit, J. S., Kullmann, J. S., Wolf, O. T., et al. (2011). Dose-dependent effects of endotoxin on

neurobehavioral functions in humans. *PLoS ONE*, 6(12), e28330. PubMed PMID: 22164271.

45. Vasconcelos, A. R., Yshii, L. M., Viel, T. A., et al. (2014). Intermittent fasting attenuates lipopolysaccharide-induced neuroinflammation and memory impairment. *Journal of Neuroinflammation*, 11, 85. PubMed PMID: 24886300.

46. Fisher, D. R., Poulose, S. M., Bielinski, D. F., & Shukitt-Hale, B. (2014). Serum metabolites from walnut-fed aged rats attenuate stress-induced neurotoxicity in BV-2 microglial cells. *Nutritional Neuroscience*, PubMed PMID: 25153536.

47. Karlsen, A., Paur, I., Bøhn, S. K., et al. (2010). Bilberry juice modulates plasma concentration of NF-kappaB related inflammatory markers in subjects at increased risk of CVD. *European Journal of Nutrition*, 49(6), 345–355. PubMed PMID: 20119859.

48. Umoh, F. I., Kato, I., Ren, J., et al. (2016). Markers of systemic exposures to products of intestinal bacteria in a dietary intervention study. *European Journal of Nutrition*, 55(2), 793–798. PubMed PMID: 25903259.

49. Capó, X., Martorell, M., Llompart, I., et al. (2014). Docosahexanoic acid diet supplementation attenuates the peripheral mononuclear cell inflammatory response to exercise following LPS activation. *Cytokine*, 69(2), 155–164. PubMed PMID: 24954162.

50. Ferguson, J. F., Mulvey, C. K., Patel, P. N., et al. (2014). Omega-3 PUFA supplementation and the response to evoked endotoxemia in healthy volunteers. *Molecular Nutrition & Food Research*, 58(3), 601–613. PubMed PMID:24190860.

51. Barbosa, V. M., Miles, E. A., Calhau, C., et al. (2010). Effects of a fish oil containing lipid emulsion on plasma phospholipid fatty acids, inflammatory markers, and clinical outcomes in septic patients: A randomized, controlled clinical trial. *Critical Care : The Official Journal of the Critical Care Forum*, 14(1), R5. PubMed PMID: 20085628.

52. Vors, C., Pineau, G., Drai, J., et al. (2015). Postprandial endotoxemia linked with chylomicrons and lipopolysaccharides handling in obese versus lean men: A lipid dose-effect trial. *The Journal of Clinical Endocrinology and Metabolism*, 100(9), 3427–3435. PubMed PMID: 26151336.

53. Morel, F. B., Dai, Q., Ni, J., et al. (2015). α-Galacto-oligosaccharides dose-dependently reduce appetite and decrease inflammation in overweight adults. *The Journal of Nutrition*, 145(9), 2052–2059. PubMed PMID: 26180243.

54. Roberts, J. D., Suckling, C. A., Peedle, G. Y., et al. (2016). An exploratory investigation of endotoxin levels in novice long distance triathletes, and the effects of a multi-strain probiotic/prebiotic, antioxidant intervention. *Nutrients*, 8(11), pii: E733. PubMed PMID: 27869661.

55. Villar-García, J., Hernández, J. J., Güerri-Fernández, R., et al. (2015). Effect of probiotics (Saccharomyces boulardii) on microbial translocation and inflammation in HIV-treated patients: A double-blind, randomized, placebo-controlled trial. *Journal of Acquired Immune Deficiency Syndromes*, 68(3), 256–263. PubMed PMID: 25469528.

56. Li, A., Dong, L., Duan, M. L., et al. (2013). Emodin improves lipopolysaccharide-induced microcirculatory disturbance in rat mesentery. *Microcirculation*, 20(7), 617–628. PubMed PMID: 23551520.

57. Hamzeh, N., Li, L., Barkes, B., et al. (2016). The effect of an oral anti-oxidant, N-Acetyl-cysteine, on inflammatory and oxidative markers in pulmonary sarcoidosis. *Respiratory Medicine*, 112, 106–111. PubMed PMID: 26831541.

58. Schaller, G., Pleiner, J., Mittermayer, F., Posch, M., Kapiotis, S., & Wolzt, M. (2007). Effects of N-acetylcysteine against systemic and renal hemodynamic effects of endotoxin in healthy humans. *Critical Care Medicine*, 35(8), 1869–1875. PubMed PMID: 17568325.

59. Aschauer, S., Gouya, G., Klickovic, U., et al. (2014). Effect of systemic high dose vitamin C therapy on forearm blood flow reactivity during endotoxemia in healthy human subjects. *Vascular Pharmacology*, 61(1), 25–29. PubMed PMID: 24512733.

60. Hernandez, M. L., Wagner, J. G., Kala, A., et al. (2013). Vitamin E, γ-tocopherol, reduces airway neutrophil recruitment after inhaled endotoxin challenge in rats and in healthy volunteers. *Free Radical Biology & Medicine*, 60, 56–62. PubMed PMID: 23402870.

61. Song, J. H., Lee, J. W., Shim, B., et al. (2013). Glycyrrhizin alleviates neuroinflammation and memory deficit induced by systemic lipopolysaccharide treatment in mice. *Molecules : A Journal of Synthetic Chemistry and Natural Product Chemistry*, 18(12), 15788–15803. PubMed PMID: 24352029.

62. Ni, Y. F., Kuai, J. K., Lu, Z. F., et al. (2011). Glycyrrhizin treatment is associated with attenuation of lipopolysaccharide-induced acute lung injury by inhibiting cyclooxygenase-2 and inducible nitric oxide synthase expression. *The Journal of Surgical Research*, 165(1), e29–e35. PubMed PMID: 21074783.

63. Lee, J. S., Song, J. H., Sohn, N. W., & Shin, J. W. (2013). Inhibitory effects of ginsenoside

Rb1 on neuroinflammation following systemic lipopolysaccharide treatment in mice. *Phytotherapy Research : PTR, 27*(9), 1270–1276. PubMed PMID: 23042638.

64. Lee, Y. J., Choi, D. Y., Yun, Y. P., et al. (2013). Epigallocatechin-3-gallate prevents systemic inflammation-induced memory deficiency and amyloidogenesis via its anti-neuroinflammatory properties. *The Journal of Nutritional Biochemistry, 24*(1), 298–310. PubMed PMID: 22959056.

65. Roe, A. L., Warren, G., Hou, G., et al. (1998). The effect of high dose endotoxin on CYP3A2 expression in the rat. *Pharmaceutical Research, 15*(10), 1603–1608. PubMed PMID: 9794504.

66. Cheng, P. Y., Wang, M., & Morgan, E. T. (2003). Rapid transcriptional suppression of rat cytochrome P450 genes by endotoxin treatment and its inhibition by curcumin. *The Journal of Pharmacology and Experimental Therapeutics, 307*(3), 1205–1212. PubMed PMID: 14557382.

36

Alcohol

SUMMARY

- Presence in population: In the United States, 16.3 million adults (18 years and older) had an alcohol use disorder (AUD) in 2014, and an estimated 679,000 adolescents (12–17 years old) had an AUD;[1] approximately 88,000 people die of alcohol related causes annually[2]
- Major diseases: Alcohol dependence, cirrhosis, kidney failure, cancer, pancreatitis, cardiovascular disease, injuries

- Primary sources: Direct consumption
- Best measure: Blood, breathalyzer
- Best intervention: Avoidance; the most important nutrients for those who abuse alcohol include the minerals magnesium, selenium, and zinc; the vitamins A, B-complex, and C; and nutrients glutamine, carnitine, and free-form amino acids

DESCRIPTION

Ingestion of toxins has direct and/or indirect effects on the body depending on the specific toxin consumed. Exposure to environmental toxins, such as mercury and persistent organic pollutants (POPs), and nutritional deficiencies, such as vitamin D, vitamin K_2, and iodine, also detract from health. However, in these cases, the clinical applications are straightforward: decrease exposure to toxins and optimize intake of nutrients. Other toxins, such as alcohol, are not as straightforward. Although alcohol (ethanol) can be directly toxic, with resulting symptoms occurring quickly and transiently, toxicity is dose-dependent and small amounts may actually be beneficial. Excess is clearly a serious clinical problem in North America with a prevalence of lifetime alcohol abuse of 17.8% and a prevalence of 12-month alcohol abuse of 4.7%. In addition, alcohol dependence has a lifetime prevalence of 12.5% and a 12-month prevalence of 3.8%.[3] On the other hand, teetotalers do not live as long and have a higher incidence of several diseases compared with those who consume light to moderate amounts of alcohol. This suggests that some alcohol is valuable; however, the research regarding the beneficial amount of alcohol is unclear and complicated.

TOXICITY

The health-damaging effects of excessive alcohol are substantial. The most toxic effects of alcohol are not due to ethanol itself but its first metabolic product, acetaldehyde. Acetaldehyde is responsible for many of the unpleasant symptoms associated with alcohol intake, including nausea, sweating, vomiting, flushing, and increased heart rate. Acetaldehyde has been shown to promote cancer by interfering with the replication of DNA and by inhibiting the body's ability to repair damaged DNA.[4] Alcohol use increases the risk of developing a variety of cancers, including cancers of the colon, liver, breast, throat, mouth, and upper respiratory tract.[5] Box 36.1 shows some of the major consequences and health effects that may occur from chronic alcohol abuse.

The diverse toxic effects of alcohol result not only from the variation in the levels of breakdown products but also from the depletion of glutathione (GSH). This results in the upregulation of gamma glutamyl transferase

BOX 36.1   Consequences of Alcoholism (Listed Alphabetically)

Increased Mortality
- 10–12 year decrease in life expectancy
- Death rate double in men, triple in women
- Major factor in the four leading causes of death in men between the ages of 25 and 44: accidents, homicides, suicides, cirrhosis
- Suicide rate increased sixfold

Health Effects
- Abstinence and withdrawal syndromes
- Angina
- Arrhythmias
- Cancer of mouth, pharynx, larynx, esophagus increased
- Cerebellar degeneration
- Cerebral atrophy
- Coagulation disorders
- Esophagitis, gastritis, ulcer
- Hypertension
- Hypoglycemia
- Intoxication
- Liver fatty degeneration and cirrhosis
- Metabolic damage to every cell
- Myocardial degeneration
- Myopathy
- Nutritional diseases
- Osteoporosis
- Pancreatitis
- Protein synthesis decreased
- Psychiatric disorders
- Rosacea, spider veins
- Testosterone decreased
- Triglycerides increased, serum and liver

Effects on Fetus
- Fetal alcohol syndrome
- Growth retardation
- Mental retardation
- Teratogenicity

Data from Hymen, S. E., & Cassem, N. H. (1997). Alcoholism. In D. C. Dale & D. D. Federman (Eds.), *Scientific American medicine* (III:1–12, 13). New York, NY: Scientific American.

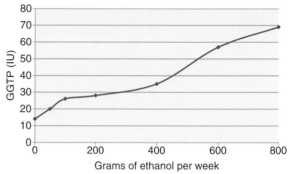

FIG. 36.1 GGTP increases with amount of ethanol consumption. (Data from Nagaya, T., Yoshida, H., Takahashi, H., Matsuda, Y., & Kawai M. [1999]. Dose–response relationships between drinking and serum tests in Japanese men aged 40–59 years. *Alcohol, 17*[2], 133–138.)

(GGT) to provide more GSH, likely for phase II conjugation, as well as to neutralize oxidative stress. Cellular GGT metabolizes extracellular GSH, allowing the precursor cysteine to be reutilized for *de novo* synthesis of intracellular GSH. Elevations of GGT within the "normal" range are strongly associated with several chronic diseases, including diabetes, coronary heart disease, hypertension, stroke, dyslipidemia, chronic kidney disease, and cancer.[6]

There are some major limitations in the use of GGT as a measure of excessive alcohol consumption:
1. GGT also elevates after exposure to other chemicals, especially POPs and several prescription drugs.
2. Genetics and nutrient availability will affect GGT's sensitivity to alcohol consumption.
3. Some chronic imbibers (upward of nine drinks per day) have GGT in the "normal" range.

Individuals have great variation in their ability to produce GSH in response to toxic and oxidative challenges. Nonetheless, GGT is most beneficial when baseline levels are determined on an individual basis. In a uniform population, GGT will increase in direct proportion to alcohol consumption as shown in Fig. 36.1. In a nonuniform population, 40 g of ethanol per day will elevate GGT ~15% whereas 60 g/d for 5 weeks in young men will almost double GGT from 27 to 52 u/L. However, there is a lot of individual variation. In general, GGT goes back to "normal" after abstinence for 1 month.

Research is lacking regarding what value of GGT is indicative of excessive alcohol consumption for an individual. One study evaluating abstinent/relapse status in alcohol-dependent patients showed a cutoff level of 50u/L GGT exhibited specificity of 100% and sensitivity varying from 56% to 100%.[7] A review of the research between alcohol and POP exposure shows that GGT levels above 30u/L clearly indicates too much chemical exposure.

However, GGT levels as low as 20 to 25 u/L may be significant.

SOURCES

A standard alcoholic beverage in the United States is equivalent to:

- 12 ounces of beer (5% alcohol content)
- 8 ounces of malt liquor (7% alcohol content)
- 5 ounces of wine (12% alcohol content)
- 1.5 ounces of 80 proof distilled spirits or liquor (e.g., vodka, gin, rum, whiskey, tequila; 40% alcohol content)

Other sources of alcohol include herbal extracts, mouthwash, food sources such as vanilla extract, hand sanitizer, some liquid medicines, hairspray, and perfume.

BODY BURDEN

Blood alcohol content (BAC) is typically expressed in milligrams per deciliter (mg/dL). Fifteen milliliters of pure alcohol (the equivalent of 1 ounce of whiskey, 4 ounces of wine, or 10 ounces of beer) raise the blood level of alcohol by 25 mg/dL in a 70 kg person. After the consumption of one drink, an individual's blood alcohol concentration (BAC) peaks within 30 to 45 minutes. When an individual consumes more alcohol than the body can eliminate, alcohol accumulates in the blood and the BAC increases. A blood level of 100 mg/dL is equal to a 0.1% BAC. The amount of alcohol measured on the breath is generally accepted as proportional to the amount of alcohol present in the blood at a rate of 1:2100. However, this rate can vary from person to person and moment to moment. Table 36.1 describes the physical effects of varying levels of blood alcohol.

Detoxification/Excretion Processes

It was long believed that, regardless of the amount of alcohol consumed, the rate of alcohol metabolism was constant at 16% per hour.[8] However, recent developments show several factors influence the rate of alcohol elimination, including gender,[9] body composition and lean body mass,[10] liver volume, food and food composition,[11] ethnicity,[12] genetic polymorphisms in alcohol metabolizing enzymes,[13] and polymorphisms in the promoter regions of the genes for these enzymes. It is now understood that the rate of change in the concentration of alcohol depends on the concentration of alcohol and the kinetic constants Km and Vmax, i.e., Michaelis-Menten kinetics.[14]

TABLE 36.1 Physical Effects of Varying Levels of Blood Alcohol

Blood Level (mg/dL)	Effect
<50	No significant motor dysfunction
100	Mild intoxication—decreased inhibitions, slight visual impairment, slight muscular incoordination, slowing of reaction time Legally intoxicated in most jurisdictions
150	Ataxia, dysarthria, slurring of speech, nausea and vomiting
350	Marked muscular incoordination, blurred vision, approaching stupor
500	Coma and death

The primary metabolic processes that regulate the rate of alcohol catabolism in normal individuals are:[15]

1. The rate of ethanol absorption,
2. The concentration and activity of liver alcohol dehydrogenase (ADH) and aldehyde dehydrogenase (ALDH), and
3. The reduced nicotinamide adenine dinucleotide (NADH)/oxidized nicotinamide adenine dinucleotide (NAD$^+$) ratio in the liver mitochondria.

The availability and regeneration of NAD$^+$ are the dominant rate-limiting factors for ethanol oxidation. Ethanol is converted to acetaldehyde by ADH, with NAD$^+$ as a necessary cofactor. Acetaldehyde is converted by ALDH to acetate, most of which is converted to long-chain fatty acids.[16] The aldehyde product of ethanol metabolism is believed to be responsible for many of the harmful effects of alcohol consumption and for the addictive process itself. Higher than normal blood aldehyde levels have been found in alcoholics and their relatives after alcohol consumption.[17] This suggests either increased ADH activity or depressed ALDH activity in people susceptible to alcohol dependence. Other enzymes including cytochrome P450 2E1 (CYP2E1) and catalase also break down alcohol to acetaldehyde. CYP2E1 metabolizes alcohol in the liver, and its formation is induced by chronic heavy alcohol consumption.[18,19]

All of these factors result in alcohol not having a half-life for detoxification such as found in other toxicants.

Nutritional Factors. Nutritional factors have a significant effect on the metabolism and the toxicity of alcohol. For example, zinc is a required cofactor for both ADH and ALDH. However, ALDH is more sensitive to zinc deficiency, which, when present, results in greater aldehyde levels after alcohol consumption and resultant increased toxicity.[20] Low serum zinc levels are also associated with impaired alcohol metabolism, a predisposition to cirrhosis, impaired testicular function, and other complications of alcohol abuse. Vitamin A deficiency appears to work synergistically with zinc deficiency to produce the major complications of alcoholism.[21]

Evidence suggests that a thiamine deficiency results in a greater intake of alcohol, and that thiamine deficiency may be a predisposing factor for alcoholism.[22] Hypomagnesemia (which is induced by alcohol) is strongly linked to delirium tremens[23] and may be the major reason why increased cardiovascular disease occurs in alcoholics.[24] Alcohol ingestion also increases intestinal permeability to endotoxins and macromolecules, allowing increased toxic and antigenic effects.[25]

Genetic Factors. There is evolving research showing that populations susceptible to alcoholism have significant genetic variation in the activity of ADH and ALDH, such as found in individuals of Otomi Mexican Indian ancestry.[26] Variants of the ADH enzyme and/or the ALDH enzyme affect the way an individual metabolizes alcohol into acetaldehyde or acetaldehyde into acetate. For example, individuals with an inactive ALDH2 allele are poor eliminators of acetaldehyde. The resulting accumulation of acetaldehyde produces unpleasant effects from alcohol (e.g., nausea, vomiting, flushing, increased heart rate), and consequently, these individuals consume little to no alcohol.[27,28] About 15% to 40% of the East Asian population has an inactive ALDH2 allele that leads to acetaldehyde levels that are 5- to 20-fold higher than those with an active ALDH allele.[29] Lower rates of alcohol dependence have been associated with certain genetic variants including the ADH1B*2, ADH1B*3, ADH1C*1, and ALDH2*2 alleles.[30]

Other Unexpected Concerns With Alcohol

Several unexpected problems with alcoholic beverages exist beyond their ethanol content. For example, some alcohol beverages contain surprisingly high levels of fluoride, which might be problematic for those sensitive to fluorides or who are already being exposed to excessive amounts of fluoride through water, toothpaste, dental applications, environmental exposure, etc.

Aluminum and plastic containers (BPA) pose other concerns surrounding increased exposure to exogenous toxins. Artificial flavors, artificial colors (e.g., caramel coloring, FD&C Blue 1, FD&C Red 40, FD&C Yellow 5), and artificial sweeteners increase chemical exposure. Genetically modified grains used as sources of alcoholic beverages (e.g., beer, bourbon, whiskey) may also have damaging effects. Pesticides, herbicides, and POPs may also contaminate grains used in the production of alcoholic beverages. Sulfites are commonly used as preservatives in wine and have been shown to cause allergic reactions (anaphylaxis), asthma, flushing, and cramping.[31] Wine also contains biogenic amines, such as histamine, and salicylates that have been associated with several symptoms including sneezing, rhinitis, pruritus, headaches, and asthma.[32] Calcium disodium EDTA (preservative), carrageenan (emulsifier, stabilizer, thickening agent), and propylene glycol (flavor enhancer) may also be found in alcoholic beverages and should be avoided.

Benefits

Research has clearly documented that light to moderate alcohol consumption provides protection from vascular and all-cause mortality, ischemic stroke, peripheral arterial disease, congestive heart failure, and recurrence of ischemic events.[33] In addition, consuming alcohol has been shown to improve the efficacy of triple drug therapy (omeprazole, 20 mg twice daily, clarithromycin, 500 mg twice daily, and amoxicillin, 1000 mg twice daily) in the treatment of *Helicobacter pylori* (*H. pylori*). Eradication was dose dependent: 70.1% in teetotalers, 79.3% in users of 4 to 16 g of ethanol a day, and nearly 100% in users of 18 to 60 g daily.[34]

The generally recommended amount of "safe" alcohol consumption in healthy individuals is two standard drinks for a man and up to one drink for a nonpregnant woman.[35] The form of alcohol does have an effect, with wine (which contains antiinflammatory antioxidants like resveratrol) being clearly better than spirits or beer.[36] However, there is huge individual variation in the level of alcohol consumption that can quickly transition from modestly helpful to seriously damaging.

Clinical Significance

There are several standards for diagnosing when a patient is consuming too much alcohol. The following are indicative of serious alcohol dependence:

- Serious symptoms when alcohol is withdrawn: tremulousness, convulsions, hallucinations, delirium
- Alcoholic binges, benders (48 or more hours of drinking associated with failure to meet usual obligations), or blackouts
- Evidence of alcohol-induced illnesses: cirrhosis, gastritis, pancreatitis, myopathy, polyneuropathy, cerebellar degeneration
- Physical signs of excess alcohol consumption: alcohol odor on breath, flushed face, tremor, ecchymoses
- Psychological/social signs of excess alcohol consumption: depression, loss of friends, arrest for driving while intoxicated, surreptitious drinking, drinking before breakfast, frequent accidents, unexplained work absences

INTERVENTION

Alcohol may be considered a "toxin of choice" and, as such, exposure can be managed by the individual. There is evidence that small amounts of alcohol may be beneficial, so limiting toxin exposure is the primary intervention. Setting limits, alternating alcoholic and nonalcoholic drinks, drinking slowly, and eating before and/or while drinking may also lower risks associated with alcohol consumption.

Carnitine has been shown to inhibit alcohol-induced fatty liver disease and reduces serum triglycerides and aspartate aminotransferase (AST) levels while elevating HDL cholesterol.[37,38] Antioxidant administration, either before or simultaneously with ethanol intake, inhibits lipoperoxide formation and prevents fatty infiltration of the liver.[39] Alcoholics are typically deficient in most of the B vitamins.[40] Alcohol also decreases the absorption and utilization by the liver, and/or increases the urinary excretion of many B vitamins, especially folic acid.[41] Ethanol has been shown to interfere with essential fatty acid (EFA) metabolism and as a result may produce symptoms of EFA deficiency in excess.[42] Glutamine supplementation (1 g/day) has been shown to reduce voluntary alcohol consumption in uncontrolled human studies and experimental animal studies.[43,44] Silymarin has been shown to be effective in the treatment of the full spectrum of alcohol-related liver disease from relatively mild to serious cirrhosis.[45] Silymarin can also improve immune function in patients with cirrhosis.[46]

There is a direct correlation between leukocyte ascorbic acid levels (a good index of actual body ascorbic acid status), the rate of ethanol clearance from the blood, and the activity of hepatic ADH.[47] Evidence suggests that ascorbic acid, a strong reducing agent, can function as an electron donor similar to NAD in ethanol metabolism, thereby increasing the conversion of ethanol to acetaldehyde and the further catabolism of acetaldehyde.[48] Less understood, but with promising evolving research, are N-acetylcysteine (NAC) and curcumin. Early research shows that curcumin decreases the rate of alcohol absorption, decreases blood aldehyde levels, and decreases the normally resultant elevation in GGT.[49] Animal research has shown that NAC provides substantial protection from acetaldehyde poisoning, the efficacy of which was improved by coadministration of vitamin D and thiamin.[50]

The research is clear that light to moderate alcohol consumption is healthful, and excessive alcohol is extremely damaging to health. The challenge is that the transition between healthful effects and toxic effects has huge variation based on genetics, nutritional status, and environmental toxin load. Perhaps one of the beneficial reasons of light to moderate alcohol consumption (separate from the antioxidant benefits of wine and the HDL elevation from ethanol) is the increased level of GSH that results from the induction of GGT. Technically, the elevation in tissue GSH is more likely due to the decreased depletion secondary to antioxidant effects rather than increased production. Although most of the GSH is used to detoxify alcohol and its metabolites, some may be left over, resulting in increased oxidative protection within cells, especially mitochondria. However, as soon as alcohol breaches a threshold level, which varies according to diet and genetics, cytoplasmic and mitochondrial GSH levels plunge, resulting in metabolic dysfunction and disease. Safer ways to increase GSH production include supplementation with NAC, alpha-lipoic-acid[51] whey protein powder,[52] and S-adenosyl L-methionine (SAMe),[53] as well as meditation[54] and exercise.[55]

GGT may be a useful tool to provide individualized recommendations and guidance. Elevation of GGT (above about 30 u/L) is associated with substantial increased risk of sick days, disease (especially obesity, diabetes, and myocardial infarction) and all-cause mortality, an association which has been reported in research since 1974.[56] Early research shows promise in using glutathione transferase (GSTA1) as a measure for advising patients on their alcohol consumption, as GSTA1 has been shown

TABLE 36.2   Compounds and Symptoms Associated with Alcohol Use

Constituent	Toxic Substances	Affects/Disease
Pure Ethanol	Low toxicity at moderate dosages	Health benefits including reduction in cardiovascular disease
Alcohol	Acetaldehyde	Nausea, sweating, vomiting, flushing, tachycardia Cancer, DNA damage
Wine/Ciders	Sulfites (e.g., sulfur dioxide, potassium bisulfite, sodium bisulfite), biogenic amines (histamine), salicylates	Sulfites: allergic reactions (anaphylaxis), asthma, cramping, flushing Biogenic amines/salicylates: asthma, allergic reactions
Plastic containers	BPA	Neurological symptoms, hypertension, fetotoxic
Aged alcohols	Aldehydes/Ketones	Form reactive advanced lipoxidation (ALE) or glycoxidation (AGE) end products that contribute to aging, atherosclerosis, microvascular disease, interfere with protein and cellular function; ketoacidosis
Ales	Esters	Irritation of the eyes, nose, pharynx

to be a sensitive and reliable marker in ethanol-induced hepatic injury.[57]

One-hundred percent United States Department of Agriculture (USDA) organic beer, wine, and spirits contain no added chemicals and no genetically modified ingredients. Alcohol in glass containers reduces exposure to chemicals such as BPA, and clear alcohols, such as organic vodka, organic tequila, and organic gin, eliminate exposure to artificial colors, artificial sweeteners, and artificial flavors. Table 36.2 provides a summary of toxins associated with alcohol and the symptoms that may result from the ingestion of these toxins.

At this time, the safest recommendation is to follow the general guidelines of 1 drink (1 to 2 ounces) of ethanol per day for women and up to 2 drinks (2 to 3 ounces) for men. For those unwilling to accept such limits, or wanting to explore their limits, GGT monitoring might be a useful clinical tool for providing guidance.

REFERENCES

1. Substance Abuse and Mental Health Services Administration (SAMHSA). *2014 National Survey on Drug Use and Health (NSDUH). Table 5.8A – substance dependence or abuse in the past year among persons aged 18 or older by demographic characteristics: numbers in thousands, 2013 and 2014.* Available at: http://www.samhsa.gov/data/sites/default/files/NSDUH-DetTabs2014/NSDUH-DetTabs2014.htm#tab5-8a.
2. Centers for Disease Control and Prevention (CDC). *Alcohol and public health: alcohol-related disease impact (ARDI).* Available at https://nccd.cdc.gov/DPH_ARDI/default/default.aspx. (Accessed 10 November 2017).
3. Hasin, D. S., Stinson, F. S., Ogburn, E., & Grant, B. F. (2007). Prevalence, correlates, disability, and comorbidity of DSM-IV alcohol abuse and dependence in the United States: Results from the National Epidemiologic Survey on Alcohol and Related Conditions. *Archives of General Psychiatry, 64*(7), 830–842.
4. Seitz, H. K., & Becker, P. (2007). Alcohol metabolism and cancer risk. *Alcohol Research and Health: The Journal of the National Institute on Alcohol Abuse and Alcoholism, 30*(1), 36–47.
5. Bagnardi, V., Blangiardo, M., La Vecchia, C., & Corrao, G. (2001). Alcohol consumption and the risk of cancer: A meta-analysis. *Alcohol Research and Health: The Journal of the National Institute on Alcohol Abuse and Alcoholism, 25*(4), 263–270.
6. Lee, D. H., et al. (2008). Can persistent organic pollutants explain the association between serum gamma-glutamyltransferase and type 2 diabetes? *Diabetologia, 51*(3), 402–407.
7. Dixit, S., & Singh, P. (2015). Usefulness of gamma glutamyl transferase as reliable biological marker in objective corroboration of relapse in alcohol dependent patients. *Journal of Clinical and Diagnostic Research : JCDR, 9*(12), VC1–VC4.
8. Wilkinson, P. K., Sedman, A. J., Sakmar, E., Kay, D. R., & Wagner, J. G. (1977). Pharmacokinetics of ethanol after oral administration in the fasting state. *Journal of Pharmacokinetics and Biopharmaceutics, 5*(3), 207–224.

9. Baraona, E., Abittan, C. S., Dohmen, K., Moretti, M., et al. (2001). Gender differences in pharmacokinetics of alcohol. *Alcoholism, Clinical and Experimental Research*, 25(4), 502–507.

10. Liangpunsakul, S., Crabb, D. W., & Qi, R. (2010). Relationship between alcohol intake, body fat, and physical activity – a population-based study. *Annals of Epidemiology*, 20(9), 670–675.

11. Ramchandani, V. A., Kwo, P. Y., & Li, T. K. (2001). Effect of food and food composition on alcohol elimination rates in healthy men and women. *Journal of Clinical Pharmacology*, 41(12), 1345–1350.

12. Dohmen, K., Baraona, E., Ishibashi, H., Pozzato, G., et al. (1996). Ethnic differences in gastric sigma-alcohol dehydrogenase activity and ethanol first pass metabolism. *Alcoholism, Clinical and Experimental Research*, 20(9), 1569–1576.

13. Agarwal, D. P. (2001). Genetic polymorphisms of alcohol metabolizing enzymes. *Pathologie-Biologie*, 49(9), 703–709.

14. Matsumoto, H., & Fukui, Y. (2002). Pharmacokinetics of ethanol: A review of the methodology. *Addiction Biology*, 7, 5–14.

15. Murray, M. (2012). Alcohol dependence. In J. Pizzorno & M. Murray (Eds.), *Textbook of natural medicine*. Elsevier.

16. Goldstein, D. B. (1983). *Pharmacology of ethanol*. New York, NY.: Oxford University Press.

17. Tipton, K. F., Heneman, G. T. M., & McCrodden, J. M. (1983). Metabolic and nutritional aspects of alcohol. *Biochemical Society Transactions*, 11, 59–61.

18. Lieber, C. S. (1994). Metabolic consequences of ethanol. *The Endocrinologist*, 4(2), 127–139.

19. Cederbaum, A. I. (2012). Alcohol Metabolism. *Clinics in Liver Disease*, 16(4), 667–685. doi:10.1016/j.cld.2012.08.002.

20. Das, I., Burch, R. E., & Hahn, H. K. (1984). Effects of zinc deficiency on ethanol metabolism and alcohol and aldehyde dehydrogenase activities. *The Journal of Laboratory and Clinical Medicine*, 104, 610–617.

21. Scholmerich, J., Lohle, E., Kottgen, E., & Gerok, W. (1983). Zinc and vitamin A deficiency in liver cirrhosis. *Hepato-Gastroenterology*, 30, 119–125.

22. Zimatkin, S. M., & Zimatkina, T. I. (1996). Thiamine deficiency as predisposition to, and consequence of, increased alcohol consumption. *Alcohol and Alcoholism: International Journal of the Medical Council on Alcoholism*, 31, 421–427.

23. Jermain, D. M., Crimson, M. L., & Nisbet, R. B. (1992). Controversies over the use of magnesium sulfate in delirium tremens. *The Annals of Pharmacotherapy*, 26, 650–652.

24. Abbott, L., Nadler, J., & Rude, R. K. (1994). Magnesium deficiency in alcoholism. *Alcoholism, Clinical and Experimental Research*, 18, 1076–1082.

25. Worthington, B. S., Meserole, L., & Syrotuck, J. A. (1978). Effect of daily ethanol ingestion on intestinal permeability to macromolecules. *Digestive Diseases*, 23, 23–32.

26. Montano Loza, A. J., Ramirez Iglesias, M. T., Perez Diaz, I., et al. (2006). Association of alcohol-metabolizing genes with alcoholism in a Mexican Indian (Otomi) population. *Alcohol*, 39(2), 73–79.

27. Harada, S. (2001). Classification of alcohol metabolizing enzymes and polymorphisms – specificity in Japanese. *Nihon Arukoru Yakubutsu Igakkai Zasshi*, 36(2), 85–106.

28. Kang, T. S., Woo, S. W., Park, H. J., Lee, Y., & Roh, J. (2009). Comparison of genetic polymorphisms of CYP2E!, ADH2, ALDH2 genes involved in alcohol metabolism in Koreans and four other ethnic groups. *Journal of Clinical Pharmacy and Therapeutics*, 34(2), 225–230.

29. Eng, M. Y., Luczak, S. E., & Wall, T. L. (2007). ALDH2, ADH1B, and ADH1C genotypes in Asians: A literature review. *Alcohol Research and Health: The Journal of the National Institute on Alcohol Abuse and Alcoholism*, 30(1), 22–27.

30. Wall, T. L., Luczak, S. E., & Hiller-Sturmhofel, S. (2016). Biology, genetics, and environment: Underlying factors influencing alcohol metabolism. *Alcohol Research: Current Reviews*, 38(1), 59–68.

31. Vally, H., de Klerk, N., & Thompson, P. J. (2000). Alcoholic drinks: Important triggers for asthma. *The Journal of Allergy and Clinical Immunology*, 105(3), 462–467.

32. Vally, H., & Thompson, P. J. (2003). Allergic and asthmatic reactions to alcoholic drinks. *Addiction Biology*, 8(1), 3–11.

33. U.S. Department of Agriculture. *Scientific Report of the 2015 Dietary Guidelines Advisory Committee, Part D*. Chapter 2, Table D2.3, p. 43. Available at: http://health.gov/dietaryguidelines/2015-scientific-report/pdfs/scientific-report-of-the-2015-dietary-guidelines-advisory-committee.pdf.

34. Baena, J. M., López, C., Hidalgo, A., Rams, F., Jiménez, S., García, M., et al. (2002). Relation between alcohol consumption and the success of Helicobacter pylori eradication therapy using omeprazole, clarithromycin and amoxicillin for 1 week. *European Journal of Gastroenterology and Hepatology*, 14(3), 291–296.

35. Di Minno, M. N., Franchini, M., Russolillo, A., Lupoli, R., Iervolino, S., & Di Minno, G. (2011). Alcohol dosing

and the heart: Updating clinical evidence. *Seminars in Thrombosis and Hemostasis, 37*(8), 875–884. Epub 2011 Dec 23.

36. Lippi, G., Franchini, M., Favaloro, E. J., & Targher, G. (2010). Moderate red wine consumption and cardiovascular disease risk: Beyond the "French paradox". *Seminars in Thrombosis and Hemostasis, 36*(1), 59–70. Epub 2010 Apr 13.

37. Sachan, D. S., Rhew, T. H., & Ruark, R. A. (1984). Ameliorating effects of carnitine and its precursors on alcohol-induced fatty liver. *The American Journal of Clinical Nutrition, 39*, 736–744.

38. Hosein, E. A., & Bexton, B. (1975). Protective action of carnitine on liver lipid metabolism after ethanol administration to rats. *Biochemical Pharmacology, 24*, 1859–1863.

39. Suematsu, T., Matsumura, T., Sato, N., et al. (1981). Lipid peroxidation in alcoholic liver disease in humans. *Alcoholism, Clinical and Experimental Research, 5*, 427–430.

40. Baines, M. (1978). Detection and incidence of B and C vitamin deficiency in alcohol-related illness. *Annals of Clinical Biochemistry, 15*, 307–312.

41. McMartin, K. E., Collins, T. D., & Bairnsfather, L. (1986). Cumulative excess urinary excretion of folate in rats after repeated ethanol treatment. *The Journal of Nutrition, 116*, 1316–1325.

42. Horrobin, D. F. (1980). A biochemical basis for alcoholism and alcohol-induced damage including the fetal alcohol syndrome and cirrhosis: Interference with essential fatty acid and prostaglandin metabolism. *Medical Hypotheses, 6*, 929–942.

43. Rogers, L. L., & Pelton, R. B. (1955). Glutamine in the treatment of alcoholism. *The Journal of Biological Chemistry, 214*, 503–506.

44. Ravel, J. M., Felsing, B., Lansford, E., et al. (1955). Reversal of alcohol toxicity by glutamine. *The Journal of Biological Chemistry, 214*, 497–502.

45. Ferenci, P., Dragosics, B., & Dittrich, H. (1989). Randomized controlled trial of Silymarin treatment in patients with cirrhosis of the liver. *Journal of Hepatology, 9*, 105–113.

46. Deak, G., Muzes, G., & Lang, I. (1990). Immunomodulator effect of silymarin therapy in chronic alcoholic liver diseases. *Orvosi Hetilap, 131*, 1291–1292, 1295-1296.

47. Yunice, A. A., & Lindeman, R. D. (1977). Effect of ascorbic acid and zinc sulphate on ethanol toxicity and metabolism. *Proceedings of the Society for Experimental Biology and Medicine, 154*, 146–150.

48. Yunice, A. A., Hsu, J. M., Fahmy, A., & Henry, S. (1984). Ethanol-ascorbate interrelationship in acute and chronic alcoholism in the guinea pig. *Proceedings of the Society for Experimental Biology and Medicine, 177*, 262–271.

49. Shimatsu, A., Kakeya, H., Imaizumi, A., et al. (2012). Clinical application of "curcumin", a multi-functional substance. *Anti-Aging Medicine, 9*(1), 43–51.

50. Sprince, H., Parker, C. M., Smith, G. G., & Gonzales, L. J. (1975). Protective action of ascorbic acid and sulfur compounds against acetaldehyde toxicity: Implications in alcoholism and smoking. *Agents and Actions, 5*(2), 164–173.

51. Jariwalla, R. J., et al. (2008). Restoration of blood total glutathione status and lymphocyte function following alpha-lipoic acid supplementation in patients with HIV infection. *The Journal of Alternative and Complementary Medicine: Research on Paradigm, Practice, and Policy, 14*(2), 139–146.

52. Micke, P., et al. (2001). Oral supplementation with whey proteins increases plasma glutathione levels of HIV-infected patients. *European Journal of Clinical Investigation, 31*(2), 171–178.

53. Lieber, C. S., & Packer, L. (2002). S-Adenosylmethionine: Molecular, biological, and clinical aspects—an introduction. *The American Journal of Clinical Nutrition, 76*(5), 1148S–1150S.

54. Sharma, H., et al. (2008). Gene expression profiling in practitioners of SudarshanKriya. *Journal of Psychosomatic Research, 64*(2), 213–218.

55. Rundle, A. G., et al. (2005). Preliminary studies on the effect of moderate physical activity on blood levels of glutathione. *Biomarkers: Biochemical Indicators of Exposure, Response, and Susceptibility to Chemicals, 10*(5), 390–400.

56. Whitfield, J. B. (2001). Gamma Glutamyl Transferase. *Critical Reviews in Clinical Laboratory Sciences, 38*(4), 263–355.

57. Chang, Y. C., Liu, F. P., Ma, X., Li, M. M., Li, R., et al. (2016 May 18). Glutathione S-transferase A1 – a sensitive marker of alcoholic injury on primary hepatocytes. *Human and Experimental Toxicology*, [Epub ahead of print].

37

Marijuana
(Cannabis sativa *L.*, Cannabis indica *L.)*

SUMMARY

- Presence in population: 43% of US adults have tried marijuana; 13% of US adults report being current marijuana users; 22.2 million are past-month users
- Major diseases: Bronchial irritation, decreased motivation, learning difficulties, accidental injuries
- Primary sources: Direct consumption of marijuana; oils or extracts contaminated with solvents; dried flower buds may be contaminated by pesticides

- Best measure: Urine test for 11-nor-delta(9)-carboxy-tetrahydrocannabinol-9-carboxylic acid (a metabolic byproduct of delta-9-tetrahydrocannabinol [THC]); plasma analysis for acute intoxication
- Best intervention: Avoidance; organic marijuana if possible; CO_2 extracts safest

DESCRIPTION

Cannabis (marijuana) is the most commonly used illicit drug in the United States and is considered by many to be the illicit drug with the least risk. As of January 2016, 24 states and the District of Columbia have legalized the medical use of marijuana, and four states and the District of Columbia have legalized the recreational use of marijuana. Decriminalization of marijuana in 13 states, coupled with legalization of recreational and medicinal use, has contributed to a significant increase in the use of marijuana. The percentage of Americans who say they have tried marijuana has steadily increased from 4% in 1969 to 43% in 2016.[1]

Cannabis production is a multibillion-dollar industry in the United States, and legal US markets for cannabis are projected to reach $11 billion by 2019.[2] Growers have a financial incentive to maximize yield regardless of risks placed on employees, customers, or the surrounding environment. The federal status of cannabis as an illegal Schedule I drug has prevented all but a few researchers from conducting field and laboratory studies.

In an unregulated production environment, millions of people are at risk for exposure to harmful chemicals. Toxicity of marijuana may be the result of cannabinoids and/or contaminants such as solvents, pesticides, and heavy metals, which may explain some of the discrepancies in the research. The purpose of this chapter is to examine the toxicity of pure cannabis and explore how contaminants introduced through production and extraction may affect the safety of cannabis use.

TOXICITY

Pure Marijuana

More than 480 compounds have been extracted from the plant resin of cannabis, of which 65 are cannabinoids. The most abundant compounds found in cannabis include delta-9-tetrahydrocannabinolic acid (THCA), cannabidiolic acid (CBDA), cannabigerolic acid (CBGA) and their decarboxylated derivatives THC, cannabidiol (CBD), and cannabigerol (CBG).[3] The cannabinoids are converted into their more active decarboxylated counterparts by heat (e.g., smoking, baking), light, or natural degradation. THC is the most psychoactive component of cannabis and appears to alter mood and cognition by potentiating the effects of glycine receptors and through the activation of CB1 receptors on presynaptic axons suppressing neurotransmitter release.[4,5] The potency of THC in marijuana increased 66%, from 3.08% potency in 1992 to 5.11% potency in 2002.[6,7]

Toxic reactions to marijuana are defined here as any effects that result in physical or psychological damage, are subjectively experienced as unpleasant by the user, or interfere with adequate social functioning.[8,9] Pure THC has low toxicity, and modest use has minimal long-term physical or psychological effects. Acute intoxication reactions occur rapidly and transiently and include nausea, anxiety, paranoia, short-term memory loss, confusion, and disorientation.[10] The concentration of active ingredient, the quantity used, and the tolerance of the user determine the degree of intoxication.

Conflicting studies exist regarding the toxicity of pure marijuana. Compounds, such as THC, have been shown to be detrimental in some cases and beneficial in others. THC appears to have antitumor properties such as apoptosis, as well as tumor-promoting properties such as increasing reactive oxygen species.[11] THC inhibits the biosynthesis of macromolecules and reduces the level of histone gene expression.[12] In addition, THC disrupts all phases of gonadal function by blocking gonadotropin-releasing hormone (GnRH) release. This results in decreased luteinizing hormone (LH) and follicle-stimulating hormone (FSH) levels, which are responsible for reduced testosterone production by the Leydig cells of the testis.[13] Studies evaluating the toxicity of marijuana have several limitations, including nonassessment of dose response, small sample sizes, limited number of heavy marijuana users in the studies, unregulated mode of use, and failure to adjust for tobacco smoking.[14] In addition, cannabis is often used with other drugs, creating a much more complex scenario when trying to determine toxicity.

The mode of use (e.g., smoked in a cigarette, pipe, or filtered water pipe, vaporized, or ingested) may significantly influence the toxicity of marijuana and the corresponding damaging effects. The most common form of marijuana use is inhalation of the smoke. Individuals who use marijuana in the form of blunt or blunt-cigar forms have more severe risk profiles and a greater number of disorder symptoms.[15] Cannabis smoke has been shown to contain many hazardous compounds, including ammonia, cyanide, heavy metals, carbon monoxide, mutagens, carcinogens, and polycyclic aromatic hydrocarbons.[16] The tar from a cannabis cigarette contains higher concentrations of the carcinogens benzanthracenes and benzpyrenes than tobacco smoke does.[17] Vaporization (commonly referred to as "vaping") as a method of using cannabis has been shown to reduce respiratory exposure to toxic particulates.[18] However, limited research is available on the long-term potential harms and benefits of cannabis vaping.

Contaminants

Pesticides. During the 1970s, the majority of marijuana produced in the United States was grown in outdoor areas, primarily in southwestern regions where the weather was warmer and drier. Over time, as law enforcement practices improved, many of these outdoor operations became more vulnerable to detection, which resulted in an increase in indoor marijuana-growing operations. Indoor growing operations provide a year-round growing season and an environment that can be tightly controlled and monitored. However, like any other agricultural product, cannabis requires nutrients for growth (i.e., fertilizers) and must be protected from pests (i.e., pesticides).

Many growers of cannabis resort to over-the-counter insecticides, acaricides, and fungicides to protect their crops. Because the chemicals are regulated by the US Environmental Protection Agency (EPA) and cannabis is illegal under federal law, there are no pesticides registered for use on cannabis in the United States. In other words, all pesticide use on cannabis is currently illegal and understudied.[19] The absence of approved pesticides for cannabis may result in exposure to otherwise more hazardous pesticides or higher residue levels for both consumers and workers.[20] There have been no studies performed showing how pesticides used on marijuana could affect consumers or whether or not their use is safe.

A variety of pesticides have been observed in both medical- and street-grade marijuana products. Anticoagulant rodenticides and insecticides have been found at some marijuana cultivation sites.[21] Seized and legally produced marijuana have been shown to contain pesticide residues of diazinon, tebuconazole, ethephon, and teflubenzuron.[22] One study found the pest repellant DEET, a compound that the EPA considers safe when used topically, in all medical-grade marijuana samples tested.[23] The Los Angeles City Attorney's office acquired and tested three medical cannabis samples in 2009 and found elevated levels of bifenthrin in two out of the three samples, with one sample found to contain more than 1600 times the legal digestible limit of bifenthrin.[21] When present on the product, cannabis smoke has been shown to contain significant amounts of pesticide residues. Filtration has a significant effect on the total pesticide residues consumed, with the greatest quantity found in smoke from hand-held glass pipes (60.3%–69.5%), followed by unfiltered water pipes (42.2%–59.9%), and with the lowest quantity found in smoke from filtered water pipes (0.08%–10.9%).[25] In addition, during heating, pyrolysis products may form, which may interact either with the pesticides themselves or with the pyrolysis products of the pesticides to form more toxic materials.[26] Table 37.1 shows a number of other pesticides detected in marijuana samples.

Solvents. Various methods of cannabis oil extraction are used to concentrate active ingredients for use as direct oral or topical application. Many of the common methods used to extract the oil require the use of organic solvents (e.g., benzene, hexane, naphtha, petroleum ether, butane) that pose a risk of chemical contamination.[27] Hexane and benzene may have neurotoxic effects, and naphtha and petroleum ether are considered potential carcinogens. Marijuana flowers (buds) are infused with a hydrocarbon, which extracts THC and other cannabinoids when the mixture is placed under extreme pressure. The marijuana concentrate that forms is laced with the solvent and requires heat to evaporate and remove the residual solvent. The result is a hash oil concentrate containing 80% to 90% THC. Studies have shown significant residues of petroleum hydrocarbons in extracts produced by organic solvents.[28]

"Dabbing" refers to the use of butane-extracted marijuana products that provide higher THC content compared with flower cannabis.[29] Studies have shown that these cannabis concentrates contain considerable amounts of residual solvent and pesticide contamination.[30]

Alternative methods of extraction involve the use of safer solvents such as ethanol or avoiding organic solvents altogether by using olive oil. Some manufacturers are now using supercritical CO_2 to extract volatile oils from cannabis. This process preserves the integrity of the oils and avoids the use of harmful solvents, providing a safe and ecofriendly approach. Although limited research is available regarding the effectiveness of these methods, nontoxic solvents are advised to avoid potential residues that are harmful to health.

Heavy Metals. Metals such as mercury, cadmium, and chromium are widely dispersed in the environment and contaminate water supplies and agricultural soils to a certain degree. Cannabis has been shown to hyperaccumulate metals such as cadmium and copper from contaminated soils.[31] Cannabis has also been intentionally contaminated with metals to increase the market weight and enhance profits. In 2008, 150 people in Germany developed lead poisoning as the result of using cannabis that was adulterated with powdered lead.[32] Glass particles have also been found in cannabis, likely with the same intention of increasing weight and profits.[33]

TABLE 37.1 Pesticides Detected in Marijuana Samples

Sample	Pesticides Detected	Supplemental Info
1	414 ng/g methamidophos	Discontinued use in commercial settings in 2009
2	2496 ng/g DEET	89% more DEET present compared with medical samples
3	120 ng/g DEET 1385 ng/g chlorpyrifos	Chlorpyrifos: EPA released proposal in Oct. 2015 to revoke its use
4	6527 ng/g chlorpyrifos 449 ng/g DEET 72 ng/g fenamiphos sulfone	Fenamiphos sulfone: restricted-use pesticide due to its high acute toxicity
5	178 ng/g carbaryl 691 ng/g DEET 71 ng/g malathion	Carbaryl: "likely" to be carcinogenic to humans Malathion: mosquito control, low risk to human health

From UCT Research & Development Team. (2015). Potency and pesticide content in medical vs. recreational marijuana. Retrieved from http://www.amchro.com/uct/Potency_and_Pesticide_Content_in_Medical_vs._Recreational_Marijuana_0_6101-02-01.pdf. UCT, LTD. 2731 Bartram Rd, Bristol, PA 19007.

Microbial. Cannabis is also subject to contamination by several microbes including pathogenical fungi, bacteria, and plant viruses. The growing and drying of marijuana plants in residential buildings increases water vapor in the indoor environment, contributing to the formation of mycotoxin-producing fungi.[34] *Penicillium* spp. have been shown to be the predominant indoor species with increasing fungal spore concentrations associated with movement or removal of marijuana plants.[35] Powdered cannabis can become contaminated with fecal pathogens, molds (especially *Aspergillus fumigates*), and aflatoxins during cultivation, harvesting, drying, storage, and distribution.[36] Cannabis may be contaminated with human pathogens such as hepatitis A,[37] hepatitis B,[38] and salmonella.[39] Several studies have linked chronic pulmonary aspergillosis with the medical or recreational use of cannabis, especially in immunocompromised individuals.[40,41,42] In countries such as Canada and the Netherlands, medical cannabis is irradiated to control the bioburden of potential microbial contaminants. Treatment of cannabis with gamma-irradiation does not cause changes in the THC and CBD content and is the recommended method of decontamination.[43]

Synthetic Cannabinoids. Although there is limited research on synthetic cannabinoids (SCBs; "Spice," "K2," "herbal incense"), reports of adverse effects include tachycardia, hypertension, tachypnea, chest pain, heart palpitations, hallucinations, racing thoughts, and seizures.[44] The most common clinical signs of intoxication are neurological, including agitation, central nervous system depression/coma, and delirium/toxic psychosis.[45] Effects of SCBs may occur because they are direct agonists of the cannabinoid receptors, or the effects may be the result of unknown contaminants typically found in synthetic marijuana.[46] There have been reports of acute renal failure associated with the use of SCBs.[47] The toxicity of SCBs is significantly greater than the toxicity of cannabis, and the relative health hazard of SCBs is also higher than that of cannabis.[48]

BODY BURDEN

Detectable amounts of THC can remain in the body for days to weeks after use. Detection times can vary based upon dose, route of administration, metabolism, and characteristics of the screening mechanisms. Cannabinoids can be detected in saliva, blood, urine, hair, and nails.[49]

After inhalation, THC and other cannabinoids are rapidly absorbed from the lungs and quickly reach high concentration in the blood. THC levels increase rapidly, peak before the end of smoking, and dissipate quickly. Effects from smoking marijuana are felt almost immediately and last about 1 to 3 hours.

Ingestion of marijuana or its constituents in foods or beverages delivers significantly less THC into the bloodstream because it must first pass through the digestive system. It is estimated that liver metabolism reduces the oral bioavailability of THC by 4% to 12%.[50] Effects of ingested marijuana appear within 30 to 60 minutes and can last for several hours afterward.

Urine is the preferred method of testing because of higher concentration and longer detection time of metabolites as well as ease of sample collection. THC has a half-life of 1.3 days for infrequent users and between 5 to 13 days for frequent users.[51] 11-nor-delta(9)-carboxy-tetrahydrocannabinol-9-carboxylic acid (THCCOOH) is an oxidized byproduct of THC that can be used to measure marijuana use. THCCOOH is detectable (using a screening cut-off of 50 ng/mL) in urine for 2 to 4 days after smoking one marijuana cigarette, and more frequent use will be detectable for almost 1 month.[52]

Detoxification/Excretion Processes

THC is eliminated quickly from plasma and widely distributed to tissues such as the spleen, liver, lungs, and adipose tissue. The liver metabolizes THC using hydroxylation and oxidation reactions catalyzed by cytochrome P450 enzymes.[53] CYP2C9 and CYP3A4 are the major enzymes involved in the hydroxylation of cannabinoids in liver microsomes.[54,55] The majority of cannabis (65%) is excreted in the feces, and about 20% is excreted in urine.[56] THC is excreted in the urine mainly as the glucuronic acid conjugate THCCOOH. THCCOOH has a half-life between 30 and 44 hours, and the majority of cannabis is excreted within 5 days after use.[57]

Clinical Significance

Epidemiological evidence over the past 20 years shows that heavy cannabis use increases the risk of accidents, can produce dependence, and has been associated with poor social outcomes and mental health in adulthood.[58] Long-term daily use has been associated with decreased motivation, impairment in ability to learn, and reductions in sexual desire.[59,60] Daily heavy inhalation can produce bronchial irritation and may lead to long-term pulmonary damage secondary to the associated hydrocarbon residue.[61]

Marijuana smoke has been shown to be mutagenic in the Ames test and in tissue culture.[62] Smoking marijuana can lead to symptoms of airway obstruction;[63] squamous metaplasia;[64] impairment of psychomotor performance; increased incidence of schizophrenia;[65] cancer of the mouth, jaw, tongue, and lung; and nonlymphoblastic leukemia in children of marijuana smoking mothers.[66] However, a large population-based study showed that, after adjusting for sex, education, birth year, alcohol consumption, and cigarette smoking, marijuana use was not associated with the development of oral squamous cell carcinoma.[67] Although marijuana smoke has been shown to contain carcinogenic compounds, a link between marijuana use and lung cancer has been inconclusive.[68]

A meta-analysis evaluating the nonacute neurocognitive effects of chronic marijuana users showed some decreased effects in ability to learn and remember new information but no effect on other measured cognitive abilities.[69] No significant abstinence syndrome has been seen after the discontinuation of marijuana, and death from marijuana overdose is still considered virtually impossible.

INTERVENTION

Marijuana may be considered a "toxin of choice" and, as such, exposure can be managed by the individual. Avoidance is the primary intervention. Studies have shown little value in the treatment of cannabis dependence with selective serotonin reuptake inhibitor (SSRI) antidepressants, mixed action antidepressants, atypical antidepressants (bupropion), anxiolytics (buspirone), and norepinephrine reuptake inhibitors.[70] At this time, no medication is approved for the treatment of intoxication, withdrawal, or cannabis use disorder (CUD).[71]

For individuals with CUD, interventions begin with abstinence as well as psychosocial treatment. N-acetyl-cysteine (NAC) has proven to be beneficial in the treatment of cannabis addiction by attenuating the pathophysiological processes associated with CUD, including oxidative stress, apoptosis, mitochondrial dysfunction, neuroinflammation, and glutamate and dopamine dysregulation.[72,73] NAC (1200 mg twice daily) has also demonstrated increased odds of abstinence in cannabis-dependent adolescents.[74]

BENEFITS

Over the last several years, cannabinoids have shown promise in the management and treatment of several conditions. In a cancer context, cannabinoids have many palliative effects including alleviating nausea and vomiting induced by chemotherapy,[75] treatment of cancer-associated pain,[76] appetite stimulation, and attenuation of wasting.[77] Cannabinoids have also been shown to have potential antitumor effects by modulating key cell-signaling pathways.[78] CBD induces apoptosis of glioma cells *in vitro* and tumor regression *in vivo* through activation of caspases and reactive oxygen species in tumor cells.[79] THC has been shown to induce apoptosis in prostate cancer cells in a dose-dependent manner.[80] CBD, CBG, cannabichromene, cannabidiol acid, and THC have all shown antitumor activities, with CBD being a potent inhibitor of breast cancer cell growth.[81] Cannabinoids have also shown promise in the treatment of skin cancer,[82] pancreatic cancer,[83] and lymphoma.[84]

CBD has shown promise as an anticonvulsant in the treatment of seizures.[85,86] CBD reduces glutamate release, which may be a potential antiseizure mechanism.[87] Two recent papers demonstrated a reduction in seizure frequency in pediatric patients with refractory seizures treated with a high CBD:THC ratio.[88,89]

Many other conditions may be improved with the use of cannabinoids, including symptoms of multiple sclerosis,[90] headaches (migraines),[91] autoimmune conditions,[92] neuropathic pain,[93] and inflammatory conditions (by downregulating cytokine and chemokine production).[94]

CONCLUSION

The toxicity of marijuana is difficult to establish as a result of several confounding factors. Contaminants, mode of use, and prevalence of cannabis use in combination with other drugs complicate the ability to isolate and determine the toxicity of pure marijuana. The lack of research on cannabis agricultural practice as well as the limited long-term studies on the health effects of marijuana have resulted in a great deal of controversy surrounding cannabis use. At this time, evidence of the potentially damaging effects of marijuana and the toxicity associated with pure marijuana is contradictory. Table 37.2 provides a summary of symptoms and conditions that may occur as a result of toxins associated with marijuana use. It may take several years of research to

TABLE 37.2 Toxins and Symptoms Associated With Cannabis Use

Constituent Pure THC	Toxins Low Toxicity	Effects/Diseases
Smoking dried cannabis flower buds	PAHs, ammonia, cyanide, heavy metals, carbon monoxide, mutagens, carcinogens	Cancer, COPD, impairment of psychomotor performance, toxic metal poisoning
Pesticide contamination	Pyrethrums Organophosphates Carbamates Organochlorines (e.g., DDT – removed from the market)	Cancer (particularly non-Hodgkin's lymphoma, leukemia, brain, prostate, kidney) Pyrethrums: Difficulty breathing, nasal irritation, headache, nausea, tremors, convulsions Organophosphates: neurobehavioral alterations
Solvent contamination	Benzene, hexane, naphtha, petroleum ether, butane	Neurotoxins, cancer

associate trace pesticide residues with human health effects and several more years to develop standardized rules, regulations, and procedures on the growth, manufacturing, handling, and distribution of cannabis.

Conflicting research makes it difficult to provide recommendations on the use of marijuana in any form. For individuals who decide to smoke marijuana, consuming organically grown cannabis reduces the risk of exposure to pesticides and other topical contaminants. Using a filtered water pipe also reduces inhaled contaminants. For those who ingest cannabis orally, organically grown, supercritical CO_2 extracted oils appears to be the best guidance to provide patients.

REFERENCES

1. Gallup. (2016). In U.S., 45% Say They Have Tried Marijuana. Available at http://news.gallup.com/poll/214250/say-tried/marijuana.aspxbi. (Accessed 10 November 2017).
2. Arcview Market Research 2014 The State of Legal Marijuana Markets 3rd ed San Francisco, CA ArcView Market Research.
3. Happyana, N., Agnolet, S., Muntendam, R., Van Dam, A., et al. (2013). Analysis of cannabinoids in laser-microdissectedtrichomes of medicinal Cannabis sativa using LCMS and cryogenic NMR. Phytochemistry, 87, 51–59.
4. Wilson, R., & Nicoll, R. (2002). Endocannabinoid signaling in the brain. Science, 296(5568), 678–682.
5. Hejazi, N., Zhou, C., Oz, M., Sun, H., Ye, J. H., & Zhang, L. (2006). Delta-9-tetrahydrocannabinol and endogenous cannabinoid anandamide directly potentiate the function of glycine receptors. Molecular Pharmacology, 69(3), 991–997.
6. ElSohly, M. A., Ross, S. A., Mehmedic, Z., et al. (2000). Potency trends of delta-9-THC and other cannabinoids in confiscated marijuana from 1980-1997. Journal of Forensic Sciences, 45, 24–30.
7. National Center for the Development of Natural Products. Quarterly Report Potency Monitoring Project, May 9, 2003-August 8, 2003. NIDA Marijuana Project. University, Miss: Research Institute of Pharmaceutical Sciences, School of Pharmacy, University of Mississippi; 2003.
8. Smith, D. E. & Mehl C. (1970). An analysis of marijuana toxicity. Clinical Toxicology, 3(1), 101–105.
9. Smith, D. E. (1968). The acute and chronic toxicity of marijuana. Journal of Psychedelic Drugs, 2(1), 37–47.
10. Weil, A. (1970). Adverse reactions to marijuana – classification and suggested treatment. The New England Journal of Medicine, 282, 997–1000.
11. Hashibe, M., Ford, D. E., & Zhang, Z. F. (2002). Marijuana smoking and head and neck cancer. Journal of Clinical Pharmacology, 42(Suppl. 11), 103S–107S.
12. Zimmerman, S., & Zimmerman, A. M. (1990). Genetic effects of marijuana. The International Journal of Addictions, 25(1A), 19–33.
13. Harclerode, J. (1984). Endocrine effects of marijuana in the male: preclinical studies. NIDA Research Monograph, 44, 46–64.
14. Hashibe, M., Straif, K., Tashkin, D. P., Morgenstren, H., Greenland, S., & Zhang, Z. F. (2005). Epidemiologic review of marijuana use and cancer risk. Alcohol, 35(3), 265–275.
15. Cohn, A., Johnson, A., Ehlke, S., & Villanti, A. (2016). Characterizing substance use and mental health profiles of cigar, blunt, and non-blunt marijuana users from the National Survey of drug Use and Health. Drug and Alcohol Depend, 160, 105–111.
16. Moir, D., Rickert, W., Levasseur, G., Larose, Y., et al. (2008). A comparison of mainstream and sidestream

marijuana and tobacco cigarette smoke produced under two machine smoking conditions. *Chemical Research in Toxicology*, 21(2), 494–502.

17. Wu, T. C., Scott, R., Burnett, S., et al. (1988). Pulmonary hazards of smoking marijuana as compared with tobacco. *The New England Journal of Medicine*, 318, 347–351.

18. Tashkin, D. P. (2015). How beneficial is vaping cannabis to respiratory health compared to smoking? *Addiction*, 110(11), 1706–1707.

19. Thomson, J. (2012). Medical marijuana cultivation and policy gaps. *California Research Bureau*. Available at http://library.humboldt.edu/humco/holdings/CAMP/CRB_Pesticides_on_Medical_Marijuana_Report.pdf. (Accessed on 27 March 2017).

20. Stone, D. (2014). Cannabis, pesticides and conflicting laws: the dilemma for legalized states and implications for public health. *Regulatory toxicology and pharmacology: RTP*, 69(3), 284–288.

21. Thompson, C., Sweitzer, R., Gabriel, M., Purcell, K., Barrett, R., & Poppenga, R. (2014). Impacts of rodenticide and insecticide toxicants from marijuana cultivation sites on fisher survival rates in the sierra national forest, CA. *Conserv Letter*, 7, 91–102.

22. Perez-Parada, A., Alonso, B., Rodriguez, C., Besil, N., et al. (2016). Evaluation of three multiresidue methods for the determination of pesticides in marijuana (Cannabis sativa L) with liquid chromatography-tandem mass spectrometry. *Chromatographia*, 79(17), 1069–1083.

23. UCT Part Numbers. Pennsylvania. (2015). *Potency and Pesticide Content in Medical vs Recreational Marijuana.* Available at https://sampleprep.unitedchem.com/media/at_assets/tech_doc_info/Potency_and_Pesticide_Content_in_Medical_vs._Recreational_Marijuana.pdf. (Accessed 27 March 2017).

24. Skeet, N. (2009). *City attorney explains medical marijuana issue on NBC*, http://lacityorgatty.blogspot.com/2009/10/city-attorney-explains-medical.html.

25. Sullivan, N., Elzinga, S., & Raber, J. (2013). Determination of pesticide residues in cannabis smoke. *Journal of toxicology*, 3, 1–6.

26. Lorenz, W., Bahadir, M., & Korte, F. (1987). Thermolysis of pesticide residues during tobacco smoking. *Chemosphere*, 16(2–3), 521–522.

27. Rosenthal, E., & Downs, D. (2014). *Beyond buds: marijuana extracts – hash, vaping, dabbing, edibles, and medicines.* [ebook]: Quick American Archives.

28. Romano, L., & Hazekamp, A. (2013). Cannabis oil: chemical evaluation of an upcoming cannabis based medicine. *Cannabinoids.*, 1(1), 1–11.

29. Miller, B. L., Stogner, J. M., & Miller, J. M. (2016). Exploring butane hash oil use: a research note. *Journal of Psychoactive Drugs*, 48(1), 44–49.

30. Raber, J. C., Elzinga, S., & Kaplan, C. (2015). Understanding dabs: contamination concerns of cannabis concentrates and cannabinoid transfer during the act of dabbing. *The Journal of Toxicological Sciences*, 40(6), 797–803.

31. Kozlowski, R. (1995). Interview with Professor R. Kozlowski, director of the Institute of Natural Fibers. *Journal of the International Hemp Association*, 2(2), 86–87.

32. Busse, F., Omidi, L., Timper, K., et al. (2008). Lead poisoning due to adulterated marijuana. *The New England Journal of Medicine*, 358(15), 1641–1642.

33. Cole, C., Jones, L., McVeigh, J., Kicman, A., et al. (2011). Adulterants in illicit drugs: a review of empirical evidence. *Drug Testing and Analysis*, 3(2), 89–96.

34. Miller, J. D., & Johnson, L. (2012). Consequences of large-scale production of marijuana in residential buildings. *Indoor and Built Environ*, 21, 595–600.

35. Martyny, J., Serrano, K., Scaeffer, J., & Van Dyke, M. (2013). Potential exposures associated with indoor marijuana growing operations. *Journal of occupational and environmental hygiene*, 10(11), 622–639.

36. Cundell, T. (2015). Microbiological attributes of powdered cannabis. *Am Pharm Bus Tech*, July 31.

37. Alexander, T. (1987). Hepatitis outbreak linked to imported pot. *Sinsemilla Tips*, 7(3), 22.

38. Cates, W., & Warren, J. W. (1975). Hepatitis B in Nuremburg, Germany. *JAMA: The Journal of the American Medical Association*, 234, 930–934.

39. Taylor, D. N., Washsmuth, I. K., Shangkuan, Y. H., Schmidt, E. V., et al. (1981). Salmonellosis associated with marijuana. *The New England Journal of Medicine*, 306, 1249–1253.

40. Chusid, M. J., Gelfand, J. A., Nutter, C., & Fauci, A. S. (1975). Pulmonary aspergillosis, inhalation of contaminated marijuana smoke, and chronic granulation disease. *Ann Intern Med*, 82, 61–64.

41. Cescon, D. W., Page, S., Richardson, M. J., Moore, S., et al. (2008). Invasive allergic bronchopulmonary aspergillosis associated with marijuana use in a man with colorectal cancer. *Journal of Clinical Oncology* 26(13), 2214–2215.

42. Gargani, Y., Bishop, P., & Denning, D. W. (2011). Too many moldy joints: marijuana and chronic pulmonary aspergillosis. *Mediterranean Journal of Hematology and Infectious Diseases*, 3, e2011005. Open Journal System.

43. Hazekamp, A. (2016). Evaluating the effects of gamma-irradiation for decontamination of medicinal cannabis. *Frontiers in Pharmacology*, Apr 27 7, 108.

44. Wells, D. L., & Ott, C. A. (2011). The 'new" marijuana. *Ann of Pharmacother*, *45*(3), 414–417.

45. Riederer, A. M., Campleman, S. L., Carlson, R. G., Boyer, E. W., et al. (2016). Acute poisonings from synthetic cannabinoids – 50 US toxicology investigators consortium registry sites, 2010-2015. *MMWR. Morbidity and Mortality Weekly Report*, *65*(27), 692–695.

46. Mills, B., Yepes, A., & Nugent, K. (2015). Synthetic cannabinoids. *The American journal of the medical sciences*, *350*(1), 59–62.

47. Gudsoorkar, V. S., & Perez, J. A., Jr. (2015). A new differential diagnosis: synthetic cannabinoids-associated acute renal failure. *Methodist DeBakey Cardiovascular Journal*, *11*(3), 189–191. PubMed PMID: 26634029.

48. Bonnet, U., & Mayler, H. (2015). Synthetic cannabinoids: spread, addiction biology, and current perspective of personal health hazard. *Fort der Neurol-Psych*, *83*(4), 221–231.

49. Manno, J. E., Manno, B. R., Kemp, P. M., Alford, D. D., et al. (2001). Temporal indication of marijuana use can be estimated from plasma and urine concentrations of delta-9-tetrahydrocannabinol, 11-hydroxy-delta-9-tetrahydrocannabinol, and 11-nor-delta-9-tetrahydrocannabinol-9-carboxylic acid. *Journal of Analytical Toxicology*, *25*, 538–549.

50. Owens, S. M., McBay, A. J., Reisner, H. M., & Perez-Reyes, M. (1981). 125I radioimmunoassay of delta-9-tetrahydrocannibinol in blood and plasma with a solid-phase second-antibody separation method. *Clinical Chemistry*, *27*, 619–624.

51. Smith-Kielland, A., Skuterud, B., & Morland, J. (1999). Urinary excretion of 11-nor-9-carboxy-delta9-tetrahydrocannabinol and cannabinoids in frequent and infrequent drug users. *Journal of Analytical Toxicology*, *23*, 323–332.

52. Vandevenne, M., Vandenbussche, H., & Verstraete, A. (2000). Detection time of drug abuse in urine. *Acta Clinica Belgica*, *55*(6), 323–333.

53. Sharma, P., Murthy, P., & Bharath, M. M. (2012). Chemistry, metabolism, and toxicology of cannabis: clinical implications. *Iranian journal of psychiatry*, *7*(4), 149–156.

54. Watanabe, K., Yamaori, S., Funahashi, T., Kimura, T., & Yamamoto, I. (2007). Cytochrome P450 enzymes involved in the metabolism of tetrahydrocannabinols and cannabinol by human hepatic microsomes. *Life Sciences*, *80*(15), 1415–1419.

55. Stout, S. M., & Cimino, N. M. (2014). Exogenous cannabinoids as substrates, inhibitors, and inducers of human drug metabolizing enzymes: a systematic review. *Drug Metabolism Reviews*, *46*(1), 86–95.

56. Lemberger, L., Axelrod, J., & Kopin, I. J. (1971). Metabolism and disposition of delta-9-tetrahydrocannabinol in man. *Pharmacological Reviews*, *23*, 371–380.

57. Goulle, J. P., Saussereau, E., & Lacroix, C. (2008). Delta-9-tetrahydrocannabinol pharmacokinetics. *Annales Pharmaceutiques Francaises*, *66*, 232–244.

58. Hall, W. (2015). What has research over the past two decades revealed about the adverse health effects of recreational cannabis use? *Addiction*, *110*(1), 19–35.

59. Pope, H. G., Gruber, A. J., Hudson, J. I., & Huestis, M. A. (2002). Yergelun-Todd D. Cognitive measures in long-term cannabis users. *Journal of Clinical Pharmacology*, *42*(Suppl. 1), 41S–47S.

60. Bolla, K. I., Brown, K., Eldreth, D., Tate, K., & Cadet, J. L. (2002). Dose-related neurocognitive effects of marijuana use. *Neurology*, *59*(9), 1337–1343.

61. Bloom, J. W., Kaltenborn, W., Paoletti, P., Camilli, A., & Lebowitz, M. (1987). Respiratory effects of non-tobacco cigarettes. *British Medical Journal (Clinical Research Ed.)*, Dec 12 *295*.

62. Nahas, G., & Latour, C. (1992). The human toxicity of marijuana. *The Medical Journal of Australia*, *156*(7), 495–497.

63. Tashkin, D. P., Baldwin, G. C., Sarafian, T., Dubinett, S., & Roth, M. D. (2002). Respiratory and immunologic consequences of marijuana smoking. *Journal of Clinical Pharmacology*, *42*(Suppl. 11), 715–815.

64. Zhang, Z. F., Morgenstern, H., Spitz, M. R., Tashkin, D. P., Yu, G. P., Marshall, J. R., et al. (1999). Marijuana use and increased risk of squamous cell carcinoma of the head and neck. *Cancer Epidemiology, Biomarkers & Prevention: a Publication of the American Association for Cancer Research Cosponsored by the American Society of Preventive Oncology*, *8*(12), 1071–1078.

65. Kelley, M., Wan, C., Broussard, B., Crisafio, A., Cristofaro, S., et al. (2016). Marijuana use in the immediate 5-year premorbid period is associated with increased risk of onset of schizophrenia and related psychotic disorders. *Schizophrenia research*, *171*(1), 62–67.

66. Robison, L. L., Buckley, J. D., Daigle, A. E., Wells, R., Benjamin, D., et al. (1989). Maternal drug use and risk of childhood nonlymphoblastic leukemia among offspring. An epidemiologic investigation implicating marijuana a report from the Children's Cancer Study Group). *Cancer*, *63*(10), 1904–1911.

67. Rosenblatt, K. A., Daling, J. R., Chen, C., Sherman, K. J., & Schwartz, S. M. (2004). Marijuana use and risk of oral squamous cell carcinoma. *Cancer Research*, *64*(11), 4049–4054.

68. Hashibe, M., Morgenstern, H., Cui, Y., et al. (2006). Marijuana use and the risk of lung and upper aerodigestive tract cancers: results of a population-based case-control study. *Cancer Epidemiol Biomark Prev Publ Am Assoc Cancer Res Cosponsored Am Soc Prev Oncol*, *15*(10), 1829–1834.

69. Grant, I., Gonzalez, R., Carey, C. L., Natarajan, L., & Wolfson, T. (2003). Non-acute (residual) neurocognitive effects of cannabis use: a meta-analytic study. *Journal of the International Neuropsychological Society*, *9*(5), 679–689.

70. Marshall, K., Gowing, L., Ali, R., & Le Foll, B. (2014). Pharmacotherapies for cannabis dependence. *The Cochrane Database of Systematic Reviews*, (12), CD008940.

71. Gorelick, D. A. (2016). Pharmacological treatment of cannabis-related disorders: a narrative review. *Current Pharmaceutical Design*, Aug 22, [Epub ahead of print].

72. Deepmala, Slattery, J., Kumar, N., Delhey, L., et al. (2015). Clinical trials of N-acetylcysteine in psychiatry and neurology: a systematic review. *Neuroscience and Biobehavioral Reviews*, *55*, 294–321.

73. Asevedo, E., Mendes, A. C., Berk, M., & Brietzke, E. (2014). Systematic review of N-acetylcysteine in the treatment of addictions. *Revista Brasileira de Psiquiatria*, *36*(2), 168–175.

74. Gray, K. M., Carpenter, M. J., Baker, N. L., DeSantis, S. M., et al. (2012). A double-blind randomized controlled trial of N-acetylcysteine in cannabis-dependent adolescents. *The American Journal of Psychiatry*, *169*(8), 805–812.

75. Guzman, M. (2003). Cannabinoids: potential anticancer agents. *Nature Reviews. Cancer*, *3*(10), 745–755.

76. Pertwee, R. G. (2009). Emerging strategies for exploiting cannabinoid receptor agonists as medicines. *British Journal of Pharmacology*, *156*(3), 397–411. PubMed PMID: 19226257.

77. Pertwee, R. G., Howlett, A. C., Abood, M. E., Alexander, S. P., et al. (2010). International Union of Basic and Clinical Pharmacology. LXXIX. Cannabinoid receptors and their ligands: beyond CB1 and CB2. *Pharmacological Reviews*, *62*(4), 588–631. PubMed PMID: 21079038.

78. Bifulco, M., Laezza, C., Pisanti, S., & Gazzerro, P. (2006). Cannabinoids and cancer: pros and cons of an antitumor strategy. *British Journal of Pharmacology*, *148*(2), 123–135.

79. Massi, P., Vaccani, A., Bianchessi, S., Costa, B., et al. (2006). The non-psychoactive cannabidiol triggers caspase activation and oxidative stress in human glioma cells. *Cellular and Molecular Life Sciences*, *63*(17), 2057–2066. PubMed PMID:16909207.

80. Ruiz, L., Miguel, A., & Diaz-Laviada, I. (1999). Delta9-tetrahydrocannabinol induces apoptosis in human prostate PC-3 cells via a receptor-independent mechanism. *FEBS Letters*, *458*(3), 400–404. PubMed PMID: 10570948.

81. Ligresti, A., Moriello, A. S., Starowicz, K., Matias, I., et al. (2006). Antitumor activity of plant cannabinoids with emphasis on the effect of cannabidiol on human breast carcinoma. *The Journal of Pharmacology and Experimental Therapeutics*, *318*(3), 1375–1387. PubMed PMID: 16728591.

82. Blazquez, C., Carracedo, A., Barrado, L., Real, P. J., et al. (2006). Cannabinoid receptors as novel targets for the treatment of melanoma. *FASEB Journal*, *20*(14), 2633–2635. PubMed PMID: 17065222.

83. Fogli, S., Nieri, P., Chicca, A., Adinolfi, B., et al. (2006). Cannabinoid derivatives induce cell death in pancreatic MIA PaCa-2 cells via a receptor-independent mechanism. *FEBS Letters*, *580*(7), 1733–1739. PubMed PMID: 16500647.

84. Flygae, J., Gustafsson, K., Kimby, E., et al. (2005). Cannabinoid receptor ligands mediate growth inhibition and cell death in mantle cell lymphoma. *FEBS Letters*, *579*(30), 6885–6889. PubMed PMID: 16337199.

85. Consroe, P., & Wolkin, A. (1977). Cannabidiol – antiepileptic drug comparisons and interactions in experimentally induced seizures in rats. *The Journal of Pharmacology and Experimental Therapeutics*, *201*(1), 26–32.

86. Hess, E. J., Moody, K. A., Geffrey, A. L., Pollack, S. F., et al. (2016). Cannabidiol as a new treatment for drug-resistant epilepsy in tuberous sclerosis complex. *Epilepsia*, Oct 3, [Epub ahead of print].

87. Sylantyev, S., Jensen, T. P., Ross, R. A., & Rusakov, D. A. (2013). Cannabinoid- and lysophosphatidylinositol-sensitive receptor GPR55 boosts neurotransmitter release at central synapses. *Proceedings of the National Academy of Sciences of the United States of America*, *110*(13), 5193–5198. PubMed PMID: 23472002.

88. Porter, B. E., & Jacobson, C. (2013). Report of a parent survey of cannabidiol-enriched cannabis use in pediatric treatment-resistant epilepsy. *Epilepsy and Behavior: E&B*, *29*(3), 574–577. PubMed PMID: 24237632.

89. Press, C. A., Knupp, K. G., & Chapman, K. E. (2015). Parental reporting of response to oral cannabis extracts for the treatment of refractory epilepsy. *Epilepsy and Behavior: E&B*, *45*, 49–52. PubMed PMID: 25845492.

90. De Lago, E., Moreno-Martet, M., Cabranes, A., et al. (2012). Cannabinoids ameliorate disease progression in a model of multiple sclerosis in mice, acting

preferentially through CB1 receptor-mediated anti-inflammatory effects. *Neuropharmacology, 62*(7), 2299–2308. PubMed PMID: 22342378.

91. Baron, E. P. (2015). Comprehensive review of medicinal marijuana, cannabinoids, and therapeutic implications in medicine and headache: what a long strange trip it's been… *Headache, 55*(6), 885–916. PubMed PMID: 26015168.

92. Katchan, V., David, P., & Shoenfeld, Y. (2016). Cannabinoids and autoimmune disease: a systematic review. *Autoimmunity Reviews, 15*(6), 513–528. PubMed PMID: 26876387.

93. Klein, T. W., & Newton, C. A. (2007). Therapeutic potential of cannabinoid-based drugs. *Advances in Experimental Medicine and Biology, 601*, 395–413. PubMed PMID: 17713029.

94. Nagarkatti, P., Pandey, R., Rieder, S. A., et al. (2009). Cannabinoids as novel anti-inflammatory drugs. *Future Medicinal Chemistry, 1*(7), 1333–1349. PubMed PMID: 20191092.

38

High Fructose Corn Syrup

SUMMARY

- Presence in population: The average American consumes approximately 25 lbs of high fructose corn syrup (HFCS) each year[1]
- Major diseases: Diabetes, obesity, metabolic syndrome, hyperlipidemia, cardiovascular disease
- Primary sources: Sugar-sweetened beverages (e.g., juice, soda, sports drinks), processed foods and

  beverages, baked goods (e.g., breads, pastries, cookies), dairy products (e.g., yogurt, eggnog, ice cream, flavored milks), canned foods (e.g., canned fruits, sauces, soups), cereals, and energy bars
- Best measure: Diet diary, serum level of glucose, glucose tolerance test (GTT) lipid panel
- Best intervention: Dietary modification

DESCRIPTION

HFCS is a fructose-glucose liquid sweetener introduced in the 1970s and used in many foods and beverages as an alternative to sucrose (table sugar). Because HFCS is derived from corn (an abundant agricultural raw material), is stable in acidic foods and beverages, and requires only simple dilution before use, it is readily accepted by the food industry and has become one of the most successful food ingredients in modern history.[2]

Significant scientific debate and controversy exist concerning fructose, sucrose, and HFCS regarding their metabolism, endocrine response, and health effects. Considering sucrose and HFCS contain the same number of calories, approximately the same amount of fructose and glucose, the same level of sweetness, and are absorbed equally in the digestive tract, it is not surprising that many studies have shown that there are no metabolic or endocrine response differences between sucrose and HFCS related to obesity or any other adverse health outcome.[3,4,5] However, a number of studies have shown HFCS to be a contributing factor to energy overconsumption, weight gain, and a rise in the prevalence of obesity.[6,7,8]

Some of the controversy revolves around the selection of the name "high-fructose" corn syrup because HFCS contains about the same amount fructose as sucrose. In addition, several studies were performed comparing pure fructose versus pure glucose, and although there are metabolic differences between the two monosaccharides, neither are consumed independently to any appreciable degree in the human diet. Although fructose is present in fruits, honey, and other carbohydrate sources, the major source of fructose in the US diet is HFCS.[9] That said, the increase in HFCS consumption in the United States has coincided with the increased incidence of obesity, diabetes, cardiovascular disease, and metabolic syndrome.

TOXICITY

Toxicity of HFCS not only includes the potential negative health consequences associated with consuming the sweetener (discussed later), but also includes contaminants resulting from the processing and manufacturing of the product. HFCS is produced by the chemical and enzymatic hydrolysis of corn starch to corn syrup, followed by the isomerization of some of the glucose in corn syrup to fructose. Corn starch consists of amylose and amylopectin, which require heat, caustic soda, and/or hydrochloric acid as well as three different enzymes to convert the starch into glucose and fructose. Alpha-amylase (an enzyme produced from *Bacillus* spp.) hydrolyzes long-chain carbohydrates of corn starch to short-chain dextrins and oligosaccharides, and glucoamylase (an enzyme produced from fungi such as *Aspergillus*) breaks down the dextrins and oligosaccharides into glucose syrup (i.e., corn syrup). The alpha-amylase and glucoamylase used in this process are often genetically modified to improve their heat stability.[10] To produce HFCS, a third enzyme, glucose isomerase, is used to isomerize the glucose from the glucose syrup into a mixture of 90% fructose and 10% glucose (HFCS-90). Finally, after clarification and removal of impurities, HFCS-90 is blended with glucose syrup to dilute the solution for use in manufacturing foods and beverages. The predominant syrups of commerce contain 42% (HFCS-42) or 55% (HFCS-55) fructose.

Residuals from chemicals used in the manufacturing HFCS can ultimately make their way into the end-product. Several chemicals are involved in the production of HFCS, including caustic soda, hydrochloric acid, enzymes (alpha-amylase, glucoamylase, glucose isomerase), filter aid, powdered carbon, calcium chloride, and magnesium sulfate.[11] Caustic soda and hydrochloric acid used in the production of HFCS are often produced by the mercury cell chlor-alkali industry and are used throughout the corn wet-milling process to adjust the pH of the product. Each year the chlor-alkali industry reports unaccounted mercury losses to the Environmental Protection Agency (EPA).[12] A study performed in 2004 found that 9 of 20 samples of HFCS had detectable mercury levels ranging between 0.065 µg to 0.570 µg of mercury/g of HFCS, providing an average daily mercury exposure of between 0 to 28.4 µg (similar to dental amalgam).[13] Table 38.1 lists total mercury detected in selected commercial products containing HFCS.

Current international food standards allow 1 µg mercury/g of caustic soda, and there is no standard for mercury in food-grade hydrochloric acid.[14] The use of mercury-grade caustic soda or hydrochloric acid in the manufacturing process of HFCS may very well lead to mercury contamination of food products. Testing foods containing HFCS for mercury contamination may be warranted.

SOURCES

In 2015, the average American consumed approximately 25 lbs of HFCS[1] and 40.5 lbs of refined cane and beet sugar.[15] As can be seen in Fig. 38.1, sugar consumption increased over the last two centuries. Exposure to HFCS

TABLE 38.1   **Total Mercury Detected in Commercial Products Containing HFCS**

Product	Total Hg Detected (ppt)	Laboratory Detection Limit (ppt)
Quaker Oatmeal To Go	350	80
Jack Daniels Barbeque Sauce	300	100
Hershey's Chocolate Syrup	257	50
Kraft Original Barbeque Sauce	200	100
Nutri-grain Strawberry Cereal Bar	180	80
Manwich Bold Sloppy Joe	150	80
Market Pantry Grape Jelly	130	80
Smucker's Strawberry Jelly	100	80
Frosted Blueberry Pop Tarts	100	80

HFCS: high fructose corn syrup
Hg: mercury
ppt: parts per trillion
Modified from Wallinga, D., Sorensen, J., Mottl, P., & Yablon, B. (2009). Not so sweet: Missing mercury and high fructose corn syrup. *Institute for Agriculture and Trade Policy.* Retrieved from https://www.iatp.org/documents/not-so-sweet-missing-mercury-and-high-fructose-corn-syrup

escalated as soft drink consumption increased globally from 9.5 gallons per person per year in 1997 to 11.4 gallons in 2010.[16] Sugar-sweetened beverages, including carbonated soft drinks, fruit drinks, sports drinks, energy and vitamin water drinks, sweetened iced tea, cordials, and lemonades are the largest contributor to added sugar in the United States.[17] HFCS can also be found in processed food products such as baked goods (e.g., breads, pastries, cookies), dairy products (e.g., yogurt, eggnog, ice cream, flavored milks), canned foods (e.g., canned fruits, sauces, soups), cereals, and energy bars.

BODY BURDEN

HFCS reaches the small intestine predominantly as a monosaccharide, as the minor amount of polysaccharide glucose in HFCS is quickly broken down to free glucose by salivary and intestinal amylases.[18] Although HFCS contains the same monosaccharides as sucrose, the linkage between fructose and glucose in sucrose needs to be cleaved to initiate digestion, whereas the monosaccharides are free and unlinked in HFCS. Single-sugar carbohydrates, such as glucose, do not require digestion to be absorbed.

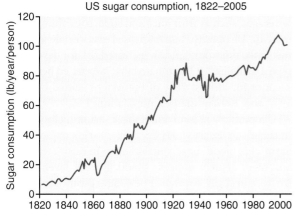

US sugar consumption, 1822–2005

FIG. 38.1 Sugar consumption in the U.S. (Added sugars: glucose, sucrose, high fructose corn syrup, and maple syrup). (From Guyenet, S. and Landen, J. [2012, February 18]. *By 2606, the U.S. diet will be 100 percent sugar.* Retrieved from http://wholehealthsource.blogspot.com/2012/02/by-2606-us-diet-will-be-100-percent.html.)

Glucose is absorbed in the small intestine primarily by active transport using the sodium-dependent glucose transporter (SGLT1). However, during sugar-rich meals, this transport becomes saturated and a diffusive process provides a major pathway for absorption. This diffusive absorption is facilitated by glucose transporter type 2 (GLUT2), a receptor normally found in the basolateral membrane, which inserts into the apical membrane within minutes in response to a high-sugar meal.[19] Fructose is absorbed through the sodium independent GLUT5 transporter.[20]

In a Western diet high in sugar, there is a constant elevation of GLUT2 in the apical membrane, which further increases the absorption of glucose. Artificial sweeteners likely have this same effect and may also lead to increased absorption of any natural sugars present in the diet (Fig. 38.2). GLUT2 may also act as a glucose sensor in the brain, a hypothesis suggested by data showing an increased intake among those with a GLUT2 genetic variant in both diabetic and healthy populations.[21] Flavonoids, particularly quercetin, may have some role in reducing the absorption of glucose by inhibiting GLUT2.[22]

Disaccharides, such as sucrose and lactose, require small intestinal surface enzymes for hydrolysis to monosaccharides. Sucrose is composed of 50% glucose and 50% fructose, whereas HFCS is composed of 55% fructose

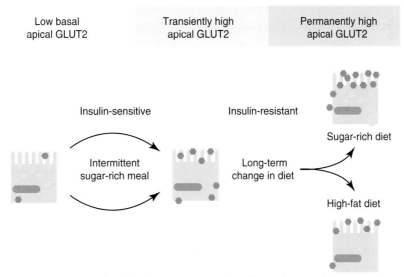

FIG. 38.2 Permanent apical GLUT2 elevation due to insulin resistance in response to poor diet. (Modified from Kellett, G. L., Brot-Laroche, E., Mace, O. J., & Leturque, A. [2008]. Sugar absorption in the intestine: The role of GLUT2. *Annual Review of Nutrition, 28,* 35–54.)

and 45% glucose (HFCS-55, the form typically used in beverages) or 42% fructose and 58% glucose (HFCS-42, the form typically used in baked goods, canned fruits, soups, dairy products, and other manufactured foods).[23] Digestive enzymes, such as lactase-phlorizin hydrolase and sucrase isomaltase, are anchored to the mucosal surface of the small intestine where the soluble sugars in the lumen are hydrolyzed to free glucose, galactose, and fructose, which are absorbed rapidly from the lumen.[24] Fructose is passively absorbed further down the small intestine than glucose, but compared with sucrose and glucose, absorption of fructose is small. Inside cells, fructose is phosphorylated to fructose-1-phosphate, which is then cleaved by aldolase to trioses that form the building blocks for the synthesis of triglycerides and phospholipids.[25] Because fructose must be changed to glucose in the liver to be utilized by the body, blood glucose levels do not rise as rapidly after fructose consumption as they do with other simple sugars. Fructose does not stimulate insulin secretion from pancreatic beta-cells,[26] tends to blunt insulin responses compared with glucose,[27,28,29] and may enhance the sensitivity to insulin.[30] However, simultaneous ingestion of glucose with fructose increases fructose absorption, suggesting that the pair of monosaccharides might be absorbed by the disaccharidase-related transport system as if they were the product of the enzymatic hydrolysis of sucrose.[31] In addition, although pure fructose does not increase plasma glucose or insulin, consumption of HFCS does increase plasma glucose and insulin, likely due to the glucose moiety.[32]

Detoxification/Excretion Processes

Refined sugars are quickly absorbed into the bloodstream, causing a rapid rise in blood sugar. The body's response to this is to greatly increase the secretion of insulin by the pancreas. The excessive secretion of insulin drives blood sugar down and often leads to hypoglycemia. In response to the rapid fall in blood glucose levels, the adrenal glands secrete epinephrine (adrenaline), which causes a rapid increase in the blood glucose level. In time, the adrenal glands become "exhausted" by the repeated stress and cannot mount an appropriate response. This lack of response leads to reactive hypoglycemia. If blood sugar control mechanisms are further stressed, the body will eventually become insensitive to insulin, and the reactive hypoglycemia will turn into diabetes.

Clinical Significance

HFCS and sucrose have similar metabolic and endocrine responses, and therefore similar adverse clinical effects when consumed in large quantities. Studies have shown that HFCS and sucrose produce similar responses of glucose, insulin, leptin, ghrelin, energy intake, and appetite ratings.[4,33,34,35] Higher consumption of sugar-sweetened beverages, such as fruit juice and soda, contributes to an increase in obesity,[36] an increased risk for developing metabolic syndrome, and an increased risk for developing type 2 diabetes.[37] It is estimated that sweetened beverages account for at least 20% of the weight gained between 1977 and 2007 in the U.S. population.[38]

Certainly, there is no doubt that consuming foods high in sugar (i.e., sucrose, HFCS, maple syrup, or honey) is harmful to blood sugar control. Sugars in sugar-sweetened beverages acutely increase blood glucose levels,[39] and fructose in sugar-sweetened beverages promotes hepatic lipogenesis and insulin resistance.[40] Fructose from HFCS may further increase cardiovascular disease risk by promoting dyslipidemia,[41] depositing visceral fat, and increasing hepatic de novo lipogenesis and hypertension due to hyperuricemia.[42,43] In addition, fructose may promote the formation of advanced glycation end-products that appear to play a role in the aging process, the development of atherosclerosis, and in the pathogenesis of diabetic renal, vascular, and ocular complications.[44]

HFCS is a rapidly absorbable carbohydrate and contributes to a higher glycemic load, leading to inflammation, insulin resistance, and impaired beta-cell function.[45] Epidemiologically, diabetes mellitus has been linked to the Western lifestyle and is uncommon in cultures consuming a more "primitive" diet.[46] A thorough review of diabetes mellitus I and II and their associated health consequences is more extensive and requires more time and space than available in this chapter. Briefly, diabetes is a chronic disorder of carbohydrate, fat, and protein metabolism characterized by fasting elevations of blood glucose levels and an increased risk of heart disease, stroke, kidney disease, and loss of nerve function. Diabetes can occur when the pancreas does not secrete enough insulin or if the cells of the body become resistant to insulin; hence, blood sugar cannot get into cells, which then leads to serious complications. Elevated insulin levels are associated with elevations in cholesterol, triglycerides, blood pressure, and risk of death from cardiovascular disease. In addition, type 2 diabetes is associated with reduced hippocampal volume,[47] cognitive impairment,[48] depression,[49] increased risk of Alzheimer's disease,[50] inflammation and neurodegeneration in brain tissues and brain astrocytes resulting from the accumulation of reactive oxygen species (ROSs) in neuronal cells,[51] retinopathy,[52] peripheral polyneuropathy,[53] increased viral susceptibility through the increase of NF-κβ binding and TNF-alpha expression,[54] and decreased neutrophil function.[55]

As cultures switch from their native diets to the "foods of commerce," their rate of diabetes increases, eventually reaching the same proportions seen in Western societies.[56] More than half of the carbohydrates consumed in the United States are in the form of sugars added to processed foods as sweetening agents.[57] Evidence shows that women who consumed one or more sugar-sweetened soft drink(s) per day had a relative risk of type 2 diabetes of 1.83 (95% confidence interval) compared with those who consumed less than one sugar-sweetened beverage per month.[58] Independent of obesity status, it is estimated that consumption of sugar-sweetened beverages would result in 1.8 million excess events of type 2 diabetes in the United States over the next 10 years.[59]

In addition to the direct health effects of HFCS, clinical consequences may also result from mercury contamination of foods containing HFCS that has been contaminated with mercury. Considering mercury is toxic at any level, the cumulative effect of these sources increases the potential for mercury toxicity. Mercury is a potent neurotoxin, and effects of long-term mercury exposure include learning disabilities, parkinsonism, insomnia, respiratory failure, and neurological malfunction.[60,61]

INTERVENTION

A combination of diet and exercise has been shown to be a powerful tool for improving glycemic control.[62,63,64] Studies have shown that onions and garlic have demonstrated blood sugar–lowering action.[65,66] A number of whole foods–based diets have been shown effective in the treatment and even reversal of type 2 diabetes. One example is the high complex carbohydrate, high plant fiber (HCF) diet popularized by James Anderson, MD. This approach has substantial support and validation in the scientific literature as effective in the treatment of diabetes mellitus.[67,68,69,70] It is high in cereal grains, legumes, and root vegetables, and restricts simple sugar and fat intake. The positive metabolic effects of the HCF diet include reduced postprandial hyperglycemia and delayed hypoglycemia,

increased tissue sensitivity to insulin, reduced cholesterol and triglyceride levels with increased high-density lipoprotein (HDL) cholesterol levels, and progressive weight reduction. Although adequate, improvements to the HCF diet can be made by further reducing carbohydrates and consuming organic, mostly plant-based, unprocessed foods when possible.

In addition to lifestyle changes, several nutritional supplements have been shown to improve insulin resistance and reduce hyperglycemia. Chromium and omega-3-fatty acids have been shown to improve glucose tolerance, lower insulin levels, decrease total cholesterol and triglyceride levels, and increase HDL cholesterol levels.[71,72] Biotin supplementation has been shown to enhance insulin sensitivity and increase the activity of glucokinase, the enzyme responsible for the first step in the utilization of glucose by the liver.[73] Zinc is involved in virtually all aspects of insulin metabolism (synthesis, secretion, and utilization), and supplementation with zinc has a protective effect against beta cell destruction and improves insulin levels.[74]

REFERENCES

1. United States Department of Agriculture. Economic Research Service. Table 52 – High fructose corn syrup: estimated number of per capita calories consumed daily, by calendar year. Available at https://www.ers.usda.gov/webdocs/DataFiles/53304/table52.xls?v=42951. (Accessed November 16, 2016.)
2. Buck, A. W. (2001). High fructose corn syrup. In L. O. Nabors (Ed.), *Alternative sweeteners* (3rd ed., pp. 391–411). New York, NY: Marcel Dekker.
3. Stanhope, K. L., Griffen, S. C., Bair, B. R., et al. (2008). Twenty-four-hour endocrine and metabolic profiles following consumption of high-fructose corn syrup-, sucrose-, fructose-, and glucose-sweetened beverages with meals. *The American Journal of Clinical Nutrition, 87*(5), 1194–1203.
4. Yu, Z., Lowndes, J., & Rippe, J. (2013). High-fructose corn syrup and sucrose have equivalent effects on energy-regulating hormones at normal human consumption levels. *Nutrition Research, 33*(12), 1043–1052.
5. Melanson, K. J., Zukley, L., Lowndes, J., Nguyen, V., Angelopoulos, T. J., & Rippe, J. M. (2007). Effects of high-fructose corn syrup and sucrose consumption on circulating glucose, insulin, leptin, and ghrelin and on appetite in normal-weight women. *Nutrition, 23*(2), 103–112.
6. Ludwig, D. S., Peterson, K. E., & Gortmaker, S. L. (2001). Relation between consumption of sugar

sweetened drinks and childhood obesity: A prospective, observational analysis. *Lancet, 357*, 505–508.

7. Bray, G. A., Nielsen, S. J., & Popkin, B. M. (2004). Consumption of high-fructose corn syrup in beverages may play a role in the epidemic of obesity. *The American Journal of Clinical Nutrition, 79*, 537–543.

8. Elliot, S. S., Keim, N. L., Stern, J. S., Teff, K., & Havel, P. J. (2002). Fructose, weight gain, and the insulin resistance syndrome. *The American Journal of Clinical Nutrition, 76*, 911–922.

9. Hein, G. L., Storey, M. L., White, J. S., & Lineback, D. R. (2005). Highs and lows of high fructose corn syrup. *Nutrition Today, 40*(6), 253.

10. Parker, K., Salas, M., & Mwosu, V. (2010). High fructose corn syrup: Production, uses and public health concerns. *Biotech Molecular Biology Reviews, 5*(5), 71–78.

11. Lurgi Life Science GmbH. (1999). *High-fructose syrup production-process and economics. Proceedings of International Conference on Value-Added Products for the Sugar Industry*. Baton Rouge.

12. United States Environmental Protection Agency Mercury Cell ChlorAlkali Plants: National Emissions Standards for Hazardous Air Pollutants (NESHAP). Available at https://www.epa.goc/stationary-sources-air-pollution/mercury-cell-chloralkali-plants-national-emissions-standards. (Accessed November 10, 2017.)

13. Dufault, R., LeBlanc, B., Schnoll, R., Cornett, C., et al. (2009). Mercury from chlor-alkali plants: Measured concentrations in food product sugar. *Environmental Health, 8*, 2. doi:10.1186/1476-069X-8-3.

14. Joint FAO/WHO Expert Committee on Food Additives. (2004: Geneva, Switzerland) *Evaluation of certain food additives: sixty-third report of the Joint FAO/WHO Expert Committee on Food Additives*. Available at http://whqlibdoc.who.int/trs/WHO_TRS_928.pdf. (Accessed November 10, 2017.)

15. United States Department of Agriculture. Economic Research Service. Table 51 – Refined cane and beet sugar: estimated number of per capita calories consumed daily, by calendar year. Available at https://www.ers.usda.gov/webdocs/DataFiles/53304/table51.xls?v=42951. (Accessed on November 16, 2016.)

16. Basu, S., McKee, M., Galea, G., & Stuckler, D. (2013). Relationship of soft drink consumption to global overweight, obesity, and diabetes: A cross-national analysis of 75 countries. *American Journal of Public Health, 103*(11), 2071–2077.

17. Johnson, R. K., Appel, L. J., Brands, M., et al. (2009). Dietary sugars intake and cardiovascular health: A scientific statement from the American Heart Association. *Circulation, 120*(11), 1011–1020.

18. White, J. S. (2008). Straight talk about high-fructose corn syrup: What it is and what it ain't. *The American Journal of Clinical Nutrition, 88*(6), 1716S–1721S.

19. Kellett, G. L., Brot-Laroche, E., Mace, O. J., et al. (2008). Sugar absorption in the intestine: The role of GLUT2. *Annual Review of Nutrition, 28*, 35–54.

20. Schorin, M. D. (2005). High fructose corn syrups part 1: Composition, consumption and metabolism. *Nutrition Today, 40*, 248–252.

21. Eny, K. M., Wolever, T. M., Fontaine-Bisson, B., et al. (2008). Genetic variant in the glucose transporter type 2 is associated with higher intakes of sugars in two distinct populations. *Physiological Genomics, 33*(3), 355–360.

22. Kwon, O., Eck, P., Chen, S., et al. (2007). Inhibition of the intestinal glucose transporter GLUT2 by flavonoids. *FASEB Journal : Official Publication of the Federation of American Societies for Experimental Biology, 21*(2), 366–377.

23. White, J. S., Foreyt, J. P., Melanson, K. J., & Angelopoulos, T. J. (2010). High-fructose corn syrup: Controversies and common sense. *American Journal of Lifestyle Medicine, 4*, 515–520.

24. Robayo-Torres, C. C., Quezada-Calvillo, R., & Nichols, B. L. (2006). Disaccharide digestion: Clinical and molecular aspects. *Clinical Gastroenterology and Hepatology, 4*(3), 276–287.

25. Mayes, P. A. (1993). Intermediary metabolism of fructose. *The American Journal of Clinical Nutrition, 58*, 754S–765S.

26. Rodin, J. (1991). Effects of pure sugar vs mixed starch fructose loads on food intake. *Appetite, 17*(3), 213–219.

27. Vozzo, R., Baker, B., Wittert, G. A., et al. (2002). Glycemic, hormone, and appetite responses to monosaccharide ingestion in patients with type 2 diabetes. *Metabolism: Clinical and Experimental, 51*, 949–957.

28. Kong, M. F., Chapman, I., Goble, E., et al. (1999). Effects of oral fructose and glucose on plasma GLP-1 and appetite in normal subjects. *Peptides, 20*, 545–551.

29. Wei, W., & Melanson, K. J. (2006). Metabolic and appetitive responses to test drinks sweetened by fructose or glucose in overweight males. *Obesity, 14*, A218.

30. Koivisto, V. A., & Yki-Jarvinen, H. (1993). Fructose and insulin sensitivity in patients with type 2 diabetes. *Journal of Internal Medicine, 233*, 145–153.

31. Riby, J. E., Fujisawa, T., & Kretchmer, N. (1993). Fructose absorption. *The American Journal of Clinical Nutrition, 58*, 748S–53S.

32. Melanson, K., Angelopoulos, T. J., Nguyen, V., Zukley, L., Lowndes, J., & Rippe, J. M. (2008). High-fructose

corn syrup, energy intake, and appetite regulation. *The American Journal of Clinical Nutrition, 88*(6), 1738S–1744S.

33. Soenen, S., & Westerterp-Plantenga, M. S. (2007). No differences in satiety or energy intake after high-fructose corn syrup, sucrose, or milk preloads. *The American Journal of Clinical Nutrition, 86*, 1586–1594.

34. Monsivais, P., Perrigue, M., & Drewnowski, A. (2007). Sugars and satiety: Does the type of sweetener make a difference? *The American Journal of Clinical Nutrition, 86*, 116–123.

35. Zuckley, L., Lowndes, J., Nguyen, V., et al. (2007). Consumption of beverages sweetened with high fructose corn syrup and sucrose produce similar levels of glucose, leptin, insulin, and ghrelin in obese females. *Experimental Biology, 538*, 9 (abstr).

36. Cutler, D., Glaeser, E., & Shapiro, J. (2003). Why have Americans become more obese? *The Journal of Economic Perspectives : A Journal of the American Economic Association, 17*(3), 93–118.

37. Hu, F. B., & Malik, V. S. (2010). Sugar-sweetened beverages and risk of obesity and type 2 diabetes: Epidemiologic evidence. *Physiology and Behavior, 100*(1), 47–54.

38. Woodward-Lopez, G., Kao, J., & Ritchie, L. (2011). To what extent have sweetened beverages contributed to the obesity epidemic? *Public Health Nutrition, 14*(3), 499–509.

39. Atkinson, F. S., Foster-Powell, K., & Brand-Miller, J. C. (2008). International tables of glycemic index and glycemic load values: 2008. *Diabetes Care, 31*, 2281–2283.

40. Stanhope, K. L. (2012). Role of fructose-containing sugars in the epidemics of obesity and metabolic syndrome. *Annual Review of Medicine, 63*, 329–343.

41. Mock, K., Sundus, L., Benedito, V. A., & Tou, J. C. (2017). High-fructose corn syrup-55 consumption alters hepatic lipid metabolism and promotes triglyceride accumulation. *J Nutritional Biochem, 39*, 32–39.

42. Nguyen, S., Choi, H. K., Lustig, R. H., & Hsu, C. Y. (2009). Sugar-sweetened beverages, serum uric acid, and blood pressure in adolescents. *The Journal of Pediatrics, 154*(6), 807–813.

43. Stanhope, K. L., Schwarz, J. M., Keim, N. L., et al. (2009). Consuming fructose-sweetened, not glucose-sweetened, beverages increases visceral adiposity and lipids and decreases insulin sensitivity in overweight/obese humans. *The Journal of Clinical Investigation, 119*(5), 1322–1334.

44. Gaby, A. R. (2005). Adverse effects of dietary fructose. *Alternative Medicine Review : A Journal of Clinical Therapeutic, 10*(4), 294–306.

45. Schulze, M. B., Liu, S., Rimm, E. B., Manson, J. E., Willett, W. C., & Hu, F. B. (2004). Glycemic index, glycemic load, and dietary fiber intake and incidence of type 2 diabetes in younger and middle-aged women. *The American Journal of Clinical Nutrition, 80*, 348–356.

46. Burkitt, D., & Trowell, H. (1981). *Western diseases: their emergence and prevention.* Cambridge, MA: Harvard University Press.

47. Gold, S. M., Dziobek, I., et al. (2007). Hippocampal damage and memory impairments as possible early brain complications of type 2 diabetes. *Diabetologia, 50*(4), 711–719.

48. Bruehl, H., Rueger, M., Dziobek, I., et al. (2007). Hypothalamic-pituitary-adrenal axis dysregulation and memory impairments in type 2 diabetes. *The Journal of Clinical Endocrinology and Metabolism, 92*(7), 2439–2445.

49. Kivimaki, M., Tabak, A. G., et al. (2009). Hyperglycemia, type 2 diabetes, and depressive symptoms: The British Whitehall II study. *Diabetes Care, 32*(10), 1867–1869.

50. Irie, F., Fitzpatrick, A. L., Lopez, O. L., et al. (2008). Enhanced risk for Alzheimer disease in persons with type 2 diabetes and APOE epsilon4: The Cardiovascular Health Study Cognition Study. *Archives of Neurology, 65*(1), 89–93.

51. Kumar, P., Raman, T., Swain, M. M., Mishra, R., & Pal, A. (2016). Hyperglycemia-induced oxidative-nitrosative stress induces inflammation and neurodegeneration via augmented tuberous sclerosis complex-2 (TSC-2) activation in neuronal cells. *Molecular Neurobiology*. [epub ahead of print].

52. Wyngaarden, J. B., Smith, L. H., & Bennett, J. C. (Eds.), (1992). *Cecil textbook of medicine.* Philadelphia, PA: WB Saunders.

53. Campbell, P. J., & Carlson, M. G. (1993). Impact of obesity on insulin action in NIDDM. *Diabetes, 42*, 405–410.

54. Aljada, A., Friedman, J., Ghanim, H., et al. (2006). Glucose ingestion induces an increase in intranuclear nuclear factor kappaB, a fall in cellular inhibitor kappaB, and an increase in tumor necrosis factor alpha messenger RNA by mononuclear cells in healthy human subjects. *Metabolism: Clinical and Experimental, 55*(9), 1177–1185.

55. Turina, M., Fry, D. E., & Polk, H. C., Jr. (2005). Acute hyperglycemia and the innate immune system: Clinical, cellular, and molecular aspects. *Critical Care Medicine, 33*(7), 1624–1633.

56. Vahouny, G., & Kritchevsky, D. (1982). *Dietary fiber in health and disease.* New York, NY: Plenum Press.

57. National Research Council. (1989). *Diet and Health. Implications for reducing chronic disease risk.* Washington, DC: National Academy Press.

58. Schulze, M. B., Manson, J. E., Ludwig, D. S., Colditz, G. A., et al. (2004). Sugar-sweetened beverages, weight gain, and incidence of type 2 diabetes in young and middle-aged women. *JAMA: The Journal of the American Medical Association, 292*(8), 927–934.

59. Imamura, T., O'Connor, L., Ye, Z., et al. (2015). Consumption of sugar sweetened beverages, artificially sweetened beverages, and fruit juice and incidence of type 2 diabetes: Systematic review, meta-analysis, and estimation of population attributable fraction. *BMJ (Clinical Research Ed.), 351*, h3576.

60. Carta, P., et al. (2003). Sub-clinical neurobehavioral abnormalities associated with low level of mercury exposure through fish consumption. *Neurotoxicology, 24*, 617–623.

61. Björnberg, K. A., et al. (2005). Transport of methylmercury and inorganic mercury to the fetus and breast-fed infant. *Environmental Health Perspectives, 113*(10), 1381–1385.

62. Panagiotakos, D. B., Tzima, N., Pitsavos, C., et al. (2007). The association between adherence to the Mediterranean diet and fasting indices of glucose homoeostasis: The ATTICA Study. *Journal of the American College of Nutrition, 26*(1), 32–38, 17353581.

63. Panagiotakos, D. B., Chrysohoou, C., Pitsavos, C., et al. (2006). Association between the prevalence of obesity and adherence to the Mediterranean diet: The ATTICA study. *Nutrition, 22*(5), 449–456, 16457990.

64. Martínez-González, M. A., de la Fuente-Arrillaga, C., Nunez-Cordoba, J. M., et al. (2008). Adherence to Mediterranean diet and risk of developing diabetes: Prospective cohort study. *BMJ (Clinical Research Ed.), 336*(7657), 1348–1351, 18511765.

65. Sheela, C. G., & Augusti, K. T. (1993). Antidiabetic effects of S-allyl cysteine sulphoxide isolated from garlic (Allium sativum, Linn.). *Indian Journal of Experimental Biology, 30*, 523–526.

66. Sharma, K. K., Gupta, R. K., Gupta, S., & Samuel, K. C. (1977). Antihyperglycemic effect of onion: Effect on fasting blood sugar and induced hyperglycemia in man. *The Indian Journal Medical Research, 65*, 422–429.

67. Anderson, J. (1988). Nutrition management of diabetes mellitus. In R. Goodheart & V. R. Young (Eds.), *Modern nutrition in health and disease* (pp. 1201–1229). Philadelphia PA: Lea and Febiger.

68. Anderson, J. W., & Ward, K. (1979). High-carbohydrate, high-fiber diets for insulin-treated men with diabetes mellitus. *The American Journal of Clinical Nutrition, 32*, 2312–2321.

69. Anderson, J. W. (1977). High polysaccharide diet studies in patients with diabetes and vascular disease. *Cereal Foods World, 22*, 12–22.

70. Jenkins, D. J. A., Wolever, T. M. S., Bacon, S., et al. (1980). Diabetic diets: High carbohydrate combined with high fiber. *The American Journal of Clinical Nutrition, 33*, 1729–1733.

71. Baker, B. (1996). Chromium supplements tied to glucose control. *Family Practice News, 15*, 5.

72. Schmidt, E. B., & Dyerberg, J. (1994). Omega-3-fatty acids. Current status in cardiovascular medicine. *Drugs, 47*, 405–424.

73. Maebashi, M., Makino, Y., Furukawa, Y., et al. (1993). Therapeutic evaluation of the effect of biotin on hyperglycemia in patients with non-insulin dependent diabetes mellitus. *Journal of Clinical Biochemistry and Nutrition, 114*, 211–218.

74. Hegazi, S. M. (1992). Effect of zinc supplementation on serum glucose, insulin, glucagon, glucose-6-phosphatase, and mineral levels in diabetics. *Journal of Clinical Biochemistry and Nutrition, 12*, 209–215.

39

Salt

SUMMARY

- Presence in population: The mean intake of sodium in the global population is estimated at 3.9 g/day, with consumption of salt averaging 8.7 g/day in the United States
- Major diseases: Hypertension, stroke, cardiovascular disease, metabolic acidosis
- Primary sources: In the United States, 75% of sodium is added to food during the manufacturing process and 20% is discretionary, often added as condiments (sodium chloride, soy sauce, fish sauce, bouillon)

- Best measure: Net endogenous acid production (NEAP), renal net acid excretion rate (NAE), 24-hour urinary sodium excretion, 24-hour urinary chlorine excretion
- Best intervention: Avoidance—regulations for food manufacturers being implemented; nutritional supplementation with alkali salts (potassium citrate/bicarbonate, magnesium citrate, sodium bicarbonate)

DESCRIPTION

Although sodium chloride is a necessary constituent of a healthy diet, contemporary Western diets contain excessive amounts, leading to direct physiological effects and indirect disease-inducing adaptations. Because the Western diet provides far more acid precursors than base precursors, the resulting physiological adaptations result in increased risk for many common diseases. Although salt has a neutral pH, the physiological adaptations aggravate the excess acidity of the Western diet. A blood pH constantly at the lower end of the normal range has been termed *latent acidosis*. The term *acidosis* is often used interchangeably with the term *acidemia*. However, *acidemia* refers to a blood pH of less than 7.35, whereas *acidosis* refers to a process, or a trend toward acidemia, without the blood necessarily reaching a pH of less than 7.35. Diet-induced acidosis results in small decreases in blood pH and plasma bicarbonate, often within the range considered to be normal. Of

greater clinical significance is the decrease in pericellular and cellular pH and disease-inducing adaptations needed to maintain blood pH.

Nutrition has long been known to strongly influence acid-base balance in human subjects. Sodium is an essential nutrient required for normal human physiology, but excess sodium is a risk factor for cardiovascular disease, osteoporosis, and kidney stone formation. When salt (NaCl) is added to the diet, it becomes a condiment, not a requirement, and when consumed acutely in large quantities, NaCl increases the risk for many diseases. Excess sodium intake is one of the top two dietary risk factors contributing to the global burden of disease.[1]

TOXICITY

The toxicity of salt is both direct—typically because of the sodium—and indirect, related to its substantial contribution to diet-induced acidosis.

Direct Toxicity

Hypernatremia may occur from dehydration, treatment with sodium chloride, or acute ingestion of large amounts of salt. The neurotoxic mechanism of hypernatremia may be the result of the inhibition of glucose metabolism with ensuing loss of adenosine triphosphate (ATP) and the increased uptake of extracellular neuroactive amino acids (glutamate) and reduced intracellular Ca^{2+}.[2] In salt-sensitive hypertension, increased oxidative stress, perhaps via the activation of reduced nicotinamide-adenine dinucleotide phosphate oxidase, elevates arterial pressure through central sympathoexcitation.[3]

Dietary salt has been shown to interfere with the regulatory mechanisms of both the innate and the adaptive immune systems, enhancing proinflammatory responses by inducing IFN-gamma production and reducing the activation of interleukin (IL)-4 and IL-13 macrophages.[4,5]

Indirect Toxicity

Approximately 50% of the acidity-induction from a Western diet is related to excessive salt consumption.[6] A positive NEAP diet results in increased urinary levels of calcium, nitrogen, and bone matrix protein excretion. Aldosterone is associated with the regulation of salt and potassium homeostasis and has profound effects on acid-base balance. During acidosis, circulating aldosterone levels are increased, and the hormone acts in concert with angiotensin II and other factors to stimulate renal acid secretion.[7] Glucocorticoid and mineralocorticoid activities increase significantly in response to acidosis. Mineralocorticoids act centrally to increase salt appetite, sympathetic drive, and vasopressin release, resulting in hypertension.[8]

Metabolic acidosis has dual effects on urinary Na^+ excretion. The early natriuresis results from decreased Na^+ reabsorption in the proximal tubule and serum- and glucocorticoid-regulated kinase 1 (SGK1)-related decreased epithelial sodium channels (ENaC) activity in the distal tubule and collecting duct. Aldosterone-induced upregulation of the cortical NaCl cotransporter (NCC), SGK1, and ENaC likely contributes to the antinatriuretic phase of metabolic acidosis.[9] This adaptation prevents Na^+ wasting and volume depletion during chronic acid insult.

Acidosis results in an increase in urinary calcium (Ca) excretion because of reduced renal tubular reabsorption of filtered Ca. Urinary Ca excretion has been shown to be directly proportional to NAE.[10] Over time, the kidneys' ability to excrete daily net acid loads declines. To mitigate the increasing baseline metabolic acidosis, there is an increased utilization of base stores (bone, skeletal muscle), which results in increased calciuria and net losses of body calcium.[8] In addition, blood P_{CO_2} decreases as the respiratory system adapts to long-term metabolic acidosis.

SOURCES

In industrialized countries, approximately 75% of the salt in the diet comes from that added to food during the manufacturing process, with 15% to 20% a result of adding salt to food when cooking or at the table, and the remainder naturally occurring in food.[11] In low-income countries, most salt is discretionary, often consumed as condiments (e.g., soy sauce, fish sauce, bouillon). Mean intake of sodium in a global population is estimated at 3.95 g/day (equivalent to 10.06 g/day of salt), and in the United States, the average intake of sodium is 3.4 g/day (equivalent to 8.7 g/day of salt).[12] Diets of natural foods without added salt contain 500 to 800 mg of sodium per day.[13]

Salt (sodium chloride, NaCl) consumption, phosphoric acid–containing soft drinks, and diets high in animal and grain protein are common causes of diet-induced acidosis. The deficiency of potassium alkali salts, as a result of the significant decrease in consumption of plant foods, combined with the exchange of these salts for sodium chloride, have resulted in a significant shift in the acid-base balance, increasing the net systemic acid load.

BODY BURDEN

Direct Measures of Salt Consumption

Both 24-hour urinary sodium excretion and 24-hour urinary chlorine excretion are effective measures of daily salt consumption. The Fantus test is an easily performed office procedure that measures urinary chloride and is a reliable estimate of dietary sodium chloride consumption. A complete description of the methodology and interpretation can be found in the *Textbook of Natural Medicine*.[14]

Assessment of Indirect Effects of Salt

The diet net acid load can be estimated by the steady-state NAE. NAE is measured by quantifying the amount of acids in the form of ammonium and titratable acid in the urine and subtracting the amount of bicarbonate.[15] NEAP is another method used to estimate the acid load of the diet. NEAP represents the amount of net acid produced daily by the metabolic system and can be measured by either estimating the acid or base production from the constituents of the diet or by quantifying the inorganic constituents of diet, urine, and stool and of the total organic anion content of the urine (calculated as the sum of urinary inorganic sulfate and organic acid salts minus dietary organic anions less fecal organic anions).[16] NEAP is closely linked to NAE, and the values are often considered equivalent. Although analyzed NAE appears to be the closest approximation of "true" NEAP, several algorithms have been developed to estimate NEAP from dietary components (Table 39.1).

Acid-base balance is carefully regulated by pulmonary and renal responses to control pH. However, when pH regulation malfunctions, hydrogen ions begin to accumulate, causing metabolic acidosis. Studies have shown a strong connection between NaCl intake and acid-base balance, with high-salt diets causing a decrease in pH and moderate metabolic acidosis.[17,18] In healthy humans, diets containing sodium chloride independently predict systemic acid-base status, and as the load increases, so does the degree of

hyperchloremic metabolic acidosis.[19] In other words, the severity of low-grade metabolic acidosis is proportional to the sodium chloride content of the diet.

In response to acidosis, the kidney implements adaptive processes to restore the acid-base balance. These include the removal of the nonmetabolizable anions, the conservation of citrate, the enhancement of kidney ammoniagenesis, and urinary excretion of ammonium ions, resulting in the lowering of urinary pH, hypocitraturia, hypercalciuria, and nitrogen and phosphate wasting.[20]

Chronic metabolic acidosis in human beings is characterized by increased renin-angiotensin-aldosterone (RAA) activity, cortisol secretion, and nitrogen wasting.[21] The mineralocorticoid aldosterone activates similar signaling and effector mechanisms in the kidney and the brain, including the mineralocorticoid receptor, the serum- and glucocorticoid-induced kinase SGK1, the ubiquitin ligase NEDD4-2, and the epithelial sodium channels.[22] Aldosterone increases renal salt retention as well as sodium appetite, which in some cases sustains the pathophysiological response.

TABLE 39.1 Algorithms to Determine Net Endogenous Acid Production (NEAP)

Algorithm	Formula for Estimated NEAP (mEq/d)
Remer and Manz[51]	PRAL (mEq/d) + OA$_{est}$ (mEq/d) PRAL = 0.4888 × protein (g/d) + 0.0366 × P (mg/d) − 0.025 × K (mg/d) − 0.0263 × Mg (mg/d) − 0.0125 × Ca (mg/d) OA$_{est}$ (mEq/d) = body surface area × 41/1.73 Body surface area (m^2) = 0.007184 − height (cm)$^{0.725}$ − weight (kg)$^{0.425}$
Sebastian et al.[52]	Sulfuric acid (mEq/d) + organic acids (mEq/d) − bicarbonate (mEq/d) Sulfuric acid based on cysteine and methionine content of protein (U.S. Dept. of Agriculture database), assuming fractional intestinal absorption rate of 75%, and complete metabolism to sulfuric acid Organic acids = 32.9 + 0.15 × diet unmeasured anion content (which equals Na$^+$ + K$^+$ + Ca^{2+} + Mg^{2+} − Cl$^-$ − P$_i$) Bicarbonate = 0.95 × (Na$^+$) + 0.80 × (K$^+$) + 0.25 × (Ca^{2+}) + 0.32 × (Mg^{2+}) − 0.95 × (Cl$^-$) − 0.63 × (P$_i$) (all in mEq/d)
Frassetto et al.[53]	[0.91 × protein (g/d)] − [0.57 × K (mEq/d)] + 21 or [54.5 × protein (g/d)/K (mEq/d)] − 10.2
Renal net acid excretion analyzed[10]	TA + NH$_4$ − HCO$_3$ (24h urine, all in mEq/d)

PRAL: potential renal acid load
OAest: estimated urinary organic anions
TA: titratable acid
NH4: ammonium
HCO3: bicarbonate
Data from Frassetto, L. A., Lanham-New, S. A., Macdonald, H. M., Remer, T., Sebastian, A., Tucker, K. L., Tylavsky, F. A. (2007). Standardizing terminology for estimating the diet dependent net acid load to the metabolic system. *The Journal of Nutrition, 137*, 1491–1492.

Detoxification/Excretion Processes

The primary method of excretion of sodium chloride is through the kidneys. The typical half-life is 15 hours, but it may be longer in those with hypertension.[23]

Clinical Significance

Chronic excessive sodium ingestion, in genetically susceptible individuals, is an important etiological factor in essential hypertension, and positive correlations have been found between dietary salt intake and the incidence of stroke and gastric cancer.[24] Studies have reported a J-shaped association between sodium intake and cardiovascular disease (CVD) and mortality, with an increased risk at sodium intakes below 2.6 g/day and above 5.0 g/day and lowest risk associated with moderate sodium intake.[25] A J-shaped association has also been found between urinary sodium excretion and major cardiovascular events and death.[26]

There is evidence linking a high-salt diet with stomach cancer, kidney stones, and osteoporosis.[27] Fig. 39.1 describes the effects of salt intake on calcium metabolism and its implications for kidney stone formation, hypertension, and bone health.

Acidification increases cellular calcium levels, impairs lymphocyte proliferation, encourages tumor cell growth, impairs mitochondrial function, increases the rate of bone resorption through the activation of osteoclasts, and reduces insulin sensitivity.[28] In addition, chronic metabolic acidosis decreases insulin-like growth factor 1 (IGF-1)[29]; induces a decrease in thyroid hormone secretion, resulting in a mild form of hypothyroidism[30]; and increases serum 1,25(OH)$_2$ vitamin D concentration, leading to decreased parathyroid hormone (PTH) concentration.[31] Therefore dietary acidosis has been linked to osteoporosis, renal stone formation,[32] cancer, muscle wasting (sarcopenia),[33] hypertension,[34] diabetes, and metabolic syndrome.[35]

INTERVENTION

The optimal intake of sodium chloride and the concept that a low-grade metabolic alkalosis may be the optimal acid-base state for humans are somewhat controversial. Excessive salt consumption needs to be addressed at the behavioral level. Mitigation of the harmful effects of excessive salt consumption can be achieved by 1) greatly reducing content of energy-dense, nutrient-poor foods and potassium-poor, acid-producing cereal grains; 2) increasing consumption of potassium-rich net base-producing fruits and vegetables; and 3) supplementing with alkalizing agents.[36]

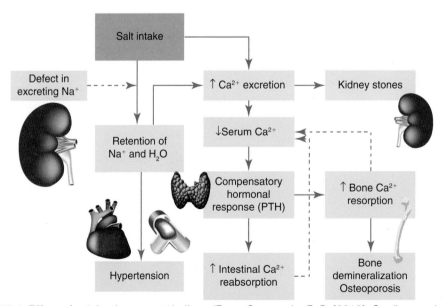

FIG. 39.1 Effect of salt intake on metabolism. (From Cappuccio, F. P. [2013]. Cardiovascular and other effects of salt consumption. *Kidney International Supplements*, 3[4], 312–315.)

Supplementation with alkali salts has been shown to cause clinical improvements in diet-induced acidosis.[37] Increased intake of dietary sources of potassium alkaline salts from fruits and vegetables may be beneficial for postmenopausal women at risk for osteoporosis by preventing the increased excretion of urine calcium associated with high-salt diets.[38] Dietary supplementation with potassium bicarbonate neutralizes dietary acid load, resulting in improved calcium and phosphorous balances, reduced bone resorption rates, improved nitrogen balance, and mitigation of the normally occurring age-related decline in growth hormone secretion, all without restricting dietary sodium chloride.[39]

Epidemiological evidence suggests that hip fracture incidence in older women correlated with animal protein intake as a result of the acid load from sulfur-containing amino acids.[40] Studies have shown plant food intake tends to be protective against hip fracture, and that hip fracture incidence correlates inversely with the ratio of plant-to-animal food intake.[41] In older patients, a restriction of sodium intake along with a higher intake of potassium, magnesium, and citrate reduces urinary risk factors for stone formation and prevents the loss of bone mass and the incidence of hypertension.[42]

Increased brain oxidative stress may elevate arterial pressure through central sympathoexcitation in salt-sensitive hypertension.[43] Alpha lipoic acid (ALA) has been shown to attenuate the oxidative stress in the hypothalamic paraventricular nucleus, thereby decreasing the sympathetic activity and arterial pressure in high salt–induced hypertension. This may be the result of ALA suppressing the activation of the renin-angiotensin system and restoring the balance between pro- and anti-inflammatory cytokines.[44]

Use of salt replacers (potassium partly replacing sodium) may help to decrease sodium intake and reduce blood pressure. Reductions in sodium intake have been shown to reduce blood pressure with no adverse effect on blood lipids, catecholamine levels, or renal function.[45] Perhaps the most well-known study confirming the benefits of a low-salt diet on hypertension is the Dietary Approaches to Stop Hypertension (DASH) trial. The DASH trial showed that reducing dietary intake of salt from "normal" (8 g per day) to intermediate (6 g per day) or low (4 g per day) intake levels lowered blood pressure in both hypertensive and normotensive individuals.[46] Long-term follow-up of individuals who participated in the low-salt arm of the Trial of Hypertension Prevention I and II had a 25%

reduction of cardiovascular events despite receiving no further dietary advice after completing the study.[47]

Although the risk of developing a cardiovascular event is highest among individuals with hypertension, a shift in the entire blood pressure distribution, including normotensives, even of a moderate amount, would avert a greater number of events than just the treatment of those in the extreme end of the blood pressure distribution.[6] A reduction in salt intake has been shown to reduce cardiovascular events, including chronic kidney disease, by as much as 23% (i.e., 1.25 million deaths worldwide).[48] A 2013 Cochrane Review showed that modest reduction in salt intake for 4 or more weeks causes significant and, from a population viewpoint, important falls in blood pressure in both hypertensive and normotensive individuals.[49] When applied on a population-wide basis, salt restriction may reduce the prevalence of hypertension by about 17%.[50]

REFERENCES

1. Eyles, H., Shields, E., Webster, J., & Ni Mhurchu, C. (2016). Achieving the WHO sodium target: Estimation of reductions required in the sodium content of packaged foods and other sources of dietary sodium. *The American Journal of Clinical Nutrition, 104*(2), 470–479.
2. Morland, C., Pettersen, M. N., & Hassel, B. (2016). Hyperosmolar sodium chloride is toxic to cultured neurons and causes reduction of glucose metabolism and ATP levels, and increase in glutamate uptake, and a reduction in cytosolic calcium. *Neurotoxicology, 54,* 34–43.
3. Fujita, M., Ando, K., Nagae, A., & Fujita, T. (2007). Sympathoexcitation by oxidative stress in the brain mediates arterial pressure elevation in salt-sensitive hypertension. *Hypertension, 50*(2), 360–367.
4. Min, B., & Fairchild, R. L. (2015). Over-salting ruins the balance of the immune menu. *The Journal of Clinical Investigation, 125*(11), 4002–4004.
5. Binger, K. J., Gebhardt, M., Heinig, M., Rintisch, C., et al. (2015). High salt reduces the activation of IL-4 and IL-13-stimulated macrophages. *The Journal of Clinical Investigation, 125*(11), 4223–4238.
6. Frassetto, L. A., Morris, R. C., Jr., & Sebastian, A. (2007). Dietary sodium chloride intake independently predicts the degree of hyperchloremic metabolic acidosis in healthy humans consuming a net acid-producing diet. *American Journal of Physiology – Renal Physiology, 293,* F521–F525.

7. Wagner, C. A. (2014). Effect of mineralocorticoids on acid-base balance. *Nephron. Physiology*, *128*(1–2), 26–34.

8. Oki, K., Gomez-Sanchez, E. P., & Gomez-Sanchez, C. E. (2012). Role of mineralocorticoid action in the brain in salt-sensitive hypertension. *Clinical and Experimental Pharmacology and Physiology*, *39*(1), 90–95.

9. Faroqui, S., Sheriff, S., & Amlal, H. (2006). Metabolic acidosis has dual effects on sodium handling by rat kidney. *American Journal of Physiology – Renal Physiology*, *291*(2), F322–F331.

10. Lemann, J., Jr. (1999). Relationship between urinary calcium and net acid excretion as determined by dietary protein and potassium: A review. *Nephron*, *81*(Suppl. 1), 18–25.

11. Cappuccio, F. (2016). SY 09-1 Lowering salt intake and cardiovascular risk reduction: What is the evidence? *Journal of Hypertension*, *34*(Suppl. 1), e184.

12. Powles, J., Fahimi, S., Micha, R., et al. (2013). Global, regional and national sodium intakes in 1990 and 2010: A systemic analysis of 24h urinary sodium excretion and dietary surveys worldwide. *BMJ Open*, *3*(12), e003733.

13. Campbell, N. (2016). SY 09-4 Public policies to reduce salt in processed foods: How they may correlate with improvement in blood pressure control and reduced cardiovascular mortality. *Journal of Hypertension*, *34*(Suppl. 1), e185.

14. Powell, D. W. (2013). Fantus Test. In J. Pizzorno & T. Murray (Eds.), *Textbook of natural medicine*. Elsevier.

15. Frasetto, L., & Sebastian, A. (1996). Age and systemic acid-base equilibrium: Analysis of published data. *The Journals of Gerontology. Series A, Biological Sciences and Medical Sciences*, *51*, B91–B99.

16. Lennon, E. J., Lemann, J., Jr., & Litzow, J. R. (1966). The effects of diet and stool composition on the net external acid balance of normal subjects. *The Journal of Clinical Investigation*, *45*, 1601–1607.

17. Sharma, A. M., & Distler, A. (1994). Acid-base abnormalities in hypertension. *The American Journal of the Medical Sciences*, *307*(Suppl. 1), S112–S115.

18. Sharma, A. M., Kribben, A., Schattenfroh, S., Cetto, C., & Distler, A. (1990). Salt sensitivity in humans is associated with abnormal acid-base regulation. *Hypertension*, *16*(4), 407–413.

19. Frassetto, L. A., Morris, R. C., Jr., & Sebastian, A. (2007). Dietary sodium chloride intake independently predicts the degree of hyperchloremic metabolic acidosis in healthy humans consuming a net acid-producing diet. *American Journal of Physiology – Renal Physiology*, *293*(2), F521–F525.

20. Adeva, M. M., & Souto, G. (2011). Diet-induced metabolic acidosis. *Clinical Nutrition : Official Journal of the European Society of Parenteral and Enteral Nutrition*, *30*(4), 416–421.

21. Henger, A., Tutt, P., Riesen, W. F., Hulter, H. N., & Krapf, R. (2000). Acid-base and endocrine effects of aldosterone and angiotensin II inhibition in metabolic acidosis in human patients. *The Journal of Laboratory and Clinical Medicine*, *136*(5), 379–389.

22. Fu, Y., & Vallon, V. (2014). Mineralocorticoid-induced sodium appetite and renal salt retention: Evidence for common signaling and effector mechanisms. *Nephron. Physiology*, *128*(1–2), 8–16.

23. Dahl, L. K., Smilay, M. S., Silver, L., & Spraragen, S. (1962). Evidence for a Prolonged Biological Half-Life of Na22 in Patients with Hypertension. *Circulation Research*, *X*, 313–320.

24. Battarbee, H. D., & Meneely, G. R. (1978). The toxicity of salt. *CRC Critical Reviews in Toxicology*, *5*(4), 355–376.

25. O'Donnell, M. (2016). SY 09-2 Salt intake: How much should we reduce? *Journal of Hypertension*, *34*(Suppl. 1), e184.

26. O'Donnell, M., Mente, A., Rangarajan, S., et al. (2014). Urinary sodium and potassium excretion, mortality, and cardiovascular events. *The New England Journal of Medicine*, *371*, 612–623.

27. Cappuccio, F. P. (2013). Cardiovascular and other effects of salt consumption. *Kidney International Supplements*, *3*(4), 312–315.

28. Pizzorno, J., Frassetto, L. A., & Katzinger, J. (2010). Diet-induced acidosis: Is it real and clinically relevant? *The British Journal of Nutrition*, *103*(8), 1185–1194.

29. Challa, A., Chan, W., Krieg, R. J., Thabet, M. A., Liu, F., et al. (1993). Effect of metabolic acidosis on the expression of insulin-like growth factor and growth hormone receptor. *Kidney International*, *44*, 1224–1227.

30. Brungger, M., Hulter, H. N., & Krapf, R. (1997). Effect of chronic metabolic acidosis on thyroid hormone homeostasis in humans. *American Journal of Physiology – Renal Physiology*, *272*, F648–F653.

31. Krapf, R., Vetsch, R., Vetsch, W., & Hulter, H. N. (1992). Chronic metabolic acidosis increases the serum concentrations of 1,25-dihydroxyvitamin D in humans by stimulating its production rate. Critical role of acidosis-induced renal hypophosphatemia. *The Journal of Clinical Investigation*, *90*(6), 2456–2463.

32. Trinchieri, A., et al. (2006). Effect of potential renal acid load of foods on urinary citrate excretion in calcium renal stone formers. *Urological Research*, *34*(1), 1–7.

33. Mitch, W. E., Medina, R., Grieber, S., et al. (1994). Metabolic acidosis stimulates muscle protein degradation by activating the adenosine

triphosphate-dependent pathway involving ubiquitin and proteasomes. *The Journal of Clinical Investigation*, *93*, 2127–2133.

34. Zhang, L. (2009). Diet-dependent net acid load and risk of incident hypertension in United States women. *Hypertension*, *54*(4), 751–755.

35. Maalouf, N. M., et al. (2007). Low urine pH: A novel feature of the metabolic syndrome. *Clinical Journal of the American Society of Nephrology : CJASN*, *2*(5), 883–888.

36. Frassetto, L. A., Morris, R. C., Jr., Sellmeyer, D. E., & Sebastian, A. (2008). Adverse effects of sodium chloride on bone in the aging human population resulting from habitual consumption of typical American diets. *The Journal of Nutrition*, *138*(2), 419S–422S.

37. Della-Guardia, L., Roggi, C., & Cena, H. (2016). Diet-induced acidosis and alkali supplementation. *International Journal of Food Sciences and Nutrition*, *67*(7), 754–761.

38. Sellmeyer, D. E., Schloetter, M., & Sebastian, A. (2002). Potassium citrate prevents increased urinary calcium excretion and bone resorption induced by a high sodium chloride diet. *The Journal of Clinical Endocrinology and Metabolism*, *87*(5), 2008–2012.

39. Frassetto, L., Morris, R. C., Jr., Sellmeyer, D. E., Todd, K., & Sebastian, A. (2001). Diet, evolution and aging-the pathophysiologic effects of the post-agricultural inversion of the potassium-to-sodium and base-to-chloride ratios in human diet. *European Journal of Nutrition*, *40*(5), 200–213.

40. Frassetto, L. A., Todd, K. M., Morris, R. C., Jr., & Sebastian, A. (2000). Worldwide incidence of hip fracture in elderly women: Relation to consumption of animal and vegetable foods. *The Journals of Gerontology. Series A, Biological Sciences and Medical Sciences*, *55*(10), M585–M592.

41. Sellmeyer, D. E., Syone, K. L., Sebastian, A., & Cummings, S. R. (2001). A high ratio of dietary animal to vegetable protein increases the rate of bone loss and the risk of fracture in postmenopausal women. Study of Osteoporotic Fractures Research Group. *The American Journal of Clinical Nutrition*, *73*(1), 118–122.

42. Prezioso, D., Strazzullo, P., Lotti, T., Bianchi, G., Borghi, L., et al. (2015). Dietary treatment of urinary risk factors for renal stone formation. A review of CLU Working Group. *Archivio Italiano Di Urologia, Andrologia: Organo Ufficiale [Di] Societa Italiana Di Ecografia Urologica E Nefrologica*, *87*(2), 105–120.

43. Fujita, M., & Fujita, T. (2016). The role of CNS in the effects of salt on blood pressure. *Current Hypertension Reports*, *18*(2), 10.

44. Su, Q., Liu, J. J., Cui, W., Shi, X. L., Guo, J., et al. (2016). Alpha lipoic acid supplementation attenuates reactive oxygen species in hypothalamic paraventricular nucleus and sympathoexcitation in high salt-induced hypertension. *Toxicology Letters*, *241*, 152–158.

45. Aburto, N. J., Ziolkovska, A., Hooper, L., Elliot, P., Cappuccio, F. P., & Meerpohl, J. J. (2013). Effect of lower sodium intake on health: Systematic review and meta-analyses. *BMJ (Clinical Research Ed.)*, *346*, f1326.

46. Sacks, F. M., Svetkey, L. P., Vollmer, W. M., Appel, L. J., et al. (2001). Effects on blood pressure of reduced dietary sodium and the Dietary Approaches to Stop Hypertension (DASH) diet. DASH-Sodium Collaborative Research Group. *The New England Journal of Medicine*, *344*(1), 3–10.

47. Cook, N., Cutler, J., Buring, J., et al. (2007). Long term effects of dietary sodium reduction on cardiovascular disease outcomes: Observational follow-up of the trials of hypertension prevention (TOHP). *BMJ (Clinical Research Ed.)*, *334*, 885–888.

48. He, F. J., & MacGregor, G. A. (2011). Salt reduction lowers cardiovascular risk: Meta-analysis of outcome trials. *Lancet*, *378*, 380–383.

49. He, F. J., Li, J., & Macgregor, G. A. (2013). Effect of longer term modest salt reduction on blood pressure: Cochrane systematic review and meta-analysis of randomized trials. *BMJ (Clinical Research Ed.)*, *346*, f1325.

50. Beevers, D. G. (2002). The epidemiology of salt and hypertension. *Clinical Autonomic Research*, *12*(5), 353–357.

51. Remar, T., & Manz, F. (1994). Estimation of the renal net acid excretion by adults consuming diets containing variable amounts of protein. *The American Journal of Clinical Nutrition*, *59*, 1356–1361.

52. Sebastian, A., Frassetto, L. A., Sellmeyer, D. E., et al. (2002). Estimation of the net acid load of the diet of ancestral pre-agricultural Homo sapiens and their hominid ancestors. *The American Journal of Clinical Nutrition*, *76*, 1308–1316.

53. Frassetto, L. A., Todd, K. M., Morris, R. C., Jr., et al. (1998). Estimation of net endogenous noncarbonic acid production in humans from diet potassium and protein contents. *The American Journal of Clinical Nutrition*, *68*, 576–583.

40

Smoking
Cigarettes and E-Cigarettes

SUMMARY

- Presence in population: In 2015, about 15 out of every 100 US adults aged 18 years or older smoked cigarettes, equating to an estimated 36.5 million adults[1]
- Major diseases: Cancer, cardiovascular disease, chronic obstructive pulmonary disease (COPD)
- Primary sources: Cigarettes and e-cigarettes containing nicotine

- Best measure: Urinary cotinine, hair nicotine
- Best intervention: Smoking cessation using various techniques, including nicotine replacement therapy (gum, patches), hypnosis, acupuncture, and behavioral modification

DESCRIPTION

Tobacco production is a multibillion-dollar industry in the United States, with farms producing nearly 800 million pounds of tobacco in 2012.[2] Cigarette smoking is the leading cause of preventable disease and death in the United States, accounting for more than 480,000 deaths annually.[3] In 2015, approximately 15 out of every 100 US adults aged 18 years or older smoked cigarettes, equating to an estimated 36.5 million adults.[4]

TOXICITY

The tobacco alkaloid (S)-(-)nicotine is the primary addictive agent in mainstream cigarette smoke.[5] Nicotine acts on nicotinic cholinergic receptors in the brain to release dopamine, glutamate, acetylcholine, serotonin, and gamma aminobutyric acid to sustain addiction.[6] The amount of active ingredient, the quantity used, tolerance of the user, speed of delivery, and epigenetic variations determine the degree of intoxication and addiction potential.[7] The mode of use (e.g., smoked in a cigarette, pipe, filtered water pipe, topical patch, snuff, vape) may significantly influence the toxicity of nicotine.

The most common form of tobacco use is inhalation of the smoke.[8] Filter type, paper permeability, tobacco weight, and tip dilution may not influence tobacco-specific chemicals as much as manufacturers suggest.[9] Polycyclic aromatic hydrocarbons (PAHs) have long been recognized as the primary carcinogens in tobacco smoke and contribute to 90% of indoor PAH levels in the homes of smokers.[10,11] The major PAH carcinogen in tobacco smoke is benzoapyrene (BAP), which is transformed by cytochrome P450 into the carcinogenic BAP epoxide. Tobacco smoke contains more than 5000 chemicals, of which more than 50 substances have been identified as carcinogens.[12] Nine of these other toxicants occur in mainstream cigarette smoke and have been classified by the International Agency of Research on Cancer (IARC) as Group 1 carcinogens, indicating the agent is carcinogenic to humans. The nine agents reported are benzene, cadmium, arsenic, nickel, chromium, 2-naphthyl-amine, vinyl chloride, 4-aminobiphenyl, and beryllium.[13]

Several other compounds are present in tobacco and tobacco smoke as either probably or possibly carcinogenic to humans. Cigarette smoke contains many volatile compounds, including the reactive aldehydes, crotonaldehyde, and acrolein.[14] Formaldehyde is generated from saccharides used as tobacco ingredients, and different sugars increase mainstream formaldehyde to different extents.[15] Acetaldehyde, although on the "generally recognized as safe" (GRAS) list for foods, is classified as a possible human carcinogen by the IARC.[16] Ammonia and ammonia-forming compounds are endogenous constituents of tobacco.[17] Phenols are present as a result of heating polyphenols present in the tobacco plant and have significant genotoxic, cardiotoxic, and carcinogenic properties.[18] Tobacco-specific nitrosamines (TSNAs) may be some of the most significant compounds associated with negative health effects from tobacco cigarettes because of their strong carcinogenicity.[19]

Cross-contamination with numerous pesticides and fertilizers increases the harmful effects of tobacco and tobacco smoking.[20,21] In addition, during heating, pyrolysis products form that may interact either with the pesticides or with the pyrolysis products of the pesticides themselves, forming more toxic materials.[22]

Various mechanisms of toxicity have been reported. Many of the diseases associated with cigarette smoking are associated with changes in the levels of cytokines such as interleukin-6 (IL-6). Cigarette smoke is thought to contribute to mitochondrial damage and cardiovascular dysfunction from an increase in reactive oxygen species (ROS) as well as the uncoupling of oxidative phosphorylation (OXPHOS).[23] In a setting of cigarette smoking, free radicals may arise from 1) the gas or tar phase of cigarette smoke,[24] 2) circulating or *in situ* activated macrophages and neutrophils,[25] and 3) endogenous sources of ROS.[26]

Cigarette smoke inhibits the L-arginine nitric oxide synthase pathway, as do cadmium[27] and arsenic (two common components of cigarette smoke), leading to elevated levels of asymmetrical dimethylarginine (ADMA).[28,29] Smoking has also been shown to increase advanced glycation end-product (AGE) formation, which may contribute to an increased risk of developing cardiovascular disease and cancers.[30] TSNAs are also metabolized into reactive electrophiles, which react with nucleophilic centers of DNA and proteins, activating oncogenes.[31]

Vaporizers/Electrically Heated Cigarette Smoking Systems

Vaporizers have become a popular alternative to smoking traditional cigarettes as a method of delivering nicotine without some of the highly toxic chemicals released in tobacco smoke. Vaporization (vaping) as a method of using tobacco has been shown to reduce respiratory exposure to toxic particulates by as much as 90%.[32] A study evaluating air constituents from smoking found that using electrically heated cigarette smoking systems (EHCSS, or e-cigarettes) reduced concentrations of environmental tobacco smoke by 99%, levels similar to those in a smoke-free environment.[33] Smokers who switched to e-cigarettes for 5 days experienced slight drops in blood pressure and heartrate and had small, but statistically significant, improvements in forced vital capacity (FVC) and forced expiratory volume in one second (FEV_1).[34]

Extracts of tobacco, commonly called *Natural Extracts of Tobacco (NET)*, used for e-cigarettes are produced by a process of solvent extraction and steeping, and have been found to contain acetaldehyde, formaldehyde, phenols, and nitrates.[35] A cytotoxicity study of four NET samples found that the aerosol of these liquids had cytotoxic effects on cultured cells.[36] Although vaporization appears to produce "cleaner" smoke, limited research is available on the long-term potential harms and benefits, and further investigation, including the adverse effects of cross-contamination of toxicants, is warranted.

SOURCES

Tobacco smoking includes cigarettes, cigars, pipes, vaping, and any other smoked tobacco product. In 2016, approximately 258 billion cigarettes were sold in the United States, and about 13 billion cigars were sold in the United States in 2014.[37]

BODY BURDEN

In the gas phase of environmental tobacco, nicotine deposits primarily in the buccal cavity and upper respiratory tract. Gaseous nicotine deposits rapidly in the respiratory tract; however, the rate and magnitude of nicotine deposition depends on the fraction of the free base form found in the smoke particle phase, because only the free base form can volatize to the gas phase.[38]

Cotinine can be used as a biomarker of tobacco smoke exposure, because urinary measurement of cotinine is highly correlated with the amount of nicotine intoxication or use.[39] Hair nicotine may provide a more accurate and reliable measure of longer-term tobacco smoke exposure.[40,41]

Urinary analysis of 8-oxo-7,8-dihydro-2′-deoxyguanosine (8-oxodG) and 8-hydroxy-2′-deoxyguanosine (8OHdG) are indicative of damaged nuclear or mitochondrial DNA. 8-oxodG is a good marker for assessing oxidative damage, risk of atherosclerosis, cancer risk, and other disease complications.[42] 8-oxodG is used to estimate exposure to cancer-causing agents, such as tobacco smoke, and is significantly determined by toxin exposure.[43] For example, smokers have up to 300% more 8-oxodG than nonsmokers, and those living in polluted cities have almost twice the levels of those living in rural settings.[44,45] 8-OHdG increases in direct proportion to the number of cigarettes smoked as well and is commercially available.[46,47]

Levels of cotinine in residents of the United States have been studied in nonsmokers as part of the ongoing National Health and Nutritional Examination Survey (NHANES) trial and published by the Centers for Disease Control and Prevention (CDC) in their Exposure Report.[48] Table 40.1 summarizes the cotinine findings published in the January 2017 updated tables to the Fourth Report.

Detoxification/Excretion Processes

Most toxicants are metabolized through a combination of phase I and phase II activities, and the relationship between the phases is important in determining toxicity. When fast bioactivation is followed by slow elimination, toxicity may increase. One example of this is the interaction between smoking and polymorphisms in acetylation genes (e.g., N-acetyl transferase [NAT]2 genetic polymorphisms). Many of the toxic compounds in smoke are activated to more reactive compounds by phase I. Therefore a very active phase I combined with a low phase II is likely to increase the risk of harm.

Nicotine is intensively metabolized in the liver by CYP2A6 and oxidized into cotinine, the main nicotine metabolite. The half-life of nicotine is approximately 2 hours, but the half-life of cotinine averages 16 hours.[49] The clearance of nicotine is highly variable and is determined by genetic, racial, and hormonal (gender) factors.[50] Asians and African Americans tend to metabolize nicotine more slowly than Hispanics and Caucasians,[51] and women have a faster rate of nicotine metabolism than men.[52]

Acetylation. Acetylation by N-acetyl transferases (NAT) generally reduces the toxicity of a substrate, but it may also increase toxicity. This is also a good example of the wide individual variability in phase II detoxification activity. The slow acetylator phenotype is found in 52% to 68% of individuals of western European descent and only 10% to 15% of Japanese individuals.[53] An increased risk of breast cancer in smokers has been shown, with an odds ratio (OR) of 1.49 for slow genotypes.[54,55,56] Clinically, a 40% increased risk of bladder cancer has been shown for those with the low-activity genotype for NAT2, especially when exposed to carcinogens such as cigarette smoke.[57,58] Indeed, smokers with NAT2 slow phenotypes have a significantly increased risk of bladder cancer (OR 1.6), with increasing risk associated the number of cigarettes smoked per day.[59]

Quinone Reductase. Quinone reductase detoxifies quinones produced by phase I enzymes metabolizing auto exhaust, cigarette smoke, and any burned organic materials. Generally, quinone reductases produce hydroxyquinones, which are more easily excreted. Smokers with a deficiency in NAD(P)H-quinone oxidoreductase 1 (NQO1) in combination with marginal vitamin C deficiency are at a higher risk for developing myelodysplastic syndromes and oxidative stress.[60]

Clinical Significance

Cigarette smoking is considered by conventional public health agencies as the leading cause of preventable disease

TABLE 40.1	Serum Cotinine Levels in Nonsmokers—CDC Fourth Report, January 2017 Update, in ng/mL					
Toxicant	Smoking Status	Mean	75th %	90th %	95th %
Cotinine	Nonsmokers	*	0.059	0.356	1.30

*Not calculated; proportion of results below limit of detection was too high to provide a valid result

and death in the United States, accounting for more than 480,000 deaths annually.[61] (It is the position of the authors of this textbook that cigarette smoking has been superseded by total toxic load—of which cigarette smoking is a significant component in those who smoke—as the leading cause of preventable death and disease.) More than 16 million Americans live with a smoking-related disease.[2] Cigarette smoking has been associated with several chronic health conditions, including cancer, cardiovascular disease, and COPD.

Androgen Effects. Common causes of androgen deficiency include age, systemic or autoimmune disease, elevated cortisol, tobacco use, and environmental toxicity.[62] Cigarette smoking has been shown to impair testosterone synthesis in men.[63] Cotinine, however, inhibits testosterone breakdown, and studies show that male smokers have higher total testosterone and free testosterone levels than do nonsmokers.[64,65]

Cardiovascular Disease. Cigarette smoking is a significant risk factor for cardiovascular disease and myocardial infarction globally.[66,67] Statistical evidence reveals a threefold to fivefold increase in the risk of coronary artery disease in smokers compared with nonsmokers. The more cigarettes smoked and the longer the number of years a person has smoked, the greater the risk of dying from a heart attack or stroke. Overall, the average smoker dies 7 to 8 years sooner than nonsmokers.

The combustion of tobacco and other contaminants increases oxidative stress, damaging the cardiovascular system.[68] Many of these chemicals are carried in the bloodstream on low density lipoprotein (LDL) cholesterol, where they either directly damage the lining of the arteries or oxidize the LDL molecule (oxLDL), which then damages the arteries.[69] Exposure of human plasma to the gas phase of cigarette smoke produces oxLDL, which strongly correlates with cardiovascular disease.[70] An elevated cholesterol level makes the effect of smoking on the cardiovascular system even worse, because more cigarette toxins will be carried through the vascular system. Smoking also contributes to elevated cholesterol, presumably by damaging feedback mechanisms in the liver, which control how much cholesterol is being created.[71] Smoking promotes platelet aggregation and elevated fibrinogen levels, two other significant independent risk factors for heart disease and strokes.[72,73] In experimental models, PAHs found in the tar fraction

of cigarette smoke have been shown to accelerate atherosclerosis.[74] In addition, cigarette smoking is a contributing factor to high blood pressure.[75]

Passive exposure to cigarette smoke is also damaging. Evidence links environmental (secondhand or passive) smoke to heart disease mortality and morbidity.[76] More than 37,000 coronary heart disease deaths occur annually in the United States as a result of exposure to environmental smoke. A metaanalysis of 10 epidemiological studies indicates a consistent dose-response effect related to exposure.[77] Individuals exposed to secondhand smoke have higher homocysteine and fibrinogen (biomarkers of cardiovascular disease risk) levels than nonsmokers.[78,79] Pathophysiological and biochemical data after short- and long-term environmental tobacco smoke exposure show changes in endothelial and platelet function, arterial stiffness, atherosclerosis, heart rate variability, increased infarct size, and exercise capacity similar to those associated with active smoking.[80]

Cancer. Cigarette smoking is a major cause of cancer death in the United States. Cigarette smokers have a total overall cancer death rate twice that of nonsmokers. The greater the number of cigarettes smoked, the greater the risk.

For active smoking, a modest increase in breast cancer risk is observed in women who began smoking before the age of 17 years (RR, 1.19; 95% CI, 1.03–1.37).[81] Female smokers have a twofold to threefold increased incidence of cervical cancer and/or cervical dysplasia compared with nonsmokers.[82,83,84] Several theories have been postulated to explain this association, including the following: 1) Smoking may depress immune functions, allowing a sexually transmitted agent to promote abnormal cellular development, leading to the onset of cervical dysplasia; 2) there may be unrecognized associations between smoking and sexual behavior[85]; 3) smoking induces vitamin C deficiency[86]; and 4) vaginal or endometrial cells may concentrate carcinogenic compounds from inhaled smoke and secrete these compounds.

Two specific nicotine-derived nitrosamines, nicotine-derived nitrosamine ketone (NNK) and N-nitrosonornicotine (NNN), have been shown to induce oral tumors when applied to the rat oral cavity, and NNK in tobacco smoke induces lung cancer.[87] Excessive exposure to PAHs from cigarette smoke increases the risk of lung cancer through the formation of reactive metabolites that cause DNA mutations, alteration of gene expression profiles, and tumorigenesis.[88]

Epidemiological evidence shows a strong positive association between smoking and several cancers, including bladder cancer,[89] esophageal cancer,[90] pancreatic cancer,[91] head and neck cancer,[92] liver cancer,[93] and colorectal cancer.[94]

Depression. Cigarette smoking is a significant risk factor for depression.[95] Central to the effect of nicotine is the stimulation of adrenal hormone and cortisol secretion. Elevated cortisol levels are a well-recognized feature of depression.[96] Cortisol activates tryptophan oxygenase, resulting in less tryptophan being delivered to the brain. Because the level of serotonin in the brain is dependent on the amount of tryptophan delivered to the brain, cortisol ultimately results in reductions in the level of serotonin and melatonin.[97] Cigarette smoking is associated with various morphological changes in the brain that may contribute to depression. In studies comparing smokers with nonsmokers, smokers with psychiatric illness, including major depressive disorder (MDD), had decreased cortical thickness.[98,99] Smoking also lowers vitamin D levels, which increases the rate of depression.[100]

Graves' Disease. A statistically significant correlation exists between smoking and Graves' disease, especially with ophthalmic complications.[101] The group at the highest increase in risk for severe endocrine ophthalmopathy are those who already have some eye manifestation and who continue to smoke.[102,103] Gene polymorphisms in GSTP1, CYP1A1, and TP53 may be associated with smoking-related Graves' disease susceptibility.[104]

Macular Degeneration. Smoking has consistently been shown to be associated with macular degeneration.[105,106] Because oxidant exposure is a major factor in macular degeneration, the increased risk of macular degeneration in both male and female smokers is not surprising.[107,108,109] In a 12-year study of 31,843 registered female nurses, those who currently smoked 25 or more cigarettes per day had a relative risk of 2.4 for age-related macular degeneration compared with those who had never smoked.[110] Past smokers of 25 cigarettes or more per day still had a twofold increased risk relative to never-smokers. Risk did not return to the control levels until after quitting smoking for 15 years.

Male Infertility. Sperm is extremely sensitive to free radicals, because it is dependent on the integrity and

fluidity of their cell membrane for proper function. Cigarette smoking is a common source of oxidants and is associated with decreased sperm counts, decreased sperm motility, lower semen volume, decreased sperm concentration, and an increased frequency of abnormal sperm.[111,112,113] In one study, men who smoked one pack of cigarettes a day received either 0, 200, or 1000 mg of vitamin C daily, and after 1 month of therapy, sperm quality improved proportional to the level of vitamin C supplementation.[114]

Menopause. Cigarette smoking significantly increases the risk of early menopause.[115] Smokers have approximately double the risk of menopause between the ages of 44 and 55, and former smokers had a lowered risk, showing there could be a partial reversal of the effect.[116] Women who quit smoking for longer than 5 years had significantly lower odds, severity, and frequency of hot flashes than women who continued to smoke (OR, 0.36, 0.62, 0.63).[117]

Metabolic Syndrome/Obesity. Smoking has been associated with higher body mass index, larger waist circumference, and greater fat percentage and may promote visceral fat accumulation in morbidly obese male patients.[118,119] Women who actively smoke have increased central adiposity, as indicated by higher waist circumference and waist-to-hip ratio measurements compared with nonsmokers.[120] A large, cross-sectional, population-based study demonstrated a direct positive association between higher pack-years of smoking to a higher waist-to-hip ratio and an inverse association with the duration since quitting.[121] Heavy smoking increases the risk of developing metabolic syndrome, and this is related to the number of cigarettes smoked per day.[122,123,124]

Pelvic Inflammatory Disease. Studies have shown that cigarette smokers have an elevated risk of pelvic inflammatory disease (PID) of 1.7 (95% CI, 1.1–2.5), and former cigarette smokers have an elevated risk of 2.3 (95% CI, 1.3–4.2) without a dose-response relationship.[125] Women who smoked 10 or more cigarettes a day had a higher risk than those who smoked less.[126]

Peptic Ulcer. Smoking is related to an increased frequency of peptic ulcers, a decreased response to peptic ulcer therapy, and an increased mortality related to peptic ulcers. This may be the result of decreased pancreatic bicarbonate secretion (an important neutralizer of gastric acid), increased reflux of bile salts into the stomach, and/ or acceleration of gastric emptying into the duodenum.[127] Bile salt reflux induced by smoking appears to be the most likely factor responsible for the increased peptic ulcer rate in smokers. Cigarette smoke and its active ingredients cause mucosal cell death, inhibit cell renewal, interfere with the mucosal immune system, and decrease blood flow in the gastrointestinal (GI) mucosa.[128] The psychological aspects of smoking are also important, because the chronic anxiety and psychological stress associated with smoking appear to worsen ulcer activity.

Periodontal Disease. Tobacco smoking is associated with increased susceptibility to severe periodontal disease and tooth loss,[129,130,131] and a dose-dependent relationship exists with the amount of cigarette consumption.[132] Smokers have greater odds for more severe bone loss than nonsmokers, with the OR increasing from 3.25 for light smoking to 7.28 for heavy users.[133] Smoking also negatively affects treatment of periodontal disease.[134]

Respiratory Disease. COPD continues to be one of the leading causes of cigarette smoke–related death worldwide.[135] Compared with 2.9% among never-smokers, the prevalence of COPD among current smokers is 14.1% and is 7.1% among former smokers.[136] The risk of airflow obstruction (forced expiratory volume in 1 second/forced vital capacity <0.7) is strongly associated with number of cigarettes smoked and starting to smoke at a young age.[137] Approximately 80% of all COPD-related deaths can be attributed to smoking, and smokers are 12 to 13 times more likely to die of COPD than nonsmokers.[138] The use of long-acting anticholinergics in COPD increases pulmonary retention of pathogenical smoke constituents and therefore may increase cardiovascular disease in patients who continue to smoke.[139]

INTERVENTION

Smoking is a modifiable behavior, and various measures including nicotine-containing skin patches or chewing gum, acupuncture, and hypnosis have all been shown to provide some benefit in helping patients to quit smoking. In a systematic review of the efficacy of interventions intended to help people stop smoking, most therapies, including physician recommendation, behavioral modification techniques (e.g., relaxation, rewards and punish-ment, avoiding trigger situations), and acupuncture have shown a disappointing 2% to 3% cessation rate.[140]

Trials have shown hypnosis to have a success rate of 23% in reducing or quitting cigarette smoking when combined with nicotine patches.[141] Nicotine replacement therapy (gum or patch) alone is effective in about 10% to 20% of smokers who seek help in quitting, with higher abstinence rates associated with higher doses of nicotine.[142] However, relapse rates were similar after 1 year postcessation.

Many of the harmful effects of tobacco smoking are a result of free radical damage, particularly to epithelial cells. Smoking greatly reduces ascorbic acid levels, thereby potentiating its damaging effects.[143] Smokers require at least twice as much vitamin C as nonsmokers.[144] Carotenes and flavonoids have been shown to greatly reduce some of the toxic effects of smoking.[145,146] Black tea may also help protect smokers from cigarette smoke–induced oxidative damage.[147] In an animal model, smoking-induced oxidative stress and the associated inflammatory, profibrotic, and atherogenic cardiovascular markers were attenuated by pomegranate juice.[148]

Antioxidants such as vitamin C and vitamin E at modest daily dosages of 500 mg and 400 International Units (IU) have been shown to protect women smokers from DNA damage.[149] In animal studies, high doses of vitamin C (15 mg vitamin C/animal/day) provided protection against smoke-induced protein damage and lipid peroxidation.[150] Curcumin protects against DNA damage from PAHs in human epithelial cells.[151] Quercetin has been shown to enhance the protective effects of beta-carotene for DNA from PAHs.[152] Epicatechins have been shown in mucosal cell cultures to protect against DNA damage.[153]

Topically, resveratrol can decrease cigarette smoke–induced ROS and carbonyl formation in human keratinocytes, providing a good defense against cigarette smoke–induced skin damage.[154]

REFERENCES

1. Centers for Disease Control and Prevention. (2016). Cigarette Smoking Among Adults – United States, 2005-2015. *MMWR. Morbidity and Mortality Weekly Report*, 65(44), 1205–1211. (Accessed 22 December 2016).
2. U.S. Department of Agriculture. (2014). *2012 Census of Agriculture: United States Summary and State Data.* Vol

1;Part 51. Washington: US Department of Agriculture, National Agricultural Statistics Service. https://agcensus.usda.gov/Publications/2012/Full_Report/Volume_1,_Chapter_1_US/usv1.pdf. (Accessed 25 April 2017).

3. U.S. Department of Health and Human Services. (2014). *The Health Consequences of Smoking – 50 Years of Progress: A Report of the Surgeon General*. Atlanta: U.S. Department of Health and Human Services. Centers for Disease Control and prevention, National Center for Chronic Disease Prevention and Health Promotion, Office on Smoking and Health. (Accessed 22 December 2016).

4. Centers for Disease Control and Prevention. (2016). Cigarette Smoking Among Adults – United States, 2005-2015. *MMWR. Morbidity and Mortality Weekly Report, 65*(44), 1205–1211. (Accessed 22 December 2016).

5. No authors listed. (2014). Nicotine and health. *Drug and Therapeutics Bulletin, 52*(7), 78–81. PubMed PMID: 25012148.

6. Benowitz, N. L. (2009). Pharmacology of nicotine: Addiction, smoking-induced disease, and therapeutics. *Annual Review of Pharmacology and Toxicology, 49*, 57–71. PubMed PMID: 18834313.

7. Carter, L. P., Stitzer, M. L., Henningfield, J. E., et al. (2009). Abuse liability assessment of tobacco products including potential reduced exposure products. *Cancer Epidemiology, Biomarkers and Prevention: A Publication of the American Association for Cancer Research, Cosponsored by the American Society of Preventive Oncology, 18*(12), 3241–3262. PubMed PMID: 19959676.

8. Giovino, G. A., Mirza, S. A., Samet, J. M., et al. (2012). Tobacco use in 3 billion individuals from 16 countries: An analysis of nationally representative cross-sectional household surveys. *Lancet, 380*(9842), 668–679. PubMed PMID: 22901888.

9. Harris, J. E. (2001). Smoke yields of tobacco-specific nitrosamines in relation to FTC tar level and cigarette manufacturer: Analysis of the Massachusetts Benchmark Study. *Public Health Reports, 116*(4), 336–343. PubMed PMID: 12037262.

10. Choi, H., Harrison, R., et al. (2010). *Polycyclic aromatic hydrocarbons. WHO guidelines for indoor air quality: Selected pollutants*. Geneva.: World Health Organization.

11. Bostrom, C. E., Gerde, P., Hanberg, A., et al. (2002). Cancer risk assessment, indicators, and guidelines for polycyclic aromatic hydrocarbons in the ambient air. *Environmental Health Perspectives, 110*(Suppl. 3), 451–488. PubMed PMID: 12060843.

12. Borgerding, M., & Klus, H. (2005). Analysis of complex mixtures – cigarette smoke. *Experimental and Toxicologic Pathology, 57*(Suppl. 1), 43–73. PubMed PMID: 16092717.

13. Smith, C. J., Livingston, S. D., & Doolittle, D. J. (1997). An international literature survey of "IARC Group I carcinogens" reported in mainstream cigarette smoke. *Food and Chemical Toxicology : An International Journal Published for the British Industrial Biological Research Association, 35*(10–11), 1107–1130. PubMed PMID: 9463546.

14. Counts, M. E., Hsu, F. S., Laffoon, S. W., Dwyer, R. W., & Cox, R. H. (2004). Mainstream smoke constituent yields and predicting relationships from a worldwide market sample of cigarette brands: ISO smoking conditions. *Regulatory Toxicology and Pharmacology: RTP, 39*, 111–134.

15. Baker, R. R. (2006). The generation of formaldehyde in cigarettes – overview and recent experiments. *Food and Chemical Toxicology : An International Journal Published for the British Industrial Biological Research Association, 44*(11), 1799–1822. PubMed PMID: 16859820.

16. *International Agency of Research on Cancer (IARC) Monographs Acetaldehyde*. http://monographs.iarc.fr/ENG/Monographs/vol71/mono71-11.pdf. (Accessed 25 April 2017).

17. Callicutt, C. H., Cox, R. H., Hsu, F., Kinser, R. D., et al. (2006). The role of ammonia in the transfer of nicotine from tobacco to mainstream smoke. *Regulatory Toxicology and Pharmacology, 46*(1), 1–17. PubMed PMID: 16875767.

18. *Food and Drug Administration (FDA) Guidance for Industry: reporting harmful and potentially harmful constituents in tobacco products and tobacco smoke under section 904(a)(3) of the Federal Food, Drug, and Cosmetic Act*. http://www.fda.gov/downloads/TobaccoProducts/GuidanceComplianceRegulatoryInformation/UCM297828.pdf. (Accessed 25 April 2017).

19. Hecht, S. S. (1998). Biochemistry, biology, and carcinogenicity of tobacco-specific N-nitrosamines. *Chemical Research in Toxicology, 11*(6), 559–603. PubMed PMID: 9625726.

20. Yang, F., Bian, Z., Chen, X., et al. (2014). Analysis of 118 pesticides in tobacco after extraction with the modified QuEChRS method by LC-MS-MS. *Journal of Chromatographic Science, 52*(8), 788–792. PubMed PMID: 23888004.

21. Rahman, M. A., Chowdhury, A. Z., Moniruzzaman, M., et al. (2012). Pesticide residues in tobacco leaves from the Kushtia district in Bangladesh. *Bulletin of*

Environmental Contamination and Toxicology, 89(3), 658–663. PubMed PMID: 22782359.

22. Lorenz, W., Bahadir, M., & Korte, F. (1987). Thermolysis of pesticide residues during tobacco smoking. *Chemosphere, 16*(2–3), 521–522.

23. Ambrose, J. A., & Barua, R. S. (2004). The pathophysiology of cigarette smoking and cardiovascular disease: An update. *Journal of the American College of Cardiology, 43*(10), 1731–1737.

24. Pryor, W. A., Stone, K., Zang, L. Y., & Bermudez, E. (1998). Fractionation of aqueous cigarette tar extracts: Fractions that contain the tar radical cause DNA damage. *Chemical Research in Toxicology, 11*(5), 441–448. PubMed PMID: 9585474.

25. Powell, J. T. (1998). Vascular damage from smoking: Disease mechanisms at the arterial wall. *Vascular Medicine (London, England), 3*(1), 21–28. PubMed PMID: 9666528.

26. Barua, R. S., Ambrose, J. A., Srivastava, S., et al. (2003). Reactive oxygen species are involved in smoking-induced dysfunction of nitric oxide biosynthesis and upregulation of endothelial nitric oxide synthase: An in-vitro demonstration in human coronary artery endothelial cells. *Circulation, 107*(18), 2340–2347. PubMed PMID: 12707237.

27. Kolluru, G. K., Tamilarasan, K. P., Geetha Priya, S., et al. (2006). Cadmium induced endothelium dysfunction: Consequence of defective migratory pattern of endothelial cells in association with poor nitric oxide availability under cadmium challenge. *Cell Biology International, 30*(5), 427–438.

28. Zhang, W. Z., Venardos, K., Chin-Dusting, J., et al. (2006). Adverse effects of cigarette smoke on NO bioavailability: Role of arginine metabolism and oxidative stress. *Hypertension, 48*(2), 278–285.

29. Bhatnagar, A. (2006). Environmental cardiology: Studying mechanistic links between pollution and heart disease. *Circulation Research, 99*(7), 692–705.

30. Yamagishi, S., Matsui, T., & Nakamura, K. (2008). Possible involvement of tobacco-derived advanced glycation end products (AGEs) in an increased risk for developing cancers and cardiovascular disease in former smokers. *Medical Hypotheses, 71*(2), 259–261.

31. Hoffmann, D., Rivenson, A., Chung, F. L., & Hecht, S. S. (1991). Nicotine-derived N-nitrosamines (TSNA) and their relevance in tobacco carcinogenesis. *Critical Reviews in Toxicology, 21*(4), 305–311. PubMed PMID: 2069715.

32. Tricker, A. R., Schorp, M. K., Urban, H. J., et al. (2009). Comparison of environmental tobacco smoke (ETS) concentrations generated by an electrically heated cigarette smoking system and a conventional cigarette. *Inhalation Toxicology, 21*(1), 62–77. PubMed PMID: 18951229.

33. Frost-Pineda, K., Zedler, B. K., et al. (2008). Environmental tobacco smoke (ETS) evaluation of a third-generation electrically heated cigarette smoking system (EHCSS). *Regulatory Toxicology and Pharmacology, 52*(2), 118–121. PubMed PMID: 18639603.

34. D'Ruiz, C. D., O'Connell, G., Graff, D. W., & Yan, X. S. (2017). Measurement of cardiovascular and pulmonary function endpoints and other physiological effects following partial or complete substitution of cigarettes with electronic cigarettes in adult smokers. *Regulatory Toxicology and Pharmacology, 87*, 36–53. PubMed PMID: 28476553.

35. Farsalinos, K. E., Gillman, I. G., Melvin, M. S., et al. (2015). Nicotine levels and presence of selected tobacco-derived toxins in tobacco flavoured electronic cigarette refill liquids. *International Journal of Environmental Research and Public Health, 12*(4), 3439–3452. PubMed PMID: 25811768.

36. Farsalinos, K. E., Romagna, G., Allifranchini, E., et al. (2013). Comparison of the cytotoxic potential of cigarette smoke and electronic cigarette vapour extract on cultured myocardial cells. *International Journal of Environmental Research and Public Health, 10*(10), 5146–5162. PubMed PMID: 24135821.

37. Centers for Disease Control and Prevention (CDC). *Economic trends in tobacco.* https://www.cdc.gov/tobacco/data_statistics/fact_sheets/economics/econ_facts/. (Accessed 25 April 2017).

38. Pankow, J. F., Tavakoli, A. D., Luo, W., & Isabelle, L. M. (2003). Percent free base nicotine in the tobacco smoke particulate matter of selected commercial and reference cigarettes. *Chemical Research in Toxicology, 16*(8), 1014–1018. PubMed PMID: 12924929.

39. Berny, C., Boyer, J. C., Capolaghi, B., et al. (2002). Biomarkers of tobacco smoke exposure. *Annales de Biologie Clinique, 60*(3), 263–272. PubMed PMID: 12050041.

40. Al-Delaimy, W. K., Crane, J., & Woodward, A. (2002). Is the hair nicotine level a more accurate biomarker of environmental tobacco smoke exposure than urine cotinine? *Journal of Epidemiology and Community Health, 56*(1), 66–71. PubMed PMID: 11801622.

41. Al-Delaimy, W. K. (2002). Hair as a biomarker for exposure to tobacco smoke. *Tobacco Control, 11*(3), 176–182. PubMed PMID: 12198265.

42. Wu, L. L., Chiou, C. C., Chang, P. Y., et al. (2004). Urinary 8-OHdG: A marker of oxidative stress to

DNA and a risk factor for cancer, atherosclerosis, and diabetes. *Clinica Chimica Acta*, *339*(1–2), 1–9. PubMed PMID: 14687888.

43. Valavanidis, A., Vlachogianni, T., & Fiotakis, C. (2009). 8-hydroxy-2'-deoxyguanosine (8-OHdG): A critical biomarker of oxidative stress and carcinogenesis. *Journal of Environmental Science and Health. Part C, Environmental Carcinogenesis & Ecotoxicology Reviews*, *27*(2), 120–139.

44. Yano, T., Shoji, F., Baba, H., et al. (2009). Significance of the urinary 8-OHdG level as an oxidative stress marker in lung cancer patients. *Lung Cancer (Amsterdam, Netherlands)*, *63*(1), 111–114.

45. Buthbumrung, N., Mahidol, C., Navasumrit, P., et al. (2008). Oxidative DNA damage and influence of genetic polymorphisms among urban and rural schoolchildren exposed to benzene. *Chemico-Biological Interactions*, *172*, 185–194.

46. Lu, C. Y., Ma, Y. C., Chen, P. C., Wu, C. C., & Chen, Y. C. (2014). Oxidative stress of office workers relevant to tobacco smoking and inner air quality. *International Journal of Environmental Research and Public Health*, *11*(6), 5586–5597. PubMed PMID:24865395.

47. Chiang, H. C., Huang, Y. K., Chen, P. F., Chang, C. C., Wang, C. J., Lin, P., et al. (2012). 4-(Methylnitrosamino)-1-(3-pyridyl)-1-butanone is correlated with 8-hydroxy-2'-deoxyguanosine in humans after exposure to environmental tobacco smoke. *The Science of the Total Environment*, *414*, 134–139. PubMed PMID: 22138374.

48. Centers for Disease Control and Prevention. (January 2017). *National Report on Human Exposure to Environmental Chemicals: Updated Tables*. Available at www.cdc.gov/exposurereport/pdf/FourthReport_UpdatedTables_Volume1_Jan2017.pdf. (Accessed 25 October 2017).

49. Hukkanen, J., Jacob, P., 3rd, & Benowitz, N. L. (2005). Metabolism and disposition kinetics of nicotine. *Pharmacological Reviews*, *57*(1), 79–115. PubMed PMID: 15734728.

50. Benowitz, N. L. (2008). Clinical pharmacology of nicotine: Implications for understanding, preventing, and treating tobacco addiction. *Clinical Pharmacology and Therapeutics*, *83*(4), 531–541. PubMed PMID: 18305452.

51. Perez-Stable, E. J., Herrera, B., et al. (1998). Nicotine metabolism and intake in black and white smokers. *JAMA: The Journal of the American Medical Association*, *280*(2), 152–156. PubMed PMID: 9669788.

52. Benowitz, N. L., Lessov-Schlaggar, C. N., Swan, G. E., & Jacob, P., 3rd. (2006). Female sex and oral contraceptive use accelerate nicotine metabolism.

Clinical Pharmacology and Therapeutics, *79*(5), 480–488. PubMed PMID: 16678549.

53. Boukouvala, S., & Fakis, G. (2005). Arylamine N-acetyltransferases: What we learn from genes and gemones. *Drug Metabolism Reviews*, *37*(3), 511–564.

54. Ambrosone, C. B., Kropp, S., Yang, J., et al. (2008). Cigarette smoking, N-acetyltransferase 2 genotypes, and breast cancer risk: Pooled analysis and meta-analysis. *Cancer Epidemiology, Biomarkers and Prevention: A Publication of the American Association for Cancer Research, Cosponsored by the American Society of Preventive Oncology*, *17*(1), 15–26.

55. Ambrosone, C. B., et al. (1996). Cigarette smoking, N-acetyltransferase 2 genetic polymorphisms, and breast cancer risk. *JAMA: The Journal of the American Medical Association*.

56. Baumgartner, K. B., et al. (2009). N-acetyltransferase 2 genotype modification of active cigarette smoking on breast cancer risk among Hispanic and non-Hispanic white women. *Toxicological Sciences*, *112*(1), 211–220.

57. Garcia-Closas, M., Malats, N., & Silverman, D. (2005). NAT2 slow acetylation, GSTM1 null genotype, and risk of bladder cancer: Results from the Spanish Bladder Cancer Study and meta-analyses. *Lancet*, *366*(9486), 649–659.

58. Zhu, Z., Zhang, J., Jiang, W., et al. (2015). Risks on N-acetyltransferase 2 and bladder cancer: A meta-analysis. *OncoTargets and Therapy*, *8*, 3715–3720. PubMed PMID: 26715854.

59. Lubin, J. H., Kogevinas, M., Siverman, D., et al. (2007). Evidence for an intensity-dependent interaction of NAT2 acetylation genotype and cigarette smoking in the Spanish Bladder Cancer Study. *International Journal of Epidemiology*, *36*(1), 236–241. PubMed PMID: 17510079.

60. Das, A., Dey, N., Ghosh, A., Das, T., & Chatterjee, I. B. (2011). NAD(P)H: Quinone oxidoreductase 1 deficiency conjoint with marginal vitamin C deficiency causes cigarette smoke induced myelodysplastic syndromes. *PLoS ONE*, *6*(5), e20590. PubMed PMID: 21655231.

61. U.S. Department of Health and Human Services. (2014). *The Health Consequences of Smoking – 50 Years of Progress: A Report of the Surgeon General*. Atlanta: U.S. Department of Health and Human Services. Centers for Disease Control and prevention, National Center for Chronic Disease Prevention and Health Promotion, Office on Smoking and Health. (Accessed 22 December 2016).

62. Clark, B. J., & Cochrum, R. K. (2007). The steroidogenic acute regulatory protein as a target of

endocrine disruption in male reproduction. *Drug Metabolism Reviews*, 39(2–3), 353–370.

63. Kavitharaj, N. K., & Vijayammal, P. L. (1999). Nicotine administration induced changes in the gonadal function in male rats. *Pharmacology*, 58(1), 2–7.

64. Zhao, J., Leung, J. Y., Lin, S. L., & Schooling, C. M. (2016). Cigarette smoking and testosterone in men and women: A systematic review and meta-analysis of observational studies. *Preventive Medicine*, 85, 1–10. PubMed PMID: 26763163.

65. Wang, W., Yang, X., Liang, J., et al. (2013). Cigarette smoking has a positive and independent effect on testosterone levels. *Hormones (Athens, Greece)*, 12(4), 567–577. PubMed PMID: 24457405.

66. U.S. Department of Health and Human Services. (1988). *The Surgeon General's report on nutrition and health*. Rocklin, CA: Prima.

67. Teo, K. K., Ounpuu, S., Hawken, S., et al. (2006). Tobacco use and risk of myocardial infarction in 52 countries in the INTERHEART study: A case-controlled study. *Lancet*, 368(9536), 647–658.

68. Pryor, W. A., & Stone, K. (1993). Oxidants in cigarette smoke. Radicals, hydrogen peroxide, peroxynitrate, and peroxynitrite. *Annals of the New York Academy of Sciences*, 686, 12–27. PubMed PMID: 8512242.

69. Yokode, M., Kita, T., Arai, H., et al. (1988). Cholesterol ester accumulation in macrophages incubated with low density lipoprotein pretreated with cigarette smoke extract. *Proceedings of the National Academy of Sciences of the United States of America*, 85(7), 2344–2348. PubMed PMID: 3353382.

70. Frei, B., Forte, T. M., Ames, B. N., & Cross, C. E. (1991). Gas phase oxidants of cigarette smoke induce lipid peroxidation and changes in lipoprotein properties in human blood plasma. Protective effects of ascorbic acid. *The Biochemical Journal*, 277(Pt. 1), 133–138. PubMed PMID: 1854329.

71. Imamura, H., Tanaka, K., & Hirae, C. (1996). Relationship of cigarette smoking to blood pressure and serum lipids and lipoproteins in men. *Clinical and Experimental Pharmacology and Physiology*, 23, 397–402.

72. Fusegawa, Y., Goto, S., Handa, S., et al. (1999). platelet spontaneous aggregation in platelet-rich plasma is increased in habitual smokers. *Thrombosis Research*, 93(6), 271–278. PubMed PMID: 10093968.

73. Kannel, W. B., D'Agostino, R. B., & Belanger, A. J. (1987). Fibrinogen, cigarette smoking, and risk of cardiovascular disease: Insights from the Framingham Study. *American Heart Journal*, 113(4), 1006–1010. PubMed PMID: 3565227.

74. Penn, A., & Snyder, C. (1988). Arteriosclerotic plaque development is 'promoted' by polynuclear aromatic hydrocarbons. *Carcinogenesis*, 9(12), 2185–2189. PubMed PMID: 3142695.

75. Levenson, J., Simon, A. C., & Cambien, F. A. (1987). Cigarette smoking and hypertension. *Arteriosclerosis (Dallas, Tex.)*, 7, 572–577.

76. Faught, B. E., Flouris, A. D., & Cairney, J. (2009). Epidemiological evidence associating secondhand smoke exposure with cardiovascular disease. *Inflammation and Allergy Drug Targets*, 8(5), 321–327. PubMed PMID: 20025577.

77. Kritz, H., Schmid, P., & Sinzinger, H. (1995). Passive smoking and cardiovascular risk. *Archives of Internal Medicine*, 155, 1940–1948.

78. Clark, J. D., 3rd, Wilkinson, J. D., LeBlanc, W. G., et al. (2008). Inflammatory markers and secondhand tobacco smoke exposure among U.S. workers. *American Journal of Industrial Medicine*, 51(8), 626–632. PubMed PMID: 18481260.

79. Venn, A., & Britton, J. (2007). Exposure to secondhand smoke and biomarkers of cardiovascular disease risk in never-smoking adults. *Circulation*, 115(8), 990–995. PubMed PMID: 17296856.

80. Barnoya, J., & Glantz, S. A. (2005). Cardiovascular effects of secondhand smoke: Nearly as large as smoking. *Circulation*, 111(20), 2684–2698. PubMed PMID: 15911719.

81. Egan, K. M., Stampfer, M. J., Hunter, D., Hankinson, S., et al. (2002). Active and passive smoking in breast cancer: Prospective results from the Nurses' Health Study. *Epidemiology (Cambridge, Mass.)*, 13(2), 138–145. PubMed PMID: 11880753.

82. Clarke, E., Morgan, R., & Newman, A. (1982). Smoking as a risk factor in cancer of the cervix: Additional evidence from a case-control study. *American Journal of Epidemiology*, 115, 59–66.

83. Lyon, J., Gardner, J., West, D., et al. (1983). Smoking and carcinoma in situ of the uterine cervix. *American Journal of Public Health*, 73, 558–562.

84. Marshall, J., Graham, S., Byers, T., Swanson, M., & Brasure, J. (1983). Diet and smoking in the epidemiology of cancer of the cervix. *Journal of the National Cancer Institute*, 70, 847–851.

85. Clarke, E., Hatcher, J., McKeown-Eyssen, G., & Liekrish, G. (1985). Cervical dysplasia: Association with sexual behavior, smoking, and oral contraceptive use. *American Journal of Obstetrics and Gynecology*, 151, 612–616.

86. Pelleter, O. (1977). Vitamin C and tobacco. *International Journal for Vitamin and Nutrition Research*, 16, 147–169.

87. Hecht, S. S., & Hoffmann, D. (1988). Tobacco-specific nitrosamines, an important group of carcinogens in tobacco and tobacco smoke. *Carcinogenesis, 9*(6), 875–884. PubMed PMID: 3286030.

88. Moorthy, B., Chu, C., & Carlin, D. J. (2015). Polycyclic aromatic hydrocarbons: From metabolism to lung cancer. *Toxicological Sciences, 145*(1), 5–15. PubMed PMID: 25911656.

89. Masaoka, H., Matsuo, K., Ito, H., Wakai, K., et al. (2016). Cigarette smoking and bladder cancer risk: An evaluation based on a systematic review of epidemiologic evidence in the Japanese population. *Japanese Journal of Clinical Oncology, 46*(3), 273–283. PubMed PMID: 26941372.

90. Oze, I., Matsuo, K., Ito, H., et al. (2012). Cigarette smoking and esophageal cancer risk: An evaluation based on a systematic review of epidemiological evidence among the Japanese population. *Japanese Journal of Clinical Oncology, 42*(1), 63–73. PubMed PMID: 22131340.

91. Matsuo, K., Ito, H., Wakai, K., et al. (2011). Cigarette smoking and pancreas cancer risk: An evaluation based on a systematic review of epidemiologic evidence in the Japanese population. *Japanese Journal of Clinical Oncology, 41*(11), 1292–1302. PubMed PMID: 21971423.

92. Koyanagi, Y. N., Matsuo, K., Ito, H., et al. (2016). Cigarette smoking and the risk of head and neck cancer in the Japanese population: A systematic review and meta-analysis. *Japanese Journal of Clinical Oncology, 46*(6), 580–595. PubMed PMID: 27369767.

93. Tanaka, K., Tsuji, I., Wakai, K., et al. (2006). Cigarette smoking and liver cancer risk: An evaluation based on a systematic review of epidemiologic evidence among Japanese. *Japanese Journal of Clinical Oncology, 36*(7), 445–456. PubMed PMID: 16782973.

94. Mizoue, T., Inoue, M., Tanaka, K., et al. (2006). Tobacco smoking and colorectal cancer risk: An evaluation based on a systematic review of epidemiologic evidence among the Japanese population. *Japanese Journal of Clinical Oncology, 36*(1), 25–39. PubMed PMID: 16423841.

95. Bakhshaie, J., Zvolensky, M. J., & Goodwin, R. D. (2015). Cigarette smoking and the onset and persistence of depression among adults in the United States: 1994-2005. *Comprehensive Psychiatry, 60*, 140–148. PubMed PMID: 25882595.

96. Peterson, C. (1988). Explanatory style as a risk factor for illness. *Cognitive Therapy and Research, 12*, 117–130.

97. Altar, C., Bennett, B., Wallace, R., et al. (1983). Glucocorticoid induction of tryptophan oxygenase. *Biochemical Pharmacology, 32*, 979–984.

98. Zorlu, N., Cropley, V. L., Zorlu, P. K., et al. (2017). Effects of cigarette smoking on cortical thickness in major depressive disorder. *Journal of Psychiatric Research, 84*, 1–8. PubMed PMID: 27669406.

99. Jorgensen, K. N., Skjaervo, I., et al. (2015). Cigarette smoking is associated with thinner congulate and insular cortices in patients with severe mental illness. *Journal of Psychiatry and Neuroscience, 40*(4), 241–249. PubMed PMID: 25672482.

100. Ren, W., Gu, Y., Zhu, L., et al. (2016). The effect of cigarette smoking on vitamin D level and depression in male patients with acute ischemic stroke. *Comprehensive Psychiatry, 65*, 9–14. PubMed PMID: 26773985.

101. Winsa, B., & Karlsson, A. (1993). Grave's disease, endocrine ophthalmopathy and smoking. *Acta Endocrinologica, 128*, 156–160.

102. Bartalena, L., Bogazzi, F., Tanda, M. L., et al. (1995). Cigarette smoking and the thyroid. *European Journal of Endocrinology, 133*, 507–512.

103. Shine, B., Fells, P., Edwards, O. M., & Weetman, O. P. (1990). Association between Graves' ophthalmopathy and smoking. *Lancet, 335*, 1261–1263.

104. Bufalo, N. E., Santos, R. B., Cury, A. N., Andrade, R. A., Morari, J., et al. (2008). Genetic polymorphisms associated with cigarette smoking and the risk of Graves' disease. *Clinical Endocrinology, 68*(6), 982–987. PubMed PMID: 17980001.

105. Chakravarthy, U., Wong, T. Y., Fletcher, A., et al. (2010). Clinical risk factors for age-related macular degeneration: A systematic review and meta-analysis. *BMC Ophthalmology, 10*, 31. PubMed PMID: 21144031.

106. Thornton, J., Edwards, R., et al. (2005). Smoking and age-related macular degeneration: A review of association. *Eye (Lond), 19*(9), 935–944. PubMed PMID: 16151432.

107. Olson, R. J. (1991). Supplemental antioxidant vitamins and minerals in patients with macular degeneration. *Journal of the American College of Nutrition, 10*, 550, Abstract 52.

108. Christen, W. G., et al. (1996). A prospective study of cigarette smoking and risk of age-related macular degeneration in men. *JAMA: The Journal of the American Medical Association, 276*, 1147–1151.

109. Beatty, S., Koh, H., Phil, M., Henson, D., & Boulton, M. (2000). The role of oxidative stress in the pathogenesis of age-related macular degeneration. *Survey of Ophthalmology, 45*(2), 115–134. PubMed PMID: 11033038.

110. Seddon, J. M., Willett, W. C., Speizer, F. E., & Hankinson, S. E. (1996). A prospective study

of cigarette smoking and age-related macular degeneration in women. *JAMA: The Journal of the American Medical Association, 276*(14), 1141–1146. PubMed PMID: 8827966.

111. Kulikauskas, V. D., Blaustein, D., & Ablin, D. (1984). Cigarette smoking and its possible effects on sperm. *Fertility and Sterility, 44*, 526–528.

112. Sharma, R., Harley, A., Agarwal, A., & Esteves, S. C. (2016). Cigarette smoking and semen quality: A new meta-analysis examining the effect of the 2010 World Health Organization laboratory methods for the examination of human semen. *European Urology, 70*(4), 635–645. PubMed PMID: 27113031.

113. Asare-Anane, H., Bannison, S. B., Ofori, E. K., et al. (2016). Tobacco smoking is associated with decreased semen quality. *Reproductive Health, 13*(1), 90. PubMed PMID: 27496053.

114. Dawson, E., Harris, W., & Powell, L. (1991). Effect of vitamin C supplementation on sperm quality of heavy smokers. *FASEB Journal : Official Publication of the Federation of American Societies for Experimental Biology, 5*, A915.

115. Hayatbakhsh, M. R., Clavarino, A., et al. (2012). Cigarette smoking and age of menopause: A large prospective study. *Maturitas, 72*(4), 346–352. PubMed PMID: 22695707.

116. Midgette, A. S., & Baron, J. A. (1990). Cigarette smoking and the risk of natural menopause. *Epidemiology (Cambridge, Mass.), 1*, 474–480.

117. Smith, R. L., Flaws, J. A., & Gallicchio, L. (2015). Does quitting smoking decrease the risk of midlife hot flashes? A longitudinal analysis. *Maturitas, 82*(1), 123–127. PubMed PMID: 26149340.

118. Chatkin, R., Chatkin, J. M., Spanemberg, L., et al. (2015). Smoking is associated with more abdominal fat in morbidly obese patients. *PLoS ONE, 10*(5), e0126146. PubMed PMID: 25978682.

119. Mizuno, O., Okamoto, K., Sawada, M., et al. (2005). Obesity and smoking: Relationship with waist circumference and obesity-related disorders in men undergoing a health screening. *Journal of Atherosclerosis and Thrombosis, 12*(4), 199–204. PubMed PMID: 16141623.

120. Akbartabartoori, M., Lean, M. E., & Hankey, C. R. (2005). Relationships between cigarette smoking, body size and body shape. *International Journal of Obesity (2005), 29*(2), 236–243. PubMed PMID: 15505632.

121. Canoy, D., Wareham, N., Luben, R., Welch, A., et al. (2005). Cigarette smoking and fat distribution in 21,828 British men and women: A population-based study. *Obesity Research, 13*(8), 1466–1475. PubMed PMID: 16129730.

122. Nakanishi, N., Takatorige, T., & Suzuki, K. (2005). Cigarette smoking and the risk of the metabolic syndrome in middle-aged Japanese male office workers. *Industrial Health, 43*(2), 295–301. PubMed PMID: 15895844.

123. Wilsgaard, T., & Jacobsen, B. K. (2007). Lifestyle factors and incident metabolic syndrome. The Tromso Study 1979-2001. *Diabetes Research and Clinical Practice, 78*(2), 217–224. PubMed PMID: 17448561.

124. Chiolero, A., Jacot-Sadowski, I., et al. (2007). Association of cigarettes smoked daily with obesity in a general adult population. *Obesity, 15*(5), 1311–1318.

125. Marchbanks, P., Lee, N. C., & Peterson, H. B. (1990). Cigarette smoking as a risk factor for pelvic inflammatory disease. *American Journal of Obstetrics and Gynecology, 162*, 639–644. PubMed PMID: 2316564.

126. Scholes, D. (1992). Current cigarette smoking and risk of acute pelvic inflammatory disease. *American Journal of Public Health, 82*, 1352–1355. PubMed PMID: 1415858.

127. Anda, R. F., Williamson, D. F., Escobedo, L., et al. (1992). Self-perceived stress and the risk of peptic ulcer disease. *Archives of Internal Medicine, 152*, 829.

128. Li, L. F., Chan, R. L., Lu, L., Shen, J., et al. (2014). Cigarette smoking and gastrointestinal diseases: The causal relationship and underlying molecular mechanisms (review). *International Journal of Molecular Medicine, 34*(2), 372–380. PubMed PMID: 24859303.

129. Carranza, F. (1984). *Glickman's clinical periodontology.* Philadelphia, PA: WB Saunders.

130. Schenkein, H. A., Gunsolley, J. C., & Koertge, T. E. (1995). Smoking and its effects on early-onset periodontitis. *Journal of the American Dental Association, 126*, 1107–1113.

131. Kaldahl, W. B., et al. (1996). Levels of cigarette consumption and response to periodontal therapy. *Journal of Periodontology, 67*, 675–681.

132. Shereef, M., Sanara, P. P., et al. (2015). The effect of cigarette smoking on the severity of periodontal diseases among adults of Kothamangalam Town, Kerala. *Journal of Pharmacy & Bioallied Sciences, 7*(Suppl. 2), S648–S651. PubMed PMID: 26538936.

133. Grossi, S. G., Genco, R. J., Machtei, E. E., Ho, A. W., et al. (1995). Assessment of risk for periodontal disease. II. Risk indicators for alveolar bone loss. *Journal of Periodontology, 66*(1), 23–29. PubMed PMID: 7891246.

134. Ryder, M. I. (2007). The influence of smoking on host responses in periodontal infections. *Periodontology 2000, 43*, 267–277. PubMed PMID: 17214844.

135. U.S. Government Printing Office; Washington D.C. (2008). Smoking-attributable mortality, years of potential life lost, and productivity losses – United States, 2000-2004. *MMWR. Morbidity and Mortality Weekly Report*, 1226–1228.

136. Cunningham, T. J., Ford, E. S., Rolle, I. V., et al. (2015). Associations of self-reported cigarette smoking with chronic obstructive pulmonary disease and co-morbid chronic conditions in the United States. *COPD*, 12(3), 276–286. PubMed PMID: 25207639.

137. Kurmi, O. P., Li, L., Wang, J., Millwood, I. Y., Chen, J., et al. (2015). COPD and its association with smoking in the Mainland China: A cross-sectional analysis of 0.5 million men and women from ten diverse areas. *International Journal of Chronic Obstructive Pulmonary Disease*, 10, 655–665. PubMed PMID: 25848242.

138. U.S. Department of Health and Human Services. (2014). *The Health Consequences of Smoking – 50 Years of Progress: A Report of the Surgeon General*. Atlanta: U.S. Department of Health and Human Services. Centers for Disease Control and prevention, National Center for Chronic Disease Prevention and Health Promotion, Office on Smoking and Health. (Accessed 25 April 2017).

139. Van Dijk, W. D., Heijdra, Y., et al. (2010). Interaction in COPD experiment (ICE): A hazardous combination of cigarette smoking and bronchodilation in chronic obstructive pulmonary disease. *Medical Hypotheses*, 74(2), 277–280. PubMed PMID: 19800175.

140. Law, M., & Tang, J. L. (1995). An analysis of the effectiveness of interventions intended to help people stop smoking. *Archives of Internal Medicine*, 155, 1933–1941.

141. Carmody, T. P., Duncan, C., Simon, J. A., Solkowitz, S., et al. (2008). Hypnosis for smoking cessation: A randomized trial. *Nicotine and Tobacco Research*, 10(5), 811–818. PubMed PMID: 18569754.

142. Daughton, D. M., Fortmann, S. P., et al. (1999). The smoking cessation efficacy of varying doses of nicotine patch delivery systems 4 to 5 years post-quit day. *Preventive Medicine*, 28(2), 113–118. PubMed PMID: 10048102.

143. Pelletier, O. (1968). Smoking and vitamin C levels in humans. *The American Journal of Clinical Nutrition*, 21, 1259–1267.

144. National Research Council. (1989). *Recommended dietary allowances* (10th ed.). Washington, DC: National Academy Press.

145. Prerovsky, I., & Hladovec, J. (1979). Suppression of the desquamating effect of smoking on the human endothelium by hydroxyethylrutosides. *Blood Vessels*, 16, 239–240.

146. Burton, G., & Ingold, K. (1984). Beta-carotene. An unusual type of lipid antioxidant. *Science*, 224, 569–573.

147. Misra, A., Chattopadhyay, R., et al. (2003). Black tea prevents cigarette smoke-induced oxidative damage of proteins in guinea pigs. *The Journal of Nutrition*, 133(8), 2622–2628. PubMed PMID: 12888648.

148. Al Hariri, M., Zibara, K., Farhat, W., et al. (2016). Cigarette smoking-induced cardiac hypertrophy, vascular inflammation, and injury are attenuated by antioxidant supplementation in an animal model. *Frontiers in Pharmacology*, 7, 397. PubMed PMID: 27881962.

149. Mooney, L. A., Madsen, A. M., Tang, D., et al. (2005). Antioxidant vitamin supplementation reduces benzo(a)pyrene-DNA adducts and potential cancer risk in female smokers. *Cancer Epidemiology, Biomarkers and Prevention: A Publication of the American Association for Cancer Research, Cosponsored by the American Society of Preventive Oncology*, 14(1), 237–242.

150. Panda, K., Chattopadhyay, R., et al. (2000). Vitamin C prevents cigarette smoke-induced oxidative damage in vivo. *Free Radical Biology & Medicine*, 29(2), 115–124. PubMed PMID: 10980400.

151. Zhu, W., Cromie, M. M., Cai, Q., et al. (2014). Curcumin and vitamin E protect against adverse effects of benzo[a]pyrene in lung epithelial cells. *PLoS ONE*, 9(3), e92992.

152. Chang, Y. Z., Lin, H. C., Chan, S. T., & Yeh, S. L. (2012). Effects of quercetin metabolites on the enhancing effect of β-carotene on DNA damage and cytochrome P1A1/2 expression in benzo[a]pyrene-exposed A549 cells. *Food Chemistry*, 133(2), 445–450.

153. Baumeister, P., Reiter, M., Kleinsasser, N., et al. (2009). Epigallocatechin-3-gallate reduces DNA damage induced by benzo[a]pyrene diol epoxide and cigarette smoke condensate in human mucosa tissue cultures. *European Journal of Cancer Prevention*, 18(3), 230–235.

154. Sticozzi, C., Cervellati, F., Muresan, X. M., et al. (2014). Resveratrol prevents cigarette smoke-induced keratinocytes damage. *Food & Function*, 5(9), 2348–2356. PubMed PMID: 25088477.

41

Wheat
Gluten/Zonulin

SUMMARY

- Presence in population: Celiac disease (CD) affects up to 1% of the US population (roughly 3 million people); perhaps as much as 50% of the population experiences uncontrolled increased gut permeability in a dose-dependent response to gluten intake
- Major diseases: Nonceliac gluten sensitivity (NCGS), autoimmune disease (e.g., CD, lupus, rheumatoid arthritis, type 1 diabetes), cancer (e.g., brain, breast, lung, pancreatic)
- Primary sources: Gluten grains (e.g., wheat, rye, barley, spelt) and products manufactured from gluten grains (e.g., bread, pasta, crackers, cookies, beer, cereal)
- Best measure: Antitransglutaminase IgA antibodies, total serum IgA, lactulose/mannitol test, serum zonulin, serum haptoglobin (HP), biopsy to confirm diagnosis of CD
- Best intervention: Complete avoidance of gluten; supplementation to repair intestinal permeability (e.g., probiotics, quercetin, L-glutamine, N-acetyl-glucosamine)

DESCRIPTION

The gastrointestinal (GI) system is the primary gateway by which the external environment interacts with the body.[1] The largest mucosal surface in the body, the GI tract is responsible for the digestion and absorption of nutrients from food, but its effect extends well beyond the gut. The GI tract contains an extraordinary number of immune cells that must defend against pathogens and toxins (to which the body is exposed to on a continuous basis), while allowing for tolerance to food and commensal bacteria—a balancing act that can have systemic consequences.

The role of digestion is to first separate food into its components by mechanical homogenization and chemical breakdown, followed by absorption of the smaller carbohydrates, lipids, proteins, vitamins, minerals, and other nutrients through a variety of passive and active processes.

Tight junctions play a significant role in the regulation of intestinal permeability and adapt to a variety of developmental, physiological, and pathological circumstances.[2] Together with the gut-associated lymphoid tissue (GALT) and the neuroendocrine network, the intestinal epithelial barrier, with its intercellular tight junctions, controls the equilibrium between tolerance and immunity to nonself-antigens. In some individuals, the resistance of dietary gluten to complete digestion leads to large oligopeptides crossing into the enterocyte, triggering an autoimmune response (i.e., CD).[3] Zonulin is a protein modulator of intercellular tight junctions that has been shown to induce a significant and reversible increase in gastroduodenal and small intestinal permeability, and is involved in tolerance/immune response balance.[4] The hybridization of wheat has increased the amount of the highly reactive α-9 gliadin epitope in modern varieties, which is now consumed multiple times per day in a typical diet.[5] This ongoing recurrent exposure chronically disrupts the tolerance/immune response balance, leading to much of the chronic disease burden now suffered by Western societies.

TOXICITY

Abnormal permeability refers to a measurable increase in passage of small water-soluble compounds across the paracellular pathway of the small intestine. Intracellular enterocyte and tight junction proteins regulate the rate of movement and permeability through this pathway (Fig. 41.1).[6] Tight junctions are involved in passive absorption of nutrients, surveillance of gut microbial content, defense against some infectious agents, and transport of leukocytes into the gut.

Factors known to alter intestinal permeability include infection, inflammatory cytokines, nutrient transporter activation, and noxious environmental toxicants. In addition, the composition of the gut microbiota is a major factor associated with intestinal permeability. Exposure of the small intestine to bacteria, independent of the virulence of the microorganisms, triggers the release of zonulin, causing disengagement of the protein zonula occludens 1 from the tight junction complex between the mucosal cells.[7] This opens the space between cells in the GI mucosa, allowing water to flush into the gut, washing out the microorganisms and toxins. This opening also dramatically increases gut permeability. The zonulin-driven opening of the paracellular pathway may represent a defensive mechanism that aids the innate immune system against bacterial colonization of the small intestine. However, increased intestinal permeability also provides an underlying mechanism in the pathogenesis of allergic, inflammatory, and autoimmune diseases (i.e., most chronic diseases). The tight junctions formerly considered static structures are now being shown to be dynamic and adapt to a variety of developmental, physiological, pathological, and dietary circumstances.

Gliadin

Certainly, in patients with CD, gluten consumption causes increased permeability. However, a recent *in vitro* study suggests that wheat germ agglutinin (WGA) may have some ability to damage GI epithelium by unique mechanisms.[8] Gluten contains gliadin polypeptides, which are prolamins, a group of plant storage proteins found in the seeds of cereal grains of the grass genus *Triticum*: wheat (gliadin), barley (hordein), rye (secalin), corn (zein), sorghum (kafirin), and oats (avenin). Storage proteins account for about 50% of the total protein in mature cereal grains. Gliadins are characterized by a high content of glutamine and proline, and along with gluten, give bread the ability to rise properly during baking.

Under normal physiological conditions, competent tight junctions limit the passage of gliadin and prevent access of gliadin to GALT.[9] In genetically susceptible individuals, ingestion of gliadin has cytotoxic effects, activates the immune system, and upregulates inflammation. The increase in intestinal permeability in response to gliadin is time- and dose-dependent. This opening is rapid and reversible, except in those with CD. The increased permeability caused by gliadin in susceptible individuals is adequate to increase inflammation and disease even where there is no immunological reaction.

There are at least 50 toxic epitopes (i.e., antigenic determinants) in gluten peptides exerting cytotoxic, immunomodulatory, and gut-permeating activities. The three main types of gliadin (α, γ, and ω) are distinguished based on their amino acid sequences, all of which are reactive in celiac patients, with the alpha form being the strongest. As seen in Fig. 41.2, each of the various peptide sequences in gliadin has different toxic activities: cytotoxic, immunomodulatory, zonulin release, and interleukin (IL)-8 release.[10] The 33-mer gliadin fragment is the most immunogenic peptide, likely because it harbors six overlapping epitopes.

There is a wide range in response among those reacting to gliadin, from minimal changes in the intestinal

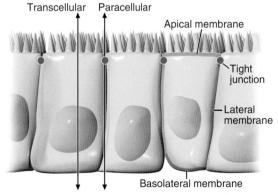

FIG. 41.1 Structure of the mucosal barrier with pathways of epithelial permeability.

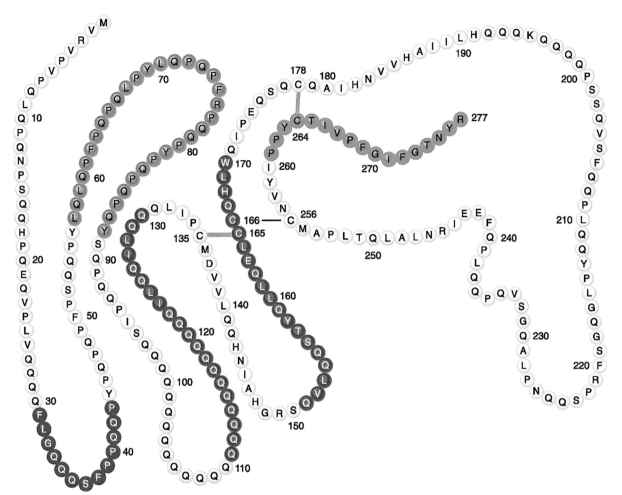

FIG. 41.2 Immunologically active peptide sequence in α-gliadin. Mapping of α-gliadin motifs exerting cytotoxic activity (red), immunomodulatory activity (light purple), zonulin release and gut-permeating activity (blue), and CXCR3-IL-8 release in CD patients (dark green). (From Fasano, A. [2011]. Zonulin and its regulation of intestinal barrier function: The biological door to inflammation, autoimmunity, and cancer. *Physiology Review, 91*[1], 151–75.)

epithelium and no obvious symptoms to severe damage of the intestinal lining or autoimmune reactions throughout the body. Further complicating the clinical picture is that CD may develop soon after wheat is introduced into the diet (i.e., infants), or significant symptoms and pathology may not manifest until adulthood. Although there are several mechanisms by which gliadin consumption causes disease in susceptible individuals, the most significant include substantial and diverse nutritional deficiencies due to loss of absorptive area in the small intestine, loss of enterocyte discrimination of molecules that can enter the body as a result of impaired pericellular junctions, and increased activation of the inflammatory and immune systems in response to gliadin and other molecules passing through the pericellular junctions. In any given patient, one or more of these mechanisms may be involved. These diverse mechanisms help explain the surprisingly dissimilar range and severity of disease caused or aggravated by the consumption of wheat in susceptible individuals.

Zonulin

Zonulin release is also stimulated by contact with gliadin (alpha-gliadin is the most effective). The enterocytes that release zonulin occur in the jejunum and distal ileum but not in the colon. When exposed to gliadin, zonulin receptor-positive IEC6 and Caco2 cells release zonulin, leading to the rearrangement of the cell cytoskeleton, the loss of occluding-ZO1 protein-protein interaction, and an increase in intestinal permeability to macromolecules.[11] Chemokine receptor CXCR3 is the receptor for specific gliadin peptides that cause zonulin release and subsequent increase in intestinal permeability (Fig. 41.3).[12] *In vitro* research with chemokine receptor CXCR3 transfectants found that several peptides from gliadin, especially 33-mer, bind to the receptor. Zonulin and CXCR3 are overexpressed in the intestinal mucosa of patients with CD and autoimmune disease. Several major diseases have been associated with elevated zonulin in the blood including cancers (e.g., brain, breast, lung, ovarian, pancreatic), autoimmune disease (e.g., multiple sclerosis [MS], rheumatoid arthritis [RA], systemic lupus erythematosus [SLE]), and diseases of the nervous system (e.g., schizophrenia, dementia, chronic inflammatory demyelinating polyneuropathy).

Haptoglobin

It was discovered that human zonulin is prehaptoglobin-2 (pre-HP2), and earlier researchers knew it was an inactive precursor for HP2.[13] HP, identified as a marker of inflammation several decades ago, is an α-2–globulin found in human plasma at a concentration of 82 to 236 mg/dL. It is an acute phase plasma protein whose primary role appears to be to bind the free hemoglobin released when erythrocytes are damaged, thus decreasing the oxidative damage of the freed iron.[14] It is composed of four polypeptide chains: two α chains and two β chains connected by disulfide bridges. Human HP occurs primarily as three major phenotypes: HP1-1, HP2-1, and HP2-2. The phenotypes are differentiated by the presence of an α-1 chain (HP1-1) or an α-2 chain (HP2-2) with a combination of α-1 and α-2 chains distinguishing HP2-1.[15] The population distribution of these phenotypes and their association with CD is shown in Table 41.1.

The genotypes have very different affinity for iron and significant disease associations. HP1-1 has the strongest and HP2-2 the weakest affinity for hemoglobin. HP1 is the original form, evolving about 800 million years ago. HP2 is a mutation found only in humans, and is believed to have occurred in India about 2 million years ago (Fig. 41.4). Some conditions such as cancer and coronary artery disease can raise HP in plasma, yet diseases such as jaundice and cirrhosis can significantly lower the total amount of HP. A small portion of individuals either has no haptoglobin (HP0) or has uncommon variations on the three main types. Most HP0 is due to acquired ahaptoglobinemia (<1.0% of the population has a genetic polymorphism that results in nonproduction). HP0 is very common in Western Africa (as high as 47%) and other areas where hemolytic diseases, such as malaria, are common.

Gliadin causes release of zonulin in the 80% of the population with HP2. Although HP1-1 has much lower chance of immunological reaction, the probability is still not zero. There is growing recognition of the nonimmunological reaction to wheat, which is now being identified as NCGS. Table 41.2 provides an estimate of the percent of the North American population in each HP category along with clinical responses and clinical recommendations. Considering the significant underdiagnosis of these conditions, research suggests the information is an accurate reflection of occurrence.

The research is clear that the mechanism of action is highly dependent on haptoglobin type, the type of grain eaten, the frequency and dosage of gliadin, and other factors such as digestive function and gut microbiota.

Gut Microbiota

Unhealthy bowels are a source of metabolic endotoxins from both "normal" and "abnormal" gut bacteria. When the microorganisms die, endotoxins are secreted and released into the surrounding environment. Technically only lipopolysaccharides (LPS) from gram-negative bacteria are known as endotoxins; however, it is clinically relevant in this context to use a broader definition including anything harmful released by gut bacteria. Endotoxins bind to toll-like receptors (TLRs) on other cells (including microglia), initiating an adaptive immune response and a signaling cascade that leads to activation of proinflammatory genes.[16] Impaired digestive function along with gut-derived microbial toxins trigger both the onset and maintenance of chronic low-grade inflammation.[17] This, in turn, enhances intestinal permeability, increasing the translocation of microbiome-derived LPS to the bloodstream and resulting in a two- to threefold increase in serum LPS concentration, which can reach a threshold

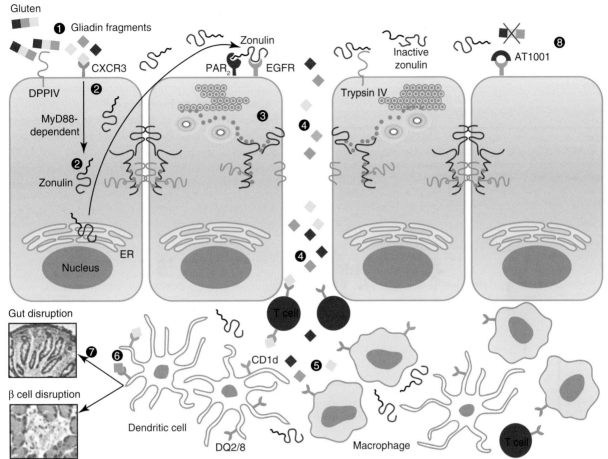

FIG. 41.3 (1) Gliadin release of zonulin to open tight junctions and activate immune system. The production of specific gliadin-derived peptides by digestive enzymes causes CXCR3-mediated, MyD88-dependent zonulin release (2) and subsequent transactivation of EGFR by PAR2 leading to small intestine tight junction (TJ) disassembly (3). The increased intestinal permeability allows nonself antigens (including gliadin) to enter the lamina propria (4), where they are presented by HLA-DQ,-DR molecules. (5) The presentation of one or more gliadin peptides leads to abrogation of oral tolerance (switch to Th1/Th17 response) and a marked increase in peripheral immune responses to gliadin. Furthermore, gliadin-loaded dendritic cells migrate from the small intestine to mesenteric and/or pancreatic lymph nodes (6) where they present gliadin-derived antigens. This presentation leads to migration of CD4–CD8–γδ and CD4–CD8+ αβ T cells to the target organ (gut and/or pancreas) where they cause inflammation (7). Implementation of a gluten-free diet or treatment with the zonulin inhibitor AT1001 (8) prevents the activation of the zonulin pathway and therefore of the autoimmune process targeting the gut or pancreatic β cells. (From Fasano, A. [2011]. Zonulin and its regulation of intestinal barrier function: the biological door to inflammation, autoimmunity, and cancer. *Physiology Review, 91*[1], 151–175.)

TABLE 41.1 **Haptoglobin Type: Prevalence and Associated Risk of Celiac Disease**		
HP Phenotype	% in Healthy US Population	% in CD Patients
HP1-1	14.5	7.1
HP2-1	48.2	35.7
HP2-2	37.3	57.2

Data from Koch, W., Latz, W., Eichinger, M., Roguin, A., Levy AP, Schömig A, Kastrati A. (2002). Genotyping of the common haptoglobin Hp ½ polymorphism based on PCR. *Clinical Chemistry, 48*(9), 1377–1382.

called "metabolic endotoxemia" (ME). ME may trigger TLR4-mediated inflammatory activation, eliciting a chronic low-grade proinflammatory and prooxidative stress.[18,19] ME is associated with the development of several chronic conditions, including obesity, cardiovascular disease, diabetes/insulin resistance, neuroinflammation, and nonalcoholic fatty liver disease.[20]

Persons with CD and those on a gluten-free diet (GFD) are both found to have microbiome imbalance. Bifidobacteria levels are lower in patients with CD, whereas gram-negative *Enterobacteriaceae* (*Bacteroides* and *Escherichia coli*) were higher.[21,22] This increase in

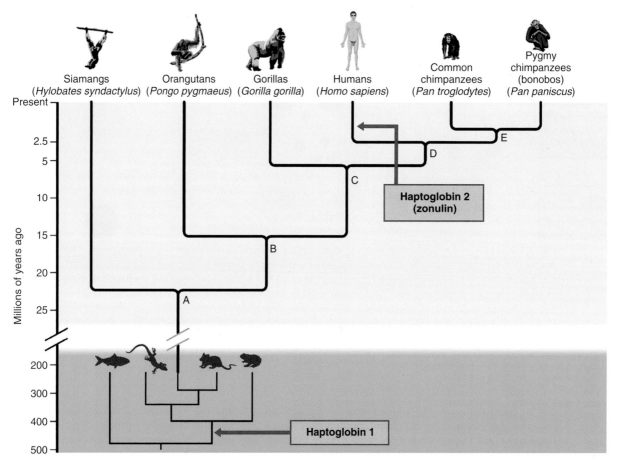

FIG. 41.4 Evolutionary development of haptoglobin. The appearance of the gene encoding HP1 has been mapped to ~450 million years ago, soon after the split between bony fish, reptiles, and mammals. HP2 appeared much later, 500,000 years after, then chimpanzee and human split 2.5 million years ago. (From Fasano, A. [2011]. Zonulin and its regulation of intestinal barrier function: the biological door to inflammation, autoimmunity, and cancer. *Physiology Review, 91*[1], 151–175.)

TABLE 41.2 Summary of Clinical Responses to Wheat and Clinical Recommendations

Response to Wheat	% Pop.	Characteristics	Intervention
Safe	34%	HP1-1; no grain antibodies	None needed
Inconsistent, dose-dependent response (some research is labeling severe form nonceliac gluten sensitivity—NCGS)	43%	HP2-1; low to elevated blood zonulin	Limit wheat, rye, barley; optimize protein digestion; reseed with Bifidobacteria and other healthy gut bacteria
Immune reactions to grains	15%	Antibodies to some grain proteins	Avoid all grains
Celiac disease	3%	HP2-1 or HP2-2; elevated antibodies to gliadin; HLA-DQ2 or DQ8	Strictly avoid wheat, rye, barley; may need to avoid other grains as well
Autoimmune disease	5%	HP2-1 or HP2-2; elevated antiself antibodies	Strictly avoid all allergens

Enterobacteriaceae will enhance the level of LPS in the hepatic portal circulation. In addition, individuals on a GFD for 1 month experienced a reduction of beneficial bifidobacteria, *Bifidobacterium longum,* and *Lactobacillus,* yet the level of Enterobacteriaceae increased in accordance with the reduction in polysaccharides entering the intestines.[23] This proinflammatory microbiome may explain why a GFD does not always result in rapid intestinal healing.

SOURCES

Gluten is a class of storage proteins present in wheat, rye, and barley but not other grains such as rice, corn, and oats. Gluten sensitivity has become quite common, and the incidence continues to increase. Interestingly, the amount of wheat consumed today is far less than the amount consumed in the 19th century. The average American consumed 225 pounds of wheat flour per person in 1880 vs. 132.5 pounds of wheat flour per person in 2011.[24]

BODY BURDEN

NCGS can be identified with a simple antigliadin antibody test. To screen for CD, serological tests are an excellent starting point and may be followed by a biopsy of the small intestine for a definitive diagnosis. To fully understand a patient's response to gluten, the key laboratory tests are HP type, serum zonulin, HLA type, antibodies to wheat proteins, and antiself antibodies. The presence of antigliadin or antiendomysium antibodies clearly indicates a more severe condition. Antitransglutaminase IgA antibodies currently have the highest sensitivity and specificity for CD, ranging from 85% to 98.5% and 95% to 99%, respectively.[25] Most reports place both values at or above 95% if the human recombinant-based test is used.[26] Total serum IgA should be measured, as individuals who have both a selective IgA deficiency as well as CD will not otherwise be identified.[26] Genetic testing for HLA-DQ2 and DQ8 have poor positive predictive value but are considered up to 100% sensitive, and are therefore able to assist in ruling out CD.[27] The progression of immunological reaction to gliadin to autoimmune disease appears dependent on several factors, especially human leukocyte antigen (HLA) class.

It should also be noted that some patients may have "latent" CD, defined as positive serological testing, but a normal biopsy. These individuals are at risk for developing CD. Finally, quite separate from CD, many patients have wheat and/or gluten intolerances. These patients may have antibodies to wheat or gluten (but not autoantibodies), and a therapeutic trial of a GFD typically provides relief of ongoing health complaints.

Detoxification/Excretion Processes

Although most dietary proteins are digested into simple amino acids, dipeptides, and tripeptides by GI proteases, gluten proteins are not completely digested and remain in the GI tract. The resistance of gluten peptides to GI digestion, specifically the immunotoxic gliadin 33-mer peptide, ensures that a significant amount of the ingested gluten peptides is excreted in feces with excretion time estimated to be between 2 and 4 days.[28] Gluten amino peptides can also be detected in urine as early as 4 to 6 hours after gluten intake and can remain detectable for 1 to 2 days after ingestion.[29]

Altered intestinal barrier function permits increased dietary antigen transport across the intestinal barrier and subsequent exposure of these antigens to the mucosal immune system, leading to the development of antigen-specific responses. One study found increased intestinal permeability of all subjects with adverse reactions to food, and the severity of the clinical symptoms correlated with the degree of permeability as measured by a lactulose/mannitol test.[30]

Laboratory assessment of paracellular intestinal permeability is evaluated primarily using the lactulose/mannitol test. After drinking a measured amount of these two sugars, the amount recovered in the urine indicates the degree of absorption of each and can be used as an index of permeability. Monosaccharides, such as mannitol (or L-rhamnose), are absorbed through the transcellular pathway and reflect the degree of absorption of small molecules. Disaccharides, such as lactulose (or cellobiose), are absorbed through the paracellular junction complex, which corresponds to the permeability of larger molecules.[31] The efficacy of treatment may also be monitored with this same test. Intracellular intestinal permeability can often be identified by finding low secretory IgA levels.

Clinical Significance

Although clinical symptoms of malabsorption, such as a low body mass index (BMI), were thought to be common among individuals with CD, research shows that only a minority (5%) are underweight. Most individuals with CD have a normal BMI or are overweight, making these indicators unreliable.[32] Common complaints include nonspecific abdominal pain or bloating, nausea, diarrhea, belching, vomiting, fat in the stool, indigestion, and heartburn. At least half of the individuals with CD have no GI-related symptoms but present with fatigue, subfertility, osteoporosis, joint pain, unexplained iron deficiency, autoimmune disease, or dermatitis herpetiformis (a skin condition found exclusively in celiac patients).[33]

The intestinal barrier controls the equilibrium between tolerance and immunity to nonself-antigens. The upregulation of zonulin alters intestinal barrier function and may lead to immune-mediated diseases such as MS, ankylosing spondylitis, IgA nephropathy, nonalcoholic steatohepatitis (NASH), Crohn's disease, and CD.[34] Altered intestinal permeability appears to play a role in a number of digestive diseases, including CD, inflammatory bowel disease (IBD), and food allergy/sensitivity, and may actually precede these illnesses.[35] Inflammation in the gut may also be associated with osteoporosis, which is commonly seen in both celiac and Crohn's disease patients.[36]

Intestinal colonization with pathogenical or immunogenic microbes such as yeast, gram-negative bacteria, protozoa, and amoebas can provoke an immune response that cross-reacts with human body tissues, inducing systemic inflammatory disease as well as tissue-specific inflammation. Autoimmune conditions associated with cross-reacting antibodies include RA, myasthenia gravis, pernicious anemia, and autoimmune thyroiditis. Although CD is often thought of as a food sensitivity/allergy, it is better understood as an autoimmune disease. What sets it apart from other autoimmune diseases is that some of the genes involved, the target autoantigen, and the environmental trigger are all known. In genetically susceptible individuals, consumption of gluten triggers an immune-mediated enteropathy, marked by the production of highly disease-specific IgA and IgG autoantibodies to tissue transglutaminase. Research indicates that gliadin may increase susceptibility to type 1 diabetes.[37,38] Some evidence suggests a possible association between CD and SLE[39] as well as other systemic autoimmune diseases.[40]

Non-Celiac Gluten Sensitivity. NCGS, described in the literature in 1978,[41] is a syndrome of symptoms that occur after gluten ingestion and are relieved by gluten avoidance in individuals who do not have CD. Both CD and NCGS share many of the same symptomatic manifestations but do not share positive biopsies or CD antibodies (Table 41.3).[42]

Diagnosis of NCGS is primarily done by elimination/challenge testing with gluten-containing foods. Elevated antigliadin IgG levels can be diagnostic but are only found to be positive in less than 60% of all NCGS individuals.[43]

Celiac Disease. The prevalence of CD has been found to be significantly greater than previously estimated, affecting up to 1% of the US population or roughly 3 million people.[44] However, several studies have shown that most cases of CD remain undiagnosed. A report from the UK estimated that only one out of every nine cases of CD has been diagnosed (i.e., eight out of nine

TABLE 41.3 Comparison of Symptomatic (Nondisease) Manifestations of Wheat Allergy, Nonceliac Gluten Sensitivity, and Celiac Disease

System	Symptoms	Wheat Sensitivity (non-IgE)	NCGS	CD
Gastrointestinal	Abdominal Pain		X	X
	Constipation	(Alternating with diarrhea)	X	X
	Diarrhea	X	X	X
	Nausea		X	
	Vomiting		X	
Neurological	Ataxia			X
	Brain fog	X	X	X
	Dizziness	X		
	Fatigue	X	X	X
	Headache	X		X
	Musculoskeletal pain		X	X
	Paresthesias		X	X
	Psychiatric		X	X
Misc	Asthma	X		
	Rhinitis/sinusitis	X		
	Rash/pruritus	X	X	
	Dermatitis herpetiformis			X
	Weight loss		X	X

remain undiagnosed),[45] and a study of the prevalence of CD in the United States showed 82% of individuals were unaware they had CD at the time of diagnosis. The absence of CD is not synonymous with the absence of a gliadin reaction. Symptoms most commonly appear during the first 3 years of life, after cereals are introduced into the diet. A second peak incidence occurs during the third decade. Although CD is often thought of as a disease diagnosed early in life, more diagnoses are made in adulthood than childhood. It is not unusual for individuals to experience symptoms for 4.5 to 9 years before a confirmed diagnosis. Studies suggest that, in some patients diagnosed with IBS, CD may be the underlying cause, with an odds ratio (OR) of ~4.0 for those with IBS.[46,47,48] A screening of more than 13,000 individuals found that those with digestive complaints such as constipation, diarrhea, and/or abdominal pain had a 1:56 chance of having CD, a risk increase of more than twofold that of the general population.[49]

CD is associated with an increased risk for other digestive disturbances, such as pancreatic insufficiency, lactose intolerance,[50] and increased intestinal permeability.[51] Research has shown an increased incidence of hypo- and achlorhydria in both dermatitis herpetiformis and CD, but no correlation was demonstrated between atrophic gastritis or achlorhydria and small-intestinal villous atrophy.[52] Pancreatic exocrine insufficiency is common in CD, and supplementation with pancreatic enzymes is very effective in reducing symptoms (19/20 with persistent diarrhea experienced improvement).[53] The fact that CD can develop later in adult life provides further support for the importance of effective digestion. As people age, their production of hydrochloric acid and pancreatic digestive enzymes decreases, thus increasing the amount of gliadin exposed to enterocytes.

Type 1 Diabetes. The effects of gut inflammation associated with altered permeability are not restricted to the digestive system. For example, animal models of type 1 diabetes have shown that intestinal permeability, with resultant inflammation, plays a role in the autoimmune destruction of pancreatic islet cells. There appears to be a link between antibodies to Glo-3a (a wheat-related protein), zonulin upregulation, and islet cell autoimmunity in children at increased risk for type 1 diabetes.[54] In individuals who went on to develop type 1 diabetes, elevated serum zonulin was detected in 70% of subjects during the pretype 1 diabetes phase and preceded the onset of disease by 3.5 ± 0.9 years.[55] Increased lactulose permeability (with normal mannitol) appears to precede the detectable clinical onset of disease, suggesting that the small intestine participates in the pathogenesis of the disease. Composition of the gut microbiota combined with gluten intake affects intestinal integrity, which affects the development of diabetes (Fig. 41.5).[56]

Other. Circulating zonulin concentration is associated with obesity and insulin resistance, and has been shown to increase with BMI, waist-to-hip ratio, fasting insulin, fasting triglycerides, and uric acid.[57] In obese individuals, plasma zonulin, but not HP level, was proportional to the total bacteria count in feces,

suggesting that zonulin may be the maker of gut mucosa inflammation.[58]

Zonulin is also associated with the development and/ or progression of chronic inflammatory lung and neurological disease. Blockade of zonulin reduces the severity of acute lung injury by reducing capillary leak, diminishing accumulation of polymorphonuclear leukocytes (PMNs) in the interstitial and alveolar components and attenuating levels of proinflammatory mediators.[59] There is some evidence that the expression of zonulin correlates with the aggressiveness of gliomas and may indicate the degree of disturbance of the blood-brain barrier and blood vessel

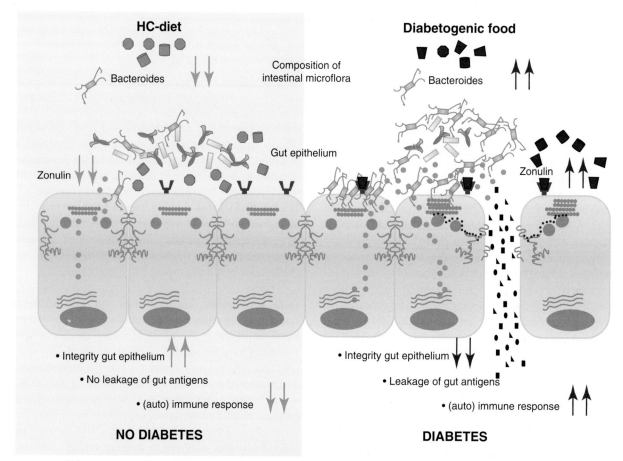

FIG. 41.5 Diet affects the composition of the intestinal microflora, and gluten interaction influences diabetes development. (From Visser, J., Rozing, J., Sapone, A., Lammers K, & Fasano A. [2009]. Tight junctions, intestinal permeability, and autoimmunity: Celiac disease and type 1 diabetes paradigms. *Annals of the New York Academy of Sciences, 1165*, 195–205.)

TABLE 41.4 Major Diseases Associated With Zonulin

Autoimmune Diseases	• Ankylosing spondylitis • Asthma • Celiac disease • Inflammatory bowel disease • Multiple sclerosis • Rheumatoid arthritis • Systemic lupus erythematosus • Type 1 diabetes
Diseases of the Nervous System	• Chronic inflammatory demyelinating polyneuropathy • Schizophrenia
Cancers	• Brain cancer • Breast cancer • Glioma • Lung adenocarcinoma • Ovarian cancer • Pancreatic cancer

walls.[60] Table 41.4 provides a summary of conditions associated with zonulin.

INTERVENTION

Complete gluten-avoidance remains the mainstay of treatment. Most celiac-related symptoms resolve with this approach, although some degree of increased gut permeability may remain. Additionally, at least temporary avoidance of lactose is often helpful, given the relative lactase deficiency that often accompanies the gluten-induced enteropathy.[61] Species falling in the genus *Triticum* are almost certain to be harmful to gliadin-sensitive patients. Although the hybridization of wheat to higher concentrations of gluten has clearly aggravated the problem, this does not mean that so called "ancient" wheats are safe for those who react to gliadin. *Triticum spelta* (spelt or spelta), *Triticum polonicum* (Polish wheat or kamut), and *Triticum monococcum* (einkorn or small spelt) still contain gliadin and must also be avoided. They may be acceptable in modest dosages for those who are wheat intolerant but do not react immunologically.

As the reaction to gliadin is based on specific peptide sequences, it seems logical to assume other foods may have similar sequences.[62] For example, several studies have found a high incidence of reaction to dairy products, especially casein, in celiac patients.[63] Fig. 41.6 shows the cross reactivity of affinity-purified α-gliadin 33-mer polyclonal antibodies to gliadin with other food antigens.[64]

The clinician must consider the nongliadin proteins in wheat that can also be allergenic. For example, alpha-amylase has been documented as a second route of allergic sensitization.[65] Alpha-amylase inhibitors are also found in rice, which might explain the reason avoidance of all grains helps those who have developed immunological reactions to gliadin, as antibodies to other wheat constituents at the same time would seem likely. Although oats, rice, and corn do not have gliadin, clinical experience has shown that celiac patients still suffering symptoms have improved when these other grass-family grains are also removed. It is unclear if this is a result of cross-contamination from storage and processing in facilities that have been used for wheat, or a result of antibodies to other amino acid sequences.

Even while on a GFD, stores of several nutrients are known to be lacking. A double-blind trial of celiac patients showed that a combination of folic acid (0.8 mg), B6 (3 mg), and B12 (0.5 mg) lowered homocysteine as well as improved anxiety and depressed mood, compared with placebo.[66] Other potential nutritional deficiencies include iron, zinc, calcium, copper, fat-soluble vitamins, and dietary fiber.[67,68]

Celiac patients should be assessed and treated for pancreatic insufficiency. Low fecal elastase-1, a marker for pancreatic insufficiency, is common among individuals with CD. Even when following a GFD, celiac patients with chronic diarrhea are likely to have low fecal elastase—another indication of pancreatic insufficiency.[69] Proteolytic enzyme replacement may provide benefit for these patients.

Although genetics is clearly the most dominant factor in gliadin susceptibility, breastfed babies have a decreased risk of developing CD.[70,71] This protection is more complete when infants continue to be breastfed after dietary gluten is introduced. Most likely this strategy is only effective in those who are not HP2-2. The risk of CD is greater when gluten is introduced in the diet in large amounts than when introduced in small or medium amounts. Early introduction of cow's milk also increases risk of CD.[72] One cell culture study found that several different *Bifidobacterium* strains counteract the inflammatory effects of gliadin-derived peptides in intestinal epithelial cells by decreasing its activation of enterocytes.[73]

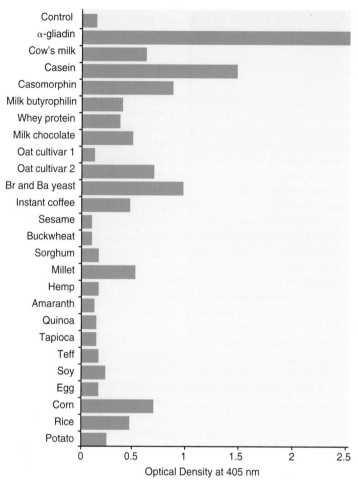

FIG. 41.6 Cross-reactivity of antigliadin antibodies with other food antigens. *Ba yeast,* Baker's yeast; *Br yeast,* brewer's yeast. (Modified from Vojdani, A., & Tarash, I. [2013]. Cross-reaction between gliadin and different food and tissue antigens. *Food and Nutrition Sciences, 4*[1], 20–32.)

Commensal bacteria have a very significant effect on intestinal integrity. A nonspecific strain of *Bifidobacterium lactis* prevented and reduced cellular damage to epithelial cells from gliadin and prevented increased intestinal permeability. The authors speculated that it might be due to protease activity in the bifidobacteria that can break down the gliadin proteins.[74] The specific probiotic *Bifidobacterium longum* (BB536) culture has been found to prevent damage to intestinal cells and to increase production of tight junction cell proteins, improving intestinal integrity. In a trial of patients with ulcerative colitis (UC), BB536 was shown not only to induce remission but also upregulate gene expression of tight junction

molecules (claudin-1 and zonula occludens-1) known to be key to selective permeability.[75] In a laboratory setting, *B. longum* IATA ES1 successfully hydrolyzed gliadin proteins, producing peptides that were typically of far lower molecular mass (around 2500 Daltons instead of 30,000 Daltons). Bifidobacteria also prevented inflammation of intestinal cells from gliadin. The cultures with bifidobacteria produced approximately 20% less NFκβ, about 40% less TNF-α, and 100% less IL-1β.[76] NFκβ is the main trigger for inflammation and is aided in proinflammation by both TNF-α and IL-1β. The fact that bifidobacteria downregulate all three proinflammatory compounds shows the power of this probiotic to reverse inflammation. Another study with *B. longum* CECT 7347 showed that this strain was also able to alleviate the toxic reactions of gliadin to the intestinal lining.[77]

The combination of prebiotics and probiotics (synbiotic therapy) has been shown to help UC patients achieve greater improvement in quality of life and inflammatory markers than either therapy alone.[78] A double-blind randomized clinical trial demonstrated that the use of probiotics reduced the rate of postoperative septicemia through reductions in serum zonulin concentration in patients undergoing colectomy for colorectal cancer.[79]

Other nutrients have also been shown to stimulate regeneration of intestinal mucosa. L-glutamine, which has long been recognized as the primary amino acid source for intestinal cells, has been shown to regulate intercellular junction integrity.[80] N-acetyl glucosamine (NAG) provides a substrate for the glycosaminoglycans that are normally broken down in a leaky gut and has shown benefit in children with IBD.[81] Zinc deficiency has been shown to disrupt tight junctions, alter membrane permeability, impair immune function, and cause intestinal ulceration.[82] Antioxidants, including vitamin C, vitamin E, beta-carotene, grape seed extract, and milk thistle extract, protect the GI system from oxidant damage and help with hepatic detoxification of compounds associated with intestinal dysfunction. Quercetin appears to be critical to intestinal integrity. In addition to quercetin's antioxidant and antiinflammatory benefits, it is involved in the assembly of several tight junction proteins (zonula occludens [ZO]-2, occludin, claudin-1, and claudin-4).[83,84] Quercetin also helps stabilize mast cells, which are important regulators of intestinal function and tight junction integrity.[85]

The discovery of the zonulin pathway enables an opportunity for both diagnostic and therapeutic applications to be developed. The strategy to facilitate repair of the damaged intestinal mucosa involves three steps: 1) stop the damage by avoiding known GI toxins; 2) reestablish a healthy microbial flora; and 3) stimulate regeneration. In addition, reestablishing the zonulin-dependent intestinal barrier function may provide a mechanism by which processes such as autoimmune disease, inflammatory conditions, and neoplastic disorders may be halted in their development and possibly reversed.[86]

There is promising evidence supporting the use of the zonulin inhibitor AT1001 in the prevention of autoimmune diseases such as type 1 diabetes and CD. Pretreatment with AT1001 has been shown to prevent the loss of intestinal barrier function, the appearance of autoantibodies, and the onset of disease. It has also been shown to protect against the insult of pancreatic islets and therefore of the insulitis responsible for the onset of type 1 diabetes.[87] The protective effects of AT1001 were also demonstrated in a small study of 20 patients on a GFD randomized to a 3-day AT1001 treatment (12 mg once daily) or placebo with a 2.5 g oral gluten challenge on the second day.[88] In the placebo group, a significant 70% increase in intestinal permeability was observed after the gluten challenge, compared with no changes in permeability in the AT1001-treated group. In addition, AT1001 has been shown to reduce proinflammatory cytokine production and GI symptoms in CD patients exposed to gluten.[89]

REFERENCES

1. Jones, David (2006). *The textbook of functional medicine.* Copyright, Gig Harbor, WA: The Institute for Functional Medicine. Quote in Chapter 28, Thomas Sult.
2. Fasano, A. (2000). Regulation of intercellular tight junctions by zonula occludens toxin and its eukaryotic analogue zonulin. *Annals of the New York Academy of Sciences, 915,* 214–222. PubMed PMID: 11193578.
3. Mowat, A. M. (2003). Coeliac disease –a meeting point for genetics, immunology, and protein chemistry. *Lancet, 361*(9365), 1290–1292. PubMed PMID: 12699968.
4. Wang, W., Uzzau, S., Goldblum, S. E., & Fasano, A. (2000). Human zonulin, a potential modulator of intestinal tight junctions. *Journal of Cell Science, 113*(Pt. 24), 4435–4440. PubMed PMID: 11082037.
5. van den Broeck, H. C., de Jong, H. C., Salentijn, E. M., Dekking, L., Bosch, D., Hamer, R. J., Gilissen, L. J. W. J., van der Meer, I. M., Smulders, M. J. M. (2010). Presence of celiac disease epitopes in modern and old hexaploid wheat varieties: Wheat breeding may have contributed to increased prevalence of celiac disease. *TAG. Theoretical and Applied Genetics. Theoretische und angewandte Genetik, 121*(8), 1527–1539. PubMed PMID: 20664999.
6. Groschwitz, K. R., & Hogan, S. P. (2009). Intestinal barrier function: Molecular regulation and disease pathogenesis. *The Journal of Allergy and Clinical Immunology, 124*(1), 3–20. PubMed PMID: 19560575.
7. El Asmar, R., Panigrahi, P., Bamford, P., Berti, I., Not, T., Coppa, G. V., Catassi, C., Fasano, A. (2002). Host-dependent zonulin secretion causes the impairment of the small intestine barrier function after

bacterial exposure. *Gastroenterol, 123*(5), 1607–1615. PubMed PMID: 12404235.

8. Dalla Pellegrina, C., Perbellini, O., Scupoli, M. T., Tomelleri, C., Zanetti, C., Zoccatelli, G., Fusi, M., Peruffo, A., Rizzi, C., Chignola, R. (2009). Effects of wheat germ agglutinin on human gastrointestinal epithelium: Insights from an experimental model of immune/epithelial cell interaction. *Toxicology and Applied Pharmacology, 237*(2), 146–153. PubMed PMID: 19332085.

9. Schneeberger, E. E., & Lynch, R. D. (2004). The tight junction: A multifunctional complex. *American Journal of Physiology. Cell Physiology, 286*(6), C1213–C1228. PubMed PMID: 15151915.

10. Kasarda, D. D. (2001). *Grains in relation to celiac (coeliac) disease. Cereal Foods World, 46*, 209–210. U.S.: Department of Agriculture, Agricultural Research Service. http://wheat.pw.usda.gov/ggpages/topics/celiac.html. (Accessed 17 June 2013).

11. Drago, S., El Asmar, R., Di Pierro, M., Grazia Clemente, M., Tripathi, A., Sapone, A., Thakar, M., Iacono, G., Carroccio, A., D'Agate, C., Not, T., Zampini, L., Catassi, C., Fasano, A. (2006). Gliadin, zonulin and gut permeability: Effects on celiac and non-celiac intestinal mucosa and intestinal cell lines. *Scandinavian Journal of Gastroenterology, 41*(4), 408–419. PubMed PMID: 16635908.

12. Lammers, K. M., Lu, R., Brownley, J., Lu, B., Gerard, C., Thomas, K., Rallabhandi, P., Shea-Donohue, T., Tamiz, A., Alkan, S., Netzel-Arnett, S., Antalis, T., Vogel, S. N., Fasano, A. (2008). Gliadin induces an increase in intestinal permeability and zonulin release by binding to the chemokine receptor CXCR3. *Gastroenterology, 135*(1), 194–204. PubMed PMID: 18485912.

13. Tripathi, A., Lammers, K. M., Goldblum, S., Shea-Donohue, T., Netzel-Arnett, S., Buzza, M. S., Antalis, T. M., Vogel, S. N., Zhao, A., Yang, S., Arrietta, M. C., Meddings, J. B., Fasano, A. (2009). Identification of human zonulin, a physiological modulator of tight junctions, as prehaptoglobin-2. *Proceedings of the National Academy of Sciences of the United States of America, 106*(39), 16799–16804. PubMed PMID: 19805376.

14. Asleh, R., Marsh, S., Shilkrut, M., Binah, O., Guetta, J., Lejbkowicz, F., Enav, B., Shehadeh, N., Kanter, Y., Lache, O., Cohen, O., Levy, N. S., Levy, A. P. (2003). Genetically determined heterogeneity in hemoglobin scavenging and susceptibility to diabetic cardiovascular disease. *Circulation Research, 92*(11), 1193–1200. PubMed PMID: 12750308.

15. Koch, W., Latz, W., Eichinger, M., Roguin, A., Levy, A. P., Schömig, A., Kastrati, A. (2002). Genotyping of the common haptoglobin Hp ½ polymorphism based on PCR. *Clinical Chemistry, 48*(9), 1377–1382. PubMed PMID: 12194911.

16. Aderem, A., & Ulevitch, R. J. (2000). Toll-like receptors in the induction of the innate immune response. *Nature, 406*(6797), 782–787. PubMed PMID: 10963608.

17. Laugerette, F. 1., Vors, C., Peretti, N., Michalski, M. C. (2011). Complex links between dietary lipids, endogenous endotoxins and metabolic inflammation. *Biochimie, 93*(1), 39–45. PubMed PMID: 20433893.

18. Suganami, T., Tanimoto-Koyama, K., Nishida, T., Itoh, M., Yuan, X., Mizuarai, S., Kotani, H., Yamaoka, S., Miyake, K., Aoe, S., Kamei, Y., Ogawa, Y. (2007). Role of the Toll-like receptor 4/NF-kappaB pathway in saturated fatty acid-induced inflammatory changes in the interaction between adipocytes and macrophages. *Arteriosclerosis, Thrombosis, and Vascular Biology, 27*(1), 84–91. PubMed PMID: 17082484.

19. Cani, P. D., Amar, J., Iglesias, M. A., Poggi, M., Knauf, C., Bastelica, D., Neyrinck, A. M., Fava, F., Tuohy, K. M., Chabo, C., Waget, A., Delmée, E., Cousin, B., Sulpice, T., Chamontin, B., Ferrières, J., Tanti, J. F., Gibson, G. R., Casteilla, L., Delzenne, N. M., Alessi, M. C., Burcelin, R. (2007). Metabolic endotoxemia initiates obesity and insulin resistance. *Diabetes, 56*(7), 1761–1772. PubMed PMID: 17456850.

20. Everard, A., & Cani, P. D. (2013). Diabetes, obesity and gut microbiota. *Best Practice & Research. Clinical Gastroenterology, 27*(1), 73–83. PubMed PMID: 23768554.

21. De Palma, G., Nadal, I., Medina, M., Donat, E., Ribes-Koninckx, C., Calabuig, M., Sanz, Y. (2010). Intestinal dysbiosis and reduced immunoglobulin-coated bacteria associated with coeliac disease in children. *BMC Microbiology, 10*, 63. PubMed PMID: 20181275.

22. Nadal, I., Donat, E., Ribes-Koninckx, C., Calabuig, M., & Sanz, Y. (2007). Imbalance in the composition of the duodenal microbiota of children with coeliac disease. *Journal of Medical Microbiology, 56*(Pt. 12), 1669–1674. PubMed PMID:18033837.

23. Sanz, Y. (2010). Effects of a gluten-free diet on gut microbiota and immune function in healthy adult humans. *Gut Microbes, 1*(3), 135–137. PubMed PMID: 21327021.

24. United States Department of Agriculture (USDA) Economic Resource Service. (2016). *Wheat's role in the U.S. diet.* Retrieved October 28, 2016, from www.ers.usda.gov/topics/crops/wheat/wheats-role-in-the-us-diet.aspx.

25. Mikesh, L. M., Crowe, S. E., Bullock, G. C., Taylor, N. E., Bruns, D. E. (2008). Celiac disease

refractory to a gluten-free diet? *Clinical Chemistry*, *54*(2), 441–444. PubMed PMID: 18223137.

26. Hill, I. D. (2005). What are the sensitivity and specificity of serologic tests for celiac disease? Do sensitivity and specificity vary in different populations? *Gastroenterology*, *128*(4 Suppl. 1), S25–S32. PubMed PMID: 15825123.

27. Hadithi, M., von Blomberg, B. M., Crusius, J. B., Bloemena, E., Kostense, P. J., Meijer, J. W., Mulder, C. J., Stehouwer, C. D., Peña, A. S. (2007). Accuracy of serologic tests and HLA-DQ typing for diagnosing celiac disease. *Annals of Internal Medicine*, *147*(5), 294–302. PubMed PMID: 17785484.

28. Comino, I., Real, A., Vivas, S., Síglez, M. Á., Caminero, A., Nistal, E., Casqueiro, J., Rodríguez-Herrera, A., Cebolla, A., Sousa, C. (2012). Monitoring of gluten-free diet compliance in celiac patients by assessment of gliadin 33-mer equivalent epitopes in feces. *The American Journal of Clinical Nutrition*, *95*(3), 670–677. PubMed PMID: 22258271.

29. Moreno, M. L., Cebolla, A., Munoz-Suano, A., Carrillo-Carrion, C., Comino, I., Pizarro, Á., León, F., Rodríguez-Herrera, A., Sousa, C. (2017). Detection of gluten immunogenic peptides in the urine of patients with coeliac disease reveals transgressions in the gluten-free diet and incomplete mucosal healing. *Gut*, *66*(2), 250–257. PubMed PMID: 26608460.

30. Ventura, M. T., Polimeno, L., & Amoruso, A. C. (2006). Intestinal permeability in patients with adverse reactions to food. *Digestive and Liver Disease*, *38*(10), 732–736. PubMed PMID: 16880015.

31. Dastych, M., Dastych, M., Jr., Novotná, H., Cíhalová, J. (2008). Lactulose/mannitol test and specificity, sensitivity, and area under curve of intestinal permeability parameters in patients with liver cirrhosis and Crohn's disease. *Digestive Diseases and Sciences*, *53*(10), 2789–2792. PubMed PMID: 18320320.

32. Hopper, A. D., Hadjivassiliou, M., Butt, S., Sanders, D. S. (2007). Adult coeliac disease. *BMJ (Clinical Research Ed.)*, *335*(7619), 558–562. PubMed PMID: 17855325.

33. Harrison, M. S., Wehbi, M., & Obideen, K. (2007). Celiac disease: More common than you think. *Cleveland Clinic Journal of Medicine*, *74*(3), 209–215. PubMed PMID: 17375801.

34. Fasano, A., & Shea-Donohue, T. (2005). Mechanisms of disease: The role of intestinal barrier function in the pathogenesis of gastrointestinal autoimmune diseases. *Nature Clinical Practice. Gastroenterology and Hepatology*, *2*(9), 416–422. PubMed PMID: 16265432.

35. Meddings, J. (2008). The significance of the gut barrier in disease. *Gut*, *57*(4), 438–440. PubMed PMID: 18334657.

36. Tilg, H., Moschen, A. R., & Kaser, A. (2008). Gut, inflammation and osteoporosis: Basic and clinical concepts. *Gut*, *57*(5), 684–694. PubMed PMID: 18408105.

37. Krause, I., Anaya, J. M., Fraser, A., Barzilai, O., Ram, M., Abad, V., Arango, A., García, J., Shoenfeld, Y. (2009). Anti-infectious antibodies and autoimmune-associated autoantibodies in patients with type I diabetes mellitus and their close family members. *Annals of the New York Academy of Sciences*, *1173*, 633–639. PubMed PMID: 19758209.

38. Joshi, A. S., Varthakavi, P. K., Bhagwat, N. M., Chadha, M. D., Mittal, S. S. (2014). Coeliac autoimmunity in type I diabetes mellitus. *Arab Journal of Gastroenterology*, *15*(2), 53–57. PubMed PMID: 25097046.

39. Dahan, S., Shor, D. B., Comanesther, D., Tekes-Manova, D., Shovman, O., Amital, H., Cohen, A. D. (2016). All disease begins in the gut: Celiac disease co-existence with SLE. *Autoimmunity Reviews*, *15*(8), 848–853. PubMed PMID: 27295421.

40. Fasano, A. (2006). Systemic autoimmune disorders in celiac disease. *Current Opinion in Gastroenterology*, *22*(6), 674–679. PubMed PMID: 17053448.

41. Ellis, A., & Linaker, B. D. (1978). Non-coeliac gluten sensitivity? *Lancet*, *1*, 1358–1359. PubMed PMID: 78118.

42. Lundin, K., & Alaedini, A. (2012). Non-celiac gluten sensitivity. *Gastrointestinal Endoscopy Clinics of North America*, *22*, 723–734. PubMed PMID: 23083989.

43. Watkins, R. D., & Zawahir, S. (2017). Celiac disease and nonceliac gluten sensitivity. *Pediatric Clinics of North America*, *64*, 563–576. PubMed PMID: 28502438.

44. Rubio-Tapia, A., Ludvigsson, J. F., Brantner, T. L., Murray, J. A., Everhart, J. E. (2012). The prevalence of celiac disease in the United States. *The American Journal of Gastroenterology*, *107*(10), 1538–1544. PubMed PMID: 22850429.

45. Van Heel, D. A., & West, J. (2006). Recent advances in coeliac disease. *Gut*, *55*(7), 1037–1046. PubMed PMID: 16766754.

46. Card, T. R., Siffledeen, J., West, J., & Fleming, K. M. (2013). An excess of prior irritable bowel syndrome diagnoses or treatments in celiac disease: Evidence of diagnostic delay. *Scandinavian Journal of Gastroenterology*, *48*(7), 801–807. PubMed PMID: 23697749.

47. Cristofori, F., Fontana, C., Magista, A., Capriati, T., Indrio, F., Castellaneta, S., Cavallo, L., Francavilla, R. (2014). Increased prevalence of celiac disease among pediatric patients with irritable bowel syndrome: A 6-year prospective cohort study. *JAMA Pediatrics*, *168*(6), 555–560. PubMed PMID: 24756157.

48. Ford, A. C., Chey, W. D., Talley, N. J., Malhotra, A., Spiegel, B. M., Moayyedi, P. (2009). Yield of diagnostic tests for celiac disease in individuals with symptoms suggestive of irritable bowel syndrome: Systematic review and meta-analysis. *Archives of Internal Medicine*, *169*(7), 651–658. PubMed PMID: 19364994.

49. Fasano, A., Berti, I., Gerarduzzi, T., Gerarduzzi, T., Not, T., Colletti, R. B., Drago, S., Elitsur, Y., Green, P. H., Hill, I. D., Pietzak, M., Ventura, A., Thorpe, M., Kryszak, D., Fornaroli, F., Wasserman, S. S., Murray, J. A., Horvath, K. (2003). Prevalence of celiac disease in at-risk and not-at-risk groups in the Unites States: A large multicenter study. *Archives of Internal Medicine*, *163*(3), 286–292. PubMed PMID: 12578508.

50. Ojetti, V., Nucera, G., Migneco, A., Gabrielli, M., Lauritano, C., Danese, S., Zocco, M. A., Nista, E. C., Cammarota, G., De Lorenzo, A., Gasbarrini, G., Gasbarrini, A. (2005). High prevalence of celiac disease in patients with lactose intolerance. *Digestion*, *71*(2), 106–110. PubMed PMID: 15775678.

51. Vilela, E. G., Torres, H. O., Ferrari, M. L., Lima, A. S., Cunha, A. S. (2008). Gut permeability to lactulose and mannitol differs in treated Crohn's disease and celiac disease patients and healthy subjects. *Brazilian Journal of Medical and Biological Research = Revista brasileira de pesquisas medicas e biologicas*, *41*(12), 1105–1109. PubMed PMID: 19148373.

52. Gillberg, R., Kastrup, W., Mobacken, H., Stockbrügger, R., Ahren, C. (1985). Gastric morphology and function in dermatitis herpetiformis and in coeliac disease. *Scandinavian Journal of Gastroenterology*, *20*(2), 133–140. PubMed PMID: 3992169.

53. Evans, K. E., Leeds, J. S., Morley, S., & Sanders, D. S. (2010). Pancreatic insufficiency in adult celiac disease: Do patients require long-term enzyme supplementation? *Digestive Diseases and Sciences*, *55*(10), 2999–3004. PubMed PMID: 20458623.

54. Simpson, M., Mojibian, M., Barriga, K., Scott, F. W., Fasano, A., Rewers, M., Norris, J. M. (2009). An exploration of Glo-3a antibody levels in children at increased risk for type 1 diabetes mellitus. *Pediatric Diabetes*, *10*(8), 563–572. PubMed PMID: 19622083.

55. Sapone, A., de Magistris, L., Pietzak, M., Clemente, M. G., Tripathi, A., Cucca, F., Lampis, R., Kryszak, D., Carteni, M., Generoso, M., Iafusco, D., Prisco, F., Laghi, F., Riegler, G., Carratu, R., Counts, D., Fasano, A. (2006). Zonulin upregulation is associated with increased gut permeability in subjects with type 1 diabetes and their relatives. *Diabetes*, *55*(5), 1443–1449. PubMed PMID: 16644703.

56. Visser, J., Rozing, J., Sapone, A., Lammers, K., Fasano, A. (2009). Tight junctions, intestinal permeability, and autoimmunity: Celiac disease and type 1 diabetes paradigms. *Annals of the New York Academy of Sciences*, *1165*, 195–205. PubMed PMID: 19538307.

57. Moreno-Navarette, J. M., Sabater, M., Ortega, F., Ricart, W., & Fernandez-Real, J. M. (2012). Circulating zonulin, a marker of intestinal permeability, is increased in association with obesity-associated insulin resistance. *PLoS ONE*, *7*(5), e37160. PubMed PMID: 22629362.

58. Zak-Golab, A., Kocelak, P., Aptekorz, M., Zientara, M., Juszczyk, L., Martirosian, G., Chudek, J., Olszanecka-Glinianowicz, M. (2013). Gut microbiota, microinflammation, metabolic profile, and zonulin concentration in obese and normal weight subjects. *International Journal of Endocrinology*, *2013*, 674106. PubMed PMID: 23970898.

59. Rittirsch, D., Flierl, M. A., Nadeau, B. A., Day, D. E., Huber-Lang, M. S., Grailer, J. J., Zetoune, F. S., Andjelkovic, A. V., Fasano, A., Ward, P. A. (2013). Zonulin as prehaptoglobin2 regulates lung permeability and activates the complement system. *American Journal of Physiology. Lung Cellular and Molecular Physiology*, *304*(12), L863–L872. PubMed PMID: 23564505.

60. Skardelly, M., Armbruster, F. P., Meixensberger, J., & Hilbig, H. (2009). Expression of zonulin, c-kit, and glial fibrillary acidic protein in human gliomas. *Translational Oncology*, *2*(3), 117–120. PubMed PMID: 19701495.

61. Ojetti, V., Gabrielli, M., Migneco, A., Lauritano, C., Zocco, M. A., Scarpellini, E., Nista, E. C., Gasbarrini, G., Gasbarrini, A. (2008). Regression of lactose malabsorption in coeliac patients after receiving a gluten-free diet. *Scandinavian Journal of Gastroenterology*, *43*(2), 174–177. PubMed PMID: 17917999.

62. Darewicz, M., Dziuba, J., & Minkiewicz, P. (2007). Computational characterization and identification of peptides for in silico detection of potentially coeliac-toxic proteins. *Food Science and Technology International*, *13*(2), 125–133.

63. Kristjansson, G., Venge, P., & Hallgren, R. (2007). Mucosal reactivity to cow's milk protein in coeliac disease. *Clinical and Experimental Immunology*, *147*(3), 449–455. PubMed PMID: 17302893.

64. Vojdani, A., & Tarash, I. (2013). Cross-reaction between gliadin and different food and tissue antigens. *Food Science & Nutrition*, *4*(1), 20–32.

65. James, J. M., Sixbey, J. P., Helm, R. M., annon, G. A., Burks, A. W. (1997). Wheat alpha-amylase inhibitor: A second route of allergic sensitization. *The Journal of Allergy and Clinical Immunology*, *99*(2), 239–244. PubMed PMID: 9042052.

66. Hallert, C., Svensson, M., Tholstrup, J., Hultberg, B. (2009). Clinical trial: B Vitamins improve health in

coeliac patients living on a gluten-free diet. *Alimentary Pharmacology and Therapeutics, 29*(8), 811–816. PubMed PMID: 19154566.

67. Henri-Bhargava, A., Melmed, C., Glikstein, R., Schipper, H. M. (2008). Neurologic impairment due to vitamin E and copper deficiencies in celiac disease. *Neurology, 71*(11), 860–861. PubMed PMID: 18779515.

68. Kupper, C. (2005). Dietary guidelines and implementation for celiac disease. *Gastroenterology, 128*(4 Suppl. 1), S121–S127. PubMed PMID: 15825119.

69. Leeds, J. S., Hopper, A. D., Hurlstone, D. P., Edwards, S. J., McAlindon, M. E., Lobo, A. J., Donnelly, M. T., Morley, S., Sanders, D. S. (2007). Is exocrine pancreatic insufficiency in adult coeliac disease a cause of persisting symptoms? *Alimentary Pharmacology and Therapeutics, 25*(3), 265–271. PubMed PMID: 17269988.

70. Persson, L. A., Ivarsson, A., & Hernell, O. (2002). Breast-feeding protects against celiac disease in childhood—epidemiological evidence. *Advances in Experimental Medicine and Biology, 503*, 115–123. PubMed PMID: 12026010.

71. Ivarsson, A., Hernell, O., Stenlund, H., Persson, L. A. (2002). Breast-feeding protects against celiac disease. *The American Journal of Clinical Nutrition, 75*(5), 914–921. PubMed PMID: 11976167.

72. Faellstroem, S. P., Winberg, J., & Andersen, H. J. (1965). Cow's milk induced malabsorption as a precursor of gluten intolerance. *Acta Paediatrica Scandinavica, 54*, 101–115. PubMed PMID: 14334544.

73. Laparra, J. M., & Sanz, Y. (2010). Bifidobacteria inhibit the inflammatory response induced by gliadins in intestinal epithelial cells via modifications of toxic peptide generation during digestion. *Journal of Cellular Biochemistry, 109*(4), 801–807. PubMed PMID: 20052669.

74. Lindfors, K., Blomqvist, T., Juuti-Uusitalo, K., Stenman, S., Venäläinen, J., Mäki, M., Kaukinen, K. (2008). Live probiotic Bifidobacterium lactis bacteria inhibit the toxic effects induced by wheat gliadin in epithelial cell culture. *Clinical and Experimental Immunology, 152*(3), 552–558. PubMed PMID: 18422736.

75. Takeda, Y., Nakase, H., Namba, K., Inoue, S., Ueno, S., Uza, N., Chiba, T. (2009). Upregulation of T-bet and tight junction molecules by Bifidobacterium longum improves colonic inflammation of ulcerative colitis. *Inflammatory Bowel Diseases, 15*(11), 1617–1618. PubMed PMID: 19161180.

76. Laparra, J. M., & Sanz, Y. (2010). Bifidobacteria inhibit the inflammatory response induced by gliadins in intestinal epithelial cells via modifications of toxic

peptide generation during digestion. *Journal of Cellular Biochemistry, 109*(4), 801–807. PMID: 20052669.

77. Olivares, M., Laparra, M., & Sanz, Y. (2012). Oral administration of Bifidobacterium longum CECT 7347 modulates jejunal proteome in an in vivo gliadin-induced enteropathy animal model. *Journal of Proteomics, 77*, 310–320. PubMed PMID: 23023000.

78. Fujimori, S., Gudis, K., Mitsui, K., Seo, T., Yonezawa, M., Tanaka, S., Tatsuguchi, A., Sakamoto, C. (2009). A randomized controlled trial on the efficacy of synbiotic versus probiotic or prebiotic treatment to improve the quality of life in patients with ulcerative colitis. *Nutrition, 25*(5), 520–525. PubMed PMID: 19201576.

79. Liu, Z. H., Huang, M. J., Zhang, X. W., Wang, L., Huang, N. Q., Peng, H., Lan, P., Peng, J. S., Yang, Z., Xia, Y., Liu, W. J., Yang, J., Qin, H. L., Wang, J. P. (2013). The effects of perioperative probiotic treatment on serum zonulin concentration and subsequent postoperative infectious complications after colorectal cancer surgery: A double-center and double-blind randomized clinical trial. *The American Journal of Clinical Nutrition, 97*(1), 117–126. PubMed PMID: 23235200.

80. Li, N., & Neu, J. (2009). Glutamine deprivation alters intestinal tight junctions via a PI3-K/Akt mediated pathway in Caco-2 cells. *The Journal of Nutrition, 139*(4), 710–714. PubMed PMID: 19211824.

81. Salvatore, S., Heuschkel, R., Tomlin, S., Davies, S. E., Edwards, S., Walker-Smith, J. A., French, I., Murch, S. H. (2000). A pilot study of N-acetyl glucosamine, a nutritional substrate for glycosaminoglycan synthesis, in paediatric chronic inflammatory bowel disease. *Alimentary Pharmacology and Therapeutics, 14*(12), 1567–1579. PubMed PMID: 11121904.

82. Amasheh, M., Andres, S., Amasheh, S., Fromm, M., Schulzke, J. D. (2009). Barrier effects of nutritional factors. *Annals of the New York Academy of Sciences, 1165*, 267–273. PubMed PMID: 19538315.

83. Suzuki, T., & Hara, H. (2009). Quercetin enhances intestinal barrier function through the assembly of zonula [corrected] occludens-2, occludin, and claudin-1 and the expression of claudin-4 in Caco-2 cells. *The Journal of Nutrition, 139*(5), 965–974. PubMed PMID: 19297429.

84. Amasheh, M., Schlichter, S., Amasheh, S., Mankertz, J., Zeitz, M., Fromm, M., Schulzke, J. D. (2008). Quercetin enhances epithelial barrier function and increases claudin-4 expression in Caco-2 cells. *The Journal of Nutrition, 138*(6), 1067–1073. PubMed PMID: 18492835.

85. Bischoff, S. C., & Krämer, S. (2007). Human mast cells, bacteria, and intestinal immunity. *Immunological Reviews, 217*, 329–337. PubMed PMID: 17498069.

86. Fasano, A. (2011). Zonulin and its regulation of intestinal barrier function: The biological door to inflammation, autoimmunity, and cancer. *Physiological Reviews, 91*(1), 151–175. PubMed PMID: 21248165.

87. Watts, T., Berti, I., Sapone, A., Gerarduzzi, T., Not, T., Zielke, R., Fasano, A. (2005). Role of the intestinal tight junction modulator zonulin in the pathogenesis of type 1 diabetes in BB diabetic-prone rats. *Proceedings of the National Academy of Sciences of the United States of America, 102*(8), 2916–2921. PubMed PMID: 15710870.

88. Paterson, B. M., Lammers, K. M., Arrieta, M. C., Fasano, A., & Meddings, J. B. (2007). The safety, tolerance, pharmacokinetic and pharmacodynamic effects of single doses of AT-1001 in coeliac subjects: A proof of concept study. *Alimentary Pharmacology and Therapeutics, 26*(5), 757–766. PubMed PMID: 17697209.

89. Kelly, C. P., Green, P. H., Murray, J. A., DiMarino, A. J., Arsenescu, R. I., Colatrella, A. M., Leffler, D. A., Alexander, D. A., Jacobstein, D., Leon, F., Jiang, J., Fedorak, R. N. (2009). M2048 safety, tolerability and effects on intestinal permeability of larazotide acetate in celiac disease: Results of a phase IIB 6-week gluten-challenge clinical trial. *Gastro, 136*(5), A–474.

42

Neurotoxicity

SUMMARY

- Presence in population: Multiple neurotoxic compounds are present in all persons
- Major diseases:
  - Children: Attention deficit hyperactivity disorder (ADHD), autism spectrum disorders, IQ loss
  - Adults: Cognitive decline, dementia (including Alzheimer's disease [AD]), headache, mood disorders, motor neuron and parkinsonism disorders
- Primary sources: Indoor and outdoor air, food, personal care products
- Best measure: Direct assessment of toxicants, computerized neurocognitive/neuropsychiatric testing, balance testing, single photon emission computerized tomography (SPECT) scans
- Best intervention: Avoidance, reduction of toxic burden, reduction of oxidative damage, and reversal of neuroinflammation with Mediterranean-style diet and botanical agents

INTRODUCTION

A great number of commonly present environmental toxicants adversely affect the central and peripheral nervous systems, especially in fetuses and children. These adverse effects are a result of both direct and indirect action, result in cognitive, mood, and movement disorders, and have been linked to the major chronic neurological diseases. Initial reports of neurotoxic actions were primarily focused on pesticides, solvents, and heavy metals that possess direct neurotoxic activity and can easily cross the blood-brain barrier. More recent research has focused on the oxidative damage caused by virtually all toxic environmental compounds, with the resulting neuroinflammation that is secondary to oxidative damage.

Neurological Cell Types

The nervous system is made up of more than 100 billion neurons, along with neuroglia (astrocytes, oligodendrocytes, and microglia), ependymal, and mesenchymal cells (that make the capillaries). The neurons carry unidirectional electrical signals along the length of their cell body (axon), stimulating a release of neurotransmitter chemicals. These excitatory or inhibitory neurotransmitters inform the connecting neuron of which message to send along its length. Neurons vary in length and are insulated with a myelin sheath, allowing the impulse to travel rapidly without unintentional excitation of adjoining neurons. Although neurons often receive the most attention, their function is dependent on their glial support network, composed of astrocytes (astroglia), oligodendrocytes, and microglia.

425

For every one neuron, there can be up to 10 astrocytes that help protect them and maintain the blood-brain barrier, preventing potentially damaging substances from getting to the neuron. The astrocytes enclose the capillaries, separating the neurons from the capillary walls. They play a role in maintaining sodium, potassium, and calcium ions in the extracellular fluid at levels that allow for proper transmission of electrical signals along the body (axon) of the neuron.

Astrocytes contain the enzyme glutamine synthetase, which combines ammonia with glutamate to form glutamine, keeping elevated ammonia levels from damaging the neurons. They also take up glutamate from the synaptic gap, protecting the neural cells against excitotoxic damage. They produce brain-derived neurotrophic factor (BDNF) proteins known to promote neuronal growth or survival. They can remove methylmercury from the extracellular spaces and will produce more metallothionein to cope with the presence of mercury. Astrocytes respond to insufficient oxygen, high or low blood sugar, or toxin presence. In response to such stress, they become enlarged and "activated," a classic sign of toxic insult to the brain.

Oligodendrocytes produce layers of myelin to wrap the neurons. The number of oligodendrocytes increases with insufficient oxygen, viral infections, or other stress situations.

Microglia provide surveillance for the neurons. However, when the brain is injured through toxins, trauma, viral or bacterial infections, or stroke, these cells release cytokines that produce an inflammatory response that leads to neuronal degeneration.[1] Compounds produced by the astroglia can help mediate this inflammatory response.

It has been postulated that neurotoxin-induced effects are a result of both age- and toxin-induced damage.[2] Although toxic insult may result in neuronal death in a specific region of the brain, the other neurons that are not injured continue to carry the function of that area. As normal neuronal attrition occurs through aging, the remaining functioning cells dwindle in number until they are unable to maintain proper functioning. Fortunately, the brain does regenerate through stimulation by BDNF, albeit quite slowly at 1% per year.

BASIC MECHANISMS OF NEUROTOXICITY

Neurotoxins may selectively impair the following:
1. The propagation and transmission of electrical impulses along nerve axons

NERVOUS SYSTEM AS A TARGET

The nervous system is a unique target for toxic agents in several ways:
1. Once the neurons are killed from toxin exposure, they are not replaced. When enough cells are damaged, neurological effects are noted.
2. The blood-brain barrier does not block nonpolar substances or items that are actively transported. This allows solvents, chlorinated pesticides, and other nonpolar lipophilic compounds that are also neurotoxic entry into the neuronal environment.
3. The normal function of the nervous system requires the action of a complex integrated network of many specialized cells. Therefore damage to even a small portion of the nervous system sometimes can result in marked effects on function.
4. The neurological systems have a limited supply of antioxidant compounds, especially glutathione, that can be rapidly depleted in the presence of high levels of reactive oxygen and nitrogen molecules.
5. Because of high lipid content (one-half of which is myelin) in the brain, there is an accumulation and storage of lipophilic xenobiotics.
6. Neurons have high surface areas and therefore increased exposure to toxins.
7. Neuroinflammation is fairly easy to start and very difficult to alleviate.

2. Neurotransmitter activity
3. The maintenance of the myelin sheath, which contains about half the total lipid content of the brain
4. Cell constituents, including microtubules and mitochondria
5. Neuroglial functioning, resulting in neuroinflammation
6. Antioxidant levels and antioxidant enzyme activity
7. Production of BDNF

Direct Neurotoxicity

The Centers for Disease Control and Prevention (CDC) Fourth Report has documented chlorinated, organophosphate, and pyrethroid pesticides to be ubiquitous among US residents.[3] Organochlorine pesticides (OCP) impair the sodium channels in the neurons, preventing proper transmission of the nerve impulse. Dichlorodiphenyldichloroethylene (DDE), a metabolite of dichlorodiphenyltrichloroethane (DDT), is biologically persistent (half-life of 2–10 years) and accumulative and is found in virtually everyone but is often found in higher levels in older individuals, as can be seen in Fig. 42.1.

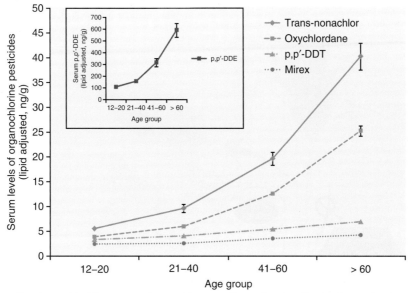

FIG. 42.1 Chlorinated POPs accumulate with age. (From Serdar, B., LeBlanc, W. G., Norris, J. M., & Dickinson, L. M. [2014]. Potential effects of polychlorinated biphenyls [PCBs] and selected organochlorine pesticides [OCPs] on immune cells and blood biochemistry measures: A cross-sectional assessment of the NHANES 2003 to 2004 data. *Environmental Health, 13,* 114.)

Chlorinated pesticides are fat soluble and are therefore readily transported across the blood-brain barrier. Pyrethroid pesticides, currently one of the most commonly used classes of insecticides, affect the neurons in the same way as the chlorinated pesticides. One pyrethroid insecticide metabolite, 3-phenoxybenzoic acid, has been found ubiquitously in the CDC report. Organophosphate pesticides interrupt transmission by inhibiting acetylcholinesterase in the synaptic clefts (Fig. 42.2). Several of their metabolites are found ubiquitously in US residents, primarily through the consumption of nonorganic fruits and vegetables.[4,5]

Solvents are fat soluble and therefore readily cross the blood-brain barrier. Once in the brain, they diminish the axonal transmission of electrical impulses along the neurons. This results in a depression of global central nervous system (CNS) functioning and was previously referred to as *chronic toxic encephalopathy*, the best example of which is alcohol-induced inebriation. Long-term solvent exposure has been associated with personality changes, memory impairment, and neurological deficits as well as chronic neurodegenerative diseases.[6]

Indirect Neurotoxicity: Oxidative Damage and Neuroinflammation

All of the environmental pollutants have demonstrated prooxidant activity, with the most toxic compounds causing the most oxidative damage. These toxicants also typically deplete the level of reduced glutathione in the brain tissue and inhibit the function of the antioxidant enzymes. Both reactive oxygen and reactive nitrogen species (ROS and RNS) can directly oxidize and damage DNA, protein, and lipids in the brain, leading to neurodegeneration. Neurons are directly affected by this oxidative stress, as are the glial cells. Oxidative stress activates the glial cells, leading to an increased production and release of the proinflammatory chemicals interleukin 1β (IL-1β), interleukin 6 and 10 (IL-6, IL-10), gamma-interferon (iFN-γ), and tumor necrosis factor alpha (TNF-α) (Fig. 42.3).

The resulting neuroinflammation is a key component in the pathobiology of headaches and chronic pain[7]; cognitive decline[8,9]; mood disorders[10]; traumatic brain injury[11]; and neurodegenerative diseases, including AD,[12] ADHD,[13] amyotrophic lateral sclerosis (ALS),[14] autism,[15]

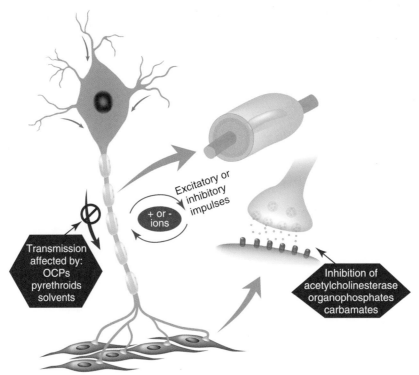

FIG. 42.2 Mechanisms of transmission disruption by solvents and pesticides.

multiple sclerosis,[16] bipolarity,[17] seizures,[18] and parkinsonism[19] (Box 42.1). Persons with neurodegenerative diseases have high levels of these same proinflammatory chemicals, including IL-1β, TNF, IL-10, IL-6, transforming growth factor β and γ-interferon.[20] Neuroinflammation has been shown to be present in parkinsonism and appears to be responsible for all the nondopamine depletion–related manifestations.[21] Activated glial cells and mast cells both appear to be responsible for the release of the proinflammatory chemical soup that fuels neuroinflammation. Glial cell activation has been implicated in the pathogenesis of epilepsy, AD and Parkinson's disease (PD), multiple sclerosis, motor neuron diseases (ALS), stroke, and mood disorders.[22] Mast cells are present in the brain and, when activated, release most of the same proinflammatory compounds as do the glial cells. Together, they start and feed the flame of neuroinflammation.[23]

Neuroinflammation is triggered by traumatic brain injury,[24] endotoxicity (circulating levels of

---

BOX 42.1   Causes and Effects of Neuroinflammation

Causes	Effects
• Traumatic brain injury	• Headaches
• Endotoxicity	• Chronic pain
• Elevated blood sugar	• Cognitive decline
• Stress	• Mood disorders
• Environmental pollutants	• Traumatic brain injury
• Vehicular exhaust	• Alzheimer's disease
• Organophosphate	• ADHD
pesticides	• ALS
• Metals	• Autism
	• Multiple sclerosis
	• Bipolarity
	• Seizures
	• Parkinsonism

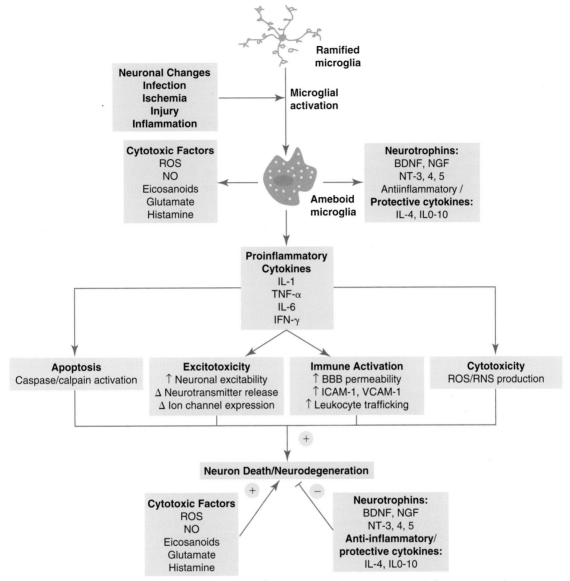

FIG. 42.3 Common mechanisms of microglial activation with resultant proinflammatory release. (From Smith, J. A., Das, A., Ray, S. K., & Banik, N. L. [2012]. Role of proinflammatory cytokines released from microglia in neurodegenerative diseases. *Brain Research Bulletin, 87*[1], 10–20.)

lipopolysaccharides),[25] elevated blood sugar (glycation end products),[26] stress,[27] and a host of environmental toxicants such as air pollutants,[28] heavy metals,[29] and organophosphate pesticides.[30] Vehicular exhaust produces particulate matter (PM) in a range of sizes, all of which carry a variety of polycyclic aromatic hydrocarbons.

DISEASE MANIFESTATION

Cognition and Executive Function Decline

- Vehicular exhaust
- Phthalates
- Organophosphate pesticides

- Heavy metals
- Polychlorinated biphenyls (PCBs)

The fear of losing cognitive function has been growing over the last decade and is approaching the same level as fear of cancer.[31] Although declining cognition has been associated with aging, it appears that our modern age may hold a great deal of blame. Based on a meta-analysis of simple reaction time measurements, it was estimated that the IQ of the general population is 14 points lower now than it was during the reign of Queen Victoria.[32] Between 1950 and 2000, the average world IQ dropped 0.86 points, with a further drop of 1.28 projected for the years 2000 to 2050.[33]

Prenatal Exposures

- Organophosphate pesticides
- Phthalates
- Methylmercury
- PCBs

Prenatal exposure to different common environmental compounds has been clearly linked to reduced cognitive function and IQ in children. Some of these compounds are nonpersistent, including organophosphate pesticides, phthalates, and air pollutants, which requires daily exposure to cause problems. *In utero* exposure to organophosphate pesticides has been associated with slower motor speed and worse motor coordination, visuospatial performance, and visual memory when the children reached the age of 6 to 8 years.[34] This translated to a developmental delay equivalent of 1.5 to 2 years. Although dietary exposure is the greatest source of organophosphates for children, the children most affected in this study were born to mothers who worked in greenhouses where organophosphates were routinely used. Maternal urinary phthalate levels in late pregnancy are associated with reduced scores on both the Mental Development Index and Psychomotor Index for their daughters by age 2 years.[35] The most significant correlations were found for maternal levels of the low-molecular-weight phthalate metabolites mono-n-butyl, mono-isobutyl, and monobenzyl—phthalates that are commonly used in nail polish and other personal care products. Maternal levels of these phthalates were also associated with a 6.7- to 7.6-point drop in IQ in their offspring by age 7 years.[36] Women with higher exposure to combustion-related air pollution, specifically polycyclic aromatic hydrocarbons, during pregnancy were three times more likely to have children with reduced verbal IQ at age 7 years.[37]

Prenatal exposure to the more persistent methylmercury during the second trimester resulted in poorer performance on the Peabody Picture Vocabulary Test and the Wide Range Assessment of Visual Motor Abilities test by the age of 3 years.[38] This was even more significant because maternal fish intake was associated with improved performance on those same tests. Methylmercury is such a potent neurotoxin that it not only negates the beneficial effect of fish oils on the developing brain; it causes a reduction in brain function as well. Children with a cord-blood mercury level of 7.5 ug/L or more were four times more likely to have an IQ score below 80.[39]

The greatest damage of PCBs to the neurological system appears to happen *in utero*, during the time of initial neurological development. Neonatal exposure of mice to PCBs results in long-term neurological problems, including diminished learning and memory function as well as spontaneous behavior that gets worse as they age[40] (Table 42.1). Several studies have looked at the effect of *in utero* exposure on humans as well and have uncovered similar problems. Children who were exposed *in utero* to PCBs from their mothers' fish consumption exhibited problems with intellectual functioning.[41]

TABLE 42.1   Neurological Problems Associated With Prenatal Exposure to Environmental Pollutants

Disease	PAH/PM	PHTH	Solvents	PCB	OCP	OP	Cd	Pb	Hg
ADHD	X	X		X					X
Autism	X	X	X	X					
Cognitive problems		X				X			X
Reduction in IQ	X	X (7 pt)		X			X		
Mood disorders	X			X					

Cd, Cadmium; *Hg*, mercury; *OCP*, organochlorine pesticides; *OP*, organophosphate pesticides; *PAH/PM*, polycyclic aromatic hydrocarbon and particulate matter; *Pb*, lead; *PCB*, polychlorinated biphenyls; *PHTH*, phthalates.

Studying mother-infant pairs in Germany revealed that *in utero* exposures to PCBs affect the mental and motor neurological development of human children.[42] Studies in Michigan, North Carolina, and Taiwan have shown that children exposed to PCBs have increased cognitive defects, poorer gross motor function, and decreased visual recognition memory.[43] By age 11 years, the Michigan children with prenatal PCB exposure continued to show greater rates of impulsivity; poorer concentration; and poorer verbal, pictorial, and auditory working memory.[44] These children also have lower IQ levels than children who were not exposed *in utero* and have increased rates of hyperactivity, with both of these problems persisting as they grow.[45,46,47] A study of Inuit preschoolers with both prenatal and postnatal PCB exposures revealed that prenatal exposure to PCB 153 was associated with increased states of unhappiness and anxiety.[48]

Prenatal exposure to PCBs have also been associated with reduced neurological function in children.[49] PCBs are even more persistent than methylmercury and are also found in high levels in some seafood, primarily sardines[50] and farmed salmon.[51] Cord blood PCB levels have also been associated with diminished attentiveness and impulse control in boys by age 8 years.[52]

As can be seen in Fig. 42.4, women who breastfeed have lower levels of PCBs. This may help explain why breastfeeding decreases the risk of breast cancer. Unfortunately, this means that breastfed infants have increased levels of PCBs.

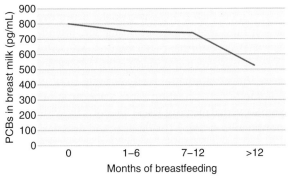

FIG. 42.4 Breastfeeding decreases the level of PCBs in women. (Data from Bjermo, H., Darnerud, P. O., Lignell, S., Pearson, M., Rantakokko, P., Nälsén, C., Enghardt Barbieri, H., Kiviranta, H., Lindroos, A. K., Glynn, A. [2013]. Fish intake and breastfeeding time are associated with serum concentrations of organochlorines in a Swedish population. *Environment International*, *51*, 88–96.)

Postnatal Exposures

- Vehicular exhaust
- Lead
- Cadmium
- Mercury
- Arsenic
- PCBs

Postnatal exposure to PM less than 2.5 μm in diameter ($PM_{2.5}$) from vehicular exhaust is the greatest threat to cognitive function for all ages. A group of Spanish researchers carefully studied the effects of a wide range of $PM_{2.5}$ sources on 2618 school children whose average age was 8.5 years.[53] The $PM_{2.5}$ readings were taken both inside and outside of their schools rather than in their homes, allowing the study to focus on the effect of classroom air quality on learning. Computerized testing for working memory and attentiveness, done at the same time as the air sampling, revealed a clear negative association between cognitive development and traffic-related $PM_{2.5}$. Children in Mexico City with no apparent risk factors for cognitive deficits living in areas with high $PM_{2.5}$ levels exhibited neuroinflammation and cognitive deficiencies,[54] confirming the role of toxicant-induced neuroinflammation in cognitive decline.[55] A study on the effects of traffic-related pollution on the cognitive function of older men (with an average age of 71 years) used black carbon (BC) as a marker for vehicular exhaust instead of $PM_{2.5}$.[56] The findings were consistent with the studies on children: the greater the exposure to vehicular exhaust (either inside or outside), the lower the scores on mental functioning. Men who had the highest levels of BC exposure had a mental decline that equaled 1.9 years of aging. A study of older women showed almost the same results, although $PM_{2.5}$ was measured instead of BC. Women between the ages of 70 and 81 with higher long-term exposure to $PM_{2.5}$ and $PM_{2.5-10}$ exhibited a cognitive decline equivalent to 2 years of aging.[57]

Although indoor and outdoor exposures to vehicular exhaust are the greatest factor in neuroinflammation and cognitive decline, the second greatest factor is toxic metals. Even though the blood lead level (BLL) is lower in the United States than it has been in decades, lead remains in the environment and is still associated with cognitive decline in children and adults.

Children's BLLs under the current CDC level of less than 5 μg/dL are still capable of causing a decline in IQ score. A 2003 article showed that children with BLLs between 1 and 10 µg/dL lost 1.37 IQ points for every 1 ug/dL of lead, while those above 10 ug/dl only lost 0.46 IQ points for each 1 ug/dL increase.[58] This resulted in a 7.4 IQ point loss in children with BLLs with a BLL of 10 µg/dL while each additional 10 ug/dL increase of BLL only increased IQ loss by 4.6 points. The IQ loss in children with BLLs below 10 µg/dL were confirmed in a subsequent study of 6-year-old children[59] and from children in seven international population studies.[60] IQ loss with BLLs above 1.71 µg/dL has also been found in a study of Italian adolescents. In this study, a doubling of the BLL equated to a 2.4-point reduction in IQ. The researchers stated that for each 0.19 µg/dL increase in BLL, one IQ point was lost.[61] In a North Carolina study, BLLs as low as 2 µg/dL were associated with poorer performance in the classroom for school-aged children.[62] Among Hispanic children in Chicago public schools with BLLs below 10 µg/dL, increasing BLL values were inversely associated with math and reading scores.[63] Children with BLLs of 0 to 4 µg/L did not exhibit math and reading problems, but children with BLLs of 5 to 9 µg/dL did. Lead-associated decline of cognitive function in children has been shown to persist into adulthood,[64] giving the current state of municipal water lead contamination the potential for significant consequences for future adults in those areas.

Cumulative lead burden in adults, measured via bone lead fluoroscopic assessment, has been associated with decreased cognition,[65] whereas current BLLs have shown no association.[66] Increasing levels of tibial lead were inversely related to impaired language, processing speed, hand-eye coordination, executive functioning, verbal memory, verbal learning, and visual memory.[67] As the tibial lead concentration rose, hand-eye coordination diminished. Women in the Nurses' Health Study also showed increased cognitive decline with increasing tibial lead levels.[68] Every increase in tibial lead of 1 standard deviation was associated with a functional decline equivalent to 0.33 years of aging. Patellar lead was associated in the Normative Aging Study with poorer scores on the Mini Mental State Examination (MMSE) in males.[69] This lead-related decline in MMSE scoring was more pronounced among men who also had GSTP1 alleles that reduced the functioning of that particular glutathione transferase enzyme.[70] Although the presence of the GSTP1 variant was not associated with cognitive decline itself, when found in those with higher patellar lead, its presence accelerated the cognitive decline equivalently to 3 years of aging. Computerized neurobehavioral testing, easily done in a clinical setting, shows clear cognitive declines associated with bone lead burden[71] but shows no correlation with BLLs.[72]

Cadmium exposure in children has been associated with a variety of neurological problems. A cohort of mother-child pairs was followed from pregnancy through the child's fifth birthday, comparing urinary cadmium levels with measurements of the children's IQ.[73] The urinary cadmium levels in the mothers ranged from 0.13 to 2.0 µg/L, with a mean of 0.63 µg/L. A doubling of the mother's urinary cadmium level caused a reduction in their child's verbal IQ, performance IQ, and full-scale IQ. Children's urinary cadmium level at the age of 5 years was associated with reduced performance IQ and with behavior problems. Data on children aged 6 to 15 years from the National Health and Nutritional Examination Survey (NHANES) was used to assess neurodevelopmental associations with urinary cadmium levels.[74] When the researchers compared those children in the highest NHANES quartile for urinary cadmium with those in the lowest, a threefold increased risk for the child requiring special education and a 3.21-fold risk of the child having learning disabilities were revealed. When the NHANES data on adults was used to assess the association of cadmium and neuroperformance, higher urinary cadmium was associated with a reduction in attention and perception.[75] Table 42.2 summarizes common neurological health problems associated with environmental pollutants.

Methylmercury exposure from eating high-mercury fish is associated with diminished visuospatial processing and memory.[76] Amazonian children with hair mercury levels of more than 10 µg/g have poorer neuropsychological (NP) test results for motor function, attention, and visuospatial performance.[77] Dentists also perform significantly worse on neurobehavioral tests measuring motor speed (finger tapping), visual scanning (trail making), visuomotor coordination and concentration (digit symbol), verbal memory, visual memory, and visuomotor coordination speed.[78] The dentists and dental assistants with statistically significant declines on multiple tests had higher mean blood mercury levels of 3.32 µg/L (versus those dentists with an average of 2.29 µg/L), with a mean blood mercury of 1.98 µg/L (versus those dental assistants with an average of 1.03 µg/L).[79] Those with a polymorphism in the coproporphyrinogen oxidase gene, making mercury-induced porphyria more likely, not only had worse performance on neurobehavioral testing but also had greater depression, highlighted by feelings of

TABLE 42.2   Common Neurological Health Problems Associated With Environmental Pollutants

Problem	PAH/PM	PHTH	Solvents	PCB	OCP	OP	Cd	Pb	Hg
Poor cognition	X		X	X	X	X	X	X	X
Lower IQ							X	X	
Special education need							X		
Memory problems			X	X	X			X	X
Depression	X	X	X		X	X	X	X	
Irritability/excitability			X						X
Tremors						X			
Balance problems			X			X			
Insomnia								X	
Fatigue			X		X	X		X	X
Headache			X			X			X

Cd, Cadmium; *Hg,* mercury; *OCP,* organochlorine pesticides; *OP,* organophosphate pesticides; *PAH/PM,* polycyclic aromatic hydrocarbons; *Pb,* lead; *PCB,* polychlorinated biphenyls; *PHTH,* phthalates.

worthlessness. Diminished complex information processing was found in fish-consuming corporate executives, whose average blood mercury was 7.2 μg/L, falling within the 90th percentile for fish-consuming Asian Americans in the CDC Fourth Report. These blood mercury levels were also found commonly in the group of internal medicine patients in San Francisco.[80] The effect of blood mercury on neurobehavioral function was also assessed among participants of the Baltimore Memory Study.[81] The mean blood mercury level of this study group was 2.76 μg/L (CDC total 90th percentile, >50th percentile for Asian Americans). As blood mercury increased from that level, significant decrements in memory were found.

Residents in Cochran and Palmer counties in Texas, where the groundwater arsenic averaged 6.32 μg/L, were assessed for NP functioning as part of an ongoing epidemiological study on cognitive aging among rural inhabitants.[82] An MMSE along with multiple computer-based tests of cognitive function (attention, language, visuospatial, constructive ability, delayed recall, word association, and verbal fluency) were performed on the study subjects. The test results of individuals from areas with higher groundwater arsenic were then compared with those with lower groundwater arsenic levels. Both current and long-term exposure to groundwater arsenic were significantly related to poorer scores in language, visuospatial skills, and executive functioning. Long-term exposure (but not current exposure) to low-level ground water arsenic were also associated with poorer scores in global cognition, processing speeds, and immediate memory.

Sport anglers who annually consumed at least 24 lb. of fish caught in Lake Michigan had much higher serum levels of PCB and DDE than non–fish eaters (<6 lb yearly) and had more memory and learning problems than nonanglers.[83] Hundreds of residents in Perry County, TN, exposed to PCBs from a gas pipeline were found to have significantly slower reaction times (for both simple and choice reactions), faster sway speeds, diminished color discrimination and visual performances, and constricted visual fields. They also had diminished scores on digit symbols, vocabulary, verbal recall, and embedded memory.[84]

Mood

- Vehicular exhaust
- Phthalates
- Pesticides
- Heavy metals

Depression is one of the most common worldwide health problems[85] and has been directly linked to both systemic and neural inflammation.[86] Exposure to elevated levels of $PM_{2.5}$ have been directly linked to the development of major depressive disorder (MDD) in previously healthy individuals.[87] Each 10 μg/m^3 increase in $PM_{2.5}$ increased the risk of developing MDD by 43%, which would increase the risk of the average resident of the greater Los Angeles area by more than 86%. The increased risk of developing depression severe enough to warrant the use of antidepressant medications was found for both 12- and 36-month exposure ranges. Not surprisingly, persons with chronic health problems that are often accompanied by systemic inflammation had even higher rates of developing MDD. In elderly populations, exposure to elevated levels of PM_{10} ($PM_{2.5}$ exposure was not measured), nitrogen dioxide (NO_2), and ozone over a 3-day period were associated with depression.[88] The cleaner the air, the happier these elderly Koreans were.

Severe depression, resulting in attempted suicide, is also associated with urban air pollutants. A study in Vancouver, British Columbia, found a seasonal association between air pollutants and suicide attempts, with increased risk during the cold months with higher pollution.[89] Total PM, carbon monoxide, NO_2, and sulfur dioxide (SO_2) were all positively associated with increased suicide attempts the following day. The greatest association was for males during the cold periods, who were almost 25% more likely to commit suicide the day after pollution spiked. Similar results were found in Korea, where spikes of both PM_{10} and $PM_{2.5}$ resulted in increased suicide attempts within 2 days.[90] Those persons with cardiovascular disease, with systemic inflammation as a hallmark, had even greater risk.

Repeated organophosphate pesticide exposures have been linked to an increased risk of depression. Individuals who had an acute poisoning episode from organophosphate pesticides are highly likely (more than a threefold risk) to develop depression years after the actual poisoning occurred.[91] This finding was also noted among Colorado farmers 3 years after an acute organophosphate poisoning incident even after adjusting for health, decreased income, and debt.[92] Their depression was dominated by being bothered by things and the feeling that everything was an effort. Cumulative exposure to a variety of insecticides and fungicides (including organophosphates, dieldrin, and phenoxy acid herbicides and fumigants) has also been linked to increased risk for depression.[93]

Interestingly, genotypically or phenotypically reduced activity of paraoxonase 1 (PON1), the enzyme that metabolizes organophosphates, is independently associated with depression and bipolar disorder.[94] It has previously been shown that persons with genotypically reduced PON1 activity were far more likely to experience neurotoxic effects from organophosphate exposure.[95] In fact, the neurotoxicity risk from underfunctioning PON1 (OR 2.8) was almost identical to the risk of organophosphate neurotoxicity in persons who had traumatic brain injury (OR 2.9).[96] Traumatic brain injury is highlighted by neuroinflammation, and PON1 is both a powerful antioxidant and antiinflammatory agent.

Low-molecular-weight phthalates, commonly found in liquid personal care products, have also been linked to depression. US residents older than 60 years who participated in the 2006 to 2012 NHANES trial and had higher urine levels of two common phthalates (mono-carboxypropyl-phthalates and mono-n-butyl phthalate) were more than twice as likely to be depressed as those with lower phthalate levels.[97] Assessment of the effect of phthalates on mood in younger individuals has not been performed.

BLLs can be predictive of problems with mood disorders in adults. Adults with BLLs higher than 1.7 µg/dL (the current CDC 50th percentile) were more likely to have problems with depression and panic.[98] When their BLLs reached 3.0 µg/dL, the risk for depression increased 2.3-fold and the risk for panic quintupled. Tibial lead burden (a marker for cumulative lead burden) has also been associated with increased risk for both depression and phobic anxiety in women participating in the Nurses' Health Study.[99] US residents participating in the NHANES trial with higher levels of cadmium were 48% more likely to have depression, whereas those with higher mercury levels had lower risk for depressive problems.[100]

DISEASES

This section discusses neurological diseases associated with environmental pollutants. Table 42.3 summarizes the link between various pollutants and neurological disorders.

Attention Deficit Hyperactive Disorder

- PCBs
- Lead
- Mercury
- Pesticides
- Air pollutants
- Phthalates

ADHD is one of the most common childhood health problems and has increased from affecting 3% to 8% of children in 2002 to between 7% and more than 13% in 2016.[101] This disorder is typically dominated by either inattention or hyperactivity and impulsivity that interferes with functioning or development. Children with ADHD are at increased risk for conduct disorder, antisocial behavior, and drug abuse in later life, and ADHD is associated with impairments in academic, social, and occupational functioning.[102,103] Both prenatal and postnatal

TABLE 42.3 **Neurological Diseases Associated With Environmental Pollutants**

Disease	PAH/PM	PHTH	Solvents	OCP	OP / PYR	Pb	Hg
ADHD	X				X	X	
ALS							
Alzheimer's	X			X	X		
Autism	X	X	X		X		
OCD/CD						X	
Parkinson's disease			X (TCE)	X	X	X	
Neuroinflammation	X		X		X	X	X

CD, Conduct disorder; *Hg,* mercury; *OCD,* obsessive compulsive disorder; *OCP,* organochlorine pesticides; *OP,* organophosphate pesticides; *PAH/PM,* polycyclic aromatic hydrocarbons and particulate matter; *Pb,* lead; *PHTH,* phthalates; *PYR,* pyrethroid; *TCE,* trichloroethylene.

exposures to a range of persistent and nonpersistent toxicants have been shown to increase the risk of ADHD.

Prenatal Exposures

- PCBs
- Methylmercury
- Air pollutants
- Phthalates

The studies on prenatal PCB exposure to children previously mentioned[44,45,46,47] revealed a strong association between maternal PCB exposure, primarily through fish consumption, and increased risk for her child to have inattentiveness and impulse control issues. Massachusetts children whose mothers resided near a harbor contaminated with PCBs were 76% more likely to have ADHD-related learning problems by age 11 years.[104]

Prenatal methylmercury exposure from maternal intake of high-mercury fish increases the risk for their children to exhibit ADHD.[105] When maternal hair mercury was used as a biomarker instead of cord blood mercury, a clear association with ADHD was also found.[106] Women with a hair mercury level above 1 µg/g during pregnancy were more likely to have a child with elevated inattentiveness and impulsivity.

Air pollutants, primarily cigarette smoke and vehicular exhaust, also increase ADHD risk for children. Prenatal exposure to both cigarette smoke[107,108] and maternal alcohol consumption confer a high risk for developing ADHD.[109] Traffic-related air pollution, previously noted to cause cognitive problems in adults, also leads to ADHD in children. Assessment of prenatal exposure to polycyclic aromatic hydrocarbons by maternal personal air monitors and PAH-DNA adducts in cord blood show positive association with attention problems.[110] These same children also had more problems with both anxiety and depression. Japanese children whose mothers were exposed to higher levels of vehicular exhaust during gestation had an increased risk for behavioral problems by the age of 9 years.[111] The most common behavioral problems in those exposed to vehicular exhaust prenatally were attention problems and both delinquent and aggressive behavior.

Prenatal exposure to high-molecular-weight phthalates is associated with delinquent and aggressive behavior in 8-year-old Taiwanese children.[112] The strongest association was with maternal urinary levels of mono-ethylhexyl phthalate (MEHP) and mono-ethyloxyhexyl phthalate (MEOHP), metabolites of diethylhexyl phthalate found in many commercial products, including plastic food coverings.

Postnatal Exposures

- Lead
- Pesticides and herbicides
- Vehicular exhaust

Data from the 1999 to 2002 NHANES trial that included 4700 children between the ages of 4 to 15 years provided great insight into the connection between blood lead and ADHD rates.[105] The BLLs in these children fit into five quintiles: first (<detection limit–0.7 µg/dL), second (0.8–1.0), third (1.1–1.3), fourth (1.4–2.0), and fifth (>2.0)—all well under the current CDC threshold level of 5.0 µg/dL and therefore presumably without health risk. However, those in the third quintile had double the risk of developing ADHD compared with those with BLLs of 0.7 µg/dL or less. The ADHD risk for those in the fourth quintile was 2.7, and for those with BLLs higher than 2.0 µg/dL the risk quadrupled (OR 4.1). Chinese children with a BLL between 5 and 10 µg/dL had an ADHD risk of 4.9, and those whose BLL was more than

10 µg/dL had a risk factor of 6.0.[106] Several other studies have confirmed the high risk of impulsivity-dominated ADHD in children as a result of exposure to lead.[113,114,115,116]

Arctic children with a BLL between 1.6 and 2.7 µg/dL (the CDC 50th percentile) showed a lower risk and were only 52% more likely to have inattentive ADHD, 86% more likely to have oppositional defiant disorder (ODD) or conduct disorder (CD), and five times more likely to have hyperactive/impulsive ADHD. When their BLL crested at 2.7 µg/dL (CDC 90th percentile for children aged 6–11 years), the risk for hyperactive/impulsive ADHD shot up to more than sevenfold. BLLs above 1.6 µg/dL in children have also been strongly linked to increased risk for ADHD, ODD, and CD.[117] Tis lower risk compared with children within the United States may be related to the protective role of fish oils in ADHD.[118]

Both of the most commonly used insecticides, pyrethroids and organophosphates, have been associated with the development of ADHD. Pyrethroids are commonly used as residential and commercial insecticides and have demonstrated the ability to cause ADHD-like behavior in animals.[119] Children between the ages of 6 and 15 years with detectable urinary levels of pyrethroid metabolites were twice as likely to have a diagnosis of ADHD.[120] Metabolites of pyrethroids have been measured in the NHANES trial, providing a means to assess their association with behavioral disorders. When the NHANES data was compared with parental reporting of ADHD-like behavior, no significant association was found.[121] However, when the same data was used and compared with that for children who had been diagnosed with ADHD, the findings were clear. Children with detectable levels of 3-phenoxybenzoic acid (3-PBA) were 2.42 times more likely to have been diagnosed with ADHD than those with nondetectable 3-PBA. The findings were stronger for boys than girls. A significant association between parent-reported ADHD symptoms and a different pyrethroid metabolite were documented in a study of Canadian children as well.[122] In this study, organophosphate pesticide metabolites were also assessed, and a significant association with high scores on the Strengths and Difficulties Questionnaire was found. Data from the 2000 to 20004 NHANES revealed a significant association between an organophosphate metabolite, dimethylalkylphosphate (DMAP), and the diagnosis of ADHD.[123]

Parents in the Red River Valley of Minnesota who regularly used glyphosate were more than three times more likely to have children with ADD/ADHD problems.[124]

Children with higher exposure to vehicular exhaust during their first year of life, through living very close to busy roadways, increased their risk of hyperactivity by age 7 years by 70%.[125]

Autism Spectrum Disorder

Autism spectrum disorder (ASD) is a group of complex neurodevelopmental disorders characterized by repetitive and characteristic patterns of behavior and difficulties with social communication and interaction. A wide range of symptoms and disability levels are present from early childhood and affect daily functioning. Some individuals with ASD are fully able to perform all activities of daily living, whereas others require substantial support to perform basic activities. In the Diagnostic and Statistical Manual of Mental Disorders, fifth edition (DSM-5, published in 2013), ASD includes Asperger syndrome, childhood disintegrative disorder, and pervasive developmental disorders not otherwise specified (PDD-NOS). A diagnosis of ASD includes an assessment of intellectual disability and language impairment. The latest analysis from the CDC estimates that 1 in 68 children has ASD, with boys being four times more likely than girls to be affected.

Neuroinflammation is known to be present in ASD, although the role of neuroinflammation in the severity and progression of this disorder is not defined.[15,126] Although the cause of ASD is still unclear, the role of environmental toxicants in increasing the risk for this disorder has been repeatedly shown. For example, insurance claim data covering one-third of the US population was reviewed to see if there was an association with known toxicant-induced disorders and ASD. Congenital malformations of the reproductive system, known to be environmentally induced, were used as a surrogate for environmental toxicant exposures. It was found that males with congenital reproductive malformations were 283% more likely to also have the diagnosis of ASD. A study of 192 twins was done to determine the roles of genetics and environment on the development of ASD.[127] These researchers found that environmental factors carried 55% of the etiological weight, whereas genetics only accounted for 37%.

Maternal exposure to environmental chemicals and body burden has also been associated. Chemical intolerance, also known as *chemical sensitivity*, is present in persons overburdened with environmental chemicals. Using the Quick Environmental Exposure and Sensitivity Inventory (QEESI), a validated measurement of chemical reactivity,[128] it was found that mothers of children with ASD or ADHD had significantly higher scores than mothers with neurotypical children.[129] Mothers with chemical sensitivity were three times more likely to have a child with autism and 2.3 times more likely to have a child with ADHD. Solvent burden is commonly found in persons with chemical sensitivity, and it has been found in women who are occupationally exposed to solvents as well as asphalt.[130] The risk of being a parent of an ASD child increased by a factor of 7.3 for occupational exposure to lacquers, 4.7 for varnish, 2.7 for xylene, 3.1 for solvents, and 6.9 for asphalt. A study in San Francisco revealed that women occupationally exposed to toxicants have a significantly higher risk of having a child with ASD.[131] Women exposed to disinfectants at work were four times more likely to have a child with ASD, whereas those exposed to exhaust and combustion byproducts were 12 times more likely. Mothers of children with ASD were also significantly less likely to be knowledgeable and aware of environmental toxicants and have higher exposure to them than mothers of neurotypical children.[132] They were also more likely to have exposures to polybrominated diphenyl ether flame retardants, PCBs, bisphenol A, and dioxins through use of canned foods, plastics, microwaved foods, and proximity to waste incinerators, old electronics, and textiles.

Prenatal Exposures

- Air pollutants
- PCBs
- Phthalates

Between 2010 and 2015, six articles were published on the relationship between air pollution and ASD. The first was a case-control led study with 383 children with ASD and 2829 control children who had speech and language impairment from North Carolina and West Virginia.[133] Exposures to ambient levels of metals, particulates, and volatile organic compounds were assessed via pollutant data on the area were the child's parents lived during pregnancy. Significant associations were found between ASD risk and exposure to the polycyclic aromatic hydrocarbon quinolone (OR 1.4), styrene (OR 1.8), and methylene chloride (OR 1.4). The second study was a population-based study with 304 children with ASD and 259 neurotypical controls from California.[134] Mothers living close to freeways during the third trimester were 2.22 times more likely to have a child with ASD. After delivery, those mother-child pairs that lived close to freeways had an 86% greater risk for the child to develop

ASD. The same group of researchers published the third study with 279 autistic children and 245 neurotypical controls to attempt to identify which of the common components of vehicular exhaust (nitrogen dioxide, PM_{10}, and $PM_{2.5}$) increased autism risk.[135] Exposure to NO_2 increased the risk of autism by 81%, whereas exposure to PM_{10} and $PM_{2.5}$ both doubled the risk of autism. Postnatal exposure to NO_2, PM_{10}, and $PM_{2.5}$ also more than doubled the risk for autism.

The fourth study compared 7603 children with autism with 76,030 matched controls from Los Angeles county in relation to the ambient levels of ozone and $PM_{2.5}$ that their respective mothers were exposed to while pregnant.[136] Daily exposure to increasing levels of ozone and $PM_{2.5}$ were both significantly associated with increasing risks of autism. The fifth study involved 325 children with ASD and 22,101 neurologically normal children of participants in the Nurses' Health Study.[137] Perinatal exposures to toxicants previously associated with autism were tracked and compared with their neurological status. Perinatal exposure to mercury doubled the risk for autism, whereas manganese, lead, and nickel exposures increased the risk by 50%, 60%, and 70%, respectively. Exposure to methylene chloride increased autism risk by 80%, and diesel exhaust exposure doubled the risk. The sixth article also studied children of participants in the Nurses' Health Study, this time with 245 children with ASD and 1522 controls.[138] Exposure to $PM_{2.5}$ levels for 9 months before conception and through each trimester were assessed in relation to ASD diagnosis. ASD risk increased by 57% for each interquartile range increase of ambient $PM_{2.5}$. The association was weak for the 9 months before conception but quite strong all three trimesters of pregnancy, with the third trimester being the strongest.

A large cohort of mother-child pairs with either ASD or intellectual dysfunction (ID) from southern California for whom second trimester blood samples were available were assessed for PCB levels.[139] Comparing prenatal PCB levels of 545 mother-child pairs with ASD, 144 with ID for whom no known etiology was present, and 413 population controls revealed a strong correlation between these disorders and PCBs (Table 42.4). PCB levels in the children (postnatal exposures) showed no correlation with either diagnosis. However, levels of PCB 138 and 153 were highly correlated with each other, indicating that they originated from the same source.

The presence of low-molecular-weight phthalate metabolites in a mother's urine during her third trimester

TABLE 42.4	Adjusted Odds Ratio for ASD and ID for Children Whose Mother Had PCBs in the 4th Quartile	
	ASD AOR Q4	**ID AOR Q4**
PCB 138/158	1.79	2.41
PCB 153	1.82	1.76
PCB 170	1.48	1.42
PCB 180	1.49	1.35

of pregnancy have been significantly correlated to the child having greater problems with social cognition, social awareness, and social communications by the age of 7 years.[140] Low-molecular-weight phthalates are present in many personal care products, including nail polish and all fragrances.

Postnatal Exposures

- Insecticides
- Phthalates
- Air pollution
- Persistent Organic Pollutants (POPs)

The possible association of both prenatal and postnatal exposure to organophosphate pesticides and ASD was assessed in group of 531 Latino farmworker children in California. The researchers found that both prenatal and postnatal exposures to organophosphate pesticides (measured by urinary dialkyl phosphate metabolites) were associated with an increased risk of being diagnosed with a pervasive personality disorder by the time they were 2 years of age.[141] When the sources of organophosphate pesticides were studied, those children who lived closer than 60 meters to an agricultural field had the highest levels of urinary metabolites, with peak values in the spring and summer. Importantly, the researchers also found a clear positive association with the number of servings of produce the children had.[142] For children not living in an agricultural area, this would be the greatest source of organophosphate pesticide exposure.

High-molecular-weight phthalates are found in solid plastic items such as food wrap, shower curtains, and polyvinyl chloride products. In a Swedish study that followed families over a 5-year period and focused on the home environment and health, researchers found a connection between vinyl flooring and the diagnosis of autism, Asperger's, and Tourette's syndromes.[143] In addition to increased rates of these diagnoses in children whose parents had vinyl flooring in the bedroom, risk

was also associated with parental smoking, condensation on the windows, and reduced ventilation in the home.

A group of 284 children with ASD in the San Francisco Bay area was compared with more than 600 neurologically normal children to see if there was any difference in air pollutant exposures between the two groups.[144] The researchers found that children living in the San Francisco Bay area with higher levels of atmospheric mercury were 92% more likely to have been diagnosed with ASD. Areas with the highest vinyl chloride levels increased ASD risk by 75%, high cadmium levels by 54%, trichlorethylene by 47%, nickel by 46%, and diesel exhaust by 44%. Another study in California compared 279 children with ASD with 245 neurotypical controls and found that those with ASD were far more likely to be living in areas with high vehicular exhaust.[134] During the first year of life, exposure to either NO_2, $PM_{2.5}$, or PM_{10} all more than doubled the child's risk of developing ASD. In a large cohort of more than 49,000 Taiwanese children, those with the highest exposure to nitrogen dioxide had a 340% increased risk of developing ASD.[145] In addition to the increased risk from NO_2, each 10 parts per billion (PPB) increase in ambient ozone increased ASD risk by 54%, and each 10 PPB increase in CO levels increased the risk of autism by 37%.

Serum levels of polybrominated diphenyl ethers (PBDE), polychlorinated biphenyls (PCBs), chlorinated pesticides, and solvents were measured in a group of children with ASD as well as controls.[146] Although pesticide and solvent levels did not differ between the groups, the ASD group had significantly more children with detectable levels of PCBs and PBDEs (p = 0.0359 and p = 0.00730, respectively). Among the ASD group, PCB 138 was detected 1.5 times more frequently than in controls.

Alzheimer's Disease

- Air pollution
- Pesticides

AD is a progressive, disabling disease with no known cure that accounts for 60% to 80% of dementia problems in the elderly and is the sixth leading cause of death in the United States.[147] Between 2014 and 2015, the number of AD-related deaths increased more than 15% (from 25.4–29.4 per 100,000), far higher than any of the other leading causes of death. It is characterized by the gradual decline of memory and other cognitive function, leading to complete incapacity and death typically within 3 to 9 years after diagnosis. The most common form of AD is late onset (LOAD), which has both genetic and environmental causes. An estimated 47 million people are affected by AD worldwide, and this is expected to increase to more than 131 million by 2050.[148] The development of AD is associated with neuroinflammation, the deposition of β-amyloid plaques, and tau tangles. Persistent activation of glial cells, a hallmark of neuroinflammation, is now considered a key abnormality in AD.[149] Oxidative stress[150] and mitochondrial dysfunction[151] are also keynotes of both AD and parkinsonism. The increased deposition of β-amyloid, both inside the mitochondria and extracellularly, arises from both overproduction of β-amyloid and decreased degradation. Apolipoprotein E, a cholesterol carrier in the brain, works to clear amyloid deposits from the parenchyma of the brain; however, at least 40% of all AD patients have a genetic deletion of the APOe4 gene that produces this protein. The classic neurofibrillary tangles of tau protein occur because of hyperphosphorylation of tau.

Air pollution, already shown to begin and fuel neuroinflammation, has also been implicated in increased levels of amyloid deposits and tau protein formation. PM can penetrate throughout the body, including the brain, where it is closely linked to inflammation. Postmortem assessment of the brains of cognitively intact persons revealed that those who lived in areas of higher vehicular air pollution had greater inflammatory markers and β-amyloid in their frontal cortex and hippocampus (those areas needed for memory function) along with their olfactory lobe.[152]

Children living in the metropolitan area of Mexico City with both prenatal and postnatal exposure to high levels of $PM_{2.5}$ have been found to have increased hyperphosphorylation of tau along with increased levels of β-amyloid.[153] Children also exhibited decreased cognitive function (attention, memory, and IQ) and decreased olfactory sense. Children with APOe4 had greater problems, especially with olfaction.[154] They also had higher levels of antibodies against basic myelin protein, myelin oligodendrocyte glycoprotein, and certain chemicals.[155] Interestingly, providing some of these children with 30 grams of cocoa daily (containing 680 mg of flavonoids) for an average of only 10 days provided some improvement in their memory function.[156]

Cognitive decline in adults, often a precursor to AD, related to vehicular exhaust was reviewed earlier in this chapter. More than 95,000 Taiwanese adults older than 65 years were followed for 9 years to see if there was any association between $PM_{2.5}$ and ozone levels and their neurological function. Over the follow-up period, those exposed to higher $PM_{2.5}$ levels were 38% more likely to develop AD, whereas those with higher ozone exposure had more than twice the rates of AD as those living in areas of lower pollution.[157]

Pesticide use and exposure has also been associated with higher risks for developing AD. A large study in southern Spain encompassed 17,420 subjects whose hospital records were reviewed between 1998 and 2005. The subjects were classified according to the agricultural pesticide usage in the regions that they lived in. Persons living in regions with higher pesticide use were more than twice as likely to develop AD and 87% more likely to commit suicide.[158] After adjustments, a group of 1924 individuals older than 70 years provided 67 persons with AD, who were matched with controls. Their residential history was collected and matched with documentation of agricultural spraying in those areas since 1970. Although herbicides showed no association with development of AD, insecticide exposure (organophosphates) was associated with a statistically significant 62% increase in AD.[159] A study of 1507 elderly French individuals revealed that those who had been occupationally exposed to pesticides in their younger years were 2.39 times more likely to develop AD than individuals in other occupations.[160] The largest prospective study to look at the relationship between pesticide use and AD was done in Cache County, Utah. More than 3000 individuals older than 65 years were enrolled and screened for dementia at baseline and classified according to pesticide exposure levels.[161] Cognitive function was reassessed after 3, 7, and 10 years. After adjusting for various factors, including APOE4 allele status, it was found that those with higher pesticide exposures were 38% more likely to have dementia and 42% more likely to develop AD. When just organophosphates and organochlorine pesticides were singled out, it was found that chlorinated pesticide exposure increased AD risk by 49%, and organophosphate use increased it by 53%. In addition, two recent studies have found that persons with AD have higher blood levels of the chlorinated pesticide DDE, and one of them also showed higher levels of β-hexachlorocyclohexane and dieldrin.[162,163]

Parkinson's Disease

- Pesticides
- Lead

Parkinson's disease (PD) is the second most common neurodegenerative disorder experienced by seniors. It is present in only 1% to 2% of 50-year-olds, but is found in 5% of those 85 years or older. Familial genetics appear to account for only 5% to 10% of all cases of PD,[164] although several genetic markers have been associated with increased risk.[165] PD is characterized by the presence of four major hallmarks: cogwheel rigidity, resting tremor, bradykinesia, and postural instability. These problems occur after a loss of 60% to 70% of dopaminergic neurons in the substantia nigra pars compacta (SNpc) and in the presence of Lewy bodies. This degeneration has been linked to oxidative stress,[166,167] mitochondrial dysfunction,[168,169] and neuroinflammation,[170,171] all of which are known to be caused by environmental toxicants. The common non–dopamine-related symptoms in those with PD include olfactory dysfunction, depression, reduced cognition, and sleep disturbances, many of which are secondary to neuroinflammation.

The first chemical compound shown to cause parkinsonism was meperidine 1-methyl-4-phenyl-l,2,3,6-tetrahydropyridine (MPTP), a contaminant of synthetic heroin, which rapidly induced irreversible PD after intravenous administration.[172,173] MPTP exposure produces lesions in the SNpc, visible on positron emission tomography (PET) scans, in both humans and primates. MPTP is metabolized in glial cells to become 1-methyl-4-phenylpyridinium (MPP+), which then inhibits complex 1 in the mitochondria of SNpc dopaminergic cells primarily through oxidative damage.[174] MPP+ has also demonstrated the ability to induce nitric oxide synthase, a critical step in the development of neuroinflammation.[175] Environmentally induced PD has also been demonstrated in welders who are exposed to airborne manganese.[176]

Pesticide exposures and farming have been repeatedly associated with developing PD along with rural living and well water use.[177,178,179] A recent review of 39 case control studies, four cohort studies, and three cross-sectional studies confirmed the association between herbicide and insecticide use and PD risk.[180] A larger review of 104 studies confirmed the association of PD and farming and confirmed increased PD risk with exposure to herbicides, solvents, and any type of pesticide.[181] The highest PD risk was for persons occupationally exposed to paraquat or maneb/mancozeb, whose risk for this disorder doubled. In a twin study, those with exposure to trichloroethylene (TCE), a common groundwater contaminant, had a PD risk more than six times higher than their nonexposed sibling.[182] Although many of the studies looked at persons who worked around pesticides, a population-based cohort study in California looked instead at persons who used organophosphate pesticides in their homes. When comparing the 357 PD cases with 807 controls, the researchers found that any household pesticide use increased the odds of developing PD by 47%.[183] When just the organophosphate pesticides were separated out, it was found that use of these insecticides increased PD risk by 71% (95% CI, 1.21, 2.41). Those individuals with a genotypically underfunctioning paraoxonase 1 enzyme, necessary to break down organophosphates, can have up to a threefold higher risk of developing PD after OP exposure than those with functioning PON1.[184]

Glutathione transferases (GSTs) are detoxification enzymes involved in the liver phase II conjugation of glutathione with pesticides and a wide variety of environmental toxins. GSTs are polymorphic and typically result in reduced GST function. Among individuals with pesticides exposure, those with the GSTP1 variation that reduced GSTP function were more likely to develop PD than persons with fully functioning GSTP.[185] Another study found a greater susceptibility to PD in males with a deletion of the GSTM1 gene,[186] whereas the deletion of GSTT1 increased the risks to males of both PD and motor neuron disease.

Cumulative lead burden, as assessed by bone lead levels, is also associated with a twofold greater risk of developing PD.[187,188] As the tibial lead burden increased in PD patients, the cognitive functioning of these individuals significantly declined.[189] Although blood lead values do not predict the risk of either PD or cognitive decline, they do predict the risk for other neurological dysfunctions in adults, including walking speed, balance, hearing, and mood, which can also be found in persons with parkinsonism.

ASSESSMENT

Specific Assessment of Neurotoxicity

Neuropsychological Testing. NP testing, sometimes referred as *neurocognitive testing*, is capable of detecting early signs of neurotoxic damage in the absence of other neurological signs and is therefore considered the most sensitive means of detecting neurotoxic effects.[190] NP assessment uses objective, standardized psychometric tests that measure and quantify aspects of psychological functioning such as intellectual level, memory, attention, language, planning, and visuospatial and verbal reasoning.

NP testing has shown reliability and validity and compares the individual result with age-appropriate population samples. Having the ability to compare individual results with what is typically found in healthy persons of the same age group allows the testing to differentiate toxicant-induced CNS dysfunction from age-related dysfunction.[191] This form of testing is done with a computer and can be done in they physician's office or online, making it readily available for clinicians and patients. It also has the benefit of being low cost and noninvasive. Four of the most commonly used NP tests are as follows:

- The **Finger-Tapping Test** (also called *simple reaction time test*). Using a keyboard, with prompts from the computer screen, the subject uses one finger—first from the dominant hand and then the nondominant hand—to hit the space bar as many times as they can in a set amount of time. This test assesses psychomotor speed (also called *visuomotor speed*).
- The **Symbol Digit Substitution Test** (also called the *Symbol Digit Coding Test*). The computer screen displays two lines of boxes, one above the other. One set of boxes contains numbers, and, either above or below that, another set contains symbols. When the computer screen prompts the beginning of the test, the subject must match the numbers to the appropriate symbols. This test reveals an individual's processing speed and several cognitive functions, including visual scanning, visual perception, visual memory, and motor function.
- The **Verbal Memory Test** uses a sequence of 15 words that are first shown one at a time on the computer screen. They are then randomly repeated twice with 15 other distracter words. The subject must correctly identify the original 15. This test measures how well one can recognize, remember, and retrieve words, a test of verbal memory.
- The **Continuous Performance Test** measures sustained attention, vigilance, and choice reaction time. For this test, the computer initially reveals a single letter. Then it reveals a random list of letters, including the original letter, one at a time, asking the subject to hit the space bar only when the original letter appears.

NP tests have revealed adverse neurological effects from a variety of common environmental toxicants, including organophosphate pesticides, solvents, brominated flame retardants (polybrominated diphenyl ethers), air pollutants, and heavy metals (Table 42.5).

Balance Testing. Equilibrium dysfunction is common in solvent-induced neurotoxicity and is so well known that law enforcement officers typically use basic tests of balance to identify drivers who have acute toxic encephalopathy from alcohol ingestion. Balance dysfunction has been shown to be present even in solvent workers who do not fit the definition of solvent-induced encephalopathy.[192,193] Basic Romberg assessment methods are typically used, although balance testing (posturographic) machines have been used in studies, which have revealed a number of other environmental toxicants that lead to balance problems. Posturographic assessments have revealed that children with a BLL below 5 μg/dL exhibit balance disorders.[194] Individuals living in areas with high levels

NP Test Area	OP	PCB	VOC	PM2.5 PAH	Ozone	Hg	Pb	Cd	As
Composite memory						X			
Verbal memory	X	PN / X	X	X		X	X		X
Visual memory	PN	PN / X	X		X	X	X		
Psychomotor speed	X		X						
Reaction time	X		X						
Complex attention					X			X	X
Processing speed			X		X		X		X
Executive Function	X	PN				X	X		X
Working memory	X		X	X					
Sustained attention		PN		PN / X					
Simple attention		PN		PN / X		X			
Motor speed	PN	PN			X	X			

TABLE 42.5 **Deficiencies in Neuropsychological Testing According to Toxicant**

PN = Prenatal exposure. OP, organophosphate pesticides, VOC, volatile organic compounds, PM2.5 particulate mater less than 2.5 microns, PAH polycyclic aromatic hydrocarbons.

of hydrogen sulfide gas,[195] PCBs,[196] and TCE[197] in the water or air have exhibited measurable balance disorders. Interior exposure to aerosol insecticide spraying[198] and residential exposures to molds[199] and new building materials[200] have also demonstrated increased postural sway.

SPECT Scans. SPECT can, on persons with both solvent and organophosphate pesticide-induced toxic encephalopathy, reveal a serious reduction in blood flow and metabolism, primarily in the frontal and temporal lobes. More than 91% of individuals with these SPECT scan abnormalities also have vestibular function deficits (measurable with posturography).[201]

General Assessment of Neurological Defects

The Mini Mental State Examination and Beck's depression index are readily available, simple, quick, noninvasive, and low-cost methods to determine whether an individual's cognition is impaired or they have depression. However, they are not able to differentiate the cause of such impairments.

Visual contrast sensitivity (VCS) testing is another low-cost, noninvasive, and simple test to show abnormalities of neurological function. Although it has gained popularity as a measurement of neurotoxicity (and is readily available online for this purpose), it is actually nonspecific for neurotoxicity, because abnormalities are found in a wide range of eye disorders and common chronic diseases. However, VCS abnormalities have been found in solvents workers,[202,203] children exposed prenatally to solvents,[204] smokers, and persons spending a lot of time in estuaries contaminated with *Pfiesteria*.[205]

INTERVENTION

Avoidance

Most of the environmental pollutants previously listed that are known to cause neurotoxicity are nonpersistent pollutants and can therefore be addressed initially by reducing one's exposure to them. Office workers in buildings that comply with green building practices are exposed to lower levels of total air pollutants and consequently have better cognitive function scores than workers in conventionally built office buildings.[206] Although not everyone has the opportunity to work in less toxic environments, the use of high-efficiency air purifiers are able to significantly reduce the level of

vehicular exhaust pollutants indoors.[207] Lifestyle choices have also demonstrated the ability to rapidly reduce one's exposure to phthalates.[208] Pesticide exposure can also be reduced dramatically by making smart dietary choices and avoiding the residential use of pesticides.[209] PCBs and chlorinated pesticides are biologically persistent and can be passed from mother to child, as can the heavy metals. However, ongoing exposure to the heavy metals and PCBs should be curtailed as well.

Diet

Both cognitive decline and depression have been linked to increased inflammation and are associated with elevated high-sensitivity C-reactive protein (CRP-hs) and IL-6.[210] The Mediterranean diet appears to be the most powerful anti-inflammatory diet currently available, and individuals with higher compliance to the Mediterranean diet have lower levels of CRP-hs and IL-6,[211] as well as better cognition and mood.[212] Adherence to the Mediterranean diet has been shown to reduce depression and cognitive decline and diminish the risk for developing AD.[213,214,215] The Mediterranean diet is composed of high vegetable and fruit intake, olive oil, legumes, fish, red wine, and whole grains with limited dairy and red meat. Many of these individual components alone have also demonstrated benefit.

Olive oil itself is highly antiinflammatory,[216] and individuals with a higher intake of olive oil have better cognition, memory, and motor function.[217,218] Higher intakes of vitamin E and beta carotene, from increased intakes of whole foods in the diet, appear to be protective against the development of PD.[219] Elevated blood levels of tocopherol and tocotrienols are associated with a lower risk of cognitive impairment in older adults, and supplementation with vitamin E appears to slow the progression of AD.[220,221]

Between the red wine and the high intake of fruits and vegetables, the Mediterranean diet has a high number of polyphenolic compounds. Resveratrol, in red wine, has demonstrated neuroprotective ability in cases of traumatic brain injury (a major cause of neuroinflammation) and stroke.[222] Polyphenols not only have powerful antioxidant activity but also reduce the circulating levels of proinflammatory cytokines.[223] Although not part of a conventional Mediterranean diet, the anthocyan polyphenolic compounds present in blueberries appear to be some of the most powerful when it comes to reducing CNS oxidative stress and inflammation and reversing age-related cognitive declines.[224,225,226] In an animal model, blueberry consumption was actually able to reduce ischemia-induced brain damage.[227] Red wine is a part of the Mediterranean diet, and the polyphenols in grape skins are able to reduce CNS oxidative stress and inflammation in animals exposed to ethanol.[228] In a mouse model of beta amyloid deposition, proanthocyans from grape seeds prevented neuronal apoptosis in proportion to the amount of anthocyans given.[229] These same compounds have demonstrated the ability to prevent both methylmercury and cadmium-induced neurotoxicity as well.[230,231]

Pycnogenol, another popular polyphenolic compound, has also demonstrated effectiveness in preventing neuroinflammation from the Parkinson's-inducing compound MPTP.[232] Carotenoids have been shown to reduce neuroinflammation, improve cognition and vision, and reduce the risk of AD.[233,234,235] Walnuts, a common component of the Mediterranean diet, have the ability to reduce neuroinflammation and specifically inhibit lipopolysaccharide induction of neuroinflammation.[236] Finally, fish oil, abundantly present in the Mediterranean diet, alleviates neuroinflammation[25] and prevents cognitive decline.[237]

Supplementation

Certain botanical compounds have demonstrated an ability to reduce neuroinflammation and improve neurological functioning that was caused by environmental pollutants.

Milk thistle (*Silybum marianum*) is best known for its liver-protecting ability but has recently been shown to prevent PD development from two compounds known to cause this debilitating condition. Silibinin, one of the main active flavone compounds in milk thistle, has demonstrated an ability to prevent neuroinflammation by suppressing the activation of glial cells in animals exposed to MPTP.[238] In MPTP-exposed animals, silibinin also stabilizes mitochondrial membranes and prevents loss of dopaminergic neurons in exposed animals and attenuates motor deficits.[239] When used in animals exposed to manganese, silibinin was able to attenuate the oxidative stress in the brain caused by manganese chloride.[240]

Green tea, and its major catechin component epigallocatechin gallate (EGCG) have demonstrated the ability to prevent the development of PD in animals exposed to MPTP when the animals were fed green tea before exposure.[241] Daily consumption of green tea has been shown to reduce the risk of cognitive decline in older adults by 74%.[242]

With regard to turmeric (*Curcuma longa*), in animal studies, lead levels in the liver, kidneys, and brain were all reduced with curcumin, and a dramatic reversal of the oxidative stress caused by lead has been noted. Curcumin also reversed cognitive defects in lead-poisoned animals who were challenged to find their way through a water maze. The animals given curcumin not only had higher levels of glutathione in their brains, but they retained better spatial memory and had faster escape times from the maze.[243] Curcumin has exhibited multiple benefits against mercury. At a dose of 80 mg/kg, it was shown to reduce peroxide levels, increase glutathione, and restore the activity of catalase, glutathione peroxidase, and superoxide dismutase.[244] Exposure to mercury both before and after consumption of curcumin also reduced levels of mercury in the liver, kidney, and brain, matching its ability to reduce lead levels in these same tissues.

Interestingly, the combination of many of the previously discussed dietary and supplement components, along with avoidance of significant sources of dietary toxicants and increasing exercise, has been shown to help a few individuals with AD.[245]

REFERENCES

1. Medlin, J. (1996). Environmental toxins and the brain. *Environmental Health Perspectives*, 104(8), 822–823.
2. Calne, D. B., Eisen, A., McGeer, E., & Spencer, P. (1986). Alzheimer's disease, Parkinson's disease, and motoneurone disease: Abiotrophic interaction between ageing and environment? *Lancet*, 2(8515), 1067–1070. PubMed PMID: 2877227.
3. Centers for Disease Control and Prevention. (January 2017). *National Report on Human Exposure to Environmental Chemicals: Updated Tables*. Available at www.cdc.gov/exposurereport/. Accessed 25 October 2017.
4. Curl, C. L., Fenske, R. A., & Elgethun, K. (2003). Organophosphorus pesticide exposure of urban and suburban preschool children with organic and conventional diets. *Environmental Health Perspectives*, 111(3), 377–382. PubMed PMID: 12611667.
5. Bradman, A., Quirós-Alcalá, L., Castorina, R., et al. (2015). Effect of organic diet intervention on pesticide exposures in young children living in low-income urban and agricultural communities. *Environmental Health Perspectives*, 123(10), 1086–1093. PubMed PMID: 25861095.

6. Dick, F. D. (2006). Solvent neurotoxicity. *Occupational and Environmental Medicine*, *63*(3), 221–226, 179. PubMed PMID: 16497867.

7. Gu, Y., Yang, D. K., Spinas, E., et al. (2015). Role of TNF in mast cell neuroinflammation and pain. *Journal of Biological Regulators and Homeostatic Agents*, *29*(4), 787–791. Review. PubMed PMID: 26753638.

8. Reis, P. A., Alexandre, P. C., D'Avila, J. C., et al. (2016). Statins prevent cognitive impairment after sepsis by reverting neuroinflammation, and microcirculatory/ endothelial dysfunction. *Brain, Behavior, and Immunity*, pii: S0889-1591(16)30496-2. PubMed PMID: 27833044.

9. Bilbo, S. D., Smith, S. H., & Schwarz, J. M. (2012). A lifespan approach to neuroinflammatory and cognitive disorders: A critical role for glia. *Journal of Neuroimmune Pharmacology: The Official Journal of the Society on NeuroImmune Pharmacology*, *7*(1), 24–41. PubMed PMID: 21822589.

10. Leonard, B. E. (2014). Impact of inflammation on neurotransmitter changes in major depression: An insight into the action of antidepressants. *Progress in Neuro-Psychopharmacology and Biological Psychiatry*, *48*, 261–267. PubMed PMID: 24189118.

11. Cherry, J. D., Tripodis, Y., Alvarez, V. E., et al. (2016). Microglial neuroinflammation contributes to tau accumulation in chronic traumatic encephalopathy. *Acta Neuropathologica Communications*, *4*(1), 112. PubMed PMID: 27793189.

12. Fuster-Matanzo, A., Llorens-Martín, M., Hernández, F., & Avila, J. (2013). Role of neuroinflammation in adult neurogenesis and Alzheimer disease: Therapeutic approaches. *Mediators of Inflammation*, *2013*, 260925. PMID: 23690659.

13. Hariri, M., Djazayery, A., Djalali, M., et al. (2012). Effect of n-3 supplementation on hyperactivity, oxidative stress and inflammatory mediators in children with attention-deficit-hyperactivity disorder. *Malaysian Journal of Nutrition*, *18*(3), 329–335. PubMed PMID: 24568073.

14. Hooten, K. G., Beers, D. R., Zhao, W., & Appel, S. H. (2015). Protective and toxic neuroinflammation in amyotrophic lateral sclerosis. *Neurotherapeutics*, *12*(2), 364–375. PubMed PMID: 25567201.

15. Di Marco, B., Bonaccorso, C. M., Aloisi, E., et al. (2016). Neuro-inflammatory mechanisms in developmental disorders associated with intellectual disability and autism spectrum disorder: A neuro-immune perspective. *CNS and Neurological Disorders Drug Targets*, *15*(4), 448–463. PubMed PMID: 26996174.

16. Nguyen, L. T., Ramanathan, M., Weinstock-Guttman, B., et al. (2003). Sex differences in in vitro pro-inflammatory cytokine production from peripheral blood of multiple sclerosis patients. *Journal of the Neurological Sciences*, *209*(1–2), 93–99. PubMed PMID: 12686409.

17. Pantović-Stefanović, M., Petronijević, N., Dunjić-Kostić, B., et al. (2016). sVCAM-1, sICAM-1, TNF-α, and IL-6 levels in bipolar disorder type I: Acute, longitudinal, and therapeutic implications. *The World Journal of Biological Psychiatry*, 1–34. PubMed PMID: 27841086.

18. de Vries, E. E., van den Munckhof, B., Braun, K. P., et al. (2016). Inflammatory mediators in human epilepsy: A systematic review and meta-analysis. *Neuroscience and Biobehavioral Reviews*, *63*, 177–190. PubMed PMID: 26877106.

19. Tansey, M. G., & Goldberg, M. S. (2010). Neuroinflammation in Parkinson's disease: Its role in neuronal death and implications for therapeutic intervention. *Neurobiology of Disease*, *37*(3), 510–518. PubMed PMID: 19913097.

20. Nagatsu, T., Mogi, M., Ichinose, H., & Togari, A. (2000). Changes in cytokines and neurotrophins in Parkinson's disease. *Journal of Neural Transmission. Supplementum*, *60*, 277–290. PubMed PMID: 11205147.

21. Machado, V., Zöller, T., Attaai, A., & Spittau, B. (2016). Microglia-mediated neuroinflammation and neurotrophic factor-induced protection in the MPTP mouse model of Parkinson's disease—lessons from transgenic mice. *International Journal of Molecular Sciences*, *17*(2), PubMed PMID: 26821015.

22. Skaper, S. D., Facci, L., & Giusti, P. (2014). Neuroinflammation, microglia and mast cells in the pathophysiology of neurocognitive disorders: A review. *CNS and Neurological Disorders Drug Targets*, *13*(10), 1654–1666. PubMed PMID: 25470401.

23. Smith, J. A., Das, A., Ray, S. K., & Banik, N. L. (2012). Role of pro-inflammatory cytokines released from microglia in neurodegenerative diseases. *Brain Research Bulletin*, *87*(1), 10–20. PubMed PMID: 22024597.

24. Mietto, B. S., Mostacada, K., & Martinez, A. M. (2015). Neurotrauma and inflammation: CNS and PNS responses. *Mediators of Inflammation*, *2015*, 251204. PubMed PMID: 25918475.

25. Shi, Z., Ren, H., Huang, Z., et al. (2016). Fish oil prevents lipopolysaccharide-induced depressive-like behavior by inhibiting neuroinflammation. *Molecular Neurobiology*. [Epub ahead of print] PubMed PMID: 27815837.

26. Pugazhenthi, S., Qin, L., & Reddy, P. H. (2016). Common neurodegenerative pathways in obesity, diabetes, and Alzheimer's disease. *Biochimica et Biophysica Acta*, pii: S0925-4439(16)30097-7. PubMed PMID: 27156888.

27. Steptoe, A., Hamer, M., & Chida, Y. (2007). The effects of acute psychological stress on circulating inflammatory factors in humans: A review and meta-analysis. *Brain, Behavior, and Immunity*, 21(7), 901–912. Review. PubMed PMID: 17475444.

28. Levesque, S., Surace, M. J., McDonald, J., & Block, M. L. (2011). Air pollution & the brain: Subchronic diesel exhaust exposure causes neuroinflammation and elevates early markers of neurodegenerative disease. *Journal of Neuroinflammation*, 8, 105. PubMed PMID: 21864400.

29. Monnet-Tschudi, F., Zurich, M. G., Boschat, C., Corbaz, A., & Honegger, P. (2006). Involvement of environmental mercury and lead in the etiology of neurodegenerative diseases. *Reviews on Environmental Health*, 21(2), 105–117. PubMed PMID: 16898674.

30. Banks, C. N., & Lein, P. J. (2012). A review of experimental evidence linking neurotoxic organophosphorus compounds and inflammation. *Neurotoxicology*, 33(3), 575–584. Review. PubMed PMID: 22342984.

31. Harris Interactive. (February 2011). *What America Thinks MetLife Foundation Alzheimer's Survey*. Available at https://www.metlife.com/assets/cao/foundation/alzheimers-2011.pdf. Accessed 16 November 2016.

32. Woodley, M. A., te Nijenhuis, J., & Murphy, R. (2013). Were the Victorians cleverer than us? The decline in general intelligence estimated from a meta-analysis of the slowing of simple reaction time. *Intelligence*, 41(4), 843–850.

33. Lynn, R., & Harvey, J. (2008). The decline of the world's IQ. *Intelligence*, 36, 112–120.

34. Harari, R., Julvez, J., Murata, K., Barr, D., et al. (2010). Neurobehavioral deficits and increased blood pressure in school-age children prenatally exposed to pesticides. *Environmental Health Perspectives*, 118(6), 890–896. PubMed PMID: 20185383.

35. Doherty, B. T., Engel, S. M., Buckley, J. P., et al. (2016). Prenatal phthalate biomarker concentrations and performance on the Bayley Scales of Infant Development-II in a population of young urban children. *Environmental Research*, 152, 51–58. PubMed PMID: 27741448.

36. Factor-Litvak, P., Insel, B., Calafat, A. M., et al. (2014). Persistent associations between maternal prenatal exposure to phthalates on child IQ at age 7 years. *PLoS ONE*, 9(12), e114003. PubMed PMID: 25493564.

37. Jedrychowski, W. A., Perera, F. P., Camann, D., et al. (2015). Prenatal exposure to polycyclic aromatic hydrocarbons and cognitive dysfunction in children. *Environmental Science and Pollution Research International*, 22(5), 3631–3639. PubMed PMID: 25253062.

38. Oken, E., Radesky, J. S., Wright, R. O., et al. (2008). Maternal fish intake during pregnancy, blood mercury levels, and child cognition at age 3 years in a US cohort. *American Journal of Epidemiology*, 167(10), 1171–1181. PubMed PMID: 18353804.

39. Jacobson, J. L., Muckle, G., Ayotte, P., et al. (2015). Relation of prenatal methylmercury exposure from environmental sources to childhood IQ. *Environmental Health Perspectives*, 123(8), 827–833. PubMed PMID:25757069.

40. Eriksson, P., & Fredriksson, A. (1998). Neurotoxic effects in adult mice neonatally exposed to 3,3′4,4″5-pentachlorobiphenyl or 2,3,3′4,4′-pentachlorobiphenyl. Changes in brain nicotinic receptors and behaviour. *Environmental Toxicology and Pharmacology*, 5, 17–27.

41. Jacobson, S., Fein, G., Jacobson, J., Schwartz, P., & Dowler, J. (1985). The effect of intrauterine PCB exposure on visual recognition memory. *Child Development*, 56, 853–860.

42. Walkowiak, J., Wiener, J. A., Fastabend, A., et al. (2001). Environmental exposure to polychlorinated biphenyls and quality of the home environment: Effects on psychodevelopment in early childhood. *Lancet*, 358, 1602–1607.

43. Jacobson, J. L., & Jacobson, S. W. (1997). Evidence for PCBs as neurodevelopmental toxicant in humans. *Neurotoxicology*, 18(2), 415–424.

44. Jacobson, J. L., & Jacobson, S. W. (2003). Prenatal exposure to polychlorinated biphenyls and attention at school age. *The Journal of Pediatrics*, 143(6), 780–788.

45. Chen, Y.-C. J., Guo, Y.-L., Hsu, C.-C., & Rogan, W. J. (1992). Cognitive development of Yu-Cheng ('Oil disease') children prenatally exposed to heat-degraded PCBs. *JAMA: The Journal of the American Medical Association*, 268(22), 3213–3218.

46. Chen, Y.-C. J., Yu, M.-L. M., Rogan, W. J., et al. (1994). A 6-year follow-up of behavior and activity disorders in the Taiwan Yu-Cheng children. *American Journal of Public Health*, 84(3), 415–421.

47. Lai, T.-J., Liu, X., Guo, Y. L., et al. (2002). A cohort study of behavior problems and intelligence in children with high prenatal polychlorinated biphenyl

exposure. *Archives of General Psychiatry, 59*(11), 1061–1066.

48. Plusquellec, P., Muckle, G., Dewailly, E., et al. (2010). The relation of environmental contaminants exposure to behavioral indicators in Inuit preschoolers in Arctic Quebec. *Neurotoxicology, 31*(1), 17–25.

49. Suzuki, K., Nakai, K., Sugawara, T., et al. (2010). Neurobehavioral effects of prenatal exposure to methylmercury and PCBs, and seafood intake: Neonatal behavioral assessment scale results of Tohoku study of child development. *Environmental Research, 110*(7), 699–704. PubMed PMID: 20673887.

50. Antunes, P., Amado, J., Vale, C., & Gil, O. (2007). Influence of the chemical structure on mobility of PCB congeners in female and male sardine (Sardina pilchardus) from Portuguese coast. *Chemosphere, 69*(3), 395–402. PubMed PMID: 17573094.

51. Hamilton, M. C., Hites, R. A., Schwager, S. J., et al. (2005). Lipid composition and contaminants in farmed and wild salmon. *Environmental Science & Technology, 39*(22), 8622–8629. PubMed PMID: 16323755.

52. Sagiv, S. K., Thurston, S. W., Bellinger, D. C., et al. (2012). Neuropsychological measures of attention and impulse control among 8-year-old children exposed prenatally to organochlorines. *Environmental Health Perspectives, 120*(6), 904–909. PubMed PMID: 22357172.

53. Basagaña, X., Esnaola, M., Rivas, I., et al. (2016). Neurodevelopmental deceleration by urban fine particles from different emission sources: A longitudinal observational study. *Environmental Health Perspectives, 124*(10), 1630–1636. PubMed PMID: 27128166.

54. Calderón-Garcidueñas, L., Mora-Tiscareño, A., Ontiveros, E., et al. (2008). Air pollution, cognitive deficits and brain abnormalities: A pilot study with children and dogs. *Brain and Cognition, 68*(2), 117–127. PubMed PMID: 18550243.

55. Calderón-Garcidueñas, L., Villarreal-Calderon, R., Valencia-Salazar, G., et al. (2008). Systemic inflammation, endothelial dysfunction, and activation in clinically healthy children exposed to air pollutants. *Inhalation Toxicology, 20*(5), 499–506. PubMed PMID: 18368620.

56. Power, M. C., Weisskopf, M. G., Alexeeff, S. E., et al. (2011). Traffic-related air pollution and cognitive function in a cohort of older men. *Environmental Health Perspectives, 119*(5), 682–687. PubMed PMID: 21172758.

57. Weuve, J., Puett, R. C., Schwartz, J., et al. (2012). Exposure to particulate air pollution and cognitive decline in older women. *Archives of Internal Medicine, 172*(3), 219–227. doi:10.1001/archinternmed.2011.683. PubMed PMID: 22332151.

58. Canfield, R. L., Henderson, C. R., Jr., Cory-Slechta, D. A., et al. (2003). Intellectual impairment in children with blood lead concentrations below 10 microg per deciliter. *The New England Journal of Medicine, 348*(16), 1517–1526. PubMed PMID:12700371.

59. Jusko, T. A., Henderson, C. R., Lanphear, B. P., et al. (2008). Blood lead concentrations < 10 microg/dL and child intelligence at 6 years of age. *Environmental Health Perspectives, 116*(2), 243–248. PubMed PMID: 18288325.

60. Lanphear, B. P., Hornung, R., Khoury, J., et al. (2005). Low-level environmental lead exposure and children's intellectual function: An international pooled analysis. *Environmental Health Perspectives, 113*(7), 894–899. PubMed PMID: 16002379.

61. Lucchini, R. G., Zoni, S., Guazzetti, S., et al. (2012). Inverse association of intellectual function with very low blood lead but not with manganese exposure in Italian adolescents. *Environmental Research, 118*, 65–71. PubMed PMID: 22925625.

62. Miranda, M. L., Kim, D., Galeano, M. A., et al. (2007). The relationship between early childhood blood lead levels and performance on end-of-grade tests. *Environmental Health Perspectives, 115*(8), 1242–1247. PubMed PMID: 17687454.

63. Blackowicz, M. J., Hryhorczuk, D. O., Rankin, K. M., et al. (2016). The impact of low-level lead toxicity on school performance among Hispanic subgroups in the Chicago public schools. *International Journal of Environmental Research and Public Health, 13*(8), PubMed PMID: 27490560.

64. Mazumdar, M., Bellinger, D. C., Gregas, M., et al. (2011). Low-level environmental lead exposure in childhood and adult intellectual function: A follow-up study. *Environmental Health: A Global Access Science Source, 10*, 24. PubMed PMID: 21450073.

65. Shih, R. A., Glass, T. A., Bandeen-Roche, K., et al. (2006). Environmental lead exposure and cognitive function in community-dwelling older adults. *Neurology, 67*(9), 1556–1562. PubMed PMID: 16971698.

66. van Wijngaarden, E., Winters, P. C., & Cory-Slechta, D. A. (2011). Blood lead levels in relation to cognitive function in older U.S. adults. *Neurotoxicology, 32*(1), 110–115. PubMed PMID: 21093481.

67. Bandeen-Roche, K., Glass, T. A., Bolla, K. I., et al. (2009). Cumulative lead dose and cognitive function in older adults. *Epidemiology (Cambridge, Mass.), 20*(6), 831–839. PubMed PMID: 19752734.

68. Power, M. C., Korrick, S., Tchetgen, E. J., et al. (2014). Lead exposure and rate of change in cognitive function in older women. *Environmental Research*, *129*, 69–75. PubMed PMID: 24529005.

69. Wright, R. O., Tsaih, S. W., Schwartz, J., Spiro, A., 3rd, McDonald, K., Weiss, S. T., et al. (2003). Lead exposure biomarkers and mini-mental status exam scores in older men. *Epidemiology (Cambridge, Mass.)*, *14*(6), 713–718. PubMed PMID: 14569188.

70. Eum, K. D., Wang, F. T., Schwartz, J., et al. (2013). Modifying roles of glutathione S-transferase polymorphisms on the association between cumulative lead exposure and cognitive function. *Neurotoxicology*, *39*, 65–71. PubMed PMID: 2395864.

71. Dorsey, C. D., Lee, B. K., Bolla, K. I., et al. (2006). Comparison of patella lead with blood lead and tibia lead and their associations with neurobehavioral test scores. *Journal of Occupational and Environmental Medicine*, *48*(5), 489–496. PubMed PMID: 16688005.

72. Krieg, E. F., Jr., Chrislip, D. W., Crespo, C. J., et al. (2005). The relationship between blood lead levels and neurobehavioral test performance in NHANES III and related occupational studies. *Public Health Reports*, *120*(3), 240–251. PubMed PMID: 16134563.

73. Kippler, M., Tofail, F., Hamadani, J. D., et al. (2012). Early-life cadmium exposure and child development in 5-year-old girls and boys: A cohort study in rural Bangladesh. *Environmental Health Perspectives*, *120*(10), 1462–1468. PubMed PMID: 22759600.

74. Ciesielski, T., Weuve, J., Bellinger, D. C., et al. (2012). Cadmium exposure and neurodevelopmental outcomes in U.S. children. *Environmental Health Perspectives*, *120*(5), 758–763. PubMed PMID: 22289429.

75. Ciesielski, T., Bellinger, D. C., Schwartz, J., et al. (2013). Associations between cadmium exposure and neurocognitive test scores in a cross-sectional study of US adults. *Environmental Health: A Global Access Science Source*, *12*, 13. PubMed PMID: 23379984.

76. Grandjean, P., Weihe, P., Debes, F., et al. (2014). Neurotoxicity from prenatal and postnatal exposure to methylmercury. *Neurotoxicology and Teratology*, *43*, 39–44. PubMed PMID: 24681285.

77. Grandjean, P., White, R. F., Nielsen, A., Cleary, D., & de Oliveira Santos, E. C. (1999). Methylmercury neurotoxicity in Amazonian children downstream from gold mining. *Environmental Health Perspectives*, *107*(7), 587–591. PubMed PMID: 10379006.

78. Ngim, C. H., Foo, S. C., Boey, K. W., & Jeyaratnam, J. (1992). Chronic neurobehavioral effects of elemental mercury in dentists. *British Journal of Industrial Medicine*, *49*, 782–790. PubMed PMID: 1463679.

79. Echeverria, D., Woods, J. S., Heyer, N. J., et al. (2006). The association between a genetic polymorphism of coproporphyrinogen oxidase, dental mercury exposure and neurobehavioral response in humans. *Neurotoxicology and Teratology*, *28*(1), 39–48. Epub 2005 Dec 15. PubMed PMID: 16343843.

80. Masley, S. C., Masley, L. V., & Gaultieri, C. T. (2012). Effect of mercury levels and seafood intake on cognitive function in middle-aged adults. *Integrated Medicine*, *11*(3), 32–39.

81. Weil, M., Bressler, J., Parsons, P., et al. (2005). Blood mercury levels and neurobehavioral function. *JAMA: The Journal of the American Medical Association*, *293*(15), 1875–1882. PubMed PMID: 15840862.

82. O'Bryant, S. E., Edwards, M., Menon, C. V., et al. (2011). Long-term low-level arsenic exposure is associated with poorer neuropsychological functioning: A Project FRONTIER study. *International Journal of Environmental Research and Public Health*, *8*(3), 861–874. PubMed PMID: 21556183.

83. Schantz, S., Gasior, D., Polverejan, E., et al. (2001). Impairments of memory and learning in older adults exposed to polychlorinated biphenyls via consumption of Great Lakes fish. *Environmental Health Perspectives*, *109*(6), 605–611.

84. Kilburn, K. H. (2000). Visual and neurobehavioral impairment associated with polychlorinated biphenyls. *Neurotoxicology*, *21*(4), 489–500.

85. Moussavi, S., Chatterji, S., Verdes, E., et al. (2007). Depression, chronic diseases, and decrements in health: Results from the World Health Surveys. *Lancet*, *370*(9590), 851–858. PubMed PMID: 17826170.

86. Anisman, H., & Hayley, S. (2012). Inflammatory factors contribute to depression and its comorbid conditions. *Science Signaling*, *5*(244), pe45. PubMed PMID: 23033537.

87. Kim, K. N., Lim, Y. H., Bae, H. J., et al. (2016). Long-term fine particulate matter exposure and major depressive disorder in a community-based urban cohort. *Environmental Health Perspectives*, *124*(10), 1547–1553. PubMed PMID: 27129131.

88. Lim, Y. H., Kim, H., Kim, J. H., et al. (2012). Air pollution and symptoms of depression in elderly adults. *Environmental Health Perspectives*, *120*(7), 1023–1028. PubMed PMID: 22514209.

89. Szyszkowicz, M., Willey, J. B., Grafstein, E., Rowe, B. H., & Colman, I. (2010). Air pollution and emergency department visits for suicide attempts in vancouver, Canada. *Environmental Health Insights [Electronic Resource]*, *4*, 79–86. PubMed PMID: 21079694.

90. Kim, C., Jung, S. H., Kang, D. R., et al. (2010). Ambient particulate matter as a risk factor for suicide. *The*

American Journal of Psychiatry, 167(9), 1100–1107. PubMed PMID: 20634364.

91. Beseler, C. L., Stallones, L., Hoppin, J. A., et al. (2008). Depression and pesticide exposures among private pesticide applicators enrolled in the Agricultural Health Study. *Environmental Health Perspectives, 116*(12), 1713–1719. doi:10.1289/ehp.11091. PubMed PMID: 19079725.

92. Beseler, C. L., & Stallones, L. (2008). A cohort study of pesticide poisoning and depression in Colorado farm residents. *Annals of Epidemiology, 18*(10), 768–774. PubMed PMID: 18693039.

93. Beard, J. D., Umbach, D. M., Hoppin, J. A., et al. (2014). Pesticide exposure and depression among male private pesticide applicators in the agricultural health study. *Environmental Health Perspectives, 122*(9), 984–991. PubMed PMID: 24906048.

94. Bortolasci, C. C., Vargas, H. O., Souza-Nogueira, A., et al. (2014). Lowered plasma paraoxonase (PON)1 activity is a trait marker of major depression and PON1 Q192R gene polymorphism-smoking interactions differentially predict the odds of major depression and bipolar disorder. *Journal of Affective Disorders, 159*, 23–30. PubMed PMID: 24679385.

95. Costa, L. G., Giordano, G., Cole, T. B., et al. (2013). Paraoxonase 1 (PON1) as a genetic determinant of susceptibility to organophosphate toxicity. *Toxicology, 307*, 115–122. PubMed PMID: 22884923.

96. Lee, B. W., London, L., Paulauskis, J., Myers, J., & Christiani, D. C. (2003). Association between human paraoxonase gene polymorphism and chronic symptoms in pesticide-exposed workers. *Journal of Occupational and Environmental Medicine, 45*(2), 118–122. PubMed PMID: 12625227.

97. Kim, K. N., Choi, Y. H., Lim, Y. H., & Hong, Y. C. (2016). Urinary phthalate metabolites and depression in an elderly population: National Health and Nutrition Examination Survey 2005-2012. *Environmental Research, 145*, 61–67. PubMed PMID: 26624239.

98. Bouchard, M. F., Bellinger, D. C., Weuve, J., et al. (2009). Blood lead levels and major depressive disorder, panic disorder, and generalized anxiety disorder in US young adults. *Archives of General Psychiatry, 66*(12), 1313–1319. PubMed PMID: 19996036.

99. Eum, K. D., Korrick, S. A., Weuve, J., et al. (2012). Relation of cumulative low-level lead exposure to depressive and phobic anxiety symptom scores in middle-age and elderly women. *Environmental Health Perspectives, 120*(6), 817–823. PubMed PMID: 22538241.

100. Berk, M., Williams, L. J., Andreazza, A. C., et al. (2014). Pop, heavy metal and the blues: Secondary analysis of persistent organic pollutants (POP), heavy metals and depressive symptoms in the NHANES National Epidemiological Survey. *BMJ Open, 4*(7), e005142. PubMed PMID: 25037643.

101. Centers for Disease Control and Prevention. *State-based Prevalence Data of Parent Reported ADHD Diagnosis by a Health Care Provider.* Available at http://www.cdc.gov/ncbddd/adhd/prevalence.html. (Accessed 21 November 2016).

102. Costello, E. J., Mustillo, S., Erkanli, A., et al. (2003). Prevalence and development of psychiatric disorders in childhood and adolescence. *Archives of General Psychiatry, 60*(8), 837–844. PubMed PMID: 12912767.

103. Barkley, R. A. (2002). Major life activity and health outcomes associated with attention-deficit/hyperactivity disorder. *The Journal of Clinical Psychiatry, 63*(Suppl. 12), 10–15. Review. PubMed PMID: 12562056.

104. Sagiv, S. K., Thurston, S. W., Bellinger, D. C., et al. (2010). Prenatal organochlorine exposure and behaviors associated with attention deficit hyperactivity disorder in school-aged children. *American Journal of Epidemiology, 171*(5), 593–601. PubMed PMID: 20106937.

105. Braun, J. M., Kahn, R. S., Froehlich, T., et al. (2006). Exposures to environmental toxicants and attention deficit hyperactivity disorder in U.S. children. *Environmental Health Perspectives, 114*(12), 1904–1909. PubMed PMID: 17185283.

106. Wang, H. L., Chen, X. T., Yang, B., et al. (2008). Case-control study of blood lead levels and attention deficit hyperactivity disorder in Chinese children. *Environmental Health Perspectives, 116*(10), 1401–1406. PubMed PMID: 18941585.

107. Desrosiers, C., Boucher, O., Forget-Dubois, N., et al. (2013). Associations between prenatal cigarette smoke exposure and externalized behaviors at school age among Inuit children exposed to environmental contaminants. *Neurotoxicology and Teratology, 39*, 84–90. PubMed PMID: 23916943.

108. Kovess, V., Keyes, K. M., Hamilton, A., et al. (2015). Maternal smoking and offspring inattention and hyperactivity: Results from a cross-national European survey. *European Child and Adolescent Psychiatry, 24*(8), 919–929. PubMed PMID: 25413602.

109. Han, J. Y., Kwon, H. J., Ha, M., et al. (2015). The effects of prenatal exposure to alcohol and environmental tobacco smoke on risk for ADHD: A large population-based study. *Psychiatry Research, 225*(1–2), 164–168. PubMed PMID: 25481018.

110. Perera, F. P., Tang, D., Wang, S., et al. (2012). Prenatal polycyclic aromatic hydrocarbon (PAH) exposure and child behavior at age 6-7 years. *Environmental Health Perspectives*, *120*(6), 921–926. PubMed PMID: 22440811.

111. Yorifuji, T., Kashima, S., Diez, M. H., et al. (2016). Prenatal exposure to outdoor air pollution and child behavioral problems at school age in Japan. *Environment International*, pii: S0160-4120(16)30811-X. PubMed PMID: 27890345.

112. Lien, Y. J., Ku, H. Y., Su, P. H., et al. (2015). Prenatal exposure to phthalate esters and behavioral syndromes in children at 8 years of age: Taiwan Maternal and Infant Cohort Study. *Environmental Health Perspectives*, *123*(1), 95–100. PubMed PMID: 25280125.

113. Choi, W. J., Kwon, H. J., Lim, M. H., et al. (2016). Blood lead, parental marital status and the risk of attention-deficit/hyperactivity disorder in elementary school children: A longitudinal study. *Psychiatry Research*, *236*, 42–46. PubMed PMID: 26774190.

114. Hong, S. B., Im, M. H., Kim, J. W., et al. (2015). Environmental lead exposure and attention deficit/hyperactivity disorder symptom domains in a community sample of South Korean school-age children. *Environmental Health Perspectives*, *123*(3), 271–276. PubMed PMID: 25280233.

115. Kim, S., Arora, M., Fernandez, C., et al. (2013). Lead, mercury, and cadmium exposure and attention deficit hyperactivity disorder in children. *Environmental Research*, *126*, 105–110. PubMed PMID: 24034783.

116. Goodlad, J. K., Marcus, D. K., & Fulton, J. J. (2013). Lead and Attention-Deficit/Hyperactivity Disorder (ADHD) symptoms: A meta-analysis. *Clinical Psychology Review*, *33*(3), 417–425. PubMed PMID: 23419800.

117. Boucher, O., Jacobson, S. W., Plusquellec, P., et al. (2012). Prenatal methylmercury, postnatal lead exposure, and evidence of attention deficit/hyperactivity disorder among Inuit children in Arctic Québec. *Environmental Health Perspectives*, *120*(10), 1456–1461. PubMed PMID: 23008274.

118. Sagiv, S. K., Thurston, S. W., Bellinger, D. C., et al. (2012). Prenatal exposure to mercury and fish consumption during pregnancy and attention-deficit/hyperactivity disorder-related behavior in children. *Archives of Pediatrics and Adolescent Medicine*, *166*(12), 1123–1131. PubMed PMID: 23044994.

119. Talts, U., Fredriksson, A., & Eriksson, P. (1998). Changes in behavior and muscarinic receptor density after neonatal and adult exposure to bioallethrin. *Neurobiology of Aging*, *19*(6), 545–552. PubMed PMID: 10192213.

120. Richardson, J. R., Taylor, M. M., Shalat, S. L., et al. (2015). Developmental pesticide exposure reproduces features of attention deficit hyperactivity disorder. *FASEB Journal: Official Publication of the Federation of American Societies for Experimental Biology*, *29*(5), 1960–1972. PubMed PMID: 25630971.

121. uirós-Alcalá, L., Mehta, S., & Eskenazi, B. (2014). Pyrethroid pesticide exposure and parental report of learning disability and attention deficit/hyperactivity disorder in U.S. children: NHANES 1999-2002. *Environmental Health Perspectives*, *122*(12), 1336–1342. PubMed PMID: 25192380.

122. Oulhote, Y., & Bouchard, M. F. (2013). Urinary metabolites of organophosphate and pyrethroid pesticides and behavioral problems in Canadian children. *Environmental Health Perspectives*, *121*(11–12), 1378–1384. PubMed PMID: 24149046.

123. Bouchard, M. F., Bellinger, D. C., Wright, R. O., & Weisskopf, M. G. (2010). Attention-deficit/hyperactivity disorder and urinary metabolites of organophosphate pesticides. *Pediatrics*, *125*(6), e1270–e1277. PubMed PMID: 20478945.

124. Garry, V. F., Harkins, M. E., Erickson, L. L., et al. (2002). Birth defects, season of conception, and sex of children born to pesticide applicators living in the Red River Valley of Minnesota, USA. *Environmental Health Perspectives*, *110*(Suppl. 3), 441–449. PubMed PMID: 12060842.

125. Newman, N. C., Ryan, P., Lemasters, G., et al. (2013). Traffic-related air pollution exposure in the first year of life and behavioral scores at 7 years of age. *Environmental Health Perspectives*, *121*(6), 731–736. PubMed PMID: 23694812.

126. Costa, L. G., Cole, T. B., Coburn, J., et al. (2014). Neurotoxicants are in the air: Convergence of human, animal, and in vitro studies on the effects of air pollution on the brain. *BioMed Research International*, *2014*, 736385. PubMed PMID: 24524086.

127. Hallmayer, J., Cleveland, S., Torres, A., et al. (2011). Genetic heritability and shared environmental factors among twin pairs with autism. *Archives of General Psychiatry*, *68*(11), 1095–1102. PubMed PMID: 21727249.

128. Andersson, M. J., Andersson, L., Bende, M., et al. (2009). The idiopathic environmental intolerance symptom inventory: Development, evaluation, and application. *Journal of Occupational and Environmental Medicine*, *51*(7), 838–847. PubMed PMID: 19542897.

129. Heilbrun, L. P., Palmer, R. F., Jaen, C. R., et al. (2015). Maternal chemical and drug intolerances: potential risk factors for autism and attention deficit hyperactivity disorder (ADHD). *Journal of the American Board of*

Family Medicine: JABFM, 28(4), 461–470. PubMed PMID: 26152436.

130. McCanlies, E. C., Fekedulegn, D., Mnatsakanova, A., et al. (2012). Parental occupational exposures and autism spectrum disorder. *Journal of Autism and Developmental Disorders, 42*(11), 2323–2334. PubMed PMID: 22399411.

131. Windham, G. C., Sumner, A., Li, S. X., et al. (2013). Use of birth certificates to examine maternal occupational exposures and autism spectrum disorders in offspring. *Autism Research: Official Journal of the International Society for Autism Research, 6*(1), 57–63. PubMed PMID: 23361991.

132. Kim, S. M., Han, D. H., Lyoo, H. S., et al. (2010). Exposure to environmental toxins in mothers of children with autism spectrum disorder. *Psychiatry Investigation, 7*(2), 122–127. PubMed PMID: 20577621.

133. Kalkbrenner, A. E., Daniels, J. L., Chen, J. C., et al. (2010). Perinatal exposure to hazardous air pollutants and autism spectrum disorders at age 8. *Epidemiology (Cambridge, Mass.), 21*(5), 631–641. PubMed PMID: 20562626.

134. Volk, H. E., Hertz-Picciotto, I., Delwiche, L., et al. (2011). Residential proximity to freeways and autism in the CHARGE study. *Environmental Health Perspectives, 119*(6), 873–877. PubMed PMID: 21156395.

135. Volk, H. E., Lurmann, F., Penfold, B., et al. (2013). Traffic-related air pollution, particulate matter, and autism. *JAMA Psychiatry, 70*(1), 71–77. PubMed PMID: 23404082.

136. Becerra, T. A., Wilhelm, M., Olsen, J., et al. (2013). Ambient air pollution and autism in Los Angeles county, California. *Environmental Health Perspectives, 121*(3), 380–386. PubMed PMID: 23249813.

137. Roberts, A. L., Lyall, K., Hart, J. E., et al. (2013). Perinatal air pollutant exposures and autism spectrum disorder in the children of Nurses' Health Study II participants. *Environmental Health Perspectives, 121*(8), 978–984. Erratum in: Environ Health Perspect. 2014 Jun;122(6):A152. PubMed PMID: 23816781.

138. Raz, R., Roberts, A. L., Lyall, K., et al. (2015). Autism spectrum disorder and particulate matter air pollution before, during, and after pregnancy: A nested case-control analysis within the Nurses' Health Study II Cohort. *Environmental Health Perspectives, 123*(3), 264–270. PubMed PMID: 25522338.

139. Lyall, K., Croen, L. A., Sjödin, A., et al. (2017). Polychlorinated biphenyl and organochlorine pesticide concentrations in maternal mid-pregnancy serum samples: Association with autism spectrum disorder and intellectual disability. *Environmental

Health Perspectives, 125*(3), 474–480. PubMed PMID: 27548254.

140. Miodovnik, A., Engel, S. M., Zhu, C., et al. (2011). Endocrine disruptors and childhood social impairment. *Neurotoxicology, 32*(2), 261–267. PubMed PMID: 21182865.

141. Eskenazi, B., Marks, A. R., Bradman, A., et al. (2007). Organophosphate pesticide exposure and neurodevelopment in young Mexican-American children. *Environmental Health Perspectives, 115*(5), 792–798. PubMed PMID: 17520070.

142. Bradman, A., Castorina, R., Barr, D. B., et al. (2011). Determinants of organophosphorus pesticide urinary metabolite levels in young children living in an agricultural community. *International Journal of Environmental Research and Public Health, 8*(4), 1061–1083. PubMed PMID: 21695029.

143. Larsson, M., Weiss, B., Janson, S., et al. (2009). Associations between indoor environmental factors and parental-reported autistic spectrum disorders in children 6-8 years of age. *Neurotoxicology, 30*(5), 822–831. PubMed PMID: 19822263.

144. Windham, G. C., Zhang, L., Gunier, R., et al. (2006). Autism spectrum disorders in relation to distribution of hazardous air pollutants in the San Francisco bay area. *Environmental Health Perspectives, 114*(9), 1438–1444. PubMed PMID: 16966102.

145. Jung, C. R., Lin, Y. T., & Hwang, B. F. (2013). Air pollution and newly diagnostic autism spectrum disorders: A population-based cohort study in Taiwan. *PLoS ONE, 8*(9), e75510. PubMed PMID: 24086549.

146. Boggess, A., Faber, S., Kern, J., & Kingston, H. M. (2016). Mean serum-level of common organic pollutants is predictive of behavioral severity in children with autism spectrum disorders. *Scientific Reports, 6,* 26185. PubMed PMID: 27174041.

147. Xu, J., Murphy, S. L., Kochanek, K. D., & Arias, E. (2016). Mortality in the United States, 2015. *NCHS Data Brief,* (267), 1–8. PubMed PMID: 27930283.

148. Prince, M., Wimo, A., Guerchet, M., et al. *World Alzheimer Report 2015. The Global Impact of Dementia: An Analysis of Prevalence, Incidence, Cost and Trends. Alzheimer's Disease International.* https://www.alz.co.uk/research/WorldAlzheimerReport2015.pdf. (Accessed 8 December 2016).

149. Bronzuoli, M. R., Iacomino, A., Steardo, L., & Scuderi, C. (2016). Targeting neuroinflammation in Alzheimer's disease. *Journal of Inflammation Research [Electronic Resource], 9,* 199–208. PubMed PMID: 27843334.

150. Zhao, Y., & Zhao, B. (2013). Oxidative stress and the pathogenesis of Alzheimer's disease. *Oxidative

Medicine and Cellular Longevity, 2013, 316523. doi:10.1155/2013/316523. Review. PubMed PMID: 23983897.

151. Picone, P., Nuzzo, D., Caruana, L., et al. (2014). Mitochondrial dysfunction: Different routes to Alzheimer's disease therapy. *Oxidative Medicine and Cellular Longevity, 2014*, 780179. PubMed PMID:25221640.

152. Calderón-Garcidueñas, L., Reed, W., Maronpot, R. R., Henríquez-Roldán, C., et al. (2004). Brain inflammation and Alzheimer's-like pathology in individuals exposed to severe air pollution. *Toxicologic Pathology, 32*(6), 650–658. PubMed PMID: 15513908.

153. Calderón-Garcidueñas, L., Avila-Ramírez, J., Calderón-Garcidueñas, A., et al. (2016). Cerebrospinal fluid biomarkers in highly exposed PM2.5 urbanites: The risk of Alzheimer's and Parkinson's diseases in young Mexico City residents. *Journal of Alzheimer's Disease, 54*(2), 597–613. PubMed PMID: 27567860.

154. Calderón-Garcidueñas, L., Mora-Tiscareño, A., Franco-Lira, M., et al. (2015). Decreases in short term memory, IQ, and altered brain metabolic ratios in urban apolipoprotein ε4 children exposed to air pollution. *Journal of Alzheimer's Disease, 45*(3), 757–770. doi:10.3233/JAD-142685. PubMed PMID: 25633678.

155. Calderón-Garcidueñas, L., Vojdani, A., Blaurock-Busch, E., Busch, Y., et al. (2015). Air pollution and children: Neural and tight junction antibodies and combustion metals, the role of barrier breakdown and brain immunity in neurodegeneration. *Journal of Alzheimer's Disease, 43*(3), 1039–1058. PubMed PMID: 25147109.

156. Calderón-Garcidueñas, L., Mora-Tiscareño, A., Franco-Lira, M., et al. (2013). Flavonol-rich dark cocoa significantly decreases plasma endothelin-1 and improves cognition in urban children. *Frontiers in Pharmacology, 4*, 104. PubMed PMID: 23986703.

157. Jung, C. R., Lin, Y. T., & Hwang, B. F. (2015). Ozone, particulate matter, and newly diagnosed Alzheimer's disease: A population-based cohort study in Taiwan. *Journal of Alzheimer's Disease: JAD, 44*(2), 573–584. PubMed PMID: 25310992.

158. Parrón, T., Requena, M., Hernández, A. F., & Alarcón, R. (2011). Association between environmental exposure to pesticides and neurodegenerative diseases. *Toxicology and Applied Pharmacology, 256*(3), 379–385. PubMed PMID: 21601587.

159. Gauthier, E., Fortier, I., Courchesne, F., et al. (2001). Environmental pesticide exposure as a risk factor for Alzheimer's disease: A case-control study. *Environmental Research, 86*(1), 37–45. PubMed PMID: 11386739.

160. Baldi, I., Lebailly, P., Mohammed-Brahim, B., et al. (2003). Neurodegenerative diseases and exposure to pesticides in the elderly. *American Journal of Epidemiology, 157*(5), 409–414. PubMed PMID: 12615605.

161. Hayden, K. M., Norton, M. C., Darcey, D., Cache County Study Investigators, et al. (2010). Occupational exposure to pesticides increases the risk of incident AD: The Cache County study. *Neurology, 74*(19), 1524–1530. PubMed PMID: 20458069.

162. Richardson, J. R., Roy, A., Shalat, S. L., et al. (2014). Elevated serum pesticide levels and risk for Alzheimer disease. *JAMA Neurology, 71*(3), 284–290. PubMed PMID: 24473795.

163. Singh, N., Chhillar, N., Banerjee, B., et al. (2013). Organochlorine pesticide levels and risk of Alzheimer's disease in north Indian population. *Human and Experimental Toxicology, 32*(1), 24–30. doi:10.1177/0960327112456315. PubMed PMID: 22899726.

164. Dauer, W., & Przedborski, S. (2003). Parkinson's disease: Mechanisms and models. *Neuron, 39*(6), 889–909. Review. PubMed PMID: 12971891.

165. Abeliovich, A., & Flint Beal, M. (2006). Parkinsonism genes: Culprits and clues. *Journal of Neurochemistry, 99*(4), 1062–1072. PubMed PMID: 16836655.

166. Hopes, L., Grolez, G., Moreau, C., et al. (2016). Magnetic resonance imaging features of the nigrostriatal system: Biomarkers of Parkinson's disease stages? *PLoS ONE, 11*(4), e0147947. PubMed PMID: 27035571.

167. Bolner, A., Micciolo, R., Bosello, O., & Nordera, G. P. (2016). A panel of oxidative stress markers in Parkinson's disease. *Clinical Laboratory, 62*(1–2), 105–112. PubMed PMID: 27012039.

168. Grünewald, A., Rygiel, K. A., Hepplewhite, P. D., et al. (2016). Mitochondrial DNA depletion in respiratory chain-deficient Parkinson disease neurons. *Annals of Neurology, 79*(3), 366–378. doi:10.1002/ana.24571. PubMed PMID: 26605748.

169. Schapira, A. H., Cooper, J. M., Dexter, D., et al. (1990). Mitochondrial complex I deficiency in Parkinson's disease. *Journal of Neurochemistry, 54*(3), 823–827. PubMed PMID: 2154550.

170. Alam, Q., Alam, M. Z., Mushtaq, G., et al. (2016). Inflammatory process in Alzheimer's and Parkinson's diseases: Central role of cytokines. *Current Pharmaceutical Design, 22*(5), 541–548. Review. PubMed PMID: 26601965.

171. Machado, V., Zöller, T., Attaai, A., & Spittau, B. (2016). Microglia-mediated neuroinflammation and neurotrophic factor–induced protection in the MPTP

mouse model of Parkinson's disease—lessons from transgenic mice. *International Journal of Molecular Sciences, 17*(2), pii:E151. PubMed PMID: 26821015.

172. Davis, G. C., Williams, A. C., Markey, S. P., et al. (1979). Chronic Parkinsonism secondary to intravenous injection of meperidine analoques. *Psychiatry Research, 1,* 249–254.

173. Langston, J. W., Ballard, P., Tetrud, J. W., & Irwin, I. (1983). Chronic Parkinsonism in humans due to a product of Meperidine-analog synthesis. *Science, 21,* 979–980.

174. Cleeter, M. W., Cooper, J. M., & Schapira, A. H. (1992). Irreversible inhibition of mitochondrial complex I by 1-methyl-4-phenylpyridinium: Evidence for free radical involvement. *Journal of Neurochemistry, 58*(2), 786–789. PubMed PMID: 1729421.

175. Liberatore, G. T., Jackson-Lewis, V., Vukosavic, S., et al. (1999). Inducible nitric oxide synthase stimulates dopaminergic neurodegeneration in the MPTP model of Parkinson disease. *Nature Medicine, 5*(12), 1403–1409. PubMed PMID: 10581083.

176. Perl, D. P., & Olanow, C. W. (2007). The neuropathology of manganese-induced Parkinsonism. *Journal of Neuropathology and Experimental Neurology, 66*(8), 675–682. Review. PubMed PMID: 17882011.

177. Gorell, J. M., Johnson, C. C., Rybicki, B. A., et al. (1998). The risk of Parkinson's disease with exposure to pesticides, farming, well water, and rural living. *Neurology, 50*(5), 1346–1350. PubMed PMID: 9595985.

178. Breckenridge, C. B., Berry, C., Chang, E. T., et al. (2016). Association between Parkinson's disease and cigarette smoking, rural living, well-water consumption, farming and pesticide use: Systematic review and meta-analysis. *PLoS ONE, 11*(4), e0151841. PubMed PMID: 27055126.

179. Ho, S. C., Woo, J., & Lee, C. M. (1989). Epidemiologic study of Parkinson's disease in Hong Kong. *Neurology, 39,* 1314–1318.

180. van der Mark, M., Brouwer, M., Kromhout, H., et al. (2012). Is pesticide use related to Parkinson disease? Some clues to heterogeneity in study results. *Environmental Health Perspectives, 120*(3), 340–347. PubMed PMID: 22389202.

181. Pezzoli, G., & Cereda, E. (2013). Exposure to pesticides or solvents and risk of Parkinson disease. *Neurology, 80*(22), 2035–2041. PubMed PMID: 23713084.

182. Goldman, S. M., Quinlan, P. J., Ross, G. W., et al. (2012). Solvent exposures and Parkinson disease risk in twins. *Annals of Neurology, 71*(6), 776–784. PubMed PMID: 22083847.

183. Narayan, S., Liew, Z., Paul, K., et al. (2013). Household organophosphorus pesticide use and Parkinson's disease. *International Journal of Epidemiology, 42*(5), 1476–1485. PubMed PMID: 24057998.

184. Lee, P. C., Rhodes, S. L., Sinsheimer, J. S., et al. (2013). Functional paraoxonase 1 variants modify the risk of Parkinson's disease due to organophosphate exposure. *Environment International, 56,* 42–47. PubMed PMID: 23602893.

185. Menegon, A., Board, P., Blackbum, A., et al. (1998). Parkinson's disease, pesticides and glutathione transferase polymorphisms. *Lancet, 352,* 1342–1346.

186. Stroombergen, M. C., & Waring, R. H. (1999). Determination of glutathione S-transferase mus and theta polymorphism in neurological disease. *Human and Experimental Toxicology, 18*(3), 141–145.

187. Coon, S., Stark, A., Peterson, E., et al. (2006). Whole-body lifetime occupational lead exposure and risk of Parkinson's disease. *Environmental Health Perspectives, 114*(12), 1872–1876. PubMed PMID: 17185278.

188. Weisskopf, M. G., Weuve, J., Nie, H., et al. (2010). Association of cumulative lead exposure with Parkinson's disease. *Environmental Health Perspectives, 118*(11), 1609–1613. PubMed PMID: 20807691.

189. Weuve, J., Press, D. Z., Grodstein, F., et al. (2013). Cumulative exposure to lead and cognition in persons with Parkinson's disease. *Movement Disorders: Official Journal of the Movement Disorder Society, 28*(2), 176–182. PubMed PMID: 23143985.

190. Ross, S. M., McManus, I. C., Harrison, V., & Mason, O. (2013). Neurobehavioral problems following low-level exposure to organophosphate pesticides: A systematic and meta-analytic review. *Critical Reviews in Toxicology, 43*(1), 21–44. PubMed PMID: 23163581.

191. Gualtieri, C. T., & Johnson, L. G. (2006). Reliability and validity of a computerized neurocognitive test battery, CNS Vital Signs. *Archives of Clinical Neuropsychology, 21*(7), 623–643. PubMed PMID: 17014981.

192. Niklasson, M., Möller, C., Odkvist, L. M., et al. (1997). Are deficits in the equilibrium system relevant to the clinical investigation of solvent-induced neurotoxicity? *Scandinavian Journal of Work, Environment and Health, 23*(3), 206–213. PubMed PMID: 9243731.

193. Zamyslowska-Szmytke, E., & Sliwinska-Kowalska, M. (2011). Vestibular and balance findings in nonsymptomatic workers exposed to styrene and dichloromethane. *International Journal of Audiology, 50*(11), 815–822. PubMed PMID: 21929376.

194. Pawlas, N., Broberg, K., Skerfving, S., & Pawlas, K. (2014). Disturbance of posture in children with very low lead exposure, and modification by VDR FokI

genotype. *Annals of Agricultural and Environmental Medicine*, 21(4), 739–744. PubMed PMID: 25528913.

195. Kilburn, K. H., Thrasher, J. D., & Gray, M. R. (2010). Low-level hydrogen sulfide and central nervous system dysfunction. *Toxicology and Industrial Health*, 26(7), 387–405. PubMed PMID: 20504829.

196. Kilburn, K. H. (2000). Visual and neurobehavioral impairment associated with polychlorinated biphenyls. *Neurotoxicology*, 21(4), 489–499. PubMed PMID: 11022858.

197. Kilburn, K. H. (2002). Is neurotoxicity associated with environmental trichloroethylene (TCE)? *Archives of Environmental Health*, 57(2), 113–120. PubMed PMID: 12194155.

198. Kilburn, K. H. (2004). Effects of onboard insecticide use on airline flight attendants. *Archives of Environmental Health*, 59(6), 284–291. PubMed PMID: 16238162.

199. Kilburn, K. H. (2009). Neurobehavioral and pulmonary impairment in 105 adults with indoor exposure to molds compared to 100 exposed to chemicals. *Toxicology and Industrial Health*, 25(9–10), 681–692. PubMed PMID: 19793776.

200. Killburn, K. H. (2000). Indoor air effects after building renovation and in manufactured homes. *The American Journal of the Medical Sciences*, 320(4), 249–254. PubMed PMID: 11061350.

201. Callender, T. J., Morrow, L., Subramanian, K., et al. (1993). Three-dimensional brain metabolic imaging in patients with toxic encephalopathy. *Environmental Research*, 60(2), 295–319. PubMed PMID: 8472660.

202. Gong, Y., Kishi, R., Kasai, S., et al. (2003). Visual dysfunction in workers exposed to a mixture of organic solvents. *Neurotoxicology*, 24(4–5), 703–710. PubMed PMID: 12900083.

203. Boeckelmann, I., & Pfister, E. A. (2003). Influence of occupational exposure to organic solvent mixtures on contrast sensitivity in printers. *Journal of Occupational and Environmental Medicine*, 45(1), 25–33. PubMed PMID: 12553176.

204. Till, C., Westall, C. A., Koren, G., Nulman, I., & Rovet, J. F. (2005). Vision abnormalities in young children exposed prenatally to organic solvents. *Neurotoxicology*, 26(4), 599–613. PubMed PMID: 16054697.

205. Moe, C. L., Turf, E., Oldach, D., et al. (2001). Cohort studies of health effects among people exposed to estuarine waters: North Carolina, Virginia, and Maryland. *Environmental Health Perspectives*, 109(Suppl. 5), 781–786. PubMed PMID: 11677189.

206. Allen, J. G., MacNaughton, P., Satish, U., et al. (2016). Associations of cognitive function scores with carbon dioxide, ventilation, and volatile organic compound exposures in office workers: A controlled exposure study of green and conventional office environments. *Environmental Health Perspectives*, 124(6), 805–812. PubMed PMID: 26502459.

207. McCarthy, M. C., Ludwig, J. F., Brown, S. G., et al. (2013). Filtration effectiveness of HVAC systems at near-roadway schools. *Indoor Air*, 23(3), 196–207. PubMed PMID: 23167831.

208. Sathyanarayana, S., Alcedo, G., Saelens, B. E., et al. (2013). Unexpected results in a randomized dietary trial to reduce phthalate and bisphenol A exposures. *Journal of Exposure Science and Environmental Epidemiology*, 23(4), 378–384. PubMed PMID: 23443238.

209. Lu, C., Barr, D. B., Pearson, M. A., & Waller, L. A. (2008). Dietary intake and its contribution to longitudinal organophosphorus pesticide exposure in urban/suburban children. *Environmental Health Perspectives*, 116(4), 537–542. PubMed PMID: 18414640.

210. Tully, P. J., Baumeister, H., Bengel, J., et al. (2015). The longitudinal association between inflammation and incident depressive symptoms in men: The effects of hs-CRP are independent of abdominal obesity and metabolic disturbances. *Physiology and Behavior*, 139, 328–335. PubMed PMID: 25460540.

211. Schwingshackl, L., & Hoffmann, G. (2014). Mediterranean dietary pattern, inflammation and endothelial function: A systematic review and meta-analysis of intervention trials. *Nutrition, Metabolism, and Cardiovascular Diseases*, 24(9), 929–939. PubMed PMID: 24787907.

212. Milaneschi, Y., Bandinelli, S., Penninx, B. W., et al. (2011). Depressive symptoms and inflammation increase in a prospective study of older adults: A protective effect of a healthy (Mediterranean-style) diet. *Molecular Psychiatry*, 16(6), 589–590. PubMed PMID: 21042319.

213. Rienks, J., Dobson, A. J., & Mishra, G. D. (2013). Mediterranean dietary pattern and prevalence and incidence of depressive symptoms in mid-aged women: Results from a large community-based prospective study. *European Journal of Clinical Nutrition*, 67(1), 75–82. PubMed PMID: 23212131.

214. Gardener, S., Gu, Y., Rainey-Smith, S. R., AIBL Research Group, et al. (2012). Adherence to a Mediterranean diet and Alzheimer's disease risk in an Australian population. *Translational Psychiatry [Electronic Resource]*, 2, e164. doi:10.1038/tp.2012.91. PubMed PMID: 23032941.

215. Singh, B., Parsaik, A. K., Mielke, M. M., et al. (2014). Association of Mediterranean diet with mild cognitive

impairment and Alzheimer's disease: A systematic review and meta-analysis. *Journal of Alzheimer's Disease, 39*(2), 271–282. PubMed PMID: 24164735.

216. Schwingshackl, L., Christoph, M., & Hoffmann, G. (2015). Effects of olive oil on markers of inflammation and endothelial function: A systematic review and meta-analysis. *Nutrients, 7*(9), 7651–7675. PubMed PMID: 26378571.

217. Martínez-Lapiscina, E. H., Clavero, P., Toledo, E., et al. (2013). Virgin olive oil supplementation and long-term cognition: The PREDIMED-NAVARRA randomized, trial. *The Journal of Nutrition, Health and Aging, 17*(6), 542–552. PubMed PMID: 23732551.

218. Pitozzi, V., Jacomelli, M., Catelan, D., et al. (2012). Long-term dietary extra-virgin olive oil rich in polyphenols reverses age-related dysfunctions in motor coordination and contextual memory in mice: Role of oxidative stress. *Rejuvenation Research, 15*(6), 601–612. PubMed PMID: 22950431.

219. Miyake, Y., Fukushima, W., Tanaka, K., Fukuoka Kinki Parkinson's Disease Study Group, et al. (2011). Dietary intake of antioxidant vitamins and risk of Parkinson's disease: A case-control study in Japan. *European Journal of Neurology, 18*(1), 106–113. PubMed PMID: 20491891.

220. Mangialasche, F., Solomon, A., Kåreholt, I., et al. (2013). Serum levels of vitamin E forms and risk of cognitive impairment in a Finnish cohort of older adults. *Experimental Gerontology, 48*(12), 1428–1435. PubMed PMID: 24113154.

221. Dysken, M. W., Guarino, P. D., Vertrees, J. E., et al. (2014). Vitamin E and memantine in Alzheimer's disease: Clinical trial methods and baseline data. *Alzheimer's & Dementia, 10*(1), 36–44. PubMed PMID: 23583234.

222. Lopez, M. S., Dempsey, R. J., & Vemuganti, R. (2015). Resveratrol neuroprotection in stroke and traumatic CNS injury. *Neurochemistry International, 89*, 75–82. PubMed PMID: 26277384.

223. Gemma, C., Mesches, M. H., Sepesi, B., et al. (2002). Diets enriched in foods with high antioxidant activity reverse age-induced decreases in cerebellar beta-adrenergic function and increases in proinflammatory cytokines. *The Journal of Neuroscience : The Official Journal of the Society for Neuroscience, 22*(14), 6114–6120. PubMed PMID: 12122072.

224. Shukitt-Hale, B., Galli, R. L., Meterko, V., et al. (2005). Dietary supplementation with fruit polyphenolics ameliorates age-related deficits in behavior and neuronal markers of inflammation and oxidative stress. *Age, 27*(1), 49–57. PubMed PMID: 23598603.

225. Shukitt-Hale, B., Lau, F. C., Carey, A. N., et al. (2008). Blueberry polyphenols attenuate kainic acid-induced decrements in cognition and alter inflammatory gene expression in rat hippocampus. *Nutritional Neuroscience, 11*(4), 172–182. PubMed PMID: 18681986.

226. Papandreou, M. A., Dimakopoulou, A., Linardaki, Z. I., et al. (2009). Effect of a polyphenol-rich wild blueberry extract on cognitive performance of mice, brain antioxidant markers and acetylcholinesterase activity. *Behavioural Brain Research, 198*(2), 352–358. PubMed PMID: 19056430.

227. Sweeney, M. I., Kalt, W., MacKinnon, S. L., et al. (2002). Feeding rats diets enriched in lowbush blueberries for six weeks decreases ischemia-induced brain damage. *Nutritional Neuroscience, 5*(6), 427–431. PubMed PMID: 12509072.

228. Mukherjee, S., Das, S. K., & Vasudevan, D. M. (2015). Protective role of extracts of grape skin and grape flesh on ethanol-induced oxidative stress, inflammation and histological alterations in rat brain. *Archives of Physiology and Biochemistry, 121*(4), 142–151. PubMed PMID: 26376104.

229. He, Q., Yang, S. Y., Wang, W., et al. (2016). Proanthocyanidins affects the neurotoxicity of Aβ25-35 on C57/bl6 mice. *European Review for Medical and Pharmacological Sciences, 20*(4), 679–684. PubMed PMID: 26957270.

230. Yang, H., Xu, Z., Liu, W., et al. (2012). Effect of grape seed proanthocyanidin extracts on methylmercury-induced neurotoxicity in rats. *Biological Trace Element Research, 147*(1–3), 156–164. doi:10.1007/s12011-011-9272-x. PubMed PMID: 22116679.

231. Dong, C. (2015). Protective effect of proanthocyanidins in cadmium induced neurotoxicity in mice. *Drug Research, 65*(10), 555–560. PubMed PMID: 25463594.

232. Khan, M. M., Kempuraj, D., Thangavel, R., & Zaheer, A. (2013). Protection of MPTP-induced neuroinflammation and neurodegeneration by Pycnogenol. *Neurochemistry International, 62*(4), 379–388. doi:10.1016/j.neuint.2013.01.029. PubMed PMID: 23391521.

233. Zhang, X. S., Zhang, X., Wu, Q., et al. (2014). Astaxanthin offers neuroprotection and reduces neuroinflammation in experimental subarachnoid hemorrhage. *The Journal of Surgical Research, 192*(1), 206–213. PubMed PMID: 24948541.

234. Johnson, E. J. (2014). Role of lutein and zeaxanthin in visual and cognitive function throughout the lifespan. *Nutrition Reviews, 72*(9), 605–612. PubMed PMID: 25109868.

235. Sachdeva, A. K., & Chopra, K. (2015). Lycopene abrogates Aβ(1-42)-mediated neuroinflammatory cascade in an experimental model of Alzheimer's disease. *The Journal of Nutritional Biochemistry, 26*(7), 736–744. PubMed PMID: 25869595.

236. Fisher, D. R., Poulose, S. M., Bielinski, D. F., & Shukitt-Hale, B. (2014). Serum metabolites from walnut-fed aged rats attenuate stress-induced neurotoxicity in BV-2 microglial cells. *Nutritional Neuroscience,* [Epub ahead of print] PubMed PMID: 25153536.

237. Famenini, S., Rigali, E. A., Olivera-Perez, H. M., et al. (2016). Increased intermediate M1-M2 macrophage polarization and improved cognition in mild cognitive impairment patients on ω-3 supplementation. *FASEB Journal: Official Publication of the Federation of American Societies for Experimental Biology,* pii: fj.201600677RR. PubMed PMID: 27677546.

238. Lee, Y., Chun, H. J., Lee, K. M., Jung, Y. S., & Lee, J. (2015). Silibinin suppresses astroglial activation in a mouse model of acute Parkinson's disease by modulating the ERK and JNK signaling pathways. *Brain Research, 1627,* 233–242. PubMed PMID: 26434409.

239. Lee, Y., Park, H. R., Chun, H. J., & Lee, J. (2015). Silibinin prevents dopaminergic neuronal loss in a mouse model of Parkinson's disease via mitochondrial stabilization. *Journal of Neuroscience Research, 93*(5), 755–765. PubMed PMID: 25677261.

240. Chtourou, Y., Fetoui, H., Sefi, M., et al. (2010). Silymarin, a natural antioxidant, protects cerebral cortex against manganese-induced neurotoxicity in adult rats. *Biometals: An International Journal on the Role of Metal Ions in Biology, Biochemistry, and Medicine, 23*(6), 985–996. PubMed PMID: 20503066.

241. Levites, Y., Weinreb, O., Maor, G., Youdim, M. B., & Mandel, S. (2001). Green tea polyphenol (-)-epigallocatechin-3-gallate prevents N-methyl-4-phenyl-1,2,3,6-tetrahydropyridine-induced dopaminergic neurodegeneration. *Journal of Neurochemistry, 78*(5), 1073–1082. PubMed PMID: 11553681.

242. Noguchi-Shinohara, M., Yuki, S., Dohmoto, C., et al. (2014). Consumption of green tea, but not black tea or coffee, is associated with reduced risk of cognitive decline. *PLoS ONE, 9*(5), e96013. PubMed PMID: 24828424.

243. Dairam, A., Limson, J. L., Watkins, G. M., et al. (2007). Curcuminoids, curcumin, and demethoxycurcumin reduce lead-induced memory deficits in male Wistar rats. *Journal of Agricultural and Food Chemistry, 55*(3), 1039–1044. PubMed PMID: 17263510.

244. Agarwal, R., Goel, S. K., & Behari, J. R. (2010). Detoxification and antioxidant effects of curcumin in rats experimentally exposed to mercury. *Journal of Applied Toxicology: JAT, 30*(5), 457–468. PubMed PMID: 20229497.

245. Bredesen, D. E. (2014). Reversal of cognitive decline: A novel therapeutic program. *Aging [Electronic Resource], 6*(9), 707–717. PubMed PMID: 25324467.

43

Immunotoxicity

SUMMARY

- Presence in population: High
- Major disease: Allergies, asthma, chronic infections, autoimmunity, chemical sensitivity
- Primary sources: Urban air pollution, phthalates, polychlorinated biphenyls (PCBs), pesticides, mercury, solvents

- Best measure: Case history
- Best intervention: Avoidance, depuration, Mediterranean diet (MD), cruciferous vegetables, probiotics

OVERVIEW/INTRODUCTION

The human immune system is a complex balance of specialized cells, immune tissues and organs, chemical messengers, and antibodies that work in concert to protect the host against pathogenical invaders, remove damaged tissues, and eliminate cancerous cells. Imbalances of the immune system can result in allergies, inability to destroy invading pathogens (resulting in chronic infections), autoimmunity, poor regeneration, and cancer.

A considerable body of research now shows widespread and increasing immune dysfunction. According to the United States Centers for Disease Control and Prevention (CDC), the rates of food allergy increased 18% among children between 1997 and 2007.[1] The rates of asthma, one of the classic manifestations of allergy, has consistently increased from 3.1% of the population in 1980 to 5.5% in 1996 and then to 8.4% in the year 2010.[2] The net incidence of autoimmune diseases is also increasing at the alarming rate of 19% per year.[3] During the same time frame, a new disorder, chemical sensitivity, displaying adverse mental, physical, or emotional reactions to ambient levels of chemicals, started occurring and is now found in up to 20% of clinical patient populations.[4,5,193] All of these conditions share similar cytokine pictures secondary to exposure to common environmental pollutants.[6]

BASIC MECHANISMS

For environmental pollutants to cause dysfunction in such a complex system, toxic compounds must be constantly present and must exert a number of different immunotoxic effects simultaneously. Many of these are summarized in Box 43.1.

In an animal model, the consumption of PCB-containing fat resulted in diminished mitogen response, decreased phagocytosis, diminished numbers of CD8+ cells, and thymic atrophy.[7,8,9] Mobile home dwellers exposed to formaldehyde were found to have lower numbers of T and B cells and diminished mitogen response to phytohemaglutinin.[10] Mold exposure has also been shown to reduce mitogen responsiveness in humans.[11] Dichlorodiphenyl-trichloroethane (DDT) and dichlorodiphenyldichloroethylene (DDE) exposure leads to apoptosis of peripheral blood mononuclear cells and reduced mitogen-induced lymphocyte response to concanavalin A.[12,13,14] Immune disruption by common toxicants can also be synergistically enhanced by certain lifestyle choices. Mice fed a protein-deficient diet exhibited immunotoxic effects when exposed to levels of DDT that were not immunotoxic to animals fed adequate protein.[15] Emotional stress was also shown to lead to the same phenomenon. When animals were stressed, they exhibited humoral immune deficiency at levels of DDT that would not cause such an effect in nonstressed animals.

Macrophages and dendritic cells, often referred to as *antigen-presenting cells (APC),* are critical for the development of naive T-cells into either Th1 or Th2 cells. Once a pathogen passes through the epithelial layer of the body (skin or mucus-secreting epithelial lining of the lungs or gut), it should be ingested by a macrophage. These macrophages include Kupffer cells (liver), alveolar macrophages (lung), mesangial macrophages (kidney), and glial cells (brain). After ingesting the pathogen, the macrophage will display the antigenic signature of the pathogen and send a chemical messenger, interleukin 1 (IL-1), to notify the T-helper cells (that have CD4 phenotype markings) of the pathogen's presence. From there, they will develop into Th1 and Th2 cells (based on the cytokine they produce).

The cytokines produced by each of these T-helper cells modulate other T-helper type activities. The production of interferon (IFN)-gamma from Th1 inhibits Th2-associated functions, whereas production of IL-4 and IL-10 from Th2 cells inhibits Th1 functions.[16] Th1 dominance is found in some individuals with tissue-specific autoimmunity (arthritis, diabetes), but not in everyone with those diseases. Th2 dominance appears to lead to increased rates of allergy and systemic autoimmunity (systemic lupus erythematosus [SLE]),[17] both of which are commonly seen in persons with chemical overburden. Reduction of Th1 function typically results in reduced cell-mediated immunity, which shows up clinically as recurrent and chronic infections by protozoan parasites (*Pneumocystis* and *Toxoplasma*), fungi (*Candida*), viruses (Epstein Barr virus [EBV], cytomegalo virus CMV, varicella, herpes), and certain bacteria (mycobacteria, listeria).[18] Th3 cells help maintain homeostasis between Th1 and Th2 cells, whereas Th17 cells

appear to downregulate the production of both Th1 and Th2 cytokines, which serves to enhance the inflammatory state.[19] Fig. 43.1 illustrates T-helper cell differentiation.

Summary of Th Cell Functions

Th1. Th1 produces IFN-γ, tumor necrosis factor (TNF)-β, interleukin (IL)-2, IL-10, and lymphotoxin, which then stimulates the cell-mediated immune responses against viral and bacterial pathogens and tumor cells through activation of macrophages and cytotoxic T-cells. IFN-γ, among its other actions, activates macrophages and stimulates natural killer (NK) cell and lymphokine-activated killer activities. IL-1 also affects the temperature regulatory centers in the hypothalamus and helps induce a fever; it also induces slow-wave sleep through the sleep regulatory center.[20]

Th2. Th2 produces IL-4, IL-5, IL-10, IL-13, IL-21, and IL-31, which stimulate B cells to produce the antibodies immunoglobulin (Ig) M, IgG1, IgA, and IgE (stimulating humoral immune response).[11]

Th3 (Regulatory T-cells). Th3 produces IL-10, transforming growth factor-beta (TGF-β), and IL-35. Th3 cells can regulate Th1 and Th2 cell function to suppress autoimmunity and inflammation (via IL-10 and TGF-β).[21]

Th17. Th17 produces IL-17, IL-17A, IL-17-F, IL-21, and IL-26, which enhance inflammation (including neuroinflammation) and cause autoimmune tissue damage.[22,23] Th17 cells have been linked to rheumatoid arthritis, systemic lupus erythematosus, multiple sclerosis (MS), gastritis, asthma, psoriasis, systemic sclerosis, chronic inflammatory bowel disease, and allograft rejection, many of which are strongly linked to environmentally toxic compounds.[24]

Glutathione, T-cell Homeostasis, and Immunotoxicity

Glutathione (L-g-glutamyl-L-cysteinyl-glycine) is the most abundant nonprotein thiol (a sulfhydryl group bonded to a carbon-containing group) in mammalian cells. Reduced glutathione (GSH) is a tripeptide made up of glycine, cysteine, and glutamate acts as a reducing agent within cells by maintaining tight control of the redox status. It is also a powerful antioxidant with a special affinity for lipid peroxides, an action facilitated by the enzyme glutathione peroxidase. GSH is 85% to 90% freely distributed in the cytosol of the cell but is also found in

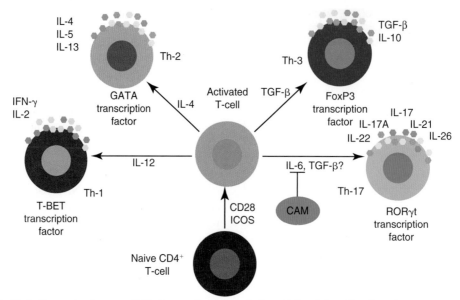

FIG. 43.1 General scheme of T-helper cell differentiation. Naive CD4+ T cells, after activation by T-cell receptor and costimulatory molecules, such as CD28 and inducible T-cell costimulator (ICOS), can differentiate into four effector T-helper cells: Th1, Th2, Th3, or Th17 cells. These cells produce different cytokines, which have specialized immunoregulatory functions. IFN produced by Th1 cells is important in the regulation of antigen presentation and cellular immunity. IL-4, IL-5, and IL-13 produced by Th2 cells regulate B-cell responses, important mediators of allergic diseases. TGF and IL-10 are produced by Th3 cells to regulate Th1 and Th2 cells. Th17 cells regulate inflammatory responses by expressing IL-17, IL-21, IL-22, and IL-26. CAM protocols can be implemented to reduce the level of proinflammatory cytokine IL-6, thereby inhibiting the conversion of activated T cells into pathogenic Th17 cells. (From Vojdani, A., Lambert, J., Kellerman, G. [2011]. The role of Th17 in neuroimmune disorders: Target for CAM therapy. Part I. *Evidence-Based Complementary and Alternative Medicine, 2011*, 927294.)

the mitochondria, the peroxisomes, the nuclear matrix, and the endoplasmic reticulum.[25] In the mitochondria, it is found mostly in the inner mitochondrial membrane, where it protects the membrane against depolarization from xenobiotic toxicants.[26] GSH production is dependent on adequate cysteine levels and the proper function of the enzymes glutamate cysteine ligase (GCL) and glutathione synthase (GS).[27]

GSH is also involved in many distinct physiological reactions; it contributes to cellular signaling, biotransformation of xenobiotics (through the activity of the enzyme glutathione transferase), and thiol disulfide exchange reactions; acts as an important reservoir of cysteine; and is essential for the proper functioning of the immune system. In fact, both *in vivo* and *in vitro* testing have shown that the glutathione content in APCs determines whether the immune system will be primarily

Th1 or Th2 dominant.[28] Low GSH levels lead to an increase in Th2 dominance, whereas higher GSH levels promote Th1 immune response.[29]

All of the immunotoxic pollutants presented in this chapter reduce glutathione levels, including mercury,[30] lead,[31] perfluorocarbons,[32] phthalates,[33] toluene and benzene,[34] PCBs,[35] chlorinated pesticides,[36] organophosphate pesticides,[37] particulate matter,[38] tobacco smoke,[39] and diesel exhaust particles (DEP) (Fig. 43.2).[40] In animal models, the endocrine-disrupting chemicals benzophenone, 0-octylphenol, and tributyltin reduce GSH levels in the APC, resulting in a reduction of APC-produced IL-12 and an enhancement of IL-10. This imbalance results in a Th2 dominance and increased inflammation.[41] The addition of supplemental N-acetyl cysteine (NAC) boosted GSH levels and cancelled the Th2 dominance in this animal model. When acetaminophen, known to

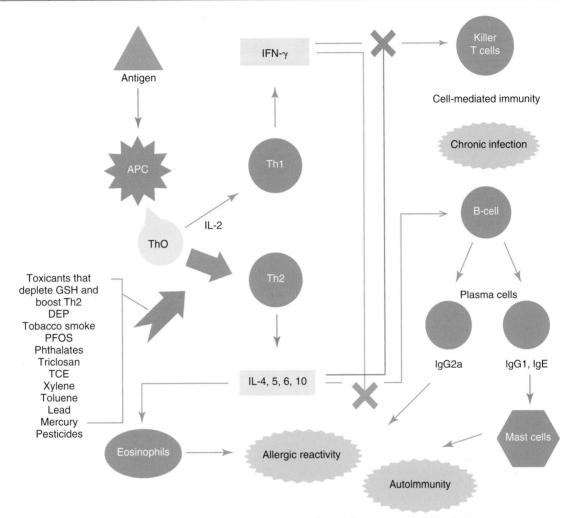

FIG. 43.2 Effect of common glutathione-reducing pollutants on Th1/Th2 balance.

deplete hepatic GSH stores, is given to animals, the same Th2 dominance is seen.[42] In this animal model, elevated levels of IL-6 were noted, which does enhance IL-17 production, although research has not yet been done to establish the effect of low GSH on Th17 activity.

HIV-positive individuals have low GSH levels[43] in addition to a serious imbalance of Th1/Th2 function. HIV-positive individuals have significantly lower levels of the Th1 cytokines IL-1b, IL-12, IFN-γ, and TNF-α, along with elevated Th2 cytokines.[44] In a trial in HIV-positive and HIV-negative individuals, liposomal glutathione was used to see if supplementation would replete GSH levels and reverse the immune imbalance. The researchers found that HIV-positive persons who took

liposomal glutathione for 13 weeks not only had increased levels of GSH but also had increased production of Th1 cytokines (IL-1b, IL-12, IFN-γ, and TNF-α) and a reduction of the immunosuppressive cytokines IL-10 and TGF-β.

All the environmental pollutants listed in Box 43.2 that have demonstrated the ability to alter cytokine production and immune function have also been shown to deplete GSH levels, primarily through oxidative stress.

Immunotoxicity

The classic picture of immunotoxicity is reduced cell-mediated immunity leading to chronic infections (reduced Th1 function), allergies and asthma (increased

---

BOX 43.2 Environmental Pollutants That Lead to Th1 Reduction and Th2 Dominance

Diesel exhaust particles (DEP)[241,242]
Polycyclic aromatic hydrocarbons[243]
$PM_{2.5}$[244,245]
Lead[246,247]
Mercury (thimerosal and methylmercury)[248,249]
Tributyl tin[250]
Organophosphate pesticides[251]
DDT/DDE[252]
Broad leaf chlorophenoxy herbicides[253]
Trichloroethylene in drinking water[254]
PCB 118[255]
Benzene[256]
Bisphenol A[257]
Bisphenol A (prenatal exposure)[258]
Phthalates[259]
Dioxin[260]
Toluene diisocyanate (from indoor building materials)[261]
Trimellitic anhydride (from indoor building materials)[39]
Perfluorooctanesulfonate (PFOS)[262]
Gas stove in the home[263]
Maternal agricultural work[68]

BOX 43.3 Environmental Pollutants That Increase Th17 Activity

Particulate matter[264]	Trichloroethylene[268]
Diesel exhaust[265]	PCBs[269]
Cigarette smoke[266]	Paraquat[270]
Bisphenol A[267]	

DISEASE MANIFESTATION

Allergies

- Vehicular exhaust
- Environmental tobacco smoke (ETS)
- Chemicals from indoor building materials
- Perfluorocarbons
- Phthalates
- Organophosphate pesticides
- Solvents and cleaning supplies
- Lead
- Chlorinated pesticides and PCBs
- Mold

As previously mentioned, allergic disorders, including asthma, have been increasing in frequency across the globe for the last few decades. In addition to asthma, increasing rates of atopic dermatitis,[46] allergic rhinitis (hay fever),[47,48,49] atopic conjunctivitis,[50] and eosinophilic esophagitis[51] have all been noted. The incidence of food allergies resulting in emergency department visits for anaphylaxis has dramatically increased in the same time period.[52] The rates of celiac disease doubled between 1974 and 1989[53] (from 1:501–1:219), with another increase between 2000 and 2010.[54] New allergies, such as latex sensitivity, have also become common.[55] Although atopic disorders are typically found in higher levels in persons with a family history of atopy, environmental chemical burden is often the trigger.

Th2 function), chemical sensitivity, and autoimmunity (overactive Th2 or Th17 activity).[45] The first manifestation of immunotoxicity often seen in a case history is the development of asthma and allergies. Multiple environmental toxicants are associated with increased incidences of allergic reactivity to the environment and to foods (see Box 43.2). The chemicals that lead the way in causing atopic reactions include both organophosphate and chlorinated pesticides, solvents, and combustion by-products, including tobacco smoke and diesel exhaust.

Because Th17 cells are a relatively new finding in the field of immunology, there are far fewer studies that have explored the connection between environmental pollutants and IL-17. However, a handful of common environmental pollutants have demonstrated the ability to enhance Th17 activity by increasing levels of IL-17 (Box 43.3).

It should be noted that, except for dioxin and maternal agriculture work in Box 43.2 and paraquat in Box 43.3, the rest of the compounds listed in both tables are common contaminants in the air, food, and water for most individuals.

Outdoor Air Pollutants

Vehicular exhaust. Vehicular exhaust emissions have been clearly linked to the increasing rates of allergy and asthma. In areas where outdoor levels of CO, PM_{10}, and $PM_{2.5}$ are elevated, indoor levels are similarly found to be higher and are associated with higher rates of allergic rhinitis and asthma.[56] Traffic-related air pollutants increase the risk of 1-year-old children becoming allergic to both foods and airborne allergens.[57] As the children continue to be exposed to vehicular exhaust, their risk of developing food allergies by age 4 years increases by 230%, far higher than their risk of having pollen allergies by that age (83% increase).[58] PM$_{2.5}$ appears to hold the greatest association with the development of allergic rhinitis.[59] In Taiwanese children, exposure to CO and nitrogen oxides were significantly associated with greater allergic reactivity.[60] For German children, PM$_{2.5}$ levels were significantly associated with sneezing and rhinitis.[61] Children in Korea with the highest total NO$_2$ and particulate count (measured as black carbon) were 67% and 60% more likely to have allergic rhinitis.[62] A review of hospital admissions in Oklahoma City revealed that spikes in NO$_2$ levels preceded increased pediatric hospitalizations for asthma.[63] Children living within 200 meters of a major roadway are far more likely to have symptoms of allergic rhinitis than those living 200 to 500 meters away.[64] The children living more than 500 meters from busy roadways had the lowest rates of sneezing, runny or stuffy nose, and itchy and watery eyes. Truck traffic is specifically associated with allergic rhinitis; children living close to higher truck traffic are more than twice as likely to have this problem.[65] For Swiss adults living by roadways, the number of cars on the proximal roads predicts their rates of pollen allergies.[66] Multiple studies have demonstrated a clear association between vehicular exhaust and asthma in both children and adults.[67,68,69,70] Children living in areas with denser traffic were 250% more likely to present to a local emergency department with asthma.[71] The spike of asthmatic symptoms in children rises with daily spikes of vehicular pollution and can persist for up to 2 days after a spike.[72] When exposure to high traffic was combined with mycotoxin (mold contamination) exposure in the home, the risk for asthma went from a 75% increase to 5.85-fold increase.[73]

Diesel exhaust particles. Persons living close to roadways with high diesel truck traffic appear to have the highest risk for allergic disorders. Prior to 2015 almost 75% of all vehicles in France were diesel, but that number has since dropped to below 50%.[74] In the United States, the sale of diesel vehicles increased by almost 40% in 2010 alone. Although diesel engines used to be mainly found in large trucks, earth-moving equipment, ships, buses, locomotives, and power generators, they are now commonly found in passenger vehicles worldwide. Exposure to DEP leads to increased rates of allergy and asthma, along with elevated production of antigen-specific IgE and histamine. DEP interferes with immune system regulation by suppressing NF-κB, reducing NF-κB cytokine production.[75] DEP reduces levels of the antiviral cytokine IFN-γ and IFN-γ mRNA more potently than either dexamethasone or cyclosporine A.[76] DEP also dramatically diminished NK cell function in human volunteers.[77,78] This reduction of Th1 function, resulting in diminished cell-mediated immunity, is the likely reason that DEP exposure increases the rates of respiratory infections.[79,80,81,82] NK function is diminished by 21% in women who live within 150 meters of a busy roadway.[83] Exposure to cigarette smoke also reduces IFN-γ[84] and NK cell activity.[85]

DEP exposure in animals results in increased allergen-specific Th2/Th17 cells in the lungs, which enhances allergic reactivity (Fig. 43.3).[70] Not surprisingly, when mice were exposed to egg albumin after DEP exposure, they produced more IgE to ovalbumin than did mice who were not exposed to DEP.[86] Human volunteers exposed to DEP showed a significant reduction in IFN-γ production after exposure, indicating a reduction in Th1 response. In another human study, the levels of mRNA for cytokine production (IL-4, IL-5, IL-6, IL-10, IL-13) were increased after DEP exposure, revealing elevated Th2 and Th17 responses.[87] The researchers also found elevated levels of IL-4 in the nasal lavage fluid after exposure.[88] In atopic individuals with null GSTT1 genotypes, DEP exposure resulted in even higher IL-5 production.[89] Other studies have confirmed the increase in Th2 cytokine production after DEP exposure and have shown that this exposure leads to increased reactivity to ragweed,[90] cedar pollen,[91] birch pollen,[92] and egg protein.[93] Simultaneous exposure to DEP and allergens leads to more rapid development of allergic reactivity to those allergens than would occur without DEP presence.[94]

DEP exposure and increased cedar pollen levels have been linked with a dramatic increase in Japanese cedar pollinosis (cedar allergy).[95] The incidence of cedar pollen allergies appears to increase along with diesel-related particulate matter levels and the number of diesel vehicles in use.[96] Between 1951 and 1988, the number of diesel cars registered in Japan increased from 20,000 to 7,600,000. Japanese men living on a busy roadway with truck traffic are 53% more likely to develop cedar allergy.[97] In areas with the same pollen count, more than 13% of those living by busy roadways became allergic, yet only 5% of those living by less-trafficked roads were reactive.[98] Children exposed to higher levels of DEP are 40% more likely to have allergic rhinitis by the age of 3 years.[77] Recognizing the increased use of diesel engines and the increase in atopic response with DEP exposure, it is quite

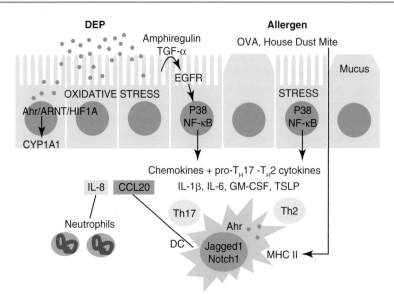

FIG. 43.3 Mechanistic insights into DEP effects on asthma pathogenesis. Lung epithelial cells recognize polycyclic aromatic hydrocarbons present in diesel exhaust particles (DEP) via the aryl hydrocarbon receptor (AhR), promoting cytochrome P450 family 1A1 (CYP1A1) mediated detoxification. Failure to detoxify results in oxidative stress and release of repair cytokines (amphiregulin, TGF-α), which signal through the epidermal growth factor receptor (EGFR), p38 mitogen-activated protein kinase, and NF-κB to induce secretion of chemokines, as well as cytokines involved in Th17 and Th2 differentiation thymic stromal lymphopoietin (TSLP). DEP promotes allergic airway inflammation by upregulating the expression of the Jagged1/Notch1 pathway in dendritic cells (DC) in an AhR-dependent manner in concert with allergens. (From Brandt, E. B., Biagini Myers, J. M., Ryan, P. H., Khurana Hershey, G. K. [2015]. Air pollution and allergic diseases. *Current opinion in pediatrics, 27*[6]:724–735.)

possible that diesel exhaust is a major factor in the worldwide increase in asthma.

Indoor Air Pollutants

Mold. Mold presence in the home is strongly associated with increased rates of asthma, rhinitis, and eczema.[99,100,101] In addition to indoor microbial volatile organic compounds, several chemical pollutants found primarily in indoor air have also been linked to increased allergic reactivity. Children raised in homes where the mothers reported "sick building" symptoms (Box 5.2, chapter 5—Indoor Air Pollution), commonly associated with increased chemical levels, were far more likely to have atopic dermatitis and adverse food reactions.[102] Environmental tobacco smoke (ETS) is often considered to be the biggest indoor air pollutant that leads to higher rates of allergy and asthma.[103]

Tobacco smoke. ETS reduces Th1 response and enhances Th2 response through greater production of IL-4, IL-5, and other proinflammatory cytokines that lead to increases in allergic reactivity and IgE levels.[104,105] The degree of allergic reactivity from ETS appears to be dependent on how well the glutathione transferase enzymes are working. Persons with null genotypes for either glutathione transferase (GST) M1 or P1 have far higher rates of allergic reactivity from ETS than whose GSTs are genotypically functional.[106]

Building and yard chemicals. Other indoor air pollutants associated with increasing rates of atopy include synthetic carpets, new wall covering, recent painting, new furniture, pesticide treatment, and plasticizers.[107,108,109] Lead exposures have been associated with increased IgE in humans[110,111] and increased food allergy,[112] whereas prenatal exposures to both PCBs and chlorinated pesticides have also been shown to increase IgE levels.[113,114] Prenatal exposure to PCBs and dioxins also increase a child's risk for becoming asthmatic within the first year of life.[115] Herbicide and pesticide exposure around the home[116] and the presence of phosphorous flame retardants in indoor dust all increase the risk of both asthma and allergic rhinitis.[117]

Solvents. Children exposed to indoor solvents (from cleaning supplies, building materials, paints, and ETS) have an enhanced Th2 immune response and are much more likely to become reactive to milk and egg whites.[118] The solvents leading to this proallergic state include toluene, o-xylene, m-xylene, p-xylene, ethyl toluene, ethyl benzene, and chlorobenzene. Homeowners using cleaning sprays once weekly were 49% more likely to have symptoms, whereas those using the sprays four times weekly were more than twice as likely to be diagnosed with asthma.[119] Although housecleaning is rarely thought of as a "toxic" profession, residential cleaners are more than three times more likely to become asthmatic.[120] The greatest associations with the development of asthma were found with kitchen cleaning and furniture polishing.

Perfluorocarbons. Perfluorooctanesulfonate (PFOS), the key ingredient in Scotchguard for fabrics and carpeting, is found ubiquitously in US residents, with a mean urinary level of 20.7 µg/L.[121] All Scotchguard-treated materials in the home, such as carpeting, upholstery, and clothing, release these PFOS into the home air. Exposing mice to PFOS resulted in a reduction of IFN-γ and IL-2 production, yet IL-4 and IL-5 production was increased, tipping the immune system to a Th2 dominance.[122] Prenatal exposure to these fluorocarbons resulted in mice being born with higher IgE levels and increased allergic reactivity.[123]

Phthalates. Phthalate compounds are added to plastics to make them more flexible, yet are weakly bound to the plastics and easily released into the surrounding environment. High-molecular-weight (HMW) phthalate-containing products (shower curtains, raincoats, toys, polyvinyl chloride flooring, furniture polishes, plastic food wrap, etc.) release these plasticizers into the environment, where they will be carried by the dust throughout the home.[124] Low-molecular-weight (LMW) phthalates are typically found in liquid personal care products such as fragrances and nail polish, and are inhaled from the fumes. Three different HMW phthalates have been associated with higher rates of allergic and respiratory problems. The presence of butyl benzyl phthalate (BBzP) in house dust is associated with rhinitis and eczema, whereas di-ethylhexyl phthalate (DEHP) is associated

with asthma.[125] Another HMW phthalate metabolite, monobenzyl phthalate (MBzP), is also associated with higher levels of asthma in adults, but not in children.[126] DEHP is in all vinyl chloride products, and BBzP is in both vinyl and carpet tiles and in some artificial leather products. Phthalates have been shown to induce Th2 immune responses with increased Th2 cytokine production, as well as increases in IgE and IgG.[127]

Trichloroethylene. Because trichloroethylene (TCE) has contaminated so many groundwater sites in the United States, the National Exposure Registry has been tracking adverse health effects for persons exposed to TCE. When Wistar rats were given water with TCE levels similar to what homeowners in those areas were ingesting, the animals produced increased levels of the Th2 cytokine and IL-4 and developed type 1 allergic reactivity.[128] Currently, more than 4000 individuals living in homes supplied with TCE-contaminated well water, all near Superfund sites, are being monitored for health outcomes. As the cumulative exposure level increases, these homeowners exhibit significantly more problems with respiratory allergies, asthma, emphysema, stroke, and hearing impairment.[129]

Autoimmunity From Toxicant Exposures

- Vehicular exhaust
- Heavy metals (predominantly mercury)
- PCBs
- Pesticides
- TCE
- Lead
- Organophosphate pesticides

In the last 30 years, the incidence and prevalence of autoimmune diseases has been steadily rising (Fig. 43.4).[3] Currently rheumatic, endocrine, gastrointestinal, and neurological autoimmune diseases are increasing annually at the rate of 7.1%, 6.3%, 6.2%, and 3.7%, respectively. Comparing rates of specific autoimmune diseases from the 1990's to the present reveals that the greatest jumps are found in celiac disease, type 1 diabetes, and myasthenia gravis.

Particulate Matter, Diesel Exhaust, BPA, Trichlorloethylene, Cigarette Smoke, PCBs, and Paraquat. Autoimmunity is associated with an increased Th17 immune response, as previously noted. Published research has already shown that particulate matter, diesel exhaust,

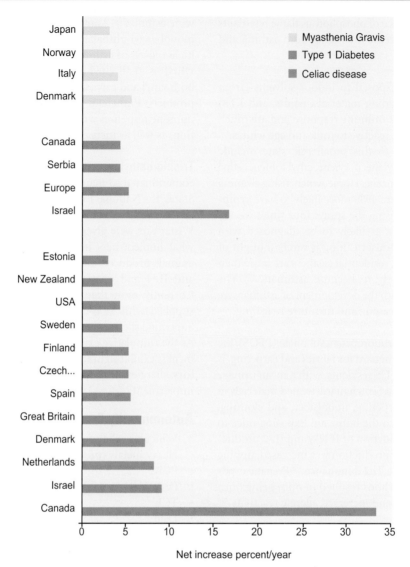

FIG. 43.4 The net percentage increase per year of three autoimmune diseases in specific surveyed countries. (From Lerner, A., Jeremias, P., & Matthias, T. [2015]. The world incidence and prevalence of autoimmune disease is increasing. *International Journal of Celiac Disease, 3*[4], 151–155.)

BPA, trichlorloethylene, cigarette smoke, PCBs, and paraquat have been linked to increased Th17 conditions (see Box 43.3). In the 2003 to 2004 National Health and Nutritional Examination Survey (NHANES), individuals with the highest levels of PCBs were more than four times more likely to have elevated antinuclear antibodies (ANA) than individuals with the lowest levels.[130] Most of those have also been clearly linked to increased rates of autoimmune disorders.

Mercury. Although not yet associated with increasing Th17 levels, women in the NHANES 1999 to 2004 study with highest versus lowest quartiles of hair and blood mercury were either 410% (hair levels) or 232% (blood levels) more likely to have elevated antinuclear antibody (ANA) levels.[131] Individuals with higher levels of mercury exposure are also more likely to have elevated ANA levels.[132,133] Animals exposed simultaneously to mercury and TCE developed autoimmune hepatitis, whereas those exposed to only one of those two compounds for 8 weeks failed to show this pathology.[134]

Chlordane. Chlordane is a persistent organochlorine pesticide that has been a primary termiticide in North America for decades. Even when applied according to directions, chlordane persists in the home for many decades, exposing the occupants to the compound.[27] Such individuals were compared with 118 nonchlordane-exposed persons using immune markers.[135] Although this study was done before the specific markers for Th1, Th2, and Th17 were in use, abnormalities in cell-mediated immune function and autoimmunity were noted. Eleven of the twelve chlordane-containing–home dwellers tested for antibody levels had elevated autoantibodies, eight of whom were positive for anti–smooth muscle antibody and four of whom had positive ANA.

Chlorpyrifos. Twelve persons who were residentially exposed to the chlorpyrifos had an elevated antibody level between 1 and 4.5 years after the exposure occurred.[136] The most common autoimmune antibodies found were anti–smooth muscle, which causes autoimmune hepatitis (OR 3.99); antiparietal cell, leading to diminished hydrochloric acid production (OR 9.7); and antithyroid and antimyelin antibodies. Animals exposed simultaneously to mercury and TCE developed autoimmune hepatitis, whereas those exposed to only one of those two compounds for 8 weeks failed to show this pathology.[137]

Formaldehyde. Four groups of patients with long-term formaldehyde exposure (mobile home dwellers, office workers in closed buildings, persons who had been removed from their formaldehyde exposure for 1 year, and persons with occupational exposure) demonstrated similar autoantibody production.[138] Mobile home dwellers had a 144-fold higher risk for anti–parietal cell antibodies than non–mobile home dwellers, and office workers were 40.5-fold more likely to have antiparietal antibodies. Levels of anti–smooth muscle, antimitochondrial, and anti–brush border were also higher in those with formaldehyde exposure.

Systemic Lupus Erythematosus
Oil Field Waste, Solvents, and Others. Systemic lupus erythematosus (SLE) has long been associated with numerous pharmaceutical compounds,[139] so its association with environmental chemicals should not be a surprise.

SLE rates in the US population vary from 14.6 (males) to 50.8 cases (females)/100,000. African Americans generally show a higher prevalence of 53 cases/100,000 males and 168 cases/100,000 females. However, in the Newton neighborhood of Gainesville, Georgia, where the homes are close to local industry, the rates of SLE are far higher. The lupus rate in this African American community is 1000 cases per 100,000 persons, a sixfold elevation over national statistics.[140] Even higher rates of 872 per 100,000 persons were found in a two-block area of Hobbs, New Mexico, where oil field waste had previously been stored.[141] Residents on these two blocks in Hobbs were compared with residents in another small New Mexican town that had not hosted oil wells. The residents of Hobbs had higher-than-normal exposures to benzene, xylene, toluene, pristine, phytane, polycyclic aromatic hydrocarbons, and mercury. Detectable blood levels of phytane were found in five individuals in the study, all of whom had SLE.

Mercury. The residents of Hobbs also had higher blood mercury levels than the controls. Hobbs residents exposed to oil field waste were almost 11 times more likely to have rheumatic disease and more than 19 times as likely to have diagnosed SLE. The exposed residents also had greater neurological problems (dizziness, lightheadedness, balance disorder, extreme fatigue, sleep disorders, and lack of concentration and balance) and respiratory problems (shortness of breath, wheezing, cough, chronic bronchitis) and were more than 15 times more likely to have experienced stroke or angina. In a different study, higher urinary mercury levels were positively associated with elevated antifibrillarin antibodies, a common finding in persons with systemic sclerosis, another autoimmune connective tissue disorder.[142]

Hair Dye. Regular, repeated exposures to hair dye has also been associated with increased rates of lupus.[143,144] Artists who regularly use paints or dyes or work who develop film are almost four times more likely to develop SLE, whereas those who regularly apply nail polish have a 10-fold greater risk.[145]

Trichloroethylene. Persons exposed to TCE from contaminated municipal drinking water have higher rates of SLE.[146] Exposure to TCE via drinking water can also increase the risk of developing scleroderma by 2.5-fold in men.[147]

Smoking, PCBs, and Pesticides. Being an active smoker increased the risk for developing SLE to 6.69, whereas the risk for those who had previously quit smoking was still elevated, at 3.62.[148] Taiwanese women who had been exposed to PCB-contaminated cooking oil in the 1980s (Yucheng disease) and survived were found to have far higher rates of SLE 24 years later than nonexposed women.[149] Data from the Women's Health Initiative Observational Study revealed that participants who self-reported residential or workplace use of pesticides were twice as likely to have been diagnosed with either rheumatoid arthritis (RA) or SLE.[150]

Particulate Matter. Elevated levels of urban $PM_{2.5}$ exposure have been associated with circulating levels of anti-dsDNA, a classic marker for SLE.[151] Persons exposed to higher levels of $PM_{2.5}$ in Quebec were more likely to have SLE or one of the other autoimmune connective tissue disorders (Sjogren's syndrome, scleroderma, polymyositis, or dermatomyositis).[152] PM_{10}, NO_2, and CO have all been shown to be risk factors for juvenile onset SLE, with each 13.4 $\mu g/m^3$ increase in PM_{10} increasing disease risk by 34%.[153]

Rheumatoid Arthritis

RA rates are 37% higher in persons living less than 50 meters from highways than in those living more than 150 meters away. When individual vehicular exhaust components were assessed for risk, $PM_{2.5}$ showed no association, but ozone levels did (accounting for a 26% increase in risk). Other studies have confirmed the lack of RA risk related to $PM_{2.5}$ in adults, but $PM_{2.5}$ levels can increase the risk of juvenile RA by 60%.[154] Women in the 1999 to 2002 NHANES trial with blood PCB levels in the second, third, and fourth quartiles had more than twice the risk of RA as those with PCBs in the first quartile.[155] Hair and blood cadmium, nickel, and lead levels are found to be significantly higher in those with RA than in healthy controls.[156]

Type 1 Diabetes

Type 1 diabetes mellitus (T1DM) risk is found to be increased by exposure to several different common pollutants. T1DM animal models exposed to levels of $PM_{2.5}$ commonly present in Taiwan were found to have increased inflammation and higher glycosylated hemoglobin levels than the same T1DM animals exposed to nonpolluted air.[157] When the same animal models are exposed to DEP,

even greater pancreatic damage is seen to occur.[158] Italian children exposed to higher levels of PM_{10} also had a slightly elevated risk for developing T1DM.[159]

Antithyroid Antibodies

Antithyroid antibodies are clearly linked with blood mercury levels. In the 2007 to 2008 NHANES, women with blood mercury levels above 1.81 $\mu g/L$ (just above the CDC 75th percentile) were 2.2 times more likely to have positive antithyroglobulin antibodies than those with blood mercury levels below 0.40 $\mu g/L$ (the female mean level is 0.69 $\mu g/L$).[160] In women who eat fish once weekly, 1.81 $\mu g/L$ matches the 75% value, whereas in women who eat fish 1.5 times weekly, the geometrical mean is 2.04 $\mu g/L$.[161] The average blood mercury for those consuming fish twice weekly or more is 2.70 $\mu g/L$, making it quite likely that individuals choosing mercury-containing fish over animal flesh are at greater risk for autoimmune thyroiditis. Individuals living in areas with higher PCB contamination have increased levels of both ANA and antithyroperoxidase antibodies (TPOab).[162] Increasing levels of both PCBs and DDE in Akwesasne Mohawk youth are significantly positively linked to levels of TPOab.[163]

Neurological Autoimmune Disorders

A study of 298 persons working with chemicals in a computer manufacturing industry showed greater reduction in cellular immunity and increased autoimmune markers compared with controls.[164] The most commonly found autoantibody was against myelin basic protein, which corresponded with the self-reporting of headaches, mental status changes, and peripheral neuropathies. Flight crew members also show greater frequency of having multiple antineurological antibodies, including antimyelin basic protein and antiglial fibrillary acidic protein.[165] Multiple antineural antibodies are also found in Faroese children with higher blood mercury levels.[166] Guillain-Barré has been noted in persons exposed to organophosphate pesticides.[167,168] MS is found 42% more frequently in those with exposure to higher levels of urban PM_{10}[169] and in persons who have ever smoked (32% increase in incidence).[170] Individuals exposed to passive cigarette smoke who have the human leukocyte antigen (HLA) genetic predisposition to autoimmunity have a 7.7-fold increased risk of developing multiple sclerosis (MS).[171] MS rates are also higher in areas with higher lead contamination in the soil.[172]

Infections

A diminished Th1 response will reduce the ability to respond to bacterial, viral, and fungal invasion, typically resulting in chronic infections. In cases of severe cytokine reduction, the typical fever and myalgia symptoms of influenza that are normally produced by cytokines and lymphokines will not be present. This often leaves the individual believing that they have a highly efficient immune system when, in fact, their cell-mediated immunity (CMI) response is quite poor. Diminished Th1 function has been found in persons with chronic cytomegalovirus,[173] chronic hepatitis C,[174] respiratory syncytial virus,[175] HIV,[176] and Lyme neuroborreliosis.[177]

Herpes Zoster. Herpes zoster has been shown to be present in persons with a diminished Th1 and increased Th2 cytokine picture.[178] Residents in Aberdeen, North Carolina, with a Superfund site containing chlorinated pesticides, solvents, and metals, had a significantly elevated risk (RR 2.0) for herpes zoster. The authors hypothesized that the incidence of herpes zoster could be used as a marker for immunotoxicity.[179] The second-phase study of residents showed both elevated serum DDE and significantly reduced mitogen-induced lymphocyte proliferation response in those living near the site.[180] A review of the data from the NHANES (years 2003–2004 and 2009–2010) found an association between urinary arsenic levels and seronegativity for zoster, indicating a lack of immunity.[181] The average urinary arsenic for those with immunity to zoster was 6.57 µg As/L, whereas those with more than 7.5 µg/L had an increased risk of seronegativity that reached an 87% increase for individuals with the highest urinary arsenic content. These values are just above the CDC 50th percentile of 5.68 µg/L and well under the 75th percentile of 12.4 µg As/L.[151] In addition, long-term chemical exposure has been linked to chronic Epstein-Barr viral infections.[182]

Childhood Infections. Although lactational PCB exposure showed no association with neurological disorders, it is associated with an increased risk of infections. The effect of prenatal and lactational exposure to PCBs on the child's immune system was studied in Dutch preschool children. At the age of 42 months, their blood was measured for total PCBs, along with immune markers. PCB serum levels in the children were associated with a higher prevalence of recurrent middle-ear infections,

chicken pox, and a lower prevalence of allergic reactions. Higher dioxin levels were associated with a higher prevalence of coughing, chest congestion, and phlegm.[183] In arctic Inuit children, prenatal exposure to DDE, hexachlorobenzene (HCB), and dieldrin increased the risk of otitis media, with higher exposure levels (including lactational PCB exposure) making it more likely that the infections will become recurrent.[184] Prenatal exposure to PCBs, DDE, and HCB were also found to lead to cord blood lymphocytes having a very low TNF-α after mitogenic stimulation.[185] Childre n exposed to ETS are also more likely to be plagued by recurrent ear infections than other children without that exposure.[186]

Although an elevation of Th2 function should enhance overall humoral immunity, several environmental toxicants actually lead to lower levels of specific antipathogen antibodies. Children aged 6 to 11 years participating in the 2003 to 2004 NHANES trial demonstrated an overall inverse relationship between blood mercury and antimeasles antibody levels.[187] Faroese children with proper immunizations, but who also had prenatal exposure to PCBs, demonstrated an inverse relationship between serum PCB levels and antidiptheria antibodies.[188] Each doubling of serum PCB concentration corresponded with a 20% drop in antibody levels, resulting in some 5-year-olds having antibody levels that are insufficient to prevent infection. Among the same population, children whose mothers had the highest serum levels of perfluorocarbons had lower levels of antidiptheria antibodies than other children.[189]

Chemical Sensitivity

Chemical sensitivity (CS), also termed *multiple chemical sensitivity (MCS)*, *environmental illness (EI)*, *idiopathic environmental intolerance (IEI)*,[190] and *toxicant-induced loss of tolerance*,[191,192] is a modern medical phenomenon that is now present in up to 20% of the population.[4,5,193] Individuals with CS experience adverse physical, mental, or emotional symptoms after being exposed to ambient levels of common environmental chemicals. Although CS is not solely related to immune system dysregulation, immunological abnormalities are consistently found in this population,[194] along with evidence of limbic kindling or neural sensitization.[195,196]

The first published definition for MCS came from Cullen in 1987, who described it as an acquired disorder that developed after an identifiable chemical exposure.[197] He further defined it as being defined by recurrent symptoms, affecting multiple organ systems, and occurring after demonstrable exposures to chemically unrelated compounds at doses far lower than those known to be harmful to the general population. In 1999, a consensus statement was published providing the following definition for CS[198]:

1. The symptoms are reproducible with repeated chemical exposure.
2. The condition is chronic.
3. Chemical exposures are at low levels (i.e., lower than previously or commonly tolerated).
4. The symptoms improve or resolve when the chemical incitants are removed.
5. Responses occur to multiple chemically unrelated substances.
6. Symptoms involve multiple organ systems.

Pesticides and Solvents. The most common chemical exposures that initiate CS are pesticides[199] and solvents, each accounting for 28% of incidence.[200] The next two most common exposures are new construction and gasoline or other petroleum products. Persons with CS have a higher prevalence of genetic polyporphisms in several detoxification enzymes, including paraoxonase 1 (PON1) and GSTM1, reducing their ability to adequately break down organophosphate pesticides or solvents.[201,202] Not surprisingly, persons with CS are often found to have detectable levels of solvents in their serum.

Two studies have reported elevated production of T-cell–derived antigen-binding molecules (TABM) in persons who report chemical intolerance.[203,204] TABM levels increase in proportion to the level of chemical exposures and correspondingly stimulate the production of TGF-β resulting in neurogenic inflammation. Persons with CS are found to have multiple cytokine imbalances that are mostly proinflammatory,[202] and allergic reactivity is the third most common comorbidity in this group.[205]

When taking a health history of adults who have developed CS, one typically finds asthma or allergies (including food allergies) present years before chemical reactions occur.[206] However, CS is now being found in very young children, who will generally not have a history of atopy before the development of CS but will usually have it concomitantly. Individuals with CS also typically exhibit increased lymphocyte imbalances, higher levels of antichemical antibodies (e.g., antibenzene, antitrimellitic anhydride, antiformaldehyde, antiisocyanate, and antiphthalic anhydride), and autoantibodies

(antithyroid, antimyelin basic protein, and antiparietal antibodies).[207,208,209]

ASSESSMENT

The best assessment methodology for identifying toxicant-induced immunological dysregulation is a good case history. The presence of allergies, asthma, and autoimmunity are commonplace but should be considered an indicator of immunotoxicity. Individuals who develop CS in their adult years typically have a history of allergy or asthma that began decades before the MCS appeared. CS is a clear indication of both chemical overexposure and immune dysregulation. When a chronological exposure history (see Chapter 52—Assessment) is compared with a chronological history of the initiation and exacerbation of chemical reactivity and the overall health history, the association between chemical burden and other health problems becomes clear. The clinician is also often able to identify which exposures are most responsible for the health problems and offer solutions for avoidance.

INTERVENTION

Avoidance

Avoidance of toxicant exposure is always the first step in environmental medicine. With urban air pollution and other indoor additions to the total airborne load, the first step in avoidance should be focused on indoor air. This begins with elimination of offgassing products in the home (especially phthalate and PFOS-containing products and solvent-containing cleaners), the use of high-quality furnace filters, and electric air purification units in the home. Removing shoes before entering the home will also reduce the amount of particulate matter (PM) and polycyclic aromatic hydrocarbons (PAH) tracked into the home. In a national study of persons with CS, the most effective therapies were removal of everything from the both bedroom and the rest of the home that emits chemical vapors.[210] Although 94% of those responding found benefit from a clean bedroom or clean home, 82% also found benefit from indoor air purifiers.

The use of electrostatic pleated air filters, rated at least a minimum efficiency rating value (MERV) 7, on home heating, ventilating and air conditioning (HVAC) units can dramatically reduce the levels of PM in the home.[211] The less costly and more commonly used filters with MERV ratings below 6 only reduce PM by less than 10%.

MERV 7 filters will aid in reducing the circulating dust in the home, which carries the majority of the semi-volatile indoor air pollutants. Although HVAC units have a limit to their ability to force air through a filter, dedicated high-quality air purifiers do a far superior job.[212] The use of home air purifiers in a community with high outdoor air pollution demonstrated the ability to reduce inflammatory markers in residents.[213] This study used both sham (units with no filters installed) and fully functional air purifiers, which only reduced indoor PM about 60%, yet the high-sensitivity C-reactive protein (hsCRP) levels dropped by more than 30%. Even the use of face masks showed dramatic improvement in endothelial function in persons in the highly polluted city of Beijing.[214] The use of high-quality indoor air purifiers that will remove small particulates from the air will not only reduce PM in the air but also take care of the most common route of exposure for indoor phthalates, lead, and perfluorocarbons.

Individuals living in areas with arsenic or TCE groundwater contamination should use reverse-osmosis filters for all drinking and cooking water.

Mercury intake can be eliminated by avoiding high-mercury fish and removal—by an ecological dentist—of mercury-containing fillings. Those with a body burden of mercury can use either dimercaptosuccinic acid (DMSA) or 2,3-dimercaptopropane-1-sulfonate (DMPS) to reduce body burdens. Lead can also be mobilized from soft tissue body stores with the use of DMSA.

These topics are more fully addressed in Chapter 60.

Depuration (Cleansing)

Depuration techniques to reduce total body load have proven to be highly effective for individuals with auto-immunity, CS, and allergy. A 10-year retrospective study of 112 individuals who underwent 18 days of a comprehensive naturopathic depuration protocol consisting of low-temperature sauna, hydrotherapy, and retrograde colonic irrigation were assessed via anonymous questionnaires and chart review. Of the 112 individuals, 16 had presented with chief complaints of autoimmune illnesses, 34 with CS, and 7 with allergy. The autoimmune disorders included Hashimoto's thyroiditis, RA, psoriatic arthritis, mixed connective tissue disorder, fibrositis, polyarteritis nodosa, silicone-related connective tissue disorder, MS, and SLE.[215] All were asked to rate their chief complaint after cleansing as either worse, no change, slight change, moderate to good improvement, or great improvement. Their ratings are reported on Table 43.1.

Although 21 of 23 individuals with a chief complaint of CS achieved significant improvement, 100% of those with an autoimmune disease did. In fact, of the 15 individuals who had autoimmunity severe enough to want to stop work for a month and undergo a 5-day-per-week depuration program that typically lasted 8 hours each day, 13 reported great improvement. By comparison, 5 out of 7 of those with a chief complaint of allergies reported good improvement and only 1 of 7 reported great results.

TABLE 43.1 Self-Reported Results of 18 Days of Naturopathic Depuration on Chemical Sensitivity, Allergy, and Autoimmunity

Complaint	Worse	No Change	Slight	Moderate/Good	Great	Total
Chemical Sensitivity	0	2	1	8	13	24
Allergy	0	0	1	5	1	7
Thyroiditis	0	0	0	0	1	1
Rheumatoid arthritis	0	0	0	0	2	2
Psoriatic arthritis	0	0	0	1	0	1
Mixed connective tissue disorder	0	0	0	0	2	2
Fibrositis	0	0	0	0	1	1
Polyarteritis nodosa	0	0	0	0	1	1
Silicone-related CTD	0	0	0	0	4	4
Multiple sclerosis	0	0	0	1	1	2
SLE	0	0	0	0	1	1
Total	0	2	2	15	27	46
Percent	0%	4.3%	4.3%	32.6%	58.7%	100%

Dietary Intervention

- MD
- Wild caught, small fish
- Cruciferous vegetables
- Turmeric
- Green tea

Mediterranean Diet. The MD appears to be the most powerful antiinflammatory diet currently available. Individuals with higher compliance to the MD have lower levels of IL-6, one of the cytokines implicated in the stimulation of Th17 activity.[216] Women whose diet more closely adhered to the MD provided allergy protection to their children.[217] By 6.5 years of age, children of the women who ate a more Mediterranean-style diet were 78% less like to have problems with persistent wheeze and 45% less likely to have a diagnosed allergic disorder. A study of 10- to 12-year-old boys in Athens, Greece, revealed that although urban living increased the risk of asthma by 78%, those urban dwellers who consumed an MD had a 29% reduction in overall asthma risk.[218] Mexican children with greater adherence to the MD were 40% less likely to have asthma, 59% less likely to have allergic rhinitis, and 37% less likely to have itchy or watery eyes.[219] Children who consumed fast food more than three times weekly and who did not include fruit in their diet were far more likely to have wheeze.[220] Not only is the MD effective at preventing allergy and asthma, but it is also therapeutic. When asthmatic children changed their diet to align with the MD for a year, the incidence of a serious asthmatic attack dropped dramatically, use of corticosteroids was cut by 60%, and bronchodilator use dropped by 75%.[221]

The MD involves a high intake of olive oil, which is known to be highly antiinflammatory.[222] The MD also calls for the moderately high intake of fish, which has demonstrated effectiveness at dropping the risk of allergic rhinitis by 44% in Japanese women.[223] The intake of fish oil by pregnant women dropped the risk of their children having food allergy by 67% and asthma risk by 65%.[224]

Brassica Family. The brassica family of vegetables contain several sulfur-containing compounds that are highly beneficial against toxicant-induced damage. Sulforaphane, one of the main sulfur compounds in the brassica family, activates the transcription factor NrF2, which in turn restores Th1 immune function through increased production of GSH.[225] Persons with low GSTM1

function are at far greater risk for developing allergies after exposure to combustion by-products than those with good glutathione transferase activity.[138] Sulforaphane is known to boost glutathione transferase activity and has demonstrated the ability to block the DEP-induced cytokine disruption that results in Th2 and Th17 dominance.[226] Volunteers who consumed a broccoli sprout beverage with high sulforaphane content were significantly protected from the proallergic effects of DEP.[227]

Curcumin. Curcumin, in the spice turmeric (*Curcuma longa*), also enhances glutathione transferase activity and has demonstrated effectiveness at preventing toxicant-induce immunotoxicity. In animal models, turmeric reduces Th2 dominance and restores Th1 function[228] and prevents DEP-induced increases in systolic blood pressure, C-reactive protein, and TNF-α.[229]

Green Tea. Green tea, another common botanical compound with glutathione-enhancing properties, has also shown immunomodulating activity. The main catechin in green tea, epigallocatechin gallate (EGCG), lowers Th17 activity and reduces autoimmune damage in animal models.[230]

Supplement Intervention

- NAC
- Vitamin A
- Vitamin D
- Probiotics

N-acetyl cysteine. NAC is well known for its ability to increase GSH levels and has similarly demonstrated usefulness against toxicant-induced immune damage. Human volunteers who took 1800 mg of NAC daily were partially protected against airway responsiveness upon exposure to diesel exhaust.[231] In animal models, NAC supplementation had demonstrated the ability to block the development of allergen-specific IgE after exposure to DEP.[232]

Vitamins A and D. Daily supplementation of 25,000 IU of vitamin A in women for 4 months significantly decreased concentration of IL-17 and TGF-β.[233] 1,25-dihydroxycholecalciferol vitamin D reduces proinflammatory cytokines (including Th17), stimulates antiinflammatory cytokines, and promotes Th3 regulatory function.[234]

Probiotics. Although the MD promotes the development of a healthy and antiinflammatory microbiome,[235] supplementation with probiotics is also beneficial. Individuals who have Japanese cedar pollinosis who participated in a double-blind study were given fermented milk with either placebo yogurt or a combination of *Lactobacillus GG/Lactobacillus gasseri*. After 9 weeks, those taking the probiotic mixture exhibited a significant reduction in allergic symptoms.[236] Those consuming the probiotic-containing fermented milk for 10 weeks were also rewarded with a microbiome shift (increased bacteroides and reduced firmicutes) similar to what is seen in persons consuming a MD.[237] A 13-week double-blind trial with *Bifidobacterium longum* (BB536) on another group of Japanese adults with cedar pollinosis revealed that BB536 relieved allergic symptoms and suppressed elevation of cedar-specific IgE.[238] A second study with BB536 on Japanese adults with cedar pollinosis confirmed the benefit of this probiotic to reduce allergic symptoms and reduce allergy medication use.[239] The daily use of *Lactobacillus plantarum* in fermented citrus juice for 8 weeks in another group of individuals with cedar allergy gave very similar results, showing that at least three different probiotics can be beneficial in reducing pollen allergies.[240]

REFERENCES

1. *Centers for Disease Control and Prevention National Center for Health Statistics: Food Allergy Among U.S. Children: Trends in Prevalence and Hospitalizations.* Available at https://www.cdc.gov/nchs/products/databriefs/db10.htm. (Accessed 20 January 2017).
2. Centers for Disease Control and Prevention. *Data Statistics, and Surveillance: Asthma Surveillance Data.* Available at https://www.cdc.gov/asthma/asthmadata.htm. (Accessed 3 January 2017).
3. Lerner, A., Jeremias, P., & Matthias, T. (2015). The world incidence and prevalence of autoimmune disease is increasing. *International Journal of Celiac Disease, 3*(4), 151–155.
4. Genuis, S. J. (2010). Sensitivity-related illness: The escalating pandemic of allergy, food intolerance and chemical sensitivity. *The Science of the Total Environment, 408*(24), 6047–6061. PubMed PMID: 20920818.
5. Katerndahl, D. A., Bell, I. R., Palmer, R. F., & Miller, C. S. (2012). Chemical intolerance in primary care settings: Prevalence, comorbidity, and outcomes. *Annals of Family Medicine, 10*(4), 357–365. PubMed PMID: 22778124.
6. Vojdani, A., Ghoneum, M., & Brautbar, N. (1992). Immune alteration associated with exposure to toxic chemicals. *Toxicology and Industrial Health, 8*(5), 239–254. PubMed PMID: 1455435.
7. Fournier, M., Degas, V., Colborn, T., Omara, F. O., Denizeau, F., Potworowski, E. F., et al. (2000). Immunosuppression in mice fed on diets containing beluga whale blubber from the St. Lawrence Estuary and the Arctic populations. *Toxicology Letters, 112-113*, 311–317.
8. Davis, D., & Safe, S. (1990). Immunosuppressive activities of polychlorinated biphenyls in C57BL/6N mice: Structure-activity relationships as Ah receptor agonist and partial antagonists. *Toxicology, 63*, 97–111.
9. Tan, Y., Li, D., Song, R., Lawrence, D., & Carpenter, D. O. (2003). Ortho-substituted PCBs kill thymocytes. *Toxicological Sciences, 76*, 328–337.
10. Thrasher, J. D., Vojdani, A., Cheung, G., & Heuser, G. (1987). Evidence for formaldehyde antibodies and altered cellular immunity in subjects exposed to formaldehyde in mobile home. *Archives of Environmental Health, 42*(6), 347–351.
11. Gray, M. R., Thrasher, J. D., Crago, R., Madison, R. A., Arnold, L., Campbell, A. W., et al. (2003). Mixed mold mycotoxicosis: Immunological changes in humans following exposure in water-damaged buildings. *Archives of Environmental Health, 58*(7), 410–420. PubMed PMID: 15143854.
12. Perez-Maldonado, I. N., Diaz-Barriga, F., de la Fuente, H., et al. (2004). DDT induces apoptosis in human mononuclear cells in vitro and is associated with increased apoptosis in exposed children. *Environmental Research, 94*(1), 38–46.
13. Perez-Maldonado, I. N., Athanasiadou, M., Yanez, L., Gonzalez-Amaro, R., et al. (2006). DDE-induced apoptosis in children exposed to the DDT metabolite. *The Science of the Total Environment, 370*(2–3), 343–351.
14. Vine, M. R., Stein, L., Weigle, K., Schroeder, J., et al. (2001). Plasma 1,1-dichloro-2,2(p-chlorophenyl) ethylene (DDE) levels and immune response. *American Journal of Epidemiology, 153*, 53–63.
15. Banerjee, B. D. (1999). The influence of various factors on immune toxicity assessment of pesticide chemicals. *Toxicology Letters, 107*, 21–31.
16. Mosmann, T. R., Li, L., & Sad, S. (1997). Functions of CD8 T-cell subsets secreting different cytokine patterns. *Seminars in Immunology, 9*(2), 87–92. PubMed PMID: 9194219.
17. Kidd, P. (2003). Th1/Th2 balance: The hypothesis, its limitations, and implications for health and disease. *Alternative Medicine Review: A Journal of Clinical Therapeutic, 8*(5), 223–246.

18. Rose, N. R., & Margolick, J. B. (1992). The Immunological assessment of immunotoxic effects in man. In D. S. Newcombe, N. R. Rose, & J. C. Bloom (Eds.) *Clinical Immunotoxicology.* New York: Raven Press.

19. Pène, J., Chevalier, S., Preisser, L., Vénéreau, E., Guilleux, M. H., Ghannam, S., et al. (2008). Chronically inflamed human tissues are infiltrated by highly differentiated Th17 lymphocytes. *The Journal of Immunology: Official Journal of the American Association of Immunologists, 180*(11), 7423–7430. PubMed PMID: 18490742.

20. Zhang, Y., Zhang, Y., Gu, W., He, L., & Sun, B. (2014). Th1/Th2 cell's function in immune system. *Advances in Experimental Medicine and Biology, 841*, 43–65. PubMed PMID: 25261204.

21. Sakaguchi, S. (2011). Regulatory T cells: History and perspective. *Methods in Molecular Biology, 707*, 3–17. PubMed PMID: 21287325.

22. Wynn, T. A. (2005). T(H)-17: A giant step from T(H)1 and T(H)2. *Nature Immunology, 6*(11), 1069–1070. PubMed PMID: 16239919.

23. Cheung, P. F., Wong, C. K., & Lam, C. W. (2008). Molecular mechanisms of cytokine and chemokine release from eosinophils activated by IL-17A, IL-17F, and IL-23: Implication for Th17 lymphocytes-mediated allergic inflammation. *The Journal of Immunology: Official Journal of the American Association of Immunologists, 180*(8), 5625–5635. PubMed PMID: 18390747.

24. Vojdani, A., & Lambert, J. (2011). The Role of Th17 in Neuroimmune Disorders: Target for CAM Therapy. Part I. *Evidence-based Complementary and Alternative Medicine, 2011*, 927294. PubMed PMID: 19622600.

25. Forman, H. J., Zhang, H., & Rinna, A. (2008). Glutathione: Overview of its protective roles, measurement, and biosynthesis. *Molecular Aspects of Medicine, 113*, 234–258. PubMed PMID: 18796312.

26. Bondy, S. C., & McKee, M. (1991). Disruption of the potential across the synaptosomal plasma membrane and mitochondria by neurotoxic agents. *Toxicology Letters, 58*, 13–21. PubMed PMID: 1897003.

27. Lu, S. C. (2009). Regulation of glutathione synthesis. *Molecular Aspects of Medicine, 30*, 42–59. PubMed PMID: 18601945.

28. Peterson, J. D., Herzenberg, L. A., Vasquez, K., & Waltenvaugh, C. (1998). Glutathione levels in antigen-presenting cells modulate Th1 versus Th2 response patterns. *Proceedings of the National Academy of Sciences of the United States of America, 95*, 3071–3076. PubMed PMID: 9501217.

29. Fraternale, A., Paoletti, M. F., Dominici, S., Buondelmonte, C., Caputo, A., Castaldello, A., et al. (2011). Modulation of Th1/Th2 immune responses to HIV-1 Tat by new pro-GSH molecules. *Vaccine, 29*(40), 6823–6829. PubMed PMID: 21816192.

30. Strenzke, N., Grabbe, J., Plath, K. E. S., Rohwer, J., Wolff, H. H., & Gibbs, B. F. (2001). Mercuric chloride enhances immunoglobulin E-dependent mediator release from human basophils. *Toxicology and Applied Pharmacology, 164*, 257–263. PubMed PMID 11485386.

31. Ahamed, M., Akhtar, M. J., Verma, S., Kumar, A., & Siddiqui, M. K. (2011). Environmental lead exposure as a risk for childhood aplastic anemia. *Bioscience Trends, 5*(1), 38–43. PubMed PMID: 21422599.

32. Hu, X. Z., & Hu, D. C. (2009). Effects of perfluorooctanoate and perfluorooctane sulfonate exposure on hepatoma Hep G2 cells. *Archives of Toxicology, 83*(9), 851–861. PubMed PMID: 19468714.

33. Zhou, D., Wang, H., Zhang, J., Gao, X., Zhao, W., & Zheng, Y. (2010). Di-n-butyl phthalate (DBP) exposure induces oxidative damage in testes of adult rats. *Systems Biology in Reproductive Medicine, 56*(6), 413–419. PubMed PMID: 20883123.

34. Wetmore, B. A., Struve, M. F., Gao, P., Sharma, S., Allison, N., et al. (2008). Genotoxicity of intermittent co-exposure to benzene and toluene in male CD-1 mice. *Chemico-Biological Interactions, 173*(3), 166–178. PubMed PMID: 18455711.

35. Hassoun, E. A., & Periandri-Steinberg, S. (2010). Assessment of the roles of antioxidant enzymes and glutathione in 3,3',4,4',5-Pentachlorobiphenyl (PCB 126)-induced oxidative stress in the brain tissues of rats after subchronic exposure. *Toxicological and Environmental Chemistry, 92*(2), 301. PubMed PMID: 20161674.

36. Jang, T. C., Jang, J. H., & Lee, K. W. (2016). Mechanism of acute endosulfan intoxication-induced neurotoxicity in Sprague-Dawley rats. *Arhiv Za Higijenu Rada I Toksikologiju, 67*(1), 9–17. PubMed PMID: 27092634.

37. Bebe, F. N., & Panemangalore, M. (2003). Exposure to low doses of endosulfan and chlorpyrifos modifies endogenous antioxidants in tissues of rats. *Journal of Environmental Science and Health. Part. B, Pesticides, Food Contaminants, and Agricultural Wastes, 38*(3), 349–363. PubMed PMID: 12716052.

38. Weichenthal, S., Crouse, D. L., Pinault, L., Godri-Pollitt, K., Lavigne, E., Evans, G., et al. (2016). Oxidative burden of fine particulate air pollution and risk of cause-specific mortality in the Canadian Census Health and Environment Cohort (CanCHEC). *Environmental Research, 146*, 92–99. PubMed PMID: 26745732.

39. Reddy, S., Finkelstein, E. I., Wong, P. S., Phung, A., Cross, C. E., & van der Vliet, A. (2002). Identification of glutathione modifications by cigarette smoke. *Free Radical Biology & Medicine, 33*(11), 1490–1498. PubMed PMID: 12446206.

40. Banerjee, A., Trueblood, M. B., Zhang, X., Manda, K. R., Lobo, P., et al. (2009). N-acetylcysteineamide (NACA) prevents inflammation and oxidative stress in animals exposed to diesel engine exhaust. *Toxicology Letters, 187*(3), 187–193. PubMed PMID: 19429263.

41. Kato, T., Tada-Oikawa, S., Takahashi, K., Saito, K., Wang, L., Nishio, A., et al. (2006). Endocrine disruptors that deplete glutathione levels in APC promote Th2 polarization in mice leading to the exacerbation of airway inflammation. *European Journal of Immunology, 36*(5), 1199–1209. PubMed PMID: 16598818.

42. Masubuchi, Y., Sugiyama, S., & Horie, T. (2009). Th1/Th2 cytokine balance as a determinant of acetaminophen-induced liver injury. *Chemico-Biological Interactions, 179*(2–3), 273–279. PubMed PMID: 19014921.

43. Morris, D., Ly, J., Chi, P. T., Daliva, J., Nguyen, T., Soofer, C., et al. (2014). Glutathione synthesis is compromised in erythrocytes from individuals with HIV. *Frontiers in Pharmacology, 5*, 73. PubMed PMID: 24782776.

44. Tudela, E. V., Singh, M. K., Lagman, M., Ly, J., Patel, N., Ochoa, C., et al. (2014). Cytokine levels in plasma samples of individuals with HIV infection. *Austin Journal of Clinical Immunology, 1*(1), 1003.

45. Rea, W. J. (1992). *Chemical Sensitivities* (Vol. 1). Boca Raton, FL.: CRC Press.

46. Christiansen, E. S., Kjaer, H. F., Eller, E., Bindslev-Jensen, C., Høst, A., Mortz, C. G., et al. (2016). The prevalence of atopic diseases and the patterns of sensitization in adolescence. *Pediatric Allergy and Immunology: Official Publication of the European Society of Pediatric Allergy and Immunology, 27*(8), 847–853. PubMed PMID: 27591739.

47. Codispoti, C. D., LeMasters, G. K., Levin, L., Reponen, T., Ryan, P. H., Biagini Myers, J. M., et al. (2015). Traffic pollution is associated with early childhood aeroallergen sensitization. *Annals of Allergy, Asthma and Immunology, 114*(2), 126–133. PubMed PMID: 25499550.

48. Sih, T., & Mion, O. (2010). Allergic rhinitis in the child and associated comorbidities. *Pediatric Allergy and Immunology: Official Publication of the European Society of Pediatric Allergy and Immunology, 21*(1 Pt. 2), e107–e113. PubMed PMID: 19664013.

49. Sly, R. M. (1999). Changing prevalence of allergic rhinitis and asthma. *Annals of Allergy, Asthma and Immunology, 82*(3), 233–248. PubMed PMID: 10094214.

50. Shaker, M., & Salcone, E. (2016). An update on ocular allergy. *Current Opinion in Allergy and Clinical Immunology, 16*(5), 505–510. PubMed PMID: 27490123.

51. Hill, D. A., Dudley, J. W., & Spergel, J. M. (2016). The prevalence of eosinophilic esophagitis in pediatric patients with IgE-mediated food allergy. *The Journal of Allergy and Clinical Immunology. In Practice*, pii: S2213-2198(16)30578-5. PubMed PMID: 28042003.

52. Motosue, M. S., Bellolio, M. F., Van Houten, H. K., Shah, N. D., & Campbell, R. L. (2017). Increasing emergency department visits for anaphylaxis, 2005-2014. *The Journal of Allergy and Clinical Immunology. In Practice, 5*(1), 171–175.e3. PubMed PMID: 27818135.

53. Catassi, C., Kryszak, D., Bhatti, B., Sturgeon, C., Helzlsouer, K., Clipp, S. L., et al. (2010). Natural history of celiac disease autoimmunity in a USA cohort followed since 1974. *Annals of Medicine, 42*(7), 530–538. PubMed PMID: 20868314.

54. Ludvigsson, J. F., Rubio-Tapia, A., van Dyke, C. T., Melton, L. J., 3rd, Zinsmeister, A. R., Lahr, B. D., et al. (2013). Increasing incidence of celiac disease in a North American population. *The American Journal of Gastroenterology, 108*(5), 818–824. PubMed PMID: 23511460.

55. Garabrant, D. H., & Schweitzer, S. (2002). Epidemiology of latex sensitization and allergies in health care workers. *The Journal of Allergy and Clinical Immunology, 110*(2 Suppl.), S82–S95. PubMed PMID: 12170248.

56. Jeong, S. H., Kim, J. H., Son, B. K., Hong, S. C., Kim, S. Y., Lee, G. H., et al. (2011). Comparison of air pollution and the prevalence of allergy-related diseases in Incheon and Jeju City. *Korean Journal of Pediatrics, 54*(12), 501–506. PubMed PMID: 22323906.

57. Sbihi, H., Allen, R. W., Becker, A., Brook, J. R., Mandhane, P., Scott, J. A., et al. (2015). Perinatal Exposure to Traffic-Related Air Pollution and Atopy at 1 Year of Age in a Multi-Center Canadian Birth Cohort Study. *Environmental Health Perspectives, 123*(9), 902–908. PubMed PMID: 25826816.

58. Gruzieva, O., Bellander, T., Eneroth, K., Kull, I., Melén, E., Nordling, E., et al. (2012). Traffic-related air pollution and development of allergic sensitization in children during the first 8 years of life. *The Journal of Allergy and Clinical Immunology, 129*(1), 240–246. PubMed PMID: 22104609.

59. Fuertes, E., Brauer, M., MacIntyre, E., Bauer, M., Bellander, T., von Berg, A., et al. (2013). Childhood allergic rhinitis, traffic-related air pollution, and variability in the GSTP1, TNF, TLR2, and TLR4 genes: Results from the TAG Study. *The Journal of Allergy and Clinical Immunology*, 132(2), 342–352.e2. PubMed PMID: 23639307.

60. Chung, H. Y., Hsieh, C. J., Tseng, C. C., & Yiin, L. M. (2016). Association between the First Occurrence of Allergic Rhinitis in Preschool Children and Air Pollution in Taiwan. *International Journal of Environmental Research and Public Health*, 13(3), pii: E268. PubMed PMID: 26927153.

61. Morgenstern, V., Zutavern, A., Cyrys, J., Brockow, I., Gehring, U., Koletzko, S., et al. (2007). Respiratory health and individual estimated exposure to traffic-related air pollutants in a cohort of young children. *Occupational and Environmental Medicine*, 64(1), 8–16. PubMed PMID: 16912084.

62. Kim, H. H., Lee, C. S., Yu, S. D., Lee, J. S., Chang, J. Y., Jeon, J. M., et al. (2016). Near-road exposure and impact of air pollution on allergic diseases in elementary school children: A cross-sectional study. *Yonsei Medical Journal*, 57(3), 698–713. PubMed PMID: 26996571.

63. Magas, O. K., Gunter, J. T., & Regens, J. L. (2007). Ambient air pollution and daily pediatric hospitalizations for asthma. *Environmental Science and Pollution Research International*, 14(1), 19–23. PubMed PMID: 17352124.

64. Porebski, G., Woźniak, M., & Czarnobilska, E. (2014). Residential proximity to major roadways is associated with increased prevalence of allergic respiratory symptoms in children. *Annals of Agricultural and Environmental Medicine*, 21(4), 760–766. PubMed PMID: 25528916.

65. Shirinde, J., Wichmann, J., & Voyi, K. (2015). Allergic rhinitis, rhinoconjunctivitis and hayfever symptoms among children are associated with frequency of truck traffic near residences: A cross sectional study. *Environmental Health: A Global Access Science Source*, 14, 84. PubMed PMID: 26503217.

66. Wyler, C., Braun-Fahrländer, C., Künzli, N., Schindler, C., Ackermann-Liebrich, U., Perruchoud, A. P., et al. (2000). Exposure to motor vehicle traffic and allergic sensitization. The Swiss Study on Air Pollution and Lung Diseases in Adults (SAPALDIA) Team. *Epidemiology (Cambridge, Mass.)*, 11(4), 450–456. PubMed PMID: 10874554.

67. Middleton, N., Yiallouros, P., Nicolaou, N., Kleanthous, S., Pipis, S., Zeniou, M., et al. (2010). Residential exposure to motor vehicle emissions and the risk of wheezing among 7-8 year-old schoolchildren: A city-wide cross-sectional study in Nicosia, Cyprus. *Environmental Health: A Global Access Science Source*, 9, 28. PubMed PMID: 20565827.

68. Gehring, U., Wijga, A. H., Brauer, M., Fischer, P., de Jongste, J. C., Kerkhof, M., et al. (2010). Traffic-related air pollution and the development of asthma and allergies during the first 8 years of life. *American Journal of Respiratory and Critical Care Medicine*, 181(6), 596–603. PubMed PMID: 19965811.

69. Brauer, M., Hoek, G., Smit, H. A., de Jongste, J. C., Gerritsen, J., Postma, D. S., et al. (2007). Air pollution and development of asthma, allergy and infections in a birth cohort. *The European Respiratory Journal*, 29(5), 879–888. PubMed PMID: 17251230.

70. Modig, L., Torén, K., Janson, C., Jarvholm, B., & Forsberg, B. (2009). Vehicle exhaust outside the home and onset of asthma among adults. *The European Respiratory Journal*, 33(6), 1261–1267. PubMed PMID: 19251785.

71. Pereira, G., De Vos, A. J., & Cook, A. (2009). Residential traffic exposure and children's emergency department presentation for asthma: A spatial study. *International Journal of Health Geographics*, 8, 63. PubMed PMID: 19930672.

72. Spira-Cohen, A., Chen, L. C., Kendall, M., Lall, R., & Thurston, G. D. (2011). Personal exposures to traffic-related air pollution and acute respiratory health among Bronx schoolchildren with asthma. *Environmental Health Perspectives*, 119(4), 559–565. Erratum in: Environ Health Perspect. 2011 Apr;119(4):564. PubMed PMID: 21216722.

73. Ryan, P. H., Bernstein, D. I., Lockey, J., Reponen, T., Levin, L., Grinshpun, S., et al. (2009). Exposure to traffic-related particles and endotoxin during infancy is associated with wheezing at age 3 years. *American Journal of Respiratory and Critical Care Medicine*, 180(11), 1068–1075. PubMed PMID: 19745206.

74. French 2017 car registrations up, diesel share below 50 pct https://www.reuters.com/article/france-autos/french-2017-car-registrations-up-diesel-share-below-50-pct-idUSL8N1OW0DC (Accessed 12 February 2018).

75. Sarkar, S., Song, Y., Sarkar, S., Kipen, H. M., Laumbach, R. J., Zhang, J., et al. (2012). Suppression of the NF-κB pathway by diesel exhaust particles impairs human antimycobacterial immunity. *The Journal of Immunology: Official Journal of the American Association of Immunologists*, 188(6), 2778–2793. PubMed PMID: 22345648.

76. Ohtani, T., Nakagawa, S., Kurosawa, M., Mizuashi, M., Ozawa, M., & Alba, S. (2005). Cellular basis of the

role of diesel exhaust particles in inducing Th-2 dominant response. *The Journal of Immunology: Official Journal of the American Association of Immunologists*, 174(4), 2412–2419. PubMed PMID: 15699178.

77. Pawlak, E. A., Noah, T. L., Zhou, H., Chehrazi, C., Robinette, C., Diaz-Sanchez, D., et al. (2016). Diesel exposure suppresses natural killer cell function and resolution of eosinophil inflammation: A randomized controlled trial of exposure in allergic rhinitics. *Particle and Fibre Toxicology*, 13(1), 24. PubMed PMID: 27154411.

78. Müller, L., Chehrazi, C. V., Henderson, M. W., Noah, T. L., & Jaspers, I. (2013). Diesel exhaust particles modify natural killer cell function and cytokine release. *Particle and Fibre Toxicology*, 10, 16. PubMed PMID: 23618096.

79. Castranova, V., Ma, J. Y., Yang, H. M., Antonini, J. M., Butterworth, L., et al. (2001). Effect of exposure to diesel exhaust particles on the susceptibility of the lung to infection. *Environmental Health Perspectives*, 109(Suppl. 4), 609–612. PubMed PMID: 11544172.

80. Yin, X. J., Dong, C. C., Ma, J. Y., Antonini, J. M., Roberts, J. R., et al. (2005). Sustained effect of inhaled diesel exhaust particles on T-lymphocyte-mediated immune responses against Listeria monocytogenes. *Toxicological Sciences*, 88(1), 73–81. PubMed PMID: 16107554.

81. Takano, H., Yanagisawa, R., & Inoue, K. (2007). Components of diesel exhaust particles diversely enhance a variety of respiratory diseases related to infection or allergy: Extracted organic chemicals and the residual particles after extraction differently affect respiratory diseases. *Journal of Clinical Biochemistry and Nutrition*, 40(2), 101–107. PubMed PMID: 18188411.

82. Yang, H. M., Antonini, J. M., Barger, M. W., Butterworth, L., Roberts, B. R., Ma, J. K., et al. (2001). Diesel exhaust particles suppress macrophage function and slow the pulmonary clearance of Listeria monocytogenes in rats. *Environmental Health Perspectives*, 109(5), 515–521. PubMed PMID: 11401764.

83. Williams, L. A., Ulrich, C. M., Larson, T., Wener, M. H., Wood, B., Campbell, P. T., et al. (2009). Proximity to traffic, inflammation, and immune function among women in the Seattle, Washington, area. *Environmental Health Perspectives*, 117(3), 373–378. PubMed PMID: 19337511.

84. Feng, Y., Kong, Y., Barnes, P. F., Huang, F. F., Klucar, P., et al. (2011). Exposure to cigarette smoke inhibits the pulmonary T-cell response to influenza virus and Mycobacterium tuberculosis. *Infection and Immunity*, 79(1), 229–237. PubMed PMID: 20974820.

85. Hogan, A. E., Corrigan, M. A., O'Reilly, V., Gaoatswe, G., O'Connell, J., et al. (2011). Cigarette smoke alters the invariant natural killer T cell function and may inhibit anti-tumor responses. *Clinical Immunology (Orlando, Fla.)*, 140(3), 229–235. PubMed PMID: 21684213.

86. Takafuji, S., Suzuki, S., Koizumi, K., Tadokoro, K., Miyamoto, T., Ikemori, R., et al. (1987). Diesel-exhaust particulates inoculated by the intranasal route have and adjunctive activity for IgE production in mice. *The Journal of Allergy and Clinical Immunology*, 79, 639–645. PubMed PMID: 2435776.

87. Diaz-Sanchez, D., Tsien, A., Casillas, A., Dotson, A. R., & Saxon, A. (1996). Enhanced nasal cytokine production in human beings after an in vivo challenge with diesel exhaust particles. *The Journal of Allergy and Clinical Immunology*, 98, 114–123. PubMed PMID: 8765825.

88. Sasaki, Y., Ohtani, T., Ito, Y., Mizuashi, M., Nakagawa, S., et al. (2009). Molecular events in human T cells treated with diesel exhaust particles or formaldehyde that underlie their diminished interferon-gamma and interleukin-10 production. *International Archives of Allergy and Immunology*, 148(3), 239–250. PubMed PMID: 18849615.

89. Carlsten, C., Blomberg, A., Pui, M., Sandstrom, T., Wong, S. W., Alexis, N., et al. (2016). Diesel exhaust augments allergen-induced lower airway inflammation in allergic individuals: A controlled human exposure study. *Thorax*, 71(1), 35–44. Erratum in: Thorax. 2016 Apr;71(4):385. PubMed PMID: 26574583.

90. Diaz-Sanchez, D., Tsien, A., Fleming, J., & Saxon, A. (1997). Combined diesel exhaust particulate and ragweed allergen challenge markedly enhances human in vivo nasal ragweed-specific IgE and skews cytokine production to a T helper cell 2-type pattern. *The Journal of Immunology: Official Journal of the American Association of Immunologists*, 158(5), 2406–2413. PubMed PMID: 9036991.

91. Maejima, K., Tamura, K., Nakajima, T., Taniguchi, Y., Saito, S., & Takenaka, H. (2001). Effects of the inhalation of diesel exhaust, Kanto loam dust, or diesel exhaust without particles on immune responses in mice exposed to Japanese cedar (Cryptomeria japonica) pollen. *Inhalation Toxicology*, 13(11), 1047–1063. PubMed PMID: 11696873.

92. Lubitz, S., Schober, W., Pusch, G., Effner, R., Klopp, N., et al. (2010). Polycyclic aromatic hydrocarbons from diesel emissions exert proallergic effects in birch pollen

allergic individuals through enhanced mediator release from basophils. *Environmental Toxicology*, 25(2), 188–197. PubMed PMID: 19382185.

93. Nilsen, A., Hagemann, R., & Eide, I. (1997). The adjuvant activity of diesel exhaust particles and carbon black on systemic IgE production to ovalbumin in mice after intranasal instillation. *Toxicology*, 124(3), 225–232. PubMed PMID: 9482124.

94. Nel, A. E., Diaz-Sanchez, D., Ng, D., Hiura, T., & Saxon, A. (1998). Enhancement of allergic inflammation by the interaction between diesel exhaust particles and the immune system. *The Journal of Allergy and Clinical Immunology*, 102(4 Pt. 1), 539–554. PubMed PMID: 9802360.

95. Muranaka, M., & Yamamoto, K. (2002). Epidemiological studies supporting that airborne diesel-exhaust particles caused the outbreak of Japanese cedar pollinosis in Japan. *(Japanese) Igaku No Ayumi*, 200, 401–406.

96. Konishi, S., Ng, C. F., Stickley, A., Nishihata, S., Shinsugi, C., Ueda, K., et al. (2014). Particulate matter modifies the association between airborne pollen and daily medical consultations for pollinosis in Tokyo. *The Science of the Total Environment*, 499, 125–132. PubMed PMID: 25181044.

97. Sakurai, Y., Nakamura, K., Teruya, K., Shimada, N., Umeda, T., Tanaka, H., et al. (1998). Prevalence and risk factors of allergic rhinitis and cedar pollinosis among Japanese men. *Preventive Medicine*, 27(4), 617–622. PubMed PMID: 9672957.

98. Ishizaki, T., Koizumi, K., Ikemori, R., Ishiyama, Y., & Kushibiki, E. (1987). Studies of prevalence of Japanese cedar pollinosis among the residents in a densely cultivated area. *Annals of Allergy*, 58(4), 265–270. PubMed PMID: 3565861.

99. Choi, H., Schmidbauer, N., & Bornehag, C. G. (2017). Volatile organic compounds of possible microbial origin and their risks on childhood asthma and allergies within damp homes. *Environment International*, 98, 143–151. PubMed PMID: 27838117.

100. Baxi, S. N., Portnoy, J. M., Larenas-Linnemann, D., Phipatanakul, W., & Environmental Allergens Workgroup. (2016). Exposure and health effects of fungi on humans. *The Journal of Allergy and Clinical Immunology. In Practice*, 4(3), 396–404. PubMed PMID: 26947460.

101. Thacher, J. D., Gruzieva, O., Pershagen, G., Melén, E., Lorentzen, J. C., Kull, I., et al. (2016). Mold and dampness exposure and allergic outcomes from birth to adolescence: Data from the BAMSE cohort. *Allergy*, PubMed PMID: 27925656.

102. Gustafsson, D., Andersson, K., Fagerlund, I., & Kjellman, N. I. (1996). Significance of indoor environment for the development of allergic symptoms in children followed up to 18 months of age. *Allergy*, 51(11), 789–795. PubMed PMID: 8947336.

103. Gilmour, M. I., Jaakkola, M. S., London, S. J., Nel, A. E., & Rogers, C. A. (2006). How exposure to environmental tobacco smoke, outdoor air pollutants, and increased pollen burdens influence the incidence of asthma. *Environmental Health Perspectives*, 114(4), 627–633. PubMed PMID: 16581557.

104. Singh, S. P., Mishra, N. C., Rir-Sima-Ah, J., Campen, M., Kurup, V., et al. (2009). Maternal exposure to secondhand cigarette smoke primes the lung for induction of phosphodiesterase-4D5 isozyme and exacerbated Th2 responses: Rolipram attenuates the airway hyperreactivity and muscarinic receptor expression but not lung inflammation and atopy. *The Journal of Immunology: Official Journal of the American Association of Immunologists*, 183(3), 2115–2121. PubMed PMID: 19596983.

105. Diaz-Sanchez, D., Rumold, R., & Gong, H., Jr. (2006). Challenge with environmental tobacco smoke exacerbates allergic airway disease in human beings. *The Journal of Allergy and Clinical Immunology*, 118(2), 441–446. PubMed PMID: 16890770.

106. Gilliland, F. D., Li, Y. F., Gong, H., Jr., & Diaz-Sanchez, D. (2006). Glutathione s-transferases M1 and P1 prevent aggravation of allergic responses by secondhand smoke. *American Journal of Respiratory and Critical Care Medicine*, 174(12), 1335–1341. PubMed PMID: 17023730.

107. Jaakkola, J. J., Parise, H., Kislitsin, V., Lebedeva, N. I., & Spengler, J. D. (2004). Asthma, wheezing, and allergies in Russian schoolchildren in relation to new surface materials in the home. *American Journal of Public Health*, 94(4), 560–562. PubMed PMID: 15054004.

108. Thrasher, J. D., Madison, R., & Broughton, A. (1993). Immunologic abnormalities in humans exposed to chlorpyrifos: Preliminary observations. *Archives of Environmental Health*, 48(2), 89–93. PubMed PMID: 7682805.

109. Bornehag, C. G., Sundell, J., Weschler, C. J., Sigsgaard, T., Lundgren, B., Hasselgren, M., et al. (2004). The association between asthma and allergic symptoms in children and phthalates in house dust: A nested case-control study. *Environmental Health Perspectives*, 112(14), 1393–1397. PubMed PMID: 15471731.

110. Kim, J. H., Chang, J. H., Choi, H. S., Kim, H. J., & Kang, J. W. (2016). The association between serum lead and total immunoglobulin E levels according to

allergic sensitization. *American Journal of Rhinology & Allergy*, 30(2), e48–e52. PubMed PMID: 26980386.

111. Lutz, P. M., Wilson, T. J., Ireland, J., Jones, A. L., Gorman, J. S., Gale, N. L., et al. (1999). Elevated immunoglobulin E (IgE) levels in children with exposure to environmental lead. *Toxicology*, 134(1), 63–78. PubMed PMID: 10413189.

112. Mener, D. J., Garcia-Esquinas, E., Navas-Acien, A., Dietert, R. R., Shargorodsky, J., & Lin, S. Y. (2015). *International Forum of Allergy & Rhinology*, 5(3), 214–220. PubMed PMID: 25524712.

113. Grandjean, P., Poulsen, L. K., Heilmann, C., Steuerwald, U., & Weihe, P. (2010). Allergy and sensitization during childhood associated with prenatal and lactational exposure to marine pollutants. *Environmental Health Perspectives*, 118(10), 1429–1433. PubMed PMID: 20562055.

114. Reichrtová, E., Ciznár, P., Prachar, V., Palkovicová, L., & Veningerová, M. (1999). Cord serum immunoglobulin E related to the environmental contamination of human placentas with organochlorine compounds. *Environmental Health Perspectives*, 107(11), 895–899. PubMed PMID: 10544157.

115. Stølevik, S. B., Nygaard, U. C., Namork, E., Haugen, M., Kvalem, H. E., Meltzer, H. M., et al. (2011). Prenatal exposure to polychlorinated biphenyls and dioxins is associated with increased risk of wheeze and infections in infants. *Food and Chemical Toxicology : An International Journal Published for the British Industrial Biological Research Association*, 49(8), 1843–1848. PubMed PMID: 21571030.

116. Salam, M. T., Li, Y. F., Langholz, B., Gilliland, F. D., & Children's Health Study. (2004). Early-life environmental risk factors for asthma: Findings from the Children's Health Study. *Environmental Health Perspectives*, 112(6), 760–765. PubMed PMID: 15121522.

117. Araki, A., Saito, I., Kanazawa, A., Morimoto, K., Nakayama, K., Shibata, E., et al. (2014). Phosphorus flame retardants in indoor dust and their relation to asthma and allergies of inhabitants. *Indoor Air*, 24(1), 3–15. PubMed PMID: 23724807.

118. Lehmann, I., Rehwagen, M., Diez, U., Seiffart, A., Rolle-Kampczyk, U., et al., Leipzig Allergy Risk Children Study. (2001). Enhanced in vivo IgE production and T cell polarization toward the type 2 phenotype in association with indoor exposure to VOC: Results of the LARS study. *International Journal of Hygiene and Environmental Health*, 204(4), 211–221. PubMed PMID: 11833293.

119. Zock, J. P., Plana, E., Jarvis, D., Antó, J. M., Kromhout, H., Kennedy, S. M., et al. (2007). The use of household cleaning sprays and adult asthma: An international longitudinal study. *American Journal of Respiratory and Critical Care Medicine*, 176(8), 735–741. PubMed PMID: 17585104.

120. Zock, J. P., Kogevinas, M., Sunyer, J., Almar, E., Muniozguren, N., Payo, F., et al. (2001). Spanish working group of the European Community Respiratory Health Survey. Asthma risk, cleaning activities and use of specific cleaning products among Spanish indoor cleaners. *Scandinavian Journal of Work, Environment and Health*, 27(1), 76–81. PubMed PMID: 11266151.

121. Centers for Disease Control and Prevention. *National Report on Human Exposure to Environmental Chemicals: Updated tables, 2017*. Available at http://www.cdc.gov/exposurereport/. (Accessed 9 January 2012).

122. Zheng, L., Dong, G. H., Zhang, Y. H., Liang, Z. F., Jun, Y. H., & He, Q. C. (2011). Type 1 and type 2 cytokines imbalance in adult male C57BL/6 mice following a 7-day oral exposure to perfluorooctanesulfonate (PFOS). *Journal of Immunotoxicology*, 8(1), 30–38. PubMed PMID: 21299352.

123. Wang, I. J., Hsieh, W. S., Chen, C. Y., Fletcher, T., Lien, G. W., et al. (2011). The effect of prenatal perfluorinated chemicals exposures on pediatric atopy. *Environmental Research*, 111(6), 785–791. PubMed PMID: 21601844.

124. Crinnion, W. J. (2010). Toxic effects of the easily avoidable phthalates and parabens. *Alternative Medicine Review: A Journal of Clinical Therapeutic*, 15(3), 190–196. Review. PubMed PMID: 21155623.

125. Bornehag, C. G., Sundell, J., Weschler, C. J., Sigsgaard, T., et al. (2004). The association between asthma and allergic symptoms in children and phthalates in house dust: A nested case-control study. *Environmental Health Perspectives*, 112, 1393–1397. PubMed PMID: 15471731.

126. Hoppin, J. A., Jaramillo, R., London, S. J., Bertelsen, R. J., Salo, P. M., Sandler, D. P., et al. (2013). Phthalate exposure and allergy in the U.S. population: Results from NHANES 2005-2006. *Environmental Health Perspectives*, 121(10), 1129–1134. PubMed PMID: 23799650.

127. Bornehag, C. G., & Nanberg, E. (2009). Phthalate exposure and asthma in chidren. *International Journal of Andrology*, 33, 1–13. PubMed PMID: 20059582.

128. Seo, M., Yamagiwa, T., Kobayashi, R., Ikeda, K., et al. (2008). Augmentation of antigen-stimulated allergic responses by a small amount of trichloroethylene ingestion from drinking water. *Regulatory Toxicology and Pharmacology*, 52(2), 140–146. PubMed PMID: 18721841.

129. Burg, J. R., & Gist, G. L. (1999). Health effects of environmental contaminant exposure: An intrafile comparison of the trichloroethylene subregistry. *Archives of Environmental Health, 54*(4), 231–241. PubMed PMID: 10433181.

130. Gallagher, C. M., McElroy, A. E., Smith, D. M., Golightly, M. G., & Meliker, J. R. (2013). Polychlorinated biphenyls, mercury, and antinuclear antibody positivity, NHANES 2003-2004. *International Journal of Hygiene and Environmental Health, 216*(6), 721–727. PubMed PMID: 23419585.

131. Somers, E. C., Ganser, M. A., Warren, J. S., Basu, N., Wang, L., Zick, S. M., et al. (2015). Mercury Exposure and Antinuclear Antibodies among Females of Reproductive Age in the United States: NHANES. *Environmental Health Perspectives, 123*(8), 792–798. PubMed PMID: 25665152.

132. Silva, I. A., Nyland, J. F., Gorman, A., Perisse, A., Ventura, A. M., Santos, E. C., et al. (2004). Mercury exposure, malaria, and serum antinuclear/antinucleolar antibodies in Amazon populations in Brazil: A cross-sectional study. *Environmental Health: A Global Access Science Source, 3*(1), 11. PubMed PMID: 15522122.

133. Gardner, R. M., Nyland, J. F., Silva, I. A., Ventura, A. M., de Souza, J. M., & Silbergeld, E. K. (2010). Mercury exposure, serum antinuclear/antinucleolar antibodies, and serum cytokine levels in mining populations in Amazonian Brazil: A cross-sectional study. *Environmental Research, 110*(4), 343–354. PubMed PMID: 20176347.

134. Gilbert, K. M., Rowley, B., Gomez-Acevedo, H., & Blossom, S. J. (2011). Coexposure to mercury increases immunotoxicity of trichloroethylene. *Toxicological Sciences, 119*(2), 281–292. PubMed PMID: 21084432.

135. McConnachie, P. R., & Zahalsky, A. C. (1992). Immune alterations in humans exposed to the termiticide technical chlordane. *Archives of Environmental Health, 47*(4), 295–301. PubMed PMID: 1497384.

136. Thrasher, J. D., Madison, R., & Broughton, A. (1993). Immunologic abnormalities in humans exposed to chlorpyrifos: Preliminary observations. *Archives of Environmental Health, 48*(2), 89–93.

137. Gilbert, K. M., Rowley, B., Gomez-Acevedo, H., & Blossom, S. J. (2011). Coexposure to mercury increases immunotoxicity of trichloroethylene. *Toxicological Sciences, 119*(2), 281–292. PubMed PMID: 21084432.

138. Thrasher, J. D., Broughton, A., & Madison, R. (1990). Immune activation and autoantibodies in humans with long-term inhalation exposure to formaldehyde. *Archives of Environmental Health, 45*(4), 217–223.

139. Skaer, T. L. (1992). Medication-induced systemic lupus erythematosus. *Clinical Therapeutics, 14*(4), 496–506.

140. Kardestuncer, T., & Frumkin, H. (1997). Systemic lupus erythematosus in relation to environmental pollution: An investigation in an African American community in North Georgia. *Archives of Environmental Health, 52*(2), 85–90.

141. Dahlgren, J., Takhar, H., Anderson-Mahoney, P., Kotlerman, J., Tarr, J., & Warshaw, R. (2007). Cluster of systemic lupus erythematosus (SLE) associated with an oil field waste site: A cross sectional study. *Environmental Health: A Global Access Science Source, 6*, 8. Erratum in: Environ Health. 2007 May 17;6:15. PubMed PMID: 17316448.

142. Arnett, F. C., Fritzler, M. J., Ahn, C., & Holian, A. (2000). Urinary mercury levels in patients with autoantibodies to U3-RNP (fibrillarin). *The Journal of Rheumatology, 27*(2), 405–410. PubMed PMID: 10685806.

143. Freni-Titulaer, L., Kelley, D., Grow, A., McKinley, T., Arnett, F., & Hochberg, M. (1989). Connective tissue disease in southeastern Georgia: A case control study of etiologic factors. *American Journal of Epidemiology, 130*, 404–409.

144. Cooper, G., Dooley, M., Treadwell, E., St Clair, E., & Gilkeson, G. (2001). Smoking and use of hair treatments in relation to risk of developing systemic lupus erythematosus. *The Journal of Rheumatology, 28*(12), 2653–2656.

145. Cooper, G. S., Wither, J., Bernatsky, S., Claudio, J. O., Clarke, A., Rioux, J. D., et al. (2010). Occupational and environmental exposures and risk of systemic lupus erythematosus: Silica, sunlight, solvents. *Rheumatology (Oxford, England), 49*(11), 2172–2180. PubMed PMID: 20675707.

146. Kilburn, K. H., & Warshaw, R. H. (1992). Prevalence of symptoms of systemic lupus erythematosus (SLE) and of fluorescent antinuclear antibodies associated with chronic exposure to trichloroethylene and other chemicals in well water. *Environmental Research, 57*(1), 1–9.

147. Cooper, G. S., Makris, S. L., Nietert, P. J., & Jinot, J. (2009). Evidence of autoimmune-related effects of trichloroethylene exposure from studies in mice and humans. *Environmental Health Perspectives, 117*(5), 696–702. PubMed PMID: 19479009.

148. Ghaussy, N. O., Sibbitt, W. L., Jr., & Qualls, C. R. (2001). Cigarette smoking, alcohol consumption, and the risk of systemic lupus erythematosus: A case-control study. *The Journal of Rheumatology, 28*(11), 2449–2453.

149. Tsai, P. C., Ko, Y. C., Huang, W., Liu, H. S., & Guo, Y. L. (2007). Increased liver and lupus mortalities in 24-year follow-up of the Taiwanese people highly exposed to

polychlorinated biphenyls and dibenzofurans. *The Science of the Total Environment*, 374(2–3), 216–222. PubMed PMID: 17257654.

150. Parks, C. G., Walitt, B. T., Pettinger, M., Chen, J. C., de Roos, A. J., Hunt, J., et al. (2011). Insecticide use and risk of rheumatoid arthritis and systemic lupus erythematosus in the Women's Health Initiative Observational Study. *Arthritis Care Research*, 63(2), 184–194. doi:10.1002/acr.20335. PubMed PMID: 20740609.

151. Bernatsky, S., Fournier, M., Pineau, C. A., Clarke, A. E., Vinet, E., & Smargiassi, A. (2011). Associations between ambient fine particulate levels and disease activity in patients with systemic lupus erythematosus (SLE). *Environmental Health Perspectives*, 119(1), 43–49. PubMed PMID: 20870568.

152. Bernatsky, S., Smargiassi, A., Barnabe, C., Svenson, L. W., Brand, A., Martin, R. V., et al. (2016). Fine particulate air pollution and systemic autoimmune rheumatic disease in two Canadian provinces. *Environmental Research*, 146, 85–91. PubMed PMID: 26724462.

153. Fernandes, E. C., Silva, C. A., Braga, A. L., Sallum, A. M., Campos, L. M., & Farhat, S. C. (2015). Exposure to air pollutants and disease activity in juvenile-onset systemic lupus erythematosus patients. *Arthritis Care & Research*, 67(11), 1609–1614. PubMed PMID: 25892357.

154. Zeft, A. S., Prahalad, S., Lefevre, S., Clifford, B., McNally, B., Bohnsack, J. F., et al. (2009). Juvenile idiopathic arthritis and exposure to fine particulate air pollution. *Clinical and Experimental Rheumatology*, 27(5), 877–884. PubMed PMID: 19917177.

155. Lee, D. H., Steffes, M., & Jacobs, D. R. (2007). Positive associations of serum concentration of polychlorinated biphenyls or organochlorine pesticides with self-reported arthritis, especially rheumatoid type, in women. *Environmental Health Perspectives*, 115(6), 883–888. PubMed PMID: 17589595.

156. Afridi, H. I., Kazi, T. G., Talpur, F. N., Naher, S., & Brabazon, D. (2014). Relationship between toxic metals exposure via cigarette smoking and rheumatoid arthritis. *Clinical Laboratory*, 60(10), 1735–1745. PubMed PMID: 25651721.

157. Yan, Y. H., C-K Chou, C., Wang, J. S., Tung, C. L., Li, Y. R., Lo, K., et al. (2014). Subchronic effects of inhaled ambient particulate matter on glucose homeostasis and target organ damage in a type 1 diabetic rat model. *Toxicology and Applied Pharmacology*, 281(2), 211–220. PubMed PMID: 25454026.

158. Nemmar, A., Al-Salam, S., Beegam, S., Yuvaraju, P., Yasin, J., & Ali, B. H. (2014). Pancreatic effects of diesel exhaust particles in mice with type 1 diabetes mellitus. *Cellular Physiology and Biochemistry: International Journal of Experimental Cellular Physiology, Biochemistry, and Pharmacology*, 33(2), 413–422. PubMed PMID: 24556638.

159. Di Ciaula, A. (2016). Type I diabetes in paediatric age in Apulia (Italy): Incidence and associations with outdoor air pollutants. *Diabetes Research and Clinical Practice*, 111, 36–43. PubMed PMID: 26527558.

160. Gallagher, C. M., & Meliker, J. R. (2012). Mercury and thyroid autoantibodies in U.S. women, NHANES 2007-2008. *Environment International*, 40, 39–43. PubMed PMID: 22280926.

161. Mahaffey, K. R., Clickner, R. P., & Bodurow, C. C. (2004). Blood organic mercury and dietary mercury intake: National Health and Nutrition Examination Survey, 1999 and 2000. *Environmental Health Perspectives*, 112(5), 562–570. PubMed PMID: 15064162.

162. Cebecauer, L., Radikova, Z., Rovensky, J., Koska, Imrich, R., Ksinantova, L., et al. (2009). Increased prevalence and coincidence of antinuclear and antithyroid antibodies in the population exposed to high levels of polychlorinated pollutants cocktail. *Endocrine Regulations*, 43(2), 75–81. PubMed PMID: 19856712.

163. Schell, L. M., Gallo, M. V., Ravenscroft, J., & DeCaprio, A. P. (2009). Persistent organic pollutants and anti-thyroid peroxidase levels in Akwesasne Mohawk young adults. *Environmental Research*, 109(1), 86–92. PubMed PMID: 18995849.

164. Vojdani, A., Ghoneum, M., & Brautbar, N. (1992). Immune alteration associated with exposure to toxic chemicals. *Toxicology and Industrial Health*, 8(5), 239–254.

165. Abou-Donia, M. B., Abou-Donia, M. M., ElMasry, E. M., Monro, J. A., & Mulder, M. F. (2013). Autoantibodies to nervous system-specific proteins are elevated in sera of flight crew members: Biomarkers for nervous system injury. *Journal of Toxicology and Environmental Health. Part A*, 76(6), 363–380. PubMed PMID: 23557235.

166. Osuna, C. E., Grandjean, P., Weihe, P., & El-Fawal, H. A. (2014). Autoantibodies associated with prenatal and childhood exposure to environmental chemicals in Faroese children. *Toxicological Sciences*, 142(1), 158–166. PubMed PMID: 25124724.

167. Rajasekaran, D., Subbaraghavalu, G., & Jayapandian, P. (2009). Guillain-Barre syndrome due to organophosphate compound poison. *The Journal of the Association of Physicians of India*, 57, 714–715. PubMed PMID: 20329431.

168. London, L., Bourne, D., Sayed, R., & Eastman, R. (2004). Guillain-Barre syndrome in a rural farming district in South Africa: A possible relationship to environmental organophosphate exposure. *Archives of Environmental Health, 59*(11), 575–580. PubMed PMID: 16599005.

169. Angelici, L., Piola, M., Cavalleri, T., Randi, G., Cortini, F., Bergamaschi, R., et al. (2016). Effects of particulate matter exposure on multiple sclerosis hospital admission in Lombardy region, Italy. *Environmental Research, 145,* 68–73. PubMed PMID: 26624240.

170. Ramagopalan, S. V., Lee, J. D., Yee, I. M., Guimond, C., Traboulsee, A. L., Ebers, G. C., et al. (2013). Association of smoking with risk of multiple sclerosis: A population-based study. *Journal of Neurology, 260*(7), 1778–1781. PubMed PMID: 23455932.

171. Hedström, A. K., Bomfim, I. L., Barcellos, L. F., Briggs, F., Schaefer, C., Kockum, I., et al. (2014). Interaction between passive smoking and two HLA genes with regard to multiple sclerosis risk. *International Journal of Epidemiology, 43*(6), 1791–1798. PubMed PMID: 25324153.

172. Tsai, C. P., & Lee, C. T. (2013). Multiple sclerosis incidence associated with the soil lead and arsenic concentrations in Taiwan. *PLoS ONE, 8*(6), e65911. PubMed PMID: 23799061.

173. Vu, D., Shah, T., Ansari, J., Sakharkar, P., Yasir, Q., Naraghi, R., et al. (2014). Interferon-gamma gene polymorphism +874 A/T is associated with an increased risk of cytomegalovirus infection among Hispanic renal transplant recipients. *Transplant Infectious Disease, 16*(5), 724–732. PubMed PMID: 25208755.

174. Abayli, B., Canataroğlu, A., & Akkiz, H. (2003). Serum profile of T helper 1 and T helper 2 cytokines in patients with chronic hepatitis C virus infection. *The Turkish Journal of Gastroenterology, 14*(1), 7–11. PubMed PMID: 14593531.

175. Pinto, R. A., Arredondo, S. M., Bono, M. R., Gaggero, A. A., & Díaz, P. V. (2006). T helper 1/T helper 2 cytokine imbalance in respiratory syncytial virus infection is associated with increased endogenous plasma cortisol. *Pediatrics, 117*(5), e878–e886. PubMed PMID: 16618789.

176. Leigh, J. E., Steele, C., Wormley, F. L., Jr., Luo, W., Clark, R. A., Gallaher, W., et al. (1998). Th1/Th2 cytokine expression in saliva of HIV-positive and HIV-negative individuals: A pilot study in HIV-positive individuals with oropharyngeal candidiasis. *Journal of Acquired Immune Deficiency Syndromes and Human Retrovirology, 19*(4), 373–380. PubMed PMID: 9833746.

177. Henningsson, A. J., Tjernberg, I., Malmvall, B. E., Forsberg, P., & Ernerudh, J. (2011). Indications of Th1 and Th17 responses in cerebrospinal fluid from patients with Lyme neuroborreliosis: A large retrospective study. *Journal of Neuroinflammation, 8,* 36. PubMed PMID: 21507218.

178. Zhang, M., Wu, N., Yang, L., Zhang, J., Sun, X., Zhong, S., et al. (2011). Study on the T-helper cell 1/2 cytokine profile in blister fluid of patients with herpes zoster and its clinical significance. *The Journal of Dermatology, 38*(12), 1158–1162. PubMed PMID: 21954956.

179. Arndt, V., Vine, M. F., & Weigle, K. (1999). Environmental chemical exposures and risk of herpes zoster. *Environmental Health Perspectives, 107*(10), 835–841.

180. Vine, M. F., Stein, L., Weigle, K., Schroeder, J., Degnan, D., Tse, C. K. E., et al. (2000). Effects on the immune system associated with living near a pesticide dumpsite. *Environmental Health Perspectives, 108,* 1113–1124.

181. Cardenas, A., Smit, E., Houseman, E. A., Kerkvliet, N. I., Bethel, J. W., & Kile, M. L. (2015). Arsenic exposure and prevalence of the varicella zoster virus in the United States: NHANES (2003-2004 and 2009-2010). *Environmental Health Perspectives, 123*(6), 590–596. PubMed PMID: 25636148.

182. Stancek, D., Kosecká, G., Oltman, M., Keleová, A., & Jahnová, E. (1995). Links between prolonged exposure to xenobiotics, increased incidence of hepatopathies, immunological disturbances and exacerbation of latent Epstein-Barr virus infections. *International Journal of Immunopharmacology, 17*(4), 321–328. PubMed PMID: 7672882.

183. Weisglas-Kuperus, N., Patadin, S., Berbers, G. A. M., Sas, T. C. J., Mulder, P. G. H., Sauer, P. J. J., et al. (2000). Immunologic effects of background exposure to polychlorinated biphenyls and dioxins in Dutch preschool children. *Environmental Health Perspectives, 108,* 1203–1207.

184. Dewailly, E., Ayotte, P., Burneau, S., Gingras, S., Belles-Isles, M., & Roy, R. (2000). Susceptibility to infections and immune status in Inuit infants exposed to organochlorines. *Environmental Health Perspectives, 108,* 205–211.

185. Bilrha, H., Roy, R., Moreau, B., Belles-Isles, M., Dewailly, E., & Ayotte, P. (2003). In vitro activation of cord blood mononuclear cells and cytokine production in a remote coastal population exposed to organochlorines and methyl mercury. *Environmental Health Perspectives, 111*(16), 1952–1957.

186. Lieu, J. E., & Feinstein, A. R. (2002). Effect of gestational and passive smoke exposure on ear infections in children. *Archives of Pediatrics and Adolescent Medicine*, *156*(2), 147–154. PubMed PMID: 11814376.

187. Gallagher, C. M., Smith, D. M., & Meliker, J. R. (2011). Total blood mercury and serum measles antibodies in US children, NHANES 2003-2004. *The Science of the Total Environment*, *410-411*, 65–71. PubMed PMID: 21992842.

188. Heilmann, C., Budtz-Jørgensen, E., Nielsen, F., Heinzow, B., Weihe, P., & Grandjean, P. (2010). Serum concentrations of antibodies against vaccine toxoids in children exposed perinatally to immunotoxicants. *Environmental Health Perspectives*, *118*(10), 1434–1438. PubMed PMID: 20562056.

189. Grandjean, P., Heilmann, C., Weihe, P., Nielsen, F., Mogensen, U. B., & Budtz-Jørgensen, E. (2016 Aug 9). Serum vaccine antibody concentrations in adolescents exposed to perfluorinated compounds. *Environmental Health Perspectives*, [Epub ahead of print]; PubMed PMID: 27501995.

190. American Academy of Allergy, Asthma and Immunology (AAAAI) Board of Directors. (1999). Idiopathic environmental intolerances. . *The Journal of Allergy and Clinical Immunology*, *103*(1 Pt. 1), 36–40. PubMed PMID: 9893182.

191. Miller, C. S. (1999). Are we on the threshold of a new theory of disease? Toxicant-induced loss of tolerance and its relationship to addiction and abdiction. *Toxicology and Industrial Health*, *15*(3–4), 284–294. PubMed PMID: 10416280.

192. Miller, C., Ashford, N., Doty, R., Lamielle, M., Otto, D., et al. (1997). Empirical approaches for the investigations of toxicant-induced loss of tolerance. *Environmental Health Perspectives*, *105*(Suppl. 2), 515–519. PubMed PMID: 9167989.

193. Caress, S. M., & Steinemann, A. C. (2009). Prevalence of fragrance sensitivity in the American population. *Journal of Environmental Health*, *71*(7), 46–50. PubMed PMID: 19326669.

194. Heuser, G., Wojdani, A., & Heuser, S. (1992). *Diagnostic markers of multiple chemical sensitivity*. Board on Environmental Studies and Toxicology, Commission on Life Sciences, National Research Council. Washington, DC: National Academy Press.

195. Bell, I. R. (1994). White paper: Neuropsychiatric aspect so sensitivity to low-level chemicals: A neural sensitization model. *Toxicology and Industrial Health*, *10*(4–5), 277–312. PubMed PMID: 7778100.

196. Bell, I. R., Hardin, E. E., Baldwin, C. M., & Schwartz, G. E. (1995). Increased limbic system symptomatology

and sensitizability of young adults with chemical and noise sensitivities. *Environmental Research*, *70*(2), 84–97. PubMed PMID: 8674484.

197. Cullen, M. R. (1987). The worker with multiple chemical sensitivities: An overview. *Occupational Medicine*, *2*(4), 655–661. PubMed PMID: 3313760.

198. (1999). Multiple chemical sensitivity: A 1999 consensus. *Archives of Environmental Health*, *54*(3), 147–149. PubMed PMID: 10444033.

199. Miller, C. S., & Mitzel, H. C. (1995). Chemical sensitivity attributed to pesticide exposure versus remodeling. *Archives of Environmental Health*, *50*(2), 119–129. PubMed PMID: 7786048.

200. Caress, S. M., & Steinemann, A. C. (2003). A review of a two-phase population study of multiple chemical sensitivities. *Environmental Health Perspectives*, *111*(12), 1490–1497. PubMed PMID: 12948889.

201. McKeown-Eyssen, G., Baines, C., Cole, D. E., Riley, N., Tyndale, R. F., Marshall, L., et al. (2004). Case-control study of genotypes in multiple chemical sensitivity: CYP2D6, NAT1, NAT2, PON1, PON2 and MTHFR. *International Journal of Epidemiology*, *33*(5), 971–978. PubMed PMID: 15256524.

202. Dantoft, T. M., Elberling, J., Brix, S., Szecsi, P. B., Vesterhauge, S., & Skovbjerg, S. (2014). An elevated pro-inflammatory cytokine profile in multiple chemical sensitivity. *Psychoneuroendocrinology*, *40*, 140–150. PubMed PMID: 24485486.

203. Little, C. H., Georgiou, G. M., Shelton, M. J., Simpson, F., & Cone, R. E. (1999). Clinical and immunological responses in subjects sensitive to solvents. *Archives of Environmental Health*, *54*(1), 6–14. PubMed PMID: 10025410.

204. Khalil, Z., Georgiou, G. M., Ogedegbe, H., Cone, R. E., Simpson, F., & Little, C. H. (2000). Immunological and in-vivo neurological studies on a benzoic acid-specific T cell-derived antigen-binding molecule from the serum of a toluene-sensitive patient. *Archives of Environmental Health*, *55*(5), 304–318. PubMed PMID: 11063405.

205. De Luca, C., Scordo, M. G., Cesareo, E., Pastore, S., Mariani, S., Maiani, G., et al. (2010). Biological definition of multiple chemical sensitivity from redox state and cytokine profiling and not from polymorphisms of xenobiotic-metabolizing enzymes. *Toxicology and Applied Pharmacology*, *248*(3), 285–292. PubMed PMID: 20430047.

206. Hojo, S., Sakabe, K., Ishikawa, S., Miyata, M., & Kumano, H. (2009). Evaluation of subjective symptoms of Japanese patients with multiple chemical sensitivity using QEESI(c). *Environmental Health and Preventive Medicine*, *14*(5), 267–275. PubMed PMID: 19603254.

207. McGovern, J. J., Jr., Lazaroni, J. A., Hicks, M. F., Adler, J. C., & Cleary, P. (1983). Food and chemical sensitivity. Clinical and immunologic correlates. *Archives of Otolaryngology (Chicago, Ill.: 1960), 109*(5), 292–297. PubMed PMID: 6189475.

208. Kipen, H., Fiedler, N., Maccia, C., Yurkow, E., Todaro, J., & Laskin, D. (1992). Immunologic evaluation of chemically sensitive patients. *Toxicology and Industrial Health, 8*(4), 125–135. PubMed PMID: 1412479.

209. Heuser, G., Wojdani, A., & Heuser, S. (1992). *Multiple chemical sensitivities addendum to biologic markers in immunotoxicology* (pp. 117–138). Washington, DC: National Academy Press.

210. Gibson, P. R., Elms, A. N., & Ruding, L. A. (2003). Perceived treatment efficacy for conventional and alternative therapies reported by persons with multiple chemical sensitivity. *Environmental Health Perspectives, 111*(12), 1498–1504. PubMed PMID: 12948890.

211. Langrish, J. P., Li, X., Wang, S., Lee, M. M., Barnes, G. D., Miller, M. R., et al. (2012). Reducing personal exposure to particulate air pollution improves cardiovascular health in patients with coronary heart disease. *Environmental Health Perspectives, 120*(3), 367–372. PubMed PMID: 22389220.

212. McCarthy, M. C., Ludwig, J. F., Brown, S. G., Vaughn, D. L., & Roberts, P. T. (2013). Filtration effectiveness of HVAC systems at near-roadway schools. *Indoor Air, 23*(3), 196–207. PubMed PMID: 23167831.

213. Allen, R. W., Carlsten, C., Karlen, B., Leckie, S., van Eeden, S., Vedal, S., et al. (2011). An air filter intervention study of endothelial function among healthy adults in a woodsmoke-impacted community. *American Journal of Respiratory and Critical Care Medicine, 183*(9), 1222–1230. PubMed PMID: 21257787.

214. Langrish, J. P., Li, X., Wang, S., Lee, M. M., Barnes, G. D., Miller, M. R., et al. (2012). Reducing personal exposure to particulate air pollution improves cardiovascular health in patients with coronary heart disease. *Environmental Health Perspectives, 120*(3), 367–372. PubMed PMID: 22389220.

215. Crinnion, W. J. (1997). Results of a decade of Naturopathic treatment for environmental illnesses. *J Naturopath Med, l7*(2), 21–27.

216. Schwingshackl, L., & Hoffmann, G. (2014). Mediterranean dietary pattern, inflammation and endothelial function: A systematic review and meta-analysis of intervention trials. *Nutrition, Metabolism, and Cardiovascular Diseases, 24*(9), 929–939. PubMed PMID: 24787907.

217. Chatzi, L., Torrent, M., Romieu, I., Garcia-Esteban, R., Ferrer, C., Vioque, J., et al. (2008). Mediterranean diet in pregnancy is protective for wheeze and atopy in childhood. *Thorax, 63*(6), 507–513. PubMed PMID: 18198206.

218. Grigoropoulou, D., Priftis, K. N., Yannakoulia, M., Papadimitriou, A., Anthracopoulos, M. B., Yfanti, K., et al. (2011). Urban environment adherence to the Mediterranean diet and prevalence of asthma symptoms among 10- to 12-year-old children: The Physical Activity, Nutrition, and Allergies in Children Examined in Athens study. *Allergy and Asthma Proceedings, 32*(5), 351–358. PubMed PMID: 22195687.

219. de Batlle, J., Garcia-Aymerich, J., Barraza-Villarreal, A., Antó, J. M., & Romieu, I. (2008). Mediterranean diet is associated with reduced asthma and rhinitis in Mexican children. *Allergy, 63*(10), 1310–1316. PubMed PMID: 18782109.

220. Castro-Rodriguez, J. A., Ramirez-Hernandez, M., Padilla, O., Pacheco-Gonzalez, R. M., Pérez-Fernández, V., & Garcia-Marcos, L. (2016). Effect of foods and Mediterranean diet during pregnancy and first years of life on wheezing, rhinitis and dermatitis in preschoolers. *Allergologia et Immunopathologia, 44*(5), 400–409. PubMed PMID: 27087566.

221. Calatayud-Sáez, F. M., Calatayud Moscoso Del Prado, B., Gallego Fernández-Pacheco, J. G., González-Martín, C., & Alguacil Merino, L. F. (2016). Mediterranean diet and childhood asthma. *Allergologia et Immunopathologia, 44*(2), 99–105. PubMed PMID: 26278484.

222. Aparicio-Soto, M., Sánchez-Hidalgo, M., Rosillo, Má, Castejón, M. L., & Alarcón-de-la-Lastra, C. (2016). Extra virgin olive oil: A key functional food for prevention of immune-inflammatory diseases. *Food and Function, 7*(11), 4492–4505. PubMed PMID: 27783083.

223. Miyake, Y., Sasaki, S., Tanaka, K., Ohya, Y., Miyamoto, S., Matsunaga, I., et al. (2007). Fish and fat intake and prevalence of allergic rhinitis in Japanese females: The Osaka Maternal and Child Health Study. *Journal of the American College of Nutrition, 26*(3), 279–287. PubMed PMID: 17634174.

224. Klemens, C. M., Berman, D. R., & Mozurkewich, E. L. (2011). The effect of perinatal omega-3 fatty acid supplementation on inflammatory markers and allergic diseases: A systematic review. *BJOG: An International Journal of Obstetrics and Gynaecology, 118*(8), 916–925. PubMed PMID: 21658192.

225. Kim, H. J., Barajas, B., Wang, M., & Nel, A. E. (2008). Nrf2 activation by sulforaphane restores the age-related decrease of T(H)1 immunity: Role of dendritic cells. *The Journal of Allergy and Clinical Immunology, 121*(5), 1255–1261.e7. PubMed PMID: 18325578.

226. Ritz, S. A., Wan, J., & Diaz-Sanchez, D. (2007). Sulforaphane-stimulated phase II enzyme induction inhibits cytokine production by airway epithelial cells stimulated with diesel extract. *American Journal of Physiology. Lung Cellular and Molecular Physiology, 292*(1), L33–L39. PubMed PMID: 16905640.

227. Heber, D., Li, Z., Garcia-Lloret, M., Wong, A. M., Lee, T. Y., Thames, G., et al. (2014). Sulforaphane-rich broccoli sprout extract attenuates nasal allergic response to diesel exhaust particles. *Food and Function, 5*(1), 35–41. PubMed PMID: 24287881.

228. Shin, H. S., See, H. J., Jung, S. Y., Choi, D. W., Kwon, D. A., Bae, M. J., et al. (2015). Turmeric (Curcuma longa) attenuates food allergy symptoms by regulating type 1/type 2 helper T cells (Th1/Th2) balance in a mouse model of food allergy. *Journal of Ethnopharmacology, 175*, 21–29. PubMed PMID: 26342520.

229. Nemmar, A., Subramaniyan, D., & Ali, B. H. (2012). Protective effect of curcumin on pulmonary and cardiovascular effects induced by repeated exposure to diesel exhaust particles in mice. *PLoS ONE, 7*(6), e39554. PubMed PMID: 22745783.

230. Wu, D., Wang, J., Pae, M., & Meydani, S. N. (2012). Green tea EGCG, T cells, and T cell-mediated autoimmune diseases. *Molecular Aspects of Medicine, 33*(1), 107–118. PubMed PMID: 22020144.

231. Carlsten, C., MacNutt, M. J., Zhang, Z., Sava, F., & Pui, M. M. (2014). Anti-oxidant N-acetylcysteine diminishes diesel exhaust-induced increased airway responsiveness in person with airway hyper-reactivity. *Toxicological Sciences, 139*(2), 479–487. PubMed PMID: 24814479.

232. Whitekus, M. J., Li, N., Zhang, M., Wang, M., Horwitz, M. A., Nelson, S. K., et al. (2002). Thiol antioxidants inhibit the adjuvant effects of aerosolized diesel exhaust particles in a murine model for ovalbumin sensitization. *The Journal of Immunology : Official Journal of the American Association of Immunologists, 168*(5), 2560–2567. PubMed PMID: 11859152.

233. Farhangi, M. A., Saboor-Yaraghi, A. A., & Keshavarz, S. A. (2016). Vitamin A supplementation reduces the Th17-Treg–Related cytokines in obese and non-obese women. *Archives Endocrinology and Metabolism, 60*(1), 29–35. PubMed PMID: 26909479.

234. Bansal, A. S., Henriquez, F., Sumar, N., & Patel, S. (2012). T helper cell subsets in arthritis and the benefits of immunomodulation by 1,25(OH)$_2$ vitamin D. *Rheumatology International, 32*(4), 843–852. PubMed PMID: 21918899.

235. Gutiérrez-Díaz, I., Fernández-Navarro, T., Sánchez, B., Margolles, A., & González, S. (2016). Mediterranean diet and faecal microbiota: A transversal study. *Food and Function, 7*(5), 2347–2356. PubMed PMID: 27137178.

236. Kawase, M., He, F., Kubota, A., Hiramatsu, M., Saito, H., Ishii, T., et al. (2009). Effect of fermented milk prepared with two probiotic strains on Japanese cedar pollinosis in a double-blind placebo-controlled clinical study. *International Journal of Food Microbiology, 128*(3), 429–434. PubMed PMID: 18977549.

237. Harata, G., Kumar, H., He, F., Miyazawa, K., Yoda, K., Kawase, M., et al. (2016). Probiotics modulate gut microbiota and health status in Japanese cedar pollinosis patients during the pollen season. *European Journal of Nutrition*, PubMed PMID: 27412706.

238. Xiao, J. Z., Kondo, S., Yanagisawa, N., Takahashi, N., Odamaki, T., Iwabuchi, N., et al. (2006). Probiotics in the treatment of Japanese cedar pollinosis: A double-blind placebo-controlled trial. *Clinical and Experimental Allergy: Journal of the British Society for Allergy and Clinical Immunology, 36*(11), 1425–1435. PubMed PMID: 17083353.

239. Xiao, J. Z., Kondo, S., Yanagisawa, N., Miyaji, K., Enomoto, K., Sakoda, T., et al. (2007). Clinical efficacy of probiotic Bifidobacterium longum for the treatment of symptoms of Japanese cedar pollen allergy in subjects evaluated in an environmental exposure unit. *Allergology International, 56*(1), 67–75. PubMed PMID: 17259812.

240. Harima-Mizusawa, N., Iino, T., Onodera-Masuoka, N., Kato-Nagaoka, N., Kiyoshima-Shibata, J., Gomi, A., et al. (2014). Beneficial effects of citrus juice fermented with lactobacillus plantarum YIT 0132 on Japanese Cedar Pollinosis. *Bioscience of Microbiota, Food and Health, 33*(4), 147–155. PubMed PMID: 25379362.

241. Ohtani, T., Nakagawa, S., Kurosawa, M., Mizuashi, M., Ozawa, M., & Aiba, S. (2005). Cellular basis of the role of diesel exhaust particles in inducing Th2-dominant response. *The Journal of Immunology : Official Journal of the American Association of Immunologists, 174*(4), 2412–2419. PubMed PMID: 15699178.

242. Chang, Y., Sénéchal, S., de Nadai, P., Chenivesse, C., Gilet, J., Vorng, H., et al. (2006). Diesel exhaust exposure favors TH2 cell recruitment in nonatopic subjects by differentially regulating chemokine production. *The Journal of Allergy and Clinical Immunology, 118*(2), 354–360. PubMed PMID: 16890758.

243. Yanagisawa, R., Koike, E., Win-Shwe, T. T., Ichinose, T., & Takano, H. (2016). Low-dose benzo[a]pyrene aggravates allergic airway inflammation in mice. *Journal of Applied Toxicology: JAT, 36*(11), 1496–1504. PubMed PMID: 26918773.

244. Zhao, C., Liao, J., Chu, W., Wang, S., Yang, T., Tao, Y., et al. (2012). Involvement of TLR2 and TLR4 and Th1/Th2 shift in inflammatory responses

induced by fine ambient particulate matter in mice. *Inhalation Toxicology*, 24(13), 918–927. Erratum in: Inhal Toxicol. 2013 Feb;25(3):178. PubMed PMID: 23121301.

245. Dobreva, Z. G., Kostadinova, G. S., Popov, B. N., Petkov, G. S., & Stanilova, S. A. (2015). Proinflammatory and anti-inflammatory cytokines in adolescents from Southeast Bulgarian cities with different levels of air pollution. *Toxicology and Industrial Health*, 31(12), 1210–1217. PubMed PMID: 23771874.

246. Iavicoli, I., Marinaccio, A., Castellino, N., & Carelli, G. (2004). Altered cytokine production in mice exposed to lead acetate. *International Journal of Immunopathology and Pharmacology*, 17(2 Suppl.), 97–102. PubMed PMID: 15345199.

247. Heo, Y., Lee, W. T., & Lawrence, D. A. (1997). In vivo the environmental pollutants lead and mercury induce oligoclonal T cell responses skewed toward type-2 reactivities. *Cellular Immunology*, 179(2), 185–195. PubMed PMID: 9268502.

248. Agrawal, A., Kaushal, P., Agrawal, S., Gollapudi, S., & Gupta, S. (2007). Thimerosal induces TH2 responses via influencing cytokine secretion by human dendritic cells. *Journal of Leukocyte Biology*, 81(2), 474–482. PubMed PMID: 17079650.

249. de Vos, G., Abotaga, S., Liao, Z., Jerschow, E., & Rosenstreich, D. (2007). Selective effect of mercury on Th2-type cytokine production in humans. *Immunopharmacology and Immunotoxicology*, 29(3–4), 537–548. PubMed PMID: 18075863.

250. Kato, T., Tada-Oikawa, S., Wang, L., Murata, M., & Kuribayashi, K. (2013). Endocrine disruptors found in food contaminants enhance allergic sensitization through an oxidative stress that promotes the development of allergic airway inflammation. *Toxicology and Applied Pharmacology*, 273(1), 10–18. PubMed PMID: 24035973.

251. Fukuyama, T., Tajima, Y., Ueda, H., Hayashi, K., & Kosaka, T. (2011). Prior exposure to immunosuppressive organophosphorus or organochlorine compounds aggravates the T(H)1- and T(H)2-type allergy caused by topical sensitization to 2,4-dinitrochlorobenzene and trimellitic anhydride. *Journal of Immunotoxicology*, 8(2), 170–182. PubMed PMID: 21534883.

252. Daniel, V., Huber, W., Bauer, K., Suesal, C., Conradt, C., & Opelz, G. (2002). Associations of dichlorodiphenyltrichloroethane (DDT) 4.4 and dichlorodiphenyldichloroethylene (DDE) 4.4 blood levels with plasma IL-4. *Archives of Environmental Health*, 57(6), 541–547. PubMed PMID: 12696651.

253. Kim, H. A., Kim, E. M., Park, Y. C., Yu, J. Y., Hong, S. K., Jeon, S. H., et al. (2003). Immunotoxicological effects of Agent Orange exposure to the Vietnam War Korean veterans. *Industrial Health*, 41(3), 158–166. PubMed PMID: 12916745.

254. Seo, M., Yamagiwa, T., Kobayashi, R., Ikeda, K., Satoh, M., Inagaki, N., et al. (2008). Augmentation of antigen-stimulated allergic responses by a small amount of trichloroethylene ingestion from drinking water. *Regulatory Toxicology and Pharmacology*, 52(2), 140–146. PubMed PMID: 18721841.

255. Gaspar-Ramírez, O., Pérez-Vázquez, F. J., Pruneda-álvarez, L. G., Orta-García, S. T., González-Amaro, R., & Pérez-Maldonado, I. N. (2012). Effect of polychlorinated biphenyls 118 and 153 on Th1/Th2 cells differentiation. *Immunopharmacology and Immunotoxicology*, 34(4), 627–632. PubMed PMID: 22233178.

256. Gillis, B., Gavin, I. M., Arbieva, Z., King, S. T., Jayaraman, S., & Prabhakar, B. S. (2007). Identification of human cell responses to benzene and benzene metabolites. *Genomics*, 90(3), 324–333. PubMed PMID: 17572062.

257. Yan, H., Takamoto, M., & Sugane, K. (2008). Exposure to Bisphenol A prenatally or in adulthood promotes T(H)2 cytokine production associated with reduction of CD4CD25 regulatory T cells. *Environmental Health Perspectives*, 116(4), 514–519. PubMed PMID: 18414636.

258. Yoshino, S., Yamaki, K., Li, X., Sai, T., Yanagisawa, R., Takano, H., et al. (2004). Prenatal exposure to bisphenol A up-regulates immune responses, including T helper 1 and T helper 2 responses, in mice. *Immunology*, 112(3), 489–495. PubMed PMID: 15196218.

259. Bornehag, C. G., & Nanberg, E. (2010). Phthalate exposure and asthma in children. *International Journal of Andrology*, 33(2), 333–345. PubMed PMID: 20059582.

260. Fujimaki, H., Nohara, K., Kobayashi, T., Suzuki, K., Eguchi-Kasai, K., Tsukumo, S., et al. (2002). Effect of a single oral dose of 2,3,7,8-tetrachlorodibenzo-p-dioxin on immune function in male NC/Nga mice. *Toxicological Sciences*, 66(1), 117–124. PubMed PMID: 11861978.

261. Fukuyama, T., Ueda, H., Hayashi, K., Tajima, Y., Shuto, Y., Saito, T. R., et al. (2008). Detection of low-level environmental chemical allergy by a long-term sensitization method. *Toxicology Letters*, 180(1), 1–8. PubMed PMID: 18571882.

262. Zheng, L., Dong, G. H., Zhang, Y. H., Liang, Z. F., Jin, Y. H., & He, Q. C. (2011). Type 1 and Type 2 cytokines

imbalance in adult male C57BL/6 mice following a 7-day oral exposure to perfluorooctanesulfonate (PFOS). *Journal of Immunotoxicology, 8*(1), 30–38. PubMed PMID: 21299352.

263. Duramad, P., Harley, K., Lipsett, M., Bradman, A., Eskenazi, B., Holland, N. T., et al. (2006). Early environmental exposures and intracellular Th1/Th2 cytokine profiles in 24-month-old children living in an agricultural area. *Environmental Health Perspectives, 114*(12), 1916–1922. PubMed PMID: 17185285.

264. van Voorhis, M., Knopp, S., Julliard, W., Fechner, J. H., Zhang, X., Schauer, J. J., et al. (2013). Exposure to atmospheric particulate matter enhances Th17 polarization through the aryl hydrocarbon receptor. *PLoS ONE, 8*(12), e82545. PubMed PMID: 24349309.

265. Brandt, E. B., Kovacic, M. B., Lee, G. B., Gibson, A. M., Acciani, T. H., Le Cras, T. D., et al. (2013). Diesel exhaust particle induction of IL-17A contributes to severe asthma. *The Journal of Allergy and Clinical Immunology, 132*(5), 1194–1204.e2. PubMed PMID: 24060272.

266. Wang, H., Peng, W., Weng, Y., Ying, H., Li, H., Xia, D., et al. (2012). Imbalance of Th17/Treg cells in mice with chronic cigarette smoke exposure. *International Immunopharmacology, 14*(4), 504–512. PubMed PMID: 23044435.

267. Luo, S., Li, Y., Li, Y., Zhu, Q., Jiang, J., Wu, C., et al. (2016). Gestational and lactational exposure to low-dose bisphenol A increases Th17 cells in mice offspring. *Environmental Toxicology and Pharmacology, 47*, 149–158. PubMed PMID: 27693988.

268. Wang, G., Wang, J., Fan, X., Ansari, G. A., & Khan, M. F. (2012). Protein adducts of malondialdehyde and 4-hydroxynonenal contribute to trichloroethene-mediated autoimmunity via activating Th17 cells: Dose- and time-response studies in female MRL+/+ mice. *Toxicology, 292*(2–3), 113–122. PubMed PMID: 22178267.

269. Kuwatsuka, Y., Shimizu, K., Akiyama, Y., Koike, Y., Ogawa, F., Furue, M., et al. (2014). Yusho patients show increased serum IL-17, IL-23, IL-1β, and TNFα levels more than 40 years after accidental polychlorinated biphenyl poisoning. *Journal of Immunotoxicology, 11*(3), 246–249. PubMed PMID: 24083809.

270. Hassuneh, M. R., Albini, M. A., & Talib, W. H. (2012). Immunotoxicity induced by acute subtoxic doses of paraquat herbicide: Implication of shifting cytokine gene expression toward T-helper (T(H))-17 phenotype. *Chemical Research in Toxicology, 25*(10), 2112–2116. PubMed PMID: 22938100.

44

Endocrine Toxicity

SUMMARY

- Presence in population: Multiple endocrine disrupting chemicals are ubiquitous in modern society
- Major disease: Obesity, diabetes, infertility and reproduction problems, hormone-sensitive cancers in females and males, thyroid disorders, adrenal dysfunction
- Primary sources: Air, food, water, and personal care products
- Best measure: Urine and blood assessment of measurable toxicants or their metabolites, common diagnostic techniques for endocrine dysfunction
- Best intervention: Avoidance, depuration techniques

INTRODUCTION

The Endocrine Society (ES) has published two executive summaries on endocrine-disrupting chemicals (EDC).[1,2] These reports directly associate obesity, diabetes, female and male reproduction problems, hormone-sensitive cancers in females, prostate cancer, adrenal dysfunction, and thyroid dysfunction with EDC exposure (Table 44.1). EDCs are now defined as "exogenous agents that interfere with synthesis, secretion, transport, metabolism, binding action, or elimination of natural bloodborne hormones present in the body and are responsible for homeostasis, reproduction, and developmental process." EDCs include the biologically persistent organochlorine compounds (chlorinated pesticides and polychlorinated biphenyls [PCB] and dioxins) and polybrominated flame retardants (PBDE) as well as the nonpersistent plastics (bisphenol A [BPA]), plasticizers (phthalates), organophosphate pesticides (OPs), fungicides, and herbicides. Xenoestrogens (genistein and coumestrol) found in soy and other food have relatively low binding affinity for estrogen receptors but can be found in quite elevated levels in some individuals and are considered possible endocrine disruptors.[3] The annual cost from the reduction of IQ points, loss of intellectual ability, and attention deficit hyperactivity

disorder (ADHD) by EDCs in the European Union alone was estimated to be 163 billion euros,[4] whereas annual costs from these neurological endpoints in the United States was estimated to be $266 billion. Other estimates of annual cost related to neurological disease (not including endocrine or immune effects) burden from EDCs was listed as $217 billion in the European Union and $340 billion in the United States.[5]

Initially, endocrine disruptors were primarily believed to act by binding as ligands to hormone receptor sites. However, it is now known that these EDCs primarily act on nuclear receptors, nonnuclear steroid hormone receptors, neurotransmitter receptors, and orphan receptors, including the aryl hydrocarbon receptors (AhR). Dioxin-like action always involves AhR binding. Included in the frequently bound receptors are glucocorticoid and peroxisome proliferation-activated receptor families. In addition, many of these EDCs cause their greatest amount of endocrine disruption at small or moderate, rather than high, levels.[6,7]

The adverse health effects of EDCs appear to be a combination of many factors, including the time of exposure, which is especially critical during fetal growth, along with amount, duration, synergism, nutritional status, and other factors. Some exposure effects are only seen generationally. *In vitro* research has clearly demonstrated

TABLE 44.1 **Endocrine-Disrupting Xenobiotics and Related Disorders Listed by the Endocrine Society and Those Not Listed**

ES: EDC-Associated Diseases	• Obesity
	• Diabetes
	• Female reproduction problems
	  • Development and age at menarche
	  • Polycystic ovary syndrome
	  • Premature ovarian failure
	  • Reproductive tract anomalies
	  • Uterine leiomyomas
	  • Endometriosis
	• Male development and infertility
	• Hormone-sensitive cancers in females
	• Prostate cancer
	• Thyroid dysfunction

Disorders not listed by the ES	• Birth outcomes
	  • Miscarriages
	  • Spontaneous abortions
	  • Preterm delivery
	  • Small-for-gestational-age babies
	  • Reduced head circumference
	  • Anogenital distance
	  • Congenital anomalies
	• Disrupted steroidogenesis
	• Hypercortisolism and hypocortisolism

ES: Listed EDCs	• Organochlorine compounds (chlorinated pesticides and polychlorinated biphenyls [PCB] and dioxins) • Flame retardants (PBDE), plastics (bisphenol A), and plasticizers (phthalates) • Organophosphate pesticides • Fungicides • Herbicides
Endocrine disruptors not listed by ES as EDCs	• Solvents • Perfluorocarbons • Trihalomethanes • Vehicular air pollutants • Metals

From Diamanti-Kandarakis, E., Bourguignon, J. P., Giudice, L. C., Hauser R., Prins G. S., & Soto A. M., et al. (2009). Endocrine-disrupting chemicals: An Endocrine Society scientific statement. *Endocrine Reviews*, 30(4), 293–342; Gore, A. C., Chappell, V. A., Fenton, S. E., Flaws J. A., Nadal A., & Prins G. S., et al. (2015). EDC-2: The Endocrine Society's Second Scientific Statement on Endocrine-Disrupting Chemicals. *Endocrine Reviews*, 36(6), E1–E150.

EDC-induced epigenetic changes in germ cells that affect F1-F3 cell generations.[8-10] PCB contamination provides one of the clearest pictures of this effect in humans.

More than 2000 Taiwanese became ill after exposure to PCB-contaminated rice bran cooking oil in 1979 in what was termed "Yu Cheng" (Chinese for "oil disease"). Those exposed had used the contaminated oil for as long as 9 months, consuming a total of about 1 g of PCB. The PCB level would have included approximately 3.8 mg of the polychlorinated benzofurans (PCDFs) that are naturally made when PCBs are heated. Taiwanese males who were exposed to the PCBs before they reached the age of 20 years were later found to have significantly fewer male children than unexposed controls,[11] although the men who were exposed after the age of 20 years had 10% fewer daughters than controls (which did not achieve statistical significance). A similar finding was noted in Seveso, Italy, in parents exposed to the dioxin 2,3,7,8-Tetrachlorodibenzo-*p*-dioxin (TCDD).[12] Although this shifting of the sex of the offspring was not found with Taiwanese mothers exposed to PCBs at any age, they did experience a higher incidence of stillbirth and had more abnormal menstrual bleeding than nonexposed women.[13] *In utero* PCB exposure reduces estradiol levels in 8-year-old children and causes shorter fundal and uterine length in the girls.[14] *In utero* exposure to phthalates also appears to alter progesterone and follicle-stimulating hormone (FSH) levels in this same group of children.[15]

DISEASE MANIFESTATION

Fertility and Reproductive Outcomes

The rate of fertility has been steadily dropping since the 1950s, with the number of children per woman decreasing from 4.97 to 2.5 in the span of 60 years (Fig. 44.1). In 2009, fertility rates hit an all-time low of 102.1 children per 1000 women.[16] The rates of teen births in the United States dropped 44% between 1991 and 2007, which does not appear to be solely related to increased use of contraceptives.[17]

Female Fertility and Reproductive Outcome Effects From Endocrine-Disrupting Chemicals

• Organochlorine compounds (chlorinated pesticides, PCBs, and dioxins)
• BPA
• OPs, fungicides, and herbicides

Table 44.2 summarizes xenobiotics associated with female reproductive problems.

Chlorinated compounds. In a German fertility clinic, hexachlorocyclohexane (HCH) serum levels were significantly associated with miscarriage history and uterine fibroid presence.[18] PCB serum levels were significantly associated with endometriosis and increasing dichlorodiphenyl-trichloroethane (DDT) levels with reduced conception. Fish-consuming women who grew up on the eastern (Baltic) coast of Sweden were 2.5 times more likely to be infertile than their counterparts on the west coast (Atlantic).[19] The PCB content in Baltic fish is up to six times higher than in the same fish species caught in the Atlantic.[20] Total blood PCB levels among fish-consuming French women was associated with a 50% reduction in their ability to conceive.[21] Italian women with higher serum PCB levels were found to have experienced miscarriage more frequently than those with lower PCB levels.[22] No such association was found with either DDT or hexachlorobenzene (HCB) in those women; however, a US study showed a clear correlation with dichlorodiphenyldichloroethylene (DDE) and both preterm births and small-for-gestational-age (SGA) babies.[23] In this study, the risk increased steadily with increasing serum levels of DDE.

Eighteen infertile Canadian couples attending an *in vitro* fertilization (IVF) program were assessed for chlorinated pollutants in the serum and follicular fluid.[24] DDE, mirex, hexachloroethane, trichlorobenzene, and three different PCBs were found in more than 50% of all follicular fluid samples. Four different PCBs, DDE, and endosulfan were also found in more than 50% of all serum samples. DDE was the most common contaminant, had the highest residue, and was negatively associated with fertilization. Of the couples tested, those who failed to achieve pregnancy with IVF methods generally had higher pollutant levels than successful couples. Elevated levels of either PCB 153 (found in high levels in sardines and farmed salmon[126]) or total serum PCBs were dose-dependently associated with failed IVF.[25] In addition to PCBs, elevated levels of perfluorocarbons have been associated with female infertility.[26]

Blood levels of pentachlorophenol (PCP), a common wood preservative, have been associated with increased miscarriage rates and levels of antinuclear antibodies (ANA). Teachers exposed to PCP, lindane, and dioxins

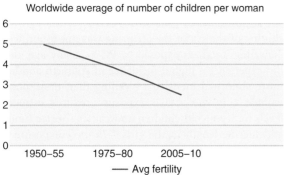

FIG. 44.1 Worldwide fertility rates 1950 to 2010. (Data from Our World In Data. (2017). *Fertility.* Retrieved from https://ourworldindata.org/fertility/.)

TABLE 44.2	Xenobiotics Associated With Female Reproductive Problems						
Pollutant	Female Infertility	IVF Failure	Miscarriage	Stillbirth	Birth Defects	Fetal Death	Small Indices
OP	X		X		X	X	X
2,4-D	X				X		
Glyphosate	X						
HCH/PCP			X				
DDT	X						X
PCB	X	X	X	X	X		
Solvents	X		X	X	X	X	X
Cigarettes	X		X	X		X	X
PAH	X					X	X
THM			X	X			X
BPA	X	X					
Metals	X	X					X

in their work environment who successfully delivered had children with significantly lower birth weights and length.[27] Elevated PCP levels were also found in 65 of 171 infertile women from a German reproductive clinic.[28] Those with elevated PCPs had significantly higher levels of FSH and stimulated cortisol and significantly lower basal levels of T3, dehydroepiandrosterone (DHEA), DHEAS, testosterone, 17-OH-progesterone, and 17-OH-pregnenolone.

Bisphenol A. In women undergoing IVF procedures, those with higher BPA levels were more likely to have implantation failure.[29] Those with urinary BPA levels in the third and fourth quartiles were 60% and 211% more likely to experience IVF failure with this procedure.

Herbicides and organophosphate pesticides. Pesticide exposure almost quadruples the risk of being infertile. A study of Ontario farmers showed an inverse association of female pesticide use with fecundity, but this association was not seen with male use.[30] Five compounds reduced the female's fecundity ratio (FR) by 24% to 49%: dicamba (FR 0.51), glyphosate (FR 0.61), 2,4-D (FR 0.71), organophosphates (FR 0.75), and thiocarbamates (FR 0.76). Female veterans with service in Vietnam had an increased risk (OR 1.46) of having children with moderate to severe birth defects compared with contemporary female veterans.[31] This study may indicate an association of phenoxy acid herbicides like 2,4-D and 2,4,5-T (the combination known as Agent Orange) in reproductive disorders, as was noted in the Ontario study with 2,4-D. Higher spontaneous abortion rates were found in Spanish greenhouse sprayers exposed to OPs, as were higher rates of depression and headaches.[32] Although these health problems were significantly associated with OP exposure, these workers were not considered OP-poisoned, because no decrease in erythrocyte acetylcholinesterase was found. A study in California farming counties showed a clear association with the timing of pesticide spraying and fetal death related to congenital anomalies.[33] In this study, when OP or carbamate pesticides were sprayed within 8 square miles of the woman's residence during the third to eighth week of pregnancy, the OR of fetal death was 1.4. When the spraying occurred within 1 square mile of the residence, the OR went to 2.2. Levels of atrazine rise and fall in the groundwater in relation to the seasonal use for this herbicide. Women exposed to atrazine levels in their drinking water during their third trimester are between 37% and 54% more likely to have SGA babies.[34]

Female Fertility and Reproductive Outcome Effects From Compounds Not Listed as Endocrine-Disrupting Chemicals by the Endocrine Society

- Solvents
- Air pollutants
- Metals
- Trihalomethanes (THMs)

Solvents. Most of the data on solvents and reproductive problems comes from persons with occupational exposure. Workplace solvent exposure has been associated with infertility (OR 1.76) and tubal-factor infertility (OR 1.95).[35] Toluene was also associated with a reduction in luteal-phase luteinizing hormone (LH) in both male and females.[36] In the laboratory workers, the greatest reduction of fertility was found in association with acetone exposure (fecundity ratio (FR) 0.72), although chronic benzene exposure was associated with abnormally long menstrual cycles.[37] Wives of men who work around organic solvents also show decreased fecundity (FR 0.36).[38] A study of Chinese female chemical plant workers revealed a threefold increased risk (OR 2.9) for spontaneous abortions.[39] Of the myriad petrochemicals they were exposed to, benzene (OR 2.5), gasoline (OR 1.8), and hydrogen sulfide (OR 2.3) all showed independent significant association with miscarriages. Pharmaceutical factory workers also have a progressively increasing risk of spontaneous abortions from multiple solvent exposures, with the greatest risk found in those who were exposed to four or more solvents.[40] Women who had any weekly exposure to toluene, trichloroethylene (TCE), or perchloroethylene (PCE) were 2.3, 3.1, and 4.7 times more likely to have their pregnancy end in spontaneous abortion.[41] The reproductive effects were present regardless of whether the women had less than 10 hours of exposure weekly or more. Pharmacy assistants also had increased risk for stillbirths and perinatal death that corresponded with solvent exposure.[42] A metaanalysis of 47 studies revealed that regular paternal exposure to solvents was significantly associated with a 30% increased risk for spontaneous abortions and a 47% increased risk for major fetal malformations.[43] This included a 2.18-fold increased risk for anencephaly, a 59% greater risk for spina bifida, and an 86% greater risk for any neural tube defect.

Nonoccupational exposure to chlorinated solvents through drinking water has been associated with reproductive problems as well. Women exposed to groundwater tetrachloroethylene (also known as PCE) contamination had increased rates of placental abruption (OR 1.35) and were more than twice as likely to have their pregnancies end in spontaneous abortion (OR 2.38).[44] Women with the greatest PCE exposures also had modest increases in breast cancer risk.[45]

Parents of children from Camp Lejeune, North Carolina, where the water is contaminated with TCE and benzene, also had higher rates of preterm delivery and SGA babies.[46] Male marines stationed at Camp Lejuene also had a 40% to 270% greater risk of developing breast cancer.[47]

Air pollutants. Smoking more than 10 cigarettes daily has been associated with reduced fertility in women (FR 0.66), with an OR for infertility at 1.64.[48] Because tobacco smoke contains high benzene and styrene levels along with heavy metals and polycyclic aromatic hydrocarbons, it is difficult to say which component has the greatest effect on fertility. Female smokers also experience higher rates of ectopic pregnancies and spontaneous abortions,[49] along with greater rates of stillbirths (OR 2.0) and infant mortality (OR 1.8).[50] Mothers who quit smoking in the first trimester showed the same rates of stillbirth and infant mortality as nonsmoking women. When Ireland banned smoking in the workplace, rates of preterm births dropped by 25%.[51]

Women living closest to busy roadways have slightly higher rates of infertility than those living further away.[52,53] Brief exposure to elevated levels of PM_{10} has been shown to increase the rates of miscarriage by up to 2.6 times.[54] Mothers with higher ambient air pollution have significantly higher levels of polycyclic aromatic hydrocarbon (PAH)-DNA adducts in their cord blood white cells.[55] Newborns with elevated PAH-DNA adducts had significantly lower birth weight, birth length, and head circumference. An inverse correlation was also seen

in this population between elevated serum cotinine levels and birth weight and length. The PAH-DNA adducts were also significantly higher in infertile men than in fertile men. Michigan residents exposed to higher levels of carbon monoxide (CO), nitrous dioxide (NO_2), ozone (O_3), and $PM_{2.5}$ had greater odds of delivering a child that is SGA.[56] Each of these air pollutants was individually associated with SGA. Each 10 µg/m³ increase in $PM_{2.5}$ results in a 13.8 g reduction in birth weight.[57]

Metals. Blood mercury levels, primarily from seafood consumption, were higher in infertile Hong Kong couples than in fertile controls (Table 44.3).[58] The values of blood mercury in these individuals is within the typical ranges found in Asian Americans in the Centers for Disease Control and Prevention's Fourth Report, in which the 50th percentile averaged 2.3 µg/L, the 75th percentile 4.32 µg/L, the 90th percentile 7.71 µg/L, and the 95th percentile 10.3 µg/L.[59] These levels are slightly more than twice the average for all persons in the National Health and Nutritional Examination Survey (NHANES) for 2011 to 2012.

In a far larger US study of 501 infertile couples who were not frequent fish consumers, a significant association was found between reduced fecundity and blood cadmium levels in women (FR 0.78) and blood lead levels in men (FR 0.85) but not with blood mercury levels for either sex.[60] Blood cadmium levels have also been significantly associated with lower birth weight, head circumference, and crown-to-heel length in daughters but not sons.[61] In women who are not occupationally exposed to lead, blood lead levels above 5 µg/dL double the risk of preterm delivery[62] and increase the rates of spontaneous abortion.[63] Each increase of 1 µg/dL of blood lead has been associated with a 9.93 g reduction of body weight, a 0.03 cm reduction of head circumference, and a 0.05 cm reduction of crown-to-heel length.[64]

TABLE 44.3   Blood Mercury Values (µg/L) in Men and Women With Infertility, Males With Abnormal Sperm Indices, Women With Unexplained Infertility, and Controls

	Infertile Group	Sperm Abnormalities	Unexplained Female Infertility	Controls (n = 26)
Males (n = 176)	8.20	8.93		6.30
Females (n = 181)	6.70		7.47	3.53

Data from Choy, C. M., Lam, C. W., Cheung, L. T., Briton-Jones C. M., Cheung L. P., & Haines C. J. (2002). Infertility, blood mercury concentrations and dietary seafood consumption: a case-control study. *BJOG, 109*(10), 1121–1125.

Trihalomethanes. Chlorination (disinfection) by-products includes four different trihalomethane (THM) compounds, chloroform, bromodichloromethane, chlorodibromomethane, and bromoform, as well as other non-THM compounds. The use of chlorinated water has been associated with an increased risk (OR 2.6) of stillbirth.[65] Although one study found no association with stillbirth and THM compounds,[66] others have reported this relationship.[67] When specific THMs were studied, the presence of high levels of bromodichloromethane was associated with the greatest incidence of spontaneous abortions.[68] Both bromodichloromethane and chloroform were associated with increased risk of stillbirth, with bromodichloromethane showing the greatest risk (OR 1.98) at the highest levels of exposure.[69]

Studies that looked at singleton live birth associations between THM content in the water showed a small but statistically significant association with low birth weight, preterm delivery, and SGA babies.[70] Women drinking chlorinated water were far more likely to deliver a child with smaller body length and smaller head circumference.[71] The risk differed with which agent was used in the municipal water treatment plant. Use of chlorine dioxide was associated with an OR of 2.0 for smaller length and 2.2 for smaller head circumference. Sodium hypochlorite use by the municipality was associated with an OR of 2.3 for small body length and 3.5 for smaller head circumference. In addition, neonatal jaundice was found more often (OR 1.7) in areas that used chlorine dioxide for water sanitation.

Xenobiotics and Birth Defects

- Living in proximity to landfills/waste sites
- Pesticides
- Chlorinated solvents

Mothers who live within 3 km of landfills have higher risk of delivering a child with neural tube defects (OR 1.86), malformations of the cardiac septa (OR 1.49), and anomalies of the great arteries and veins (OR 1.81).[72] Defects that did not reach statistical significance for those women included tracheoesophageal anomalies (OR 2.2), hypospadias (OR 1.96), and gastroschisis (OR 3.19). Not surprisingly, persons living within 3 km of hazardous waste landfills had higher rates of chromosomal anomalies (OR 1.41).[73] In contrast, one study found no differences in the rates of birth defects (which varied from OR 0.96–1.19) between in those living within 2 km of landfills with or without hazardous waste.[74] Women living within

a mile of National Priority List waste sites, state Superfund waste sites, and Toxic Release Inventory facilities were more than three times more likely to deliver children with conotruncal heart defects.[75] Women who lived in the PCB-contaminated Love Canal Emergency Declaration Area before it was evacuated had slightly fewer male children and 50% more children with congenital malformations.[76] Women exposed to PCE-contaminated groundwater had a three times greater risk of having a child with cleft palate or neural tube defects.[77] TCE is a more common contaminant in the soil and water than PCE, and Wisconsin women living near industry that emits TCE were more than three times more likely to give birth to a child with congenital heart defects.[78] Those living in an area in New York exposed to TCE through soil vapor intrusion also experienced higher rates of cardiac defects in their children and babies with lower birth weight.[79]

Children born to pesticide applicators had significantly more defects, especially circulatory and respiratory, urogenital, and musculoskeletal and integumental than children of non–pesticide appliers.[80] Differences were even seen according to geographical area and to crop selection. Birth defects were higher in western Minnesota for infants born in the spring in areas where chlorophenoxy (2,4-D and MCPA [4- chloro-2-methylphenoxy acetic acid]) herbicides and fungicides were used on wheat, sugar beets, and potatoes. The areas with high use of the chlorophenoxy herbicides had an OR of 1.86 for defects in the central nervous system, circulatory and respiratory, and urogenital and musculoskeletal systems, whereas atrazine showed an OR of 1.13 for all birth anomalies.

Dr. Jeanette Sherman published an alarming article discussing four children with multiple congenital defects.[81] Each child had ventricular, eye, and palate defects as well as growth retardation. Three of them had hydrocephaly; microcephaly; mental retardation; blindness; hypotonia; wide-spread nipples; and deformities of the teeth, external ears, and external genitalia. All of these four children had *in utero* exposure to the OP pesticide chlorpyrifos under the trade name of Dursban, whereas no other known etiological agent could be identified. The defects in these four children were rare and astoundingly quite similar to those reported in another case of *in utero* OP exposure.[82]

OP metabolites are commonly found in the North American population,[61] primarily through the consumption of nonorganic vegetables and fruits.[83] Danish mothers consuming who consumed organically grown vegetables during pregnancy were significantly less likely to have a male child with hypospadias (OR 0.36), whereas those who consumed organic dairy products were 57% less likely to have sons with this problem as well.[84]

Female Reproductive Health—Sexual Development, Endometriosis, Polycystic Ovary Syndrome, and Uterine Leiomyomas

- Phthalates
- PCB and chlorinated pesticides
- Perfluorocarbons
- BPA

Phthalate presence in young girls has been associated with both delayed menarche[85] and premature breast development (thelarche).[86] Young Puerto Rican girls with thelarche had serum di-(2-ethylhexyl) phthalate (DEHP) levels averaging 450 parts per billion (PPB), whereas those without thelarche averaged only 70 PPB. Women with endometriosis have significantly higher levels of high-molecular-weight (HMW) DEHP than controls.[87]

A review of more than 31,000 females in the 1999 to 2008 NHANES trial revealed that women with higher serum levels of persistent EDCs (half-lives >1 year) experienced menopause 2 to 4 years earlier than their counterparts with a lower persistent organic pollutant (POP) burden.[88]

In the previously mentioned German fertility clinic study, HCH serum levels were significantly associated with uterine fibroid presence, whereas PCB serum levels were significantly associated with endometriosis.[19]

Data from the 2003 to 2006 NHANES trial revealed that women with slightly higher levels (second quartile) of both perfluorooctane sulfonate (PFOS, from Scotch-guarded materials) and perfluorooctanoic acid (PFOA, from Teflon-coated pans) were three to five times more likely to have endometriosis.[89] In a case-control study of women with polycystic ovary syndrome (PCOS), serum levels of both PFOA and PFOS were also significantly associated with increased PCOS risk of more than fivefold.[90] Both obese and nonobese women with PCOS have higher serum levels of BPA than women without PCOS.[91] Not only did the BPA levels correlate with PCOS; they also correlated with elevated androgens and increased insulin resistance in those women. The same correlations between serum BPA levels, PCOS, and androgens were also found in a group of adolescent girls.[92]

Male Low Testosterone Levels

- Phthalates
- PFOS
- PBDE

Testosterone levels in males have been dropping for the last few decades, and low testosterone is linked to several sexual, psychological, and physical changes (Table 44.4). A review of the data collected through the Massachusetts Male Aging Study revealed that, in the decade between 1987 to 1997, the average testosterone level of 40-year-old men dropped from an average of 520 ng/dL to 450 ng/dL.[93] Data from the 1990s revealed 20% of men older than 60 years had clinical hypogonadism (testosterone <325 ng/dL or 11.3 nmol/L),[94] yet soon after the new millennium it was reported that 30% of men older than 40 years fit that diagnosis.[95]

Profound hypogonadism is defined as a serum testosterone below 50 ng/dL and is most common in men with prior use of anabolic steroids.[96] A number of ubiquitous pollutants have been clearly linked to men with regular hypogonadism. Maternal levels of phthalates during pregnancy have been associated with long-term hormonal imbalance in their male children up to 14 years later.[97] Maternal urinary levels of BPA and the HMW phthalate mono(2-ethylhexyl) phthalate (MEHP) were positively associated with sex hormone–binding globulin (SHBG) and inversely associated with total testosterone levels. Although maternal levels of the low-molecular-weight (LMW) mono-iso-butyl phthalate (MiBP, often found in fingernail polish) was also inversely associated with testosterone levels. The boys exposed to higher levels of phthalates *in utero* also experienced delayed puberty. Data

TABLE 44.4 Common Changes Associated With Low Testosterone

Sexual	Psychological	Physical
Decreases in:	Decreases in:	Decreases in:
Erectile ability	Cognition	Muscle mass
Morning erection	Energy	Strength
Libido	Mood	Increases in:
Ability to orgasm	Vitality	BMI
Sexual performance		Energy
		Gynecomastia

Data from Traish, A. M., Miner, M. M., Morgentaler, A., & Zitzmann, M. (2011). Testosterone deficiency. *American Journal of Medicine, 124*(7), 578–587.

from the 2011 to 2012 NHANES trial revealed that, in boys aged 6 to 12 years, adult men, and adult women, urinary levels of MEHP were associated with lower testosterone levels.[98] The clear inverse relationship between phthalates and testosterone levels has been repeatedly established across the globe.[99-101] Serum levels of PFOS are inversely associated with testosterone and estrogen in healthy men, along with increased levels of SHBG.[102] PDBE is another pollutant that is found in house dust and is also associated inversely with serum testosterone levels.[103]

Male Impaired Reproductive Ability

- Pesticides
- Metals
- Air pollutants
- Phthalates
- PCB 138

Pesticides. Argentinean farmers exhibit a significant association between OP pesticide and solvent exposures and reduced sperm values.[104] Danish organic farmers consuming at least 50% of their dairy products as organic had greater sperm levels than those not consuming organic foods.[105] Chinese males exposed to workplace OPs had significant reductions in sperm concentration and motility over nonexposed workers.[106] Young men who consumed 1.5 servings of high pesticide fruits and vegetables daily had 49% lower total sperm volume and 31% fewer morphologically normal sperm.[107] When infertile men were then checked for urinary OP metabolites it was discovered that both the sperm concentration and total sperm count were both significantly inversely associated with urinary OP metabolites, while FSH levels were positively associated.[108] Furthermore, pesticide applicators using dibromochloropropane (DBCP) have consistently showed lower sperm counts.[109] The adverse effect on sperm count was only associated with exposure in the previous year, rather than a cumulative effect of all the years exposed. Metabolites of pyrethroid pesticides, currently the most commonly used indoor pesticide, at levels found in 50% of those studied were associated with sperm aneuploidy.[110]

Metals. Lead has been implicated as a causative agent in the reduction of sperm amount and quality in both animal and human studies.[111] Lead in males reduces the likelihood of successfully fathering a child by 15%.[62] Lead-induced infertility was reversed in a firearms instructor who was able to successfully father a child after dimercaptosuccinic acid (DMSA) chelation therapy.[112] The improvement in sperm indices and conception occurred when his serum lead levels

and zinc protoporphyrin levels dropped to normal. Male fish consumers in Hong Kong with blood mercury values commonly found in fish consumers were infertile because of a high degree of abnormal sperm.[58] Higher than normal levels of blood mercury were found in 21 of 59 male partners of infertile couples seeking help in conception.[113] Increased risk of spontaneous abortions was also found in the wives of stainless steel workers (OR 3.5), possibly related to hexavalent chromium exposure.[114]

Air pollutants. Urban air pollutants from vehicular exhaust are associated with reduced fertility in males.[115,116] Men residing in an industrial town with seasonally elevated pollution levels had significantly greater reductions in sperm motility and morphology along with higher levels of sperm with abnormal chromatin compared with males in a rural district with little air pollution.[117] The air pollutants followed in this study were PM_{10} and total suspended particulates of sulfur dioxide (SO2), CO, and nitrogen oxides (NOx). PAH-DNA adducts, from nonsmoking PAH sources (outdoor air pollution), have also been positively correlated with sperm head abnormalities.[118] The levels of detectible DNA adducts from PAH compounds were significantly inversely correlated with sperm concentration, total sperm count, and sperm motility in 433 infertile Chinese males.[119] Cigarette smoking is also associated with a significant reduction in sperm density, total sperm count, number of motile sperm, and citrate concentration.[120] Nonsignificant reductions from smoking were found for percentages of normal sperm forms, sperm vitality, ejaculate volume, and fructose concentration. House dust levels of organophosphate flame retardants also alter sex hormone levels and reduce male fertility.[121]

Phthalates. A correlation was found in males attending an infertility clinic between urinary levels of the LMW plasticizer monoethyl phthalate (MEP), the metabolite of diethyl phthalate (DEP), and DNA damage in their sperm.[122] Another group of infertile men showed associations with both MiNP and MEHP levels with testosterone levels and sperm viability.[123] Elevated urinary levels of LMW phthalates (typically found in fragrances) were significantly associated with a 20% reduction in male fertility, whereas BPA levels showed no association.[124] Male partners in infertile couples with higher than average levels of methyl paraben were 81% more likely to experience failure of IVF with their partners.[125]

PCBs. Men with higher levels of PCB 138, another PCB found in high levels in sardines and farmed salmon,[126] are 38% more likely to be infertile.[25]

Erectile Dysfunction. Males exposed to solvents (mechanics, painters, and woodworkers) have a 12-fold higher risk for erectile dysfunction (ED) than nonexposed men.[127] In the same study, pesticide-exposed males (farmers, fumigators, and men involved with animal husbandry) also had a sevenfold higher risk for ED. Current and previous cigarette smokers exposed to benzene, styrene, and xylene, in addition to heavy metals and polycyclic aromatic hydrocarbons, have an 60% to 70% increased risk of ED.[128]

Obesity

- Phthalates
- BPA
- POPs
- Perfluorocarbons
- Vehicular exhaust—urban ambient air pollution

Obesity is defined as having a body mass index (BMI) of 30 or higher, whereas a BMI above 25 is considered overweight. The rates of obesity have been rising at an alarming rate for decades, especially since the late 1980s (Fig. 44.2).[129]

In 1994, only two states reported more than 17.9% of their population to be obese, yet by 2014, all but one state reported a minimum of 22% obesity, with most states (36) listing 26% or higher. Interestingly, the trends for weight gain in the United States appears to correspond with the overall chemical production in this country.[130]

Industrial chemical production and obesity rates have clearly been rising during the same time frame. The term "obesogen," now used to describe EDCs that cause weight gain, was first applied in 2006 when organotins were shown to induce weight gain in animals.[131] The previous

section of environmental pollutants that reduce testosterone levels should be kept in mind, because low testosterone results in increased BMI.

Many EDC obesogens cause weight gain by activating peroxisome proliferator-activated receptor gamma (PPAR-γ), the master regulator of adipogenesis. Activating PPAR-γ in a preadipocyte cell stimulates transformation into an adipocyte, but stimulating PPAR-γ in an active adipocyte promotes greater fat accumulation. Fetal exposure to PPAR-γ-activating EDCs increases the numbers of adipocytes present, predisposing to greater adiposity throughout life.[132]

Phthalates. Male participants in the 1999 to 2002 NHANES trial showed a significant positive correlation between urinary levels of both HMW and LMW phthalates (1-methyl-4-benzylpiperazine [MBzP], mono(2-ethyl-5-hydroxyhexyl) phthalate [MEHHP], mono(2-ethyl-5-oxohexyl) phthalate [MEOHP], and MEP) with both increasing waist circumference and insulin resistance.[133] The correlation was strongest in 20- to 59-year-old males, with MBzP causing increased belt size in all quartile levels. MEP was also found to be positively associated with waist circumference in adolescent girls.[134] In 70-year-old Swedish women, MiBP and MMP were positively related to waist circumference and truncal fat mass.[135] LMW phthalates (MnBP, MEP, and MiBP) were significantly associated with obesity in boys and adolescents in the 2007 to 2010 NHANES trial,[136] yet HMW phthalate metabolites, especially metabolites of DEHP (MEHP, MEHHP, MEOHP), were significantly associated with increased rates of obesity in all adults from the same cohort. Data

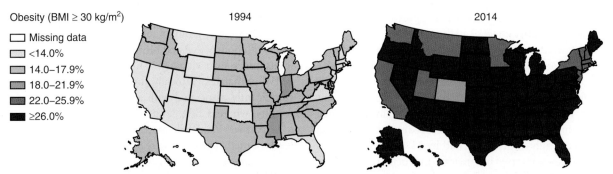

FIG. 44.2 Rates of obesity by state for 1994 and 2014. (From Centers for Disease Control and Prevention. [2017]. *Data & statistics*. Retrieved from https://www.cdc.gov/diabetes/data/.) (Accessed 28 March 2018)

from both the 1999 to 2004 and 2003 to 2008 NHANES have confirmed these findings among adult women.[137,138]

Bisphenol A. Prenatal exposure to BPA causes obesity in animals, yet may or may not in humans. One study reported that prenatal BPA exposure was associated with fat mass index, percent body fat, and waist circumference.[139] In the Center for the Health Assessment of Mothers and Children of Salinas (CHAMACOS) Study, neither prenatal BPA nor urinary BPA at age 5 years were associated with adiposity, but current BPA exposures for 9-year-old boys were associated with increased waist circumference.[140] Maternal BPA levels taken in the first trimester were not associated with childhood obesity in 4-year-old children on Crete, but their own urinary BPA was. Each 10-fold increase in urinary BPA was associated with an increased body mass index-z (BMI-z)-z score, waist circumference, and skinfold thickness.[141] In Chinese school-age children (grades 4–12), girls with an average urinary BPA of only 2 μg/L were more than twice as likely to be obese as those with lower BPA levels.[142] Adults participating in the 2003 to 2006 NHANES trial (with a mean urinary BPA level of 2.05 μg/g creatinine) whose urinary BPA levels were in the second quartile and above had increased rates of obesity.[143] This surprising finding indicates that 75% of the adults measured in those years had increased risk for being obese, with those in the second quartile having an 85% greater risk. The association held for both general and truncal obesity.

Chlorinated Compounds. Prenatal exposure to both HCB and DDE have been associated with childhood obesity. Children with the highest levels of HCB in their cord blood were more than twice as likely to be obese by age 6 years.[144] Elevated serum DDE levels found in the first trimester of pregnancy increased the risk of obesity 50% at 14 months of age.[145] Prenatal exposure to DDE from consuming sport-caught fish has also been linked to an increased risk of obesity during adulthood.[146] Elevated cord blood DDE levels increased the risk of obesity at 6.5 years of age by 67% in children of smoking mothers.[147] Also noted in this study was the positive association between prenatal PCB exposure and adiposity by age 3 years. Prenatal PCB exposure was again associated with adiposity in children by age 6.5 years in another study.[148] The greatest source of PCB exposure for the general population is from the consumption of sardines and farmed salmon, which are also contaminated with chlorinated pesticides.[149] In an interesting mouse study, reduced-POP farmed salmon filets did not cause obesity and insulin resistance in mice, whereas feeding them regular farmed salmon filets with intact POP levels did.[150]

Perfluorocarbons. Mothers with blood PFOA levels in the second and third tertiles (encompassing 66% of studied mothers) were 1.7 to 2.2 times more likely to have children with greater waist circumferences by age 8 years than mothers with the lowest tertile of serum PFOA.[151] In 8- to 10-year-old overweight children, an increase of 10 ng/mL of either PFOA or PFOS was associated with greater likelihood of insulin resistance and increased serum triglyceride levels.[152]

Air Pollutants. Children exposed prenatally and postnatally to cigarette smoke have higher BMIs by age 10 years than those who are not exposed.[153] Not only did BMI increase with the number of smokers in the home, but BMI also went up with proximity to busy roadways. Among 6- to 11-year-old children who participated in the 2001 to 2006 NHANES, those with elevated urinary PAH and naphthalene metabolites had correspondingly greater waist circumference, BMI-z scores, and obesity.[154] A different study of 5- to 11-year-old children in Southern California revealed that those with the highest exposure to traffic pollution gained almost 14% more weight each year than their less-exposed counterparts.[155] A recent longitudinal study followed 8- to 15-year-old obese or overweight Latino youth in the Los Angeles area for an average of 3.4 years to watch the effect of ambient air pollution on their health. Both $PM_{2.5}$ and NO_2 were associated with a statistically significant increase in BMI and reduced beta cell function and insulin sensitivity.[156]

The Diabetes Epidemic

- POPs as a class
- Phthalates
- Arsenic
- Polycyclic aromatic hydrocarbons
- BPA
- PCBs
- Dioxins
- Organochlorine pesticides

Diabetes is a chronic disorder of carbohydrate, fat, and protein metabolism characterized by fasting elevations of blood glucose levels and an increased risk of heart disease, stroke, kidney disease, and loss of nerve function.

Diabetes can occur when the pancreas does not secrete enough insulin or if the cells of the body become resistant to insulin. As resistance progresses, it is often accompanied by a gradual decline in beta cell activity and decreasing beta cell mass. When the pancreas can no longer sustain the excessive production of insulin needed to overcome insulin resistance, the result is diabetes.[157,158]

A study released in 2007 using NHANES data found that approximately 36% of adults in the United States had either previously diagnosed diabetes mellitus (6.7%), undiagnosed diabetes (2.9%), or impaired fasting glucose (26.6%) in the period 1999 to 2002.[159] According to the CDC, the incidence of diabetes has increased from 0.9% in 1958 to 7.2% in 2013, representing an eightfold increase.[160] It is estimated that 29.1 million people, or 9.3% of the United States population, have diabetes.[161] The diabetes epidemic is well demonstrated in Fig. 44.3. However, this may only be the tip of the iceberg, because the incidence of metabolic syndrome is even higher, and as many as 8.1 million people in the United States have diabetes that has not yet been diagnosed.

The incidence of type 2 diabetes has increased by almost 10-fold in the past half century. Beginning in the 1960s, the production of synthetic organic chemicals began to escalate along with the incidence of diabetes (Fig. 44.4). Since then, even though sugar consumption, lack of exercise, genetic predisposition, and obesity have been shown to be contributing factors, research appears

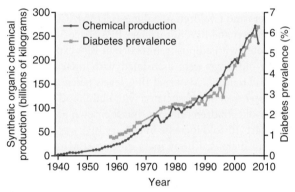

FIG. 44.4 The diabetes epidemic correlates with release of POPs into the environment. Ioannou, G. N., Bryson, C. L., & Boyko, E. J. (2007). Prevalence and trends of insulin resistance, impaired fasting glucose, and diabetes. *Journal of Diabetes and Its Complications*, *21*(6), 363–370.

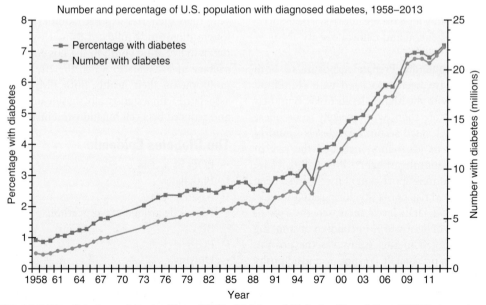

FIG. 44.3 The diabetes epidemic. (From CDC's Division of Diabetes Translation. [2017]. *Long-term trends in diabetes.* Retrieved from https://www.cdc.gov/diabetes/statistics/slides/long_term_trends.pdf.) (Accessed 28 March 2018)

to indicate that the total load of toxicants is by far the strongest contributing factor in the development of diabetes. The data is so compelling that some researchers now label these toxicants as "diabetogens."

Epidemiologically, diabetes mellitus has been linked to the Western lifestyle and is uncommon in cultures consuming a more "primitive" diet.[162] Studies have shown that when cultures switch from their native diets to the "foods of commerce," their rate of diabetes increases, eventually reaching the same proportions seen in Western societies.[163] More than half of the carbohydrates consumed in the United States are in the form of sugars added to processed foods as sweetening agents.[164] Independent of obesity status, it is estimated that consumption of sugar-sweetened beverages would result in 1.8 million excess events of type 2 diabetes in the United States over the next 10 years.[165] Although sugar consumption has increased, the increase does not correlate well with the diabetes epidemic (Fig. 44.5).[166]

A close look at Fig. 44.5 casts significant doubt on sugar consumption as the primary, or even the most important, cause. The diabetes epidemic started four decades after sugar consumption began to increase again and shows little correlation. Certainly, sugar contributes to diabetes, but if this was the primary driver, one would have expected the epidemic to start decades earlier.

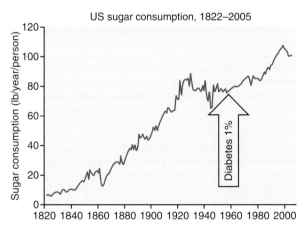

FIG. 44.5 The diabetes epidemic does not correlate with the increase in sugar consumption. (From Whole Health Source. [2017]. *By 2606, the US diet will be 100 percent sugar.* Retrieved from http://wholehealthsource.blogspot. com/2012/02/by-2606-us-diet-will-be-100-percent.html.) (Accessed 28 March 2018)

Obesity, a major risk factor for diabetes, has also been linked to the diabetes epidemic. In 2003 to 2004, 17.1% of US children and adolescents were overweight, and 66.3% of adults were either overweight or obese.[167] The prevalence of extreme obesity has also found to be increasing, especially among those with diabetes.[168] However, the obesity epidemic appears to be the result of the same causes as diabetes: diabetogens, many of which are also called obesogens. Concentrations of several prevalent phthalate metabolites showed statistically significant correlations with abdominal obesity and insulin resistance.[169]

Diabetogens: Toxicants That Disrupt Blood Sugar Control. The term *diabetogen* appears to have been coined in 1961 by G.D. Campbell of the Diabetic Clinic in King Edward VIII Hospital, Congella, Durban.[170] Campbell posted a letter in the *British Medical Journal* describing his efforts to determine the cause of an inexplicably high incidence of "connubial" diabetes in married Natal Indians. His investigative work led him to their high consumption of mustard oil, which consisted of a vegetable oil flavored with a synthetic substance containing 95% allyl isothiocyanate. He postulated that the chemical's chelation of free sulfhydryl groups in the gut resulted in a decreased availability of sulfhydryl groups, which he thought would impair carbohydrate metabolism. Although, in hindsight, he focused on the wrong molecule, his observation of food contamination as a cause of diabetes was accurate. Box 44.1 shows key diabetogens.

Persistent Organic Pollutants. Of significance is the surprising observation that obese people with low adipose levels of POPs do not have an increased risk of diabetes. In other words, if an obese person is low in POPs, the normally robust association between diabetes and obesity disappears.[171] In contrast, the diabetes epidemic does correlate with the rate of release of POPs into the environment. Individuals in the top quintile of exposure to six common POPs have a stunning 37.7-fold increased risk of diabetes—much stronger than any other known risk factor. Because many POPs block insulin receptor sites, decrease glucose transporter type-4 (GLUT-4) activity in muscles, and decrease insulin production, a causal relationship appears highly probable. Fig. 44.6 shows a very compelling association (which, of course, does not mean causation) between diabetes prevalence and production of POPs.[172-174]

More convincing is the correlation between body load of POPs and risk of metabolic syndrome as seen in Fig. 44.7. The association is synergistic. When the relationship between POP levels and diabetes risk is examined, the case becomes even more compelling. Those in the top 10% of transnonachlor, a common termiticide used in North America for decades, have a remarkable 12-fold increased risk of developing diabetes.

The highest current exposure source of chlorinated pesticides and PCBs currently comes from the consumption of sardines and farmed Atlantic salmon. An interesting association is seen when the consumption of farm salmon is compared with the rates of type 2 diabetes mellitus (T2DM) in the United States.

The direct association was actually demonstrated in animals fed filets of farmed Atlantic salmon that either had their POP content removed or left intact (Fig. 44.8). The animals fed a Western diet with Atlantic salmon filets developed visceral obesity, insulin resistance, and glucose intolerance. The animals fed the same high-fat Western diet with the reduced POP filets had lower POP body burden, accumulated less visceral fat, had lower TNF-α levels, and had better insulin sensitivity and glucose tolerance.[152]

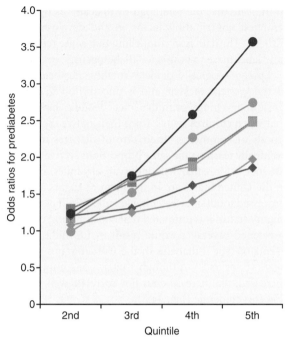

FIG. 44.6 Body load of POPs per quintile and OR for metabolic syndrome. *Black circles*, PCBs (15 congeners); *black squares*, p,p'-DDE; *white squares*, p,p'-DDT; *black diamonds*, HCB; *white diamonds*, β-HCH; *white circles*, POLL5. (From Ukropec, J., Radikova Z., Huckova M., Koska J., Kocan A., & Sebokova E., et al. [2010]. High prevalence of prediabetes and diabetes in a population exposed to high levels of an organochlorine cocktail. *Diabetologia*, *53*(5), 899–906.)

Arsenic. There is a direct correlation between the amount of arsenic in a person's body (toenail arsenic is the best measure of long-term exposure) and risk of diabetes (Fig. 44.9). In this case, the primary mechanism appears to be the result of damaged pancreatic beta cells with resultant decreased production of insulin.[175] In the Maternal-Infant Research on Environmental Chemicals (MIREC) study, women in the highest quartile of urinary arsenic were 3.7 times more likely to develop gestational diabetes than those with lower arsenic levels.[176]

Ambient Air Pollutants. A study that took place over more than 3 years of overweight and obese Latino children from Los Angeles, California, showed significant effects of elevated NO₂ and particulate matter with diameter less than 2.5 ($PM_{2.5}$) on insulin homeostasis and beta cell function that were independent of body fat percentage.[177] Epidemiological studies have also shown that a higher exposure to NO_2 and $PM_{2.5}$ is associated with a greater risk for T2DM in adults.[178-180]

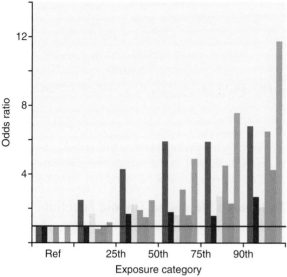

FIG. 44.7 Diabetes risk (OR) for individual POPs according to percentiles. *Blue rectangle,* PCB153; *red rectangle,* HpCDD; *yellow rectangle,* OCDD; *green rectangle,* Oxychlordane; *pink rectangle, trans*-nonachlor; *purple rectangle,* DDE. (Data from Lee DH, Lee IK, Song K, et al. (2006). A strong dose-response relation between serum concentrations of persistent organic pollutants and diabetes: results from the National Health and Examination Survey 1999-2002. *Diabetes Care, 29*(7), 1638–1644.)

Bisphenol A and Phthalates. BPA blocks insulin receptor sites, causing insulin resistance.[181] This increases not only the incidence of diabetes but also obesity, especially accumulation of visceral fat. This is well demonstrated by increasing waist size, as shown in Fig. 44.10.

In the Nurses Health Study II (mean age, 45.6 years), those with the total urinary phthalates in the highest quartiles were more than twice as likely to develop T2DM (OR 2.14).[182] Participants in the NHANES 2001 to 2008 with MiBP in the highest quartiles had higher fasting blood sugars than those with fewer phthalates.[183] MEHP demonstrates an ability to inhibit beta-oxidation of certain fatty acids by about 50% to 60% in the mitochondria.[184] This mitochondrial inhibition undoubtedly plays a role

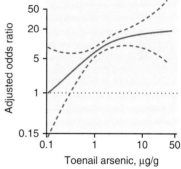

FIG. 44.9 Arsenic levels correlate with diabetes. (From Pan, W. C., Seow, W. J., Kile, M. L., Hoffman E. B., Quamruzzaman Q., & Rahman M., et al. [2013]. Association of low to moderate levels of arsenic exposure with risk of type 2 diabetes in Bangladesh. *American Journal of Epidemiology, 178,* 1563–1570.)

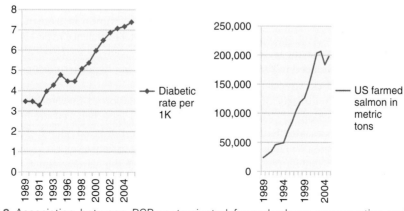

FIG. 44.8 Association between PCB-contaminated farmed-salmon consumption and rates of diabetes in the United States between 1989 and 2004.

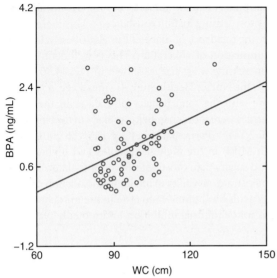

FIG. 44.10 BPA correlates with waist circumference. (From Savastano, S., Tarantino, G., D'Esposito, V., Passaretti F., Cabaro S., & Liotti A., et al. [2015]. Bisphenol-A plasma levels are related to inflammatory markers, visceral obesity and insulin-resistance: A cross-sectional study on adult male population. *Journal of Translational Medicine, 13,* 169. Reprinted under the terms and conditions of the Creative Commons Attribution (CC-BY) license (http://creativecommons.org/licenses/by/4.0/))

in phthalates causing increased rates of obesity and diabetes.[185]

Laboratory Markers. The most important and easily available laboratory test indicative of toxicant load associated with diabetes is gamma-glutamyl transferase (GGT, also known as GGTP). GGT is induced to provide more glutathione (GSH), likely for phase II conjugation, as well as to neutralize oxidative stress. This enzyme recycles GSH for detoxification of POPs and is induced in proportion to exposure. Cellular GGT metabolizes extracellular GSH, allowing precursor cysteine to be reutilized for *de novo* synthesis of intracellular GSH. Elevations of GGT within the "normal" range are strongly associated with several chronic diseases, including diabetes.[186] However, the "normal" range may be more indicative of adaptation to toxic load as opposed to a true normal. Fig. 44.11 demonstrates the predictive value of GGT and the development of diabetes. As can be seen, a strong correlation exists between GGT levels and the risk of diabetes.[187]

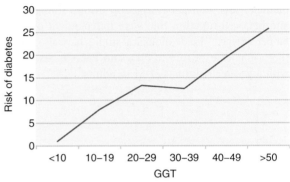

FIG. 44.11 Serum GGT (U/L) and risk of diabetes.

Not surprisingly, hemoglobin A1C (Hb A_{1c}) levels also rise along with GGT in individuals with diabetes.[188] More detailed information can be found in Chapter 54.

Xenobiotic Effects on Thyroid Function

- Organochlorine compounds (PCBs, DDT, and dioxins)
- Pesticides—chlorinated and organophosphate
- Metals (mercury and cadmium)
- Perchlorates
- Brominated flame retardants
- Perchlorate
- Phthalates

Thyroid dysfunction is the second-most common endocrine disorder.[189] Hypothyroidism is characterized by a reduction in thyroid hormone production and/or the decreased effect of thyroid hormone, thereby lowering cellular metabolism throughout the body. The prevalence of hypothyroidism ranges from 1% to 10% of adults depending on the criteria used for diagnosis. Hypothyroidism is more common in women, and data analysis has found the total prevalence to be 3.7% (TSH > 4.5 mIU/L). Individuals aged 80 years or older have a five times greater risk for hypothyroidism than those aged 12 to 49 years.[190]

The regulation of thyroid function is dependent on the feedback loop between the hypothalamus, anterior pituitary, and thyroid gland. Thyroid hormones are involved in a variety of physiological processes, including bone remodeling, cardiac function, and mental status, and have a special importance in fetal development. Thyroid hormones also regulate the rate of metabolic function of most tissues, in part by increasing the number and size of mitochondria, and by inducing transcription of enzymes of the respiratory chain and membrane sodium-potassium ATPase. Most actions of thyroid hormones result from the interaction of nuclear thyroid hormone receptors that have a preferential affinity for T3 and their specific target gene promoters.[191]

Many groups of chemicals may have thyroid-disrupting potential. Thyroid hormone–disrupting chemicals have various methods of action and, when combined, may have synergistic effects.[192-195] Thyroid activity can be adversely affected, resulting in decreased thyroid stimulating hormone (TSH) production, decreased T4 production, poor or inconsistent conversion of T4 to T3, reduced cellular response to T3, decreased absorption of iodine, and impaired mitochondrial response to T3, resulting in reduced ATP production. In addition, the function of the sodium iodide symporter (NIS) or thyroid peroxidase (TPO) can be inhibited or stimulated by chemicals, and transthyretin (TTR), a transport protein, may be a source for competitive binding of environmental chemicals. Fig. 44.12 demonstrates the mechanisms of action of several toxicants.

Organochlorines. Several animal studies confirm that exposure to PCBs or dioxin results in reduction of serum thyroid hormone levels, especially T4.[196-198] Dioxins and furans adversely affect the thyroid hormone metabolizing enzymes uridine-diphosphate-glucuronyl transferase, iodothyronine deiodinase, and sulfotransferases found in the liver and brain.[199] Hydroxylated PCBs also inhibit iodothyronine sulfotransferase activity, affecting peripheral metabolism of thyroid hormones.[200] German children

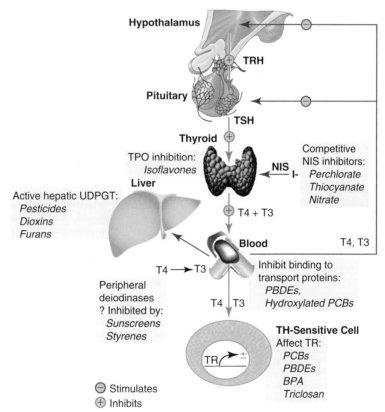

FIG. 44.12 Mechanisms of various thyroid disruptors. *I–*, Iodine; *NIS*, the sodium iodide symporter; *T3*, triiodothyronine; *T4*, thyroxine; *TH*, thyroid hormone; *TPO*, thyroperoxidase; *TR*, thyroid hormone receptor; *TRH*, thyrotropin releasing hormone; *TSH*, thyroid stimulating hormone; *UDPGT*, uridine diphosphate glucuronyltransferase. (From Pearce, E. N., & Braverman, L. E. [2009]. Environmental pollutants and the thyroid. *Best Practice & Research Clinical Endocrinology & Metabolism, 23,* 801–813.)

showed a significant positive correlation between PCB serum levels and elevation of TSH as well as a significant inverse correlation between serum PCB levels and free T4 (FT4).[201] Air Force personnel participating in operation Ranch Hand (the spraying of broad-leaf defoliants) during the Vietnam War were found to have high serum TCDD (2,3,7,8-tetrachlorodibenzo-p-dioxin, a by-product of chlorophenoxy herbicide manufacturing) levels that were significantly associated with elevated levels of TSH.[202] Thus PCBs reduce peripheral thyroid hormone levels, inducing a compensatory increase in TSH.[15,203]

PCBs, dioxins, and furans have demonstrated *in vitro* activity in binding TTR, a transport protein mechanism for thyroxine (T4), blocking the transport of thyroxine.[204] Hydroxylated PCBs bind to TTR with a stronger binding affinity than their parent compounds.[205]

Workers exposed to 2,3,7,8-TCDD have significantly higher free T4 levels.[206] Children with high perinatal exposure to polychlorinated diphenyl dioxins and furans show no change in thyroid hormone levels at age 1 or 2 years but have significantly elevated T3 levels at age 5 years.[207] While elevation of FT4 was noted at birth in babies exposed to dioxins *in utero* and through breast milk.[208] The elevation of FT4 in the exposed infants reached statistical significance at week 1 and week 11. By week 11, TSH concentrations were also statistically higher in the children receiving dioxin through breast milk. Elevated antithyroid antibodies, both antiperoxidase and antithyroglobulin, were found in workers in a PCB manufacturing plant.[209] However, no difference was found in the levels of T4 and TSH in TCDD workers than in the control group. Swedish women who consumed at least two meals of fish from the Baltic Sea each month showed a significant inverse correlation between serum PCB levels and total T3 (TT3) and an insignificant inverse correlation with total T4 (TT4).[210]

DDT was found to be higher in a group of hypothyroid Indian women than in euthyroid female controls, whereas dieldrin was significantly associated with low T4 levels.[211] Canadian newborns had significantly lower T4 concentrations in their cord blood when PCPs was also present.[212]

Polybrominated Flame Retardants. Brominated flame retardants such as polybrominated diphenyl ethers (PBDEs), pentabromophenol (PBP), and tetrabromo-bisphenol A (TBBPA) have a structural resemblance to T4 and are potent competitors for T4 binding to transthyretin (TTR).[213] PBDEs suppress the TH-regulated gene expression in humans and interfere with TH signaling.[214] Several animal studies indicate that PBDEs decrease the levels of circulating thyroid hormones,[215-217] and perinatal maternal exposure reduces thyroid hormones prenatally and postnatally.[218-221]

Organophosphate Pesticides. Individuals with acute OP pesticide poisoning have a host of hormonal alterations, including elevations of adrenocorticotropic hormone (ACTH), cortisol, and prolactin.[222] Interestingly, 31.8% of these individuals also experienced sick euthyroid syndrome with low FT3, FT4, or TSH. OP pesticide formulators have significantly low TT3 and nonsignificantly elevated TSH levels,[223] yet persons using backpack sprayers with dithiocarbamates (also acetylcholinesterase inhibitors) have increased TSH levels.[224]

Perchlorate. Newborn TSH levels in cities where 100% of the municipal drinking water was contaminated with perchlorate were significantly higher than newborns in areas with noncontaminated water.[225] Perchlorate is known to competitively inhibit iodide uptake at the sodium iodide symporter and has been used in the past in the diagnosis and treatment of thyrotoxicosis.[226] Workers in an ammonium perchlorate production plant were found to have a 38% reduction in 14-hour thyroid radioactive iodine uptake.[227]

Phthalates. Phthalates have various mechanisms of action on thyroid homeostasis, including interfering with the activity of the NIS,[228] inhibiting T3 uptake in cells,[229] and competitively binding to TTR.[230] Significant mild negative correlations were found between TT4 and FT4 and urinary phthalate monoesters in pregnant women exposed to di-n-butyl-phthalate (DBP).[231] In adult men, there is an inverse association between urinary concentration of MEHP and serum levels of FT4 and T3.[232]

Mercury. Mercury accumulates in the thyroid and reduces the uptake of iodine by binding to the sodium-iodide transporting molecule.[233] Mercury also inhibits deiodinase function in the peripheral tissues, preventing the production of T3 from T4.[234] Methylmercury, particularly when combined with an iodine or selenium deficiency, inhibits D1, the predominant deiodinase in the liver, kidney, and intestines.[235-237] Both adolescents and adults in the 2007 to 2008 NHANES had a negative association between blood mercury levels and total T3 and T4.[238] Adolescents also showed a higher risk for both antithyroglobulin and anti-TPO antibodies. Women in the same NHANES cohort with blood mercury above 1.8 µg/L (approximately the 80th percentile) were more likely to have antithyroglobuin antibodies than those with blood mercury below 0.4 µg/L.[239]

Cadmium. Increased serum cadmium levels are associated with elevated TSH and lowered FT4 levels.[240] In human neonates, cadmium in cord blood is associated with reduced TSH levels,[241] although this effect is completely blunted in animals given zinc and selenium.[242] Cadmium accumulates in the lungs, the liver, and especially the kidneys, and thyroid hyperplasia and hypertrophy are common with chronic cadmium toxicity.[243]

Xenobiotic Effects on Adrenal Function

- Alcohol
- Cigarette smoke
- Drugs
- Chlorophenols
- Organochlorine pesticides
- OPs
- Air pollution
- PCBs
- Pyrethroid pesticides
- Salt
- Toxic metals

The adrenal glands are composed of two sections: the medulla, which is responsible for producing catecholamines (e.g., epinephrine [adrenaline], norepinephrine), and the cortex, which produces a variety of steroid hormones, including glucocorticoids (e.g., cortisol), mineralocorticoids (e.g., aldosterone), and androgens. Catecholamine production is primarily regulated by sympathetic outflow from the hypothalamus. Steroidogenesis is directly controlled by ACTH secretion from the pituitary gland, which in turn is controlled by corticotrophin-releasing factor (CRF) and arginine vasopressin (AVP) secretion from the hypothalamus. Ultimately, the hypothalamus regulates all aspects of adrenal function. This cascade is known as the *hypothalamic-pituitary-adrenal axis* (HPA axis) and is self-regulated. Endogenous cortisol binds to glucocorticoid receptors in the HPA axis and acts as a potent negative regulator of HPA activity. These regulatory mechanisms

are important in determining basal levels and circadian fluctuations of cortisol levels. Although a catecholamine deficiency is quite rare, steroid deficiencies, ranging from frank adrenal failure to suboptimal steroid production, are much more common.[244]

Addison's disease is a clear example of frank adrenal failure characterized by insufficient production of all cortex hormones. Addison's disease represents 80% to 90% of all primary adrenal failure cases. More than 90% of patients with Addison's disease have adrenal autoantibodies, most commonly to the adrenal cortex and to the enzyme 21-hydroxylase.[245]

The negative effects of environmental toxicants on the adrenal gland are increasing. Research has suggested that the adrenal gland, particularly the adrenal cortex, is the most common toxicological target of all the endocrine organs.[246] Box 44.2 describes several attributes of the adrenal gland that increase its susceptibility to exposure to toxicants and toxic insult.[247] Toxic agents to the adrenal cortex include short-chain aliphatic compounds, lipidosis inducers, amphiphilic compounds, natural and synthetic steroids, and chemicals that affect hydroxylation.[248] Compounds typically produce either degenerative or proliferative changes in the zona fasciculata/reticularis, necrotic or atrophic changes in the zona glomerulosa, hypertrophic or proliferative changes in the medulla, and/or disruption of the metabolism or action of adrenocortical steroids.[249,250]

Toxicity. The rate-limiting step in steroid hormone synthesis is the movement of cholesterol across the mitochondrial membrane, from the outer to the inner membrane, mediated by the steroidogenic acute regulatory (StAR) protein, with the conversion of cholesterol to pregnenolone by cytochrome P450 side-chain cleavage (CYPscc) initiating steroidogenesis.[251] StAR mutations in humans cause congenital lipoid adrenal hyperplasia (lipoid CAH), which leads to severe deficiencies in all classes of steroid hormones and cumulative progressive increases in lipid deposits in several organs, including the adrenal glands.[252] Studies have shown that both steroidogenesis and the expression of StAR protein are inhibited by the pesticides lindane and glyphosate (Roundup™).[253,254] Spironolactone, a mineralocorticoid receptor antagonist, also inhibits StAR transcription.[255] Because many toxicants reduce StAR expression and steroidogenesis in the adrenal gland, a disruption in StAR protein expression may be the cornerstone of toxicity,

BOX 44.2   **Characteristics of the Adrenal Gland Conveying Vulnerability to Toxicity**

- High vascularity
  - Disproportionately large blood volume received per unit mass of adrenal tissue providing efficient exposures to toxicants
- Rich cholesterol and steroid content favoring capacity for uptake and storage of lipophilic agents
- Potential for lipid peroxidation both directly (via parent compound or its metabolites) and indirectly (via generation of reactive oxygen species) as a result of high adrenocortical cell membrane content of unsaturated fatty acids
- High content of enzymes of the CYP family in the adrenal cortex, which can produce the following:
  - Bioactivation of toxicants that then mediate toxicity
  - Generation of free radicals during hydroxylation reactions, which then damage adrenocortical cells and membranes
- Multiple targets, such as adrenal and systemic enzymes, transcription factors, receptors, and biochemical mediators
  - Glucocorticoid and mineralocorticoid production are most vulnerable to upstream toxicity by inhibition of any of the steroidogenic enzymes
- Functional dependence on corticosteroid binding globulin (CBG), a high-affinity binding carrier protein, that transports secreted glucocorticoids

Modified from Hinson, J. P., & Raven, P. W. (2006). Effects of endocrine-disrupting chemicals on adrenal function. *Best Practice & Research Clinical Endocrinology & Metabolism, 20*(1), 111–120.

interfering with several adrenal functions, including carbohydrate metabolism, obesity, lipid metabolism, vascular function, cardiac remodeling, immune system function, and water balance.[256]

Adrenal steroidogenesis is a vulnerable target for toxic insult. Inhibition of steroidogenic pathways is considered the major mechanism of action of toxicants on the adrenal gland. Steroidogenesis is critical for adrenocortical function and presents multiple molecular targets for toxicity, ranging from general effects on all steroidogenic tissues (e.g., via StAR protein or CYP11A1 cholesterol side-chain cleavage) through to specific targets affecting only adrenocortical function (e.g., CYP11beta/18 and glucocorticoid synthesis).[257] Virtually every step in the adrenocortical steroidogenic pathway, including the ACTH receptor, StAR, CYP 11A1 (side-chain cleavage enzyme), CYP19 (aromatase—rate-limiting step in the conversion of androgens to estrogens), CYP17A1 (17α-hydroxylase/17, 20 lyase—controls initial steps of cortisol biosynthesis, including the production of DHEA), CYP21 (steroid 21-hydroxylase—involved in the biosynthesis of aldosterone and cortisol), CYP11B1 (11β-hydroxylase—the final step in the biosynthesis of cortisol), CYP11B2 (aldosterone synthase—rate-limiting step in aldosterone synthesis), and 3-hydroxysteroid dehydrogenase-Δ-4,5 isomerase (an obligate step in in the biosynthesis of androgens, estrogens, mineralocorticoids, and glucocorticoids) are known to be potential targets. A wide range of agents directly inhibit adrenal steroidogenic enzymes, including digoxin and digitoxin (11A1 and 11B1),[258] etomidate (11A1, 11B1, 11B2, StAR, 17A1),[259] ketoconazole (17A1, 11B1, 3-hydroxysteroid dehydrogenase/isomerase),[260] nitrofurans (11B/18),[261] and the luteolytic agent azastene (3-hydroxysteroid dehydrogenase/isomerase).[262] Table 44.5 provides further examples of chemicals that induce adrenocortical toxicity and their targets in the steroidogenic pathway.[263] When interpreting toxicity data, species specificity and age dependence in the development of chemically induced adrenal lesions must be considered.

Some xenobiotics exhibit toxic effects after their metabolism and activation by adrenal cytochrome P450 enzymes. For example, 7,12-dimethylbenz[a]anthracene (DMBA), a PAH found high in tobacco smoke, is an adrenocorticolytic agent that causes hemorrhage and necrosis in the adrenal cortex, requiring metabolism by CYP1B1 for its toxic effects to occur.[264]

The generation of reactive oxygen species (ROS) is an additional mechanism by which toxicity to and from the adrenal glands may occur. Various stressors activate the HPA axis, stimulating the secretion of glucocorticoids. Glucocorticoids induce oxidative stress directly through enhanced mitochondrial respiration and oxidative phosphorylation and indirectly through interaction with nuclear genes.[265,266] ROS initiate a variety of toxic reactions, including initiation of lipid peroxidation, direct inhibition of mitochondrial respiratory chain enzymes, inactivation of glyceraldehyde-3 phosphate dehydrogenase, inhibition of membrane sodium-potassium ATPase activity, and inactivation of membrane sodium channels.[267] ROS promote an increase in HPA axis activity via reduced negative feedback, sustaining the pathophysiological response.[268]

TABLE 44.5 Chemicals that Induce Adrenocortical Toxicity and Targets in Steroidogenic Pathways

Target	Compound
ACTH receptor	Aminoglutethimide
StAR protein	Econazole, miconazole, lindane, bromocriptine, spironolactone
CYP11A1 (CYPscc)	Aminoglutethimide, bromocriptine
CYP17	Penta-, octa-, deca-brominated diphenyl ethers, tetrabromobisphenol-A, spironolactone, PCB126, ketoconazole
3-hydroxysteroid dehydrogenase-Δ-4,5 isomerase	Cyanoketone, trilostane, PCBs (101, 110, 126, 149), bromophenols, polybrominated biphenyls, 2,3,7,8-tetrabromodibenzo-p-dioxin, 2,3,7,8-tetrabromodibenzofuran, pioglitazone
17β-hydroxysteroid dehydrogenase	PCBs (101, 110, 126, 149)
CYP21	RU486, ketoconazole, flavonoids, PCB126, PAHs
CYP11B1 (CYP11β/18)	Metyrapone, mitotane (o,p-DDD), MeSO$_2$-DDE, etomidate, ketoconazole, aminoglutethimide, flavonoids, PCBs (101, 110, 126, 149), efonidipine, mibefradil
CYP19 (aromatase)	Prochloraz, imazalil, triazines, atrazine, simazine, propazine, di-, tributyl, and phenyltin chlorides, fadrozole, PCBs (101, 110, 126, 149), amoxicillin
CYP11B2 (aldosterone synthase)	Fadrozole, PCBs (101, 110, 126, 149), efonidipine, mibefradil, PAHs, amoxicillin, erythromycin

From Harvey, P. W. (2016). Adrenocortical endocrine disruption. *Journal of Steroid Biochemistry and Molecular Biology, 155*(Pt B), 199–206.

Alcohol. Alcohol produces chemical stress on the body, increases adrenal hormone output, interferes with normal brain chemistry, and interferes with normal sleep cycles. Alcohol ingestion also leads to hypoglycemia. Although many people believe that alcohol has a calming effect, a study of 90 healthy male volunteers given either a placebo or alcohol demonstrated significant increases in anxiety scores after drinking the alcohol.[269]

Chlorophenols. PCP has been used worldwide as a pesticide and wood preservative, and intermediate metabolites, such as 2,4,6-trichlorophenol (TCP), may have more toxic effects than the parent compound.[270] PCP and TCP affect production of testosterone and 17β-estradiol mediated by the inhibition of steroidogenic enzymes via decreased cellular concentration of cAMP.[271]

Cigarette smoke. Central to the effect of nicotine is the stimulation of adrenal hormone and cortisol secretion. Elevated cortisol levels are a well-recognized feature of depression,[272] and cigarette smoking is a significant risk factor in depression.[273] Cortisol activates tryptophan oxygenase, resulting in less tryptophan being delivered to the brain. Because the level of serotonin in the brain is dependent on the amount of tryptophan delivered to the brain, cortisol ultimately results in reductions in the level of serotonin and melatonin.[274] Tobacco compounds inhibit selected P450 enzymes in the glucocorticoid and sex steroid synthetic pathways, and cause direct and specific inhibition of aldosterone synthesis.[275,276]

Drugs/iatrogenic. The medical literature shows significant effects of medications causing adrenal disruption in humans. A report published in 1982 proposed that etomidate, a sedative licensed for use as an anesthetic induction agent, be considered for use as a longer-term sedative as an alternative to benzodiazepines in intensive care units.[277] Several studies were soon reported revealing that exposure to etomidate resulted in the death of several patients.[278,279] Further investigation demonstrated unpredicted chemically induced adrenal insufficiency secondary to etomidate use. It is now known that etomidate is a potent inhibitor of steroid synthesis, acting on the adrenal gland as an inhibitor of 11β-hydroxylase, a mitochondrial enzyme that converts 11-deoxycortisol to cortisol and 11-deoxycorticosterone to corticosterone.[280-282]

Ketoconazole, an antifungal agent, also inhibits 11β-hydroxylase, leading to a 2- to 50-fold increase in plasma ACTH levels.[283] In addition, ketoconazole has shown inhibitory actions on the conversion of 11-deoxycorticosterone to corticosterone, conversion of corticosterone to aldosterone, and inhibition of the microsomal enzyme C17-20-lyase, the key enzyme in androgen biosynthesis.[284]

Cushing's syndrome is an example of adrenal hyperfunction characterized by elevated cortisol levels leading to symptoms such as fatigue, weight gain, obesity, glucose intolerance, impaired ability to heal, high blood pressure, and bone loss. The most common cause of Cushing's syndrome is the long-term use of synthetic prescription corticosteroid medications.[285] Up to 20% of patients on high doses of glucocorticoids develop psychiatric disorders such as depression, mania, psychosis, or a mixed affective state, and up to 75% report psychiatric symptoms that can be reversed with cessation of glucocorticoid therapy.[286] Continuous activity leading to prolonged secretion of corticotropin-releasing hormone (CRH), norepinephrine, cortisol, and other hormones can produce anxiety, anorexia, hyperphagia, and depression. Excessive exercise, malnutrition, alcoholism, and acute trauma can all result in elevated cortisol levels. Prolonged elevations in cortisol increase epinephrine production in the adrenal gland and in the brain by enhancing phenylethanolamine-N-methyltransferase activity.[287] Thus glucocorticoids may also contribute to neuronal stress. As can be seen in Fig. 44.13, in proportion to the duration of use, glucocorticoids

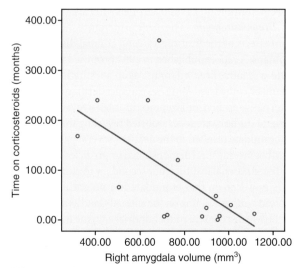

FIG. 44.13 Glucocorticoid use and amygdala volume (r =−0.597, p = 0.019). (From Brown, E. S., Woolston D. J., & Frol A. B. [2008]. Amygdala volume in patients receiving chronic corticosteroid therapy. *Biological Psychiatry, 63*[7], 705–709.)

have been shown to reduce the volume of the amygdala and hippocampus compared with healthy controls.[288] This is believed to be related to the effect of glucocorticoids on glutamate release.[289] The neuroendocrine theory of aging posits that changes in the hormonal and neurological functions that coordinate physiological adaptations to stress are significant factors in the aging process.[290]

Several other pharmaceuticals influence gene expression, adversely affecting steroidogenesis. Compared with the solvent control dimethylsulfoxide (DMSO), amoxicillin significantly increased the expression of CYP17 more than fourfold, as did cyproterone (threefold), and the β2-agonist salbutamol (more than 10-fold); in addition, the antilipidic agent clofibrate (approximately fivefold), tylosin (approximately 10-fold), erythromycin (approximately sevenfold), dexamethasone (approximately fivefold), acetaminophen (approximately fourfold), and fluoxetine (approximately fivefold) increased expression of the aldostrogenic gene CYP11B2.[291]

Organochlorine pesticides. Aliphatic compounds (3–6 carbons in length with electronegative groups on both ends) cause necrosis of the zona fasciculata and zona reticularis of the adrenals, where glucocorticoids are produced. Organochlorine pesticides (OCPs) and carbamates have caused histological changes to these areas in animal models.[292]

Dioxins and mirex (used to treat fire ants) cause direct suppression of glucocorticoid synthesis, resulting in hypoglycemia.[293] The insecticide lindane has been shown to reduce cortisol secretion, downregulate the expression of a subset of the genes encoding steroidogenic enzymes, and repress transcriptional activation of the StAR protein gene promoter.[294]

Organophosphate pesticides. Individuals with acute OP poisoning have revealed a host of hormonal alterations, including elevations of ACTH, cortisol, and prolactin.[295] Changes in hormone levels may result from the effects of neurotransmitters, from the direct effect of the toxic agent, or from stress associated with events leading to the poisoning incident.[296]

Outdoor air pollution. Diesel exhaust particles (DEP) generated by motor vehicles are a primary cause of air pollution. Two nitrophenol derivatives of DEP, 3-methyl-4-nitrophenol (PNMC) and 4-nitro-3-phenylphenol (PNMPP), accumulate in the adrenal glands, where they modulate enzyme genes responsible for the inhibition or stimulation of steroid hormones.[297] The administration of PNMC at the concentration of 10 and 100 mg/kg for

5 days in immature male rats significantly decreased the plasma levels of corticosterone and progesterone by means of inhibiting 3β-hydroxysteroid dehydrogenase-2 (3βHSD2) in the adrenal glands and altering the steroidogenesis pathway.[298]

Polychlorinated biphenyls. Polychlorinated biphenyl 126 (PCB126) increases expression of CYP11B2, stimulating basal and inducible aldosterone production (3.3-fold), and increases expression of the AT1 receptor, enhancing angiotensin II responsiveness of adrenal cells.[299] The PCB congeners (PCB101, PCB110, PCB126, and PCB149) also increase expression of the genes coding for enzymes involved in the later or final steps of steroid production, leading to excessive production of steroid hormones, including aldosterone, cortisol, and estradiol.[300]

Pyrethroid pesticides. Type I and type II pyrethroids cause adrenal activation in rats, with an increase in blood adrenaline and noradrenaline accompanying motor signs.[301]

Salt. Chronic metabolic acidosis in human beings is characterized by increased renin-angiotensin-aldosterone (RAA) activity, cortisol secretion, and nitrogen wasting.[302] Studies have shown a connection between sodium chloride intake and acid-base balance, with high-salt diets causing a decrease in pH and moderate metabolic acidosis.[303,304] In healthy humans, diets that contain sodium chloride independently predict systemic acid-base status and, as the load increases, so does the degree of hyperchloremic metabolic acidosis.[305] In other words, the severity of chronic low-grade metabolic acidosis is proportional to the sodium chloride content of the diet. The mineralocorticoid aldosterone activates signaling and effector mechanisms in the kidney and the brain, including the mineralocorticoid receptor, the serum- and glucocorticoid-induced kinase SGK1, the ubiquitin ligase NEDD4-2, and the epithelial sodium channel ENaC.[306] Aldosterone increases renal salt retention and sodium appetite, which in some cases sustains the pathophysiological response. During acidosis, circulating aldosterone levels are increased, and the hormone acts in concert with angiotensin II and other factors to stimulate renal acid secretion.[307] Glucocorticoid and mineralocorticoid activities increase significantly in response to acidosis. Mineralocorticoids act centrally to increase salt appetite, sympathetic drive, and vasopressin release, resulting in hypertension.[308]

Toxic metals. A study of occupational lead workers showed decreased secretions of corticosteroids, both glucocorticoids (17-hydroxy) and androgenic steroids (17-keto). In these persons, the lesion was apparently at the hypothalamus/pituitary level, because normal ACTH response was found with stimulation.[309] In contrast, older adults with high blood lead levels had increases in cortisol levels, suggesting that lead exposure is related to allostatic load (i.e., the "wear and tear" of chronic stress) and greater vulnerability to develop stress-related disorders as individuals get older.[310] After adjusting for confounders, pregnant women with higher blood lead levels had a reduced cortisol awakening response compared with women in the lowest quintile.[311] Animal studies also demonstrate that maternal lead itself causes permanent dysfunction of the HPA axis,[312] and rats fed lead in their drinking water showed increases in levels of the mineralocorticoid aldosterone, contributing to elevated blood pressure.[313]

Cadmium and mercury have both been shown to cause nonspecific inhibition of steroidogenesis even at very low concentrations.[314,315]

ASSESSMENT

Exposure to endocrine-disrupting xenobiotics can be assessed through case history, knowledge of the ambient pollutant levels in their geographical area, and from measurement of xenobiotics and their metabolites available from specialty laboratories.

INTERVENTION

Avoidance of all the known EDCs (both those listed by the ES and those not listed) is a critical step in avoiding and hopefully reversing the effect of these ubiquitous compounds. Avoidance of phthalates, parabens, and phenol-containing compounds is critical and has been documented to result in a reduction of the presence of these compounds in the urine.[316-319] Avoidance of indoor and outdoor air pollutants can be accomplished by the use of high-quality furnace filters and stand-alone air purification units in the home that can effectively filter out fine PM.[320,321] Water filtration in the home may provide protection against perfluorocarbons, groundwater solvents, perchlorates, and hexavalent chromium. Avoiding Atlantic salmon and sardines will reduce one's exposure to PCBs and other persistent pollutants common to these fish, but depuration techniques are needed to reduce the body burden of these compounds in the body.

REFERENCES

1. Diamanti-Kandarakis, E., Bourguignon, J. P., Giudice, L. C., et al. (2009). Endocrine-disrupting chemicals: an Endocrine Society scientific statement. *Endocrine Review, 30*(4), 293–342. PubMed PMID: 19502515.

2. Gore, A. C., Chappell, V. A., Fenton, S. E., et al. (2015). EDC-2: The Endocrine Society's Second Scientific Statement on Endocrine-Disrupting Chemicals. *Endocrine Review, 36*(6), E1–E150. PubMed PMID: 26544531.

3. Cao, Y., Calafat, A. M., Doerge, D. R., et al. (2009). Isoflavones in urine, saliva, and blood of infants: data from a pilot study on the estrogenic activity of soy formula. *Journal of Exposure Science and Environmental Epidemiology, 19*(2), 223–234. PubMed PMID: 18665197.

4. Trasande, L., Zoeller, R. T., Hass, U., et al. (2016). Burden of disease and costs of exposure to endocrine disrupting chemicals in the European Union: an updated analysis. *Andrology, 4*(4), 565–572. PubMed PMID: 27003928.

5. Attina, T. M., Hauser, R., Sathyanarayana, S., et al. (2016). Exposure to endocrine-disrupting chemicals in the USA: a population-based disease burden and cost analysis. *The Lancet Diabetes & Endocrinology, 4*(12), 996–1003. PubMed PMID: 27765541.

6. Welshons, W. V., Thayer, K. A., Judy, B. M., et al. (2003). Large effects from small exposures. I. Mechanisms for endocrine-disrupting chemicals with estrogenic activity. *Environmental Health Perspectives, 111*(8), 994–1006. PubMed PMID: 12826473.

7. Welshons, W. V., Nagel, S. C., & vom Saal, F. S. (2006). Large effects from small exposures. III. Endocrine mechanisms mediating effects of bisphenol A at levels of human exposure. *Endocrinology, 147*(6 Suppl.), S56–S69. Review. PubMed PMID: 16690810.

8. Manikkam, M., Guerrero-Bosagna, C., Tracey, R., et al. (2012). Transgenerational actions of environmental compounds on reproductive disease and identification of epigenetic biomarkers of ancestral exposures. *PLoS ONE, 7*(2), e31901. PubMed PMID: 22389676.

9. Manikkam, M., Tracey, R., Guerrero-Bosagna, C., & Skinner, M. K. (2012). Pesticide and insect repellent mixture (permethrin and DEET) induces epigenetic transgenerational inheritance of disease and sperm epimutations. *Reproductive Toxicology, 34*(4), 708–719. PubMed PMID: 22975477.

10. Skinner, M. K., Manikkam, M., Tracey, R., et al. (2013). Ancestral dichlorodiphenyltrichloroethane (DDT) exposure promotes epigenetic transgenerational inheritance of obesity. *BMC Medicine, 11*, 228. PubMed PMID: 24228800.

11. Rio Gomez, I. D., Marshall, T. K., Tsai, P., et al. (2002). Number of boys born to men exposed to polychlorinated byphenyls. *Lancet, 360*, 143–144. PubMed PMID: 12126828.

12. Mocarelli, P., Gerthoux, P. M., Ferrari, E., et al. (2000). Paternal concentrations of dioxin and sex ratio of offspring. *Lancet, 355*(9218), 1858–1863. PubMed PMID: 10866441.

13. Yu, M. L., Guo, Y. L., Hsu, C.-C., & Rogan, W. J. (2000). Menstruation and reproduction in women with polychlorinated biphenyl (PCB) poisoning: long-term follow-up interviews of the women from the Taiwan Yucheng cohort. *International Journal of Epidemiology, 29*, 672–677. PubMed PMID: 10922344.

14. Su, P. H., Huang, P. C., Lin, C. Y., et al. (2012). The effect of in utero exposure to dioxins and polychlorinated biphenyls on reproductive development in eight year-old children. *Environment International, 39*(1), 181–187. PubMed PMID: 22208758.

15. Su, P. H., Chen, J. Y., Lin, C. Y., et al. (2014). Sex steroid hormone levels and reproductive development of eight-year-old children following in utero and environmental exposure to phthalates. *PLoS ONE, 9*(9), e102788. PubMed PMID: 25207995.

16. Curtin, S. C., Abma, J. C., Ventura, S. J., & Henshaw, S. K. (2013). Pregnancy rates for U.S. women continue to drop. *NCHS Data Brief, 136*, 1–8. PubMed PMID: 24314113.

17. Hamilton, B. E., & Ventura, S. J. (2012). Birth rates for U.S. teenagers reach historic lows for all age and ethnic groups. *NCHS Data Brief, 89*, 1–8. PubMed PMID: 22617115.

18. Gerhard, I., Mongo, B., Krahe, J., & Runnebaum, B. (1999). Chlorinated hydrocarbons in infertile women. *Environmental Research, 80*, 299–310. PubMed PMID: 10330303.

19. Axmon, A., Rylander, L., Strömberg, U., & Hagmar, L. (2000). Time to pregnancy and infertility among women with a high intake of fish contaminated with persistent organochlorine compounds. *Scandinavian Journal of Work, Environment and Health, 26*(3), 199–206. PubMed PMID: 10901111.

20. Burreau, S., Zebühr, Y., Broman, D., & Ishaq, R. (2006). Biomagnification of PBDEs and PCBs in food webs from the Baltic Sea and the northern Atlantic Ocean. *The Science of the Total Environment, 366*(2–3), 659–672. PubMed PMID: 16580050.

21. Chevrier, C., Warembourg, C., Gaudreau, E., et al. (2013). Organochlorine pesticides, polychlorinated

biphenyls, seafood consumption, and time-to-pregnancy. *Epidemiology (Cambridge, Mass.)*, *24*(2), 251–260. PubMed PMID: 23348067.

22. Leoni, V., Fabiani, L., Marinelli, G., et al. (1989). PCB and other organochlorine compounds in blood of women with or without miscarriage: a hypothesis of correlation. *Ecotoxicology and Environmental Safety*, *17*(1), 1–11. PubMed PMID: 2496968.

23. Longnecker, M. P., Klebanoff, M. A., Zhou, H., & Brock, J. W. (2001). Association between maternal serum concentration of the DDT metabolite DDE and preterm and small-for-gestational-age babies at birth. *Lancet*, *358*, 110–114. PubMed PMID: 11463412.

24. Younglai, W. V., Foster, W. G., Hughes, E. G., et al. (2002). Levels of environmental contaminants in human follicular fluid, serum, and seminal plasma of couples undergoing in vitro fertilization. *Archives of Environmental Contamination and Toxicology*, *43*, 121–126. PubMed PMID: 12045882.

25. Meeker, J. D., Maity, A., Missmer, S. A., et al. (2011). Serum concentrations of polychlorinated biphenyls in relation to in vitro fertilization outcomes. *Environmental Health Perspectives*, *119*(7), 1010–1016. PubMed PMID:21345762.

26. Buck Louis, G. M., Sundaram, R., Schisterman, E. F., et al. (2013). Persistent environmental pollutants and couple fecundity: the LIFE study. *Environmental Health Perspectives*, *121*(2), 231–236. PubMed PMID: 23151773.

27. Karmaus, W., & Wolf, N. (1995). Reduced birthweight and length in the offspring of females exposed to PCDFs, PCP, and lindane. *Environmental Health Perspectives*, *103*, 1120–1125.

28. Gerhard, I., Frick, A., Monga, B., & Runnebaum, B. (1999). Pentachlorophenol exposure in women with gynecological and endocrine dysfunction. *Environmental Research*, *80*, 383–388. PubMed PMID: 10330312.

29. Ehrlich, S., Williams, P. L., Missmer, S. A., et al. (2012). Urinary bisphenol A concentrations and early reproductive health outcomes among women undergoing IVF. *Human Reproduction*, *27*(12), 3583–3592. PubMed PMID: 23014629.

30. Curtis, K. M., Savitz, D. A., & Weinberg, C. R. (1999). The effect of pesticide exposure on time to pregnancy. *Epidemiology (Cambridge, Mass.)*, *10*, 112–117. PubMed PMID: 10069244.

31. Kang, H. K., Mahan, C. M., & Lee, K. Y. (2000). Pregnancy outcomes among US women Vietnam veterans. *American Journal of Industrial Medicine*, *38*, 447–454. PubMed PMID: 10982986.

32. Parron, T., Hernandez, A. F., Pla, A., & Villanueva, E. (1996). Clinical and biochemical changes in greenhouse sprayers chronically exposed to pesticides. *Human and Experimental Toxicology*, *15*(12), 957–963. PubMed PMID: 8981099.

33. Bell, E. M., Hertz-Picciotto, I., & Beaumont, J. J. (2001). A case-control study of pesticides and fetal death due to congenital anomalies. *Epidemiology (Cambridge, Mass.)*, *12*, 148–156. PubMed PMID: 11246574.

34. Villanueva, C. M., Durand, G., Coutté, M. B., et al. (2005). Atrazine in municipal drinking water and risk of low birth weight, preterm delivery, and small-for-gestational-age status. *Occupational and Environmental Medicine*, *62*(6), 400–405. PubMed PMID: 15901888.

35. Rogan, W. J., Gladen, B. C., McKinney, J. D., et al. (1986). Neonatal effects of transplacental exposure to PCBs and DDE. *The Journal of Pediatrics*, *109*(2), 335–341. PubMed PMID: 3090217.

36. Luderer, U., Morgan, M. S., Brodkin, C. A., et al. (1999). Reproductive endocrine effects of acute exposure to toluene in men and women. *Occupational and Environmental Medicine*, *56*, 657–666. PubMed PMID: 10658543.

37. Thurston, S. W., Ryan, L., Christiani, D. C., et al. (2000). Petrochemical exposure and menstrual disturbances. *American Journal of Industrial Medicine*, *38*(5), 555–564. PubMed PMID: 11025497.

38. Sallmén, M., Lindbohm, M. L., Anttila, A., et al. (1998). Time to pregnancy among the wives of men exposed to organic solvents. *Occupational and Environmental Medicine*, *55*(1), 24–30. PubMed PMID: 9536159.

39. Xu, X., Cho, S. I., Sammel, M., et al. (1998). Association of petrochemical exposure with spontaneous abortion. *Occupational and Environmental Medicine*, *55*(1), 31–36. PubMed PMID: 9536160.

40. Taskinen, H., Lindbohm, M.-L., & Hemminki, K. (1986). Spontaneous abortions among women working in the pharmaceutical industry. *British Journal of Industrial Medicine*, *43*, 199–205. PubMed PMID: 3947584.

41. Windham, G. C., Shusterman, D., Swan, S. H., et al. (1991). Exposure to organic solvents and adverse pregnancy outcome. *American Journal of Industrial Medicine*, *20*(2), 241–259. PubMed PMID: 1951371.

42. Schaumburg, I., & Olsen, J. (1990). Congenital malformations and death among the offspring of Danish pharmacy assistants. *American Journal of Industrial Medicine*, *18*(5), 555–564. PubMed PMID: 2244628.

43. Logman, J. F., de Vries, L. E., Hemels, M. E., et al. (2005). Paternal organic solvent exposure and adverse

pregnancy outcomes: a meta-analysis. *American Journal of Industrial Medicine, 47*(1), 37–44. PubMed PMID: 15597360.

44. Carwile, J. L., Mahalingaiah, S., Winter, M. R., & Aschengrau, A. (2014). Prenatal drinking-water exposure to tetrachloroethylene and ischemic placental disease: a retrospective cohort study. *Environmental Health: A Global Access Science Source, 13*, 72. PubMed PMID: 25270247.

45. Gallagher, L. G., Vieira, V. M., Ozonoff, D., et al. (2011). Risk of breast cancer following exposure to tetrachloroethylene-contaminated drinking water in Cape Cod, Massachusetts: reanalysis of a case-control study using a modified exposure assessment. *Environmental Health: A Global Access Science Source, 10*, 47. PubMed PMID: 21600013.

46. Ruckart, P. Z., Bove, F. J., & Maslia, M. (2014). Evaluation of contaminated drinking water and preterm birth, small for gestational age, and birth weight at Marine Corps Base Camp Lejeune, North Carolina: a cross-sectional study. *Environmental Health: A Global Access Science Source, 13*, 99. PubMed PMID: 25413571.

47. Ruckart, P. Z., Bove, F. J., Shanley, E., 3rd, & Maslia, M. (2015). Evaluation of contaminated drinking water and male breast cancer at Marine Corps Base Camp Lejeune, North Carolina: a case control study. *Environmental Health: A Global Access Science Source, 14*, 74. PubMed PMID: 26376727.

48. Axmon, A., Rylander, L., Stromberg, U., & Hagmar, L. (2000). Time to pregnancy and infertility among women with a high intake of fish contaminated with persistent organochlorine compounds. *Scandinavian Journal of Work, Environment & Health, 26*(3), 199–206. PubMed PMID: 10901111.

49. Burguet, A., & Agnani, G. (2003). [Smoking, fertility and very preterm birth]. *Journal de gynécologie, obstétrique et biologie de la reproduction, 32*(1 Suppl.), 1S9–1S16.

50. Wisborg, K., Kesmodel, U., Henrikson, T. B., et al. (2001). Exposure to tobacco smoke in utero and the risk of stillbirth and death in the first year of life. *American Journal of Epidemiology, 154*, 322–327. PubMed PMID: 11495855.

51. Kabir, Z., Clarke, V., Conroy, R., et al. (2009). Low birthweight and preterm birth rates 1 year before and after the Irish workplace smoking ban. *BJOG: An International Journal of Obstetrics and Gynaecology, 116*(13), 1782–1787. PubMed PMID: 19832830.

52. Mahalingaiah, S., Hart, J. E., Laden, F., et al. (2016). Adult air pollution exposure and risk of infertility in the Nurses' Health Study II. *Human Reproduction, 31*(3), 638–647. PubMed PMID: 26724803.

53. Nieuwenhuijsen, M. J., Basagaña, X., Dadvand, P., et al. (2014). Air pollution and human fertility rates. *Environment International, 70*, 9–14. PubMed PMID: 24879367.

54. Perin, P. M., Maluf, M., Czeresnia, C. E., et al. (2010). Effects of exposure to high levels of particulate air pollution during the follicular phase of the conception cycle on pregnancy outcome in couples undergoing in vitro fertilization and embryo transfer. *Fertility and Sterility, 93*(1), 301–303. PubMed PMID: 19631320.

55. Perera, F. P., Jedrychowski, W., Rauh, V., & Whyatt, R. M. (1999). Molecular epidemiological research on the effects of environmental pollutants on the fetus. *Environmental Health Perspectives, 107*(Suppl. 3), 451–460. PubMed PMID: 10346993.

56. Le, H. Q., Batterman, S. A., Wirth, J. J., et al. (2012). Air pollutant exposure and preterm and term small-for-gestational-age births in Detroit, Michigan: long-term trends and associations. *Environment International, 44*, 7–17. PubMed PMID: 22314199.

57. Kloog, I., Melly, S. J., Coull, B. A., et al. (2015). Using Satellite-Based Spatiotemporal Resolved Air Temperature Exposure to Study the Association between Ambient Air Temperature and Birth Outcomes in Massachusetts. *Environmental Health Perspectives, 123*(10), 1053–1058. PubMed PMID: 25850104.

58. Choy, C. M., Lam, C. W., Cheung, L. T., et al. (2002). Infertility, blood mercury concentrations and dietary seafood consumption: a case-control study. *BJOG: An International Journal of Obstetrics and Gynaecology, 109*(10), 1121–1125. PubMed PMID: 12387464.

59. Centers for Disease Control and Prevention. Updated Tables, January 2017. *By National Report on Human Exposure to Environmental Chemicals.* Available at: www.cdc.gov/exposurereport/. (Accessed 17 June 2017).

60. Buck Louis, G. M., Sundaram, R., Schisterman, E. F., et al. (2012). Heavy metals and couple fecundity, the LIFE Study. *Chemosphere, 87*(11), 1201–1207. PubMed PMID: 22309709.

61. Taylor, C. M., Golding, J., & Emond, A. M. (2016). Moderate Prenatal Cadmium Exposure and Adverse Birth Outcomes: a Role for Sex-Specific Differences? *Paediatric and Perinatal Epidemiology, 30*(6), 603–611. PubMed PMID: 27778365.

62. Taylor, C. M., Tilling, K., Golding, J., & Emond, A. M. (2016). Low level lead exposure and pregnancy outcomes in an observational birth cohort study: dose-response relationships. *BMC Research Notes, 9*, 291. PubMed PMID: 27260491.

63. Hertz-Picciotto, I. (2000). The evidence that lead increases the risk for spontaneous abortion. *American Journal of Industrial Medicine, 38*(3), 300–309. PubMed PMID: 10940968.

64. Taylor, C. M., Tilling, K., Golding, J., & Emond, A. M. (2016). Low level lead exposure and pregnancy outcomes in an observational birth cohort study: dose-response relationships. *BMC Research Notes, 9,* 291. PubMed PMID: 27260491.

65. Aschengrau, A., Zierler, S., & Cohen, A. (1993). Quality of community drinking water and the occurrence of late adverse pregnancy outcomes. *Archives of Environmental Health, 48,* 105–113. PubMed PMID: 8476301.

66. Bove, F. J., Fulcomer, M. C., Klotz, J. B., et al. (1995). Public drinking water contamination and birth outcomes. *American Journal of Epidemiology, 141*(9), 850–862. PubMed PMID: 7717362.

67. Dodds, L., King, W., Allen, A. C., et al. (2004). Trihalomethanes in public water supplies and risk of stillbirth. *Epidemiology (Cambridge, Mass.), 15*(2), 179–186. PubMed PMID: 15127910.

68. Waller, K., Swan, S. H., DeLorenze, G., & Hopkins, B. (1998). Trihalomethanes in drinking water and spontaneous abortion. *Epidemiology (Cambridge, Mass.), 9,* 134–140. PubMed PMID: 9504280.

69. King, W. D., Dodds, L., & Allen, A. C. (2000). Relation between stillbirth and specific chlorination by-products in public water supplies. *Environmental Health Perspectives, 108,* 883–886. PubMed PMID: 11017894.

70. Kumar, S., Forand, S., Babcock, G., et al. (2014). Total trihalomethanes in public drinking water supply and birth outcomes: a cross-sectional study. *Maternal and Child Health Journal, 18*(4), 996–1006. PubMed PMID: 23884785.

71. Kanitz, S., Franco, Y., Patrone, V., et al. (1996). Association between drinking water disinfection and somatic parameters at birth. *Environmental Health Perspectives, 104*(5), 516–520. PubMed PMID: 8743439.

72. Dolk, H., Vrijheid, M., Armstrong, B., et al. (1998). Risk of congenital anomalies near hazardous-waste landfill sites in Europe: the EUROHAZCON study. *Lancet, 352*(9126), 423–427. PubMed PMID: 9708749.

73. Vrijheid, M., Dolk, H., Armstrong, B., et al. (2002). Chromosomal congenital anomalies and residence near hazardous waste landfill sites. *Lancet, 359*(9303), 320–322. PubMed PMID: 11830202.

74. Elliott, P., Briggs, D., Morris, S., et al. (2001). Risk of adverse birth outcomes in populations living near landfill sites. *BMJ (Clinical Research Ed.), 323*(7309), 363–368. PubMed PMID: 11509424. Erratum in: BMJ 2001 Nov 17;323(7322):1182.

75. Langlois, P. H., Brender, J. D., Suarez, L., et al. (2009). Maternal residential proximity to waste sites and industrial facilities and conotruncal heart defects in offspring. *Paediatric and Perinatal Epidemiology, 23*(4), 321–331. PubMed PMID: 19523079.

76. Austin, A. A., Fitzgerald, E. F., Pantea, C. I., et al. (2011). Reproductive outcomes among former Love Canal residents, Niagara Falls, New York. *Environmental Research, 111*(5), 693–701. PubMed PMID: 21555122.

77. Aschengrau, A., Weinberg, J. M., Janulewicz, P. A., et al. (2009). Prenatal exposure to tetrachloroethylene-contaminated drinking water and the risk of congenital anomalies: a retrospective cohort study. *Environmental Health: A Global Access Science Source, 8,* 44. PubMed PMID: 19778411.

78. Yauck, J. S., Malloy, M. E., Blair, K., et al. (2004). Proximity of residence to trichloroethylene-emitting sites and increased risk of offspring congenital heart defects among older women. *Birth Defects Research. Part A, Clinical and Molecular Teratology, 70*(10), 808–814. PubMed PMID: 15390315.

79. Forand, S. P., Lewis-Michl, E. L., & Gomez, M. I. (2012). Adverse birth outcomes and maternal exposure to trichloroethylene and tetrachloroethylene through soil vapor intrusion in New York State. *Environmental Health Perspectives, 120*(4), 616–621. PubMed PMID: 22142966.

80. Garry, V. F., Schreinemachers, D., Harkins, M. E., & Griffith, J. (1996). Pesticide appliers, biocides, and birth defects in rural Minnesota. *Environmental Health Perspectives, 104,* 394–399. PubMed PMID: 8732949.

81. Sherman, J. D. (1996). Chlorpyrifos (Dursban) associated birth defects: report of four cases. *Archives of Environmental Health, 51,* 5–8. PubMed PMID: 8629864.

82. Romero, P., Barnett, P. G., & Midtling, J. E. (1989). Congenital anomalies associated with maternal exposure to oxydemetron-methy. *Environmental Research, 50,* 256–261. PubMed PMID: 2583071.

83. Bradman, A., Quirós-Alcalá, L., Castorina, R., et al. (2015). Effect of Organic Diet Intervention on Pesticide Exposures in Young Children Living in Low-Income Urban and Agricultural Communities. *Environmental Health Perspectives, 123*(10), 1086–1093. PubMed PMID: 25861095.

84. Brantsæter, A. L., Torjusen, H., Meltzer, H. M., et al. (2016). Organic Food Consumption during Pregnancy and Hypospadias and Cryptorchidism at Birth: The Norwegian Mother and Child Cohort Study (MoBa).

Environmental Health Perspectives, 124(3), 357–364. PubMed PMID: 26307850.

85. Wolff, M. S., Pajak, A., Pinney, S. M., et al. (2017). Breast Cancer and Environment Research Program. Associations of urinary phthalate and phenol biomarkers with menarche in a multiethnic cohort of young girls. *Reproductive Toxicology, 67*, 56–64. PubMed PMID: 27851993.

86. Colon, I., Caro, D., Bourdony, C. J., & Rosario, O. (2000). Identification of phthalate esters in the serum of young Puerto Rican girls with premature breast development. *Environmental Health Perspectives, 108*, 895–900. PubMed PMID: 11017896.

87. Cobellis, L., Latini, G., De Felice, C., et al. (2003). High plasma concentrations of di-(2-ethylhexyl)-phthalate in women with endometriosis. *Human Reproduction, 18*(7), 1512–1515. PubMed PMID: 12832380.

88. Grindler, N. M., Allsworth, J. E., Macones, G. A., et al. (2015). Persistent organic pollutants and early menopause in U.S. women. *PLoS ONE, 10*(1), e0116057. PubMed PMID: 25629726.

89. Campbell, S., Raza, M., & Pollack, A. Z. (2016). Perfluoroalkyl substances and endometriosis in US women in NHANES 2003-2006. *Reproductive Toxicology, 65*, 230–235. PubMed PMID: 27544573.

90. Vagi, S. J., Azziz-Baumgartner, E., Sjödin, A., et al. (2014). Exploring the potential association between brominated diphenyl ethers, polychlorinated biphenyls, organochlorine pesticides, perfluorinated compounds, phthalates, and bisphenol A in polycystic ovary syndrome: a case-control study. *BMC Endocrine Disorders, 14*, 86. PubMed PMID: 25348326.

91. Kandaraki, E., Chatzigeorgiou, A., Livadas, S., et al. (2011). Endocrine disruptors and polycystic ovary syndrome (PCOS): elevated serum levels of bisphenol A in women with PCOS. *The Journal of Clinical Endocrinology and Metabolism, 96*(3), E480–E484. PubMed PMID: 21193545.

92. Akın, L., Kendirci, M., Narin, F., et al. (2015). The endocrine disruptor bisphenol A may play a role in the aetiopathogenesis of polycystic ovary syndrome in adolescent girls. *Acta Paediatrica, 104*(4), e171–e177. PubMed PMID: 25469562.

93. Feldman, H. A., Longcope, C., Derby, C. A., et al. (2002). Age trends in the level of serum testosterone and other hormones in middle-aged men: longitudinal results from the Massachusetts male aging study. *The Journal of Clinical Endocrinology and Metabolism, 87*(2), 589–598. PubMed PMID: 11836290.

94. Harman, S. M., Metter, E. J., Tobin, J. D., Baltimore Longitudinal Study of Aging, et al. (2001). Longitudinal effects of aging on serum total and free testosterone levels in healthy men. Baltimore Longitudinal Study of Aging. *The Journal of Clinical Endocrinology and Metabolism, 86*(2), 724–731. PubMed PMID: 11158037.

95. Allan, C. A., & McLachlan, R. I. (2004). Age-related changes in testosterone and the role of replacement therapy in older men. *Clinical Endocrinology, 60*(6), 653–670. PubMed PMID: 15163327.

96. Coward, R. M., Rajanahally, S., Kovac, J. R., et al. (2013). Anabolic steroid induced hypogonadism in young men. *The Journal of Urology, 190*(6), 2200–2205. PubMed PMID: 23764075.

97. Ferguson, K. K., Peterson, K. E., Lee, J. M., et al. (2014). Prenatal and peripubertal phthalates and bisphenol A in relation to sex hormones and puberty in boys. *Reproductive Toxicology, 47*, 70–76. PubMed PMID: 24945889.

98. Meeker, J. D., & Ferguson, K. K. (2014). Urinary phthalate metabolites are associated with decreased serum testosterone in men, women, and children from NHANES 2011-2012. *The Journal of Clinical Endocrinology and Metabolism, 99*(11), 4346–4352. PubMed PMID: 25121464.

99. Joensen, U. N., Frederiksen, H., Blomberg Jensen, M., et al. (2012). Phthalate excretion pattern and testicular function: a study of 881 healthy Danish men. *Environmental Health Perspectives, 120*(10), 1397–1403. PubMed PMID: 22832070.

100. Meeker, J. D., Calafat, A. M., & Hauser, R. (2009). Urinary metabolites of di(2-ethylhexyl) phthalate are associated with decreased steroid hormone levels in adult men. *Journal of Andrology, 30*(3), 287–297. PubMed PMID: 19059903.

101. Specht, I. O., Toft, G., Hougaard, K. S., et al. (2014). Associations between serum phthalates and biomarkers of reproductive function in 589 adult men. *Environment International, 66*, 146–156. PubMed PMID: 24583187.

102. Joensen, U. N., Veyrand, B., Antignac, J. P., et al. (2013). PFOS (perfluorooctanesulfonate) in serum is negatively associated with testosterone levels, but not with semen quality, in healthy men. *Human Reproduction, 28*(3), 599–608. PubMed PMID: 23250927.

103. Johnson, P. I., Stapleton, H. M., Mukherjee, B., et al. (2013). Associations between brominated flame retardants in house dust and hormone levels in men. *The Science of the Total Environment, 445-446*, 177–184. PubMed PMID: 23333513.

104. Oliva, A., Spira, A., & Multigner, L. (2001). Contribution of environmental factors to the risk

of male infertility. *Human Reproduction*, *16*(8), 1768–1776. PubMed PMID: 11473980.

105. Abell, A., Ernst, E., & Bonde, J. P. (1994). High sperm density among members of organic farmers association. *Lancet*, *343*, 1498. PubMed PMID: 7911193.

106. Padungtod, C., Savitz, D. A., Overstreet, J. W., et al. (2000). Occupational pesticide exposure and semen quality among Chinese workers. *Journal of Occupational and Environmental Medicine*, *42*(10), 982–992. PubMed PMID: 11039162.

107. Chiu, Y. H., Afeiche, M. C., Gaskins, A. J., et al. (2015). Fruit and vegetable intake and their pesticide residues in relation to semen quality among men from a fertility clinic. *Human Reproduction*, *30*(6), 1342–1351. PubMed PMID: 5824023.

108. Melgarejo, M., Mendiola, J., Koch, H. M., et al. (2015). Associations between urinary organophosphate pesticide metabolite levels and reproductive parameters in men from an infertility clinic. *Environmental Research*, *137*, 292–298. PubMed PMID: 25601731.

109. Glass, R. I., Lyness, R. N., Mengle, D. C., et al. (1979). Sperm count depression in pesticide applicators exposed to dibromochloropropane. *American Journal of Epidemiology*, *109*, 346–351. PubMed PMID: 453171.

110. Radwan, M., Jurewicz, J., Wielgomas, B., et al. (2015). The association between environmental exposure to pyrethroids and sperm aneuploidy. *Chemosphere*, *128C*, 42–48. PubMed PMID: 25655817.

111. Apostoli, P., Kiss, P., Porru, S., et al. (1998). Male reproductive toxicity of lead in animals and humans. ASCLEPIOS Study Group. *Occupational and Environmental Medicine*, *55*(6), 364–374. Review. PubMed PMID: 9764095.

112. Fisher-Fischbein, J., Fischbein, A., Melnick, H. D., & Bardin, C. W. (1987). Correlation between biochemical indicators of lead exposure and semen quality in a lead-poisoned firearms instructor. *JAMA: The Journal of the American Medical Association*, *257*(6), 803–805. PubMed PMID: 3806856.

113. Leung, T. Y., Choy, C. M., Yim, S. F., et al. (2001). Whole blood mercury concentrations in sub-fertile men in Hong Kong. *The Australian and New Zealand Journal of Obstetrics and Gynaecology*, *41*(1), 75–77. PubMed PMID: 11284652.

114. Hjollund, N. H., Bonde, J. P., Jensen, T. K., et al. (2000). Male-mediated spontaneous abortion among spouses of stainless steel welders. *Scandinavian Journal of Work, Environment and Health*, *26*(3), 187–192. PubMed PMID: 10901109.

115. Rengaraj, D., Kwon, W. S., & Pang, M. G. (2015). Effects of motor vehicle exhaust on male reproductive function and associated proteins. *Journal of Proteome Research*, *14*(1), 22–37. PubMed PMID: 25329744.

116. De Rosa, M., Zarrilli, S., Paesano, L., et al. (2003). Traffic pollutants affect fertility in men. *Human Reproduction*, *18*(5), 1055–1061. PubMed PMID: 12721184.

117. Selevan, S. G., Borkovec, L., Slott, V. L., et al. (2000). Semen quality and reproductive health of young Czech men exposed to seasonal air pollution. *Environmental Health Perspectives*, *108*(9), 887–894. PubMed PMID: 11017895.

118. Gaspari, L., Chang, S. S., Santella, R. M., et al. (2003). Polycyclic aromatic hydrocarbon-DNA adducts in human sperm as a marker of DNA damage and infertility. *Mutation Research*, *535*(2), 155–160. PubMed PMID: 12581533.

119. Ji, G., Yan, L., Wu, S., et al. (2013). Bulky DNA adducts in human sperm associated with semen parameters and sperm DNA fragmentation in infertile men: a cross-sectional study. *Environmental Health: A Global Access Science Source*, *12*(1), 82. PubMed PMID: 24073787.

120. Künzle, R., Mueller, M. D., Hänggi, W., et al. (2003). Semen quality of male smokers and nonsmokers in infertile couples. *Fertility and Sterility*, *79*(2), 287–291. PubMed PMID: 12568836.

121. Meeker, J. D., & Stapleton, H. M. (2010). House dust concentrations of organophosphate flame retardants in relation to hormone levels and semen quality parameters. *Environmental Health Perspectives*, *118*(3), 318–323. PubMed PMID: 20194068.

122. Duty, S. M., Singh, N. P., Silva, M. J., et al. (2003). The relationship between environmental exposures to phthalates and DNA damage in human sperm using the neutral comet assay. *Environmental Health Perspectives*, *111*(9), 1164–1169. PubMed PMID: 12842768.

123. Jurewicz, J., Radwan, M., Sobala, W., et al. (2013). Human urinary phthalate metabolites level and main semen parameters, sperm chromatin structure, sperm aneuploidy and reproductive hormones. *Reproductive Toxicology*, *42*, 232–241. PubMed PMID: 24140385.

124. Buck Louis, G. M., Sundaram, R., Sweeney, A. M., et al. (2014). Urinary bisphenol A, phthalates, and couple fecundity: the Longitudinal Investigation of Fertility and the Environment (LIFE) Study. *Fertility and Sterility*, *101*(5), 1359–1366. PubMed PMID: 24534276.

125. Dodge, L. E., Williams, P. L., Williams, M. A., et al. (2015). Paternal urinary concentrations of parabens and other phenols in relation to reproductive outcomes among couples from a fertility clinic.

Environmental Health Perspectives, 123(7), 665–671. PubMed PMID: 25767892.

126. Schecter, A., Colacino, J., Haffner, D., et al. (2010). Perfluorinated compounds, polychlorinated biphenyls, and organochlorine pesticide contamination in composite food samples from Dallas, Texas, USA. *Environmental Health Perspectives, 118*(6), 796–802. PubMed PMID: 20146964.

127. Oliva, A., Giami, A., & Multigner, L. (2002). Environmental agents and erectile dysfunction: a study in a consulting population. *Journal of Andrology, 23*(4), 546–550. PubMed PMID: 12065462.

128. Mirone, V., Imbimbo, C., Bortolotti, A., et al. (2002). Cigarette smoking as risk factor for erectile dysfunction: results from an Italian epidemiological study. *European Urology, 41*(3), 294–297. PubMed PMID: 12180231.

129. Centers for Disease Control and Prevention. *Data, Trends and Maps.* Available at: https://www.cdc.gov/obesity/data/databases.html. (Accessed 21 November 2017).

130. Baillie-Hamilton, P. F. (2002). Chemical toxins: a hypothesis to explain the global obesity epidemic. *Journal of Alternative and Complementary Medicine (New York, N.Y.), 8*(2), 185–192. PubMed PMID: 12006126.

131. Grün, F., & Blumberg, B. (2006). Environmental obesogens: organotins and endocrine disruption via nuclear receptor signaling. *Endocrinology, 147*(6 Suppl.), S50–S55. Review. PubMed PMID: 16690801.

132. Yan, Z., Zhang, H., Maher, C., et al. (2014). Prenatal polycyclic aromatic hydrocarbon, adiposity, peroxisome proliferator-activated receptor (PPAR) γ methylation in offspring, grand-offspring mice. *PLoS ONE, 9*(10), e110706. PubMed PMID: 25347678.

133. Stahlhut, R. W., van Wijngaarden, E., Dye, T. D., Cook, S., & Swan, S. H. (2007). Concentrations of urinary phthalate metabolites are associated with increased waist circumference and insulin resistance in adult U.S. males. *Environmental Health Perspectives, 115*(6), 876–882. PubMed PMID: 17589594.

134. Hatch, E. E., Nelson, J. W., Qureshi, M. M., et al. (2008). Association of urinary phthalate metabolite concentrations with body mass index and waist circumference: a cross-sectional study of NHANES data, 1999-2002. *Environmental Health: A Global Access Science Source, 7*, 27. PubMed PMID: 18522739.

135. Lind, P. M., Roos, V., Rönn, M., et al. (2012). Serum concentrations of phthalate metabolites are related to abdominal fat distribution two years later in elderly women. *Environmental Health: A Global Access Science Source, 11*, 21. PubMed PMID: 22472124.

136. Buser, M. C., Murray, H. E., & Scinicariello, F. (2014). Age and sex differences in childhood and adulthood obesity association with phthalates: analyses of NHANES 2007-2010. *International Journal of Hygiene and Environmental Health, 217*(6), 687–694. PubMed PMID: 24657244.

137. Yaghjyan, L., Sites, S., Ruan, Y., & Chang, S. H. (2015). Associations of urinary phthalates with body mass index, waist circumference and serum lipids among females: National Health and Nutrition Examination Survey 1999-2004. *International Journal of Obesity (2005), 39*(6), 994–1000. PubMed PMID: 25644057.

138. Trasande, L., Attina, T. M., Sathyanarayana, S., et al. (2013). Race/ethnicity-specific associations of urinary phthalates with childhood body mass in a nationally representative sample. *Environmental Health Perspectives, 121*(4), 501–506. PubMed PMID: 23428635.

139. Hoepner, L. A., Whyatt, R. M., Widen, E. M., et al. (2016). Bisphenol A and adiposity in an inner-city birth cohort. *Environmental Health Perspectives, 124*(10), 1644–1650. PubMed PMID: 27187982.

140. Harley, K. G., Aguilar Schall, R., et al. (2013). Prenatal and postnatal bisphenol A exposure and body mass index in childhood in the CHAMACOS cohort. *Environmental Health Perspectives, 121*(4), 514–520. PubMed PMID: 23416456.

141. Vafeiadi, M., Roumeliotaki, T., Myridakis, A., et al. (2016). Association of early life exposure to bisphenol A with obesity and cardiometabolic traits in childhood. *Environmental Research, 146*, 379–387. PubMed PMID: 26821262.

142. Li, D. K., Miao, M., Zhou, Z., et al. (2013). Urine bisphenol-A level in relation to obesity and overweight in school-age children. *PLoS ONE, 8*(6), e65399. PubMed PMID: 23776476.

143. Carwile, J. L., & Michels, K. B. (2011). Urinary bisphenol A and obesity: NHANES 2003-2006. *Environmental Research, 111*(6), 825–830. PubMed PMID: 21676388.

144. Smink, A., Ribas-Fito, N., Garcia, R., et al. (2008). Exposure to hexachlorobenzene during pregnancy increases the risk of overweight in children aged 6 years. *Acta Paediatrica, 97*(10), 1465–1469. PubMed PMID: 18665907.

145. Mendez, M. A., Garcia-Esteban, R., Guxens, M., et al. (2011). Prenatal organochlorine compound exposure, rapid weight gain, and overweight in infancy. *Environmental Health Perspectives, 119*(2), 272–278. PubMed PMID: 20923745.

146. Karmaus, W., Osuch, J. R., Eneli, I., et al. (2009). Maternal levels of dichlorodiphenyl-dichloroethylene (DDE) may increase weight and body mass index in adult female offspring. *Occupational and Environmental Medicine, 66*(3), 143–149. PubMed PMID: 19060027.

147. Verhulst, S. L., Nelen, V., Hond, E. D., et al. (2009). Intrauterine exposure to environmental pollutants and body mass index during the first 3 years of life. *Environmental Health Perspectives, 117*(1), 122–126. PubMed PMID: 19165398.

148. Valvi, D., Mendez, M. A., Martinez, D., et al. (2012). Prenatal concentrations of polychlorinated biphenyls, DDE, and DDT and overweight in children: a prospective birth cohort study. *Environmental Health Perspectives, 120*(3), 451–457. PubMed PMID: 22027556.

149. Berntssen, M. H., Maage, A., Julshamn, K., et al. (2011). Carry-over of dietary organochlorine pesticides, PCDD/Fs, PCBs, and brominated flame retardants to Atlantic salmon (Salmo salar L.) fillets. *Chemosphere, 83*(2), 95–103. PubMed PMID: 21284993.

150. Ibrahim, M. M., Fjære, E., Lock, E. J., et al. (2011). Chronic consumption of farmed salmon containing persistent organic pollutants causes insulin resistance and obesity in mice. *PLoS ONE, 6*(9), e25170. PubMed PMID: 21966444.

151. Braun, J. M., Chen, A., Romano, M. E., et al. (2016). Prenatal perfluoroalkyl substance exposure and child adiposity at 8 years of age: The HOME study. *Obesity, 24*(1), 231–237. PubMed PMID: 26554535.

152. Timmermann, C. A., Rossing, L. I., Grøntved, A., et al. (2014). Adiposity and glycemic control in children exposed to perfluorinated compounds. *The Journal of Clinical Endocrinology and Metabolism, 99*(4), E608–E614. PubMed PMID: 24606078.

153. McConnell, R., Shen, E., Gilliland, F. D., et al. (2015). A longitudinal cohort study of body mass index and childhood exposure to secondhand tobacco smoke and air pollution: the Southern California Children's Health Study. *Environmental Health Perspectives, 123*(4), 360–366. PubMed PMID: 25389275.

154. Scinicariello, F., & Buser, M. C. (2014). Urinary polycyclic aromatic hydrocarbons and childhood obesity: NHANES (2001-2006). *Environmental Health Perspectives, 122*(3), 299–303. PubMed PMID: 24380973.

155. Jerrett, M., McConnell, R., Wolch, J., et al. (2014). Traffic-related air pollution and obesity formation in children: a longitudinal, multilevel analysis. *Environmental Health: A Global Access Science Source, 13*, 49. PubMed PMID: 24913018.

156. Alderete, T. L., Habre, R., Toledo-Corral, C. M., et al. (2017). Longitudinal associations between ambient air pollution with insulin sensitivity, β-cell function, and adiposity in Los Angeles Latino children. *Diabetes, 66*, 1789. doi:10.2337/db16-1416. PubMed PMID: 28137791. pii: db161416.

157. Fonseca, V. A. (2007). Early identification and treatment of insulin resistance: impact on subsequent prediabetes and type 2 diabetes. *Clinical Cornerstone, 8 Suppl 7*, S17–S18.

158. Tabak, A. G., Jokela, M., Akbaraly, T. N., et al. (2009). Trajectories of glycaemia, insulin sensitivity, and insulin secretion before diagnosis of type 2 diabetes: an analysis from the Whitehall II study. *Lancet, 373*(9682), 2215–2221.

159. Ioannou, G. N., Bryson, C. L., & Boyko, E. J. (2007). Prevalence and trends of insulin resistance, impaired fasting glucose, and diabetes. *Journal of Diabetes and Its Complications, 21*(6), 363–370.

160. Centers for Disease Control and Prevention. *Long-term Trends in Diabetes*, April 2017. By CDC's Division of Diabetes Translation. Available at: http://www.cdc.gov/diabetes/statistics/slides/long_term_trends.pdf. (Accessed 21 November 2017).

161. Diabetes statistics USA. (https://www.cdc.gov/diabetes/data/index.html. (Accessed 28 March 2018).

162. Burkitt, D., & Trowell, H. (1981). *Western diseases: their emergence and prevention*. Cambridge, MA: Harvard University Press.

163. Vahouny, G., & Kritchevsky, D. (1982). *Dietary fiber in health and disease*. New York: Plenum Press.

164. National Research Council (1989). *Diet and Health. Implications for reducing chronic disease risk*. Washington, DC: National Academy Press.

165. Imamura, T., O'Connor, L., Ye, Z., et al. (2015). Consumption of sugar sweetened beverages, artificially sweetened beverages, and fruit juice and incidence of type 2 diabetes: systematic review, meta-analysis, and estimation of population attributable fraction. *BMJ (Clinical Research Ed.), 351*, h3576.

166. Guyenet, S., & Landen, J. (2012). *By 2606, the US Diet will be 100 Percent Sugar [website]*. Available at http://wholehealthsource.blogspot.com/2012/02/by-2606-us-diet-will-be-100-percent.html. (Accessed 21 November 2017).

167. Ogden, C. L., Carroll, M. D., Curtin, L. R., et al. (2006). Prevalence of overweight and obesity in the United States, 1999-2004. *JAMA: The Journal of the American Medical Association, 295*(13), 1549–1555.

168. Gregg, E. W., Cheng, Y. J., Narayan, K. M., et al. (2007). The relative contributions of different levels of overweight and obesity to the increased prevalence of diabetes in the United States: 1976-2004. *Preventive Medicine, 45*(5), 348–352.

169. Stahlhut, R. W., van Wijngaarden, E., Dye, T. D., et al. (2007). Concentrations of urinary phthalate metabolites are associated with increased waist circumference and insulin resistance in adult U.S. males. *Environmental Health Perspectives, 115*(6), 876–882.

170. Campbell, G. D. (1961). letter to the editor. *BMJ (Clinical Research Ed.)*, Available at http://www.ncbi.nlm.nih.gov/pmc/articles/PMC1954516/pdf/brmedj02895-0078b.pdf. (Accessed 21 November 2017).

171. Lee, D. H., Lee, I. K., Song, K., et al. (2006). A strong dose-response relation between serum concentrations of persistent organic pollutants and diabetes: results from the National Health and Examination Survey 1999-2002. *Diabetes Care, 29*(7), 1638–1644.

172. Neel, B. A., Robert, M., & Sargis, R. M. (2011). The paradox of progress: Environmental disruption of metabolism and the diabetes epidemic. *Diabetes, 60*, 1838–1848.

173. Ukropec, J., et al. (2010). High prevalence of prediabetes and diabetes in a population exposed to high levels of an organochlorine cocktail. *Diabetologia, 53*(5), 899–906.

174. Lee, D. H., et al. (2007). Association between serum concentrations of persistent organic pollutants and insulin resistance among nondiabetic adults: results from the National Health and Nutrition Examination Survey 1999-2002. *Diabetes Care, 30*(3), 622–628.

175. Liu, S., Guo, X., Wu, B., et al. (2014). Arsenic induces diabetic effects through beta-cell dysfunction and increased gluconeogenesis in mice. *Scientific Reports, 4*, 6894.

176. Shapiro, G. D., Dodds, L., Arbuckle, T. E., et al. (2015). Exposure to phthalates, bisphenol A and metals in pregnancy and the association with impaired glucose tolerance and gestational diabetes mellitus: The MIREC study. *Environment International, 83*, 63–71. PubMed PMID: 26101084.

177. Alderete, T. L., Habre, R., Toledo-Corral, C. M., et al. (2017). Longitudinal associations between ambient air pollution with insulin sensitivity, beta-cell function, and adiposity in Los Angeles Latino children. *Diabetes*, Pii:db161416. Epub ahead of print. PubMed PMID: 28137791.

178. Pearson, J. F., Bachireddy, C., Shyamprasad, S., et al. (2010). Association between fine particulate matter and diabetes prevelance in the U.S. *Diabetes Care, 33*(10), 219602201. PubMed PMID: 20628090.

179. Andersen, Z. J., Raaschou-Nielsen, O., Ketzel, M., et al. (2012). Diabetes incidence and long-term exposure to air pollution: a cohort study. *Diabetes Care, 35*(1), 92–98. PubMed PMID: 22074722.

180. Weinmayr, G., Hennig, F., Fuks, K., et al. (2015). Long term-exposure to fine particulate matter and incidence of type 2 diabetes mellitus in a cohort study: effects of total and traffic-specific air pollution. *Environmental Health: A Global Access Science Source, 14*, 53. PubMed PMID: 26087770.

181. Wang, T., Li, M., Chen, B., et al. (2012). Urinary bisphenol A (BPA) concentration associates with obesity and insulin resistance. *The Journal of Clinical Endocrinology and Metabolism, 97*(2), E223–E227.

182. Sun, Q., Cornelis, M. C., Townsend, M. K., et al. (2014). Association of urinary concentrations of bisphenol A and phthalate metabolites with risk of type 2 diabetes: a prospective investigation in the Nurses' Health Study (NHS) and NHSII cohorts. *Environmental Health Perspectives, 122*(6), 616–623. PubMed PMID: 24633239.

183. Huang, T., Saxena, A. R., Isganaitis, E., & James-Todd, T. (2014). Gender and racial/ethnic differences in the associations of urinary phthalate metabolites with markers of diabetes risk: National Health and Nutrition Examination Survey 2001-2008. *Environmental Health: A Global Access Science Source, 13*(1), 6. PubMed PMID: 24499162.

184. Winberg, L. D., & Badr, M. Z. (1995). Mechanism of phthalate-induced inhibition of hepatic mitochondrial beta-oxidation. *Toxicology Letters, 76*(1), 63–69. PubMed PMID: 7701518.

185. Stahlhut, R. W., van Wijngaarden, E., Dye, T. D., Cook, S., & Swan, S. H. (2007). Concentrations of urinary phthalate metabolites are associated with increased waist circumference and insulin resistance in adult US males. *Environmental Health Perspectives, 115*, 876–882. PubMed PMID: 17589594.

186. Lee, D. H., et al. (2008). Can persistent organic pollutants explain the association between serum gamma-glutamyltransferase and type 2 diabetes? *Diabetologia, 51*(3), 402–407.

187. Lee, D. H., Ha, M. H., Kim, J. H., et al. (2003). Gamma-glutamyltransferase and diabetes–a 4 year follow-up study. *Diabetologia, 46*(3), 359–364.

188. Gohel, M. G., & Chacko, A. N. (2013). Serum GGT activity and hsCRP level in patients with type 2 diabetes mellitus with good and poor glycemic control: An evidence linking oxidative stress, inflammation and

glycemic control. *Journal of Diabetes and Metabolic Disorders*, 12(1), 56.

189. Razvi, S., Weaver, J. U., et al. (2010). Subclinical thyroid disorders: significance and clinical impact. *Journal of Clinical Pathology*, 63(5), 379–386.

190. Aoki, Y., Belin, R. M., Clickner, R., et al. (2007). Serum TSH and total T4 in the United States population and their association with participant characteristics: National Health and Nutrition Examination Survey (NHANES 1999-2002). *Thyroid*, 17(12), 1211–1223.

191. Nussey, S. S., & Whitehead, S. A. (2001). *Endocrinology: An Integrated Approach.* Oxford: BIOS Scientific Publishers.

192. Crofton, K. M., Craft, E. S., Hedge, J. M., et al. (2005). Thyroid-hormone-disrupting chemicals: evidence for dose-dependent additivity or synergism. *Environmental Health Perspectives*, 113(11), 1549–1554.

193. Mastorakos, G., Karoutsou, E. I., Mizamtsidi, M., et al. (2007). The menace of endocrine disruptors on thyroid hormone physiology and their impact on intrauterine development. *Endocrine*, 31(3), 219–237.

194. Sanderson, J. T. (2006). The steroid hormone biosynthesis pathway as a target for endocrine-disrupting chemicals. *Toxicological Sciences*, 94(1), 3–21.

195. Langer, P., Kocan, A., Tajtakova, M., et al. (2005). Human thyroid in the population exposed to high environmental pollution by organochlorinated pollutants for several decades. *Endocrine Regulations*, 39(1), 13–20.

196. Gauger, K. J., Kato, Y., Haraguchi, K., et al. (2004). Polychlorinated biphenyls (PCBs) exert thyroid hormone-like effects in the fetal rat brain but do not bind to thyroid hormone receptors. *Environmental Health Perspectives*, 112(5), 516–523. PubMed PMID: 15064154.

197. Hallgren, S., & Darnerud, P. O. (2002). Polybrominated diphenyl ethers (PBDEs), polychlorinated biphenyls (PCBs) and chlorinated paraffins (CPs) in rats-testing interactions and mechanisms for thyroid hormone effects. *Toxicology*, 177(2–3), 227–243. PubMed PMID: 12135626.

198. Martin, L., & Klaassen, C. D. (2010). Differential effects of polychlorinated biphenyl cogeners on serum thyroid hormone levels in rats. *Toxicological Sciences*, 117(1), 36–44. PubMed PMID: 20573785.

199. Brouwer, A., Morse, D. C., Lans, M. C., et al. (1998). Interactions of persistent environmental organohalogens with the thyroid hormone system: mechanisms and possible consequences for animal and human health. *Toxicology and Industrial Health*, 14(1–2), 59–84. PubMed PMID: 9460170. Review.

200. Schuur, A. G., Brouwer, A., Bergman, A., et al. (1998). Inhibition of thyroid hormone sulfation by hydroxylated metabolites of polychlorinated biphenyls. *Chemico-Biological Interactions*, 109(1–3), 293–297. PubMed PMID: 9566753.

201. Osius, N., Karmaus, W., Kruse, H., & Witten, J. (1999). Exposure to polychlorinated biphenyls and levels of thyroid hormones in children. *Environmental Health Perspectives*, 107, 843–849. PubMed PMID: 10504153.

202. Pavuk, M., Schecter, A. J., Akhtar, F. Z., & Michalek, J. E. (2003). Serum 2,3,7,8-tetrachlorodibenzo-p-dioxin (TCDD) levels and thyroid function in Air Force veterans of the Vietnam War. *Annals of Epidemiology*, 13(5), 335–343. PubMed PMID: 12821272.

203. Schell, L. M., Gallo, M. V., Denham, M., et al. (2008). Relationship of thyroid hormone levels to levels of polychlorinated biphenyls, lead, p,p'-DDE, and other toxicants in Akwesasne Mohawk youth. *Environmental Health Perspectives*, 116(6), 806–813. PubMed PMID: 18560538.

204. Lans, M. C., Spiertz, C., Brouwer, A., & Koeman, J. H. (1994). Different competition of thyroxine binding to transthyretin and thyroxine binding globulin by hydroxy-PCBs, PCDDs and PCDFs. *European Journal of Pharmacology*, 270, 129–136. PubMed PMID: 8039542.

205. Purkey, H. E., Palaninathan, S. K., Kent, K. C., et al. (2004). Hydroxylated polychlorinated biphenyls selectively bind transthyretin in blood and inhibit amyloidogenesis: rationalizing rodent PCB toxicity. *Chemistry & Biology*, 11(12), 1719–1728. PubMed PMID: 15610856.

206. Calvert, G. M., Haring Sweeney, M., Deddens, J., & Wall, D. K. (1997). Evaluation of diabetes mellitus, serum glucose, and thyroid function among United States workers exposed to 2,3,7,8-tetrachlorodibenzo-p-dioxin. *Occupational and Environmental Medicine*, 56, 270–276. PubMed PMID: 10450245.

207. Su, P. H., Chen, J. Y., Chen, J. W., & Wang, S. L. (2010). Growth and thyroid function in children with in utero exposure to dioxin: a 5-year follow-up study. *Pediatric Research*, 67(2), 205–210. PubMed PMID: 20091939.

208. Pluim, H. J., de Vijlder, J. J., Olie, K., et al. (1993). Effects of pre- and postnatal exposure to chlorinated dioxins and furans on human neonatal thyroid hormone concentrations. *Environmental Health Perspectives*, 101(6), 504–508. PubMed PMID: 8137779.

209. Langer, P., Tajtakova, M., & Fodor, G. (1998). Increased thyroid volume and prevalence of thyroid disorders in a area heavily polluted by polychlorinated biphenyls. *European Journal of Endocrinology*, 139, 402–409. PubMed PMID: 9820616.

210. Hagmar, L., Rylander, L., Dyremark, E., Klasson-Wehler, E., & Erfurth, E. M. (2001). Plasma concentrations of persistent organochlorines in relation to thyrotropin and thyroid hormone levels in women. *International Archives of Occupational and Environmental Health*, *74*, 184–188. PubMed PMID: 11355292.

211. Rathore, M., Bhatnagar, P., Mathur, D., & Saxena, F. N. (2002). Burden of organochlorine pesticides in blood and its effect on thyroid hormones in women. *The Science of the Total Environment*, *295*(1–3), 207–215. PubMed PMID: 12186288.

212. Sandau, C. D., Ayotte, P., Dewailly, E., Duffe, J., & Norstrom, R. J. (2002). Pentachlorophenol and hyroxylated polychlorinated biphenyl metabolites in umbilical cord plasma of neonates from coastal populations in Quebec. *Environmental Health Perspectives*, *110*, 411–417. PubMed PMID: 11940460.

213. Meerts, I. A., van Zanden, J. J., Luijks, E. A., et al. (2000). Potent competitive interactions of some brominated flame retardants and related compounds with human transthyretin in vitro. *Toxicological Sciences*, *56*(1), 95–104. PubMed PMID: 10869457.

214. Zheng, J., He, C. T., Chen, S. J., Yan, X., et al. (2017). Disruption of thyroid hormone (TH) levels and TH-regulated gene expression be polybrominated diphenyl ethers (PBDEs), polychlorinated biphenyls (PCBs), and hydroxylated PCBs in e-waste recycling workers. *Environment International*, *102*, 138–144. PubMed PMID: 28245931.

215. Fowles, J. R., Fairbrother, A., Beacher-Steppan, L., & Kerkvliet, N. I. (1994). Immunologic and endocrine effects of the flame-retardant pentabromodiphenyl ether(DE-71) in C57BL/6J mice. *Toxicology*, *86*(1–2), 49–61. PubMed PMID: 8134923.

216. Zhou, T., Ross, D. G., DeVito, M. J., & Crofton, K. M. (2001). Effects of short-term in vivo exposure to polybrominated diphenyl ethers on thyroid hormones and hepatic enzyme activities in weanling rats. *Toxicological Sciences*, *61*(1), 76–82. PubMed PMID: 11294977.

217. Stoker, T. E., Laws, S. C., Crofton, K. M., et al. (2004). Assessment of DE-71, a commercial polybrominated diphenyl ether (PBDE) mixture, in the EDSP male and female pubertal protocols. *Toxicological Sciences*, *78*(1), 144–155. PubMed PMID: 14999130.

218. Kim, T. H., Lee, Y. J., Lee, E., et al. (2009). Effects of gestational exposure to decarbromodiphenyl ether on reproductive parameters, thyroid hormone levels, and neuronal development in Sprague-Dawley rats offspring. *Journal of Toxicology and Environmental Health. Part A*, *72*(21–22), 1296–1303. PubMed PMID: 20077200.

219. Kodavanti, P. R., Coburn, C. G., Moser, V. C., et al. (2010). Developmental exposure to a commercial PBDE mixture, DE-71: neurobehavioral, hormonal, and reproductive effects. *Toxicological Sciences*, *116*(1), 297–312. PubMed PMID: 20375078.

220. Lema, S. C., Dickey, J. T., Scholtz, I. R., & Swanson, P. (2008). Dietary exposure to 2,2',4,4'-tetrabromodiphenyl ether (PBDE-47) alters thyroid status and thyroid hormone-regulated gene transcription in the pituitary and brain. *Environmental Health Perspectives*, *116*(12), 1694–1699. PubMed PMID: 19079722.

221. Fernie, K. J., Shutt, J. L., Mayne, G., et al. (2005). Exposure to polybrominated diphenyl ethers (PBDEs): changes in thyroid, vitamin A, glutathione homeostasis, and oxidative stress in Americal kestrels (Falco sparverius). *Toxicological Sciences*, *88*(2), 375–383. PubMed PMID: 16120752.

222. Guven, M., Bayram, F., Unluhizarci, K., & Kelestimur, F. (1999). Endocrine changes in patients with acute organophosphorus poisoning. *Human and Experimental Toxicology*, *18*, 598–601. PubMed PMID: 10557009.

223. Zaidi, S. S., Bhatnagar, V. K., Gandhi, S. J., et al. (2000). Assessment of thyroid function in pesticide formulators. *Human and Experimental Toxicology*, *19*(9), 497–501. PubMed PMID: 11204551.

224. Steenland, K., Cedillo, L., Tucker, J., et al. (1997). Thyroid hormones and cytogenetic outcomes in backpack sprayers using ethylenebis(dithiocarbamate) (EBDC) fungicides in Mexico. *Environmental Health Perspectives*, *105*(10), 1126–1130. PubMed PMID: 9349837.

225. Brechner, R. J., Parkhurst, G. D., Humble, W. O., et al. (2000). Ammonium perchlorate contamination of Colorado River drinking water is associated with abnormal thyroid function in newborns in Arizona. *Journal of Occupational and Environmental Medicine*, *42*, 777–782. PubMed PMID: 10953814.

226. Tonacchera, M., Pinchera, A., Dimida, A., et al. (2004). Relative potencies and additivity of perchlorate, thiocyanate, nitrate, and iodide on the inhibition of radioactive iodide uptake by the human sodium iodide symporter. *Thyroid*, *14*(12), 1012–1019. PubMed PMID: 15650353.

227. Braverman, L. E., He, X., Pino, S., Cross, M., et al. (2005). The effect of perchlorate, thiocyanate, and nitrate on thyroid function in workers exposed to perchlorate long-term. *The Journal of Clinical Endocrinology and Metabolism*, *90*(2), 700–706. PubMed PMID: 15572417.

228. Breous, E., Wenzel, A., & Loos, U. (2005). The promotor of the human sodium/iodide symporter responds to certain phthalate plasticisers. *Molecular and Cellular Endocrinology*, 244(1–2), 75–78. PubMed PMID: 16257484.

229. Shimada, N., & Yamauchi, K. (2004). Characteristics of 3,5,3'-triiodothyronine (T3)-uptake system of tadpole red blood cells: effect of endocrine-disrupting chemicals on cellular T3 response. *The Journal of Endocrinology*, 183(3), 627–637. PubMed PMID: 15590988.

230. Ishihara, A., Nishiyama, N., Sugiyama, S., & Yamauchi, K. (2003). The effect of endocrine disrupting chemicals on thyroid hormone binding to Japanese quail thransthyretin and thyroid hormone receptor. *General and Comparative Endocrinology*, 134(1), 36–43. PubMed PMID: 13129501.

231. Huang, P. C., Kuo, P. L., Guo, Y. L., Liao, P. C., & Lee, C. C. (2007). Associations between urinary phthalate monoesters and thyroid hormones in pregnant women. *Human Reproduction*, 22(10), 2715–2722. PubMed PMID: 17704099.

232. Meeker, J. D., Calafat, A. M., & Hauser, R. (2007). Di(2-ethylhexyl) phthalate metabolites may alter thyroid hormone levels in men. *Environmental Health Perspectives*, 115(7), 1029–1034. PubMed PMID: 17637918.

233. Nishida, M., Yamamoto, T., Yoshimura, Y., & Kawada, J. (1986). Subacute toxicity of methylmercuric chloride and mercuric chloride on mouse thyroid. *Journal of Pharmacobio-Dynamics*, 9(4), 331–338. PubMed PMID: 3735055.

234. Tan, S. W., Meiller, J. C., & Mahaffey, K. R. (2009). The endocrine effects of mercury in humans and wildlife. *Critical Reviews in Toxicology*, 39(3), 228–269. PubMed PMID: 19280433.

235. Ellingsen, D. G., Efskind, J., Haug, E., et al. (2000). Effects of low mercury vapour exposure on the thyroid function in chloralkali workers. *Journal of Applied Toxicology : JAT*, 20(6), 483–489.

236. Soldin, O. P., O'Mara, D. M., & Aschner, M. (2008). Thyroid hormones and methylmercury toxicity. *Biological Trace Element Research*, Aug 22. [Epub ahead of print].

237. Takser, L., Mergler, D., Baldwin, M., et al. (2005). Thyroid hormones in pregnancy in relation to environmental exposure to organochlorine compounds and mercury. *Environmental Health Perspectives*, 113(8), 1039–1045.

238. Chen, A., Kim, S. S., Chung, E., & Dietrich, K. N. (2013). Thyroid hormones in relation to lead, mercury, and cadmium exposure in the National Health and Nutrition Examination Survey, 2007-2008. *Environmental Health Perspectives*, 121(2), 181–186. PubMed PMID: 23164649.

239. Gallagher, C. M., & Meliker, J. R. (2012). Mercury and thyroid autoantibodies in U.S. women, NHANES 2007-2008. *Environment International*, 40, 39–43. PubMed PMID: 22280926.

240. Osius, N., Karmaus, W., Kruse, H., & Witten, J. (1999). Exposure to polychlorinated biphenyls and levels of thyroid hormones in children. *Environmental Health Perspectives*, 107(10), 843–849. PubMed PMID: 10504153.

241. Iijima, K., Otake, T., Yoshinaga, J., et al. (2007). Cadmium, lead, and selenium in cord blood and thyroid hormone status of newborns. *Biological Trace Element Research*, 119(1), 10–18.

242. Hammouda, F., Messaoudi, I., El Hani, J., et al. (2008). Reversal of cadmium-induced thyroid dysfunction by selenium, zinc, or their combination in rat. *Biological Trace Element Research*, Aug 8. [Epub ahead of print].

243. Jancic, S. A., & Stosic, B. Z. (2014). Cadmium effects on the thyroid gland. *Vitamins and Hormones*, 94, 391–425. PubMed PMID: 24388198.

244. Arlt, W., & Allolio, B. (2003). Adrenal insufficiency. *Lancet*, 361(9372), 1881–1893. PubMed PMID: 12788587.

245. Coco, G., Dal Pra, C., Presotto, F., et al. (2006). Estimated risk for developing autoimmune Addison's disease in patients with adrenal cortex autoantibodies. *The Journal of Clinical Endocrinology and Metabolism*, 91(5), 1637–1645. PubMed PMID: 16522688.

246. Harvey, P. W., Everett, D. J., & Springall, C. J. (2007). Adrenal toxicology: a strategy for assessment of functional toxicity to the adrenal cortex and steroidogenesis. *Journal of Applied Toxicology : JAT*, 27(2), 103–115. PubMed PMID: 17265431.

247. Hinson, J. P., & Raven, P. W. (2006). Effects of endocrine-disrupting chemicals on adrenal function. *Best Practice and Research. Clinical Endocrinology and Metabolism*, 20(1), 111–120. PubMed PMID: 16522523.

248. Rosol, T. J., Yarrington, J. T., et al. (2001). Adrenal gland: structure, function, and mechanisms of toxicity. *Toxicologic Pathology*, 29(1), 41–48. PubMed PMID: 11215683.

249. Ullerås, E., Ohlsson, A., & Oskarsson, A. (2008). Secretion of cortisol and aldosterone as a vulnerable target for adrenal endocrine disruption—screening of 30 selected chemicals in the human H295R cell model. *Journal of Applied Toxicology : JAT*, 28(8), 1045–1053. PubMed PMID: 18626888.

250. Ribelin, W. E. (1984). The effects of drugs and chemicals upon the structure of the adenal gland. *Fundamental and Applied Toxicology, 4*(1), 105–119. PubMed PMID: 6692999.

251. Shi, Z., Zhang, H., Ding, L., et al. (2009). The effect of perfluorododecanoic acid on endocrine status, sex hormones and expression of steroidogenic genes in pubertal female rats. *Reproductive Toxicology, 27*(3–4), 352–359. PubMed PMID: 19429406.

252. Hasegawa, T., Zhao, L., et al. (2000). Developmental roles of the steroidogenic acute regulatory protein (StAR) as revealed by StAR knockout mice. *Molecular Endocrinology, 14*(9), 1462–1471. PubMed PMID: 10976923.

253. Walsh, L. P., & Stocco, D. M. (2000). Effects of lindane on steroidogenesis and steroidogenic acute regulatory protein expression. *Biology of Reproduction, 63*(4), 1024–1033. PubMed PMID: 10993823.

254. Walsh, L. P., McCormick, C., Martin, C., & Stocco, D. M. (2000). Roundup inhibits steroidogenesis by disrupting steroidogenic acute regulatory (StAR) protein expression. *Environmental Health Perspectives, 108*(8), 769–776. PubMed PMID: 10964798.

255. Hilscherova, K., Jones, P. D., et al. (2004). Assessment of the effects of chemicals on the expression of ten steroidogenic genes in the H295R cell line using real-time PCR. *Toxicological Sciences, 81*(1), 78–89. PubMed PMID: 15187238.

256. Arukwe, A. (2008). Steroidogenic acute regulatory (StAR) protein and cholesterol side-chain cleavage (P450scc)-regulated steroidogenesis as an organ-specific molecular and cellular target for endocrine disrupting chemicals in fish. *Cell Biology and Toxicology, 24*(6), 527–540. PubMed PMID: 18398688.

257. Harvey, P. W., & Everett, D. J. (2003). The adrenal cortex and steroidogenesis as cellular and molecular targets for toxicity: critical omissions from regulatory endocrine disruptor screening strategies for human health? *Journal of Applied Toxicology: JAT, 23*(2), 81–87. PubMed PMID: 12666151.

258. Wang, S. W., Pu, H. F., Kan, S. F., et al. (2004). Inhibitory effects of digoxin and digitoxin on corticosterone production in rat zona fasciculata-reticularis cells. *British Journal of Pharmacology, 142*(7), 1123–1130. PubMed PMID: 15249423.

259. Hahner, S., Sturmer, A., et al. (2010). Etomidate unmasks intraadrenal regulation of steroidogenesis and proliferation in adrenal cortical cell lines. *Hormone and Metabolic Research, 42*(7), 528–534. PubMed PMID: 20352599.

260. Couch, R. M., Muller, J., Perry, Y. S., & Winter, J. S. (1987). Kinetic analysis of inhibition of human adrenal steroidogenesis by ketoconazole. *The Journal of Clinical Endocrinology and Metabolism, 65*(3), 551–554. PubMed PMID: 3497939.

261. Jager, L. P., de Graaf, G. J., et al. (1997). Differential effects of nitrofurans on the production/release of steroid hormones by porcine adrenocortical cells in vitro. *European Journal of Pharmacology, 331*(2–3), 325–331. PubMed PMID: 9274996.

262. Creange, J. E., Schane, H. P., Anzalone, A. J., & Potts, G. O. (1978). Interruption of pregnancy in rats by azastene, an inhibitor of ovarian and adrenal steroidogenesis. *Fertility and Sterility, 30*(1), 86–90. PubMed PMID: 680188.

263. Harvey, P. W. (2016). Adrenocortical endocrine disruption. *The Journal of Steroid Biochemistry and Molecular Biology, 155*(Pt. B), 199–206. PubMed PMID: 25460300.

264. Lindhe, O., Granberg, L., & Brandt, I. (2002). Target cells for cytochrome p450-catalysed irreversible binding of 7,12-dimethylbenz[a]anthracene (DMBA) in rodent adrenal glands. *Archives of Toxicology, 76*(8), 460–466. PubMed PMID: 12185414.

265. Spiers, J. G., Chen, H. J., et al. (2015). Activation of the hypothalamic-pituitary-adrenal stress axis induces cellular oxidative stress. *Frontiers in Neuroscience, 8*, 456. PubMed PMID: 25646076.

266. Lee, S. R., Kim, H. K., et al. (2013). Glucocorticoids and their receptors: insights into specific roles in mitochondria. *Progress in Biophysics and Molecular Biology, 112*(1–2), 44–54. PubMed PMID: 23603102.

267. Cuzzocrea, S. (2006). Role of nitric oxide and reactive oxygen species in arthritis. *Current Pharmaceutical Design, 12*(27), 3551–3570. PubMed PMID: 17017948.

268. Asaba, K., Iwasaki, Y., et al. (2004). Attenuation by reactive oxygen species of glucocorticoid suppression on proopiomelanocortin gene expression in pituitary corticotroph cells. *Endocrinology, 145*(1), 39–42. PubMed PMID: 14576191.

269. Montiero, M. G., et al. (1990). Subjective feelings of anxiety in young men after ethanol and diazepam infusions. *The Journal of Clinical Psychiatry, 51*(1), 12–16. PubMed PMID: 2295585.

270. Eker, S., & Kargi, F. (2009). Biological treatment of 2,4,6-trichlorophenol (TCP) containing wastewater in a hybrid bioreactor system with effluent recycle. *Journal of Environmental Management, 90*(2), 692–698. PubMed PMID: 18276060.

271. Ma, Y., Liu, C., et al. (2011). Modulation of steroidogenic gene expression and hormone

synthesis in H295R celles exposed to PCP and TCP. *Toxicology*, 282(3), 146–153. PubMed PMID: 21296122.

272. Peterson, C. (1988). Explanatory style as a risk factor for illness. *Cognitive Therapy and Research*, 12, 117–130. PubMed PMID: 25882595.

273. Bakhshaie, J., Zvolensky, M. J., & Goodwin, R. D. (2015). Cigarette smoking and the onset and persistence of depression among adults in the United States: 1994-2005. *Comprehensive Psychiatry*, 60, 142–148. PubMed PMID: 25882595.

274. Altar, C., Bennett, B., Wallace, R., et al. (1983). Glucocorticoid induction of tryptophan oxygenase. Attenuation by intragastrically administered carbohydrates and metabolites. *Biochemical Pharmacology*, 32(6), 979–984. PubMed PMID: 6838662.

275. Barbieri, R. L., Friedman, A. J., & Osathanondh, R. (1989). Cotinine and nicotine inhibit human fetal adrenal 11 beta-hydroxylase. *The Journal of Clinical Endocrinology and Metabolism*, 69(6), 1221–1224. PubMed PMID: 2584357.

276. Skowronski, R. J., & Feldman, D. (1994). Inhibition of aldosterone synthesis in rat adrenal cells by nicotine and related constituents of tobacco smoke. *Endocrinology*, 134(5), 2171–2177. PubMed PMID: 8156919.

277. Edbrooke, D. L., Newby, D. M., et al. (1982). Safer sedation for ventilated patients. A new application for etomidate. *Anaesthesia*, 37(7), 765–771. PubMed PMID: 7048991.

278. Watt, I., & Ledingham, I. M. (1984). Mortality amongst multiple trauma patients admitted to an intensive therapy unit. *Anaesthesia*, 39(10), 973–981. PubMed PMID: 6496912.

279. Fellows, I. W., Bastow, M. D., et al. (1983). Adrenocortical suppression in multiple injury patients: a complication of etomidate treatment. *British Medical Journal (Clinical Research Ed.)*, 287(6408), 1835–1837. PubMed PMID: 6322902.

280. Diago, M. C., Amado, J. A., et al. (1988). Anti-adrenal action of a subanaesthetic dose of etomidate. *Anaesthesia*, 43(8), 644–645. PubMed PMID: 3421456.

281. Fry, D. E., & Griffiths, H. (1984). The inhibition by etomidate of the 11 beta-hydroxylation of cortisol. *Clinical Endocrinology*, 20(5), 625–629. PubMed PMID: 6744636.

282. Dorr, H. G., Kuhnle, U., et al. (1984). Etomidate: a selective adrenocortical 11 beta-hydroxylase inhibitor. *Klinische Wochenschrift*, 62(21), 1011–1013. PubMed PMID: 6096625.

283. Engelhardt, D., Dorr, G., et al. (1985). Ketoconazole blocks cortisol secretion in man by inhibition of adrenal 11 beta-hydroxylase. *Klinische Wochenschrift*, 63(13), 607–612. PubMed PMID: 2993735.

284. Yamakita, N., Yasuda, K., et al. (1987). Response of plasma adrenal steroids to synthetic ACTH under ketoconazole in man. *Endocrinologia Japonica*, 34(1), 29–35. PubMed PMID: 3038504.

285. Chabre, O. (2014). Cushing syndrome: physipathology, etiology, and principles of therapy. *La Presse Medicale*, 43(4 Pt. 1), 376–392. PubeMed PMD: 24656295.

286. Marques, A. H., Silverman, M. N., et al. (2009). Glucocorticoid dysregulations and their clinical correlates. From receptors to therapeutics. *Annals of the New York Academy of Sciences*, 1179, 1–18. PubMed PMID: 19906229.

287. Wurtman, R. J. (2002). Stress and the adrenocortical control of epinephrine synthesis. *Metabolism: Clinical and Experimental*, 51(6 Suppl. 1), 11–14. PubMed PMID: 12040535.

288. Brown, E. S., et al. (2008). Amygdala volume in patients receiving chronic corticosteroid therapy. *Biological Psychiatry*, 63(7), 705–709. PubMed PMID: 17981265.

289. Desai, S., Khanani, S., Shad, M. U., & Brown, E. S. (2009). Attenuation of amygdala atrophy with lamotrigine in patients receiving corticosteroid therapy. *Journal of Clinical Psychopharmacology*, 29(3), 284–287. PubMed PMID: 19440084.

290. Tosato, M., Zamboni, V., et al. (2007). The aging process and potential interventions to extend life expectancy. *Clinical Interventions in Aging*, 2(3), 401–412. PubMed PMID: 18044191.

291. Gracia, T., Hilscherova, K., et al. (2007). Modulation of steroidogenic gene expression and hormone production of H295R cells by pharmaceuticals and other environmentally active compounds. *Toxicology and Applied Pharmacology*, 225(2), 142–153. PubMed PMID: 17822730.

292. Lund, B., Bergman, A., & Brandt, I. (1988). Metabolic activation and toxicity of a DDT-metabolite, 3-methylsulphonyl-DDE, in the adrenal zona fasciculata in mice. *Chemico-Biological Interactions*, 65(1), 25–40. PubMed PMID: 3345572.

293. Jovanovich, L., Levin, S., & Khan, M. A. (1987). Significance of mirex-caused hypoglycemia and hyperlipidemia in rats. *Journal of Biochemical Toxicology*, 3, 203–213. PubMed PMID: 3508472.

294. Oskarsson, A., Ulleras, E., et al. (2006). Steroidogenic gene expression in H295R cells and the human adrenal gland: adrenotoxic effects of lindane in vitro. *Journal*

of Applied Toxicology: JAT, *26*(6), 484–492. PubMed PMID: 17080404.

295. Guven, M., Bayram, F., Unluhizarci, K., & Kelestimur, F. (1999). Endocrine changes in patients with acute organophosphorus poisoning. *Human and Experimental Toxicology*, *18*, 598–601. PubMed PMID: 10557009.

296. Satar, S., Sebe, A., et al. (2004). Endocrine effects of organophosphate antidotal therapy. *Advances in Therapy*, *21*(5), 301–311. PubMed PMID: 15727399.

297. Furuta, C., Noda, S., et al. (2008). Nitrophenols isolated from diesel exhaust particles regulate steroidogenic gene expression and steroid synthesis in the human H295R adrenocortical cell line. *Toxicology and Applied Pharmacology*, *229*(1), 109–120. PubMed PMID: 18336853.

298. Li, C., Taneda, S., et al. (2007). Effects of 3-methyl-4-nitrophenol on the suppression of adrenocortical function in immature rats. *Biological and Pharmaceutical Bulletin*, *30*(12), 2376–2380. PubMed PMID: 18057729.

299. Li, L. A., Wang, P. W., & Chang, L. W. (2004). Polychlorinated biphenyl 126 stimulates basal and inducible aldosterone biosynthesis of human adrenocortical H295R cells. *Toxicology and Applied Pharmacology*, *195*(1), 92–102. PubMed PMID: 14962509.

300. Xu, Y., Yu, R. M., et al. (2006). Effects of PCBs and MeSO2-PCBs on adrenocortical steroidogenesis in H295R human adrenocortical carcinoma cells. *Chemosphere*, *63*(5), 772–784. PubMed PMID: 16216300.

301. Cremer, J. E., & Seville, M. P. (1985). Changes in regional cerebral blood flow and glucose metabolism associated with sympoms of pyrethroid toxicity. *Neurotoxicology*, *6*(3), 1–12. PubMed PMID: 4047507.

302. Henger, A., Tutt, P., Riesen, W. F., Hulter, H. N., & Krapf, R. (2000). Acid-base and endocrine effects of aldosterone and angiotensin II inhibition in metabolic acidosis in human patients. *The Journal of Laboratory and Clinical Medicine*, *136*(5), 379–389. PubMed PMID: 11079465.

303. Sharma, A. M., & Distler, A. (1994). Acid-base abnormalities in hypertension. *The American Journal of the Medical Sciences*, *307*(Suppl. 1), S112–S115. PubMed PMID: 8141148.

304. Sharma, A. M., Kribben, A., Schattenfroh, S., Cetto, C., & Distler, A. (1990). Salt sensitivity in humans is associated with abnormal acid-base regulation. *Hypertension*, *16*(4), 407–413. PubMed PMID: 2210808.

305. Frassetto, L. A., Morris, R. C., Jr., & Sebastian, A. (2007). Dietary sodium chloride intake independently predicts the degree of hyperchloremic metabolic acidosis in healthy humans consuming a net acid-producing diet. *American Journal of Physiology – Renal Physiology*, *293*(2), F521–F525. PubMed PMID: 17522265.

306. Fu, Y., & Vallon, V. (2014). Mineralocorticoid-induced sodium appetite and renal salt retention: evidence for common signaling and effector mechanisms. *Nephron. Physiology*, *128*(1–2), 8–16. PubMed PMID: 25376899.

307. Wagner, C. A. (2014). Effect of mineralocorticoids on acid-base balance. *Nephron. Physiology*, *128*(1–2), 26–34. PubMed PMID: 25377117.

308. Oki, K., Gomez-Sanchez, E. P., & Gomez-Sanchez, C. E. (2012). Role of mineralocorticoid action in the brain in salt-sensitive hypertension. *Clinical and Experimental Pharmacology and Physiology*, *39*(1), 90–95. PubMed PMID: 21585422.

309. Fortin, M. C., Cory-Slechta, D. A., et al. (2012). Increased lead biomarker levels are associated with changes in hormonal response to stress in occupationally exposed male participants. *Environmental Health Perspectives*, *120*(2), 278–283. PubMed PMID: 22112310.

310. Souza-Talarico, J. N., Suchecki, D., et al. (2017). Lead exposure is related to hypercortisolemic profiles and allostatic load in Brazilian older adults. *Environmental Research*, *154*, 261–268. PubMed PMID: 28110240.

311. Braun, J. M., Wright, R. J., et al. (2014). Relationships between lead biomarkers and diurnal salivary cortisol indices in pregnant women from Mexico City: a cross-sectional study. *Environmental Health: A Global Access Science Source*, *13*(1), 50. PubMed PMID: 24916609.

312. Rossi-George, A., Virgolini, M. B., et al. (2009). Alterations in glucocorticoid negative feedback following maternal Pb, prenatal stress and the combination: a potential biological unifying mechanism for their corresponding disease profiles. *Toxicology and Applied Pharmacology*, *234*(1), 117–127. PubMed PMID: 18977374.

313. Goodfriend, T. L., Ball, D. L., et al. (1995). Lead increases aldosterone production by rat adrenal cells. *Hypertension*, *25*(4 Pt. 2), 785–789. PubMed PMID: 7721433.

314. Knazicka, Z., Forgacs, Z., et al. (2015). Endocrine disruptive effects of cadmium on steroidogenesis: human adrenocortical carcinoma cell line NCI-H295R as a cellular model for reproductive toxicity testing. *Journal of Environmental Science and Health. Part A, Toxic/Hazardous Substances & Environmental*

Engineering, 50(4), 348–356. PubMed PMID: 25723060.

315. Knazicka, Z., Lukac, N., et al. (2013). Effects of mercury on the steroidogenesis of human adenocarcinoma (NCI-H295R) cell line. *Journal of Environmental Science and Health. Part A, Toxic/ Hazardous Substances & Environmental Engineering, 48*(3), 348–353. PubMed PMID: 23245310.

316. Koch, H. M., Lorber, M., Christensen, K. L., et al. (2013). Identifying sources of phthalate exposure with human biomonitoring: results of a 48h fasting study with urine collection and personal activity patterns. *International Journal of Hygiene and Environmental Health, 216*(6), 672–681. PubMed PMID: 23333758.

317. Harley, K. G., Kogut, K., Madrigal, D. S., et al. (2016). Reducing phthalate, paraben, and phenol exposure from personal care products in adolescent girls: findings from the HERMOSA intervention study. *Environmental Health Perspectives, 124*(10), 1600–1607. PubMed PMID: 26947464.

318. Chen, C. Y., Chou, Y. Y., Lin, S. J., & Lee, C. C. (2015). Developing an intervention strategy to reduce phthalate exposure in Taiwanese girls. *The Science of the Total Environment, 517,* 125–131. PubMed PMID: 25725197.

319. Hagobian, T., Smouse, A., Streeter, M., et al. (2017). Randomized intervention trial to decrease bisphenol a urine concentrations in women: pilot study. *Journal of Women's Health (2002), 26*(2), 128–132. PubMed PMID: 27726525.

320. Allen, R. W., Carlsten, C., Karlen, B., et al. (2011). An air filter intervention study of endothelial function among healthy adults in a woodsmoke-impacted community. *American Journal of Respiratory and Critical Care Medicine, 183*(9), 1222–1230. PubMed PMID: 21257787.

321. McNamara, M. L., Thornburg, J., Semmens, E. O., et al. (2017). Reducing indoor air pollutants with air filtration units in wood stove homes. *The Science of the Total Environment, 592,* 488. PubMed PMID: 28320525. pii: S0048-9697(17)30623-X.

45

Mitochondrial Toxicity

SUMMARY

- Presence in population: Signs and symptoms of reduced mitochondrial function (fatigue, cognitive problems, obesity, diabetes) are commonly found in all Western populations
- Major diseases: Diabetes mellitus, metabolic syndrome, obesity, chronic neurological disorders (parkinsonism, multiple sclerosis, amyotrophic lateral sclerosis, etc.), depression, gastric cancer, glioblastoma multiforme, steatohepatitis, and cardiomyopathy
- Primary sources: Air, food, water, and personal care product pollution
- Best measure: Case history
- Best intervention: Avoidance, supplementation, depuration

OVERVIEW

Mitochondria are cellular organelles responsible for metabolizing nutrients to produce energy in the form of adenosine triphosphate (ATP). They also play a role in calcium homeostasis, programmed cell death, and the production of cellular growth substrates and free radicals. Energy production occurs via oxidative phosphorylation (OXPHOS) utilizing Krebs cycle products ($NADH^+H^+$ and $FADH^2$) and fatty acids. Mitochondria consist of an outer and inner membrane, intermembrane space, and an intracellular matrix. Along the inner membrane are five complexes that participate in proton pumping across the inner membrane, ultimately resulting in ATP production (Fig. 45.1). As OXPHOS occurs, reactive oxygen species (ROS) are produced, along with energy. In addition to providing energy for each cell, ATP levels are also necessary for the proper function of the various biotransformation pathways in the liver and bloodstream. Mitochondria are incredible organelles that, at rest, produce a person's body weight in ATP every day, which may explain why even mild dysfunction can have profound health-damaging effects.

MITOCHONDRIAL INSUFFICIENCY

Mitochondria are not only critical for cellular health and function but also for cell death or apoptosis. While under oxidative stress, mitochondria can release caspases and cytochrome C to trigger apoptosis. Mitochondria also play a role in calcium signaling[1] and neuronal health,[2,3] and may have a role in immune function as well.[4] They play a critical role in copper and iron homeostasis, heme and iron–sulfur cluster assembly, the synthesis of pyrimidines and steroids, thermogenesis, and fever response.[5]

Mitochondrial insufficiency typically occurs from oxidative stress in the cytoplasm of the cell. It is also associated with many commonly used pharmaceuticals[6] and commonly encountered xenobiotic pollutants. In addition to overall fatigue, mitochondrial dysfunction is associated with several disease states, including insulin resistance, metabolic syndrome, obesity,[7,8] diabetes,[9,10] chronic neurological disorders (parkinsonism, multiple sclerosis, amyotrophic lateral sclerosis, etc.),[11,12] depression,[13] gastric cancer,[14] glioblastoma multiforme,[15] steatohepatitis,[16] and cardiomyopathy,[17] many of which are

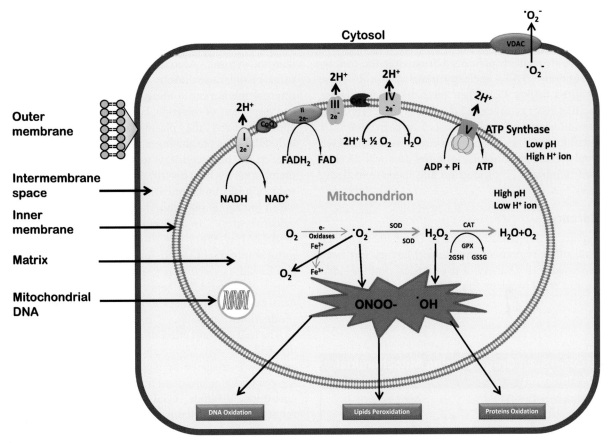

FIG. 45.1 Proton ion pumps result in the formation of adenosine triphosphate. From Mitochondrial dysfunction and oxidative stress in metabolic disorders—A step towards mitochondria based therapeutic strategies. Biochim Biophys Acta. 2016 Nov 9. pii: S0925-4439(16)30292-7. PubMed PMID: 27836629.

directly associated with same environmental pollutants that are discussed later. In fact, the aging process itself could be considered the result of progressive loss of mitochondrial function.

One of the first xenobiotic compounds found to exhibit mitochondrial damage leading to disease manifestation was 1-methyl-4-phenyl-1,2,3,6–tetrahydropyridine (MPTP), which caused rapid-onset parkinsonism.[18] MPP+, the metabolite of MPTP, accumulates in the mitochondria, leading to a body-wide inhibition of complex I of the electron transport chain. The reduction of complex I activity diminishes ATP production and reduces the activity of the plasma membrane Na/K ATPase, leading to partial neuronal depolarization. This, in turn, reduces the magnesium blockade of N-methyl-D-aspartate (NMDA)

glutamate receptors, which increases excitotoxic activity and ultimately leads to cellular death.

The CDC Fourth National Report on Human Exposure to Environmental Chemicals has measured for the presence of 246 compounds among National Health and Nutritional Examination Survey (NHANES) participants.[19] A count of all pollutants for which mean values are listed, along with a 50th percentile value, revealed that 120 of those tested would fall into this "ubiquitous" category. A PubMed search for each of those compounds and the term "and mitochondria" reveals that all 120 compounds have been shown to damage mitochondrial function in some way. This chapter reviews some of the most common pollutants that are also reported to have significant disease association.

Drugs

Some of the most common causes of mitochondrial damage are regularly prescribed drugs, over-the-counter medications (OTCs), and recreational chemicals. These are listed in Box 45.1. Their mechanisms are diverse, affecting every complex and decreasing the levels of key intramitochondrial molecules such as coenzyme Q10, glutathione (GSH), and many critical antioxidants. Even simply taking an antibiotic for a few days will decrease mitochondrial ATP production and increase oxidative stress.

Mercury

Mercury is ubiquitously found in US residents as well as all other regions of the globe. Mercury has been associated with a variety of neurological, immunological, and renal problems, and is a major mitochondrial poison. Unfortunately, 48% of cellular burden of this potent mitochondrial poison is found in the mitochondria, whereas only 38% is in the nuclei and 8% is in the cytosol.[20] Mercury-exposed cells show structural changes, including a loss of mitochondrial internal membrane folding, mitochondrial swelling, and dispersion of the endoplasmic reticulum, the Golgi apparatus, and the plasma membrane. Mercury-induced damage to the inner mitochondrial membrane appears to be secondary to GSH reduction in the membrane itself. This thiol depletion results in a reduction of mitochondrial transmembrane potential, which uncouples phosphorylation, leading to increased oxidative stress.[21] In addition to decreasing mitochondrial GSH, mercury has also been found to increase mitochondrial H_2O_2 and lipid peroxide production, and to cause cytochrome C release, stimulating apoptosis.[22] As would be expected with mitochondrial damage/alteration, there is also a reduction in ATP production (Fig. 45.2).

The feed-forward effect of mercury in the mitochondria will ultimately lead to apoptosis of the cell. Cellular apoptosis is triggered by high amounts of ROS inside the cytoplasm as indicated by a falling ratio of GSH to glutathione disulfide (GSSG). Not only does mercury result in increased levels of lipid peroxide formation, but it also leads to a reduction in available glutathione peroxidase, which if present could quench those ROS. Interestingly, mercury-induced cellular apoptosis is not prevented by antioxidant supplementation alone, making it appear that multiple mechanisms may be present.[23] Nonetheless, mitochondrial damage from cadmium and chromium is somewhat abated by antioxidant presence.

BOX 45.1   Drugs Causing Mitochondrial Dysfunction

Anticancer Drugs	**Antivirals**
Doxorubicin/Adriamycin	Azidothymidine
Cisplatin	Efavirenz
Trastuzumab	Stavadine
Arsenic trioxide	**Antibacterial**
Mitoxantrone	Chloramphenicol
Imatinib	Linezolid
Bevacizumab	Cephaloglycin
Sunitinib	Imipenem
Sorafenib	**Oral Antidiabetics**
Neurological Agents	Rosiglitazone
Valproic acid	Metformin &
Amitriptyline & Desipramine	Phenformin
Nefazodone	Troglitazone
Chlorpromazines, Haloperidol	**Drugs of Abuse**
Clozapine	Alcohol
Cardiovascular	Cocaine
Simvastatin	Methamphetamine
	Ecstasy

Data from Varga, Z. V., Ferdinandy, P., Liaudet, L., & Pacher, P. (2015). Drug-induced mitochondrial dysfunction and cardiotoxicity. *American Journal of Physiology - Heart and Circulatory Physiology, 309*(9), H1453–H1467; and Vuda, M., & Kamath, A. (2016). Drug-induced mitochondrial dysfunction: Mechanisms and adverse clinical consequences. *Mitochondrion, 31*, 63–74.

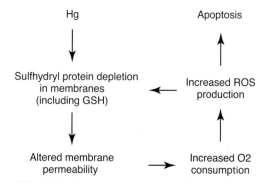

FIG. 45.2 Mercury damage to mitochondria.

Mercury damage to the immune, the neurological, and the renal system appears to be mediated, at least in part, via mitochondrial damage. Mercury increases the apoptosis of T cell and monocytes via mitochondrial damage.[24,25,26,27] Mercury disrupts the movement of neurotransmitters by damaging the synaptosomal membrane[21] and by blocking electron transport from complexes I and II.[28] Renal toxicity from mercury also appears to be mediated by mitochondrial damage.[29]

Cadmium

Cadmium causes changes in the mitochondrial membrane permeability, leads to mitochondrial swelling, and affects OXPHOS, thereby damaging mitochondria in multiple ways, like mercury.[30] Cadmium causes oxidative stress, depletes GSH stores, and stimulates the release of cytochrome c, leading to cellular apoptosis.[31,32] All of these methods of mitochondria damage appear to be responsible for cadmium-induced hepatotoxicity.[33]

Lead

In animal models, lead causes a dose-dependent decrease in the activity of mitochondrial monoamineoxidase in all regions of the brain.[34] The toxic effect of lead on mitochondrial function is heightened if alcohol is present at the same time.[35] Children with elevated blood lead levels showed a decline in the level of N-acetyl aspartate, a marker of mitochondrial metabolism, as well as choline and phosphocreatine in all regions of the brain.[36]

Arsenic and Tin

Similar to mercury and cadmium, arsenic increases intracellular ROS levels, alters the mitochondrial membrane permeability, and increases cytochrome c reductase. These changes are clearly present in the skin lesions of persons with chronic arsenic toxicity.[37] Organotins, tributyl tin, and dibutyl tin reduce natural killer cell activity by as much as 90% via a reduction of available cyclic adenosine monophosphate (AMP) secondary to mitochondrial damage.[38]

Air Pollution From Combustion

Cigarette smoke damages the inner mitochondrial membrane and leads to vacuolization of the mitochondrial matrix.[39] Although cigarette smoke is known to cause oxidative damage, vitamin C did not prevent this damage in an animal model. Smokers have 24%

lower function of complex I mitochondrial activity than nonsmokers.[40]

Diesel exhaust exposure led to a string of mitochondrial changes culminating in cellular apoptosis from the increased levels of ROS production.[41] These changes occurred in an orderly sequence beginning with depolarization of the inner mitochondrial membrane, followed by cytochrome c release, then by membrane asymmetry, and finally apoptosis. The researchers found that supplementation with N-acetyl cysteine (NAC) reversed the loss of mitochondrial function and lowered the production of ROS. Diesel exhaust includes various sizes of particulate matter (PM): coarse (2.5–10 um), fine (<2.5 um), and ultrafine (<0.1 um), all of which carry a host of polycyclic aromatic hydrocarbons (PAHs). The smallest PM, ultrafine particles ($PM_{0.1}$), easily penetrate cells throughout the body and are found inside the mitochondria.[42] The adsorbed PAH chemicals are also known to disrupt OXPHOS, prevent ATP production, and induce apoptosis.[43]

Chlorinated Compounds

Dichlorodiphenyldichloroethylene (DDE) increases production of ROS inside the cell, affecting the mitochondria by reducing the transmembrane potential, which is followed by the release of cytochrome c and leads to apoptosis.[44] This appears to be the mechanism by which DDE reduces male fertility. In an animal model, the release of cytochrome c, post DDE exposure, was blocked if NAC. Lindane causes apoptosis of testicular cells in animals after a single exposure secondary to mitochondrial damage.[45,46] Similarly, the common chlordane insecticide methoxychlor also causes testicular damage via mitochondrial damage.[47]

Dioxins are produced when organochlorine compounds are made; of these, 2,3,7,8-tetrachlorodiphenyldioxin (2,3,7,8-TCDD) is considered to be the most toxic. This dioxin damages the mitochondria both with increased ROS production and via the aryl hydrocarbon receptor which leads to reduced ATP production.[48,49,50] Dioxins are common contaminants of the chlorophenoxy acid broad-leaf herbicides 2,4-D and 2,4,5-T, which were used in southeast Asia under the name of Agent Orange. 2,4-D is still in commercially available weed-and-feed garden products and is used by railroads along with state and local municipalities to control weeds on roadsides and right-of-ways. These herbicides have also been shown to cause the loss of ATP production via mitochondrial damage.[51,52]

Pyrethroids, Organophosphates, and Other Pesticides

Commonly used pyrethroids and organophosphate pesticides have both demonstrated the ability to cause mitochondrial damage. Organophosphate pesticides cause neuronal damage via a very rapid change in transmembrane potential, preventing proper OXPHOS.[53] Permethrin damages Leydig cell mitochondria, resulting in low testosterone production, and reduced sperm count and motility.[54] Deltamethrin causes changes in the inner mitochondrial membrane and inhibits the respiratory chain between complexes II and III.[55] The mitochondrial damage from cypermethrin is only partly prevented by alpha tocopherol, indicating that only a portion of its toxic effect is via ROS production.[56] Rotenone, a natural pesticide used by many organic gardeners and farmers, is one of the compounds shown to be able to cause neurological damage, resulting in parkinsonism. Rotenone causes mitochondrial dysfunction in multiple ways, including complex I inhibition, induction of H_2O_2 production, mitochondrial membrane potential changes, and caspase-3 activity, leading to apoptosis.[57,58]

Phthalates and Plasticizers

Phthalates, specifically the high-molecular-weight mono-ethyl-hexyl phthalate (MEHP), has been shown to reduce mitochondrial succinate dehydrogenase activity and to reduce cellular ATP by 20%.[59] MEHP was the most potent inhibitor of mitochondrial activity followed by di-n-butyl phthalate (DBT) and di-mono-n-butyl phthalate (DMBT).[60] MEHP also demonstrates an ability to inhibit beta-oxidation of certain fatty acids by about 50% to 60% in the mitochondria.[61] This mitochondrial inhibition undoubtedly plays a role in phthalates, increasing rates of obesity and diabetes.[62] Phthalate inhibition of mitochondrial function is responsible for its adverse effect on Sertoli cells that leads to male infertility.[59] Phthalates have been found in significantly higher levels in infertile men where they are linked with mitochondrial depolarization along with increased levels of ROS and lipid peroxidases.[63]

Solvents

Alcohol alters mitochondrial structure and function and reduces mitochondrial protein synthesis.[64] It also increases ROS production, reduces ATP synthesis, and plays a role in the development of steatohepatitis.[65] Alcohol consumption lowers GSH levels both in the mitochondria as well as in the cytosol of the cell.[66] Trichloroethylene and its GSH-pathway metabolites are potent mitochondrial poisons.[67]

Mycotoxins

Mycotoxins isolated from the common aspergillus and penicillium mold families have been found to be toxic to mitochondria.[68] Damage (in some cases destruction) of the mitochondria have been shown with the mycotoxins ochratoxin and citrinin, which leads to renal damage.[69] Mycotoxic effects on the mitochondria are undoubtedly due in part to their effect on lowering GSH stores.[70] Hepatic damage from aspergillus aflatoxin is mediated via mitochondrial dysfunction but can be ameliorated by curcumin.[71] Vitamin E has also shown benefit in reducing mitochondrial effects from aflatoxin.[72]

ASSESSMENT

No single commonly used laboratory marker is currently available to detect mitochondrial dysfunction. Some indirect measures of mitochondrial damage are available, such as elevation of serum lactic acid when severe, and urinary organic acids and porphyrins when less severe. In persons with severe statin-induced myopathy, some will have elevated creatine kinase,[73] while others will not.[74] Oxidative stress, a clear factor in mitochondrial dysfunction,[75] can be assessed with urinary 8-OHdG[76] levels and measurements of F2-isoprostane.[77]

INTERVENTION

Nutrients

Deficiencies of iron, zinc, biotin, and pantothenic acid can enhance the normal aging-associated decay of mitochondria.[78] Vitamin E has been shown to protect mitochondria from prooxidant damage.[79] Folic acid supplementation enhanced mitochondrial Complex 1 function in children with autism.[80]

The underfunctioning of complex I in Parkinson's patients has been improved with supplementing 200 mg of coenzyme Q10 (CoQ10) four times daily.[81] In an animal model of rotenone-induced parkinsonism, animals given high doses of CoQ10 showed not only a reduction of parkinsonian symptoms but a return of complex I functioning and ATP production.[82] Giving humans higher levels of CoQ10 resulted in a reduction of the progression of parkinsonism, with those receiving the highest doses (1200 mg daily) experiencing the greatest improvements.[83] However, a follow-up study using 300 mg daily showed no improvements.[84] In two brothers with myopathic CoQ10 deficiency, the supplementation of 2 to 300 mg daily resulted in restored functioning of complexes I, II, and III.[85]

Alpha lipoic acid (ALA) at a dose of 600 mg daily has shown as beneficial for mitochondrial cytopathy.[86] Alpha lipoic acid supplementation provided a 55% increase in mitochondrial function in the first month, and continued treatment led to continued improvements. ALA has also been shown to prevent and reverse cadmium-induced enzyme damage (including GSH depletion).[87] Both R-alpha lipoic acid and acetyl-L-carnitine were able to reverse age-associated mitochondrial structural damage and provide improvement in memory.[88] L-carnitine has also demonstrated the ability to help reverse methamphetamine-induced mitochondrial damage and restore mitochondrial function.[89] S-adenosyl-l-methionine (SAMe) has demonstrated effectiveness against ethanol-induced mitochondrial damage. SAMe both restores mitochondrial GSH levels (something NAC was unable to do) and preserves mitochondrial function including ATP production.[90,91] D-ribose has also been proposed to be of assistance in restoring mitochondrial function. The use of 5,000 mg three times daily has offered relief to persons with chronic fatigue and fibromyalgia.[92]

GSH replacement has also been shown to improve mitochondrial function.[66] Clinically, liposomal GSH replacement appears to be the best method for increasing cellular GSH stores.[93] NAC, a precursor for GSH and a powerful antioxidant in its own right, has demonstrated the ability to prevent mitochondrial damage from diesel exhaust and DDE.[41,44] NAC has been shown to limit antibiotic-induced mitochondrial damage in both cell and animal models.[94]

Botanical Agents

Flavonoid molecules exhibit tissue-specific antioxidant abilities and appear to be primary active ingredients in many commonly used botanicals. Extracts of ginkgo biloba prevent a reduction of mitochondrial ATP production and protect complexes I and III.[95,96] Ginkgo is also protective against mercury-induced oxidative damage,[97] whereas acai (*Euterpe oleracea* Mart.) is able to prevent rotenone-induced mitochondrial damage.[98] Extracts of the herb *Phyllanthus fraternus*, common to the southeast region of the United States, has also been shown to protect against alcohol and carbon-tetrachloride-induced mitochondrial damage.[99,100] The common curry-spice ingredient turmeric (*Curcuma longa*) has demonstrated mitochondrial protection against oxidative damage.[101] Resveratrol has also demonstrated a protective benefit for mitochondria.[102]

Anthocyans, the dark blue pigments in berries, have demonstrated the ability to protect and restore mitochondrial function.[103] *Vaccinum myrtillus*, also known as bilberry or European blueberry, exhibited the greatest mitochondrial protecting activity of all *Vaccinum* species. Blackberry juice, in varying concentrations, exhibited the ability to reverse the suppression of mitochondrial function caused by peroxynitrites.[104] Polyphenols, the active ingredients in green tea, have also demonstrated the ability to protect, restore, and optimize mitochondrial function.[105,106]

REFERENCES

1. Duchen, M. R. (2000). Mitochondria and calcium: From cell signalling to cell death. *The Journal of Physiology*, 529(Pt. 1), 57–68. PubMed PMID: 11080251.
2. Li, Z., Okamoto, K., Hayashi, Y., & Sheng, M. (2004). The importance of dendritic mitochondria in the morphogenesis and plasticity of spines and synapses. *Cell*, 119(6), 873–887. PubMed PMID: 15607982.
3. Scaini, G., Rezin, G. T., Carvalho, A. F., Streck, E. L., Berk, M., & Quevedo, J. (2016). Mitochondrial dysfunction in bipolar disorder: Evidence, pathophysiology and translational implications. *Neuroscience and Biobehavioral Reviews*, 68, 694–713. PubMed PMID: 27377693.
4. Monlun, M., Hyernard, C., Blanco, P., Lartigue, L., & Faustin, B. (2017). Mitochondria as molecular platforms integrating multiple innate immune signalings. *Journal of Molecular Biology*, 429(1), 1–13. PubMed PMID: 27923767.
5. Meyer, J. N., Leung, M. C., Rooney, J. P., Sendoel, A., Hengartner, M. O., Kisby, G. E., et al. (2013). Mitochondria as a target of environmental toxicants. *Toxicological Sciences*, 134(1), 1–17. PubMed PMID: 23629515.
6. Varga, Z. V., Ferdinandy, P., Liaudet, L., & Pacher, P. (2015). Drug-induced mitochondrial dysfunction and cardiotoxicity. *American Journal of Physiology, Heart*

and Circulatory Physiology, 309(9), H1453–H1467. PubMed PMID: 26386112.

7. Bhatti, J. S., Bhatti, G. K., & Reddy, P. H. (2016). Mitochondrial dysfunction and oxidative stress in metabolic disorders – A step towards mitochondria based therapeutic strategies. *Biochimica et Biophysica Acta*, Nov 9. pii: S0925-4439(16)30292-7, PubMed PMID: 27836629.

8. Kim, J. A., Wei, Y., & Sowers, J. R. (2008). Role of mitochondrial dysfunction in insulin resistance. *Circulation Research*, 102, 401–414. PubMed PMID: 18309108.

9. Wada, J., & Nakatsuka, A. (2016). Mitochondrial dynamics and mitochondrial dysfunction in diabetes. *Acta Medica Okayama*, 70(3), 151–158. PubMed PMID: 27339203. Review.

10. Lamson, D. W., & Plaza, S. M. (2002). Mitochondrial factors in the pathogenesis of diabetes: a hypothesis for treatment. *Alternative Medicine Review: A Journal of Clinical Therapeutic*, 7, 94–111. PubMed PMID: 11991790.

11. Kidd, P. M. (2005). Neurodegeneration from mitochondrial insufficiency: nutrients, stem cells, growth factors and prospects for brain rebuilding using integrative management. *Alternative Medicine Review: a Journal of Clinical Therapeutic*, 10, 268–293. PubMed PMID: 16366737.

12. Beal, M. F. (2000). Limited time exposure to mitochondrial toxins may lead to chronic progressive neurodegenerative diseases. *Movement Disorders: Official Journal of the Movement Disorder Society*, 15, 434–435. PubMed PMID: 10830405.

13. Bansal, Y., & Kuhad, A. (2016). Mitochondrial dysfunction in depression. *Current Neuropharmacology*, 14(6), 610–618. PubMed PMID: 26923778. Review.

14. Ling, X. L., Fang, D. C., Wang, R. Q., Yang, S. M., & Fang, L. (2004). Mitochondrial microsatellite instability in gastric cancer and its precancerous lesions. *World Journal of Gastroenterology*, 10, 800–803. PubMed PMID: 15040020.

15. Guntuku, L., Naidu, V. G., & Yerra, V. G. (2016). Mitochondrial dysfunction in gliomas: pharmacotherapeutic potential of natural compounds. *Current Neuropharmacology*, 14(6), 567–583. PubMed PMID: 26791479.

16. Pessayre, D., Fromenty, B., & Mansouri, A. (2004). Mitochondrial injury in steatohepatitis. *Gastroenterologia Y Hepatologia*, 16, 1095–1105. PubMed PMID: 15489566.

17. Brunel-Guitton, C., Levtova, A., & Sasarman, F. (2015). Mitochondrial diseases and cardiomyopathies. *The Canadian Journal of Cardiology*, 31(11), 1360–1376. PubMed PMID: 26518446.

18. Sherer, T., Betarbet, R., & Greenamyre, J. T. (2002). Environment, mitochondria, and Parkinson's disease. *The Neuroscientist: A Review Journal Bringing Neurobiology, Neurology and Psychiatry*, 8(3), 192–197. PubMed PMID: 12061498.

19. Centers for Disease Control and Prevention: *National Report on Human Exposure to Environmental Chemicals: Updated tables*, 2017. Available at www.cdc.gov/exposurereport. (Accessed 25 April 2017).

20. Konigsberg, M., Lopez-Diazguerrero, N. E., Bucio, L., & Gutierrez-Ruiz, M. C. (2001). Uncoupling effect of mercuric chloride on mitochondria isolated from an hepatic cell line. *Journal of Applied Toxicology : JAT*, 21, 323–329. PubMed PMID: 11481667.

21. Bondy, S. C., & McKee, M. (1991). Disruption of the potential across the synaptosomal plasma membrane and mitochondria by neurotoxic agents. *Toxicology Letters*, 58, 13–21. PubMed PMID: 1897003.

22. Kahrizi, F., Salimi, A., Noorbakhsh, F., Faizi, M., Mehri, F., Naserzadeh, P., et al. (2016). Repeated administration of mercury intensifies brain damage in multiple sclerosis through mitochondrial dysfunction. *Iranian Journal of Pharmaceutical Research: IJPR*, 15(4), 834–841. PubMed PMID: 28243280.

23. Pourahmad, J., Mihajlovic, A., & O'Brien, P. J. (2001). Hepatocyte lysis induced by environmental metal toxins may involve apoptotic death signals initiated by mitochondrial injury. *Advances in Experimental Medicine and Biology*, 249–252. PubMed PMID: 11764948.

24. Makani, S., Gollapudi, S., Yei, L., Chiplunkar, S., & Gupta, S. (2002). Biochemical and molecular basis of thimerosal-induced apoptosis in T cells: a major role of mitochondrial pathway. *Genes and Immunity*, 3, 370–378. PubMed PMID: 12140745.

25. Shenker, B. J., Guo, T. L., O, I., & Shapiro, I. M. (1999). Induction of apoptosis in human T-cells by methyl mercury: temporal relationship between mitochondrial dysfunction and loss of reductive reserve. *Toxicology and Applied Pharmacology*, 157(1), 23–35. PubMed PMID: 10329504.

26. Shenker, B. J., Pankoski, L., Zekavat, A., & Shapiro, I. M. (2002). Mercury-induced apoptosis in human lymphocytes: caspase activation is linked to redox status. *Antioxidants & Redox Signaling*, 4, 379–389. PubMed PMID: 11068922.

27. Insug, O., Datar, S., Koch, C. J., Shapiro, I. M., & Shenker, B. J. (1997). Mercuric compounds inhibit human monocyte function by inducing apoptosis: evidence for formation of reactive oxygen species, development of mitochondrial membrane permeability

transition and loss of reductive reserve. *Toxicology*, *124*, 211–224. PubMed PMID: 9482123.

28. Yee, S., & Choi, B. H. (1996). Oxidative stress in neurotoxic effects of methylmercury poisoning. *Neurotoxicology*, *17*, 17–25. PubMed PMID: 8784815.

29. Weinberg, J. M., Harding, P. G., & Humes, H. D. (1982). Mitochondrial bioenergetics during the initiation of mercuric chloride-induced renal injury. *The Journal of Biological Chemistry*, *257*, 60–67. PubMed PMID: 6458618.

30. Belyaeva, E. A., Glazunov, V. V., & Korotkov, S. M. (2004). Cd2 promoted mitochondrial permeability transition: a comparison with other heavy metals. *Acta Biochimica Polonica*, *51*, 545–551. PubMed PMID: 15218548.

31. Li, M., Xia, T., Jiang, C. S., Li, L. J., Fu, J. L., & Zhou, Z. C. (2003). Cadmium directly induced the opening of membrane permeability pore of mitochondria which possibly involved in cadmium-triggered apoptosis. *Toxicology*, *194*, 19–33. PubMed PMID: 14636693.

32. Stohs, S. J., Bagchi, D., Hassoun, E., & Bagchi, M. (2000). Oxidative mechanisms in the toxicity of chromium and cadmium ions. *Journal of Environmental Pathology, Toxicology and Oncology*, *19*, 201–213. PubMed PMID: 10983887.

33. Lasfer, M., Vadrot, N., Aoudjehane, L., Conti, F., Bringuier, A. F., & Feldmann, G. (2008). Reyl-Desmars F. Cadmium induces mitochondria-dependent apoptosis of normal human hepatocytes. *Cell Biology and Toxicology*, *24*(1), 55–62. [Epub 2007 Jul 3]; PubMed PMID: 17610031.

34. Devi, C. B., Reddy, G. H., Prasanthi, R. P., Chetty, C. S., & Reddy, G. R. (2005). Developmental lead exposure alters mitochondrial monoamine oxidase and synaptosomal catecholamine levels in rat brain. *International Journal of Developmental Neuroscience*, *23*, 375–381. PubMed PMID: 15927761.

35. Verma, S. K., Dua, R., & Gill, K. D. (2005). Impaired energy metabolism after co-exposure to lead and ethanol. *Basic and Clinical Pharmacology and Toxicology*, *96*, 475–479. PubMed PMID: 15910412.

36. Meng, X. M., Zhu, D. M., Ruan, D. Y., She, J. Q., & Luo, L. (2005). Effects of chronic lead exposure on 1H MRS of hippocampus and frontal lobes of children. *Neurology*, *64*, 1644–1647. PubMed PMID: 15883337.

37. Banerjee, N., Banerjee, M., Ganguly, S., Bandyopadhyay, S., Das, J. K., Bandyopadhay, A., et al. (2008). Arsenic-induced mitochondrial instability leading to programmed cell death in the exposed individuals. *Toxicology*, *246*(2–3), 101–111. PubMed PMID: 18304716.

38. Whalen, M. M., & Loganathan, B. G. (2001). Butyltin exposure causes a rapid decrease in cyclic AMP levels in human lymphocytes. *Toxicology and Applied Pharmacology*, *171*, 141–148. PubMed PMID: 11243913.

39. Yang, Y. M., & Liu, G. T. (2003). Injury of mouse brain mitochondria induced by cigarette smoke extract and effect of vitamin C on it in vitro. *Biomedical and Environmental Sciences*, *16*, 256–266. PubMed PMID: 14631831.

40. Smith, P. R., Cooper, J. M., Govan, G. G., Harding, A. E., & Schapira, A. H. V. (1993). Smoking and mitochondrial function: A model for environmental toxins. *The Quarterly Journal of Medicine*, *86*, 657–660. PubMed PMID: 8255963.

41. Hiura, T. S., Li, N., Kaplan, R., Horwitz, M., Seagrave, J. C., & Nel, A. E. (2000). The role of a mitochondrial pathway in the induction of apoptosis by chemicals extracted from diesel exhaust particles. *The Journal of Immunology: Official Journal of the American Association of Immunologists*, *165*(5), 2703–2711. PubMed PMID: 10946301.

42. Li, N., Sioutas, C., Cho, A., Schmitz, D., Misra, C., Sempf, J., et al. (2003). Ultrafine particulate pollutants induce oxidative stress and mitochondrial damage. *Environmental Health Perspectives*, *111*(4), 455–460. PubMed PMID: 12676598.

43. Xia, T., Korge, P., Weiss, J. N., Li, N., Venkatesen, M. I., Sioutas, C., et al. (2004). Quinones and aromatic chemical compounds in particulate matter induce mitochondrial dysfunction: Implications for ultrafine particle toxicity. *Environmental Health Perspectives*, *112*(14), 1345–1358. PubMed PMID: 15471724.

44. Song, Y., Liang, X., Hu, Y., Wang, Y., Yu, H., & Yang, K. (2008). p,p'-DDE induces mitochondria-mediated apoptosis of cultured rat Sertoli cells. *Toxicology*, *253*(1–3), 53–61. PubMed PMID: 18817639.

45. Saradha, B., Vaithinathan, S., & Mathur, P. P. (2009). Lindane induces testicular apoptosis in adult Wistar rats through the involvement of Fas-FasL and mitochondria-dependent pathways. *Toxicology*, *255*(3), 131–139. PubMed PMID: 19038305.

46. Bagchi, M., & Stohs, S. J. (1993). In vitro induction of reactive oxygen species by 2,3,7,8-tetrac hlorodibenzo-p-dioxin, endrin, and lindane in rat peritoneal macrophages, and hepatic mitochondria and microsomes. *Free Radical Biology & Medicine*, *14*(1), 11–18. PubMed PMID: 7681024.

47. Latchoumycandane, C., & Mathur, P. P. (2002). Effect of methoxychlor on the antioxidant system

in mitochondrial and microsome-rich fractions of rat testis. *Toxicology, 176,* 67–75. PubMed PMID: 12062931.

48. Senft, A. P., Dalton, T. P., Nebert, D. W., Genter, M. B., Hutchinson, R. J., & Shertzer, H. G. (2002). Dioxin increases reactive oxygen production in mouse liver mitochondria. *Toxicology and Applied Pharmacology, 178,* 15–21. PubMed PMID: 11781075.

49. Senft, A. P., Dalton, T. P., Nebert, D. W., Genter, M. B., et al. (2002). Mitochondrial reactive oxygen production is dependent on the aromatic hydrocarbon receptor. *Free Radical Biology & Medicine, 33,* 1268–1278. PubMed PMID: 12398935.

50. Fisher, M. T., Nagarkatti, M., & Nagarkatti, P. S. (2005). Aryl hydrocarbon receptor-dependent induction of loss of mitochondrial membrane potential in epidydimal spermatozoa by 2,3,7,8-tetr achlorodibenzo-p-dioxin (TCDD). *Toxicology Letters, 157,* 99–107. PubMed PMID: 15836997.

51. Oakes, D. J., & Pollak, J. K. (1999). Effects of a herbicide formulation, Tordon 75D, and its individual components on the oxidative functions of mitochondria. *Toxicology, 13,* 41–52. PubMed PMID: 10499849.

52. Oakes, D. J., & Pollak, J. K. (2000). The in vitro evaluation of the toxicities of three related herbicide formulations containing ester derivatives of 2,4,5-T and 2,4-D using sub-mitochondrial particles. *Toxicology, 151,* 1–9. PubMed PMID: 11074295.

53. Carlson, K., & Ehrich, M. (1999). Organophosphorus compound-induced modification of SH-SY5Y human neuroblastoma mitochondrial transmembrane potential. *Toxicology and Applied Pharmacology, 160,* 33–42. PubMed PMID: 10502500.

54. Zhang, S. Y., Ito, Y., Yamanoshita, O., Yanagiba, Y., Kobayashi, M., Taya, K., et al. (2007). Permethrin may disrupt testosterone biosynthesis via mitochondrial membrane damage of Leydig cells in adult male mouse. *Endocrinology, 148*(8), 3941–3949. PubMed PMID: 17463061.

55. Braguini, W. L., Cadena, S. M., Carnieri, E. G., Rocha, M. E., & de Oliveira, M. B. (2004). Effects of deltamethrin on function of rat liver mitochondria and on native and synthetic model membranes. *Toxicology Letters, 152,* 191–202. PubMed PMID: 15331128.

56. Aldana, L., Tsutsumi, V., Craigmill, A., Silveira, M. I., & Gonzalez de Mejia, E. (2001). Alpha-tocopherol modulated liver toxicity of the pyrethroid cypermethrin. *Toxicology Letters, 125,* 107–116. PubMed PMID: 11701229.

57. Zhang, X., Jones, D., & Gonzalez-Lima, F. (2002). Mouse model of optic neuropathy caused by mitochondrial complex I dysfunction. *Neuroscience Letters, 326,* 97–100. PubMed PMID: 12057837.

58. Tada-Oikawa, S., Hiraku, Y., Kawanishi, M., & Kawanishi, S. (2003). Mechanism for generation of hydrogen peroxide and change of mitochondrial membrane potential during rotenone-induced apoptosis. *Life Sciences, 73,* 3277–3288. PubMed PMID: 14561532.

59. Chapin, R. E., Gray, T. J., Phelps, J. L., & Dutton, S. L. (1988). The effects of mono – (2-ethylhexyl)-phthalate on rat Sertoli cell enriched primary cultures. *Toxicology and Applied Pharmacology, 9293,* 467–479. PubMed PMID: 3353991.

60. Melnick, R. L., & Schiller, C. M. (1982). Mitochondrial toxicity of phthalate esters. *Environmental Health Perspectives, 45,* 51–56. PubMed PMID: 7140696.

61. Winberg, L. D., & Badr, M. Z. (1995). Mechanism of phthalate-induced inhibition of hepatic mitochondrial beta-oxidation. *Toxicology Letters, 76*(1), 63–69. PubMed PMID: 7701518.

62. Stahlhut, R. W., van Wijngaarden, E., Dye, T. D., Cook, S., & Swan, S. H. (2007). Concentrations of urinary phthalate metabolites are associated with increased waist circumference and insulin resistance in adult US males. *Environmental Health Perspectives, 115,* 876–882. PubMed PMID: 17589594.

63. Pant, N., Shukla, M., Kumar Patel, D., Shukla, Y., Mathur, N., Kumar Gupta, Y., et al. (2008). Correlation of phthalate exposures with semen quality. *Toxicology and Applied Pharmacology, 231*(1), 112–116. PubMed PMID: 18513777.

64. Patel, V. B., & Cunningham, C. C. (2002). Altered hepatic mitochondrial ribosome structure following chronic ethanol consumption. *Archives of Biochemistry and Biophysics, 398,* 41–50. PubMed PMID: 11811947.

65. Pessayre, D., Mansouri, A., & Fromenty, B. (2002). Nonalcoholic steatosis and steatohepatitis v. mitochondrial dysfunction in steatohepatitis. *American Journal of Physiology. Gastrointestinal and Liver Physiology, 282,* G193–G199. PubMed PMID: 11804839.

66. Guidot, D. M., & Brown, L. A. (2000). Mitochondrial glutathione replacement restores surfactant synthesis and secretion in alveolar epithelial cells of ethanol-fed rats. *Alcoholism, Clinical and Experimental Research, 24,* 1070–1076. PubMed PMID: 10924012.

67. Lash, L. H., Qian, W., Putt, D. A., Hueni, S. E., Elfarra, A. A., Krause, R. J., et al. (2001). Renal and hepatic toxicity of trichloroethylene and its glutathione-derived metabolites in rats and mice: Sex-, species-, and tissue-dependent differences. *The Journal of Pharmacology and Experimental*

Therapeutics, 297(1), 155–164. PubMed PMID: 11259540.

68. Da Lozzo, E. J., & Oliveira, M. B. (1998). Carnieri EG. Citrinin-induced mitochondrial permeability transition. *Journal of Biochemical Toxicology, 12,* 291–297. PubMed PMID: 9664235.

69. Kumar, M., Dwivedi, P., Sharma, A. K., Singh, N. D., & Patil, R. D. (2007). Ochratoxin A and citrinin nephrotoxicity in New Zealand white rabbits: And ultrastructural assessment. *Mycopathologia, 163,* 21–30. PubMed PMID: 17216328.

70. Guilford, F. T., & Hope, J. (2014). Deficient glutathione in the pathophysiology of mycotoxin-related illness. *Toxins, 6*(2), 608–623. PubMed PMID: 24517907.

71. Verma, R. J., Chakraborty, B. S., Patel, C., & Mathurai, N. (2008). Curcumin ameliorates aflatoxin-induced changes in SDH and ATPase activities in the liver and kidney of mice. *Acta Poloniae Pharmaceutica, 65,* 415–419. PubMed PMID: 19051581.

72. Xia, T., Korge, P., Weiss, J. N., Li, N., Venkatesen, M. I., Sioutas, C., et al. (2004). Quinones and aromatic chemical compounds in particulate matter induce mitochondrial dysfunction: Implications for ultrafine particle toxicity. *Environmental Health Perspectives, 112*(14), 1345–1358. PubMed PMID: 15471724.

73. Hou, T., Li, Y., Chen, W., Heffner, R. R., & Vladutiu, G. D. (2017). Histopathologic and biochemical evidence for mitochondrial disease among 279 patients with severe statin myopathy. *Journal of Neuromuscular Diseases, 4*(1), 77–87. PubMed PMID: 28269789.

74. Phillips, P. S., Haas, R. H., Bannykh, S., Hathaway, S., Gray, N. L., Kimura, B. J., et al. (2002). Statin-associated myopathy with normal creatine kinase levels. *Annals of Internal Medicine, 137*(7), 581–585. PubMed PMID: 12353945.

75. Ayala-Peña, S. (2013). Role of oxidative DNA damage in mitochondrial dysfunction and Huntington's disease pathogenesis. *Free Radical Biology & Medicine, 62,* 102–110. PubMed PMID: 23602907.

76. Valavanidis, A., Vlachogianni, T., & Fiotakis, C. (2009). 8-hydroxy-2' –deoxyguanosine (8-OHdG): A critical biomarker of oxidative stress and carcinogenesis. *Journal of Environmental Science and Health. Part C, Environmental Carcinogenesis & Ecotoxicology Reviews, 27*(2), 120–139. PubMed PMID: 19412858.

77. Santilli, F., D'Ardes, D., & Davì, G. (2015). Oxidative stress in chronic vascular disease: From prediction to prevention. *Vascular Pharmacology, 74,* 23–37. PubMed PMID: 26363473.

78. Ames, B. N., Atamna, H., & Killilea, D. W. (2005). Mineral and vitamin deficiencies can accelerate the

mitochondrial decay of aging. *Molecular Aspects of Medicine, 26,* 363–378. PubMed PMID: 16102804.

79. Gavazza, M. B., & Catala, A. (2006). The effect of alpha-tocopherol on lipid peroxidation of microsomes and mitochondria from rat testes. *Prostaglandins, Leukotrienes, and Essential Fatty Acids, 74,* 245–254. PubMed PMID: 11716353.

80. Delhey, L. M., Nur Kilinc, E., Yin, L., Slattery, J. C., Tippett, M. L., Rose, S., et al. (2017). The effect of mitochondrial supplements on mitochondrial activity in children with autism spectrum disorder. *Journal of Clinical Medicine, 6*(2), PubMed PMID: 28208802.

81. Shults, C. W., Beal, M. F., Fontaine, D., Nakano, K., & Haas, R. H. (1998). Absorption, tolerability, and effects on mitochondrial activity of oral coenzyme Q10 in parkinsonian patients. *Neurology, 50,* 793–795. PubMed PMID: 9521279.

82. Adbin, A. A., & Hamouda, H. E. (2008). Mechanism of the neuroprotective role of coenzyme Q10 with or without L-dopa in rotenone-induced parkinsonism. *Neuropharmacol, 55,* 1340–1346. PubMed PMID: 18817789.

83. Shults, C. W., Oakes, D., Kieburtz, K., Beal, M. F., Haas, R., Plumb, S., et al. (2002). Effects of coenzyme Q10 in early Parkinson disease: Evidence of slowing of the functional decline. *Archives of Neurology, 59*(10), 1541–1550. PubMed PMID: 12374491.

84. Storch, A., Jost, W. H., Vieregge, P., Spiegel, J., Greulich, W., Durner, J., et al. (2007). Randomized, double-blind, placebo-controlled trial on symptomatic effects of coenzyme Q(10) in Parkinson disease. *Archives of Neurology, 64*(7), 938–944. [Epub 2007 May 14]; PubMed PMID: 17502459.

85. Di Giovanni, S., Mirabella, M., Spinazzola, A., Crociani, P., Silvestri, G., Broccolini, A., et al. (2001). Coenzyme Q10 reverses pathological phenotype and reduces apoptosis in familial CoQ10 deficiency. *Neurology, 57*(3), 515–518. PubMed PMID: 11502923.

86. Barbiroli, B., Medori, R., Tritschler, H. J., Klopstock, T., Seibel, P., Reichmann, H., et al. (1995). Lipoic (thioctic) acid increases brain energy availability and skeletal muscle performance as shown by in vivo 31P-MRS in a patient with mitochondrial cytopathy. *Journal of Neurology, 242*(7), 472–477. PubMed PMID: 7595680.

87. Bludovska, M., Kotyzova, D., Koutensky, J., & Eybl, V. (1999). The influence of alpha-lipoic acid on the toxicity of cadmium. *General Physiology and Biophysics, 18,* 28–32. PubMed PMID: 10703716.

88. Liu, J., Head, E., Gharib, A. M., Yuan, W., Ingersoll, R. T., Hagen, T. M., et al. (2002). Memory loss in old rats is associated with brain mitochondrial decay and RNA/

DNA oxidation: partial reversal by feeding acetyl-L-carnitine and/or R-alpha -lipoic acid. *Proceedings of the National Academy of Sciences of the United States of America*, 99(4), 2356–2361. PubMed PMID: 11854529. Erratum in: Proc Natl Acad Sci U S A 2002 May 14;99(10):7184-5.

89. Virmani, A., Gaetani, F., Imam, S., Binienda, Z., & Ali, S. (2002). The protective role of L-carnitine against neurotoxicity evoked by drug of abuse, methamphetamine, could be related to mitochondrial dysfunction. *Annals of the New York Academy of Sciences*, 965, 225–232. PubMed PMID: 12105098.

90. García-Ruiz, C., Morales, A., Colell, A., Ballesta, A., Rodés, J., Kaplowitz, N., et al. (1995). Feeding S-adenosyl-L-methionine attenuates both ethanol-induced depletion of mitochondrial glutathione and mitochondrial dysfunction in periportal and perivenous rat hepatocytes. *Hepatology*, 21(1), 207–214. PubMed PMID: 7806156.

91. Colell, A., García-Ruiz, C., Morales, A., Ballesta, A., Ookhtens, M., Rodés, J., et al. (1997). Transport of reduced glutathione in hepatic mitochondria and mitoplasts from ethanol-treated rats: effect of membrane physical properties and S-adenosyl-L-methionine. *Hepatology*, 26(3), 699–708. PubMed PMID: 9303501.

92. Teitelbaum, J. (2008). Enhancing mitochondrial function with D-ribose. *Integrative Medicine*, 7, 46–51. http://www.nanotechnologystore.com/(3)Enhancing-Mitochondrial-Function-With-D-Ribose.pdf.

93. Morris, D., Guerra, C., Khurasany, M., Guilford, F., Saviola, B., Huang, Y., et al. (2013). Glutathione supplementation improves macrophage functions in HIV. *Journal of Interferon and Cytokine Research*, 33(5), 270–279. PubMed PMID: 23409922.

94. Kalghatgi, S., Spina, C. S., Costello, J. C., et al. (2013). Bactericidal antibiotics induce mitochondrial dysfunction and oxidative damage in Mammalian cells. *Science Translational Medicine*, 5(192), 192. PMID: 23825301.

95. Du, G., Willet, K., Mouithys-Michalad, A., et al. (1999). EGb 761 protects liver mitochondria against injury induced by Du G, Willet K, Mouithys-Mickalad A, Sluse-Goffart CM, Droy-Lefaix MT, Sluse FE. EGb 761 protects liver mitochondria against injury induced by in vitro anoxia/reoxygenation. *Free Radical Biology & Medicine*, 27(5–6), 596–604. PubMed PMID: 10490280.

96. Janssens, D., Remacle, J., Drieu, K., & Michiels, C. (1999). Protection of mitochondrial respiration activity by bilobalide. *Biochemical Pharmacology*, 58, 109–119. PubMed PMID: 10403524.

97. Tunali-Akbay, T., Sener, G., Salvarli, H., Sehirli, O., & Yarat, A. (2007). Protective effects of Ginkgo biloba extract against mercury (II) induced cardiovascular oxidative damage in rats. *Phytotherapy Research: PTR*, 21, 26–31. PubMed PMID: 17072828.

98. Machado, A. K., Andreazza, A. C., da Silva, T. M., Boligon, A. A., do Nascimento, V., Scola, G., et al. (2016). Neuroprotective effects of açaí (euterpe oleracea mart.) against rotenone in vitro exposure. *Oxidative Medicine and Cellular Longevity*, 2016, 8940850. PubMed PMID: 27781077.

99. Sailaja, R., & Setty, O. H. (2006). Protective effect of Phyllanthus fraternus against allyl alcohol-induced oxidative stress in liver mitochondria. *Journal of Ethnopharmacology*, 105, 201–209. PubMed PMID: 16359838.

100. Padma, P., & Setty, O. H. (1999). Protective effect of Phyllanthus fraternus against carbon tetrachloride-induced mitochondrial dysfunction. *Life Sciences*, 64, 2411–2417. PubMed PMID: 10374905.

101. Quiles, J. L., Aquilera, C., Mesa, M. D., Ramirez-Tortosa, M. C., Baro, L., & Gil, A. (1998). An ethanolic-aqueous extract of Curcuma longa decreases the susceptibility of liver microsomes and mitochondria to lipid peroxidation in atherosclerotic rabbits. *Biofactors*, 8, 51–57. PubMed PMID: 9699009.

102. de Oliveira, M. R., Nabavi, S. F., Manayi, A., Daglia, M., Hajheydari, Z., & Nabavi, S. M. (2016). Resveratrol and the mitochondria: From triggering the intrinsic apoptotic pathway to inducing mitochondrial biogenesis, a mechanistic view. *Biochimica et Biophysica Acta*, 1860(4), 727–745. PubMed PMID: 26802309.

103. Yao, Y., & Vieira, A. (2007). Protective activities of Vaccinum antioxidants with potential relevance to mitochondrial dysfunction and neurotoxicity. *Neurotoxicity*, 28, 93–100. PubMed PMID: 16956663.

104. Serraino, I., Dugo, L., Dugo, P., Mondello, L., Mazzon, E., Dugo, G., et al. (2003). Protective effects of cyanidin-3-O-glucoside from blackberry extract against peroxynitrite-induced endothelial dysfunction and vascular failure. *Life Sciences*, 73(9), 1097–1114. PubMed PMID: 12818719.

105. Mustata, G. T., Rosca, M., Biemel, K. M., Reihl, O., Smith, M. A., Viswanathan, A., et al. (2005). Paradoxical effects of green tea (Camellia sinensis) and antioxidant vitamins in diabetic rats: Improved retinopathy and renal mitochondrial defects but deterioration of collagen matrix glycoxidation and cross-linking. *Diabetes*, 54(2), 517–526. PubMed PMID: 15677510.

106. Mandel, S., & Youdim, M. B. (2004). Catechin polyphenols: Neurodegeneration and neuroprotection in neurodegenerative diseases. *Free Radical Biology & Medicine*, 37, 304–317. PubMed PMID: 15223064.

46

Respiratory Toxicity
Chronic Obstructive Pulmonary Disease and Asthma

SUMMARY

- Presence in population: Chronic obstructive pulmonary disease (COPD) is the third leading cause of death globally[1] and affects approximately 14% of adults over 40 years of age in the United States, whereas 1 in 12 people (8.4% of the US population) have asthma[2]
- Primary sources: Tobacco smoke, air pollution, environmental allergens, pesticides, toxic metals, sulfites

- Best measure: Spirometry
- Best intervention: Avoidance of known irritants, toxicant-specific elimination (smoking cessation), antioxidant support, inhaled glutathione (GSH) with N-acetyl cysteine (NAC)

DESCRIPTION
Chronic Obstructive Pulmonary Disease

COPD is a respiratory condition characterized by airflow inflammation secondary to chronically inhaled noxious particles. COPD is comprised of three separate but interconnected processes: 1) airway thickening and narrowing with expiratory airflow obstruction; 2) chronic mucus hypersecretion, resulting in chronic cough and phlegm production; and 3) emphysema (an abnormal dilation of distal airspaces combined with destruction of alveolar walls).[3] COPD affects approximately 14% of adults in the United States between the ages of 40 and 79 years.[4] The death rate attributed to COPD increased by 67%, from 40.7 deaths to 66.9 deaths per 100,000 persons, between 1980 and 2000.[5]

Asthma. Asthma is a chronic disease of the lungs characterized by repeated episodes of wheezing, breathless-ness, chest tightness, and nighttime or early morning coughing. Airflow is obstructed by inflammation, and airway hyperreactivity occurs in reaction to certain exposures, including exercise, infection, allergens, occupational exposures, and airborne irritants.[6] In 2010, it was estimated that 25.7 million people had asthma in the United States, with 18.7 million being adults aged 18 and over and 7.0 million children aged 0 to 17 years.[1] As can be seen in Table 46.1, asthma prevalence was higher for children ages 0 to 17 years, women, and for non-Hispanic black people.

There are several theories provided to explain the rising rates of asthma, including 1) increased stress on the immune system due to factors such as greater chemical pollution in the air, water, and food; 2) earlier weaning and earlier introduction of solid foods to infants; 3) food additives; and 4) genetic manipulation of plants resulting in food components with greater allergenic tendencies.

TABLE 46.1   National Current Asthma Prevalence, 2015

	Number With Current Asthma (in Thousands)	Percent of US Population With Current Asthma
Total Population	24,633	7.8%
Age		
0–4 years	935	4.7%
5–14 years	4033	9.8%
15–19 years	2107	10.2%
20–24 years	1655	7.6%
25–34 years	2916	6.8%
35–64 years	9907	8.0%
65+ years	3079	6.6%
Gender		
Male	9998	6.5%
Female	14,634	9.1%
Race/Ethnicity		
NH-White	15,244	7.8%
NH-Black	3931	10.3%
Hispanic	3665	6.6%

NH, *non-Hispanic.*
From Centers for Disease Control and Prevention. (2017). *Most recent asthma data.* Retrieved from https://www.cdc.gov/asthma/most_recent_data.htm

BASIC MECHANISMS OF TOXICITY

Most pulmonary toxicants generate reactive oxygen species (ROS), resulting in oxidative stress (OS). Mechanisms of OS from pollutants include direct generation of ROS from the surface of particles, formation of soluble compounds such as transition metals or organic compounds, altered function of mitochondria or nicotinamide adenine dinucleotide phosphate (NADPH)-oxidase, and activation of inflammatory cells capable of generating ROS and reactive nitrogen species.[7] GSH is present in high concentrations in epithelial lining fluid. Lower levels of GSH in the serum and airspaces are found with both COPD and asthma and are indicators of increased oxidative stress.[8,9]

Chronic Obstructive Pulmonary Disease

In COPD, innate immune cells, including macrophages and neutrophils, increase the levels of airway inflammation through the abnormal secretion of cytokines and chemokines that recruit and activate other immune cells and release tissue destructive proteases.[10,11] Repair and remodeling of the damaged tissue leads to thickening of the walls of the small airways. The neutrophil chemoattractant interleukin 8 (CXCL8) is secreted in the airways of COPD patients at higher levels compared with healthy controls.[12,13] Cigarette smoke increases secretion of CXCL8, which may be an important mechanism in propelling neutrophilic airway inflammation under conditions of OS and bacterial exposure.[14]

Evidence indicates that bacterial pathogens, including *Haemophilus influenza, Streptococcus pneumoniae,* and *Moraxella catarrhallis,* cause approximately 40% to 50% of acute exacerbations of COPD.[15] Bacterial proteins activate macrophages through Toll-like receptors (TLRs), which bind to ligands initiating intracellular signaling pathways leading to the upregulation of inflammatory mediators.[16,17,18] In addition, bacterial products in the tracheobronchial tree cause neutrophil influx, degranulation in the airways, and lung parenchyma, contributing to the chronic inflammation, parenchymal lung damage, and progressive small airway obstruction seen in COPD.[19,20,21] Exposure to cigarette smoke suppresses macrophage phagocytosis, which allows bacteria to persist in the airways further, aggravating COPD.[22] Potentially pathogenical bacteria (PPB) were recovered at 100 CFU/mL in 34.6% of ex-smokers with stable COPD, 0% of ex-smokers without COPD, and 6.7% of nonsmokers ($p = 0.003$).[23] COPD exacerbation is associated twice as often with distal airway infection $\geq 10^3$ CFU of pathogenical bacteria per mL and four times as often with $\geq 10^4$ CFU/mL ($p < 0.05$ for both comparisons).[24] Isolation of a new strain of pathogenical bacteria has been associated with a significantly increased risk (Relative Risk (RR) = 2.15; 95% Confidence Interval (CI), 1.83–2.53) of COPD exacerbation and further supports the causative role of bacteria in exacerbations of COPD.[25]

Asthma

Asthma can be divided into two categories, extrinsic and intrinsic. Extrinsic (allergic) asthma is considered an immunologically mediated condition with a characteristic increase in serum IgE that is often triggered by allergens suspended in the air (e.g., pollen, dust, smoke, automobile exhaust, animal dander). Intrinsic asthma is a bronchial reaction triggered by factors not related to allergies (e.g., chemicals, cold air, exercise, infection, emotional upset).

Extrinsic and intrinsic factors trigger the release of mast cell–derived chemical mediators that are responsible for the signs and symptoms of most asthma cases. These mediators include histamine; chemotactic peptides, such as eosinophilotactic factor (ECF) and high-molecular weight neutrophil chemotactic factor (NCF); proteases; glycosidases; heparin proteoglycan; leukotrienes (LTs); prostaglandins (PGs); thromboxanes (TXs); and platelet-activating factor (PAF). The modes of action vary depending on the mediator involved. The actions include bronchial smooth muscle constriction (LT, PG, and PAF), mucosal edema (histamine, LT, and PAF), vasodilation (PG), mucous plugging (histamine and LT), inflammatory cell infiltrate (NCF, ECF, LT, and PAF), and desquamation of epithelium (proteases and glycosides). LTs are the most potent chemical mediators in asthma. Asthmatics have an imbalance in arachidonic acid metabolism, leading to a relative increase in lipoxygenase products (LT and slow-reacting substance of anaphylaxis).[26] Slow-reacting substances of anaphylaxis (LTC_4, LTD_4, LTE_4) are approximately 1000 times more potent as stimulators of bronchial constriction than histamine.

ROS are produced by macrophages, neutrophils, and eosinophils in the airway and may play an important role in originating pulmonary inflammation.[27] Noninvasive markers of oxidative stress such as hydrogen peroxide, nitric oxide, and carbon monoxide released in expired air correlate with the degree of airway inflammation in asthmatic subjects.[28,29,30] Asthmatic subjects also have altered levels of lung antioxidant enzymes.[31,32]

SOURCES OF RESPIRATORY TOXICANTS
Air Pollution
Particulate Matter. Exposure to particulate matter (PM) has been associated with worse morbidity and mortality in patients with COPD, including higher exacerbation rates, aggravation of symptoms, and increased health care utilization.[33,34] Increased outdoor PM_{10} concentrations are associated with lower forced expiratory volume in one second (FEV_1) and forced vital capacity (FVC) in COPD patients presenting with urgent hospitalization.[35] In the National Emphysema Treatment Trial (NETT), $PM_{2.5}$ exposure, even under air quality standards, was associated with FEV_1 decline in subjects with severe COPD.[36] Exposure to $PM_{0.1}$ activates signaling pathways (e.g., NF-κB, NADPH oxidase) that induce inflammation, generate ROS, and lead to cell death, which may explain

the association between long-term particle accumulation and chronic inflammatory diseases such as COPD.[37]

Several studies have explored the relationship between childhood asthma and respiratory problems with exposure to vehicle exhaust.[38,39] Children in the Netherlands living within 100 m of a freeway had significantly more cough, wheeze, rhinitis, and diagnosed asthma than those living further away.[40] Among children living within 150 m of a main road, the risk of wheeze increases with increasing proximity by an odds ratio of 1.17 (95% CI 1.01–1.36) per 30-meter increment.[41] Studies of families living on busy roadways found that girls had significantly higher risk for wheezing and higher use of respiratory medication.[42,43]

Both men and women living in downtown Marseilles, France had significantly altered baseline lung function than those living in the suburbs.[44] Men living downtown also showed higher rates of bronchial hyperreactivity and symptoms of asthma. Fine and ultrafine diesel exhaust particles can reach small airways, including the alveolar/gas exchange regions of the lung, and exacerbate asthma symptoms.[45] Direct exposure to diesel exhaust has been linked to the development of asthma, which persists even after exposure ceases.[46]

Ozone. Urban joggers exposed to ozone exhibited increased markers of chronic respiratory inflammation.[47] College students exposed to high ambient ozone had more respiratory symptoms of cough, phlegm, and wheezing, as well as statistically significantly decreased lung function as exhibited by lower FEV_1 and FEF_{25-75}.[48] Men with COPD and healthy controls exposed to "worst case" ambient levels of ozone at 0.24 parts per million (PPM) showed lung dysfunction, and those with COPD who exercised during ozone exposure exhibited the worst respiratory response.[49] Asthma-related visits to the emergency room are associated with ozone levels. A study in New Jersey reported that ER visits for asthma occurred 28% more frequently when the mean ozone levels were >0.06 PPM than when they were <0.06 PPM.[50] Children exposed to higher levels of ground level ozone have greater rates of asthma and rhinitis than children in areas with less ozone.[51]

Sulfur Dioxide. Outdoor air levels of SO_2 have been associated with increased rates of asthma in French children,[52] whereas industrial exposure to SO_2 was associated with bronchial hyperresponsiveness and reduced FEV_1/FVC ratio.[53] In Taiwanese children, SO_2 levels were associated with increased incidence of contracting the flu as well as asthma.[54] In adolescents with asthma, exposure to SO_2 after ozone exposure (0.120 PPM for 45 min) resulted in a significant decrease in FEV and Vmax50 (compared with FEV and Vmax50 without ozone preexposure).[55]

Nitrogen Dioxide. Nitrogen dioxide is a powerful respiratory irritant that can lead to asthma, decreased lung function, pulmonary edema, and diffuse lung injury.[56] Emergency room visits for asthma are increased 1 to 5 days after outdoor levels of NO_2 spike.[57,58] Nitrogen dioxide exposure in individuals with allergenic tendencies increases their allergic reactivity to airborne pollens.[59,60] These individuals will then react to levels of pollen that would previously not have induced an allergic reaction.

Smoking (Tobacco and Marijuana). Smoking and exposure to environmental tobacco smoke (ETS) causes bronchial irritation, precipitates acute asthma episodes, and causes airway sensitization to several occupational allergens.[61] There is a greater prevalence of asthma among female smokers. The Canadian National Population Survey 1994 to 1995 reported that, among subjects aged 25 years or more, women had a higher prevalence of asthma compared with men, and female smokers had a 1.7-fold increase in the prevalence rate of asthma compared with female nonsmokers.[62] The risk of childhood asthma and wheezing is significantly increased in association with maternal and household smoking.[63,64,65] Smoking is strongly predictive of the development of new onset asthma in allergic adults.[66] Tobacco smoking adversely affects the health and treatment outcomes of asthma,[67] and a reduced therapeutic response to inhaled and/or oral corticosteroid treatment in asthmatic patients who smoke has been reported.[68,69] Daily heavy inhalation of marijuana can produce bronchial irritation and may lead to airway obstruction and long-term pulmonary damage secondary to the associated hydrocarbon residue.[70,71]

Continued smoking by adult asthmatics is a likely cause of irreversible airway obstruction and the development of COPD.[72] Cigarette smoking is the major risk factor for COPD and continues to be one of the leading causes of cigarette smoke–related death worldwide.[73] Exposure to cigarette smoke *in vitro* induces the release of IL-1β from human airway epithelial cells and CXCL8 from neutrophils and epithelial cells.[74,75] Elevations in IL-1β and CXCL8 are believed to play a key role in the development of the chronic inflammation associated with COPD.[76] The prevalence of COPD is 14.1% among current smokers and 7.1% among former smokers.[77] Approximately 80% of all COPD–related deaths can be attributed to smoking, and smokers are 12 to 13 times more likely to die from COPD than nonsmokers.[78] The risk of airflow obstruction is strongly associated with starting to smoke at a young age and the amount of cigarettes smoked.[79]

Occupational Agricultural Exposure

Occupational exposures in the agricultural industry are associated with numerous lung diseases, including asthma. Production agriculture leads to a variety of exposures, including organic dusts from livestock, chemical toxicants from fermentation and bacterial degradation of grain and animal wastes, pesticides, microorganisms, and bacterial endotoxins. Table 46.2 describes some of the agricultural respiratory hazards and associated diseases.[80]

Pesticides may contribute to asthma among farmers and has been associated with wheeze among US farmers.[81] For farmers, the organophosphates chlorpyrifos, malathion, and parathion have all been positively associated with wheeze.[82] Farmers are more likely to be diagnosed with nonatopic asthma than atopic asthma compared with other occupational groups,[83] although high pesticide exposure events have been associated with a doubling of both allergic and nonallergic asthma in farmers.[84] Coumaphos, heptachlor, parathion, and ethylene dibromide all have odds ratios greater than 2.0 for allergic asthma.

Asthma-like syndrome is associated with swine confinement workers and grain elevator operators, with acute symptoms occurring in as many as 50%.[85] With this condition, symptoms are more pronounced upon return to work after being away for some time. Interestingly, two studies demonstrated lower prevalence rates of asthma in farmers compared with the general population, although other respiratory conditions were increased.[86,87] Elevated risks of COPD and impaired respiratory function consistent with an obstructive syndrome have been reported in workers employed in pesticide production.[88]

Bisphenol-A. Higher urinary bisphenol-A (BPA) concentrations have been associated with chronic obstructive pulmonary disease. In a small study (50 COPD patients versus 38 controls), serum BPA was significantly higher in COPD patients (3.04 ± 3.30 ng/mL) compared with controls (0.57 ± 0.19 ng/mL).[89]

TABLE 46.2 **Agricultural Respiratory Hazards and Diseases**[73]

Category	Sources	Environments	Conditions
Organic dusts	Grain, hay, endotoxin, cotton, animal feed, animal by-products, microorganisms	Animal confinement, operations, barns, silos, harvesting and processing	Asthma, asthma-like syndrome, chronic bronchitis, hypersensitivity pneumonitis (Farmer's Lung)
Inorganic dusts	Silicates	Harvesting/tilling	Pulmonary fibrosis, chronic bronchitis
Gases	Ammonia, hydrogen sulfide, nitrous oxides, methane, carbon monoxide	Animal confinement, facilities, silos, fertilizers	Asthma-like syndrome, tracheobronchitis, silo-filler's disease, pulmonary edema
Chemicals			
Pesticides	Paraquat, organophosphates, fumigants	Applicators, field workers	Pulmonary fibrosis, pulmonary edema, bronchospasm
Fertilizers	Anhydrous ammonia	Application in fields, storage containers	Mucous membrane irritation, tracheobronchitis
Disinfectants	Chlorine, quaternary compounds	Dairy barns, hog confinement	Respiratory irritant, bronchospasm
Others			
Solvents	Diesel fuel, pesticide solutions	Storage containers	Mucous membrane irritation
Welding fumes	Nitrous oxides, ozone, metals	Welding operations	Bronchitis, metal-fume fever, emphysema
Zoonotic infections	Microorganisms	Animal husbandry, veterinary services	Anthrax, Q fever, psittacosis

From Centers for Disease Control and Prevention. (2008). Smoking-attributable mortality, years of potential life lost, and productivity losses—United States, 2000–2004. *Morbidity and Mortality Weekly Report, 57*(45), 1226–1228.

Toxic Metals

Arsenic. Chronic upper and lower respiratory problems, including dyspnea, asthma, and cough, were noted in a study from India with persons consuming groundwater with arsenic levels between 11 to 50 PPM.[90] A dose-related decrease in lung function exists with increasing levels of baseline water and urinary arsenic.[91] For every one standard deviation increase in baseline water arsenic exposure, there was a decrease in FEV_1 (-46.5 mL; p $= 0.0005$) and FVC (-53.1 mL; p < 0.01). This inverse association between arsenic exposure and FVC was consistent across sexes, remained significant in never-smokers, and was strongest in male smokers. Data on Italian men chronically exposed to low-medium arsenic levels via drinking water shows that COPD risk doubles (Hazard Ratio (HR) $= 2.54$) in those men with higher arsenic intake.[92] A retrospective study from Chile identified that those exposed to arsenic either *in utero* or early life had a lower FEV_1 (11.5%; p $= 0.04$) and FVC (12.2%; p $= 0.04$) in adulthood compared with those unexposed.[93]

Cadmium. Observational studies have demonstrated an association between cadmium and pulmonary disease. Men who worked in the manufacturing of copper-cadmium alloy had an excess of abnormalities of lung function and of radiographic changes consistent with emphysema, with the greatest abnormalities in those with the highest cumulative cadmium exposure.[94] Among participants in National Health and Nutritional Examination Survey (NHANES) III, FVC, FEV_1, FEV_1/FVC ratio, and a diagnosis of COPD were all inversely correlated with urinary cadmium concentrations in current and former smokers but not in nonsmokers.[95] Increasing concentration of serum cadmium has been associated with an increased risk of moderate-severe obstructive lung disease (OLD) (OR, 3.47; 95% CI, 1.67–7.22), as well as mild OLD (OR, 2.01; 95% CI, 1.05–3.83).[96] Pooled cross-sectional data from 5972 subjects who participated in the Korean NHANES from 2008 to 2012 demonstrated a significant association between FEV_1/FVC ratio and blood concentrations of cadmium.[97] Among current smokers, the risk of OLD was higher in subjects in the highest quartile group of cadmium concentration compared with those in the lowest quartile group (OR, 1.94; 95% CI, 1.06–3.57). In Korean men who had never smoked, a higher blood cadmium level, but within the normal range, had a dose-response relationship with COPD.[98]

Lead. Blood lead levels (BLLs) have been inversely associated with lung function leading to OLD. Korean adults whose BLLs were > 2.81 µg/dL exhibited significantly lower FEV_1/FVC ratios than those with BLLs < 2.03 µg/dL.[99] Another study utilizing the data from the Korean NHANES IV-V revealed that persons with BLLs ≥ 3.17 µg/dL had the lowest FEV_1/FVC ratios.[60] Participants in 2007 to 2010 US NHANES with OLD were also found to have significantly higher BLLs than persons without this respiratory problem (1.73 [1.02] versus 1.18 [1.0], p = .001).[59] A two to three times increased risk of developing COPD was associated with urinary lead levels ≥ 2.062 µg/L.[100]

Mold/Mycotoxins

Indoor environments contain a complex mixture of live and dead microorganisms, fragments of dead organisms, myco- and endotoxins, allergens, volatile microbial organic compounds, and other chemicals. Damp building materials contribute to the production of undesirable organisms and toxins, including 1) the growth of molds which release biological agents, toxic chemicals, and spores; 2) the growth of bacteria, which release biological agents, toxic chemicals, and spores; 3) protozoal growth; 4) virus survival; 5) the proliferation of dust mites (arachnids of many different species); 6) the proliferation of rodents and cockroaches, which can carry infectious organisms; and 7) the release of chemicals and particles from building materials.

Mold and damp building exposure is a major factor in the asthma epidemic. Studies have shown that dampness or mold in houses cause 21% of asthma in the United States and a 30% to 50% increase in asthma and asthma-related health problems.[101,102] The incidence may be higher, as one study found that 67% of adult-onset asthma

developed after working in a water-damaged office building.[103] The primary mechanisms for damp building toxicity include immunological (e.g., stimulation, suppression, autoimmunity), toxic (e.g., neurotoxicity, genotoxicity, reproductive damage), and inflammatory. The Institute of Medicine report commissioned by the Centers for Disease Control and Prevention (CDC) and released in 2004 concluded that respiratory conditions, including asthma, have sufficient evidence of causation by mold or damp buildings.[104]

Fungal allergens have the strongest correlation with asthma. The trigger appears to be glycopeptides with enzymatic properties typically found in spores, hyphae, and fungal fragments. Research supports that exposure to mold and dampness increases the risk of allergy to other allergens, such as house dust mites and pollen, and causes epigenetic modulation that upregulates many inflammatory genes.[105] Once an individual has become sensitized, they become much more reactive to even low to modest exposure.

Patients suffering from any kind of chronic respiratory condition—especially those of adult onset—should be fully evaluated for mold/damp building exposure. Symptoms such as dyspnea, wheeze, cough, respiratory infections, bronchitis, allergic rhinitis, eczema, vocal cord dysfunction, and upper respiratory tract symptoms warrant further investigation.

ASSESSMENT

Spirometry is the most common lung function tests used in the diagnosis of asthma and COPD. Spirometry measures FEV_1 and FVC. OLD can be confirmed when the ratio of FEV_1 to FVC is less than 0.70.[106] An FEV_1 of < 80% of predicted after four inhalations of a short-acting bronchodilator suggests a diagnosis of COPD. If there is an improvement in FEV_1 of more than 12% after administration of a short-acting bronchodilator, then reversible airflow obstruction is present.

Spirometry is recommended in all patients with asthma and COPD as it provides useful prognostic information and the FEV_1 can be used as a measure of severity in staging (Table 46.3).[107]

In 2011, the Global Initiative for Chronic Obstructive Lung Disease (GOLD) recommended a new COPD assessment that added chronic symptoms and exacerbation history to the traditional spirometry-based severity system.[108] However, studies have found the reclassification

TABLE 46.3	Assessment of COPD Severity by Spirometry
COPD Stage	Spirometry (Postbronchodilator)
Mild	$FEV_1 \geq 80\%$ of predicted, $FEV_1/FVC < 0.7$
Moderate	$FEV_1 \leq 50\%$ to $< 80\%$ of predicted, $FEV_1/FVC < 0.7$
Severe	$FEV_1 \leq 30\%$ to $< 50\%$ of predicted, $FEV_1/FVC < 0.7$
Very severe	$FEV_1 < 30\%$ of predicted, $FEV_1/FVC < 0.7$

to be highly variable, and more time is required to recommend the new classification system.[109,110]

A chest radiograph or computed tomography (CT) scan may be ordered to detect emphysema and rule out other pulmonary conditions.

Increased markers of inflammation and OS in the blood, urine, breath, and airspaces of smokers and COPD cases have been reported. Levels of interleukin-6 (IL-6), fibrinogen, tumor necrosis factor-alpha, and C-reactive protein are increased in COPD patients.[111] Increased inflammatory markers are associated with worse disease severity, exacerbation rates, and lung function decline.[112] Malondialdehyde (MDA), a measure of oxidative stress, is a lipid peroxidation product increased in lungs of COPD patients and is negatively correlated with lung function.[113] COPD patients have been shown to have higher plasma levels of MDA and lower levels of antioxidants compared with controls ($p < 0.01$).[114]

Specific measurement of xenobiotics and their metabolites are available from specialty laboratories. More comprehensive information regarding testing guidelines can be found in the toxin and toxicant specific chapters.

INTERVENTION

Avoidance

Avoidance of commonly known irritants is prudent. Airborne allergens such as pollen, dander, dust mites, and outdoor air pollutants are often difficult to avoid entirely. However, the primary toxic environments are in the individual's control—dietary allergens and toxins/toxicants within the home. If workplace exposure is occurring, the use of airway protection while on the job

is recommended. Smoking is a modifiable behavior, and various measures, including nicotine-containing skin patches or chewing gum, acupuncture, and hypnosis, have all been shown to provide some benefit in helping patients quit smoking (see Chapter 40 for more details).

Eliminating exposure to dogs and cats, as well as carpets, rugs, and upholstered furniture where allergens can collect is a good first step. Environmental chemicals around the home should be removed. These include: paints, solvents, new furniture, chemical cleaners, and scented candles/air fresheners, to name a few. Building materials containing formaldehyde (e.g., carpeting, cabinetry) should also be avoided. Perfume, cologne, hair spray, lotions, antiperspirant, and scented soaps and shampoos often contain a number of chemicals that should be avoided. High quality air purifiers can be used to reduce levels of PM, nitrogen oxides (NOx), and other pollutants in the indoor air.

Water-damaged buildings must be professionally remediated with the removal of all contaminated material (without spreading spores in the indoor air) as well as properly addressing the moisture source. Professional mold spore testing (International Risk Management Institute [IRMI] testing) should also be conducted before and after remediation.

Antioxidants

- Vitamins C and E
- NAC
- Glutathione
- Quercetin

Antioxidants are thought to provide important defense mechanisms by counteracting OS and reducing the formation of free radicals. Smoking greatly reduces ascorbic acid levels, thereby potentiating its damaging effects.[115] Smokers require at least twice as much vitamin C as nonsmokers.[116] In animal models, vitamin C has been shown to offer significant protection against nitrogen oxide damage in the lungs.[117] Clinical studies have demonstrated significant improvements in respiratory measures and asthma symptoms with supplementation of 1 to 2 g of vitamin C.[118] Vitamin C also prevents the secretion of histamine by white blood cells and increases the detoxification of histamine.[119]

A randomized, double-blind, placebo-controlled study of stable COPD patients found that treatment for 1 year with high-dose N-acetylcysteine (600 mg twice daily (BID)) improved small airway function and decreased exacerbation frequency.[120] A study of Chinese patients with moderate to severe COPD (the PANTHEON Study) confirmed that long-term use of NAC (600 mg BID) can prevent exacerbations.[121] Curcumin attenuates lung injury and fibrosis caused by toxicants and may play a protective role in COPD by modulating proinflammatory cytokines and reducing oxidative stress.[122,123]

GSH is involved in metabolic and biochemical reactions such as DNA synthesis and repair, protein synthesis, prostaglandin synthesis, amino acid transport, and enzyme activation. Glutathione therefore affects every system in the body, especially the nervous gastrointestinal immune and the respiratory systems. Asthmatics have reduced levels of glutathione peroxidase.[124] Supplemental selenium may reduce the production of LT by ensuring optimal activity of glutathione peroxidase in asthmatics.[125,126]

Quercetin has vitamin C–sparing effects and also helps stabilize mast cells. In addition, quercetin inhibits: histamine release from mast cells and basophils when stimulated by antigens, phospholipase A_2 in neutrophils, lipoxygenase, anaphylactic contractions of smooth muscle, and biosynthesis of slow-reacting substance of anaphylaxis (SRS-A).[127,128]

Vitamin D. Vitamin D deficiency is highly prevalent in patients with COPD and correlates with disease severity. As many as 77% of patients with GOLD stage 4 COPD exhibited deficient 25-OHD levels < 20 ng/mL.[129] Using spirometric data from NHANES, a strong dose-response relationship between serum levels of 25-OHD and pulmonary function was found with higher vitamin D levels, correlating with increased lung function.[130] The evidence suggests supplementation with vitamin D is warranted in patients with COPD.

REFERENCES

1. Minino, A. M., Xu, J., & Kochanek, K. D. (2010). Deaths: Preliminary data for 2008. *National Vital Statistics Reports: From the Centers for Disease Control and Prevention, National Center for Health Statistics, National Vital Statistics System, 59*(2), 1–52. PubMed PMID: 25073655.
2. Akinbami, L. J., Moorman, J. E., Bailey, C., et al. (2012). Trends in asthma prevalence, health care use, and mortality in the United States, 2001-2010. *NCHS Data Brief,* (94), 1–8. PubMed PMID: 22617340.
3. Forey, B. A., Thornton, A. J., & Lee, P. N. (2011). Systematic review with meta-analysis of the epidemiological evidence relating smoking to COPD, chronic bronchitis and emphysema. *BMC Pulmonary Medicine, 11,* 36. PubMed PMID:21672193.
4. Tilert, T., Dillon, C., Paulose-Ram, R., et al. (2013). Estimating the U.S prevalence of chronic obstructive pulmonary disease using pre- and post-bronchodilator spirometry: The National Health and Nutrition Examination Survey (NHANES) 2007-2010. *Respiratory Research, 14,* 103. PubMed PMID: 24107140.
5. Mannino, D. M., Homa, D. M., Akinbami, L. J., et al. (2002). Chronic obstructive pulmonary disease surveillance – United States, 1971-2000. *MMWR. Surveillance Summaries: Morbidity and Mortality Weekly Report. Surveillance Summaries, 51*(6), 1–16. PubMed PMID: 12198919.
6. National Institutes of Health. (2007). *National Asthma Education and Prevention Program Expert Panel Report 3: Guidelines for the diagnosis and management of asthma.* NIH publication No. 08-5846.
7. Rison, L., Moller, P., & Loft, S. (2005). Oxidative stress-induced DNA damage by particulate air pollution. *Mutation Research, 592*(1–2), 119–137. PubMed PMID: 16085126.
8. Drost, E. M., Skwarskin, K. M., Sauleda, J., et al. (2005). Oxidative stress and airway inflammation in severe exacerbations of COPD. *Thorax, 60*(4), 293–300. PubMed PMID: 15790984.
9. Zinellu, A., Fois, A. G., Sotgia, S., et al. (2016). Plasma protein thiols: An early marker of oxidative stress in asthma and chronic obstructive pulmonary disease. *European Journal of Clinical Investigation, 46*(2), 181–188. PubMed PMID: 26681451.
10. Hogg, J. C., Chu, F., Utokaparch, S., et al. (2004). The nature of small-airway obstruction in chronic obstructive pulmonary disease. *The New England Journal of Medicine, 350*(26), 2645–2653. PubMed PMID: 15215480.
11. Tetley, T. D. (2005). Inflammatory cells and chronic obstructive pulmonary disease. *Current Drug Targets. Inflammation and Allergy, 4*(6), 607–618. PubMed PMID: 17305517.
12. Keatings, V. M., Collins, P. D., et al. (1996). Differences in interleukin-8 and tumor necrosis factor-alpha in induced sputum from patients with chronic obstructive pulmonary disease or asthma. *American Journal of Respiratory and Critical Care Medicine, 153*(2), 530–534. PubMed PMID: 8564092.
13. Richman-Eisenstat, J. B., Jorens, P. G., et al. (1993). Interleukin-8: An important chemoattractant in sputum of patients with chronic inflammatory

airway diseases. *The American Journal of Physiology, 264*(4 Pt. 1), L413–L418. PubMed PMID: 8476069.

14. Moretto, N., Facchinetti, F., Southworth, T., et al. (2009). alpha, beta-unsaturated aldehydes contained in cigarette smoke elicit IL-8 release in pulmonary cells through mitogen-activated protein kinases. *American Journal of Physiology. Lung Cellular and Molecular Physiology, 296*(5), L839–L848. PubMed PMID: 19286926.

15. Sethi, S., & Murphy, T. F. (2001). Bacterial infection in chronic obstructive pulmonary disease in 2000: A state-of-the-art review. *Clinical Microbiology Reviews, 14*(2), 336–363. PubMed PMID: 11292642.

16. Knapp, S., Wieland, C. W., et al. (2004). Toll-like receptor 2 plays a role in the early inflammatory response to murine pneumococcal pneumonia but does not contribute to antibacterial defense. *The Journal of Immunology: Official Journal of the American Association of Immunologists, 172*(5), 3132–3138. PubMed PMID: 14978119.

17. Punturieri, A., Cooper, P., Polak, T., et al. (2006). Conserved nontypeable Haemophilus influenza-derived TLR2-binding lipopeptides synergize with IFN-beta to increase cytokine production by resident murine and human alveolar macrophages. *The Journal of Immunology: Official Journal of the American Association of Immunologists, 177*(1), 673–680. PubMed PMID: 16785566.

18. Raoust, E., Balloy, V., Garcia-Verdugo, I., et al. (2009). Pseudomonas aeruginosa LPS or flagellin are sufficient to activate TLR-dependent signaling in murine alveolar macrophages and airway epithelial cells. *PLoS ONE, 4*(10), e7259. PubMed PMID: 19806220.

19. Hiemstra, P. S., van Wetering, S., & Stolk, J. (1998). Neutrophil serine proteinases and defensins in chronic obstructive pulmonary disease: Effects on pulmonary epithelium. *The European Respiratory Journal, 12*(5), 1200–1208. PubMed PMID: 9864022.

20. Pardo, A., & Selman, M. (1999). Proteinase-antiproteinase imbalance in the pathogenesis of emphysema: The role of metalloproteinases in lung damage. *Histology and Histopathology, 14*(1), 227–233. PubMed PMID: 9987667.

21. Amitani, R., Wilson, R., et al. (1991). Effects of human neutrophil elastase and Pseudomonas aeruginosa proteinases on human respiratory epithelium. *American Journal of Respiratory Cell and Molecular Biology, 4*(1), 26–32. PubMed PMID: 1898852.

22. Bozinovski, S., Vlahos, R., Zhang, Y., et al. (2011). Carbonylation caused by cigarette smoke extract is associated with defective macrophage immunity. *American Journal of Respiratory Cell and Molecular Biology, 45*(2), 229–236. PubMed PMID: 20935190.

23. Sethi, S., Maloney, J., Grove, L., et al. (2006). Airway inflammation and bronchial bacterial colonization in chronic obstructive pulmonary disease. *American Journal of Respiratory and Critical Care Medicine, 173*(9), 991–998. PubMed PMID: 16474030.

24. Monso, E., Ruiz, J., Rosell, A., Manterola, J., et al. (1995). Bacterial infection in chronic obstructive pulmonary disease. A study of stable and exacerbated outpatients using the protected specimen brush. *American Journal of Respiratory and Critical Care Medicine, 152*(4 Pt. 1), 1316–1320. PubMed PMID: 7551388.

25. Sethi, S., Evans, N., Grant, B. J., & Murphy, T. F. (2002). New strains of bacteria and exacerbations of chronic obstructive pulmonary disease. *The New England Journal of Medicine, 347*(7), 465–471. PubMed PMID: 12181400.

26. Yen, S. S., & Morris, H. G. (1981). An imbalance of arachidonic acid metabolism in asthma. *Biochemical and Biophysical Research Communications, 103*(2), 774–779. PubMed PMID: 6800369.

27. Bowler, R. P., & Crapo, J. D. (2002). Oxidative stress in allergic respiratory diseases. *The Journal of Allergy and Clinical Immunology, 110*(3), 349–356. PubMed PMID: 12209079.

28. Horvath, I., Donnelly, L. E., Kiss, A., et al. (1998). Raised levels of exhaled carbon monoxide are associated with an increased expression of heme oxygenase-1 in airway macrophages in asthma: A new marker of oxidative stress. *Thorax, 53*(8), 668–672. PubMed PMID: 9828853.

29. Silkoff, P. E., Robbins, R. A., Gaston, B., et al. (2000). Endogenous nitric oxide in allergic airway disease. *The Journal of Allergy and Clinical Immunology, 105*(3), 438–448. PubMed PMID: 10719291.

30. Emelyanov, A., Fedoseev, G., Abulimity, A., et al. (2001). Elevated concentrations of exhaled hydrogen peroxide in asthmatic patients. *Chest, 120*(4), 1136–1139. PubMed PMID: 11591550.

31. Powell, C. V., Nash, A. A., Powers, H. J., & Primhak, R. A. (1994). Antioxidant status in asthma. *Pediatric Pulmonology, 18*(1), 34–38. PubMed PMID: 7970906.

32. Kinnula, V. L., & Crapo, J. D. (2003). Superoxide dismutases in the lung and human lung diseases. *American Journal of Respiratory and Critical Care Medicine, 167*(12), 1600–1619. PubMed PMID: 12796054.

33. Peacock, J. L., Anderson, H. R., Bremner, S. A., et al. (2011). Outdoor air pollution and respiratory health in patients with COPD. *Thorax, 66*(7), 591–596. PubMed PMID: 21459856.

34. Dominici, F., Peng, R. D., et al. (2006). Fine particulate air pollution and hospital admission for cardiovascular and respiratory diseases. *JAMA: The Journal of the American Medical Association, 295*(10), 1127–1134. PubMed PMID: 16522832.

35. Mariani, E., Bonati, E., et al. (2010). Respiratory function in subjects with chronic obstructive pulmonary disease (COPD) and atmospheric pollution in the city of Parma. Preliminary analysis. *Acta Bio-Medica: Atenei Parmensis, 81*(2), 109–114. PubMed PMID: 21305875.

36. Kariisa, M., Foraker, R., Pennell, M., et al. (2015). Short- and long-term effects of ambient ozone and fine particulate matter on the respiratory health of chronic obstructive pulmonary disease subjects. *Archives of Environmental and Occupational Health, 70*(1), 56–62. PubMed PMID: 25136856.

37. Traboulsi, H., Guerrina, N., Iu, M., et al. (2017). Inhaled pollutants: The molecular scene behind respiratory and systemic diseases associated with ultrafine particulate matter. *International Journal of Molecular Sciences, 18*(2), Pii: E243. PubMed PMID: 28125025.

38. Duhme, H., Weiland, S. K., Keil, U., et al. (1996). The association between self-reported symptoms of asthma and allergic rhinitis and self-reported traffic density on street of residence in adolescents. *Epidemiology (Cambridge, Mass.), 7*(6), 578–582. PubMed PMID: 8899382.

39. Weiland, S. K., Mundt, K. A., Ruckmann, A., & Keil, U. (1994). Self-reported wheezing and allergic rhinitis in children and traffic density on street of residence. *Annals of Epidemiology, 4*(3), 243–247. PubMed PMID: 7519948.

40. Van Vliet, P., Knape, M., de Hartog, J., Janssen, N., Harssema, H., & Brunekreef, B. (1977). Motor vehicle exhaust and chronic respiratory symptoms in children living near freeways. *Environmental Research, 74*, 122–132. PubMed PMID: 9339225.

41. Venn, A., Yemaneberhan, H., et al. (2005). Proximity of the home to roads and the risk of wheeze in an Ethiopian population. *Occupational and Environmental Medicine, 62*(6), 376–380. PubMed PMID: 15901884.

42. Oosterlee, A., Drijver, M., Lebret, E., & Brunekreef, B. (1966). Chronic respiratory symptoms in children and adults living along streets with high traffic density. *Occupational and Environmental Medicine, 53*, 241–247. PubMed PMID: 8664961.

43. Venn, A. J., Lewis, S. A., Cooper, M., et al. (2001). Living near a main road and the risk of wheezing illness in children. *American Journal of Respiratory and Critical Care Medicine, 164*(12), 2177–2180. PubMed PMID: 11751183.

44. Jammes, Y., Delpierre, S., Delvolgo, M. J., Humbert-Tena, C., & Burnet, H. (1998). Long-term exposure of adults to outdoor air pollution in associated with increased airway obstruction and higher prevalence of bronchial hyper responsiveness. *Archives of Environmental Health, 53*(6), 372–377. PubMed PMID: 9886154.

45. Alessandrini, F., Schulz, H., et al. (2006). Effects of ultrafine carbon particle inhalation on allergic inflammation of the lung. *The Journal of Allergy and Clinical Immunology, 117*(4), 824–830. PubMed PMID: 16630940.

46. Wade, J. F., & Newman, L. S. (1993). Diesel asthma, reactive airway disease following overexposure to locomotive exhaust. *Journal of Occupational Medicine, 35*(2), 149–154. PubMed PMID: 8433186.

47. Kinney, P. L., Nilsen, D. M., Lippmann, M., Brescia, M., Gordon, T., McGovern, T., et al. (1996). Biomarkers of lung inflammation in recreational joggers exposed to ozone. *American Journal of Respiratory and Critical Care Medicine, 154*(5), 1430–1435. PubMed PMID:8912760.

48. Glizia, A., & Kinney, P. L. (1999). Long-term residence in areas of high ozone: Associations with respiratory health in a nationwide sample of nonsmoking young adults. *Environmental Health Perspectives, 107*(8), 675–679. PubMed PMID: 10417367.

49. Gong, H., Shamoo, D., Anderson, K., & Linn, W. (1997). Responses of older men with and without chronic obstructive pulmonary disease to prolonged ozone exposure. *Archives of Environmental Health, 52*(1), 18–25. PubMed PMID: 9039853.

50. Weisel, C. P., Cody, R. P., & Lioy, P. J. (1995). Relationship between summertime ambient ozone levels and emergency department visits for asthma in central New Jersey. *Environmental Health Perspectives, 103*(Suppl. 2), 97–102. PubMed PMID: 7614954.

51. Kim, B. J., Kwon, J. W., Seo, J. H., Kim, H. B., Lee, S. Y., Park, K. S., et al. (2011). Association of ozone exposure with asthma, allergic rhinitis, and allergic sensitization. *Annals of Allergy, Asthma and Immunology, 107*(3), 214–219, e1. PubMed PMID: 21875539.

52. Penard-Morand, C., Charpin, D., Raherison, C., Kopferschmitt, C., Caillaud, D., Lavaud, F., et al. (2005). Long-term exposure to background air pollution related to respiratory and allergic health in schoolchildren. *Clinical and Experimental Allergy:*

Journal of the British Society for Allergy and Clinical Immunology, 35(10), 1279–1287. PubMed PMID: 16238786.

53. Abramson, M. J., Benke, G. P., Cui, J., de Klerk, N. H., Del Monaco, A., Dennekamp, M., et al. (2010). Is potroom asthma due more to sulphur dioxide than fluoride? An inception cohort study in the Australian aluminium industry. *Occupational and Environmental Medicine, 67*(10), 679–685. PubMed PMID: 20798006.

54. Liao, C. M., Hsieh, N. H., & Chio, C. P. (2011). Fluctuation analysis-based risk assessment for respiratory virus activity and air pollution associated asthma incidence. *The Science of the Total Environment, 409*(18), 3325–3333. PubMed PMID: 21663946.

55. Koenig, J. Q., Covert, D. S., Hanley, W. S., Van Belle, G., & Pierson, W. E. (1990). Prior exposure to ozone potentiates subsequent response to sulfur dioxide in adolescent asthmatic subjects. *The American Review of Respiratory Disease, 141*, 377–380. PubMed PMID: 2301855.

56. U.S. Environmental Protection Agency. *Indoor Air Quality (IAQ): Nitrogen Dioxide's Impact on Indoor Air Quality.* Available at https://www.epa.gov/indoor-air-quality-iaq/nitrogen-dioxides-impact-indoor-air-quality (Accessed 15 November 2017).

57. Pereira, G., Cook, A., De Vos, A. J., & Holman, C. D. (2010). A case-crossover analysis of traffic-related air pollution and emergency department presentations for asthma in Perth, Western Australia. *The Medical Journal of Australia, 193*(9), 511–514. PubMed PMID: 21034384.

58. Krmpoti, D., Luzar-Stiffler, V., Rakusic, N., Stipic Markovic, A., Hrga, I., & Pavlovic, M. (2011). Effects of traffic air pollution and hornbeam pollen on adult asthma hospitalizations in Zagreb. *International Archives of Allergy and Immunology, 156*(1), 62–68. PubMed PMID: 21447960.

59. Strand, V., Svartengren, M., Rak, S., Barck, C., & Bylin, G. (1998). Repeated exposure to an ambient level of NO2 enhances asthmatic response to a nonsymptomatic allergen dose. *The European Respiratory Journal, 12*(1), 6–12. PubMed PMID: 9701406.

60. Wang, J. H., Devalia, J. L., Duddle, J. M., Hamilton, S. A., & Davies, R. J. (1995). Effects of six-hour exposure to nitrogen dioxide on early phase nasal response to allergen challenge in patients with a history of seasonal allergic rhinitis. *The Journal of Allergy and Clinical Immunology, 96*(5 Pt. 1), 669–676. PubMed PMID: 7599684.

61. Jindal, S. K., & Gupta, D. (2004). The relationship between tobacco smoke and bronchial asthma. *The Indian Journal of Medical Research, 120*(5), 443–453. PubMed PMID: 15591628.

62. Chen, Y., Dales, R., et al. (1999). Increased effects of smoking and obesity on asthma among female Canadians: The National Population Health Survey, 1994-1995. *American Journal of Epidemiology, 150*(3), 255–262. PubMed PMID: 10430229.

63. Ehrlich, R. I., Du Toit, D., Jordaan, E., et al. (1996). Risk factors for childhood asthma and wheezing. Importance of maternal and household smoking. *American Journal of Respiratory and Critical Care Medicine, 154*(3 Pt. 1), 681–688. PubMed PMID: 8810605.

64. Li, Y. F., Gilliland, F. D., Berhane, K., et al. (2000). Effects of in utero and environmental tobacco smoke exposure on lung function in boys and girls with and without asthma. *American Journal of Respiratory and Critical Care Medicine, 162*(6), 2097–2104. PubMed PMID: 11112121.

65. Lux, A. L., Henderson, A. J., & Pocock, S. J. (2000). Wheeze associated with prenatal tobacco smoke exposure: A prospective, longitudinal study. ALSPAC Study Team. *Archives of Disease in Childhood, 83*(4), 307–312. PubMed PMID: 10999864.

66. Polosa, R., Knoke, J. D., Russo, C., et al. (2008). Cigarette smoking is associated with a greater risk of incident asthma in allergic rhinitis. *The Journal of Allergy and Clinical Immunology, 121*(6), 1428–1434. PubMed PMID: 18436295.

67. Jindal, S. K. (2014). Effects of smoking on asthma. *The Journal of the Association of Physicians of India, 62*(Suppl. 3), 32–37. PubMed PMID: 25327058.

68. Chaudhuri, R., Livingston, E., McMahon, A. D., et al. (2003). Cigarette smoking impairs the therapeutic response to oral corticosteroids in chronic asthma. *American Journal of Respiratory and Critical Care Medicine, 168*(11), 1308–1311. PubMed PMID: 12893649.

69. Tomlinson, J. E., McMahon, A. D., Chaudhuri, R., et al. (2005). Efficacy of low and high dose inhaled corticosteroid in smokers versus nonsmokers with mild asthma. *Thorax, 60*(4), 282–287. PubMed PMID: 15790982.

70. Bloom, J. W., Kaltenborn, W., Paoletti, P., Camilli, A., & Lebowitz, M. (1987). Respiratory effects of non-tobacco cigarettes. *British Medical Journal (Clinical Research Ed.), 295*, 1516–1518. PubMed PMID: 3122882.

71. Tashkin, D. P., Baldwin, G. C., Sarafian, T., Dubinett, S., & Roth, M. D. (2002). Respiratory and immunologic

consequences of marijuana smoking. *Journal of Clinical Pharmacology, 42*(Suppl. 11), 715–815. PubMed PMID: 12412839.

72. Jindal, S. K., & Gupta, D. (2004). The relationship between tobacco smoke and bronchial asthma. *The Indian Journal of Medical Research, 120*(5), 443–453. PubMed PMID: 15591628.

73. Centers for Disease Control and Prevention (CDC). (2008). Smoking-attributable mortality, years of potential life lost, and productivity losses – United States, 2000-2004. *MMWR. Morbidity and Mortality Weekly Report, 57*(45), 1226–1228. PubMed PMID: 19008791.

74. Mortaz, E., Henricks, P. A., Kraneveld, A. D., Givi, M. E., et al. (2011). Cigarette smoke induces the release of CXCL8 from human bronchial epithelial cells via TLRs and induction of the inflammasome. *Biochimica et Biophysica Acta, 1812*(9), 1104–1110. PubMed PMID: 21684332.

75. Mortaz, E., Adcock, I. M., Ito, K., et al. (2010). Cigarette smoke induces CXCL8 production by human neutrophils via activation of TLR9 receptor. *The European Respiratory Journal, 36*(5), 1143–1154. PubMed PMID: 19840968.

76. Barnes, P. J. (2009). The cytokine network in chronic obstructive pulmonary disease. *American Journal of Respiratory Cell and Molecular Biology, 41*(6), 631–638. PubMed PMID: 19717810.

77. Cunningham, T. J., Ford, E. S., Rolle, I. V., et al. (2015). Associations of self-reported cigarette smoking with chronic obstructive pulmonary disease and co-morbid chronic conditions in the United States. *COPD, 12*(3), 276–286. PubMed PMID: 25207639.

78. U.S. Department of Health and Human Services (2014). *The Health Consequences of Smoking – 50 Years of Progress: A Report of the Surgeon General.* Retrieved from https://www.surgeongeneral.gov/library/reports/50-years-of-progress/index.html (Accessed 25 April 2017).

79. Kurmi, O. P., Li, L., Wang, J., Millwood, I. Y., Chen, J., et al. (2015). COPD and its association with smoking in the Mainland China: A cross-sectional analysis of 0.5 million men and women from ten diverse areas. *International Journal of Chronic Obstructive Pulmonary Disease, 10*, 655–665. PubMed PMID: 25848242.

80. Kirkhorn, S. R., & Garry, V. F. (2000). Agricultural lung diseases. *Environmental Health Perspectives, 108*(Suppl. 4), 705–712. PubMed PMID: 10931789.

81. Senthilselvan, A., McDuffie, H. H., & Dosman, J. A. (1992). Association of asthma with use of pesticides. Results of a cross-sectional survey of farmers. *The American Review of Respiratory Disease, 146*(4), 884–887. PubMed PMID: 1416414.

82. Hoppin, J. A., Umbach, D. M., London, S. J., et al. (2006). Pesticides and adult respiratory outcomes in the agricultural health study. *Annals of the New York Academy of Sciences, 1076*, 343–354. PubMed PMID: 17119214.

83. Eduard, W., Omenaas, E., Bakke, P. S., et al. (2004). Atopic and non-atopic asthma in a farming and a general population. *American Journal of Industrial Medicine, 46*(4), 396–399. PubMed PMID: 15376208.

84. Hoppin, J. A., Umbach, D. M., London, S. J., et al. (2009). Pesticide use and adult-onset asthma among male farmers in the Agricultural Health Study. *The European Respiratory Journal, 34*(6), 1296–1303. PubMed PMID: 19541724.

85. Respiratory health hazards in agriculture. (1998). *American Journal of Respiratory and Critical Care Medicine, 158*(5 Pt. 2), S1–S76. PubMed PMID: 9817727.

86. Kimbell-Dunn, M., Bradshaw, L., Slater, T., et al. (1999). Asthma and allergy in New Zealand farmers. *American Journal of Industrial Medicine, 35*(1), 51–57. PubMed PMID: 9884745.

87. Dalphin, J. C., Dubiez, A., et al. (1998). Prevalence of asthma and respiratory symptoms in dairy farmers in the French province of the Doubs. *American Journal of Respiratory and Critical Care Medicine, 158*(5 Pt. 1), 1493–1498. PubMed PMID: 9817698.

88. Mamane, A., Baldi, I., Tessier, J. F., Raherison, C., & Bouvier, G. (2015). Occupational exposure to pesticides and respiratory health. *European Respiratory Review : An Official Journal of the European Respiratory Society, 24*(136), 306–319. PubMed PMID: 26028642.

89. Erden, E. S., Motor, S., Ustun, I., Demirkose, M., et al. (2014). Investigation of bisphenol A as an endocrine disruptor, total thiol, malondialdehyde, and C-reactive protein levels in chronic obstructive pulmonary disease. *European Review for Medical and Pharmacological Sciences, 18*(22), 3477–3483. PubMed PMID: 25491624.

90. Das, D., Bindhani, B., Mukherjee, B., Saha, H., Biswas, P., Dutta, K., et al. (2014). Chronic low-level arsenic exposure reduces lung function in male population without skin lesions. *International Journal of Public Health, 59*(4), 655–663. PubMed PMID: 24879317.

91. Parvez, F., Chen, Y., et al. (2013). Arsenic exposure and impaired lung function. Findings from a large population-based prospective cohort study. *American Journal of Respiratory and Critical Care Medicine, 188*(7), 813–819. PubMed PMID: 23848239.

92. D'Ippoliti, D., Santelli, E., et al. (2015). Arsenic in drinking water and mortality for cancer and chronic diseases in central Italy, 1990-2010. *PLoS ONE*, *10*(9), e0138182. PubMed PMID: 26383851.

93. Dauphine, D. C., Ferreccio, C., et al. (2011). Lung function in adults following in utero and childhood exposure to arsenic in drinking water: Preliminary findings. *International Archives of Occupational and Environmental Health*, *84*(6), 591–600. PubMed PMID: 20972800.

94. Davison, A. G., Fayers, P. M., Taylor, A. J., et al. (1988). Cadmium fume inhalation and emphysema. *Lancet*, *1*(8587), 663–667. PubMed PMID: 2895211.

95. Mannino, D. M., Holguin, F., Greves, H. M., et al. (2004). Urinary cadmium levels predict lower lung function in current and former smokers: Data from the Third National Health and Nutrition Examination Survey. *Thorax*, *59*(3), 194–198. PubMed PMID: 14985551.

96. Rokadia, H., & Agarwal, S. (2013). Serum heavy metals and obstructive lung disease: Results from the National Health and Nutrition Examination Survey. *Chest*, *143*(2), 388–397. PubMed PMID: 22911427.

97. Leem, A. Y., Kim, S. K., Chang, J., Kang, Y. A., Kim, Y. S., et al. (2015). Relationship between blood levels of heavy metals and lung function based on the Korean National Health and Nutrition Examination Survey IV-V. *International Journal of Chronic Obstructive Pulmonary Disease*, *10*, 1559–1570. PubMed PMID: 26345298.

98. Oh, C. M., Oh, I. H., Lee, J. K., et al. (2014). Blood cadmium levels are associated with a decline in lung function in males. *Environmental Research*, *132*, 119–125. PubMed PMID: 24769560.

99. Chung, H. K., Chang, Y. S., & Ahn, C. W. (2015). Effects of blood lead levels on airflow limitations in Korean adults: Findings from the 5th KNHNES 2011. *Environmental Research*, *136*, 274–279. PubMed PMID: 25460646.

100. Feng, W., Huang, X., Zhang, C., Liu, C., et al. (2015). The dose-response association of urinary metals with altered pulmonary function and risks of restrictive and obstructive lung diseases: A population-based study in China. *BMJ Open*, *5*(5), e007643. PubMed PMID: 25998037.

101. Mudarri, D., & Fisk, W. J. (2007). Public health and economic impact of dampness and mold. *Indoor Air*, *17*(3), 226–235. PubMed PMID: 17542835.

102. Fisk, W. J., Lei-Gomez, Q., & Mendell, M. J. (2007). Meta-analyses of the associations of respiratory health effects with dampness and mold in homes. *Indoor Air*, *17*(4), 284–296. PubMed PMID: 17661925.

103. Cox-Ganser, J. M., White, S. K., Jones, R., et al. (2005). Respiratory morbidity in office workers in a water-damaged building. *Environmental Health Perspectives*, *113*(4), 485–490. PubMed PMID: 15811840.

104. Institute of Medicine (U.S.). Committee on Damp Indoor Spaces and Health, Board on Health Promotion and Disease Prevention of the National Academies (2004). *Damp indoor spaces and health*. Washington, DC: National Academies Press.

105. Miller, J. D., & McMullin, D. R. (2014). Fungal secondary metabolites as harmful indoor air contaminants: 10 years on. *Applied Microbiology and Biotechnology*, *98*(24), 9953–9966. PubMed PMID: 25363558.

106. Kirenga, B. J., Schwartz, J. I., et al. (2015). Guidance on the diagnosis and management of asthma among adults in resource limited settings. *African Health Sciences*, *15*(4), 1189–1199. PubMed PMID: 26958020.

107. Shavelle, R. M., Paculdo, D. R., et al. (2009). Life expectancy and years of life lost in chronic obstructive pulmonary disease: Findings from the NHANES III follow-up study. *International Journal of Chronic Obstructive Pulmonary Disease*, *4*, 137–148. PubMed PMID: 19436692.

108. GOLD COPD Committee. (2017). *Global Strategy for the Diagnosis, Management and Prevention of COPD*. Global Initiative for Chronic Obstructive Lung Disease. http://goldcopd.org (Accessed 14 May 2017).

109. Haughney, J., Gruffydd-Jones, K., et al. (2014). The distribution of COPD in UK general practice using the new GOLD classification. *The European Respiratory Journal*, *43*(4), 993–1002. PubMed PMID: 24176990.

110. Mapel, D. W., Dalal, A. A., Johnson, P. T., et al. (2015). Application of the new GOLD COPD staging system to a US primary care cohort, with comparison to physician and patient impressions of severity. *International Journal of Chronic Obstructive Pulmonary Disease*, *10*, 1477–1486. PubMed PMID: 26251587.

111. Gan, W. Q., Man, S. F., Senthilselvan, A., & Sin, D. D. (2004). Association between chronic obstructive pulmonary disease and systemic inflammation: A systematic review and meta-analysis. *Thorax*, *59*(7), 574–580. PubMed PMID: 15223864.

112. Stockley, R. A. (2009). Progression of chronic obstructive pulmonary disease: Impact of inflammation, comorbidities and therapeutic intervention. *Current Medical Research and Opinion*, *25*(5), 1235–1245. PubMed PMID: 19335322.

113. Nadeem, A., Raj, H. G., & Chhabra, S. K. (2005). Increased oxidative stress and altered levels of

antioxidants in chronic obstructive pulmonary disease. *Inflammation, 29*(1), 23–32. PubMed PMID: 16502343.

114. Arja, C., Surapaneni, K. M., Raya, P., et al. (2013). Oxidative stress and antioxidant enzyme activity in South Indian male smokers with chronic obstructive pulmonary disease. *Respirology, 18*(7), 1069–1075. PubMed PMID: 23683270.

115. Pelletier, O. (1968). Smoking and vitamin C levels in humans. *The American Journal of Clinical Nutrition, 21,* 1259–1267. PubMed PMID: 5699721.

116. National Research Council (1989). *Recommended dietary allowances* (10th ed.). Washington, DC: National Academy Press.

117. Fewtrell, C. M. S., & Gomperts, B. D. (1977). Effect of flavone inhibitors of transport ATPase on histamine secretion from rat mast cells. *Nature, 265,* 635–636. PubMed PMID: 67562.

118. Bielory, L., & Gandhi, R. (1994). Asthma and vitamin C. *Annals Allergy, 73,* 89–96. PubMed PMID: 8067602.

119. Johnston, C. S., Martin, L. J., & Cai, X. (1992). Antihistamine effect of supplemental ascorbic acid and neutrophil chemotaxis. *Journal of the American College of Nutrition, 11,* 172–176. PubMed PMID: 1578094.

120. Tse, H. N., Raiteri, L., Wong, K. Y., et al. (2013). High-dose N-acetylcysteine in stable COPD: The 1-year, double-blind, randomized, placebo-controlled HIACE study. *Chest, 144*(1), 106–118. PubMed PMID: 23348146.

121. Zheng, J. P., Wen, F. Q., Bai, C. X., Wan, H. Y., et al. (2014). Twice daily N-acetylcysteine 600 mg for exacerbations of chronic obstructive pulmonary disease (PANTHEON): A randomized, double-blind placebo-controlled trial. *The Lancet Respiratory Medicine, 2*(3), 187–194. PubMed PMID: 24621680.

122. Venkatesan, N., Punithavathi, D., & Babu, M. (2007). Protection from acute and chronic lung diseases by curcumin. *Advances in Experimental Medicine and Biology, 595,* 379–405. PubMed PMID: 17569221.

123. Rennolds, J., Malireddy, S., Hassan, F., et al. (2012). Curcumin regulates airway epithelial cell cytokine responses to the pollutant cadmium. *Biochemical and Biophysical Research Communications, 417*(1), 256–261. PubMed PMID: 22142850.

124. Misso, N. L., Powers, K. A., Gillon, R. L., et al. (1996). Reduced platelet glutathione peroxidase activity and serum selenium concentration in atopic asthmatic patients. *Clinical and Experimental Allergy: Journal of the British Society for Allergy and Clinical Immunology, 26,* 838–847. PubMed PMID: 8842559.

125. Stone, J. (1989). Reduced selenium status of patients with asthma. *Clinical Science, 77,* 495–500. PubMed PMID: 2582721.

126. Kadrabova, J., Mad'aric, A., Kovacikova, Z., et al. (1996). Selenium status is decreased in patients with intrinsic asthma. *Biological Trace Element Research, 52,* 241–248. PubMed PMID: 8811281.

127. Hope, W. C., et al. (1983). In vitro inhibition of the biosynthesis of slow reacting substance of anaphylaxis (SRS-A) and lipoxygenase activity by quercetin. *Biochemical Pharmacology, 32,* 367–371. PubMed PMID: 6191762.

128. Foreman, J. C. (1984). Mast cells and the actions of flavonoids. *The Journal of Allergy and Clinical Immunology, 73,* 769–774. PubMed PMID: 6202730.

129. Janssens, W., Bouillon, R., Claes, B., et al. (2010). Vitamin D deficiency is highly prevalent in COPD and correlates with variants in the vitamin D-binding gene. *Thorax, 65*(3), 215–220. PubMed PMID: 19996341.

130. Black, P. N., & Scragg, R. (2005). Relationship between serum 25-hydroxyvitamin D and pulmonary function in the Third National Health and Nutrition Examination Survey. *Chest, 128*(6), 3792–3798. PubMed PMID: 16354847.

47

Cardiovascular Toxicity

SUMMARY

- Presence in population: Cardiovascular disease (CVD) remains the leading cause of mortality, with 11.5% of the US population having been diagnosed with some form of CVD
- Major diseases: Myocardial infarction, sudden cardiac death, stroke, congestive heart failure, hypertension

- Primary sources: Ambient air pollution ($PM_{2.5}$, PM_{10}, proximity to roadways), plastics, persistent organic pollutants, metals
- Best measure: Conventional cardiovascular workup and environmental exposure review
- Best intervention: Avoidance, supplementation, and depuration

OVERVIEW/INTRODUCTION

CVD is the leading cause of death in the United States, accounting for close to a quarter of all deaths.[1] CVDs include hypertension, stroke, myocardial infarction (MI), cardiac arrest, and congestive heart failure. Atherosclerosis (perhaps best described as endothelial damage) is a basic underlying mechanism present in all the CVD states. Carotid intima-media thickness (CIMT) is now established to be an excellent marker for the development of atherosclerosis and for predicting disease progression.[2] As CIMT increases, the risk of stroke increases 32% per each standard deviation, and MI risk increases 26%.

DISEASE MANIFESTATION

The American Heart Association (AHA) lists major (unavoidable) risks, modifiable risks, and contributing risks.[3] Being male of advancing age with a family history of heart disease comprise the three major risks for heart disease. The modifiable risks are smoking, high cholesterol, high blood pressure, physical inactivity, obesity, and diabetes mellitus. Contributing factors include stress and alcohol as well as diet and overall nutrition. Environmental toxicants (summarized in Box 47.1), though strongly associated with CVD, have still not been added to the list of modifiable risk factors.

Ambient Air Pollution From Vehicular Sources

Although the AHA website does not list air pollution as a main modifiable cause of heart disease, the AHA convened an expert panel that published a statement[4] in 2004 with the following conclusions:

- Short-term exposure to elevated particular matter (PM) significantly contributes to increased acute cardiovascular mortality, particularly in certain at-risk subsets of the population.
- Hospital admissions for several cardiovascular and pulmonary diseases acutely increase in response to higher ambient PM concentrations.
- Prolonged exposure to elevated levels of PM reduces overall life expectancy by a few years.

A more recent expert panel containing many of the same individuals updated their statements based on research published between 2004 and 2015.[5] Their conclusion reads in part as follows:

"There is now abundant evidence that air pollution contributes to the risk of cardiovascular disease and

549

> BOX 47.1   **Primary Toxicants Affecting Cardiovascular Health Risk Factors**
>
> Ambient air pollution from vehicular exhaust
> Tobacco smoke
> PCBs
> Bisphenol A
> Phthalates
> Metals

associated mortality, underpinned by credible evidence of multiple mechanisms that may drive this association. In light of this evidence, efforts to reduce exposure to air pollution should urgently be intensified and supported by appropriate and effective legislation."

PM causes significant oxidative damage in the tissues and organs that it reaches[6,7,8] and has been associated with increased mortality primarily from cardiovascular,[9,10] respiratory,[11] and neoplastic diseases.[12] Adsorbed to PM are multiple polycyclic aromatic hydrocarbons and volatile organic compounds, which account for some of their toxic effects.[13] Aromatic hydrocarbons, including benzo-a-pyrene, are produced from combustion of wood, tobacco, gasoline, and diesel. The main metabolite of pyrenes, 1-hydroxypyrene (1-OHP), is found higher in persons who had recently experienced an acute MI than in persons who did not have a heart attack.[14] The urinary levels of 1-OHP were also significantly associated with elevations of malondialdehyde and high-sensitivity C-reactive protein (hsCRP) and lower levels of β-carotene and superoxide dismutase activity.

Cardiovascular Mortality. Increased mortality has been associated with elevated levels of both $PM_{2.5}$ and PM_{10}. Persons living in larger cities are 15% to 17% more likely to die a premature death than people living in cities with less polluted air.[15] Cardiovascular mortality is significantly associated with $PM_{2.5}$, PM_{10}, and elemental carbon (ultrafine), along with other air pollutants (CO, NO_2, SO_2), among older individuals in the Phoenix valley (Arizona, United States).[16] In Sydney, Australia, increased mortality has been found with exposures to total PM, ozone, and NO_2.[17] When the daily mean of an individual's pollutants increased from the 10th to the 90th percentile, all-cause mortality increased 2.63% for total PM, 2.04% for ozone, and 2.66% for NO_2. Increase in the daily mean led to 2.68% increased cardiovascular mortality for total PM,

2.52% for ozone, and 2.34 for NO_2. Respiratory mortality also increased by 3.24% for PM and 7.71% for NO_2. Nonaccidental death risk, including cardiovascular-related mortality, increased 22% with each 10 $\mu g/m^3$ of $PM_{2.5}$.[18] When individual mortality risks were assessed, each 10 $\mu g/m^3$ rise of $PM_{2.5}$ increased the risk of ischemic heart disease death by 43% and fatality from an acute MI by 64%.

Living close to a major roadway alone confers increased risk of dying from an acute heart attack. By collecting data on home location/proximity from 3886 persons presenting to hospitals with an acute MI, it was found that those living between 200 and 1000 meters from a major roadway were 13% more likely to have a fatal heart attack than those living more than 1000 meters away. If they lived 100 to 200 meters from a major roadway, they were 19% more likely to die of their heart attack. Those that lived closest to high traffic (within 100 meters) had the highest risk of dying from their MI, with an odds ratio of 1.27.[19]

PM_{10} increases the levels of platelets, fibrinogen, and C-reactive protein, all of which are risk factors for CVD.[20,21] PM exposure has been associated with indicators of autonomic function of the heart including increased heart rate, decreased heart rate variability (HRV), and increased cardiac arrhythmias. Exposure to vehicular traffic exhaust alone triples the risk of experiencing an acute MI within an hour after exposure in susceptible individuals.[22]

Atherosclerosis. $PM_{2.5}$ in the Los Angeles area is among the highest in the nation with an average median range between 13.4 and 27.1 $\mu g/m^3$. $PM_{2.5}$ levels were positively associated with increased CIMT in a group of 798 residents of the Los Angeles area.[23] For each 10 $\mu g/m^3$ of $PM_{2.5}$, the CIMT increased by 5.9%. Those on lipid-lowering agents had almost triple the increase in CIMT (15.8%) from each 10 $\mu g/m^3$ rise in $PM_{2.5}$, and in women over the age of 60, CIMT increased an average of 19.2%. The national median average of $PM_{2.5}$ ranges from a low average of 4.68 to a high of 15.56, with areas such as Los Angeles basin attaining even higher levels. With the lowest average Los Angeles $PM_{2.5}$ levels at 13.4 (more than twice as high as the national low average), greater CIMT would be the norm for those residents. Those in the highest $PM_{2.5}$ levels in Los Angeles can have close to three times the CIMT as those in cleaner areas of the country.

The typical annual progression of CIMT for an urban dweller is 2.04 μm/year. But for those living within 100 m of a highway, the progression more than doubled to

5.62 μm/year. For each 10 μg/m^3 increase in both indoor and outdoor PM$_{2.5}$, CIMT progression increased by an additional 1.72 μm and 2.53 μm, respectively.[24] A group of 5660 persons without preexisting CVD from five different states in the United States (Baltimore, Maryland; Chicago, Illinois; Forsyth County, North Carolina; Los Angeles County, California; Northern Manhattan and Southern Bronx, New York; and St. Paul, Minnesota) were monitored with carotid artery ultrasounds in 2002 and again in 2005.[25] The median annual PM$_{2.5}$ exposure for this huge cohort was 16.6 μg/m^3 with an annual increase in CIMT of 14 μm/year, both far higher than national averages. Airborne PM$_{2.5}$ levels were positively correlated with progression of CIMT in all persons after adjusting for potential confounders. The researchers noted that persons with higher PM$_{2.5}$ in their indoor air had an additional 5 μm/year increase in CIMT. If their outdoor PM$_{2.5}$ stayed high, they had an additional 3.8 μm/year increase in CIMT. And for those in areas where the PM$_{2.5}$ dropped, each 1 μg/m^3 decrease was rewarded with a 2.8 μm/year reduction in normal progression of CIMT. These statistics make a very good case for utilizing a high-quality air purifier in the home.

Greater coronary artery calcification (CAC) has also been associated with exposure to high level of vehicular pollution. A group of German researchers compared electron-beam computed tomography (CT) measurements of CAC in 4494 adults with their residential proximity to major roadways.[26] Persons living within 50 meters of busy roadways had a 63% greater risk of having high CAC. Those living 51 to 100 meters away were 34% more likely to have a high CAC score, whereas those living 101 to 200 meters from a major roadway were only 8% more likely to have a high CAC.

Not surprisingly, PM$_{2.5}$ is also associated with an increase in blood pressure. After only 24 hours of moving from a suburban to an urban campus with higher PM$_{2.5}$, the average systolic blood pressure increased by 1.08 mm Hg, and the diastolic by 0.96 mm Hg in 39 healthy university students.[27]

ST-Segment Depression. The effect of air pollution on ST-depression, reflective of myocardial ischemia, was studied over a course of 10 consecutive days, with continuous electrocardiogram (ECG) monitoring, on 38 Los Angeles residents with a history of coronary artery disease.[28] Each interquartile increase of aromatic hydrocarbons (but not ozone) was associated with a 15.4%

increased risk of ST-depression. Daily counts of ST-segment depression findings were consistently associated with aromatic hydrocarbon levels and with a 2-day average of ultrafine particulate matter. ST-depression was also greater in a group of 20 men with previous (but stable) MI who were exposed to dilute diesel exhaust during moderate exercise. When they exercised with diesel exhaust particulate (DEP) exposure, their ST-depression was close to triple the depression that occurred with exercise alone.[29] Those with DEP exposure also showed a greater tendency toward clotting by having lower fibrinolytic capacity.

Oxidation of LDL. Oxidized low density lipoprotein (LDL-ox) is a well-established biomarker for the presence of subclinical atherosclerosis and plaque formation. Levels of LDL-ox greater than 117 U/L are strongly associated with increased risk of having carotid plaques.[30] LDL-ox was measured in a group of 79 nonsmoking diabetic individuals along with the amount of carbon in their airway macrophages, which is reflective of the person's daily exposure to the combustion of fossil fuels.[31] Comparing those two findings with their residential proximity to major roadways revealed that the further one lives from a busy roadway, the less oxidized LDL becomes. Each doubling of distance from a major roadway was associated with a 0.027 μm^2 decrease in macrophage carbon and a 2.9 U/L decrease in LDL-ox.

Indoor Air Pollutants

Solvent exposure in hair salons is positively associated with elevated CRP and 8-hydroxy deoxyguanosine (8-OHdG), indicating both inflammation and oxidative stress.[32] On days when the subjects were not working and therefore not exposed to the solvents, the CRP levels averaged 1.1 mg/dL and their 8-OHdG was 0.6 ng/mL, but on work days, these levels jumped to 10.9 mg/dL for CRP and 4.5 for 8-OHdG. The total airborne volatile organic compound (VOC) levels averaged 44 parts per billion (PPB) on nonworking days and 75 PPB on working days.

Reduced HRV is an established marker of cardiac autonomic dysfunction and increased risk for cardiovascular events and mortality.[33] Significant changes in markers of HRV were associated with use of indoor freshening sprays at least 1 day weekly that worsened with increased frequency of use.[34] Associations were also found between the use of cleaning sprays and other home scented products and HRV.

Tobacco smoke exposure has long been associated with increased risk of heart disease and is listed as the first modifiable risk by the AHA. Because of the known health risks of environmental tobacco smoke (ETS), many areas of the country have passed laws prohibiting smoking in workplaces, restaurants, and other areas where people are gathered. Minnesota enjoyed a 33% reduction in acute MI within 18 months of the enactment their 2002 law forbidding smoking in workplaces, restaurants, and bars.[35] Sudden cardiac death declined by 17% in the same time frame, while the rates of the major CV risk factors of hypertension, diabetes mellitus, hypercholesterolemia, and obesity either stayed constant or increased.

Persistent Organic Pollutants

Data from 1999 to 2002 National Health and Nutrition Examination Survey (NHANES) was assessed for the possible connection between persistent organic pollutant (POP) serum levels and cardiovascular illness.[36] When serum levels of 21 POPs (3 dioxins, 3 furans, 11 polychlorinated biphenyls [PCBs], and 4 chlorinated pesticides) were compared with health histories, it was found that men with detectable levels of PCBs and dioxins had increased risk of cardiovascular illnesses, whereas women showed increased risk from detectable levels of PCBs, dioxins, and chlorinated pesticides. It should be noted that simply the detection of these toxicants in the blood was sufficient to increase CV risk, as can be seen in Table 47.1, where those with PCBs in the 25th percentile had the greatest increase in risk for all but one PCB.

Interestingly, the most common dietary source for PCBs 118, 138, 153, and 180 is farmed salmon and sardines, with a lesser amount from hamburgers.[37] Because salmon is considered by some a heart-protective "functional food," this is a very concerning study.

Swedish seniors with higher levels of PCBs 206, 170, 156, 153, 138, and 118 had more carotid artery atherosclerosis than those with lower PCB levels.[38] PCBs 170 and 156 both doubled the risk, yet PCBs 206 and 153 increased the risk by 65%, 138 by 46%, and 118 by 16%. PCB serum levels found in residents of Anniston, Alabama (living by a Monsanto plant that manufactured PCBs for decades), were positively correlated with elevated blood pressure.[39] PCBs 170, 172, 178, 180, 182, 187, 196, and 203 were significantly associated with both systolic and diastolic blood pressure increases. PCBs 99, 118, 105, 138, 153, and 180 were also significantly associated with a reduced left ventricular ejection fraction in Swedish seniors participating in the prospective investigation of the vasculature in Uppsala seniors (PIVUS) study.[40]

Bisphenol A and Phthalates

Urinary bisphenol A (BPA) levels can increase 1600% with the consumption of two soy beverages stored in cans versus glass. Along with that increase in urinary BPA, systolic blood pressure also increases by approximately 4.5 mm Hg.[41] Maternal exposure to BPA appears to confer on their children an increased risk for hypertension as well.[42] Data from the 18- and 74-year-olds participating in NHANES between 2003 to 2006 were used to compare their self-reporting of cardiovascular illnesses with urinary BPA levels.[43] Table 47.2 shows the odds ratio for the presence of any of those three manifestations of cardiovascular illness, after adjusting for all other CVD risk factors.

TABLE 47.1   Odds Ratio for Cardiovascular Disease Risk for Self-Reporting Women by Quartile of Detectable Levels of PCBs

PCB	Detection %	< 25%	25th–50th %	50th–75th %	> 75%
118 (DL)	87.7	1.8	0.6	1.3	4.5
156 (DL)	71.4	2.0	2.6	9.2	10.4
138 (NDL)	87.7	6.8	1.6	3.6	13.4
153 (NDL)	90.3	3.7	3.0	3.6	10.4
170 (NDL)	88.3	2.5	3.8	3.5	9.2
180 (NDL)	92.2	1.8	2.0	2.0	4.5
187 (NDL)	82.5	5.0	3.5	5.8	7.4

DL, Dioxin-like; *NDL,* nondioxin-like.
Data from Ha, M.-H., Lee, D.-H., & Jacobs, D. R. Association between serum concentrations of persistent organic pollutants and self-reported cardiovascular disease prevalence: Results from the National Health and Nutrition Examination Survey, 1999–2002. *Environmental Health Perspectives, 115*(8), 1204–1209.

TABLE 47.2 **Odds Ratio for Myocardial Infarction, Angina, CHD, CVD, and Diabetes by each Standard Deviation of Urinary BPA**

Condition	NHANES 2003-2004	NHANES 2005-2006	Pooled— 2003–2006
Myocardial infarction	1.40	1.39	1.32
Angina	1.27	1.16	1.24
Coronary heart disease	1.60	1.33	1.42
CVD (any of above)	1.34	1.18	1.26
Diabetes	1.40	1.02	1.24

Data from U.S. Department of Health and Human Services. (2013). *Fourth national report on human exposure to environmental chemicals: Updated tables, September 2013.* Retrieved from https://www.cdc.gov/exposurereport/pdf/FourthReport_UpdatedTables_Sep2013.pdf

TABLE 47.3 **Urinary Levels of BPA from NHANES 2002 to 2006**

NHANES BPA	50th %	75th %	95th %
2003–2004	2.80 ng/mL	5.50	16.0
2005–2006	2.00	3.70	11.5
2007–2008	2.10	4.10	13.0
2009–2010	1.90	3.50	9.60

Data from U.S. Department of Health and Human Services. (2013). *Fourth national report on human exposure to environmental chemicals: Updated tables, September 2013.* Retrieved from https://www.cdc.gov/exposurereport/pdf/FourthReport_UpdatedTables_Sep2013.pdf

Based on the data in Tables 47.2 and 47.3 the 25% of the population studied with a urinary BPA level of 3.70 to 5.50 were 34% more likely to have some form of CVD, whereas those in the 95th percentile would have doubled their risk. Participants without coronary artery disease in the Metabonomics and Genomics in Coronary Artery Disease (MaGiCAD) study in the United Kingdom had a mean urinary BPA of 1.28 ng/mL, while those with severe coronary artery disease had a mean of only 1.53 ng/mL.[44] Persons with higher urinary BPA were 43% more likely to have severe CAD. Increased risk of developing CAD over a 10-year time course was also significantly linked to BPA levels by a large European study.[45] Each 4.56 ng/mL increase of urinary BPA increased the CAD risk by 13%.

Swedish seniors in the PIVUS study also showed positive association between BPA and carotid atherosclerosis with both thickness of the carotid intima and echogenicity of plaque.[46] Data from this study also revealed a positive association between carotid atherosclerosis and monomethyl phthalates (MMP), monoisobutyl phthalate (MiBP), and mono-2-ethylhexyl phthalate (MEHP).

Heavy Metals

Lead—Hypertension and Cardiovascular Death.
Lead increases blood pressure by multiple mechanisms, including renal damage and oxidative damage, and, reducing available nitric oxide, increasing circulating vasoconstrictive prostaglandins, and altering the renin-angiotensin system.[47]

Female NHANES 1988 to 1994 participants with blood lead levels (BLLs) over 4 µg/dL (fourth quartile) had a greater risk of both systolic and diastolic hypertension than those with BLLs under 1.6 µg/dL (first quartile).[48] However, in postmenopausal women, the risk for diastolic hypertension was far higher with a 4.6-fold risk between just the first and second quartiles. Women with BLLs in the third quartile had a 5.9-fold increased risk, yet those in the top 25% of BLLs had a hypertensive risk 8.1 times higher. However, a pooling of NHANES data from 2003 to 2010 only found a nonsignificant association (p <0.060) between hypertension and BLL.[49] A key challenge in considering the effects of lead is that blood levels do not reflect chronic exposure, whereas bone lead is much more strongly correlated with disease risk.

Data from the Normative Aging Study revealed a significant correlation between tibial lead, elevations in serum creatinine, and elevated blood pressure.[50] Individuals with the highest patellar lead levels had the greatest risk for developing hypertension (odds ratio (OR) 1.71).[51] The data also revealed a synergistic effect of both stress and lead on hypertension.[52] Those who reported being highly stressed had a 2.6-fold increased risk for hypertension over those with the same level of bone lead who were not stressed. Lead is such a serious toxicant that even prenatal exposure gives children an increased risk of being hypertensive.[53]

The Normative Aging Study also revealed an association between both blood and tibial lead levels and increased risk of ischemic heart disease.[54] Not surprisingly, with hypertension and ischemic heart disease linked to lead burden, cardiac mortality should not be far behind. So far, two studies have utilized data from NHANES 2 and showed mortality risk associated with lead burden. A 2002 study revealed that those individuals in the 95th percentile of BLL had a 46% greater likelihood of all-cause mortality and a 39% greater risk of dying from cardiovascular issues. After observing this cohort for 12 years, it was found that those persons whose BLLs were >3.62 µg/dL were 55% more likely to die of CVD and 25% more likely to die of all causes.[55]

Methylmercury—Hypertension and Atherosclerosis

The intake of high omega-3 fish has been associated with a reduction in cardiovascular illness for close to 30 years.[56] Unfortunately, mercury is such a powerful cardiac toxicant that its presence in fish completely negates the positive benefit of the omega-3 oils for cardiac protection.[57] Data from NHANES 1999 to 2000 showed that, for each 1.3 µg/L increase in mercury, the systolic blood pressure increased almost 2 points.[58] Residents of Minamata, Japan, where a huge spill of mercury into the bay resulted in one of the worst methylmercury poisonings ever recorded, had cardiovascular effects as a part of their mercury-induced health problems. Approximately 10 years after the bay was first contaminated with mercury, the blood pressures of the area areas fish-consuming residents began to rise.[59] Minamata residents had a 60% greater likelihood of being hypertensive during the exposure, and by 2010 they were 40% more likely to have their hypertension persist.[60]

Hair mercury is a commonly used marker for a body burden of methylmercury through the consumption of high-mercury fish. As hair mercury levels increase, the CIMT also increases, indicating carotid atherosclerosis.[61] Elevated hair mercury is also strongly associated with a 60% increase in having an acute MI, a 68% greater likelihood of having CVD, and a 56% greater risk of having coronary heart disease (CHD).[62] The authors specifically noted that "High mercury content in hair also attenuated the protective effects of high-serum docosahexaenoic acid plus docosapentaenoic acid concentration."

Cadmium and Arsenic—Cardiovascular Illness. Persons in the 1999 to 2006 NHANES trial showed a clear association between blood cadmium levels (associated with current cadmium exposure) and both stroke and heart failure.[63] A 50% increase in blood cadmium was associated with a 35% increase in the risk of stroke and a 48% increased risk for heart failure. A second group of researchers reviewed the NHANES data and gave people with high blood cadmium levels a 54% greater risk of having cardiovascular or cerebrovascular diseases.[64] Swedish adults (46–67 years of age) with blood cadmium levels in the fourth quartile were 80% more likely to have an acute coronary event and 90% more likely to have a stroke.[65]

Toenail arsenic levels, a reflection of long term exposure, in persons in the Veterans Administration Normative Aging study showed significant association with elevated blood pressure, whereas cadmium, mercury, and lead did not.[66] Higher toenail arsenic levels were associated with prolonged QT segments, a known risk factor for arrhythmia, and sudden cardiac death.[67] The STRONG heart study of Native Americans living in Arizona, Oklahoma, North Dakota, and South Dakota also found a clear association between arsenic and heart disease.[68] Those with an urinary arsenic level of 15.7 µg/g creatinine (primarily from arsenic in drinking water) were 65% more likely to have CVD, 71% more likely to have CHD, and more than three times more likely to have had a stroke than those with urinary arsenic of 5.8 µg/g creatinine.

SUMMARY LIST OF CARDIOVASCULAR ILLNESSES AND ENVIRONMENTAL TOXICANT ASSOCIATIONS

Hypertension
- PCBs increase risk of HTN
- Lead increases HTN in all persons with BLL over 1.6
- Lead increases diastolic HTN risk in postmenopausal women 4.6–8.1 times
- Lead and high stress are synergistic in increasing BP (2.6 × increase per quartile)
- Mercury increases BP
- Arsenic is associated with HTN
- BPA, including prenatal exposure, increases risk

MI Risk
- Traffic exhaust increases MI OR 2.92
- PM_{10}: each increase of 10 µg/m^3 increases risk by 15%
- $PM_{2.5}$: each increase of 10 µg/m^3 increases risk by 32%
- PAH increases risk
- PCBs increase risk 4.5–13.4 times
- BPA increase risk 30% to 40%
- Ch3Hg increases risk by 60%

SUMMARY LIST OF CARDIOVASCULAR ILLNESSES AND ENVIRONMENTAL TOXICANT ASSOCIATIONS—cont'd

Coronary Heart Disease/Atherosclerosis
- PM_{10}: each increase of 10 μg/m³ increases risk by 15%
- $PM_{2.5}$: each increase of 10 μg/m³ increases risk by 32%
- Living within 50 m of major roadway increases risk by 63%
- Living within 100 m of major roadway increases risk by 34%
- PCBs increase risk 4.5–13.4 times (angina)
- BPA increases 16% to 27% (angina)
- BPA increases CHD risk 33% to 60%
- Ch3Hg increases risk by 56%
- Arsenic (low level) increases risk by 71%

CIMT
- $PM_{2.5}$ increases growth (especially in those on statins)
- Living within 100 m of highway increases growth
- Ch3Hg increases CIMT growth
- BPA increases CIMT growth

CV Mortality
- $PM_{2.5}$: causal association
- Living close to major roadway increase risk of death from MI
- Lead increases CV mortality by 55% above 3.62 μg/dL

Heart Rate Variability Reduction
- Cleaning sprays
- Solvents

ST-Segment Depression
- $PM_{2.5}$ and PAH increase risk
- DEP increase risk
- Arsenic increase risk

Left Ventricular Ejection Fraction
- PCBs diminishes effectiveness
- Cadmium diminishes effectiveness

Stroke
- PM_{10}: each increase of 10 μg/m3 increases risk by 15%
- $PM_{2.5}$: each increase of 10 μg/m3 increases risk by 32%
- PCBs increase risk 4.5–13.4 times
- Cadmium increases risk by 35%
- Arsenic increases risk by threefold

ASSESSMENT

Standard cardiovascular assessments are usually effective in determining the presence of CVD. Family history will provide indication of excess risk due to genetics and familial lifestyle choices.

Urinary assessment of common air pollutant metabolites are currently not commercially available but would be quite beneficial at monitoring risk for the numerous health problems that vehicular exhaust is associated with. In addition, such tests could also be used to monitor the effectiveness of air purifiers and other methods to reduce one's exposure to such toxicants.

Urinary tests can reveal ongoing exposure to BPA and some phthalates and current exposure to arsenic, lead, and mercury. Urinary levels of cadmium are reflective of total body burden. Blood tests can be used to determine mercury and lead levels along with PCB presence.

INTERVENTION

Avoidance

Reducing exposure to $PM_{2.5}$ levels slows the progression of CIMT.[25] Chinese adults with CHD utilizing a high-efficiency particulate air (HEPA) face mask while walking outside reduced their $PM_{2.5}$ exposure and improved their cardiac function.[69] Wearing the mask effectively dropped the inhaled $PM_{2.5}$ from 74 μg/m³ to only 2 μg/m³ and did so without being uncomfortable for the users. When the subjects used the face masks, they also experienced a reduction in normal cardiac symptoms, less ST-segment depression, lower median blood pressure, and improved HRV. Persons living in or visiting an area with high PM levels could use similar filters to protect their cardiac function.

The use of indoor air purifiers that were only able to clear 60% of the PM in the home air rewarded the residents with a 9.4% improvement in endothelial function and a 32.6% reduction in inflammatory CRP levels.[70] Air purifier units that reduce indoor PM burden by close to 98% are commercially available and would be preferable.

Avoidance of phthalates, parabens, and phenol-containing compounds is critical and has been documented to result in a reduction of the presence of these compounds in the urine.[71,72,73,74] Avoidance of high-mercury fish as well as farmed salmon and sardines that are sources of PCBs will reduce exposure to these toxicants.

Supplementation

Fish oil supplements appear to reduce the adverse cardiac effects of particulate matter. Three grams of fish oil daily for 4 weeks prevented PM-induced HRV variability as well as ECG changes in human volunteers.[75] The exposure to elevated PM lasted for 2 hours in these volunteers, and no cardioprotection was noted in the group that used olive oil instead of fish oil.

Depuration

The use of chelation to reduce the soft-tissue burden of lead and mercury can be employed to help diminish their effect on CVDs. Intravenous calcium–edetate calcium disodium (EDTA) is used for chelation of lead burden and can itself increase nitric oxide levels, which can result in rapid temporary reduction of elevated blood pressure.[76] In persons with a previous MI, weekly infusions of EDTA and nutrients for 30 weeks resulted in significant reductions in future cardiac problems.[77] Those who received EDTA were 27% less likely to have another MI or a stroke and 28% less likely to be hospitalized for angina.

Low temperature thermal chambers (saunas) are a popular method for reducing total POP burden and have been shown to reduce risk of fatal CVD, sudden cardiac death, and CHD.[78] Repeated sauna sessions can also improve left-ventricular ejection fraction and be beneficial to individuals with chronic heart failure.[79]

REFERENCES

1. Kenneth, D., Kochanek, M. A., Sherry, L., Murphy, B. S., Jiaquan Xu, M. D., & Betzaida Tejada-Vera, M. S. (2016). Division of Vital Statistics. Deaths: Final Data for 2014. *National Vital Statistics Reports*, 4(65), 1–122. Available at https://www.cdc.gov/nchs/data/nvsr/nvsr65/nvsr65_04.pdf. (Accessed 30 March 2017).

2. Lorenz, M., Markus, H., Bots, M., Rosvall, M., & Sitzer, M. (2007). Prediction of clinical cardiovascular events with carotid intima-media thickness. A systematic review and meta-analysis. *Circulation*, 115, 459–467. PubMed PMID: 17242284.

3. *American Heart Association website. Understand Your Risks to Prevent a Heart Attack* Available at http://www.heart.org/heartorg/conditions/heartattack/understandyourriskofheartattack/understand-your-risk-of-heart-attack_ucm_002040_article.jsp (Accessed 31 March 2017).

4. Brook, R. D., Franklin, B., Cascio, W., Hong, Y., Howard, G., Lipsett, M., et al. (2004). Expert Panel on Population and Prevention Science of the American Heart Association. Air pollution and cardiovascular disease: A statement for healthcare professionals from the expert panel on population and prevention science of the American Heart Association. *Circulation*, 109(21), 2655–2671. PubMed PMID: 15173049.

5. Newby, D. E., Mannucci, P. M., Tell, G. S., Baccarelli, A. A., Brook, R. D., Donaldson, K., et al. (2015). Esc Working Group on Thrombosis, European Association for Cardiovascular Prevention and Rehabilitation.; Esc Heart Failure Association. Expert position paper on air pollution and cardiovascular disease. *European Heart Journal*, 36(2), 83–93b. PubMed PMID: 25492627.

6. Oh, S. M., Kim, H. R., Park, Y. J., Lee, S. Y., & Chung, K. H. (2011). Organic extracts of urban air pollution particulate matter (PM2.5)-induced genotoxicity and oxidative stress in human lung bronchial epithelial cells (BEAS-2B cells). *Mutation Research*, 723(2), 142–151. PubMed PMID: 21524716.

7. Frikke-Schmidt, H., Roursgaard, M., Lykkesfeldt, J., Loft, S., Nøjgaard, J. K., & Møller, P. (2011). Effect of vitamin C and iron chelation on diesel exhaust particle and carbon black induced oxidative damage and cell adhesion molecule expression in human endothelial cells. *Toxicology Letters*, 203(3), 181–189. PubMed PMID: 21421028.

8. Harrison, C. M., Pompilius, M., Pinkerton, K. E., & Ballinger, S. W. (2011). Mitochondrial oxidative stress significantly influences atherogenic risk and cytokine-induced oxidant production. *Environmental Health Perspectives*, 119(5), 676–681. PubMed PMID: 21169125.

9. Zhang, P., Dong, G., Sun, B., Zhang, L., Chen, X., Ma, N., et al. (2011). Long-term exposure to ambient air pollution and mortality due to cardiovascular disease and cerebrovascular disease in Shenyang, China. *PLoS ONE*, 6(6), e20827. PubMed PMID: 21695220.

10. Ito, K., Mathes, R., Ross, Z., Nadas, A., Thurston, G., & Matte, T. (2011). Fine particulate matter constituents

associated with cardiovascular hospitalizations and mortality in New York City. *Environmental Health Perspectives, 119*, 467–473. PubMed PMID: 21463978.

11. Guaita, R., Pichiule, M., Maté, T., Linares, C., & Díaz, J. (2011). short-term impact of particulate matter (PM₂.₅) on respiratory mortality in Madrid. *International Journal of Environmental Health Research, 21*(4), 260–274. PubMed PMID: 21644129.

12. Katanoda, K., Sobue, T., Satoh, H., Tajima, K., Suzuki, T., Nakatsuka, H., et al. (2011). An association between long-term exposure to ambient air pollution and mortality from lung cancer and respiratory diseases in Japan. *Journal of Epidemiology, 21*(2), 132–143. PubMed PMID: 21325732.

13. Yu, J. Z., Huang, X. H., Ho, S. S., & Bian, Q. (2011). Nonpolar organic compounds in fine particles: quantification by thermal desorption-GC/MS and evidence for their significant oxidation in ambient aerosols in Hong Kong. *Analytical and Bioanalytical Chemistry, 401*(10), 3125–3139. PubMed PMID: 21983947.

14. Brucker, N., Moro, A. M., Charão, M. F., Durante, J., Freitas, F., Baierle, M., et al. (2013). Biomarkers of occupational exposure to air pollution, inflammation and oxidative damage in taxi drivers. *Science of the Total Environment, 463-464*, 884–893. PubMed PMID: 23872245.

15. Peters, A., Skorkovsky, J., Kotesovec, F., Brynda, J., Spix, C., Wichmann, H. E., et al. (2000). Associations between mortality and air pollution in central Europe. *Environmental Health Perspectives, 108*(4), 282–287. PubMed PMID: 10753084.

16. Mar, T. F., Norris, G. A., Koenig, J. Q., & Larson, T. V. (2000). Associations between air pollution and mortality in Phoenix, 1995-1997. *Environmental Health Perspectives, 108*(4), 347–353. PubMed PMID: 10753094.

17. Morgan, G., Corbett, S., Wlodarczyk, J., & Lewis, P. (1998). Air pollution and daily mortality in Sydney, Australia, 1989 through 1993. *Am J Pub Health, 88*, 759–764. pubmed pmid: 9585741, PubMed PMID: 9585741.

18. Chen, H., Burnett, R. T., Copes, R., Kwong, J. C., Villeneuve, P. J., Goldberg, M. S., et al. (2016). Ambient fine particulate matter and mortality among survivors of myocardial infarction: Population-based cohort study. *Environmental Health Perspectives, 124*(9), 1421–1428. PubMed PMID: 27152932.

19. Rosenbloom, J. I., Wilker, E. H., Mukamal, K. J., Schwartz, J., & Mittleman, M. A. (2012). Residential proximity to major roadway and 10-year all-cause mortality after myocardial infarction. *Circulation, 125*(18), 2197–2203. PubMed PMID: 22566348.

20. Schwartz, J. (2001). Air pollution and blood markers of cardiovascular risk. *Environmental Health Perspectives, 109*(Suppl. 3), 405–409. PubMed PMID: 11427390.

21. Donaldson, K., Stone, V., Seaton, A., & Macnee, W. (2001). Ambient particle inhalation and cardiovascular system: potential mechanisms. *Environmental Health Perspectives, 109*(Suppl. 40), 523–527. PubMed PMID: 11544157.

22. Peters, A., Von Klot, S., Heier, M., Trentinaglia, I., Hörmann, A., Wichmann, H. E., et al. (2004). Cooperative Health Research in the Region of Augsburg Study Group. Exposure to traffic and the onset of myocardial infarction. *The New England Journal of Medicine, 351*(17), 1721–1730. PubMed PMID: 15496621.

23. Künzli, N., Jerrett, M., Mack, W. J., Beckerman, B., Labree, L., Gilliland, F., et al. (2005). Ambient air pollution and atherosclerosis in Los Angeles. *Environmental Health Perspectives, 113*(2), 201–206. PubMed PMID: 15687058.

24. Künzli, N., Jerrett, M., Garcia-Esteban, R., Basagaña, X., Beckermann, B., Gilliland, F., et al. (2010). Ambient air pollution and the progression of atherosclerosis in adults. *PLoS ONE, 5*(2), e9096. PubMed PMID: 20161713.

25. Adar, S., Sheppard, L., Vedal, S., Polak, J. F., Sampson, P. D., Diez Roux, A. V., et al. (2013). Fine particulate air pollution and the progression of carotid intima-medial thickness: a prospective cohort study from the multi-ethnic study of atherosclerosis and air pollution. *PLoS Medicine, 10*(4), e1001430. PubMed PMID: 23637576.

26. Hoffmann, B., Moebus, S., Möhlenkamp, S., Stang, A., Lehmann, N., Dragano, N., et al. (2007). Heinz Nixdorf Recall Study Investigative Group. Residential exposure to traffic is associated with coronary atherosclerosis. *Circulation, 116*(5), 489–496. PubMed PMID: 17638927.

27. Wu, S., Deng, F., Huang, J., Wang, H., Shima, M., Wang, X., et al. (2013). Blood pressure changes and chemical constituents of particulate air pollution: results from the healthy volunteer natural relocation(HVNR) study. *Environmental Health Perspectives, 121*(1), 66–72. PubMed PMID: 23086577.

28. Delfino, R., Gillen, D., Tjoa, T., Staimer, N., Polidor, A., Arhami, M., et al. (2011). Electrocardiographic ST-segment depression and exposure to traffic-related aerosols in elderly subjects with coronary artery disease. *Environmental Health Perspectives, 119*, 196–202. PubMed PMID 20965803.

29. Mills, N. L., Törnqvist, H., Gonzalez, M. C., Vink, E., Robinson, S. D., Söderberg, S., et al. (2007). Ischemic and thrombotic effects of dilute diesel-exhaust

inhalation in men with coronary heart disease. *The New England Journal of Medicine, 357*(11), 1075–1082. PubMed PMID: 17855668.

30. Wallenfeldt, K., Fagerberg, B., Wikstrand, J., & Hulthe, J. (2004). Oxidized low-density lipoprotein in plasma is a prognostic marker of subclinical atherosclerosis Development in clinically healthy men. *Journal of Internal Medicine, 256*(5), 413–420. PubMed PMID: 15485477.

31. Jacobs, L., Emmerechts, J., Hoylaerts, M. F., Mathieu, C., Hoet, P. H., Nemery, B., et al. (2011). Traffic air pollution and oxidized LDL. *PLoS ONE, 6*(1), e16200. PubMed PMID: 2128382.

32. Ma, C. M., Lin, L. Y., Chen, H. W., Huang, L. C., Li, J. F., & Chuang, K. J. (2010). Volatile organic compounds exposure and cardiovascular effects in hair salons. *Occupational Medicine, 60*(8), 624–630. PubMed PMID:20819803.

33. Dekker, J. M., Schouten, E. G., Klootwijk, P., Pool, J., Swenne, C. A., & Kromhout, D. (1997). Heart rate variability from short electrocardiographic recordings predicts mortality from all causes in middle-aged and elderly men. The Zutphen study. *American Journal of Epidemiology, 145*(10), 899–908. PubMed PMID: 9149661.

34. Mehta, A. J., Adam, M., Schaffner, E., Barthélémy, J. C., Carballo, D., Gaspoz, J. M., et al. (2012). Sapaldia Team. Heart rate variability in association with frequent use of household sprays and scented products in Sapaldia. *Environmental Health Perspectives, 120*(7), 958–964. PubMed PMID: 22538298.

35. Hurt, R. D., Weston, S. A., Ebbert, J. O., Mcnallan, S. M., Croghan, I. T., Schroeder, D. R., et al. (2012). Myocardial infarction and sudden cardiac death in Olmsted county, Minnesota, before and after smoke-free workplace laws. *Archives of Internal Medicine, 172*(21), 1635–1641. PubMed PMID: 23108571.

36. Ha, M. H., Lee, D. H., & Jacobs, D. R. (2007). Association between serum concentrations of persistent organic pollutants and self-reported cardiovascular disease prevalence: Results from the National Health and Nutrition Examination Survey, 1999-2002. *Environmental Health Perspectives, 115*(8), 1204–1209. PubMed PMID:17687448.

37. Schecter, A., Colacino, J., Haffner, D., Patel, K., Opel, M., Päpke, O., et al. (2010). Perfluorinated compounds, polychlorinated biphenyls, and organochlorine pesticide contamination in composite food samples From Dallas, Texas, USA. *Environmental Health Perspectives, 118*(6), 796–802. PubMed PMID: 20146964.

38. Lind, P. M., Van Bavel, B., Salihovic, S., & Lind, L. (2012). Circulating levels of persistent organic pollutants (pops) and carotid atherosclerosis in the elderly. *Environmental Health Perspectives, 120*(1), 38–43. PubMed PMID: 22222676.

39. Goncharov, A., Pavuk, M., Foushee, H. R., & Carpenter, D. O. (2011). Blood pressure in relation to concentrations of pcb congeners and chlorinated pesticides. *Environmental Health Perspectives, 119*(3), 319–325. PubMed PMID: 21362590.

40. Sjöberg Lind, Y., Lind, P. M., Salihovic, S., Van Bavel, B., & Lind, L. (2013). Circulating levels of persistent organic pollutants (POPs) are associated with left ventricular systolic and diastolic dysfunction in the elderly. *Environmental Research, 123*, 39–45. PubMed PMID:23562393.

41. Bae, S., & Hong, Y. C. (2015). Exposure to bisphenol a from drinking canned beverages increases blood pressure: Randomized crossover trial. *Hypertension, 65*(2), 313–319. PubMed PMID: 25489056.

42. Bae, S., Lim, Y. H., Lee, Y. A., Shin, C. H., Oh, S. Y., & Hong, Y. C. (2017). Maternal urinary bisphenol a concentration during midterm pregnancy and children's blood pressure at age 4. *Hypertension, 69*(2), 367–374. PubMed PMID: 27920131.

43. Melzer, D., Rice, N. E., Lewis, C., Henley, W. E., & Galloway, T. S. (2010). Association of urinary bisphenol a concentration with heart disease: Evidence from NHANES 2003/06. *PLoS ONE, 5*(1), e8673. PMID:20084273.

44. Melzer, D., Gates, P., Osborne, N. J., Henley, W. E., Cipelli, R., Young, A., et al. (2012). Urinary bisphenol a concentration and angiography-defined coronary artery stenosis. *PLoS ONE, 7*(8), e43378. PubMed PMID: 22916252.

45. Melzer, D., Osborne, N., Henley, W., Cipelli, R., Young, A., Money, C., et al. (2012). Urinary bisphenol a concentration and risk of future coronary artery disease in apparently healthy men and women. *Circulation, 125*(12), 1482–1490. PubMed PMID: 22354940.

46. Lind, P. M., & Lind, L. (2011). Circulating levels of bisphenol a and phthalates are related to carotid atherosclerosis in the elderly. *Atherosclerosis, 218*(1), 207–213. PubMed PMID: 21621210.

47. Vaziri, N. D. (2008). Mechanisms of lead-induced hypertension and cardiovascular disease. *American Journal of Physiology, Heart and Circulatory Physiology, 295*(2), h454–h465. PubMed PMID: 18567711.

48. Nash, D., Magder, L., Lustberg, M., Sherwin, R. W., Rubin, R. J., Kaufmann, R. B., et al. (2003). Blood lead, blood pressure, and hypertension in perimenopausal and postmenopausal women. *JAMA: The Journal of the American Medical Association, 289*(12), 1523–1532. PubMed PMID: 12672769.

49. Hara, A., Thijs, L., Asayama, K., Gu, Y. M., Jacobs, L., Zhang, Z. Y., et al. (2015). Blood pressure in relation to environmental lead exposure in the national health and nutrition examination survey 2003 to 2010. *Hypertension, 65*(1), 62–69. PubMed PMID: 25287397.

50. Tsaih, S. W., Korrick, S., Schwartz, J., Amarasiriwardena, C., Aro, A., Sparrow, D., et al. (2004). Lead, diabetes, hypertension, and renal function: The normative aging study. *Environmental Health Perspectives, 112*(11), 1178–1182. PubMed PMID: 15289163.

51. Cheng, Y., Schwartz, J., Sparrow, D., Aro, A., Weiss, S. T., & Hu, H. (2001). Bone lead and blood lead levels in relation to baseline blood pressure and the prospective development of hypertension: the normative aging study. *American Journal of Epidemiology, 153*(2), 164–171. PubMed PMID: 11159162.

52. Peters, J. L., Kubzansky, L., Mcneely, E., Schwartz, J., Spiro, A., 3rd, Sparrow, D., et al. (2007). Stress as a potential modifier of the impact of lead levels on blood pressure: The normative aging study. *Environmental Health Perspectives, 115*(8), 1154–1159. PubMed PMID: 17687441.

53. Zhang, A., Hu, H., Sánchez, B. N., Ettinger, A. S., Park, S. K., Cantonwine, D., et al. (2012). Association between prenatal lead exposure and blood pressure in children. *Environmental Health Perspectives, 120*(3), 445–450. PubMed PMID: 21947582.

54. Jain, N. B., Potula, V., Schwartz, J., Vokonas, P. S., Sparrow, D., Wright, R. O., et al. (2007). Lead levels and ischemic heart disease in a prospective study of middle-aged and elderly men: The VA normative aging study. *Environmental Health Perspectives, 115*(6), 871–875. PubMed PMID: 17589593.

55. Menke, A., Muntner, P., Batuman, V., Silbergeld, E. K., & Guallar, E. (2006). Blood lead below 0.48 micromol/l (10 microg/dl) and mortality among us adults. *Circulation, 114*(13), 1388–1394. PubMed PMID: 16982939.

56. Kromhout, D., Bosschieter, E. B., & De Lezenne Coulander, C. (1985). The inverse relation between fish consumption and 20-year mortality from coronary heart disease. *The New England Journal of Medicine, 312*(19), 1205–1209. PubMed PMID: 3990713.

57. Wennberg, M., Strömberg, U., Bergdahl, I. A., Jansson, J. H., Kauhanen, J., Norberg, M., et al. (2012). Myocardial infarction in relation to mercury and fatty acids from fish: a risk-benefit analysis based on pooled Finnish and Swedish data in men. *The American Journal of Clinical Nutrition, 96*(4), 706–713. PubMed PMID: 22894940.

58. Vupputuri, S., Longnecker, M. P., Daniels, J. L., Guo, X., & Sandler, D. P. (2005). Blood mercury level and blood pressure among us women: Results from the National Health And Nutrition Examination Survey 1999-2000.

Environmental Research, 97(2), 195–200. PubMed PMID: 15533335.

59. Inoue, S., Yorifuji, T., Tsuda, T., & Doi, H. (2012). Short-term effect of severe exposure to methylmercury on atherosclerotic heart disease and hypertension mortality in Minamata. *Science of the Total Environment, 417-418*, 291–293. PubMed PMID: 22277149.

60. Yorifuji, T., Tsuda, T., Kashima, S., Takao, S., & Harada, M. (2010). Long-term exposure to methylmercury and its effects on hypertension in Minamata. *Environmental Research, 110*(1), 40–46. PubMed PMID: 19922910.

61. Salonen, J. T., Seppänen, K., Lakka, T. A., Salonen, R., & Kaplan, G. A. (2000). Mercury accumulation and accelerated progression of carotid atherosclerosis: a population-based prospective 4-year follow-up study in men in eastern Finland. *Atherosclerosis, 148*(2), 265–273. PubMed PMID: 10657561.

62. Virtanen, J. K., Voutilainen, S., Rissanen, T. H., Mursu, J., Tuomainen, T. P., Korhonen, M. J., et al. (2005). Mercury, fish oils, and risk of acute coronary events and cardiovascular disease, coronary heart disease, and all-cause mortality in men in eastern Finland. *Arteriosclerosis, Thrombosis, and Vascular Biology, 25*(1), 228–233. PubMed PMID: 15539625.

63. Peters, J. L., Perlstein, T. S., Perry, M. J., Mcneely, E., & Weuve, J. (2010). Cadmium exposure in association with history of stroke and heart failure. *Environmental Research, 110*(2), 199–206. PubMed PMID: 20060521.

64. Agarwal, S., Zaman, T., Tuzcu, E. M., & Kapadia, S. R. (2011). Heavy metals and cardiovascular disease: Results from the National Health and Nutrition Examination Survey (NHANES) 1999-2006. *Angiology, 62*(5), 422–429. PubMed PMID: 21421632.

65. Barregard, L., Sallsten, G., Fagerberg, B., Borné, Y., Persson, M., Hedblad, B., et al. (2016). Blood cadmium levels and incident cardiovascular events during follow-up in a population-based cohort of Swedish adults: the Malmö diet and cancer study. *Environmental Health Perspectives, 124*(5), 594–600. PubMed PMID: 26517380.

66. Mordukhovich, I., Wright, R. O., Hu, H., Amarasiriwardena, C., Baccarelli, A., Litonjua, A., et al. (2012). Associations of toenail arsenic, cadmium, mercury, manganese, and lead with blood pressure in the normative aging study. *Environmental Health Perspectives, 120*(1), 98–104. PubMed PMID: 21878420.

67. Mordukhovich, I., Wright, R. O., Amarasiriwardena, C., Baja, E., Baccarelli, A., Suh, H., et al. (2009). Association between low-level environmental arsenic exposure and QT interval duration in a general population study. *American Journal of Epidemiology, 170*(6), 739–746. PubMed PMID: 19700500.

68. Moon, K. A., Guallar, E., Umans, J. G., Devereux, R. B., Best, L. G., Francesconi, K. A., et al. (2013). Association between exposure to low to moderate arsenic levels and incident cardiovascular disease: a prospective cohort study. *Annals of Internal Medicine, 159*, PubMed PMID:24061511.

69. Langrish, J. P., Li, X., Wang, S., Lee, M. M., Barnes, G. D., Miller, M. R., et al. (2012). Reducing personal exposure to particulate air pollution improves cardiovascular health in patients with coronary heart disease. *Environmental Health Perspectives, 120*(3), 367–372. PubMed PMID: 22389220.

70. Allen, R. W., Carlsten, C., Karlen, B., Leckie, S., Van Eeden, S., Vedal, S., et al. (2011). An air filter intervention study of endothelial function among healthy adults in a woodsmoke-impacted community. *American Journal of Respiratory and Critical Care Medicine, 183*(9), 1222–1230. PubMed PMID: 21257787.

71. Koch, H. M., Lorber, M., Christensen, K. L., Pälmke, C., Koslitz, S., & Brüning, T. (2013). Identifying sources of phthalate exposure with human biomonitoring: results of a 48h fasting study with urine collection and personal activity patterns. *International Journal of Hygiene and Environmental Health, 216*(6), 672–681. PubMed PMID: 23333758.

72. Harley, K. G., Kogut, K., Madrigal, D. S., Cardenas, M., Vera, I. A., Meza-Alfaro, G., et al. (2016). Reducing phthalate, paraben, and phenol exposure from personal care products in adolescent girls: findings from the HERMOSA intervention study. *Environmental Health Perspectives, 124*(10), 1600–1607. PubMed PMID: 26947464.

73. Chen, C. Y., Chou, Y. Y., Lin, S. J., & Lee, C. C. (2015). Developing an intervention strategy to reduce phthalate exposure in Taiwanese girls. *Science of the Total Environment, 517*, 125–131. PubMed PMID: 25725197.

74. Hagobian, T., Smouse, A., Streeter, M., Wurst, C., Schaffner, A., & Phelan, S. (2017). Randomized intervention trial to decrease bisphenol a urine concentrations in women: pilot study. *Journal of Women's Health (2002), 26*(2), 128–132. PubMed PMID: 27726525.

75. Tong, H., Rappold, A. G., Diaz-Sanchez, D., Steck, S. E., Berntsen, J., Cascio, W. E., et al. (2012). Omega-3 fatty acid supplementation appears to attenuate particulate air pollution-induced cardiac effects and lipid changes in healthy middle-aged adults. *Environmental Health Perspectives, 120*(7), 952–957. PubMed PMID: 22514211.

76. Foglieni, C., Fulgenzi, A., Ticozzi, P., Pellegatta, F., Sciorati, C., Belloni, D., et al. (2006). Protective effect of EDTA preadministration on renal ischemia. *BMC Nephrology, 15*(7), 5. PubMed PMID: 16536881.

77. Lamas, G. A., Goertz, C., Boineau, R., Mark, D. B., Rozema, T., Nahin, R. L., et al. (2013). Tact Investigators.. Effect of disodium EDTA chelation regimen on cardiovascular events in patients with previous myocardial infarction: the tact randomized trial. *JAMA: The Journal of the American Medical Association, 309*(12), 1241–1250. PubMed PMID: 23532240.

78. Laukkanen, T., Khan, H., Zaccardi, F., & Laukkanen, J. A. (2015). Association between sauna bathing and fatal cardiovascular and all-cause mortality events. *JAMA Internal Medicine, 175*(4), 542–548. PubMed PMID: 25705824.

79. Haseba, S., Sakakima, H., Kubozono, T., Nakao, S., & Ikeda, S. (2016). Combined effects of repeated sauna therapy and exercise training on cardiac function and physical activity in patients with chronic heart failure. *Disability and Rehabilitation, 38*(5), 409–415. PubMed PMID: 25941983.

Musculoskeletal Toxicity
Gout, Rheumatoid Arthritis, Osteoporosis

SUMMARY

- Presence in population: In 2013 to 2015, 54.4 million adults in the United States (22.7% of all adults) had doctor-diagnosed arthritis,[1] and 10.3% of the US adult population has osteoporosis
- Primary sources: Diet and lifestyle, hormonal changes, toxicants
- Best measure: Radiographs, laboratory evaluation (e.g., uric acid, ESR, CRP, ANA, RF, DEXA), urinary 8-OHdG

- Best intervention: Diet and lifestyle modification, toxic compound avoidance, gastrointestinal (GI) repair and support, joint repair and support (e.g., supplemental glucosamine), supplemental calcium, vitamin D, vitamin K2, and antioxidants

DESCRIPTION

Gout

Gout is typically caused by an increased concentration of uric acid in biological fluids and typically presents as monoarticular joint pain involving the metatarsophalangeal joint of the big toe in about 50% of cases. Gout is characterized biochemically by increased leukotriene levels and neutrophil accumulation. In persons with gout, uric acid crystals (monosodium urate monohydrate—tophi) are deposited in joints, tendons, kidneys, and other tissues where they cause considerable inflammation and damage. According to the National Health and Nutritional Examination Survey (NHANES) 2007 to 2008, hyperuricemia affects > 20% of the US population, and about 3.9% (8.3 million individuals) of American adults have gout.[2] Several diet and lifestyle factors have been implicated in the development of hyperuricemia and gout, including elevated body mass index (BMI),[3] alcohol consumption,[4] high dietary intakes of meat and seafood,[5] increased fructose consumption,[6] and exposure to xenobiotics.

Rheumatoid Arthritis

Rheumatoid arthritis (RA) is a chronic, autoimmune, inflammatory condition where antibodies develop against components of joint tissues. RA begins insidiously in the small joints and progresses to affect all joints with severe joint pain and inflammation. Dysregulated inflammatory processes in the synovium of the joint lead to the destruction of both cartilaginous and bony elements of the joint. Fatigue, low-grade fever, weakness, weight loss, joint stiffness, and vague joint pain may precede the appearance of painful, swollen joints by several weeks. The hands, feet, knees, wrists, and ankles are typically involved, often in a symmetrical fashion, and are characteristically quite warm, tender, red, and swollen. It is estimated that between 1% and 3% of the population is affected, with female patients outnumbering male patients almost three to one.[7]

The presence of circulating immune complexes is one of the major factors thought to contribute to the pathogenesis of RA. The cell-mediated, humoral, and nonspecific immune complexes lead to much of the proliferative inflammation seen in RA. Genetic susceptibility, abnormal bowel permeability, lifestyle and nutritional factors, food allergies/sensitivities (including gluten intolerance), microorganisms, and environmental toxicants have all been investigated as triggers of this autoimmune reaction.

Osteoporosis

Osteoporosis is characterized by reduction in the quantity of bone or atrophy of skeletal tissue.[8] Specifically, using the World Health Organization (WHO) criteria, osteoporosis is indicated by a T-score ≤ -2.5 at either the femoral neck or the lumbar spine, and low bone mass is indicated by a T-score between -1.0 and -2.5 at either skeletal site.[9] In 2010, based on adjusted prevalence estimates from the NHANES 2005 to 2010, it was estimated that among US adults age 50 years and older, 10.2 million (10.3%) had osteoporosis and 43.4 million (43.9%) had low bone mass, totaling 53.6 million adults or 54% of the US adult population.[10] As can be seen in Table 48.1, prevalence was significantly higher for women, increased with age, and was lowest for non-Hispanic Black people.

BASIC MECHANISMS OF TOXICITY

The classic picture of immunotoxicity included autoimmunity (increased Th2 or Th17 cytokines) in addition to reduced cell-mediated immunity (reduced Th1 function).[11] One of the major mechanisms for this cytokine imbalance resulting in autoimmunity is depletion of glutathione (GSH) (Fig. 48.1). All the environmental pollutants listed in Box 48.1 have demonstrated the ability to alter cytokine production and immune function, and have also been shown to deplete GSH levels, primarily through oxidative stress.

Both Interleukin (IL)-6 and IL-10, Th2 cytokines, have been implicated in the production of a Th17 cytokine picture. Individuals with low GSH levels have significantly lower levels of the Th1 cytokines Il-1β, IL-12, interferon (IFN)-γ, and tumor necrosis factor (TNF)-α, along with elevated Th2 cytokines.[12] In a trial of HIV-positive patients with that same cytokine picture, liposomal GSH increased production of Th1 cytokines (Il-1β, IL-12, IFN-γ, and TNF-α) and reduced IL-10 and transforming growth factor-beta (TGF-β).

TABLE 48.1   Prevalence Estimates for US Adults Over Age 50 With Osteoporosis and Low Bone Mass in 2010

	Total Population, N	Osteoporosis Prevalence % (SE)	Low Bone Mass Prevalence % (SE)
Total Population	99,048,838	10.3 (0.37)	43.9 (0.72)
Age (years)			
48–59	41,962,930	5.1 (0.60)	40.2 (1.12)
60–69	29,253,187	8.0 (0.87)	43.6 (1.18)
70–79	16,595,961	16.4 (0.94)	47.3 (1.41)
80+	11,236,760	26.2 (1.59)	52.9 (2.22)
Gender			
Male	45,897,382	4.3 (0.40)	35.2 (0.93)
Female	53,151,456	15.4 (0.63)	51.4 (0.93)
Race/Ethnicity			
NH-White	75,272,609	10.2 (0.47)	44.9 (0.89)
NH-Black	9,830,977	4.9 (0.65)	29.7 (1.51)
Mexican-American	4,595,535	13.4 (1.10)	43.2 (1.41)

Modified from Wright, N. C., Looker, A. C., Saag, K. G., Curtis, J. R., Delzell, E. S., Randall, S., Dawson-Hughes, B. (2014). The Recent Prevalence of Osteoporosis and Low Bone Mass in the United States Based on Bone Mineral Density at the Femoral Neck or Lumbar Spine. *Journal of Bone and Mineral Research: The Official Journal of the American Society for Bone and Mineral Research*, 29(11), 2520–2526.

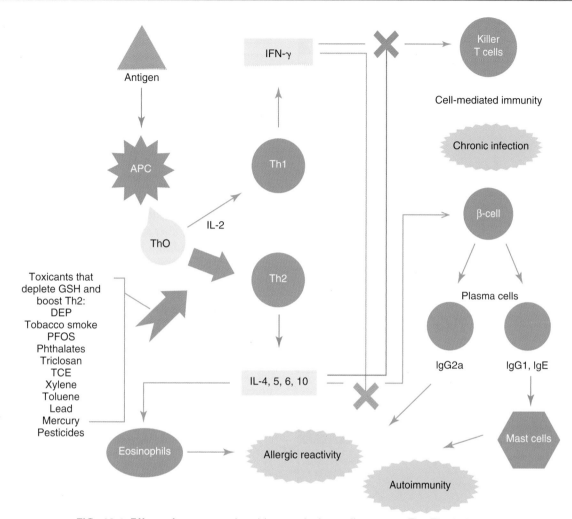

FIG. 48.1 Effect of common glutathione-reducing pollutants on Th1/Th2 balance.

Th17 cells produce IL-17, IL-17A, IL-17F, IL-21, and IL-26, which enhance inflammation (including neuro-inflammation) and cause autoimmune tissue damage.[13,14] The Th17 cells have been linked to RA, systemic lupus erythematosus, multiple sclerosis, gastritis, asthma, psoriasis, systemic sclerosis, chronic inflammatory bowel disease, and allograft rejection, many of which are strongly linked to environmentally toxic compounds.[15] Because Th17 cells are a relatively new finding in the field of immunology, there are far fewer studies that have explored the connection between environmental pollutants and IL-17. However, a handful of common environmental pollutants have demonstrated the ability to enhance Th17 activity by increasing levels of IL-17 (Box 48.2).

Although only a handful of the toxicants listed in Boxes 48.1 and 48.2 have been linked directly to RA, the research to date has been quite limited.

Abnormalities of bone resorption and bone formation play a major role in the development and progression of osteoporosis. Several factors are involved in bone growth and normal bone turnover including genetics, hormones (e.g., parathyroid hormone, 1,25-[OH]$_2$-vitamin D$_3$, calcitonin), nutritional factors, lifestyle factors (e.g., physical activity, nutrition), smoking, alcohol use, and hormone disruptors. In addition, bone tissue is highly sensitive to many types of toxic substances (e.g., toxic metals, organochlorine [OC] compounds), which affect bone composition and mineralization and produce specific

> **BOX 48.1   Environmental Pollutants That Lead to Th1 Reduction and Th2 Dominance**
>
> Diesel exhaust particles (DEP)[123,124]
> Polycyclic aromatic hydrocarbons[125]
> $PM_{2.5}$[126,127]
> Lead[128,129]
> Mercury (thimerosal and methylmercury)[130,131]
> Tributyl tin[132]
> Organophosphate pesticides[133]
> DDT/DDE[134]
> Broad leaf chlorophenoxy herbicides[135]
> Trichloroethylene in drinking water[136]
> PCB 118[137]
> Benzene[138]
> Bisphenol A (BPA)[139]
> Bisphenol A (prenatal exposure)[140]
> Phthalates[141]
> Dioxin[142]
> Toluene diisocyanate (from indoor building materials)[143]
> Trimellitic anhydride (from indoor building materials)[39]
> Perfluorooctanesulfonate (PFOS)[144]
> Gas stove in the home[145]
> Maternal agricultural work [68]

> **BOX 48.2   Environmental Pollutants That Increase Th17 Activity**
>
> Particulate matter[146]
> Diesel exhaust[147]
> Cigarette smoke[148]
> Bisphenol A[149]
> Trichloroethylene[150]
> PCBs[151]
> Paraquat[152]

bone pathologies. Indirectly, elevated body load of cadmium impairs the second hydroxylation of vitamin D in the kidneys, which is critical for bone formation.

SOURCES OF MUSCULOSKELETAL TOXICANTS

Mold

Several studies have clearly shown mold-induced immunotoxicity. In humans, chronic mold/damp building exposure increases production of multiple inflammatory measures and alters immune function mediators. The immune systems of those working in damp buildings and reacting to exposure show a 2- to 1000-fold increased production of a wide variety of inflammatory/immune mediators.[16] *In vitro* studies revealed that extracts from moist building materials caused chondrocyte damage in a dose-dependent manner.[17]

Air Pollution

RA rates are 37% higher in persons living <50 meters from highways than in those living >150 meters away. When individual vehicular exhaust components were assessed for risk, particulate matter ($PM_{2.5}$) showed no association, but ozone levels did (accounting for a 26% increase in risk). Other studies have confirmed the lack of RA risk due to $PM_{2.5}$ in adults, but $PM_{2.5}$ levels can increase risk of juvenile RA by 60%.[18]

Persistent Organic Pollutants

Epidemiological studies have reported increased prevalence of antinuclear antibodies associated with occupational exposures to persistent organic pollutants (POPs). POPs influence the immune system, which may increase the risk of autoimmune conditions such as RA.[19] POPs stored in adipose tissue can be related to differentiation, metabolism, and function in adipose tissue and may therefore be involved in the relation between obesity and osteoarthritis (OA).[20] Women in the 1999 to 2002 NHANES trial with blood polychlorinated biphenyl (PCB) levels in the second, third, and fourth quartiles had more than twice the risk of RA as those with PCBs in the first quartile.[21] The risk of hyperuricemia is increased in subjects with higher serum concentrations of OC pesticides, polychlorinated dibenzodioxins (PCDDs), and dioxin-like PCBs.[22]

Animal studies show 2,3,7,8-tetrachlorodibenzo-p-dioxin (TCDD) inhibits tibial growth,[23] and 3,3',4,4',5-pen-tachlorobiphenyl (PCB-126) impairs mineralization and reduces the collagen content in ovariectomized rats.[24] High dietary intake of OC compounds found in fatty fish may be associated with an increase in vertebral fractures. A study of Swedish fishermen's wives, who consume twice as much fish as the general population, showed a significantly increased incidence rate ratio (IRR: 2.29, 95% Confidence Interval (CI): 1.23–4.28) for vertebral fractures compared with women living on the east coast of the Baltic Sea.[25] High accidental exposure to hexachlorobenzene, a fungicide added to wheat seedlings, resulted in severe osteoporosis and small stature.[26]

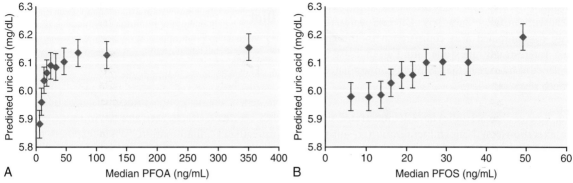

FIG. 48.2 Serum uric acid increases in proportion to body load of PFOA and PFOS. (From Steenland, K., Tinker, S., Shankar, A., & Ducatman, A. [2010]. Association of Perfluorooctanoic Acid (PFOA) and Perfluorooctane Sulfonate (PFOS) with Uric Acid among Adults with Elevated Community Exposure to PFOA. *Environmental Health Perspectives, 118*(2), 229–233.)

Perfluorocarbons. Serum uric acid increases in proportion to body load of perfluorinated hydrocarbons (PFOA and PFOS).[27,28] Fig. 48.2 demonstrates an interesting threshold effect where low levels of PFOA or PFOS show little effect initially, and then uric acid levels rapidly elevate. Urinary 24-hour uric acid levels can be used to monitor treatment efficacy (maintain under 0.8 g/day).

Metals and Metalloids

Aluminum. It was believed that aluminum was quantitatively excreted a short time after uptake, but evidence now suggests some aluminum is retained in the body, mostly in the skeleton.[29] Aluminum may interfere with normal bone function by inhibiting the influx of calcium at the osteoid/calcified-bone boundary and suppressing the secretion of parathyroid hormone (PTH).[30] Aluminum also directly reduces osteoblast numbers inducing severe, resistant osteomalacia.[31] In patients with chronic renal failure, aluminum derived from the dialysate and/or from orally administered aluminum-containing phosphate binders causes aluminum-induced bone disease (AIBD).[32] Aluminum has been significantly reduced in dialysis-dependent patients since incorporating reverse osmosis and deionization techniques to the dialysate.[33] Incidence of low-turnover osteomalacia (LTOM) and aplastic bone lesions are associated with aluminum exposure even in individuals with normal renal function.[34] Research shows individuals on long-term parenteral nutrition also experience metabolic bone disease because of aluminum contamination of parenteral nutrition solutions.[35,36,37]

Arsenic. Low-level arsenic exposure may be associated with hyperuricemia and gout. In men, the adjusted odds ratio (OR) for hyperuricemia comparing highest to lowest quartiles of total arsenic was 1.84 (95% CI, 1.26–2.68), and in women, the OR was 1.26 (95% CI, 0.77–2.07).[38]

Cadmium. The combination of osteoporosis, osteomalacia, and kidney damage was first noted in Japan in areas of high cadmium contamination from mining waste, leading to cross-contamination of rice fields.[39,40] In a nonexposed population with relatively low kidney levels of cadmium, simply having cadmium tissue levels over the mean significantly increased urinary calcium excretion.[41] An increase in urinary calcium is positively associated with cadmium burden, and hypercalciuria occurs even at relatively subtle levels of cadmium-induced tubular dysfunction.[42] Data from the 1988 to 1994 and 1999 to 2004 NHANES revealed that women over 50 with urinary cadmium over 0.50 µg/g creatinine had an increased risk of being diagnosed with osteoporosis by 43%.[43] This may be related to a reduced activation of 1,25 (OH)$_2$-vitamin D$_3$ by kidneys damaged by cadmium and increases in parathyroid hormone, which leads to decreased calcium absorption and impaired bone mineralization.[44] A doubling of urinary cadmium increases the risk of bone fractures in women by 73% and loss of height in men by 60% even at a low degree of environmental exposure.[45] In children, a doubling of urinary cadmium increased risk of bone resorption by 1.72 times.[46] In a cadmium-polluted area of China, the prevalence of osteoporosis in women over 50 years old increased from 34.0% to 51.9% with an OR = 2.09 (95% CI, 1.08–4.03) for the highly contaminated area compared with the control area.[47] Interestingly, the study found an increase in the prevalence of fracture in the cadmium-contaminated area for both sexes.

Lead. *In vivo* animal studies have demonstrated significant alterations on bone mineralization resulting in decreased bone density and increased bone turnover associated with lead exposure.[48,49] Lead has complex effects on bone cell function, including altering the plasma levels of calcitropic hormones, perturbing calcium-mediated and other sensitive signal transduction pathways, uncoupling osteoblasts and osteoclasts from normal paracrine control by interfering with hormone processes, and biochemically inhibiting enzymes resulting in altered cellular energetics.[50] In lead-intoxicated children, blood levels of 1,25-dihydroxyvitamin D_3 are reduced to levels comparable to those BL of patients with metabolic bone disease.[51]

A significant increase in blood lead level (BLL) has been detected after menopause secondary to increased bone resorption from decreasing estrogen levels.[52] The increase was higher in white women compared with black women, which is consistent with prevalence rates and supports the possibility of lead playing a significant role in postmenopausal osteoporosis.

Among patients in the highest BLL quartile (mean, 3.95 µg/dL), the prevalence of gout was 6.05% (95% CI, 4.49%–7.62%) compared with 1.76% (CI, 1.10%–2.42%) among those in the lowest quartile (mean, 0.89 µg/dL).[53] Each doubling of BLL was associated with an unadjusted OR of 1.74 (CI, 1.47–2.05) for gout and 1.25 (CI, 1.12–1.40) for hyperuricemia. Hair and blood cadmium, nickel, and lead levels are found to be significantly higher in those with RA than in healthy controls.[54]

Silica. Exposure to silica particles in dust activates the innate immune system, leading to activation of proinflammatory cytokine production, activation of adaptive immunity, autoantibody production, and tissue damage.[55] Several studies suggest an association between silicosis and RA.[56,57,58] However, a large case-controlled study of pottery, sandstone, and refractory workers did not find a statistically significant association between respiratory silica and RA.[59]

Diet
- Wheat
- Salt
- Fructose
- Alcohol

In genetically susceptible individuals, ingestion of gliadin has cytotoxic effects, activates the immune system, and upregulates inflammation. When exposed to gliadin, zonulin receptor-positive cells release zonulin, leading to the rearrangement of the cell cytoskeleton and increased intestinal permeability to macromolecules.[60] Autoimmune diseases, such as RA, have been associated with elevated zonulin. At least half of the individuals with celiac disease (CD) have no GI-related symptoms but present with fatigue, subfertility, osteoporosis, joint pain, unexplained iron deficiency, and/or autoimmune disease.[61,62] Reestablishing the zonulin-dependent intestinal barrier function may provide a mechanism by which processes such as autoimmune disease, inflammatory conditions, and neoplastic disorders may be halted in their development and possibly reversed.[63]

Dietary salt has been shown to interfere with the regulatory mechanisms of both the innate and the adaptive immune systems. Dietary salt enhances proinflammatory responses by inducing IFN-γ production and reduces the activation of IL-4 and IL-13 macrophages.[64,65] A cross-sectional study demonstrated a significant dose-dependent association between total sodium intake in the fourth quartile and a diagnosis of RA (OR 1.5; 95% CI, 1.1–2.1, p for trend = 0.02).[66]

Consumption of two or more sugar-sweetened beverages (SSB) per day is associated with a 1.78-fold increased risk of gout in men and a 3.05-fold increased risk in women.[67,68]

Alcohol increases uric acid production by accelerating purine nucleotide degradation and reduces uric acid excretion by increasing lactate production, which impairs kidney function.[69] Using a 24-hour diet recall, beer consumption was significantly associated with hyperuricemia with an adjusted OR of 1.28 for men who consumed five or more cans of beer daily compared with those who did not drink.[70]

Gut Microbiota
Individuals with RA have increased intestinal permeability to bacterial antigens as well as alterations in bacterial flora.[71,72] Intestinal colonization with pathogenical or

immunogenic microbes such as yeast, gram-negative bacteria, protozoa, and amoebas can provoke an immune response that cross-reacts with human body tissues, inducing systemic inflammatory disease as well as tissue-specific inflammation.[73] When the microorganisms die, toxins are secreted and released into the surrounding environment. These toxins bind to receptors initiating an adaptive immune response and a signaling cascade, leading to activation of proinflammatory genes.[74] Impaired digestive function along with gut-derived microbial toxins trigger both the onset and maintenance of chronic low-grade inflammation.[75]

Increased gut permeability allows increased absorption of antigens similar to proteins in joint tissues. Antibodies formed to microbial antigens could cross-react with certain self-antigens present in synovial tissues triggering an autoimmune inflammatory response. Antibodies to *Klebsiella pneumoniae, Proteus mirabilis,* and *Yersinia enterocolitica* have been shown to cross-react with collagen and other joint tissues.[76,77,78] Autoimmune conditions associated with cross-reacting antibodies include RA, ankylosing spondylitis, myasthenia gravis, pernicious anemia, and autoimmune thyroiditis. Many patients with RA have small intestinal bacterial overgrowth (SIBO), and the degree of SIBO is associated with the severity of symptoms and disease activity.[79] SIBO has also been linked to the development of bowel-associated dermatosis-arthritis syndrome, which can present as arthralgia and swelling in multiple joints.[80]

Prescription Drugs

Several prescription and over-the-counter (OTC) drugs have detrimental effects on the skeleton and increased risk of fracture. Box 48.3 lists the many pharmaceuticals associated with bone loss and drug-induced osteoporosis.

Aromatase Inhibitors/Gonadotropin-releasing Hormone (GnRH) Analogs.

Aromatase inhibitors block the enzyme aromatase, which converts androgens into estrogens. The reduction in estrogen concentration causes bone loss. Exemestane, letrozole, and anastrozole increase the rate of bone turnover and decrease bone mineral density.[81]

Gonadotropin-releasing hormone (GnRH) analogs cause a profound inhibition of estrogen and androgen synthesis. In patients treated with goserelin, bone mineral density at the lumbar spine decreased by 10.5%.[82]

BOX 48.3 Drugs Associated With Osteoporosis

Androgen deprivation therapy
Anticonvulsants
Antiretroviral therapy
Aromatase inhibitors
Calcineurin inhibitors
Glucocorticoids
Heparins
Loop diuretics
Oral anticoagulants
Ovarian suppressing agents
Proton pump inhibitors
Selective serotonin reuptake inhibitors (SSRIs)
Thiazolidinediones
Thyroid hormone

Data from Mazziotti, G., Canalis, E., & Giustina, A. (2010). Drug-induced osteoporosis: Mechanisms and clinical implications. *American Journal of Medicine, 123*(10), 877–884.

Glucocorticoids. The most common cause of drug-induced osteoporosis is the use of glucocorticoids. Glucocorticoids inhibit bone formation by impairing the replication, differentiation, and function of osteoblasts and induce apoptosis of mature osteoblasts and osteocytes.[83] There is a 17-fold increase in vertebral fracture incidence with glucocorticoid therapy, and fractures occur at higher bone mineral densities than in postmenopausal osteoporosis.[84]

Heparin. Heparin decreases bone formation, inhibits the differentiation and function of osteoblasts, and increases bone resorption by inhibiting the expression of osteoprotegerin.[85] Heparin has been associated with a 2.2% to 5% incidence of heparin-induced osteoporotic fracture.[86] An important mechanism is impairment of vitamin K–dependent metabolism.

Proton Pump Inhibitors. The absorption of calcium is dependent on being solubilized by stomach acid and ionized in the intestines. Proton pump inhibitors (PPIs) interfere with calcium absorption through the induction of hypochlorhydria and decrease intestinal absorption of calcium. In postmenopausal women, omeprazole use was a significant and independent predictor of vertebral fractures (Relative Risk (RR) = 3.50, 95% CI, 1.14–8.44).[87] Patients prescribed long-term high-dose PPI therapy showed a significantly increased risk of hip fracture (Adjusted Odds Ratio (AOR), 2.65; 95% CI, 1.80–3.90; P = .001).[88]

Selective Serotonin Reuptake Inhibitors. Selective serotonin reuptake inhibitors (SSRIs) are used in the treatment of depression and can cause bone loss. Serotonin acts on osteoblasts to inhibit their proliferation, decreasing bone formation.[89] Daily SSRI use is associated with lower bone mineral density at the hip and a trend toward lower bone mineral density at the spine in a dose-dependent manner.[90]

Thiazolidinediones. Thiazolidinediones are used in the treatment and prevention of type 2 diabetes mellitus. Thiazolidinediones interfere with insulin-like growth factor 1 (IGF-1) and may decrease bone formation, as IGF-1 enhances the differentiated function of osteoblasts and bone formation.[91] In diabetic patients treated with rosiglitazone, an increased prevalence of vertebral fractures was observed in those treated with rosiglitazone plus metformin compared with those treated with metformin alone (66.7% vs. 27.3%; p = 0.01).[92]

Thyroxine. Thyroid hormones induce the production of bone-resorbing cytokines,[93] and the suppression of thyroid-stimulating hormone (TSH) itself may cause bone loss.[94] Subclinical hyperthyroidism causes bone loss in elderly subjects and postmenopausal women.[95]

ASSESSMENT

Considering the role of reactive oxygen species in cellular dysfunction and inflammation, biomarkers of oxidative damage, such as 8-hydroxy-2'-deoxyguanosine (8-OHdG) and thiobarbituric acid reactive substances (TBARS), may be helpful to assess antioxidant status and toxicant load.[96] Studies have shown increased lipid, protein, and DNA oxidation markers, and impaired antioxidant status, confirming the role of oxidative stress in the pathogenesis of RA.[97,98] Another study showed greater baseline 8-OHdG levels among subjects with RA compared with both healthy young (p < 0.001) and elderly (p < 0.05) subjects, indicating subjects with RA have higher levels of oxidative stress than healthy individuals.[99]

INTERVENTION

- Avoidance
- Chelation to reduce metal burden
- Supplementation
  - Antioxidants
  - Calcium
  - Probiotics
  - Vitamins D and K

Avoidance of all the known toxins and toxicants is a critical step in preventing and reversing the effects of these ubiquitous compounds. Body burdens of the toxic metals can be addressed through both chelation and avoidance.

As oxidative damage is significant in arthritic processes, the addition of antioxidants in treatment is essential. In animal studies, quercetin inhibits leukocyte recruitment, TNF-α and IL-1β production, superoxide anion production, decrease of antioxidant levels, and NF-κβ activation.[100] Resveratrol has been shown to inhibit the interaction of AP-1 and NF-κβ with COX-2 promoter in human RA synovial fibroblasts.[101] Resveratrol may also have protective effects against matrix degradation and inflammation in OA-affected chondrocytes by reversing IL-1β–induced catabolic and inflammatory responses.[102] Multiple studies indicate that vitamin C is associated with a reduction in the risk of cartilage loss and OA in humans related to its capacity to reduce oxidative stress.[103,104] A clinical trial using 600 International Units (IU) of vitamin E for 10 days in patients with OA demonstrated significant benefit in pain relief.[105]

Avoiding triggers and/or restoring intestinal integrity both have the potential to halt an autoimmune process.[106] The probiotic species *Bifidobacterium longum* (BB536) has been found to prevent damage to intestinal cells and to increase production of tight junction cell proteins, improving intestinal integrity.[107] L-glutamine, which has long been recognized as the primary amino acid source for intestinal cells, has been shown to regulate intercellular junction integrity.[108] In addition to quercetin's antioxidant and antiinflammatory benefits, it also is involved in the assembly of several tight junction proteins (zonula occludens [ZO]-2, occludin, claudin-1, and claudin-4).[109,110]

Calcium

Calcium supplementation has been shown in multiple studies to be effective in reducing bone loss in postmenopausal women.[111,112] Continued calcium supplementation produces a sustained reduction in the rate of loss of total

TABLE 48.2 Recommended Dietary Allowances for Calcium

Age	Male	Female
19–50 years	1000 mg	1000 mg
51–70 years	1000 mg	1200 mg
71+ years	1200 mg	1200 mg

Data from National Institutes of Health, Office of Dietary Supplements. (2016). *Dietary supplement fact sheet.* Retrieved from http://ods.od.nih.gov/factsheets/calcium.asp.

bone mineral density and a reduction in the incidence of bone fractures.[113] The recommended dietary allowance of calcium for adults is between 1000 to 1200 mg per day (see Table 48.2).[114] A double-blind, placebo-controlled study of 301 healthy postmenopausal women—half of whom had a calcium intake lower than 400 mg per day and half an intake of 400 to 650 mg per day—was conducted to determine the effects of calcium on bone loss.[115] For 2 years, the women received placebo or either calcium carbonate or calcium citrate malate (500 mg of calcium per day). In early postmenopausal women with low calcium intake, supplementation with calcium did not affect bone loss. However, in women who had been postmenopausal for ≥ 6 years, supplementation with calcium citrate malate was more effective than calcium carbonate and actually produced small gains in bone mineral density at the femoral neck and radius and reductions in bone mineral density loss in the spine. Natural oyster shell calcium, dolomite, and bone meal products should be avoided as studies have indicated these may contain substantial amounts of lead.[116] This not only poses a risk of lead intoxication but may further aggravate osteoporosis as described earlier.

Vitamin D

Vitamin D has been shown to increase innate immunity while modulating adaptive immunity, and vitamin D deficiency is associated with an increased prevalence of autoimmune conditions including RA.[117]

Vitamin D is also essential for the intestinal absorption of calcium, and because of its diverse and expanding roles in the body, many experts consider it more of a hormone than a vitamin. Vitamin D maintains adequate serum calcium and phosphate concentrations to enable normal mineralization of bone and is required for bone growth and bone remodeling by osteoblasts and osteoclasts. Vitamin D also plays a role in neuromuscular and

immune function, modulation of cell growth, and reduction of inflammation.[118] The current recommended dietary allowance for vitamin D ranges from 600 IU/day to 800 IU/day.[119] One study using vitamin D_3 alone found that supplementation with 700 IU/day reduces the annual rate of hip fracture by nearly 60%.[120] Combining vitamin D with calcium supplementation has been shown to reduce the risk of fracture. A study of 3270 elderly women living in nursing homes showed a 43% reduction in hip fracture rate in those that received a combination of 1200 mg/day of calcium and 800 IU/day of vitamin D_3.[121] A Cochrane review concluded that a combination of vitamin D with calcium is more effective in preventing hip or any type of fracture.[122]

Other

Vitamin K_2 supplementation is critical when supplementing with vitamin D and calcium. Also, restoration of vitamin D levels may uncover a previously unrecognized vitamin A deficiency. A high potency multiple vitamin and mineral formula is recommended because bone is dependent on a constant supply of many nutrients.

REFERENCES

1. Barbour, K. E., Helmick, C. G., Boring, M., & Brady, T. J. (2017). Vital signs: prevalence of doctor-diagnosed arthritis and arthritis-attributable activity limitation – United States, 2013-2015. *MMWR. Morbidity and Mortality Weekly Report, 66*(9), 246–253. PubMed PMID: 28278145.
2. Zhu, Y., Pandya, B. J., & Choi, H. K. (2011). Prevalence of gout and hyperuricemia in the US general population: the National Health and Nutrition Examination Survey 2007-2008. *Arthritis and Rheumatism, 63*(10), 3136–3141. PubMed PMID: 21800283.
3. Aune, D., Norat, T., & Vatten, L. J. (2014). Body mass index and the risk of gout: a systematic review and dose-response meta-analysis of prospective studies. *European Journal of Nutrition, 53*(8), 1591–1601. PubMed PMID: 25209031.
4. Wang, M., Jiang, X., Wu, W., & Zhang, D. (2013). A meta-analysis of alcohol consumption and the risk of gout. *Clinical Rheumatology, 32*(11), 1641–1648. PubMed PMID: 23881436.
5. Schlesinger, N. (2005). Dietary factors and hyperuricaemia. *Current Pharmaceutical Design, 11*(32), 4133–4138. PubMed PMID: 16375734.

6. Merriman, T. R., Dalbeth, N., & Johnson, R. J. (2014). Sugar-sweetened beverages, urate, gout and genetic interaction. *Pacific Health Dialog: A Publication of the Pacific Basin Officers Training Program and the Fiji School of Medicine, 20*(1), 31–38. PubMed PMID: 25928993.

7. Gibofsky, A. (2012). Overview of epidemiology, pathophysiology, and diagnosis of rheumatoid arthritis. *The American Journal of Managed Care, 18*(13 Suppl.), S295–S302. PubMed PMID: 23327517.

8. Garnero, P., Shih, W. J., Gineyts, E., et al. (1994). Comparison of new biochemical markers of bone turnover in late postmenopausal osteoporotic women in response to alendronate treatment. *The Journal of Clinical Endocrinology and Metabolism, 79*(6), 1693–1700. PubMed PMID: 7989477.

9. Kanis, J. A., McCloskey, E. V., Johansson, H., et al. (2008). A reference standard for the description of osteoporosis. *Bone, 42*(3), 467–475. PubMed PMID: 18180210.

10. Wright, N. C., Looker, A. C., Saag, K. C., et al. (2014). The recent prevalence of osteoporosis and low bone mass in the United States based on bone mineral density at the femoral neck or lumbar spine. *Journal of Bone and Mineral Research, 29*(11), 2520–2526.

11. Rea, W. J. (1992). *Chemical sensitivities* (Vol. 1). Boca Raton, FL.: CRC Press.

12. Tudela, E. V., Singh, M. K., Lagman, M., et al. (2014). Cytokine levels in plasma samples of individuals with HIV infection. *Austin Journal of Clinical Immunology, 1*(1), 1003.

13. Wynn, T. A. (2005). T(H)-17: a giant step from T(H)1 and T(H)2. *Nature Immunology, 6*(11), 1069–1070. PubMed PMID: 16239919.

14. Cheung, P. F., Wong, C. K., & Lam, C. W. (2008). Molecular mechanisms of cytokine and chemokine release from eosinophils activated by IL-17A, IL-17F, and IL-23: implication for Th17 lymphocytes-mediated allergic inflammation. *The Journal of Immunology: Official Journal of the American Association of Immunologists, 180*(8), 5625–5635. PubMed PMID: 18390747.

15. Vojdani, A., & Lambert, J. (2011). The role of Th17 in neuroimmune disorders: target for CAM therapy. Part I. *Evidence-Based Complementary and Alternative Medicine, 2011*, 927294. PubMed PMID: 19622600.

16. Rosenblum Lichtenstein, J. H., Hsu, Y. H., Gavin, I. M., et al. (2015). Environmental mold and mycotoxin exposures elicit specific cytokine and chemokine responses. *PLoS ONE, 10*(5), e0126926. PubMed PMID: 26010737.

17. Lorenz, W., Sigrist, G., Shakibaei, M., et al. (2006). A hypothesis for the origin and pathogenesis of rheumatoid diseases. *Rheumatology International, 26*(7), 641–654. PubMed PMID: 16362367.

18. Zeft, A. S., Prahalad, S., Lefevre, S., et al. (2009). Juvenile idiopathic arthritis and exposure to fine particulate air pollution. *Clinical and Experimental Rheumatology, 27*(5), 877–884. PubMed PMID: 19917177.

19. Ahmed, S. A. (2000). The immune system as a potential target for environmental estrogens (endocrine disruptors): a new emerging field. *Toxicology, 150*(1–3), 191–206. PubMed PMID: 10996675.

20. Mullerova, D., & Kopecky, J. (2007). White adipose tissue: storage and effector site for environmental pollutants. *Physiological Research, 56*(4), 375–381. PubMed PMID: 16925464.

21. Lee, D. H., Steffes, M., & Jacobs, D. R. (2007). Positive associations of serum concentration of polychlorinated biphenyls or organochlorine pesticides with self-reported arthritis, especially rheumatoid type, in women. *Environmental Health Perspectives, 115*(6), 883–888. PubMed PMID: 17589595.

22. Lee, Y. M., Bae, S. G., Lee, S. H., et al. (2013). Persistent organic pollutants and hyperuricemia in the US general population. *Atherosclerosis, 230*(1), 1–5. PubMed PMID: 23958244.

23. Jamsa, T., Viluksela, M., Tuomisto, J. T., et al. (2001). Effects of 2,3,7,8-tetrachlorodibenzo-p-dioxin on bone in two rat strains with different aryl hydrocarbon receptor structures. *Journal of Bone and Mineral Research, 16*(10), 1812–1820. PubMed PMID: 11585345.

24. Lind, P. M., Eriksen, E. F., Sahlin, L., et al. (1999). Effects of the antiestrogenic environmental pollutant 3,3′,4,4′,5-pentachlorobiphenyl (PCB #126) in rat bone and uterus: diverging effects in ovariectomized and intact animals. *Toxicology and Applied Pharmacology, 154*(3), 236–244. PubMed PMID: 9931283.

25. Alveblom, A. K., Rylander, L., Johnell, O., & Hagmar, L. (2003). Incidence of hospitalized osteoporotic fractures in cohorts with high dietary intake of persistent organochlorine compounds. *International Archives of Occupational and Environmental Health, 76*(3), 246–248. PubMed PMID: 12690500.

26. Gocmen, A., Peters, H. A., Cripps, D. J., et al. (1989). Hexachlorobenzene episode in Turkey. *Biomedical and Environmental Sciences, 2*(1), 36–43. PubMed PMID: 2590490.

27. Steenland, K., Tinker, S., Shankar, A., & Ducatman, A. (2010). Association of perfluorooctanoic acid (PFOA)

and perfluorooctane sulfonate (PFOS) with uric acid among adults with elevated community exposure to PFOA. *Environmental Health Perspectives, 118,* 229–233. PubMed PMID: 20123605

28. Geiger, S. D., Xiao, J., & Shankar, A. (2013). Positive association between perfluoroalkyl chemicals and hyperuricemia in children. *American Journal of Epidemiology, 177*(11), 1255–1262. PubMed PMID: 23552989.

29. Priest, N. D. (2004). The biological behavior and bioavailability of aluminum in man, with special reference to studies employing aluminum-26 as a tracer: review and study update. *Journal of Environmental Monitoring, 6*(5), 375–403. PubMed PMID: 15152306.

30. Visser, W. J., & Van de Vyver, F. L. (1985). Aluminum-induced osteomalacia in severe chronic renal failure (SCRF). *Clinical Nephrology, 24*(Suppl. 1), S30–S36. PubMed PMID: 3915958.

31. Dunstan, C. R., Evans, R. A., Hills, E., et al. (1984). Effect of aluminum and parathyroid hormone on osteoblasts and bone mineralization in chronic renal failure. *Calcified Tissue International, 36*(2), 133–138. PubMed PMID: 6430496.

32. Ward, M. K., Feest, T. G., Ellis, H. A., et al. (1978). Osteomalacic dialysis osteodystrophy: evidence for a water-borne aetiological agent, probably aluminum. *Lancet, 1*(8069), 841–845. PubMed PMID: 76795

33. Jaffe, J. A., Liftman, C., & Glickman, J. D. (2005). Frequency of elevated serum aluminum levels in adult dialysis patients. *American Journal of Kidney Diseases, 46*(2), 316–319. PubMed PMID: 16112051.

34. Ott, S. M. (1985). Aluminum accumulation in individuals with normal renal function. *American Journal of Kidney Diseases, 6*(5), 297–301. PubMed PMID: 3933333.

35. Klein, G. L. (1991). The aluminum content of parenteral solutions: current status. *Nutrition Reviews, 49*(3), 74–79. PubMed PMID: 1905389.

36. Klein, G. L. (1995). Aluminum in parenteral solutions revisited – again. *The American Journal of Clinical Nutrition, 61*(3), 449–456. PubMed PMID: 7872206.

37. Popinska, K., Kierkus, J., Lyszkowska, M., et al. (1999). Aluminum contamination of parenteral nutrition additives, amino acid solutions, and lipid emulsions. *Nutrition, 15*(9), 683–686. PubMed PMID: 10467613.

38. Kuo, C. C., Weaver, V., Fadrowski, J. J., et al. (2015). Arsenic exposure, hyperuricemia, and gout in US adults. *Environment International, 76,* 32–40. PubMed PMID: 25499256.

39. Tsuritani, I., Honda, R., Ishizaki, M., et al. (1992). Impairment of vitamin D metabolism due to environmental cadmium exposure, and possible relevance to sex-related differences in vulnerability to the bone damage. *Journal of Toxicology and Environmental Health, 37*(4), 519–533. PubMed PMID: 1464907.

40. Emmerson, B. T. (1970). Ouch-ouch" disease: the osteomalacia of cadmium nephropathy. *Annals of Internal Medicine, 73*(5), 854–855. PubMed PMID: 5476215.

41. Wallin, M., Sallsten, G., Fabricius-Lagging, E., et al. (2013). Kidney cadmium levels and associations with urinary calcium and bone mineral density: a cross-sectional study in Sweden. *Environmental Health: A Global Access Science Source, 12,* 22. PubMed PMID: 23497059.

42. Buchet, J. P., Lauwerys, R., Roels, H., et al. (1990). Renal effects of cadmium body burden of the general population. *Lancet, 336*(8717), 699–702. PubMed PMID: 1975890.

43. Gallagher, C. M., Kovach, J. S., & Meliker, J. R. (2008). Urinary cadmium and osteoporosis in U.S. Women >or= 50 years of age: NHANES 1988-1994 and 1999-2004. *Environmental Health Perspectives, 116*(10), 1338–1343. PubMed PMID: 18941575.

44. Nogawa, K., Tsuritani, I., Kido, T., et al. (1987). Mechanism for bone disease found in inhabitants environmentally exposed to cadmium: decreased serum 1 alpha, 25-dihydroxyvitamin D level. *International Archives of Occupational and Environmental Health, 59*(1), 21–30. PubMed PMID: 3793241.

45. Staessen, J. A., Roels, H. A., Emelianov, D., et al. (1999). Environmental exposure to cadmium, forearm bone density, and risk of fractures: prospective population study. Public Health and Environmental Exposure to Cadmium (PheeCad) Study Group. *Lancet, 353*(9159), 1140–1144. PubMed PMID: 10209978.

46. Sughis, M., Penders, J., Haufroid, V., et al. (2011). Bone resorption and environmental exposure to cadmium in children: a cross-sectional study. *Environmental Health: A Global Access Science Source, 10,* 104. PubMed PMID: 22151692.

47. Zhu, G., Wang, H., Shi, Y., et al. (2004). Environmental cadmium exposure and forearm bone density. *Biometals: An International Journal on the Role of Metal Ions in Biology, Biochemistry, and Medicine, 17*(5), 499–503. PubMed PMID: 15688853.

48. Lee, C. M., Terrizzi, A. R., Bozzini, C., et al. (2016). Chronic lead poisoning magnifies bone detrimental effects in an ovariectomized rat model of postmenopausal osteoporosis. *Experimental and*

Toxicologic Pathology, *68*(1), 47–53. PubMed PMID: 26422677.

49. Monir, A. U., Gundberg, C. M., Yagerman, S. E., et al. (2010). The effect of lead on bone mineral properties from female adult C57/BL6 mice. *Bone*, *47*(5), 888–894. PubMed PMID: 20643234.

50. Goyer, R. A., Epstein, S., Bhattacharyya, M., et al. (1994). Environmental risk factors for osteoporosis. *Environmental Health Perspectives*, *102*(4), 390–394. PubMed PMID: 7925179.

51. Rosen, J. F., Chesney, R. W., Hamstra, A., et al. (1980). Reduction in 1,25-dihydroxyvitamin D in children with increased lead absorption. *The New England Journal of Medicine*, *302*(20), 1128–1131. PubMed PMID: 7366636.

52. Silbergeld, E. K., Schwartz, J., & Mahaffey, K. (1988). Lead and osteoporosis: mobilization of lead from bone in postmenopausal women. *Environmental Research*, *47*(1), 79–94. PubMed PMID: 3168967.

53. Krishnan, E., Lingala, B., & Bhalla, V. (2012). Low-level lead exposure and the prevalence of gout: an observational study. *Annals of Internal Medicine*, *157*(4), 233–241. PubMed PMID: 22910934.

54. Afridi, H. I., Kazi, T. G., Talpur, F. N., et al. (2014). Relationship between toxic metals exposure via cigarette smoking and rheumatoid arthritis. *Clinical Laboratory*, *60*(10), 1735–1745. PubMed PMID: 25651721.

55. Pollard, K. M. (2016). Silica, silicosis, and autoimmunity. *Frontiers in Immunology*, *7*, 97. PubMed PMID: 27014276.

56. Rosenman, K. D., Moore-Fuller, M., & Reilly, M. J. (1999). Connective tissue disease and silicosis. *American Journal of Industrial Medicine*, *35*, 375–381. PubMed PMID: 10086214.

57. Brown, L. M., Gridley, G., Olsen, J. H., et al. (1997). Cancer risk and mortality patterns among silicotic men in Sweden and Denmark. *Journal of Occupational and Environmental Medicine*, *39*, 633–638. PubMed PMID: 9253724.

58. Rosenman, K. D., & Zhu, Z. (1995). Pneumoconiosis and associated medical conditions. *American Journal of Industrial Medicine*, *27*, 107–113. PubMed PMID: 7900728.

59. Turner, S., & Cherry, N. (2000). Rheumatoid arthritis in workers exposed to silica in the pottery industry. *Occupational and Environmental Medicine*, *57*, 443–447. PubMed PMID: 10854495.

60. Drago, S., El Asmar, R., Di Pierro, M., et al. (2006). Gliadin, zonulin and gut permeability: effects on celiac and non-celiac intestinal mucosa and intestinal cell lines. *Scandinavian Journal of Gastroenterology*, *41*(4), 408–419. PubMed PMID: 16635908.

61. Harrison, M. S.,Wehbi, M., & Obideen, K. (2007). Celiac disease: more common than you think. *Cleveland Clinic Journal of Medicine*, *74*(3), 209–215. PubMed PMID: 17375801.

62. Fasano, A. (2006). Systemic autoimmune disorders in celiac disease. *Current Opinion in Gastroenterology*, *22*(6), 674–679. PubMed PMID: 17053448.

63. Fasano, A. (2011). Zonulin and its regulation of intestinal barrier function: the biological door to inflammation, autoimmunity, and cancer. *Physiological Reviews*, *91*(1), 151–175. PubMed PMID: 21248165.

64. Min, B., & Fairchild, R. L. (2015). Over-salting ruins the balance of the immune menu. *The Journal of Clinical Investigation*, *125*(11), 4002–4004. PubMed PMID: 26485281.

65. Binger, K. J., Gebhardt, M., Heinig, M., et al. (2015). High salt reduces the activation of IL-4 and IL-13-stimulated macrophages. *The Journal of Clinical Investigation*, *125*(11), 4223–4238. PubMed PMID: 26485286.

66. Salgado, E., Bes-Rastrollo, M., de Irala, J., et al. (2015). High sodium intake is associated with self-reported rheumatoid arthritis: a cross sectional and case control analysis within the SUN cohort. *Medicine*, *94*(37), e924. PubMed PMID: 26376372.

67. Choi, H. K., & Curhan, G. (2008). Soft drinks, fructose consumption, and the risk of gout in men: prospective cohort study. *BMJ (Clinical Research Ed.)*, *336*(7639), 309–312. PubMed PMID: 18244959.

68. Choi, H. K., Willett, W., & Curhan, G. (2010). Fructose-rich beverages and risk of gout in women. *JAMA: The Journal of the American Medical Association*, *304*(20), 2270–2278. PubMed PMID: 21068145.

69. Yamanaka, H. (1996). Alcohol ingestion and hyperuricemia. *Nihon Rinsho. Japanese Journal of Clinical Medicine*, *54*(12), 3369–3373. PubMed PMID: 8976122.

70. Yu, K. H., See, L. C., Huang, Y. C., et al. (2008). Dietary factors associated with hyperuricemia in adults. *Seminars in Arthritis and Rheumatism*, *37*(4), 243–250. PubMed PMID: 17570471.

71. Smith, M. D., Gibson, R. A., & Brooks, P. M. (1985). Abnormal bowel permeability in ankylosing spondylitis and rheumatoid arthritis. *The Journal of Rheumatology*, *12*(2), 299–305. PubMed PMID: 4032403.

72. Segal, A. W., Isenberg, D. A., Hajirousou, V., et al. (1986). Preliminary evidence for gut involvement in the pathogenesis of rheumatoid arthritis? *British*

Journal of Rheumatology, 25(2), 162–166. PubMed PMID: 3085760.

73. Wucherpfennig, K. W. (2001). Mechanisms for the induction of autoimmunity by infectious agents. *The Journal of Clinical Investigation, 108*(8), 1097–1104. PubMed PMID: 11602615.

74. Aderem, A., & Ulevitch, R. J. (2000). Toll-like receptors in the induction of the innate immune response. *Nature, 406*, 782–787. PubMed PMID: 10963608.

75. Laugerette, F. 1., Vors, C., Peretti, N., et al. (2011). Complex links between dietary lipids, endogenous endotoxins and metabolic inflammation. *Biochimie, 93*(1), 39–45. PubMed PMID: 20433893.

76. Rashid, T., Ebringer, A., & Wilson, C. (2017 May 8). The link between Proteus mirabilis, environmental factors and autoantibodies in rheumatoid arthritis. *Clinical and Experimental Rheumatology*, [Epub ahead of print]. PubMed PMID: 28516867.

77. Khalafpour, S., Ebringer, A., Abuljadayel, I., & Corbett, M. (1988). Antibodies to Klebsiella and Proteus microorganisms in ankylosing spondylitis and rheumatoid arthritis patients measured by ELISA. *British Journal of Rheumatology, 27*(Suppl. 2), 86 89. PubMed PMID: 3042078.

78. Ebringer, A., Cox, N. L., Abuljadayel, I., et al. (1988). Klebsiella antibodies in ankylosing spondylitis and Proteus antibodies in rheumatoid arthritis. *British Journal of Rheumatology, 27*(Suppl. 2), 72–85. PubMed PMID: 3042077.

79. Henriksson, A. E., Blomquist, L., Nord, C. E., et al. (1993). Small intestinal bacterial overgrowth in patients with rheumatoid arthritis. *Annals of the Rheumatic Diseases, 52*(7), 503–510. PubMed PMID: 8346978.

80. Patton, T., Jukic, D., & Juhas, E. (2009). Atypical histopathology in bowel-associated dermatosis-arthritis syndrome: a case report. *Dermatology Online Journal, 15*(3), 3. PubMed PMID: 19379647.

81. Khan, M. N., & Khan, A. A. (2008). Cancer treatment-related bone loss: a review and synthesis of the literature. *Current Oncology, 15*(Suppl. 1), S30–S40. PubMed PMID: 18231646.

82. Jonat, W., Kaufmann, M., Sauerbrei, W., et al. (2002). Goserelin versus cyclophosphamide, methotrexate, and fluorouracil as adjuvant therapy in premenopausal patients with node positive breast cancer: the Zoladex Early Breast Cancer Research Association Study. *Journal of Clinical Oncology : Official Journal of the American Society of Clinical Oncology, 20*(24), 4628–4635. PubMed PMID: 12488406.

83. Canalis, E., Mazziotti, G., Giustina, A., & Bilezikian, J. P. (2007). Glucocorticoid-induced osteoporosis: pathophysiology and therapy. *Osteoporosis International, 18*(10), 1319–1328. PubMed PMID: 17566815.

84. Van Staa, T. P., Laan, R. F., Barton, I. P., et al. (2003). Bone density threshold and other predictors of vertebral fracture in patients receiving oral glucocorticoid therapy. *Arthritis and Rheumatism, 48*(11), 3224–3229. PubMed PMID: 14613287.

85. Rajgopal, R., Bear, M., Butcher, M. K., & Shaughnessy, S. G. (2008). The effects of heparin and low molecular weight heparins on bone. *Thrombosis Research, 122*(3), 293–298. PubMed PMID: 17716711.

86. Lefkou, E., Khamashta, M., Hampson, G., & Hunt, B. J. (2010). Review: low-molecular-weight heparin-induced osteoporosis and osteoporotic fractures: a myth or an existing entity? *Lupus, 19*(1), 3–12. PubMed PMID: 19934178.

87. Roux, C., Briot, K., Gossec, L., et al. (2009). Increase in vertebral fracture risk in postmenopausal women using omeprazole. *Calcified Tissue International, 84*(1), 13–19. PubMed PMID: 19023510.

88. Yang, Y. X., Lewis, J. D., Epstein, S., & Metz, D. C. (2006). Long-term proton pump inhibitor therapy and risk of hip fracture. *JAMA: The Journal of the American Medical Association, 296*(24), 2947–2953. PubMed PMID: 17190895.

89. Yadav, V. K., Ryu, J. H., Suda, N., et al. (2008). Lrp5 controls bone formation by inhibiting serotonin synthesis in the duodenum. *Cell, 135*(5), 825–837. PubMed PMID: 19041748.

90. Richards, J. B., Papaioannou, A., Adachi, A. D., et al. (2007). Effect of selective serotonin reuptake inhibitors on the risk of fracture. *Archives of Internal Medicine, 167*(2), 188–194. PubMed PMID: 17242321.

91. Giustina, A., Mazziotti, G., & Canalis, E. (2008). Growth hormone, insulin-like growth factors, and the skeleton. *Endocrine Reviews, 29*(5), 535–559. PubMed PMID: 18436706.

92. Mancini, T., Mazziotti, G., Doga, M., et al. (2009). Vertebral fractures in males with type 2 diabetes treated with rosiglitazone. *Bone, 45*(4), 784–788. PubMed PMID: 19527806.

93. Lakatos, P. (2003). Thyroid hormones: beneficial or deleterious for bone? *Calcified Tissue International, 73*(3), 205–209. PubMed PMID: 14667131.

94. Mazziotti, G., Porcelli, T., Patelli, I., et al. (2010). Serum TSH values and risk of vertebral fractures in euthyroid postmenopausal women with low bone mineral density. *Bone, 46*(3), 747–751. PubMed PMID: 19892039.

95. Biondi, B., & Cooper, D. S. (2008). The clinical significance of subclinical thyroid

dysfunction. *Endocrine Reviews, 29*(1), 76–131. [Epub 2007 Nov 8]; PubMed PMID: 17991805.

96. Valavanidis, A., Vlachogianni, T., & Fiotakis, C. (2009). 8-hydroxy-2' –deoxyguanosine (8-OHdG): A critical biomarker of oxidative stress and carcinogenesis. *Journal of Environmental Science and Health. Part C, Environmental Carcinogenesis & Ecotoxicology Reviews, 27*(2), 120–139. PubMed PMID: 19412858.

97. Seven, A., Guzel, S., Aslan, M., & Hamuryudan, V. (2008). Lipid, protein, DNA oxidation and antioxidant status in rheumatoid arthritis. *Clinical Biochemistry, 41*(7–8), 538–543. PubMed PMID: 18313405.

98. Ozturk, H. S., Cimen, M. Y., Cimen, O. B., et al. (1999). Oxidant/antioxidant status of plasma samples from patients with rheumatoid arthritis. *Rheumatology International, 19*(1–2), 35–37. PubMed PMID: 10651080.

99. Rall, L. C., Roubenoff, R., Meydani, S. N., et al. (2000). Urinary 8-hydroxy-2'-deoxyguanosine (8-OHdG) as a marker of oxidative stress in rheumatoid arthritis and aging: effect of progressive resistance training. *The Journal of Nutritional Biochemistry, 11*(11–12), 581–584. PubMed PMID: 11137896.

100. Ruiz-Miyazawa, K. W., Staurengo-Ferrari, L., Mizokami, S. S., et al. (2017). Quercetin inhibits gout arthritis in mice: induction of an opioid-dependent regulation of inflammasome. *Inflammopharmacology*, PubMed PMID: 28508104.

101. Yang, C. M., Chen, Y. W., Chi, P. L., et al. (2017). Resveratrol inhibits BK-induced COX-2 transcription by suppressing acetylation of AP-1 and NF-κβ in human rheumatoid arthritis synovial fibroblasts. *Biochemical Pharmacology, 132*, 77–91. PubMed PMID: 28288820.

102. Gu, H., Jiao, Y., Yu, X., et al. (2017). Resveratrol inhibits the IL-1β-induced expression of MMP-13 and IL-6 in human articular chondrocytes via TLR4/MyD88-dependent and -independent signaling cascades. *International Journal of Molecular Medicine, 39*(3), 734–740. PubMed PMID: 28204817.

103. McAlindon, T. E., Jacques, P., Zhang, Y., et al. (1996). Do antioxidant micronutrients protect against the development and progression of knee osteoarthritis? *Arthritis and Rheumatism, 39*(4), 648–656. PubMed PMID: 8630116.

104. Chamg, Z., Huo, L., Li, P., et al. (2015). Ascorbic acid provides protection for human chondrocytes against oxidative stress. *Molecular Medicine Reports, 12*(5), 7086–7092. PubMed PMID: 26300283.

105. Machtey, I., & Ouaknine, L. (1978). Tocopherol in osteoarthritis: a controlled pilot study. *Journal of the American Geriatrics Society, 26*(7), 328–330. PubMed PMID: 350940.

106. Fasano, A., & Shea-Donohue, T. (2005). Mechanisms of disease: the role of intestinal barrier function in the pathogenesis of gastrointestinal autoimmune diseases. *Nature Clinical Practice. Gastroenterology and Hepatology, 2*(9), 416–422. PubMed PMID: 16265432.

107. Takeda, Y., Nakase, H., et al. (2009). Upregulation of T-bet and tight junction molecules by Bifidobacterium longum improves colonic inflammation of ulcerative colitis. *Inflammatory Bowel Diseases, 15*(11), 1617–1618.

108. Li, N., & Neu, J. (2009). Glutamine deprivation alters intestinal tight junctions via a PI3-K/Akt mediated pathway in Caco-2 cells. *The Journal of Nutrition, 139*(4), 710–714. PubMed PMID: 19161180.

109. Suzuki, T., & Hara, H. (2009). Quercetin enhances intestinal barrier function through the assembly of zonula [corrected] occludens-2, occludin, and claudin-1 and the expression of claudin-4 in Caco-2 cells. *The Journal of Nutrition, 139*(5), 965–974. PubMed PMID: 19297429.

110. Amasheh, M., Schlichter, S., Amasheh, S., et al. (2008). Quercetin enhances epithelial barrier function and increases claudin-4 expression in Caco-2 cells. *The Journal of Nutrition, 138*(6), 1067–1073. PubMed PMID: 18492835.

111. Heaney, R. P. (1992). Calcium in the prevention and treatment of osteoporosis. *Journal of Internal Medicine, 231*(2), 169–180. PubMed PMID: 1541941.

112. Reid, I. R. (1996). Therapy of osteoporosis: calcium, vitamin D, and exercise. *The American Journal of the Medical Sciences, 312*(6), 278–286. PubMed PMID: 8969617.

113. Reid, I. R., Ames, R. W., Evans, M. C., et al. (1995). Long-term effects of calcium supplementation on bone loss and fractures in postmenopausal women: a randomized controlled trial. *The American Journal of Medicine, 98*(4), 331–335. PubMed PMID: 7709944.

114. National Institutes of Health, Office of Dietary Supplements. (2017). *Dietary Supplement Fact Sheet.* http://ods.od.nih.gov/factsheets/calcium.asp. [Accessed 5 May 2017].

115. Dawson-Hughes, B., Dallal, G. E., Krall, E. A., et al. (1990). A controlled trial of the effect of calcium supplementation on bone density in postmenopausal women. *The New England Journal of Medicine, 323*(13), 878–883. PubMed PMID: 2203964.

116. Bourgoin, B. P., Evans, D. R., Cornett, J. R., et al. (1993). Lead content in 70 brands of dietary calcium supplements. *American Journal of Public Health, 83*(8), 1155–1160. PubMed PMID: 8342726.

117. Adorini, L., & Penna, G. (2008). Control of autoimmune diseases by the vitamin D endocrine system. *Nature Clinical Practice. Rheumatology*, 4(8), 404–412. PubMed PMID: 18594491.

118. Institute of Medicine, Food and Nutrition Board. (2010). *Dietary reference intakes for calcium and vitamin D*. Washington, DC: National Academy Press.

119. National Institutes of Health, Office of Dietary Supplements. (2017). *Dietary Supplement Fact Sheet: Vitamin D*. http://ods.od.nih.gov/factsheets/vitamind.asp. [Accessed 5 May 2017].

120. Dawson-Hughes, B., Harris, S. S., Krall, E. A., et al. (1995). Rates of bone loss in postmenopausal women randomly assigned to one of two dosages of vitamin D. *The American Journal of Clinical Nutrition*, 61(5), 1140–1145. PubMed PMID: 7733040.

121. Chapuy, M. C., Arlot, M. E., Delmas, P. D., & Meunier, P. J. (1994). Effect of calcium and cholecalciferol treatment for three years on hip fractures in elderly women. *BMJ (Clinical Research Ed.)*, 308(6936), 1081–1082. PubMed PMID: 8173430.

122. Avenell, A., Mak, J. C., O'Connell, D., & Vitamin, D. (2014). and vitamin D analogues for preventing fractures in postmenopausal women and older men. *The Cochrane Database of Systematic Reviews*, (4), CD000227, PubMed PMID: 24729336.

123. Ohtani, T., Nakagawa, S., Kurosawa, M., et al. (2005). Cellular basis of the role of diesel exhaust particles in inducing Th2-dominant response. *The Journal of Immunology: Official Journal of the American Association of Immunologists*, 174(4), 2412–2419. PubMed PMID: 15699178.

124. Chang, Y., Sénéchal, S., de Nadai, P., et al. (2006). Diesel exhaust exposure favors TH2 cell recruitment in nonatopic subjects by differentially regulating chemokine production. *The Journal of Allergy and Clinical Immunology*, 118(2), 354–360. PubMed PMID:16890758.

125. Yanagisawa, R., Koike, E., Win-Shwe, T. T., et al. (2016). Low-dose benzo[a]pyrene aggravates allergic airway inflammation in mice. *Journal of Applied Toxicology: JAT*, 36(11), 1496–1504. PubMed PMID: 26918773.

126. Zhao, C., Liao, J., Chu, W., et al. (2012). Involvement of TLR2 and TLR4 and Th1/Th2 shift in inflammatory responses induced by fine ambient particulate matter in mice. *Inhalation Toxicology*, 24(13), 918–927. Erratum in: *Inhalation Toxicology* 2013 Feb;25(3):178. PubMed PMID: 23121301.

127. Dobreva, Z. G., Kostadinova, G. S., Popov, B. N., et al. (2015). Proinflammatory and anti-inflammatory cytokines in adolescents from Southeast Bulgarian cities with different levels of air pollution. *Toxicology and Industrial Health*, 31(12), 1210–1217. PubMed PMID: 23771874.

128. Iavicoli, I., Marinaccio, A., Castellino, N., & Carelli, G. (2004). Altered cytokine production in mice exposed to lead acetate. *International Journal of Immunopathology and Pharmacology*, 17(2 Suppl.), 97–102. PubMed PMID: 15345199.

129. Heo, Y., Lee, W. T., & Lawrence, D. A. (1997). In vivo the environmental pollutants lead and mercury induce oligoclonal T cell responses skewed toward type-2 reactivities. *Cellular Immunology*, 179(2), 185–195. PubMed PMID: 9268502.

130. Agrawal, A., Kaushal, P., Agrawal, S., et al. (2007). Thimerosal induces TH2 responses via influencing cytokine secretion by human dendritic cells. *Journal of Leukocyte Biology*, 81(2), 474–482. PubMed PMID: 17079650.

131. de Vos, G., Abotaga, S., Liao, Z., et al. (2007). Selective effect of mercury on Th2-type cytokine production in humans. *Immunopharmacology and Immunotoxicology*, 29(3–4), 537–548. PubMed PMID: 18075863.

132. Kato, T., Tada-Oikawa, S., Wang, L., et al. (2013). Endocrine disruptors found in food contaminants enhance allergic sensitization through an oxidative stress that promotes the development of allergic airway inflammation. *Toxicology and Applied Pharmacology*, 273(1), 10–18. PubMed PMID: 24035973.

133. Fukuyama, T., Tajima, Y., Ueda, H., et al. (2011). Prior exposure to immunosuppressive organophosphorus or organochlorine compounds aggravates the T(H)1- and T(H)2-type allergy caused by topical sensitization to 2,4-dinitrochlorobenzene and trimellitic anhydride. *Journal of Immunotoxicology*, 8(2), 170–182. PubMed PMID: 21534883.

134. Daniel, V., Huber, W., Bauer, K., et al. (2002). Associations of dichlorodiphenyltrichloroethane (DDT) 4.4 and dichlorodiphenyldichloroethylene (DDE) 4.4 blood levels with plasma IL-4. *Archives of Environmental Health*, 57(6), 541–547. PubMed PMID: 12696651.

135. Kim, H. A., Kim, E. M., Park, Y. C., et al. (2003). Immunotoxicological effects of Agent Orange exposure to the Vietnam War Korean veterans. *Industrial Health*, 41(3), 158–166. PubMed PMID: 12916745.

136. Seo, M., Yamagiwa, T., Kobayashi, R., et al. (2008). Augmentation of antigen-stimulated allergic responses by a small amount of trichloroethylene ingestion from drinking water. *Regulatory Toxicology and Pharmacology*, 52(2), 140–146. PubMed PMID: 18721841.

137. Gaspar-Ramírez, O., Pérez-Vázquez, F. J., Pruneda-Álvarez, L. G., et al. (2012). Effect of

polychlorinated biphenyls 118 and 153 on Th1/Th2 cells differentiation. *Immunopharmacology and Immunotoxicology*, *34*(4), 627–632. PubMed PMID: 22233178.

138. Gillis, B., Gavin, I. M., Arbieva, Z., et al. (2007). Identification of human cell responses to benzene and benzene metabolites. *Genomics*, *90*(3), 324–333. PubMed PMID: 17572062.

139. Yan, H., Takamoto, M., & Sugane, K. (2008). Exposure to Bisphenol A prenatally or in adulthood promotes T(H)2 cytokine production associated with reduction of CD4CD25 regulatory T cells. *Environmental Health Perspectives*, *116*(4), 514–519. PubMed PMID: 18414636.

140. Yoshino, S., Yamaki, K., Li, X., et al. (2004). Prenatal exposure to bisphenol A up-regulates immune responses, including T helper 1 and T helper 2 responses, in mice. *Immunology*, *112*(3), 489–495. PubMed PMID: 15196218.

141. Bornehag, C. G., & Nanberg, E. (2010). Phthalate exposure and asthma in children. *International Journal of Andrology*, *33*(2), 333–345. PubMed PMID: 20059582.

142. Fujimaki, H., Nohara, K., Kobayashi, T., et al. (2002). Effect of a single oral dose of 2,3,7,8-tetrac hlorodibenzo-p-dioxin on immune function in male NC/Nga mice. *Toxicological Sciences*, *66*(1), 117–124. PubMed PMID: 11861978.

143. Fukuyama, T., Ueda, H., Hayashi, K., et al. (2008). Detection of low-level environmental chemical allergy by a long-term sensitization method. *Toxicology Letters*, *180*(1), 1–8. PubMed PMID: 18571882.

144. Zheng, L., Dong, G. H., Zhang, Y. H., et al. (2011). Type 1 and Type 2 cytokines imbalance in adult male C57BL/6 mice following a 7-day oral exposure to perfluorooctanesulfonate (PFOS). *Journal of Immunotoxicology*, *8*(1), 30–38. PubMed PMID: 21299352.

145. Duramad, P., Harley, K., Lipsett, M., et al. (2006). Early environmental exposures and intracellular Th1/Th2 cytokine profiles in 24-month-old children living in an agricultural area. *Environmental Health Perspectives*, *114*(12), 1916–1922. PubMed PMID: 17185285.

146. van Voorhis, M., Knopp, S., Julliard, W., et al. (2013). Exposure to atmospheric particulate matter enhances Th17 polarization through the aryl hydrocarbon receptor. *PLoS ONE*, *8*(12), e82545. PubMed PMID: 24349309.

147. Brandt, E. B., Kovacic, M. B., Lee, G. B., et al. (2013). Diesel exhaust particle induction of IL-17A contributes to severe asthma. *The Journal of Allergy and Clinical Immunology*, *132*(5), 1194–1204.e2. PubMed PMID: 24060272.

148. Wang, H., Peng, W., Weng, Y., et al. (2012). Imbalance of Th17/Treg cells in mice with chronic cigarette smoke exposure. *International Immunopharmacology*, *14*(4), 504–512. PubMed PMID: 23044435.

149. Luo, S., Li, Y., Li, Y., et al. (2016). Gestational and lactational exposure to low-dose bisphenol A increases Th17 cells in mice offspring. *Environmental Toxicology and Pharmacology*, *47*, 149–158. PubMed PMID: 27693988.

150. Wang, G., Wang, J., Fan, X., et al. (2012). Protein adducts of malondialdehyde and 4-hydroxynonenal contribute to trichloroethene-mediated autoimmunity via activating Th17 cells: dose- and time-response studies in female MRL+/+ mice. *Toxicology*, *292*(2–3), 113–122. PubMed PMID: 22178267.

151. Kuwatsuka, Y., Shimizu, K., Akiyama, Y., et al. (2014). Yusho patients show increased serum IL-17, IL-23, IL-1β, and TNFα levels more than 40 years after accidental polychlorinated biphenyl poisoning. *Journal of Immunotoxicology*, *11*(3), 246–249. PubMed PMID: 24083809.

152. Hassuneh, M. R., Albini, M. A., & Talib, W. H. (2012). Immunotoxicity induced by acute subtoxic doses of paraquat herbicide: implication of shifting cytokine gene expression toward T-helper (T(H))-17 phenotype. *Chemical Research in Toxicology*, *25*(10), 2112–2116. PubMed PMID: 22938100.

49

Liver Toxicity
Nonalcoholic Fatty Liver Disease and Nonalcoholic Steatohepatitis

SUMMARY

- Presence in population: In the United States, prevalence of nonalcoholic fatty liver disease (NAFLD) is estimated to be 30.0%
- Primary sources: Diet, high fructose corn syrup, persistent organic pollutants (POPs), toxic metals

- Best measure: Liver enzymes as screening, liver ultrasound, and biopsy to confirm diagnosis
- Best intervention: Diet and lifestyle modifications, avoidance of toxicants, reduction of toxic body burden

DESCRIPTION

The liver metabolizes many potentially harmful environmental contaminants and facilitates the excretion of these contaminants from the body. Eighty percent of the liver is made up of hepatocytes, which play a critical role in the amino acid and ammonia metabolism, biochemical oxidation reactions, and detoxification of a variety of drugs, vitamins, hormones, and environmental toxicants. Kupffer cells constitute most of the tissue macrophages present in the body and play a protective role against gut-derived bacterial endotoxins and microbial debris. Upon activation, Kupffer cells release cytokines, prostanoids, nitric oxide, and reactive oxygen species (ROS), which cause inflammation and can influence the noxiousness of environmental toxicants.[1]

Hepatotoxicity is the most common organ injury due to occupational and environmental chemical exposures. Variations in genetics, dietary factors, and nutrient cofactors all affect an individual's ability to metabolize chemicals effectively and efficiently. A variety of toxins and toxicants can cause liver dysfunction because of the central role this organ plays in xenobiotic metabolism. Industrial toxicants and drugs have been associated with the development of nonalcoholic fatty liver disease (NAFLD) and nonalcoholic steatohepatitis (NASH).[2]

NAFLD is characterized by fatty infiltration of the liver, primarily by triglycerides, and insulin resistance in the absence of chronic alcohol consumption. NAFLD has been described as the hepatic component of metabolic syndrome.[3] The diagnosis of NASH is established by the presence of lobular inflammation and cell injury (and in some cases progressive fibrosis) in addition to hepatocellular fat accumulation.[4] Pathophysiology involves insulin resistance, which causes steatosis, and oxidative stress, which produces lipid peroxidation and activates inflammatory cytokines, resulting in NASH.[5]

Using ultrasonographic data from National Health and Nutritional Examination Survey (NHANES) III, prevalence estimates found the age-adjusted incidence of hepatic steatosis and NAFLD in the US population to be 21.4% and 19.0%, respectively.[6] This equates to approximately 32.5 million adults with hepatic steatosis and 28.8 million adults with NAFLD. More recent analysis has found the prevalence of NAFLD to be 30.0% nationwide, making NAFLD the most common chronic liver disease in the United States.[7] Defining fatty liver as a fatty liver index score ≥ 30 shows the prevalence of NAFLD has increased

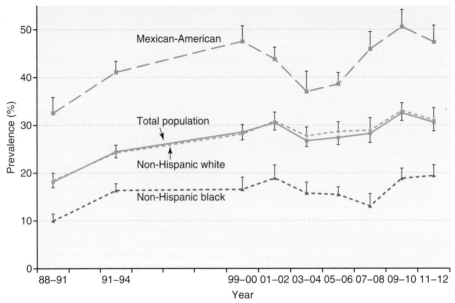

FIG. 49.1 Time trends of fatty liver prevalence in the United States population. (From Ruhl, C. E., & Everhart, J. E. [2015]. Fatty liver indices in the multiethnic United States National health and Nutrition Examination Survey. *Alimentary Pharmacology and Therapeutics, 41*[1], 65–76.)

from 18% in 1988 to 1991, to 29% in 1999 to 2000, to 31% in 2011 to 2012 (Fig. 49.1).[8] The prevalence of NAFLD increases significantly to 80% to 90% in obese adults, 90% in patients with hyperlipidemia, and 30% to 50% in diabetics, and parallels the prevalence of metabolic syndrome, insulin resistance, type 2 diabetes, and central obesity.[9,10] Having metabolic syndrome is an independent risk factor for NAFLD, and those with metabolic syndrome have a 2.37-fold risk of NAFLD compared with those without metabolic syndrome.[11] Alarmingly, NAFLD is emerging as a common pediatric disease, affecting approximately 3% to 9% of all children in the United States and up to 50% of obese children.[12]

Prevalence of NASH has been difficult to establish because a liver biopsy is required for diagnosis. In 1990, an autopsy-based cross-sectional study reported the overall prevalence of NASH in adults in North America to be 18.5% in obese and 2.7% in nonobese individuals.[13] Since that time, the rates of diabetes and obesity have steadily increased, along with the quantity and concentration of toxic compounds in the environment.[14,15,16] More recent evidence estimates the prevalence of NASH to be 12.2%, and among patients with a positive ultrasound for fatty liver, the prevalence of NASH increases to 29.9%.[17]

NAFLD and NASH disproportionally affect Mexican Americans, men, older adults, and people with diabetes and obesity (Table 49.1). However, when Mexican-American and Caucasian subjects are well matched for clinical parameters, particularly for degree of obesity, there is no significant differences in the severity of insulin resistance or steatohepatitis.[18] Aging of the population and increasing prevalence of diabetes and obesity are expected to contribute to an increase in the overall burden of liver disease in the United States. Although liver-related deaths are increased by NAFLD, cardiovascular mortality is the leading cause of death,[19] and NAFLD is an independent risk factor for cardiovascular disease.[20]

TOXICITY—MECHANISMS OF ACTION

Excess intracellular fatty acids (FAs), oxidative stress, insulin resistance with a decreased adiponectin-leptin ratio, adenosine triphosphate (ATP) depletion, metabolic endotoxemia, and mitochondrial dysfunction are all important causes of hepatocellular injury in the steatoic liver.[21] It is likely these factors are not mutually exclusive and act in a more coordinated manner. For example, mitochondrial structural defects lead to increased FA

TABLE 49.1	Prevalence of NAFLD in the US, NHANES III, 1988 to 1994			
Sex by Age	Non-Hispanic White Prevalence	Non-Hispanic Black Prevalence	Mexican American Prevalence	Total Prevalence
Men				
< 30 years	8.3	10.9	15.6	9.9
30≤40 years	15.9	12.5	25.7	16.1
40≤50 years	22.2	17.1	36.2	22.3
50≤60 years	28.0	17.4	41.4	29.3
≥60 years	28.1	22.6	33.4	27.6
Women				
< 30 years	9.5	12.0	16.5	10.6
30≤40 years	11.1	10.4	23.2	12.5
40≤50 years	15.0	14.3	34.7	16.1
50≤60 years	20.5	21.9	35.7	21.6
≥60 years	25.7	23.9	34.4	25.4

From Lazo, M., Hernaez, R., Eberhardt, M. S., Bonekamp, S., Kamel, I., Guallar, E., Koteish, A., Brancati, F. L., Clark, J. M. (2013). Prevalence of nonalcoholic fatty liver disease in the United States: The Third National Health and Nutrition Examination Survey, 1988–1994. *American Journal of Epidemiology, 178*(1), 38–45.

beta oxidation, leading to abnormal cytokine production and insulin resistance, which are crucial pathophysiologic factors in NASH.[22,23] Interleukin (IL)-6 levels are increased in NAFLD but are significantly higher in those with steatohepatitis as opposed to simple fatty liver.[24] Accumulation of intrahepatic FAs can promote the formation of reactive oxygen intermediates, which in turn can impair liver function directly or indirectly by perpetuating the inflammatory response.[25] Serum-free FAs have direct hepatotoxicity through the induction of an endoplasmic reticulum stress response and subsequent activation of the mitochondrial pathway of cell death.[26]

NAFLD is associated with decreased cellular glutathione (GSH), the major endogenous antioxidant produced in the body.[27] In addition, cytochrome P450 2E1 (CYP2E1) has emerged as an important cause of ROS overproduction, and higher hepatic CYP2E1 expression and activity have been observed in the context of obesity and NAFLD.[28] Higher levels of CYP2E1 in NAFLD may aggravate liver injury from xenobiotic compounds through the generation of harmful reactive metabolites.

SOURCES

Diet and Lifestyle

High Fructose Corn Syrup. Several studies have shown high fructose corn syrup (HFCS) to be a contributing factor to energy overconsumption, weight gain, and the rise in the prevalence of obesity.[29,30,31] Fructose in sugar-sweetened beverages promotes insulin resistance.[32] HFCS also promotes dyslipidemia,[33] increases visceral fat deposits, and increases hepatic *de novo* lipogenesis.[34] In NAFLD patients, *de novo* synthesis of FAs from glucose and fructose is dysregulated, leading to an increase in plasma-free fatty acids (FFAs) and a subsequent increase in the liver triglyceride content.[35] Fructose also provokes a hepatic stress response involving activation of c-Jun N-terminal kinases (JNK) and subsequent reduced hepatic insulin signaling.[36]

In a small-scale study, it was observed that consumption of fructose in 49 patients with NAFLD was two- to threefold higher than in 24 control subjects, and hepatic mRNA expression of fructokinase and FA synthase were increased in NAFLD patients.[37] Another study showed that 80% of patients (25 out of 31) with NAFLD consumed an excessive amount of soft drinks, totaling more than 50 g of added sugar per day.[38] In patients with NAFLD, fructose consumption was linked with lower hepatic fat content but increased hepatic fibrosis, suggesting that fructose may enhance liver inflammation.[39]

Obesity. The release of FAs from dysfunctional and insulin-resistant adipocytes results in lipotoxicity caused by the accumulation of triglyceride-derived toxic metabolites in the liver.[40] Excess adiposity is associated with increased proinflammatory cytokines, oxidative stress, and an exaggerated inflammatory response to endotoxin administration.[41]

Gut-Derived Endotoxins. Dysfunctional gut microbiota may play a role in the development of NASH and activate inflammation and endoplasmic reticulum stress.[42] Alterations in gut microbiota, increased intestinal permeability, and metabolic endotoxemia create a low-grade inflammatory state that contributes to the development of obesity and associated NAFLD.[43]

Air Particulate Matter

Toll-like receptor (TLR) activation of Kupffer cells, resident hepatic macrophages, and proinflammatory cytokine production have all been shown to play a role in the progression of NAFLD.[44] Animal studies suggest airborne pollutants may play a role in the pathogenesis of NAFLD. Mice exposed to diesel exhaust particles at 50 µg/kg bodyweight developed inflammation and oxidative DNA damage in the liver without systemic inflammation.[45] Obese, diabetic mice had increased levels of aspartate transaminase (AST) and alanine aminotransferase (ALT), enhanced steatosis, and elevated markers of oxidative stress after pulmonary exposure to diesel exhaust particles.[46] Researchers have postulated that inhaled fine particulate matter (PM) may aggravate NAFLD by crossing the alveolar membranes and entering circulation, where it accumulate in hepatic Kupffer cells and triggers toll-like receptor (TLR)4-dependent activation of cytokine release, which leads to inflammation and hepatic stellate cell collagen synthesis.[47]

Chemicals

Chloroalkenes. Vinyl chloride (VC) is metabolized by CYP2E1 forming the highly reactive genotoxic epoxide, chloroethylene oxide.[48] Occupational exposure to VC has been associated with steatohepatitis in lean Brazilian petrochemical workers,[49] and ultrasound studies demonstrated hepatomegaly, steatosis, and fibrosis in VC workers.[50]

A study of 29 dry cleaner workers exposed to 16 PPM of perchloroethylene (PCE), far less than the permissible exposure limit of 100 PPM in the United States, showed they had fatty infiltration, with mostly normal serum aminotransferase levels.[51]

Volatile Organic Compounds (VOC). Volatile organic compound (VOC) exposures, such as toluene, benzene,

styrene, and xylene, have been associated with NASH with both normal liver enzymes and abnormal liver enzymes.[52] Seventy-five percent of household painters with VOC exposures and abnormal liver enzymes had fatty liver on biopsy,[53] and 100% of toluene-exposed printers with persistent mild liver enzyme elevation had hepatic steatosis.[54]

Persistent Organic Pollutants. POPs are lipophilic in nature and can easily cross the biological membranes and accumulate in fatty tissues. Multiple animal studies show exposure to 2,3,7,8-tetrachlorodibenzo-para-dioxin (TCDD) produces toxic manifestations in the liver, including lipid accumulation, hepatocellular hypertrophy inflammatory cell infiltration, and hyperplasia,[55] as well as an increase in total hepatic FAs, triglycerides, and serum ALT levels.[56] Polychlorinated biphenyl (PCB) 153 exposure causes NAFLD with hepatic antioxidant depletion.[57]

Toxic Metals

The presence of toxic heavy metals (arsenic, mercury, cadmium, chromium, copper, nickel, lead, and zinc) has been shown to be a significant risk factor for fatty liver disease in men (Odds Ratio (OR) 1.83, 95% Confidence Interval (CI); 1.161–2.899, $p = 0.009$), especially with a body mass index (BMI) < 24 kg/m^2.[58]

Cadmium. Low urinary levels of cadmium (0.65–0.83 ug/g) are associated in NAFLD (OR 2.21) and NASH (OR 1.30).[59]

Mercury. Elevations of serum ALT, indicating NAFLD, are associated with blood mercury levels. In the NHANES 2003 to 2004 cohort, individuals with blood mercury levels in the second quartile (25th to 50th percentile) were twice as likely to have elevated ALT.[60] Data collected from the Korea National Health and Nutrition Examination Survey (KNHANES) showed that increasing blood mercury levels were associated with increases in AST, ALT, and elevated gamma-glutamyl transferase (GGTP; >56 IU/L).[61,62] The primary mechanism of mercury hepatotoxicity may be related to poisoning of cysteine-containing proteins and GSH depletion.[63]

ASSESSMENT

The "gold standard" for diagnosing and staging NAFLD is histology via biopsy of the liver.[64] However, risks and costs of liver biopsy have prompted researchers to seek noninvasive methods to diagnose and stage NAFLD. Cytokeratin (CK) 18 is a serum marker of NASH that has been the most validated. CK-18 fragments stem from apoptosis of hepatocytes and can be measured in plasma. The utility of CK-18 fragments has been validated in a multicenter study, which demonstrated that for every 50 U/L increase in the plasma level of CK-18, the likelihood of having NASH increased by 74% (OR: 1.74; 95% CI, 1.31–2.31).[65]

Conventional biomarkers of hepatotoxicity include serum ALT, AST, alkaline phosphatase (ALP), total bilirubin, gamma-glutamyltransferase (GGT), and albumin. Research indicates that several liver enzymes increase in proportionate response to the load of specific classes of toxins.

Alkaline Phosphatase

ALP is a hydrolase enzyme responsible for dephosphorylation. It is present in higher concentration in the liver, kidney, and bone. Chronic exposure of pesticides in agricultural workers was found to be associated with significantly higher activities of ALP compared with controls, and the number of years exposed to pesticides predicted higher activities of ALP.[66]

Bilirubin

Bilirubin levels increase in proportion to the level of various PCBs, which is significant as bilirubin is considered the best prognostic measure of chronic liver dysfunction.[67,68] Direct bilirubin is inversely associated with NAFLD with a significant dose-response relationship (p = <0.05) and serves as a protective biomarker, likely based on the endogenous antioxidant and cytoprotectant properties of bilirubin.[69]

Transaminase Enzymes—ALT and AST

ALT is a transaminase enzyme that catalyzes the transfer of an amino group from L-alanine to α-ketoglutarate. For men aged 18 to 20, ALT values >37 IU/L are considered elevated, whereas the cutoff for men over the age of 21 is >48 IU/L. For women aged 18 to 20, ALT values >30 IU/L are considered elevated, and ALT values >31 IU/L are considered elevated for women over the age of 21.

Unexplained elevations in ALT level have been used to signify the presence of NAFLD. Data from the NHANES III suggests that the prevalence of unexplained elevations in ALT is 7% in individuals with metabolic syndrome and 3.5% in those without metabolic syndrome.[70] However, many patients with NAFLD have normal ALT levels, and the data likely underestimates the actual frequency of NAFLD.[71]

ALT increases in a dose-dependent manner with body load of blood cadmium, lead, mercury, and PCBs within and above the normal range.[72] Exposure to polycyclic aromatic hydrocarbons causes elevations in AST and ALT.[73] When serum log-perfluorooctanoic acid (PFOA, a perfluorinated chemical) increases by one unit, serum ALT increases by 1.86 units (95% CI, 1.24–2.48; p = 0.005).[74]

The AST level may occasionally be higher than the ALT level, especially in the presence of cirrhosis, but the AST/ALT ratio is rarely greater than 2.[75] Among patients who have NAFLD without advanced fibrosis, the AST/ALT ratio is typically less than 1, but it tends to reverse as the degree of fibrosis progresses to cirrhosis.[76]

Gamma-Glutamyltransferase

Elevations of GGT directly correlate with alcohol consumption and toxic metal load (cadmium and lead).[77,78] Serum GGT, within its reference range, is also associated with organochlorine pesticides and polycyclic aromatic hydrocarbons.[79] GGT elevates by exposure to other chemicals, especially POPs and several prescription drugs. Workers with a history of alcohol consumption and high exposure to TCDD were found to have a statistically significant elevated risk for out of range GGT compared with referents.[80] GGT has been shown to be a surrogate marker of NAFLD and may be a simple and reliable marker of visceral and hepatic fat deposition and hepatic steatosis.[81,82] GGT shows significant positive association with HOMA-IR in NAFLD subjects, even after waist circumference and Hb A_{1c} are adjusted.[83]

INTERVENTION

Managing comorbidities—obesity, diabetes, and hyperlipidemia—with diet and lifestyle modifications is at the forefront of treatment. Weight loss improves liver aminotransferase levels and hepatic steatosis in proportion to the total amount of weight loss. Thirty-one obese subjects were randomized to 48 weeks of lifestyle intervention (200 minutes a week of moderate physical activity) versus standard dietary counseling alone. Participants who lost ≥ 7% of weight compared with those who lost < 7% had significant improvements in steatosis, lobular inflammation, and ballooning injury.[84] The addition of flaxseed oil may enhance these lifestyle modifications.[85]

Antioxidants, such as vitamin E and vitamin C, have shown promise. A double-blind, randomized, placebo-controlled study demonstrated that a combination of vitamin C (1000 mg/day × 6 months) and vitamin E (1000 IU/day × 6 months) resulted in statistically significant improvement in fibrosis score.[86] Treatment with silymarin plus vitamin E along with diet and lifestyle modifications reduces GGT levels and decreases noninvasive NAFLD index scores.[87] Ginger has been hypothesized to prevent NAFLD via several mechanisms, including sensitizing insulin effects, downregulation of proinflammatory cytokines, antioxidant and antidyslipidemic effects, and reducing hepatic triglyceride content.[88]

Lipotropic agents such as choline, methionine, betaine, folate, and vitamin B_{12} help promote the export of fat from the liver and may be helpful in a variety of liver conditions including chemical-induced liver disease. Supplementation with chlorella decreases toxic metals and metabolites by directly preventing absorption of toxins, increasing stool and urinary excretion of metals, and preventing enterohepatic recirculation of toxins.[89]

Bile acid therapy with ursodeoxycholic acid may be beneficial by reducing bile acid cytotoxicity and protecting hepatocytes against bile acid–induced apoptosis.[90]

REFERENCES

1. Bilzer, M., Roggel, F., & Gerbes, A. L. (2006). Role of Kupffer cells in host defense and liver disease. *Liver International, 26*(10), 1175–1186. PubMed PMID: 17105582.
2. Cotrim, H. P., Andrade, Z. A., et al. (1999). Nonalcoholic steatohepatitis: a toxic liver disease in industrial workers. *Liver, 19*(4), 299–304. PubMed PMID: 10459628.
3. Akbar, D. H., & Kawther, A. H. (2006). Nonalcoholic fatty liver disease and metabolic syndrome: what we know and what we don't know. *Medical Science Monitor, 12*(1), RA23–RA26. PubMed PMID: 16369477.
4. Neuschwander-Tetri, B. A. (2002). Evolving pathophysiological concepts in nonalcoholic steatohepatitis. *Current Gastroenterology Reports, 4*(1), 31–36. PubMed PMID: 11825539.
5. McCullough, A. J. (2002). Update on nonalcoholic fatty liver disease. *Journal of Clinical Gastroenterology, 34*(3), 255–262. PubMed PMID: 11873108.
6. Lazo, M., Hernaez, R., et al. (2013). Prevalence of nonalcoholic fatty liver disease in the United States: the Third National Health and Nutrition Examination Survey, 1988-1994. *American Journal of Epidemiology, 178*(1), 38–45. PubMed PMID: 23703888.
7. Le, M. H., Devaki, P., Ha, N. B., Jun, D. W., et al. (2017). Prevalence of nonalcoholic fatty liver disease and risk factors for advanced fibrosis and mortality in the united States. *PLoS ONE, 12*(3), e0173499. PubMed PMID: 28346543.
8. Ruhl, C. E., & Everhart, J. E. (2015). Fatty liver indices in the multiethnic United States National health and Nutrition Examination Survey. *Alimentary Pharmacology and Therapeutics, 41*(1), 65–76. PubMed PMID: 25376360.
9. Loomba, R., & Sanyal, A. J. (2013). The global NAFLD epidemic. *Nature Reviews. Gastroenterology & Hepatology, 10*(11), 686–690. PubMed PMID: 24042449.
10. Bellentani, S., Scaglioni, F., Marino, M., & Bedogni, G. (2010). Epidemiology of nonalcoholic fatty liver disease. *Digestive Diseases, 28*(1), 155–161. PubMed PMID: 20460905.
11. Tsai, C. H., Li, T. C., & Lin, C. C. (2008). Metabolic syndrome as a risk factor for nonalcoholic fatty liver disease. *Southern Medical Journal, 101*(9), 900–905. PubMed PMID: 18708987.
12. Papandreou, D., Ruosso, I., & Mavromichalis, I. (2007). Update on nonalcoholic fatty liver disease in children. *Clinical Nutrition: Official Journal of the European Society of Parenteral and Enteral Nutrition, 26*(4), 409–415. PubMed PMID: 17449148.
13. Wanless, I. R., & Lentz, J. S. (1990). Fatty liver hepatitis (steatohepatitis) and obesity: an autopsy study with analysis of risk factors. *Hepatology, 12*(5), 1106–1110. PubMed PMID: 2227807.
14. Ogden, C. L., Carroll, M. D., et al. (2006). Prevalence of overweight and obesity in the United States, 1999-2004. *JAMA: The Journal of the American Medical Association, 295*(13), 1549–1555. PubMed PMID: 16595758.
15. Carpenter, D. O. (2008). Environmental contaminants as risk factors for developing diabetes. *Reviews on Environmental Health, 23*(1), 59–74. PubMed PMID: 18557598.
16. Lee, D. H., Lee, I. K., Jin, S. H., Steffes, M., & Jacobs, D. R., Jr. (2007). Association between serum concentrations of persistent organic pollutants and insulin resistance among nondiabetic adults: results from the National Health and Nutrition Examination Survey 1999-2002. *Diabetes Care, 30*(3), 622–628. PubMed PMID: 17327331.
17. Williams, C. D., Stengel, J., Asike, M. I., et al. (2011). Prevalence of nonalcoholic fatty liver disease and nonalcoholic steatohepatitis among a largely middle-aged population utilizing ultrasound and liver

biopsy: a prospective study. *Gastroenterology*, 140(1), 124–131. PubMed PMID: 20858492.

18. Lomonaco, R., Ortiz-Lopez, C., et al. (2011). Role of ethnicity in overweight and obese patients with nonalcoholic steatohepatitis. *Hepatology*, 54(3), 837–845. PubMed PMID: 21674556.

19. Adams, L. A., Lymp, J. F., et al. (2005). The natural history of nonalcoholic fatty liver disease: a population-based cohort study. *Gastroenterology*, 129(1), 113–121. PubMed PMID: 16012941.

20. Bhatia, L. S., Curzen, N. P., Calder, P. C., & Byrne, C. D. (2012). Nonalcoholic fatty liver disease: a new and important cardiovascular risk factor? *European Heart Journal*, 33(10), 1190–1200. PubMed PMID: 22408036.

21. Neuschwander-Tetri, B. A., & Caldwell, S. H. (2003). Nonalcoholic steatohepatitis: summary of an AASLD single topic conference. *Hepatology*, 37(5), 1202–1219. PubMed PMID: 12717402.

22. Sanyal, A. J., Campbell-Sargent, C., et al. (2001). Nonalcoholic steatohepatitis: association of insulin resistance and mitochondrial abnormalities. *Gastroenterology*, 120(5), 1183–1192. PubMed PMID: 11266382.

23. Tilg, H., & Hotamisligil, G. S. (2006). Nonalcoholic fatty liver disease: cytokine-adipokine interplay and regulation of insulin resistance. *Gastroenterology*, 131(3), 934–945. PubMed PMID: 16952562.

24. Wieckowska, A., Papouchado, B. G., Li, Z., et al. (2008). Increased hepatic and circulating interleukin-6 levels in human nonalcoholic steatohepatitis. *The American Journal of Gastroenterology*, 103(6), 1372–1379. PubMed PMID: 18510618.

25. Gentile, C. L., & Pagliassotti, M. J. (2008). The role of fatty acids in the development and progression of nonalcoholic fatty liver disease. *The Journal of Nutritional Biochemistry*, 19(9), 567–576. PubMed PMID: 18430557.

26. Ibrahim, S. H., Kohli, R., & Gores, G. J. (2011). Mechanisms of lipotoxicity in NAFLD and clinical implications. *Journal of Pediatric Gastroenterology and Nutrition*, 53(2), 131–140. PubMed PMID: 21629127.

27. Merrell, M. D., & Cherrington, N. J. (2011). Drug metabolism alterations in nonalcoholic fatty liver disease. *Drug Metabolism Reviews*, 43(3), 317–334. PubMed PMID: 21612324.

28. Aubert, J., Begriche, K., et al. (2011). Increased expression of cytochrome P450 2E1 in nonalcoholic fatty liver disease: mechanisms and pathophysiological role. *Clinics and Research in Hepatology and Gastroenterology*, 35(10), 630–637. PubMed PMID: 21664213.

29. Ludwig, D. S., Peterson, K. E., & Gortmaker, S. L. (2001). Relation between consumption of sugar sweetened drinks and childhood obesity: a prospective, observational analysis. *Lancet*, 357, 505–508. PubMed PMID: 11229668.

30. Bray, G. A., Nielsen, S. J., & Popkin, B. M. (2004). Consumption of high-fructose corn syrup in beverages may play a role in the epidemic of obesity. *The American Journal of Clinical Nutrition*, 79, 537–543. PubMed PMID: 15051594.

31. Elliot, S. S., Keim, N. L., Stern, J. S., Teff, K., & Havel, P. J. (2002). Fructose, weight gain, and the insulin resistance syndrome. *The American Journal of Clinical Nutrition*, 76, 911–922. PubMed PMID: 12399260.

32. Stanhope, K. L. (2012). Role of fructose-containing sugars in the epidemics of obesity and metabolic syndrome. *Annual Review of Medicine*, 63, 329–343.

33. Mock, K., Sundus, L., Benedito, V. A., & Tou, J. C. (2017). High-fructose corn syrup-55 consumption alters hepatic lipid metabolism and promotes triglyceride accumulation. *The Journal of Nutritional Biochemistry*, 39, 32–39.

34. Stanhope, K. L., Schwarz, J. M., Keim, N. L., et al. (2009). Consuming fructose-sweetened, not glucose-sweetened, beverages increases visceral adiposity and lipids and decreases insulin sensitivity in overweight/obese humans. *The Journal of Clinical Investigation*, 119(5), 1322–1334.

35. Donnelly, K. L., Smith, C. I., et al. (2005). Sources of fatty acids stored in liver and secreted via lipoproteins in patients with nonalcoholic fatty liver disease. *The Journal of Clinical Investigation*, 115(5), 1343–1351. PubMed PMID: 15864352.

36. Basaranoglu, M., Basaranoglu, G., Sabunco, T., & Senturk, H. (2013). Fructose as a key player in the development of fatty liver disease. *World Journal of Gastroenterology*, 19(8), 1166–1172. PubMed PMID: 23482247.

37. Ouyang, X., Cirillo, P., et al. (2008). Fructose consumption as a risk factor for nonalcoholic fatty liver disease. *Journal of Hepatology*, 48(6), 993–999. PubMed PMID: 18395287.

38. Assy, N., Nasser, G., Kamayse, I., et al. (2008). Soft drink consumption linked with fatty liver in the absence of traditional risk factors. *Canadian Journal of Gastroenterology*, 22(10), 811–816. PubMed PMID: 18925303.

39. Abdelmalek, M. F., Suzuki, A., Guy, C., et al. (2010). Increased fructose consumption is associated with fibrosis severity in patients with nonalcoholic fatty liver disease. *Hepatology*, 51(6), 1961–1971. PubMed PMID: 20301112.

40. Cusi, K. (2012). Role of obesity and lipotoxicity in the development of nonalcoholic steatohepatitis: pathophysiology and clinical implications. *Gastroenterology*, 142(4), 711–725. PubMed PMID: 22326434.

41. Yang, S. Q., Lin, H. Z., Lane, M. D., et al. (1997). Obesity increases sensitivity to endotoxin liver injury: implications for the pathogenesis of steatohepatitis. *Proceedings of the National Academy of Sciences of the United States of America*, 94(6), 2557–2562. PubMed PMID: 9122234.

42. Tilg, H., & Moschen, A. R. (2010). Evolution of inflammation in nonalcoholic fatty liver disease: the multiple parallel hits hypothesis. *Hepatology*, 52(5), 1836–1846. PubMed PMID: 21038418.

43. Frazier, T. H., DiBaise, J. K., & McClain, C. J. (2011). Gut microbiota, intestinal permeability, obesity-induced inflammation, and liver injury. *JPEN. Journal of Parenteral and Enteral Nutrition*, 35(5 Suppl.), 14S–20S. PubMed PMID: 21807932.

44. Isogawa, M., Robek, M. D., et al. (2005). Toll-like receptor signaling inhibits hepatitis B virus replication in vivo. *Journal of Virology*, 79(11), 7269–7272. PubMed PMID: 15890966.

45. Folkmann, J. K., Risom, L., et al. (2007). Oxidatively damaged DNA and inflammation in the liver of dyslipidemic ApoE-/-mice exposed to diesel exhaust particles. *Toxicology*, 237(1–3), 134–144. PubMed PMID: 17602821.

46. Tomaru, M., Takano, H., Inoue, K., et al. (2007). Pulmonary exposure to diesel exhaust particles enhances fatty change of the liver in obese diabetic mice. *International Journal of Molecular Medicine*, 19(1), 17–22. PubMed PMID: 17143543.

47. Tan, H. H., Fiel, M. I., et al. (2009). Kupffer cell activation by ambient air particulate matter exposure may exacerbate nonalcoholic fatty liver disease. *Journal of Immunotoxicology*, 6(4), 266–275. PubMed PMID: 19908945.

48. Huang, C. Y., Huang, K. L., et al. (1997). The GST T1 and CYP2E1 genotypes are possible factors causing vinyl chloride induced abnormal liver function. *Archives of Toxicology*, 71(8), 482–488. PubMed PMID: 9248625.

49. Cotrim, H. P., De Freitas, L. A., et al. (2004). Clinical and histopathological features of NASH in workers exposed to chemicals with or without associated metabolic conditions. *Liver International*, 24(2), 131–135. PubMed PMID: 15078477.

50. Hsiao, T. J., Wang, J. D., Yang, P. M., Yang, P. C., & Cheng, T. J. (2004). Liver fibrosis in asymptomatic polyvinyl chloride workers. *Journal of Occupational and Environmental Medicine*, 46(9), 962–966. PubMed PMID: 15354062.

51. Brodkin, C. A., Daniell, W., et al. (1995). Hepatic ultrasonic changes in workers exposed to perchloroethylene. *Occupational and Environmental Medicine*, 52(10), 679–685. PubMed PMID: 7489059.

52. Brautbar, N., & Williams, J. (2002). Industrial solvents and liver toxicity: risk assessment, risk factors and mechanisms. *International Journal of Hygiene and Environmental Health*, 205(6), 479–491. PubMed PMID: 12455270.

53. Dossing, M., Arlien-Soborg, P., et al. (1983). Liver damage associated with occupational exposure to organic solvents in house painters. *European Journal of Clinical Investigation*, 13(2), 151–157. PubMed PMID: 6409638.

54. Guzelian, P. S., Mills, S., & Fallon, H. J. (1988). Liver structure and function in print workers exposed to toluene. *Journal of Occupational Medicine*, 30(10), 791–796. PubMed PMID: 3230426.

55. Kopec, A. K., D'Souza, M. L., Mets, B. D., Burgoon, L. D., et al. (2011). Non-additive hepatic gene expression elicited by 2,3,7,8-tetrachlorodibenzo-p-dioxin (TCDD) and 2,2',4,4',5,5'-hexachlorobiphenyl (PCB153) co-treatment in C57BL/6 mice. *Toxicology and Applied Pharmacology*, 256(2), 154–167. PubMed PMID: 21851831.

56. Boverhof, D. R., Burgoon, L. D., et al. (2006). Comparative toxicogenomic analysis of the hepatotoxic effects of TCDD in Sprague Dawley rats and C57BL/6 mice. *Toxicological Sciences*, 94(2), 398–416. PubMed PMID: 16960034.

57. Shi, X., Wahlang, B., Wei, X., et al. (2012). Metabolomic analysis of the effects of polychlorinated biphenyls in nonalcoholic fatty liver disease. *Journal of Proteome Research*, 11(7), 3805–3815. PubMed PMID: 22686559.

58. Lin, Y. C., Lian, I. B., Kor, C. T., et al. (2017). Association between soil heavy metals and fatty liver disease in men in Taiwan: a cross-sectional study. *BMJ Open*, 7(1), e014215. PubMed PMID: 28115335.

59. Hyder, O., Chung, M., Cosgrove, D., et al. (2013). Cadmium exposure and liver disease among US adults. *Journal of Gastrointestinal Surgery: Official Journal of the Society for Surgery of the Alimentary Tract*, 17(7), 1265–1273. PubMed PMID: 23636881.

60. Lin, Y. S., Ginsberg, G., Caffrey, J. L., Xue, J., Vulimiri, S. V., Nath, R. G., et al. (2014). Association of body burden of mercury with liver function test status in the U.S. population. *Environment International*, 70, 88–94. PubMed PMID: 24908642.

61. Lee, H., Kim, Y., Sim, C. S., Ham, J. O., Kim, N. S., & Lee, B. K. (2014). Associations between blood mercury levels

and subclinical changes in liver enzymes among South Korean general adults: analysis of 2008-2012 Korean national health and nutrition examination survey data. *Environmental Research*, 130, 14–19. PubMed PMID: 24525240.

62. Seo, M. S., Lee, H. R., Shim, J. Y., Kang, H. T., & Lee, Y. J. (2014). Relationship between blood mercury concentrations and serum γ-glutamyltranspeptidase level in Korean adults using data from the 2010 Korean National Health and Nutrition Examination Survey. *Clinica Chimica Acta*, 430, 160–163. PubMed PMID: 24508988.

63. Lin, T. H., Huang, Y. L., & Huang, S. F. (1996). Lipid peroxidation in liver of rats administered with methyl mercuric chloride. *Biological Trace Element Research*, 54(1), 33–41. PubMed PMID: 8862759.

64. Sanyal, A. J. (2002). American Gastroenterological Association. AGA technical review on nonalcoholic fatty liver disease. *Gastroenterology*, 123(5), 1705–1725. PubMed PMID: 12404245.

65. Feldstein, A. E., Wieckowska, A., et al. (2009). Cytokeratin-18 fragment levels as noninvasive biomarkers for nonalcoholic steatohepatitis: a multicenter validation study. *Hepatology*, 50(4), 1072–1078. PubMed PMID: 19585618.

66. Araoud, M., Neffeti, F., Douki, W., et al. (2012). Adverse effects of pesticides on biochemical and haematological parameters in Tunisian agricultural workers. *Journal of Exposure Science and Environmental Epidemiology*, 22(3), 243–247. PubMed PMID: 22377683.

67. Dufour, D. R., et al. (2000). Diagnosis and monitoring of hepatic injury. II. Recommendations for use of laboratory tests in screening, diagnosis, and monitoring. *Clinical Chemistry*, 46(12), 2050–2068. PubMed PMID: 11106350.

68. Kumar, J., et al. (2014). Persistent organic pollutants and liver dysfunction biomarkers in a population-based human sample of men and women. *Environmental Research*, 134, 251–256. PubMed PMID: 25173059.

69. Tian, J., Zhong, R., Liu, C., et al. (2016). Association between bilirubin and risk of nonalcoholic fatty liver disease based on a prospective cohort study. *Scientific Reports*, 6, 310006. PubMed PMID: 27484402.

70. Liangpunsakul, S., & Chalasani, N. (2005). Unexplained elevations in alanine aminotransferase in individuals with the metabolic syndrome: results from the third National Health and Nutrition Survey (NHANES III). *The American Journal of the Medical Sciences*, 329(3), 111–116. PubMed PMID: 15767815.

71. Mofrad, P., Contos, M. J., et al. (2003). Clinical and histologic spectrum of nonalcoholic fatty liver disease associated with normal ALT values. *Hepatology*, 37(6), 1286–1292. PubMed PMID: 12774006.

72. Cave, M., et al. (2010). Polychlorinated biphenyls, lead, and mercury are associated with liver disease in American adults: NHANES 2003-2004. *Environmental Health Perspectives*, 118(12), 1735–1742. PubMed PMID: 21126940.

73. Min, Y. S., Lim, H. S., & Kim, H. (2015). Biomarkers for polycyclic aromatic hydrocarbons and serum liver enzymes. *American Journal of Industrial Medicine*, 58(7), 764–772. PubMed PMID: 25940037.

74. Lin, C. Y., Lin, L. Y., Chiang, C. K., Wang, W. J., et al. (2010). Investigation of the associations between low-dose serum perfluorinated chemicals and liver enzymes in US adults. *The American Journal of Gastroenterology*, 105(6), 1354–1363. PubMed PMID: 20010922.

75. Bacon, B. R., Farahvash, M. J., Janney, C. G., & Neuschwander-Tetri, B. A. (1994). Nonalcoholic steatohepatitis: an expanded clinical entity. *Gastroenterology*, 107(4), 1103–1109. PubMed PMID: 7523217.

76. Angulo, P., Keach, J. C., Batts, K. P., & Lindor, K. D. (1999). Independent predictors of liver fibrosis in patients with nonalcoholic steatohepatitis. *Hepatology*, 30(6), 1356–1362. PubMed PMID: 10573511.

77. Nagaya, T., et al. (1999). Dose-response relationships between drinking and serum tests in Japanese men aged 40–59 years. *Alcohol*, 17(2), 133–138. PubMed PMID: 10064381.

78. Lee, D. H., et al. (2006). Graded associations of blood lead and urinary cadmium concentrations with oxidative-stress-related markers in the U.S. population: results from the third National Health and Nutrition Examination Survey. *Environmental Health Perspectives*, 114(3), 350–354. PubMed PMID: 16507456.

79. Lee, D. H., & Jacobs, D. R. (2009). Is serum gamma-glutamyltransferase an exposure marker of xenobiotics? Empirical evidence with polycyclic aromatic hydrocarbon. *Clinical Chemistry and Laboratory Medicine*, 47(7), 860–862. PubMed PMID: 19575547.

80. Calvert, G. M., Hornung, R. W., et al. (1992). Hepatic and gastrointestinal effects in an occupational cohort exposed to 2,3,7,8-tetrachlorodibenzo-para-d ioxin. *JAMA: The Journal of the American Medical Association*, 267(16), 2209–2214. PubMed PMID: 1348289.

81. Angulo, P. (2005). Nonalcoholic fatty liver disease. *Revista de Gastroenterologia de Mexico*, 70(Suppl. 3), 52–56. PubMed PMID: 17471859.

82. Karp, D. R., Shimooku, K., & Lipsky, P. E. (2001). Expression of gamma-glutamyl transpeptidase protects

ramos B cells from oxidation-induced cell death. *The Journal of Biological Chemistry, 276*(6), 3798–3804. PubMed PMID: 11080500.

83. Hossain, I. A., Rahman Shah, M. M., Rahman, M. K., & Ali, L. (2016). Gamma glutamyl transferase is an independent determinant for the association of insulin resistance with nonalcoholic fatty liver disease in Bangladeshi adults: association of GGT and HOMA-IR with NAFLD. *Diabetes & Metabolic Syndrome, 10*(1 Suppl. 1), S25–S29. PubMed PMID: 26482965.

84. Promrat, K., Kleiner, D. E., Niemeier, H. M., Jackvony, E., et al. (2010). Randomized controlled trial testing the effects of weight loss on nonalcoholic steatohepatitis. *Hepatology, 51*(1), 121–129. PubMed PMID: 19827166.

85. Yari, Z., Rahimlou, M., et al. (2016). Flaxseed supplementation in nonalcoholic fatty liver disease: a pilot randomized, open labeled, controlled study. *International Journal of Food Sciences and Nutrition, 67*(4), 461–469. PubMed PMID: 26983396.

86. Harrison, S. A., Torgerson, S., et al. (2003). Vitamin E and vitamin C treatment improves fibrosis in patients with nonalcoholic steatohepatitis. *The American Journal of Gastroenterology, 98*(11), 2485–2490. PubMed PMID: 14638353.

87. Aller, R., Izaola, O., et al. (2015). Effect of silymarin plus vitamin E in patients with nonalcoholic fatty liver disease. A randomized clinical pilot study. *European Review for Medical and Pharmacological Sciences, 19*(16), 3118–3124. PubMed PMID: 26367736.

88. Sahebkar, A. (2011). Potential efficacy of ginger as a natural supplement for nonalcoholic fatty liver disease. *World Journal of Gastroenterology, 17*(2), 271–272. PubMed PMID: 21246004.

89. Uchikawa, T., Kumamoto, Y., et al. (2011). Enhanced elimination of tissue methylmercury in Parachlorella beijerinckii-fed mice. *The Journal of Toxicological Sciences, 36*(1), 121–126. PubMed PMID: 21297350.

90. Paumgartner, G., & Beuers, U. (2002). Ursodeoxycholic acid in cholestatic liver disease: mechanisms of action and therapeutic use revisited. *Hepatology, 36*(3), 525–531. PubMed PMID: 12198643.

50

Renal Toxicity

SUMMARY

- Presence in population: The prevalence of chronic kidney disease (CKD) in the United States is approximately 14%[1]
- Major diseases: Diabetes, hypertension, hyperlipidemia, cardiovascular disease, pulmonary edema, pericarditis, anemia, depression, osteoporosis, and premature death
- Primary sources: The key nephrotoxic agents include cadmium, mercury, lead, fluorinated hydrocarbons, and glyphosate; in addition, toxins

of choice such as smoking, nonsteroidal antiinflammatory drugs, excessive use of salt, and phosphates in the diet also significantly contribute to kidney dysfunction.
- Best measures: Glomerular filtration rate (GFR), creatinine, sodium, potassium, protein in urine
- Best interventions: Dietary and lifestyle modifications, adequate hydration, botanicals (e.g., ginger, curcumin, ginkgo, beet juice, blueberries, gotu kola)

INTRODUCTION

The kidneys play several roles in maintaining health, including activating hormones, maintaining stable levels of key molecules in the blood, and excreting toxins. Most consider the kidneys to be second only to the liver in importance for toxin and toxicant elimination. However, considering that 20% to 25% of cardiac output goes through the kidneys, which filter the blood a remarkable 60 times per day, a case could be made that the kidneys are more important than the liver for toxin and toxicant elimination. The kidneys remove unwanted products of metabolism such as ammonia, urea, uric acid, creatinine, end products of hemoglobin metabolism, and hormone metabolites, as well as toxicants that have been made water soluble via phase II liver conversion. The kidneys are responsible for direct excretion of industrial toxicants such as metals and new-to-nature molecules. In addition, they excrete nutrients or food constituents when consumed in excess, such as salt, vitamin C, and B-vitamins.

Although the kidneys are good at removing many toxins and toxicants from the blood, some are difficult to excrete into the urine, thus they accumulate in the kidneys. As toxicant concentrations increase, a disproportionate amount of damage to the kidneys may result. Cadmium illustrates this problem well.[2,3]

Unfortunately, as a result of exposure to such a high toxic load in the modern world, loss of kidney function with aging—as can be seen in Fig. 50.1—is considered "normal."[4] A 90-year-old has only one-third to one-half the kidney function of a 20-year-old. This results in a significant decrease in an individual's ability to eliminate many toxic compounds and may help explain why most people have an increasing disease burden with aging. Once again, "normal" is not healthy.

The key environmental, dietary, and endogenous toxicants that appear to be the primary causes of the kidney dysfunction epidemic include heavy metals (cadmium, mercury, lead); persistent organic pollutants [POPs] (glyphosates and halogenated hydrocarbons—especially those that are fluorinated and released when nonstick pans are heated to the highest cooking temperatures); smoking; nonsteroidal antiinflammatory drugs (especially acetaminophen); lipopolysaccharides (LPS)

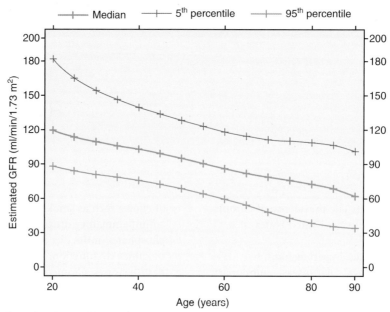

FIG. 50.1. Deterioration in kidney function with aging. (Data from Frassetto, L. A., Morris R. C. Jr., & Sebastian A. [1996]. Effect of age on blood acid-base composition in adulthood humans: role of age-related renal functional decline. *American Journal of Physiology–Renal Physiology, 271*[6 Pt 2], F1114–F1122.)

from a leaky, toxic gut; and excessive dietary salt and phosphates. These all add up to a chronic damaging load on the kidneys.

KIDNEY EXCRETION OF TOXINS AND TOXICANTS

The kidneys excrete toxic compounds via three main mechanisms: filtration through the glomeruli, passive diffusion typically from the distal tubules, and active processes where toxic compounds are transported from the blood into the urine. Note in Fig. 50.2 that some molecules are reabsorbed after being filtered by the glomeruli. This is a normal, controlled process by which the kidneys maintain blood levels of key molecules within a narrow range.

The glomeruli filter out most of the small- and medium-sized water-soluble molecules from the blood. Some are then reabsorbed, such as sodium, to ensure stable levels, maintain blood volume, and enable proper physiological body functions. The proximal tubules contain several active, energy-dependent transporters such as organic anion transporters (OATs), organic anion

transporting polypeptides (OATPs), organic cation transporters (OCTs), multidrug resistance-associated proteins (MRPs), multidrug-resistant proteins (MDRs), and multidrug and toxin extrusion proteins (MATEs) that transport specific toxicants out of the blood and, ideally, into the urine. Finally, there is passive diffusion of the more fat-soluble toxic agents across the tubules into the urine. These later processes are quite slow but may be important for some.

Several factors determine how the kidneys excrete specific toxicants. If the molecule is large or bound to protein, it does not pass through the glomeruli and has to be managed in other ways. As their fat-soluble level increases, those that are both water- and fat-soluble (the octanol/water partition coefficient) are more passively reabsorbed in the distal tubules back into the kidneys and, potentially, into the blood. The active toxicant excretion pathways have limited capacity and can be easily saturated. This limitation is used at times to add an inexpensive drug to the treatment regimen to decrease the rate at which an expensive or difficult-to-obtain drug is excreted so that higher blood levels of the medication can be attained at lower dosages. Finally, because the

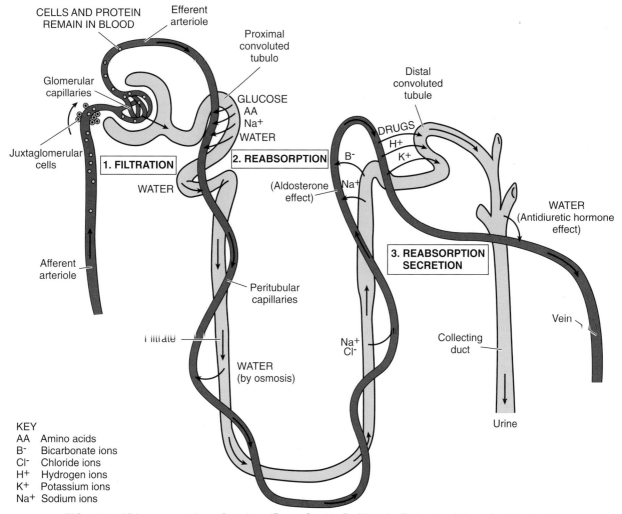

FIG. 50.2. Kidney excretion of toxins. (From Gould, B. [2011]. *Pathophysiology for the health professions* [4th ed.]. Philadelphia: Elsevier.)

body uses adenosine triphosphate (ATP) to actively pump out specific toxicants, if the kidney's mitochondria are not working well, these active processes do not work as efficiently. Worse, when the mitochondria are not working adequately, the kidneys cannot protect their own tissue, and high concentrations of toxicants can accumulate in the kidneys.

HOW THE KIDNEYS ARE DAMAGED

Damage to the kidneys can result from a variety of causes, including inadequate blood supply, dehydration, mito-

chondrial dysfunction, indirectly by toxicants that cause general tissue damage, and directly by toxicants specifically harmful to the kidney tissues. In addition, an overload of toxic compounds that may not be individually toxic can become problematic when the total load is elevated. Toxins can come from within the body, such as from an unhealthy gut, and/or externally from the many toxic metals and chemicals in the industrialized world.

Blood supply is foundational to kidney function, as most of the loss of GFR is typically due to the loss in quality and quantity of the microcirculation of the kidneys rather than glomerular damage. Many of the factors known to increase the risk of most chronic diseases include, as part of the mechanism, damage to microcirculation. Examples include smoking, poor blood sugar control (i.e., loss of microcirculation underlies the serious side effects of diabetes such as loss of vision, loss of toes, and, appropriately, accelerated decline in kidney function), elevated blood pressure, oxidative stress, elevated homocysteine, obesity, and high-fat meals, which increase absorption of endotoxins from the gut.

Some research suggests that, in addition to the factors previously mentioned, impaired microcirculation in the kidneys, not just glomerular damage, may be the primary reason for the decline in function associated with aging.[5] A significant number of the elderly have measurable loss of kidney function resulting from atherosclerosis in the arteries leading to the kidneys. Catheterization to remove the blockage significantly increases kidney function, which strongly supports the concept that glomerular dysfunction may be as much due to poor blood flow as to cellular death.[6] This decreased circulation also facilitates the accumulation of extracellular matrix (ECM) around the kidney that not only causes a buildup of scar tissue but also impairs vascular endothelial growth factor (VEGF) from helping restore blood flow. This is modeled in Fig. 50.3.

Toxic Metals

Cadmium, chromium, lead, mercury, platinum, and uranium are all nephrotoxic. Although each is significant, the most common as well as the most researched are cadmium and mercury.

Cadmium. The main sources of cadmium are tobacco smoking and conventionally grown soybeans. These crops are grown with high phosphate fertilizers that are contaminated with cadmium. Cadmium is a significant kidney toxicant. It has a worrisome half-life of more than 10 years, as it is very difficult to excrete. The kidney holds 50% of the total body burden of cadmium, which increases the nephrotoxicity. Once cadmium enters the body, much of it binds to metallothioneins. These compounds are cleared through the glomeruli but are then reabsorbed by the tubules, where they become trapped. As the metallothioneins slowly degrade, highly toxic free cadmium is constantly released. While it passively migrates into the urine, it also causes oxidative stress to the tubules. Current cadmium exposure, experienced by individuals living in the United States, has reached levels that adversely

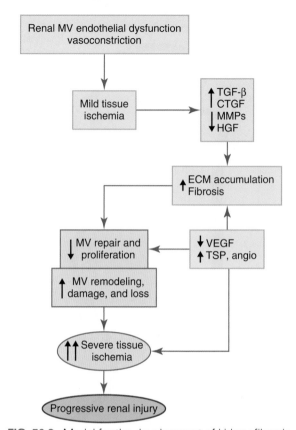

FIG. 50.3. Model for the development of kidney fibrosis.

affect kidney health in a significant proportion of the population.[7] Cadmium damage to the kidneys may help explain why it accounts for a surprising 20% of osteoporosis, as the final stage in activation of vitamin D into 1,25 OH2D3 occurs in the kidneys. As kidneys degenerate, they not only lose their ability to excrete toxicants; they are less able to perform other normal physiological functions. Cadmium exposure, especially in adults with hypertension or diabetes, is a significant risk factor in the development of CKD.[8]

Mercury. Mercury is present in the environment because of natural environmental events and/or pollution sources. The main sources of human exposure to mercury is the consumption of large fish such as tuna and, to a lesser extent, dental amalgam fillings (which are approximately 55% mercury). Kidneys have a high affinity for mercury. Within a few hours of exposure, much of the mercury that gets into blood ends up in the kidneys. Mercury damages both the glomeruli and the tubules. Proximal tubular necrosis, especially along the straight renal segments in the inner cortex and outer stripe of the outer medulla, is a prominent feature of inorganic mercury nephrotoxicity.[9] Much of the tissue damage appears to result from poisoning of the kidney mitochondria so there is not enough ATP for the cells to protect themselves from the toxicants they excrete.[10]

Lead. Renal damage is a common finding among lead workers and is also found in persons with nonoccupational low-level lead exposures. The progression to end-stage renal disease increases in direct proportion to the amount of lead in the kidneys.[11] Erythrocyte lead levels have been found to be reflective of kidney lead burden, whereas blood lead levels are positively associated with increasing serum creatinine levels in the Normative Aging Study.[12] However, it must be kept in mind that the data for the Normative Aging Study was gathered between 1961 and 1994, when blood lead levels were at their highest points in the United States. Lead damages the kidneys both from direct oxidative damage to renal cells and from lead-induced hypertension. Cumulative lead burden, assessed both via bone lead levels and the CaEDTA lead mobilization test have demonstrated a clear association between elevated body lead and renal disease.[13] Greater risks for lead-associated renal damage was noted in persons with diabetes.[14] Reducing the total body lead burden via long-term chelation with CaEDTA has proven successful in slowing the renal damage and delaying the need for dialysis.

Persistent Organic Pollutants

Persistent organic pollutants (POPs) are new-to-nature molecules specifically designed for special purposes and created to be difficult for biological systems to break down. They range from herbicides and pesticides to nonstick coatings and fire retardants. Individuals may be as contaminated with these chemicals as the environment. Because POPs are highly fat-soluble, they are particularly damaging to the kidneys. Research is still early on their long-term health effects, as many have been created relatively recently.

Many of these chemicals are classified as halogenated hydrocarbons and are so difficult to detoxify or excrete that they have half-lives measured in years to decades, such as now-banned molecules like polychlorinated biphenyls (PCBs). The following is a brief discussion of just a few POPs with serious nephrotoxicity.

Fluorinated Hydrocarbons. Tetrafluoroethylene and similar compounds are polymerized to produce polytetrafluoroethylene (PTFE) polymers such as Teflon. Other toxicants in this class include perfluorooctanoic acid (PFOA) and perfluorooctanesulfonic acid (PFOS). These compounds are used in many products such as nonstick coatings on pots and pans; waterproof, breathable clothing; and stain prevention on carpet and upholstery. Although these nonstick coatings are supposedly inert, the reality is quite different. When nonstick surfaces are heated to high temperatures on a stovetop, they emit toxic gases. The lowest temperature at which this process begins is 392° F, a temperature commonly achieved in the typical kitchen.[15] The temperature at which most oils start to smoke is high enough for the polymers to start breaking down.

Fluorinated hydrocarbons damage the kidneys by passive diffusion into the tubules, where they poison the mitochondria. The resulting damage creates inadequate energy production impairing active excretion, increases oxidative stress as the damaged mitochondria leak highly oxidative electrons and oxygen, and causes cell death producing progressive loss of kidney function.[16]

Glyphosate. The herbicide glyphosate is heavily used in conventional agriculture and around the home under names such as Roundup. Limited research is available to find definitive current measures of the amount of glyphosate or its main metabolite, aminomethylphosphonic acid (AMPA), in US water supplies. The amount in use has increased rapidly over the past 2 decades. A 2014 study commissioned by Moms Across America tested 21 drinking water samples with no apparent methodology for ensuring a representative distribution. Nonetheless, the results were alarming. Thirteen of the samples had glyphosate levels ranging from 85 to 330 PPB, and more worrisome is that 76 to 166 parts per billion (PPB) of glyphosate was found in the breast milk samples that were tested.[17]

Some researchers are speculating that glyphosates may be a significant aspect of the problems associated with genetically modified organism (GMO) foods. Glyphosate use has tripled since 1997, largely due to the increasing popularity of Roundup Ready crops (e.g., corn and soybeans).[18] These foods are genetically modified specifically to be resistant to glyphosate. This leads to an increase in the amount sprayed around them and thus an increase in contamination of the food supply, water, and breast milk.

Epidemiological research has found a strong correlation between glyphosate use and the kidney failure epidemic. Of course, association does not prove causation. Animal research shows that chronic exposure at very low dosages causes kidney damage. A 2-year study in rats' drinking water with 0.1 PPB of glyphosate resulted in cellular kidney abnormalities and significant chronic kidney deficiencies.[19] Several unpublished research projects conducted by Monsanto, some performed nearly 4 decades ago, demonstrated urinary abnormalities, hyperplasia of the urinary bladder, and significant reproductive and developmental toxicity following glyphosate exposure at various levels.[20,21,22,23]

Research conducted in Sri Lanka found that those who drank well water contaminated with glyphosate had a higher incidence of kidney failure in proportion to concentration starting at 0.7 PPB, and farmers spraying glyphosates in the fields had a 5.4-fold increased incidence of kidney disease.[24] The European standard for water contamination is 0.1 PPB, whereas the US Environmental Protection Agency (EPA) standard is an inexplicable 700 PPB.[25] As discussed elsewhere in this textbook, the toxicity of pure glyphosate and the industrial products actually used are very different, complicating the determination of its clinical significance.

Smoking

Smoking is a well-known risk factor in the development of renal dysfunction.[26,27] As the smoking dose increases, the prevalence of hypertension, serum creatinine level, urinary protein excretion, percent of global glomerulosclerosis, and the prevalence of arteriolar hyalinosis also increases.[28] Smoking damages the kidneys as a result of its cadmium content and nicotine content, which constrict the blood vessels going into the kidneys, decreasing glomerular filtration.[29] Smoking also increases the generation of reactive oxygen species and activation of fibrotic pathways in the kidneys.[30,31]

Nonsteroidal Antiinflammatory Drugs

Most nonsteroidal antiinflammatory drugs (NSAIDS) were initially available only by prescription. Later, when the patents expired, NSAIDs became available over the counter. Many of these readily available medications have long-term side effects that are not adequately appreciated. Virtually all safety studies are short term. Therefore many

toxic effects are not detected during the research and development stages, and arise later in population studies. Acetaminophen, aspirin, ibuprofen, naproxen, indomethacin, and COX-2 inhibitors have all been shown to cause kidney damage when used chronically.[32,33,34]

Chronic consumption (>3 years) of single and/or combinations of NSAIDs are known to cause irreversible analgesic nephropathy.[35] Chronic use of aspirin has an odds ratio for kidney failure of 1.5, increasing to 2.7 for chronic acetaminophen use. Note that these data are for kidney failure; loss of kidney function is much more prevalent.

Discontinuing the use of NDSAIDs results in some recovery of function, even in patients with kidney failure. After 6 months of stopping NSAIDs, those with the most damaged kidneys still had a doubling of kidney function (Fig. 50.4).[36]

Toxins from the Gut

Endogenous toxins are those originating from within an organism and are not attributable to any external or environmental factor. These include gut-derived microbial toxins, normal metabolites not properly detoxified, and poorly detoxified hormones. Substantial body load arises from endotoxins, causing significant disruption to body functions. Technically only bacterial LPS are known as endotoxins, however, it is clinically relevant in this context to use a broader definition. Endotoxins bind to

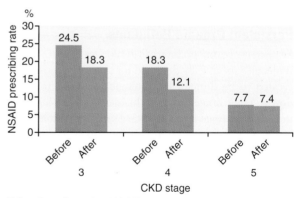

FIG. 50.4. Stopping NSAID use greatly improves function in patients with kidney failure. (From Wei, L., MacDonald, T. M., Jennings, C., Sheng, X., Flynn, R. W., & Murphy, M. J. [2013]. Estimated GFR reporting is associated with decreased nonsteroidal anti-inflammatory drug prescribing and increased renal function. Kidney International, 84[1], 174–178.)

receptors initiating an adaptive immune response and a signaling cascade, leading to activation of proinflammatory genes.[37] Impaired digestive function along with gut-derived microbial toxins trigger both the onset and maintenance of chronic low-grade inflammation.[38] This, in turn, enhances intestinal permeability and increases the translocation of microbiome-derived LPS to the bloodstream, which results in a two- to threefold increase in serum LPS concentration, which can reach a threshold named "metabolic endotoxemia" (ME). ME may trigger toll-like receptor (TLR) 4-mediated inflammatory activation, eliciting a chronic low-grade proinflammatory and prooxidative state.[39,40] Endotoxins cause direct harm to the kidneys and complicate the situation, as damaged kidneys have trouble clearing endotoxins.[41]

Further supporting the concept that a toxic gut damages the kidneys is the research showing a direct correlation between the level of indoles in the blood and loss of kidney function.[42] A long-term prospective study also found a correlation between rate of death and indole levels in dialysis patients.[43]

Excessive Salt in the Diet

Excessive salt consumption is another significant factor contributing to the degeneration of the kidneys.[44] Mean intake of sodium in a global population is estimated at 3.95 g/day (equivalent to 10.06 g/day of salt), and in the United States the average intake of sodium is 3.4 g/day (equivalent to 8.7 g/day of salt).[45] Diets of natural foods without added salt contain 500 to 800 mg sodium/day.[46]

Over the millennia, as humans have evolved as a species, salt was not readily available. Therefore we had to develop effective mechanisms for retaining salt. As shown in Fig. 50.5, humans went from an evolutionary diet that had a sodium/potassium ratio of 1 to 10 to one that is greater than 3 to 1.

Excessive salt intake appears to overload the kidneys enough to impair their ability to eliminate other toxins, especially acidic metabolic waste products. Studies have

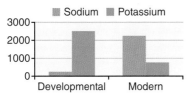

FIG. 50.5. The dramatic increase in sodium and decrease in potassium found in the modern diet.

shown a connection between NaCl intake and acid-base balance, with high-salt diets causing a decrease in pH and moderate metabolic and adaptive acidosis.[47,48] In response to acidosis, the kidney implements adaptive processes to restore the acid-base balance. These include the excretion of the nonmetabolizable anions, the conservation of citrate, the enhancement of kidney ammoniagenesis, and urinary excretion of ammonium ions, resulting in the lowering of urinary pH, hypocitraturia, hypercalciuria, and nitrogen and phosphate wasting.[49]

Excessive Phosphates in the Diet

The primary sources of "hidden" phosphates are additives used as processing aids, such as acid balancing (especially in carbonated beverages), leavening of bread, color and moisture retention, anticaking, and flavorings. As the amount of phosphorous added to prepared foods is underreported, assessing the actual amounts ingested is very difficult. Current databases underestimate the phosphorus content of processed foods by at least 25% to 30%.[50] Research suggests that a substantial portion of the population consumes more than the tolerable upper limit of 4000 mg/d and significantly more than the Recommended Dietary Allowance (RDA) of 700 mg/d for adults. As shown in Fig. 50.6, about 40% of Americans consume at least twice the RDA of phosphorous, a level known to almost double all-cause mortality.[51]

Increasing phosphate levels in the blood is one of the early signs of kidney failure.[52,53,54] Serum phosphorous levels in the "high-normal" range (≥ 4.0 mg/dL but <4.5 mg/dL) have been associated with a twofold higher risk of developing new-onset CKD and end-stage renal disease (ESRD) in the general population.[55] An observational study showed that every 0.5 mg/dL increase in serum phosphorous demonstrated a 40% greater risk for incident ESRD.[56]

Eliminating phosphates is difficult for the kidneys. Excessive intake of phosphates damages the tubules; increases fibrosis, which blocks the blood vessels; and decreases GFR. One potential mechanism linking serum phosphorous to the onset of kidney disease is increased nephrocalcinosis, where higher levels of phosphorous may directly promote vascular injury and calcifications.[57,58,59] Research has shown that excessive phosphorous consumption significantly disrupts hormonal regulation of phosphorus, calcium, and vitamin D, causing disordered mineral metabolism, osteoporosis, cardiovascular disease, and impaired kidney function.[60]

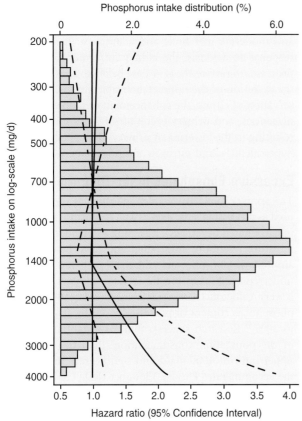

FIG. 50.6. Excessive phosphorous intake in the typical diet increases all-cause mortality. (Modified from Chang, A. R., Lazo, M., Appel, L. J., Gutiérrez, O. M., & Grams, M. E. [2014]. High dietary phosphorus intake is associated with all-cause mortality: results from NHANES III. *The American Journal of Clinical Nutrition, 99*[2], 320–327.)

PROTECTING AND REGENERATING THE KIDNEYS

The following foundational strategies are recommended for the protection and regeneration of the kidneys:
1. Decrease total toxic load on the kidneys.
2. Aggressively reduce exposure to nephrotoxins.
3. Increase microcirculation of kidneys.
4. Protect the kidneys from oxidative stress.

Decrease Total Toxic Load

Most of the causes of kidney damage can be controlled by helping people make better choices. To start, environmental chemicals around the home should be removed.

These include: paints, solvents, new furniture, chemical cleaners, and scented candles/air fresheners, to name a few. Building materials containing formaldehyde (e.g., carpeting, cabinetry) should also be avoided. Health and beauty aids can be a significant source of POPs.[61] Perfume, cologne, hair spray, lotions, antiperspirant, and scented soaps and shampoos often contain a number of chemicals that should be avoided. An air purifier can be used to help improve indoor air quality.

Some of the most immediate benefits can be seen by decreasing toxins of choice such as excessive dietary salt, excessive dietary phosphates, and drugs such as NSAIDs. Organic, mostly plant-based foods should be consumed when possible. Eating organic foods has been shown to measurably decrease POP levels within 3 days.[62]

Aggressively Decrease Exposure to Nephrotoxins

The key nephrotoxic agents include cadmium, mercury, fluorinated hydrocarbons, and glyphosate. Decreasing exposure is primarily accomplished by modifying diet and lifestyle choices. This includes eliminating or significantly reducing consumption of conventionally grown foods (e.g., soybeans grown with high-phosphate fertilizers), eliminating tobacco smoking, avoiding GMO foods, eliminating or reducing consumption of large fish (e.g., tuna), avoiding nonstick coatings on pots and pans, and avoiding clothing that is waterproof but breathable.

Improve Microcirculation of Kidneys

Beetroot Juice. Increasing blood flow to the kidneys has a huge effect on improving detoxification as well as decreasing oxidative stress. There is encouraging research evaluating the benefits of foods and nutrients that increase the production of nitrogen oxide in dilating peripheral blood vessels to increase blood flow to the tissues. One study showed an impressive, dose-dependent increase in blood flow to the kidneys of up to 26% (see Table 50.1).[63]

There is growing research on the health benefits of beetroot juice for humans, although limited research is available specifically looking at effects on kidney function. A study of adults with peripheral vascular disease found that beetroot juice clearly improved microcirculation, resulting in improved walking distance (Fig. 50.7).[64] This 18% increase in walking time certainly supports a significant improvement in blood flow.

TABLE 50.1	Beetroot Juice Increases Blood Flow to Kidneys		
	Control	BRLD[b]	BRHD[c]
Kidney	414 ± 29	447 ± 32	521 ± 32[a]

[a]$p < 0.05$ vs. Control.
[b]BRLD: beet root, low dose
[c]BRHD: beet root, high dose
From Ferguson, S. K., Hirai, D. M., Copp, S. W., Holdsworth, C. T., Allen, J. D., Jones, A. M., Musch, T. I., Poole, D. C. (2014). Dose dependent effects of nitrate supplementation on cardiovascular control and microvascular oxygenation dynamics in healthy rats. *Nitric Oxide: Biology and Chemistry/ Official Journal of the Nitric Oxide Society, 39,* 51–58.

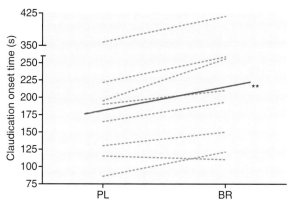

FIG. 50.7. *PL,* placebo; *BR,* beetroot. Beetroot juice improves peripheral blood supply. (From Kenjale, A. A., Ham, K. L., Stabler, T., Robbins, J. L., Johnson, J. L., VanBruggen, M., Privette, G., Yim, E., Kraus, W. E., Allen, J. D. [2011]. Dietary nitrate supplementation enhances exercise performance in peripheral arterial disease. *Journal of Applied Physiology, 110*[6], 1582–1591.)

Gotu Kola. Traditional Chinese medicine has used Gotu kola *(Centella asiatica)* to treat kidney diseases for centuries. Asiaticoside has been shown to improve microcirculation and reverse fibrosis in humans with varicose veins. Its direct benefits for the kidneys have only been shown in animals but are encouraging. In rats, gotu kola showed a protective effect from Adriamycin-induced nephropathy, resulting in dramatically improved kidney function.[65] Another study combined gotu kola with naringenin and showed decreased fibrosis formation in the kidneys.[66]

Chocolate. Dark chocolate consumption improves oxygenation of the kidneys in humans. The benefit

is directly proportional to catechin levels.[67] Animal research has shown that catechins also protect the kidneys from oxidative stress from toxic drugs like cyclosporine.[68]

Protect the Kidneys from Oxidative Stress

N-Acetylcysteine. N-acetylcysteine (NAC) is a potent antioxidant that has been shown to enhance the excretion of methylmercury. Studies demonstrate that NAC is effective at attenuating the oxidative damage caused by mercury on the kidneys by increasing the activities of superoxide dismutase (SOD), catalase (CAT), and glutathione-s-transferase (GST), and by decreasing glutathione (GSH) depletion and malondialdehyde [(MDA) the end product of lipid peroxidation] levels.[69,70]

Melatonin. In CKD, the production of melatonin is significantly impaired.[71] Melatonin has been shown to be a potent free-radical scavenger and antioxidant, which may be the reason for its benefit in CKD. Melatonin reverses mercury-induced oxidative tissue damage by increasing GSH levels and decreasing myeloperoxidase activity (an index of neutrophil infiltration).[72] Melatonin has also been shown to eliminate the deleterious effects of a high-salt diet on the kidneys via direct antioxidative effects.[73] In addition, in rats with renal ablation, melatonin retarded deterioration of the remnant kidney function and structure as well as reduced oxidative stress, hypertension, and inflammation.[74]

Blueberries. Blueberry anthocyanins specifically protect the kidneys from bowel-derived endotoxins. Fig. 50.8 shows how blueberries increase GFR in normal kidneys (but the increase is not statistically significant) and completely protect the kidneys from the dramatic lowering of GFR caused by gut toxins in those with impaired function.[75]

Quercetin. Quercetin has been shown to provide significant protective effects against mercury-induced acute kidney damage, as demonstrated by biochemical markers such as blood urea nitrogen and serum creatinine.[76] Specifically, quercetin reduced the accumulation of mercury in the kidney and protected against mercury-induced proximal tubular damage. In addition, pretreatment with quercetin significantly reduced apoptotic cell death in the kidney and increased urinary excretion of mercury and metallothionein.

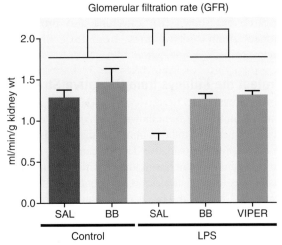

FIG. 50.8. Blueberries protect the kidneys from gut-derived toxins. (From Nair, A. R., Masson, G. S., Ebenezer, P. J., Del Piero F., & Francis J. [2014]. Role of TLR4 in lipopolysaccharide-induced acute kidney injury: Protection by blueberry. *Free Radical Biology and Medicine, 71,* 16–25.)

TABLE 50.2 Ginger Partially Restores Kidney Function in Diabetic Rats

	Kidney Function Test	
Group	Urea (mg/dL)	Creatinine (mg/dL)
Control	14.82±1.99[a]	1.72±0.26[a]
Diabetic untreated	50.61±6.82[b]	2.52±0.53[a]
Diabetic+Free	22.63±2.09[c]	2.01±0.29[a]
Diabetic+Bound	27.05±2.12[c]	2.83±0.71[a]
Diabetic+Glibenclamide	35.82±3.87[c]	2.11±0.23[a]

Values are mean±standard error of the mean (SEM) of eight rats per group. Test values down the vertical columns carrying different superscripts are significantly different ($p < 0.05$).
From Kazeem, M. I., Akanji, M. A., & Yakubu, M. T. (2015). Amelioration of pancreatic and renal derangements in streptozotocin-induced diabetic rats by polyphenol extracts of Ginger *(Zingiber officinale)* rhizome. *Pathophysiology, 22*(4), 203–209.

Curcumin. Curcumin (turmeric) has shown renoprotective benefit in diabetic nephropathy, chronic renal failure, ischemia, and in nephrotoxicity induced by cadmium, gentamicin, Adriamycin, chloroquine, iron nitrilotriacetate, sodium fluoride, hexavalent chromium, and cisplatin.[77] In fact, curcumin not only protects from damage but also maintains GFR despite the toxins.

Ginkgo Biloba. Ginkgo biloba has been shown to improve blood supply to the brain and other critical tissues. Ginkgo biloba also has the ability to protect against numerous mitochondrial toxins, which strengthens the case for its use in kidney disease, as mitochondrial damage in the kidneys mediates much of the nephrotoxicity.

Several studies have shown the benefits of ginkgo biloba on kidney function. One animal study showed improved kidney blood flow and function in hypertensive rats.[78] Another study found that ginkgo biloba protects the kidneys from glyphosate.[79] Other animal studies have shown protection of the kidneys from mercury, uranium, naphthalene, and many other toxins.[80,81,82] Ginkgo biloba also protects the kidneys from gut-derived endotoxins.[83]

Ginger (Zingiber Officinale). There is ample animal research showing that ginger *(Zingiber officinale)* not only

improves kidney function but is especially beneficial in protecting the kidney from cadmium. The primary mechanism of protection appears to be ginger's ability to decrease inflammation and oxidative damage to kidney tissue exposed to a variety of toxins. The antiinflammatory benefits of ginger in the kidney result from its antioxidant properties and the epigenetic downregulation of proinflammatory genes.[84] Ginger specifically increases activity of kidney antioxidant enzymes in obese and diabetic rats.[85]

Several animal studies have shown that ginger can protect kidneys from cadmium. One study found the antiinflammatory effects of ginger to be strong enough to prevent most of the kidney damage from cadmium.[86] Another found almost no histological kidney damage when ginger was fed along with cadmium.[87] This makes sense as much of the damage from cadmium is caused by increased oxidation.

Animal research has also shown kidney protection from alcohol, malathion, carbon tetrachloride, chromates, fructose, gentamycin, ischemia, lead, and cancer drugs.[88,89] Another study found that ginger prevented damage to the kidneys in a rat model of rheumatoid arthritis induced by injection of Complete Freund's adjuvant.[90] Table 50.2 shows restoration of kidney function in rats that already had diabetes.[91]

REFERENCES

1. Centers for Disease Control and Prevention. *Age-adjusted prevalence of CKD stages 1-4 by gender 1999-2012.* Chronic Kidney Disease (CKD) Surveillance Project website. https://nccd.cdc.gov. (Accessed 16 February 2017).

2. Shi, Z., Taylor, A. W., Riley, M., Byles, J., Liu, J., & Noakes, M. (2017). Association between dietary patterns, cadmium intake and chronic kidney disease among adults. *Clinical Nutrition: Official Journal of the European Society of Parenteral and Enteral Nutrition.* pii: S0261-5614 (16)31366-8. PubMed PMID: 28094058.

3. Wu, H., Liao, Q., Chillrud, S. N., Yang, Q., Huang, L., Bi, J., et al. (2016). Environmental exposure to cadmium: Health risk assessment and its associations with hypertension and impaired kidney function. *Scientific Reports,* 6, 29989. PubMed PMID: 27411493.

4. Frassetto, L. A., et al. (1996). Effect of age on blood acid-base composition in adulthood humans: Role of age-related renal functional decline. *The American Journal of Physiology,* 271(6 Pt. 2), F1114–F1122.

5. Chade, A. R. (2011). Renovascular disease, microcirculation, and the progression of renal injury: Role of angiogenesis. *American Journal of Physiology – Regulatory Integrative and Comparative Physiology,* 300(4), R783–R790.

6. White, C. J. (2006). Catheter-based therapy for atherosclerotic renal artery stenosis. *Circulation,* 113, 1464–1473.

7. Satarug, S., Vesey, D. A., & Gobe, G. C. (2017). Kidney cadmium toxicity, diabetes, and high blood pressure: The perfect storm. *The Tohoku Journal of Experimental Medicine,* 241(1), 65–87. PubMed PMID: 28132967.

8. Kim, N. H., Hyun, Y. Y., Lee, K. B., et al. (2015). Environmental heavy metal exposure and chronic kidney disease in the general population. *Journal of Korean Medical Science,* 30(3), 272–277. PubMed PMID: 25729249.

9. Bridges, C. C., Joshee, L., & Zalups, R. K. (2014). Aging and the disposition and toxicity of mercury in rats. *Experimental Gerontology,* 53, 31–39. PubMed PMID: 24548775.

10. Atchison, W. D., & Hare, M. F. (1994). Mechanisms of methylmercury-induced neurotoxicity. *FASEB Journal: Official Publication of the Federation of American Societies for Experimental Biology,* 8(9), 622–629. PubMed PMID: 7516300.

11. Sommar, J. N., Svensson, M. K., Björ, B. M., Elmståhl, S. I., Hallmans, G., Lundh, T., et al. (2013). End-stage renal disease and low level exposure to lead, cadmium and mercury; a population-based, prospective nested case-referent study in Sweden. *Environmental Health: A Global Access Science Source,* 12, 9. PubMed PMID: 23343055.

12. Kim, R., Rotnitsky, A., Sparrow, D., Weiss, S., Wager, C., & Hu, H. (1996). A longitudinal study of low-level lead exposure and impairment of renal function. The Normative Aging Study. *JAMA: The Journal of the American Medical Association,* 275(15), 1177–1181. PubMed PMID: 8609685.

13. Tsaih, S. W., Korrick, S., Schwartz, J., Amarasiriwardena, C., Aro, A., Sparrow, D., et al. (2004). Lead, diabetes, hypertension, and renal function: The normative aging study. *Environmental Health Perspectives,* 112(11), 1178–1182. PubMed PMID: 15289163.

14. Lin, J. L., Lin-Tan, D. T., Hsu, K. H., & Yu, C. C. (2003). Environmental lead exposure and progression of chronic renal diseases in patients without diabetes. *The New England Journal of Medicine,* 348(4), 277–286. PubMed PMID: 12540640.

15. Seidel, W. C., Scherer, K. V., Jr., Cline, D., Jr., et al. (1991). Chemical, physical, and toxicological characterization of fumes produced by heating tetrafluoroethene homo polymer and its copolymers with hexafluoropropene and perfluoro(propyl vinyl ether). *Chemical Research in Toxicology,* 4(2), 229–236.

16. Groves, C. E., Lock, E. A., & Schnellmann, R. G. (1991). Role of lipid peroxidation in renal proximal tubule cell death induced by haloalkene cysteine conjugates. *Toxicology and Applied Pharmacology,* 107(1), 54–62.

17. Honeycutt, Z., & Rowlands, H. (2014). *Glyphosate Testing Report: Findings in American Mothers' Breast Milk, Urine and Water.* Moms Across America website. Available at http://www.momsacrossamerica.com/glyphosate_testing_results. (Accessed 18 November 2015).

18. Battaglin, W. A., Thurman, E. M., Kolpin, D. W., et al. (2003). *Work plan for determining the occurrence of glyphosate, its transformation product AMPA, other herbicide compounds, and antibiotics in Midwestern United States streams, 2002:* U.S. Geological Survey Open-File Report 03-69.

19. Seralini, G. E., Clair, E., Mesnage, R., Gress, S., Defarge, N., Malatesta, M., et al. (2014). Republished study: long-term toxicity of a Roundup herbicide and a Roundup-tolerant genetically modified maize. *Environmental Sciences Europe,* 26(1), 14. PubMed PMID: 27752412.

20. IRDC. (1980). *Test article – technical glyphosate: teratology study in rats.* Unpublished report prepared by International Research and Development Corporation, Mattawan, MI. Submitted to WHO by Monsanto Ltd. (Study No. 401-054; Reference No. IR-79-018).

21. Bio/Dynamics Inc. (1981). *A three-generation reproduction study in rats with glyphosate.* Final Report. Unpublished report prepared by Bio/Dynamics Inc., Division of Biology and Safety Evaluation, East Millstone, NJ. Submitted to WHO by Monsanto Ltd. (Project No. 77-2063; BDN-77-147).

22. Bio/Dynamics Inc. (1983). *A chronic feeding study of glyphosate (Roundup technical) in mice.* Unpublished report prepared by Bio/Dynamics Inc., Division of Biology and Safety Evaluation, East Millstone, NJ. Submitted to WHO by Monsanto Ltd. (Project No. 77-2061; BDN-77-420).

23. Monsanto. (1990). *Chronic study of glyphosate administered in feed to albino rats.* Unpublished report prepared and submitted to WHO by Monsanto Ltd., Monsanto Environmental Health Laboratory, St. Louis, MO (Project No. MSL-10495).

24. Jayasumana, C., Paranagama, P., Agampodi, S., et al. (2015). Drinking well water and occupational exposure to Herbicides is associated with chronic kidney disease, in Padavi-Sripura, Sri Lanka. *Environmental Health: A Global Access Science Source, 14*, 6.

25. National Primary Drinking Water Regulations. Environmental Protection Agency. Retrieved from https://www.epa.gov/ground-water-and-drinking-water/national-primary-drinking-water-regulations. (Accessed 18 November 2016).

26. Ejerblad, E., Fored, C. M., Lindblad, P., Fryzek, J., et al. (2004). Association between smoking and chronic renal failure in a nationwide population-based case-control study. *Journal of the American Society of Nephrology, 15*, 2178–2185. PubMed PMID: 15284303.

27. Briganti, E. M., Branley, P., Chadban, S. J., Shaw, J. E., McNeil, J. J., Welborn, T. A., et al. (2002). Smoking Is associated with renal impairment and proteinuria in the normal population: The AusDiab kidney study. Australian Diabetes, Obesity and Lifestyle Study. *American Journal of Kidney Diseases, 40*(4), 704–712. PubMed PMID: 12324904.

28. Cha, Y. J., Lim, B. J., Kim, B. S., Kim, Y., Yoo, T. H., et al. (2016). Smoking-related renal histological injury in IgA nephropathy patients. *Yonsei Medical Journal, 57*(1), 209–216. PubMed PMID: 26632403.

29. Lhotta, K., Rumpelt, H. J., Konig, P., Mayer, G., & Kronenberg, F. (2002). Cigarette smoking and vascular pathology in renal biopsies. *Kidney International, 61*(2), 648–654. PubMed PMID: 11849408.

30. Pryor, W. A., & Stone, K. (1993). Oxidants in cigarette smoke – radicals, hydrogen peroxide, peroxynitrate, and peroxynitrite. *Annals of the New York Academy of Sciences, 686*, 12–28. PubMed PMID: 15145091.

31. Columbo, G., Clerici, M., Giustarini, D., Portinaro, N. M., Aldini, G., Rossi, R., et al. (2014). Pathophysiology of tobacco smoke exposure: Recent insights from comparative and redox proteomics. *Mass Spectrometry Reviews, 33*(3), 183–218. PubMed PMID: 24272816.

32. Pan, Y., Zhang, L., Wang, F., Li, X., Wang, H., & China National Survey of Chronic Kidney Disease Working Group. (2014). Status of non-steroidal anti-inflammatory drugs use and its association with chronic kidney disease: A cross-sectional survey in China. *Nephrology, 19*(10), 655–660. PubMed PMID: 25196389.

33. Gooch, K., Culleton, B. F., Manns, B. J., Zhang, J., Alfonso, H., et al. (2007). NSAID use and progression of chronic kidney disease. *The American Journal of Medicine, 120*(3), 280.e1–280.e7. PubMed PMID: 17349452.

34. Ungprasert, P., Cheungpasitporn, W., Crowson, C. S., & Matteson, E. L. (2015). Individual non-steroidal anti-inflammatory drugs and risk of acute kidney injury: A systematic review and meta-analysis of observational studies. *European Journal of Internal Medicine, 26*(4), 285–291. PubMed PMID: 25862494.

35. De Broe, M. E., & Elseviers, M. M. (2009). Over-the-counter analgesic use. *Journal of the American Society of Nephrology, 20*(10), 2098–2103.

36. Wei, L., MacDonald, T. M., Jennings, C., et al. (2013). Estimated GFR reporting is associated with decreased nonsteroidal anti-inflammatory drug prescribing and increased renal function. *Kidney International, 84*(1), 174–178.

37. Aderem, A., & Ulevitch, R. J. (2000). Toll-like receptors in the induction of the innate immune response. *Nature, 406*, 782–787.

38. Laugerette, F. 1., Vors, C., Peretti, N., et al. (2011). Complex links between dietary lipids, endogenous endotoxins and metabolic inflammation. *Biochimie, 93*(1), 39–45.

39. Suganami, T., Tanimoto-Koyama, K., et al. (2007). Role of the Toll-like receptor 4/NF-κβ pathway in saturated fatty acid-induced inflammatory changes in the interaction between adipocytes and macrophages. *Arteriosclerosis, Thrombosis, and Vascular Biology, 27*, 84–91.

40. Cani, P. D., Amar, J., Iglesias, M. A., et al. (2007a). Metabolic endotoxemia initiates obesity and insulin resistance. *Diabetes, 56*, 1761–1772.

41. McIntyre, C. W. 1., Harrison, L. E., Eldehni, M. T., et al. (2011). Circulating endotoxemia: A novel factor in systemic inflammation and cardiovascular disease in chronic kidney disease. *Clinical Journal of the American Society of Nephrology : CJASN, 6*(1), 133–141.

42. Lin, C. J., Chen, H. H., Pan, C. F., et al. (2011). p-Cresylsulfate and indoxyl sulfate level at different stages of chronic kidney disease. *Journal of Clinical Laboratory Analysis*, 25(3), 191–197.

43. Wu, I. W., Hsu, K. H., Hsu, H. J., et al. (2012). Serum free p-cresyl sulfate levels predict cardiovascular and all-cause mortality in elderly hemodialysis patients–a prospective cohort study. *Nephrology, Dialysis, Transplantation*, 27(3), 1169–1175.

44. *Personal communication Linda Frassetto, MD.*

45. Powles, J., Fahimi, S., Micha, R., et al. (2013). Global, regional and national sodium intakes in 1990 and 2010: A systemic analysis of 24h urinary sodium excretion and dietary surveys worldwide. *BMJ Open*, 3(12), e003733.

46. Campbell, N. (2016). SY 09-4 Public policies to reduce salt in processed foods: How they may correlate with improvement in blood pressure control and reduced cardiovascular mortality. *Journal of Hypertension*, 34(Suppl. 1), e185.

47. Sharma, A. M., & Distler, A. (1994). Acid-base abnormalities in hypertension. *The American Journal of the Medical Sciences*, 307(Suppl. 1), S112–S115.

48. Sharma, A. M., Kribben, A., Schattenfroh, S., Cetto, C., & Distler, A. (1990). Salt sensitivity in humans is associated with abnormal acid-base regulation. *Hypertension*, 16(4), 407–413.

49. Adeva, M. M., & Souto, G. (2011). Diet-induced metabolic acidosis. *Clinical Nutrition: Official Journal of the European Society of Parenteral and Enteral Nutrition*, 30(4), 416–421.

50. Calvo, M. S., & Uribarri, J. (2013). Contributions to total phosphorus intake: All sources considered. *Seminars in Dialysis*, 26(1), 54–61.

51. Chang, A. R., Lazo, M., Appel, L. J., Gutiérrez, O. M., & Grams, M. E. (2014). High dietary phosphorus intake is associated with all-cause mortality: Results from NHANES III. *The American Journal of Clinical Nutrition*, 99(2), 320–327.

52. Voormolen, N., Noordzij, M., Grootendorst, D. C., et al. (2007). High plasma phosphate as a risk factor for decline in renal function and mortality in pre-dialysis patients. *Nephrology, Dialysis, Transplantation*, 22, 2909–2916.

53. Norris, K. C., Greene, T., Kopple, J., et al. (2006). Baseline predictors of renal disease progression in the African American Study of Hypertension and Kidney Disease. *Journal of the American Society of Nephrology*, 17, 2928–2936.

54. Schwarz, S., Trivedi, B. K., Kalantar-Zadeh, K., et al. (2006). Association of disorders in mineral metabolism with progression of chronic kidney disease. *Clinical Journal of the American Society of Nephrology: CJASN*, 1, 825–831.

55. O'Seaghdha, C. M., Hwang, S. J., Muntner, P., Melamed, M. L., & Fox, C. S. (2011). Serum phosphorous predicts incident chronic kidney disease and end-stage renal disease. *Nephrology, Dialysis, Transplantation*, 26(9), 2885–2890.

56. Sim, J. J., Bhandari, S. K., Smith, N., Chung, J., Liu, I. L., Jacobsen, S. J., et al. (2013). Phosphorous and risk of renal failure in subjects with normal renal function. *The American Journal of Medicine*, 126(4), 311–318. PubMed PMID: 23375678.

57. Safar, M. E., Blacher, J., Pannier, B., et al. (2002). Central pulse pressure and mortality in end-stage renal disease. *Hypertension*, 39, 735–738.

58. Goodman, W. G., London, G., Amann, K., Block, G. A., et al. (2004). Vascular calcification in chronic kidney disease. *American Journal of Kidney Diseases*, 43(3), 572–579. PubMed PMID: 14981617.

59. Giachelli, C. M., Speer, M. Y., Li, X., Rajachar, R. M., & Yang, H. (2005). Regulation of vascular calcification: Roles of phosphate and osteopontin. *Circulation Research*, 96(7), 717–722. PubMed PMID: 15831823.

60. Pizzorno, L. (2014). Canaries in the Phosphate-Toxicity Coal Mines. *Integrative Medicine*, 13, 24–31.

61. Duty, S. M., et al. (2005). Personal care product use predicts urinary concentrations of some phthalate monoesters. *Environmental Health Perspectives*, 113(11), 1530–1535.

62. Curl, C. L., et al. (2003). Organophosphorus pesticide exposure of urban and suburban preschool children with organic and conventional diets. *Environmental Health Perspectives*, 111, 377–382.

63. Ferguson, S. K., Hirai, D. M., Copp, S. W., et al. (2014). Dose dependent effects of nitrate supplementation on cardiovascular control and microvascular oxygenation dynamics in healthy rats. *Nitric Oxide: Biology and Chemistry*, 39, 51–58.

64. Kenjale, A. A., Ham, K. L., Stabler, T., et al. (2011). Dietary nitrate supplementation enhances exercise performance in peripheral arterial disease. *Journal of Applied Physiology*, 110(6), 1582–1591.

65. Wang, Z., Liu, J., & Sun, W. (2013). Effects of asiaticoside on levels of podocyte cytoskeletal proteins and renal slit diaphragm proteins in Adriamycin-induced rat nephropathy. *Life Sciences*, 93(8), 352–358.

66. Meng, X. M., Zhang, Y., Huang, X. R., et al. (2015). Treatment of renal fibrosis by rebalancing TGF-β/Smad signaling with the combination of Asiatic acid and naringenin. *Oncotarget*, doi:10.18632/oncotarget.6100. [Epub ahead of print].

67. Pruijm, M., Hofmann, L., Charollais-Thoenig, J., et al. (2013). Effect of dark chocolate on renal tissue oxygenation as measured by BOLD-MRI in healthy volunteers. *Clinical Nephrology, 80*(3), 211–217.

68. Al-Malki, A. L., & Moselhy, S. S. (2011). The protective effect of epicatechin against oxidative stress and nephrotoxicity in rats induced by cyclosporine. *Human and Experimental Toxicology, 30*(2), 145–151.

69. Ekor, M., Adesanoye, O. A., & Farombi, E. O. (2010). N-acetylcysteine pretreatment ameliorates mercuric chloride-induced oxidative renal damage in rats. *African Journal of Medicine and Medical Sciences, 39*(Suppl.), 153–160. PubMed PMID: 22416658.

70. Kelly, G. S. (1998). Clinical applications of N-acetylcysteine. *Alternative Medicine Review: A Journal of Clinical Therapeutic, 3*(2), 114–127. PubMed PMID: 9577247.

71. Karasek, M., Szuflet, A., Chrzanowski, W., Zylinska, K., & Swietolawski, J. (2002). Circadian serum melatonin profiles in patients suffering from chronic renal failure. *Neuro Endocrinology Letters, 23*(Suppl. 1), 97–102. PubMed PMID: 12019361.

72. Sener, G., Sehirli, A. O., & Ayanoglu-Dulger, G. (2003). Melatonin protects against mercury (II)-induced oxidative tissue damage in rats. *Pharmacology and Toxicology, 93*(6), 290–296. PubMed PMID: 14675463.

73. Leibowitz, A., Volkov, A., Voloshin, K., Shemesh, C., Barshack, I., & Grossman, E. (2016). Melatonin prevents kidney injury in a high-salt diet-induced hypertension model by decreasing oxidative stress. *Journal of Pineal Research, 60*(1), 48–54. PubMed PMID: 26465239.

74. Quiroz, Y., Ferrebuz, A., Romero, F., Vaziri, N. D., & Rodriguez-Iturbe, B. (2008). Melatonin ameliorates oxidative stress, inflammation, proteinuria, and progression of renal damage in rats with renal mass reduction. *American Journal of Physiology – Renal Physiology, 294*(2), F336–F344. PubMed PMID: 18077597.

75. Nair, A. R., Masson, G. S., Ebenezer, P. J., et al. (2014). Role of TLR4 in lipopolysaccharide-induced acute kidney injury: Protection by blueberry. *Free Radical Biology & Medicine, 71*, 16–25.

76. Shin, Y. J., Kim, J. J., Kim, Y. J., Kim, W. H., Park, E. Y., et al. (2015). Protective effects of quercetin against HgCl2-induced nephrotoxicity in Sprague-Dawley rats. *Journal of Medicinal Food, 18*(5), 524–534. PubMed PMID: 25692400.

77. Trujillo, J., Chirino, Y. I., Molina-Jijón, E., et al. (2013). Renoprotective effect of the antioxidant curcumin: Recent findings. *Redox Biology, 1*, 448–456.

78. Mansour, S. M., Bahgat, A. K., El-Khatib, A. S., & Khayyal, M. T. (2011). Ginkgo biloba extract (EGb 761) normalizes hypertension in 2K, 1C hypertensive rats: Role of antioxidant mechanisms, ACE inhibiting activity and improvement of endothelial dysfunction. *Phytomedicine: International Journal of Phytotherapy and Phytopharmacology, 18*(8–9), 641–647.

79. Cavuşoğlu, K., Yapar, K., Oruç, E., & Yalçın, E. (2011). Protective effect of Ginkgo biloba L. leaf extract against glyphosate toxicity in Swiss albino mice. *Journal of Medicinal Food, 14*(10), 1263–1272.

80. Sener, G., Sehirli, O., Tozan, A., et al. (2007). Ginkgo biloba extract protects against mercury(II)-induced oxidative tissue damage in rats. *Food and Chemical Toxicology: An International Journal Published for the British Industrial Biological Research Association, 45*(4), 543–550.

81. Yapar, K., Cavuşoğlu, K., Oruç, E., & Yalçin, E. (2010). Protective role of Ginkgo biloba against hepatotoxicity and nephrotoxicity in uranium-treated mice. *Journal of Medicinal Food, 13*(1), 179–188.

82. Tozan, A. 1., Sehirli, O., Omurtag, G. Z., et al. (2007). Ginkgo biloba extract reduces naphthalene-induced oxidative damage in mice. *Phytotherapy Research: PTR, 21*(1), 72–77.

83. Coskun, O., Armutcu, F., Kanter, M., & Kuzey, G. M. (2005). Protection of endotoxin-induced oxidative renal tissue damage of rats by vitamin E or/and EGb 761 treatment. *Journal of Applied Toxicology: JAT, 25*(1), 8–12.

84. Kim, M. K., Chung, S. W., Kim, D. H., et al. (2010). Modulation of age-related NF-κβ activation by dietary zingerone via MAPK pathway. *Experimental Gerontology, 45*(6), 419–426.

85. Shalaby, M. A., & Saifan, H. Y. (2014). Some pharmacological effects of cinnamon and ginger herbs in obese diabetic rats. *Journal of Intercultural Ethnopharmacology, 3*(4), 144–149.

86. Onwuka, F. C., Erhabor, O., Eteng, M. U., & Umoh, I. B. (2011). Protective effects of ginger toward cadmium-induced testes and kidney lipid peroxidation and hematological impairment in albino rats. *Journal of Medicinal Food, 14*(7–8), 817–821.

87. Baiomy, A. A., & Mansour, A. A. (2015 Sep 3). Genetic and histopathological responses to cadmium toxicity in rabbit's kidney and liver: Protection by ginger (Zingiber officinale). *Biological Trace Element Research*, [Epub ahead of print].

88. Shanmugam, K. R., Ramakrishna, C. H., Mallikarjuna, K., & Reddy, K. S. (2010). Protective effect of ginger against alcohol-induced renal damage and antioxidant

enzymes in male albino rats. *Indian Journal of Experimental Biology, 48*(2), 143–149.

89. Baiomy, A. A., Attia, H. F., Soliman, M. M., & Makrum, O. (2015). Protective effect of ginger and zinc chloride mixture on the liver and kidney alterations induced by malathion toxicity. *International Journal of Immunopathology and Pharmacology, 28*(1), 122–128.

90. Ramadan, G., & El-Menshawy, O. (2013). Protective effects of ginger-turmeric rhizomes mixture on joint inflammation, atherogenesis, kidney dysfunction and other complications in a rat model of human rheumatoid arthritis. *International Journal of Rheumatic Diseases, 16*(2), 219–229.

91. Kazeem, M. I., Akanji, M. A., & Yakubu, M. T. (2015 Aug 29). Amelioration of pancreatic and renal derangements in streptozotocin-induced diabetic rats by polyphenol extracts of Ginger (Zingiber officinale) rhizome. *Pathophysiology*, doi:10.1016/j.pathophys.2015.08. 004. pii: S0928-4680(15)30009-2. [Epub ahead of print].

51

Cancer

SUMMARY

- Presence in population: In 2014, an estimated 14,740,000 people were living with cancer (of any site) in the United States
- Primary sources: Cigarette smoking, air pollution, solvents, pesticides, toxic metals
- Best measure: 8-OHdG
- Best intervention: Avoidance, antioxidants

DESCRIPTION

According to World Health Organization (WHO) estimates for 2015, cancer is the second leading cause of death globally and was responsible for 8.8 million deaths.[1] Cancer is one of the most important diseases in the world and is complicated due to being multifactorial in its incidence, distribution, causes, and effects in various populations. Carcinogenesis is considered a multistage process including induction, promotion, and progression. Induction requires an irreversible change in the cellular genome, whereas promotion is associated with prolonged and reversible alteration in gene expression. Tumor progression results in genotypic and phenotypic changes associated with tumor growth, invasion, and metastasis. Researchers have suggested that the majority of human cancers share "six essential alterations in cell physiology that collectively dictate malignant growth: self-sufficiency in growth signals, insensitivity to growth-inhibitory (antigrowth) signals, evasion of programmed cell death (apoptosis), limitless replicative potential, sustained angiogenesis, and tissue invasion and metastasis."[2] At least five coherent models of carcinogenesis have been proposed in the history of cancer research and are summarized in Table 51.1.[3]

The National Toxicology Program (NTP) produces the Report on Carcinogens (RoC) that documents chemical and biological data, which support cancer causation in animals or humans. Approximately 2500 chemicals have been evaluated.[4] Environmental risk factors including biological toxins and harmful exposures from air, food, water, pesticides, and ionizing radiation have all been associated with the development of cancer.

Toxicity—Mechanisms of Action

DNA is the only biological molecule that relies solely on repair of existing molecules rather than remanufacture. Cancer development requires the accumulation of numerous genetic changes, which are believed to occur through the presence of unrepaired DNA lesions. Combining spontaneous damage with exogenous (e.g., ultraviolet [UV] light) and endogenous (e.g., reactive oxygen species [ROS]) sources, it is estimated that close to 105 lesions per cell per day may occur.[5]

Oxidative damage has been associated with the development, progression, and mutagenesis of several mutagenic and carcinogenic processes. Oxidative DNA lesions can be efficiently repaired by base excision repair or nucleotide excision repair, but if ROS levels increase beyond the capacity of a cell's antioxidant defenses, the cell's DNA repair capacity can become overwhelmed, leading to the accumulation of DNA damage. Excess generation of ROS has been shown to induce irreversible damage to a variety of macromolecular components that

TABLE 51.1   Five Recent Nonexclusive Models of Carcinogenesis

	Model 1 "mutational"	Model 2 "genome instability"	Model 3 "nongenotoxic"	Model 4 "darwinian"	Model 5 "tissue organization"
Main focus	Chemical carcinogens, Viruses	Familiarity, Genome instability	Clonal expansion/ epigenetics	Clonal expansion/ cell selection	Microenvironment
Examples	Tobacco and lung cancer, HPV	Colon cancer, retinoblastoma	Diet, hormones	Beta-carotene, folate, chemotherapy	
Mechanisms	DNA adducts, mutations, oncogenes	CIN, MIN, MMR, Rb, BRCA1	Methylation histone acetylation	Selective advantage	Cancer precursors dependent on microenvironment of lesions

BRCA1, breast cancer 1 gene; CIN, chromosomal instability; HPV, human papillomavirus; MIN, microsatellite instability; MMR, mismatch repair; Rb, retinoblastoma

From Vineia, P., Scatzkin, A., & Potter, J. D. (2010). Models of carcinogenesis: An overview. *Carcinogenesis, 31*(10), 1703–1709.

result in genomic alterations potentiating a carcinogenic state.[6] Oxidative stress-induced mutations (e.g., point mutations, deletions, insertions, chromosomal translocations) are known to upregulate oncogenes and downregulate tumor suppressor genes.[7] Lipid peroxidation gives rise to mutagenic lipid epoxides, lipid hydroepoxides, lipid alkoxyl and peroxyl radicals, and enals (an aldehyde with a neighboring double bond).[8]

Several environmental chemicals exert carcinogenetic toxicity through oxidative stress. Exposure to organophosphate pesticides will lead to DNA oxidative damage.[9] Perfluorinated compounds, such as perfluorooctanoic acid (PFOA) and perfluorononanoic acid (PFNA) are suspected genotoxic agents responsible for oxidative DNA damage. An *in vitro* study showed that PFOA and PFNA induced DNA damage in a human lymphoblastoid cell line, and levels of 8-OHdG were increased in a dose-dependent manner with both PFOA and PFNA exposure.[10] Asbestos fibers are genotoxic to the lungs and are linked with increased levels of 8-OHdG.[11,12] Particulate matter (PM) causes significant oxidative damage in the tissues and organs to which it is distributed and has been associated with increased mortality from neoplastic diseases.[13,14] Superoxide, hydrogen peroxide, and hydroxyl radical are mutagens produced by radiation. Chronic tobacco smoke inhalation induces an intracellular oxidative environment characterized by decreased concentrations of circulating antioxidants, increased oxidation of glutathione (GSH), and increased levels of DNA damage.[15]

Chronic inflammation is associated with an increased risk of cancer through production of proinflammatory cytokines and diverse reactive oxygen/nitrogen species, which activate signaling molecules involved in carcinogenesis such as NF-κβ, inducible nitric oxide synthase, and COX-2.[16] The carcinogenetic effect of arsenic, for example, may be related to the activation of redox-sensitive transcription factors involving NF-κβ and AP-1.[17] Activation of these factors has a direct effect on cell proliferation and apoptosis.

CLINICAL SIGNIFICANCE—CANCER SITES AND ASSOCIATED TOXICANTS

Bladder Cancer

Arsenic. Worldwide, bladder cancer is the ninth-most frequent type of cancer, with an estimated 430,000 new cases diagnosed in 2012.[18] Inorganic arsenic in drinking water is classified as a Group 1 carcinogen, and observations in highly exposed populations ($\geq$100 μg/L) reveal that arsenic is an established cause of bladder cancer.[19] Mechanisms of arsenic carcinogenesis include oxidative damage,[20] epigenetic effects,[21] and interference with DNA repair.[22]

A dose-response relationship between well water arsenic levels and rates of mortality from bladder cancer has been established. In highly arsenic-exposed populations of Taiwan, age-adjusted bladder cancer mortality rates were 15.7 (< 300 μg/L arsenic), 37.8 (300–590 μg/L arsenic), and 89.1 (> 600 µg/L arsenic) per 100,000 men and 16.7, 35.1, and 91.5 per 100,000 women.[23] Compared with uncontaminated areas, men and women from a highly arsenic-contaminated region of Chile experienced mortality rates due to bladder cancer 6.0 and 8.2 times greater, respectively.[24]

Evidence remains uncertain regarding the potential risk of low-to-moderate arsenic exposure in drinking water and bladder cancer. It has been estimated that more than 350,000 people in the United States may be supplied with water containing more than 50 µg/L arsenic, and more than 2.5 million people may be supplied with water with levels above 25 µg/L.[25] Long term (> 40 years) groundwater arsenic exposure among residents in Maine was strongly associated with bladder cancer. Those with the highest arsenic exposure (> 2.2 L water/day) had more than twice the risk of developing bladder cancer (Odds Ratio (OR) 2.24; Confidence Interval (CI) 95%: 1.29, 3.89).[26] A meta-analysis suggests exposure to 10 µg/L of arsenic in drinking water may double the risk of bladder cancer, showing predicted risks for bladder cancer incidence of 2.7 [1.2–4.1]; 4.2 [2.1–6.3]; and 5.8 [2.9–8.8] for drinking water arsenic levels of 10 µg/L, 10 µg/L, and 150 µg/L, respectively.[27]

Arsenic exposure has been shown to alter methylation levels of both global DNA and gene promoters.[28] Modifications in arsenic methylation ability (defined as the ratios of monomethylarsonic acid [MMA(V)]/inorganic arsenic [primary arsenic methylation index, PMI] and dimethylarsinic acid [DMA(V)]/MMA(V) [secondary arsenic methylation index, SMI]) may provide a link between low-level arsenic exposure and bladder cancer. In subjects with a low SMI (≤ 4.8), cumulative arsenic exposure of > 12 mg/L-year are associated with an increased risk of bladder cancer (OR = 4.23, 95% CI; 1,12–16.01).[29] Thus, at low-level arsenic exposure of 50 µg/L, individuals with low SMI can accumulate > 12 mg/L-year of arsenic by drinking 1 liter of water in just 8 months. (Please see Chapter 9, Arsenic for a more complete discussion of the toxicity of mono- versus di-methylation of arsenic.)

Cadmium. A case-control study of 172 patients with bladder cancer and 359 population controls found an OR of 8.3 (95% CI 5.0–13.8) for cadmium, comparing the highest to the lowest tertile.[30] Even after adjusting for sex, age, occupational exposure to polycyclic aromatic hydrocarbons (PAHs) and smoking status, the OR remained significant (OR: 5.7; 95% CI 3.3–9.9). An experimental study demonstrated that cadmium can malignantly transform human urothelial cells,[31] and these epithelial transformations are consistent with those of a classic transitional-cell carcinoma of the bladder.[32]

Water Chlorination. Although chlorination of water supplies has had a huge public health benefit, the organic contaminants can become carcinogenic. A Canadian study examined the relationship between bladder cancer and exposure to trihalomethane (THM) chlorination by-products in public water supplies and found that the risk increases with both the duration (OR = 1.41, 95% CI 1.10–1.81 for ≥ 35 years of exposure) and concentration (OR = 1.63, 95% CI 1.08–2.46 for THM levels ≥ 50 µg/L for ≥ 35 yrs) of exposure to chlorination by-products.[33]

Tobacco Smoking. In general, tobacco is high in both arsenic and cadmium as well as the well-known carcinogenic PAHs—which help explain its role in so many cancers. Population attributable risks (PAR) of bladder cancer for tobacco smoking have been estimated to be 50% to 60% in men and 20% to 30% in women.[34] A report from the New England Bladder study suggests that the strength of the association between cigarette smoking and bladder cancer has increased. Over the course of three study periods (1994–1998, 1998–2001, and 2001–2004), the odds ratio associated with current smoking increased from 2.9 (95% CI: 2.0–4.2) to 4.2 (95% CI: 2.8–6.3) to 5.5 (95% CI: 3.5–8.9), respectively.[35] Smoking is estimated to cause approximately half of bladder cancers (former tobacco smoking – Hazard Ratio (HR): 2.22; 95% CI, 2.03–2.44; current tobacco smoking – HR: 4.1; 95% CI, 3.7–4.5),[36] likely resulting from the aromatic amines and PAHs contained in tobacco smoke and excreted in urine.[37]

Bone Cancer

Arsenic. Osteosarcoma is the eighth-most common childhood cancer and typically occurs in the long bones of the extremities—femur, tibia, and humerus.[38] A small study examining the incidence of childhood cancers in Nevada counties with low, moderate, and high levels of arsenic in the drinking water found an excess of bone cancers in 5- to 9-year-old children and 10- to 14-year-old children. The increased incidence in high exposure counties (35.9–91.5 µg/L) resulted in a greater proportion of bone cancer (14.3% of all cancer types) than the state average (8.8%).[39]

Fluoride. Two small case-control studies have shown osteosarcoma patients have higher serum fluoride concentrations compared with controls,[40,41] however, a large nationwide cross-sectional study found no such association.[42]

Brain Cancer

Pesticides and Herbicides. Research shows an association between agricultural pesticide use (chlorpyrifos and coumaphos) and an increased risk of glioma ($\geq$ 55 years on a farm OR = 3.9, 95% CI 1.8–8.6).[43] Based on a small number of cases, ORs were significantly increased for the herbicides metribuzin (OR = 3.4, 95% CI 1.2–9.7) and paraquat (OR = 11.1, 95% CI 1.2–101), and for the insecticides bufencarb (OR = 18.9, 95% CI 1.9–187), chlorpyrifos (OR = 22.6, 95% CI 2.7–191), and coumaphos (OR = 5.9, 95% CI 1.1–32). The increased risk of glioma may be due to work practices, as never immediately washing up or changing clothes after applying pesticides triples the risk of glioma.[44] Childhood brain cancers have also been evaluated for epidemiological association with chemical exposure. When comparing 45 childhood brain cancer patients with 85 friend controls (cancer-free), significant positive associations were found between brain cancer and exposure to no-pest strips in the home, termite treatment, Kwell shampoo (Lindane), flea collars on pets, diazinon use in the garden or orchard, and herbicides to control weeds in the yard (OR = 6.2).[45] In addition, compared with 108 cancer controls, significant positive associations were observed for use of pesticide bombs in the home, termite treatment, flea collars on pets, insecticide use in the garden, carbaryl in the garden, and herbicides to control weeds in the yard.

Tobacco Smoke Exposure. A meta-analysis combining 10 studies published before 2000 estimated a 22% increase in risk of childhood brain tumors with exposure to paternal tobacco smoke during pregnancy (95% CI, 1.05–1.40).[46] Children of women who smoked during pregnancy were shown to have a statistically significant 24% increase in brain tumor risk.[47] Interestingly, children with genetic polymorphisms (HR/RR for EPHX1 H139R) associated with increased activation of PAHs have a higher risk of brain tumors relative to children with a low-risk (HH) genotype when exposed to tobacco smoke during pregnancy.[48] A dose-response pattern for paternal smoking was observed among children with the EPHX1 H139R high-risk genotype only (OR [no exposure] =

1.0; OR [$\leq$ 3 hours/day] = 1.32, 95% CI: 0.52–3.34; OR [> 3 hours/day] = 3.18, 95% CI: 0.92–11.0; p[trend] = 0.07).

Lead. Positive associations have been demonstrated between lead exposure and risk of meningioma. A Finnish study found an increased risk of brain and nervous system cancer (standardized incidence ratio [SIR], 1.27; 95% CI: 0.81–2.01) in women with occupational exposure to lead.[49] A genetic susceptibility may be involved in the relationship between lead and brain tumor risk. In individuals with the ALAD2 variant allele, risk of meningioma with occupational lead exposure increased from 1.1 (95% CI: 0.3–4.5) to 5.6 (95% CI: 0.7–45.5) and 12.8 (95% CI: 1.4–120.8) for lifetime cumulative lead exposures ($\mu g/m^3$–y where y = years of exposure) of 1 to 49 $\mu g/m^3$–y, 50 to 99 $\mu g/m^3$–y, and $\geq$ 100 $\mu g/m^3$–y, respectively.[50]

Vinyl Chloride. Vinyl chloride is a human carcinogen with target organs including the liver, brain, lung, and lymphohematopoietic system.[51] Several studies have reported significant increases and mortality from cancer of the brain and central nervous system in exposed workers.[52,53]

Breast Cancer

Breast cancer is the second-most common cancer overall (1.7 million cases, 11.9%) but ranks fifth as cause of death (522,000, 6.4%) because of the relatively favorable prognosis.[54] It is the most common malignancy in women around the world, accounting for 25.1% of all cancers.[55] Breast cancer has clear associations with environmental chemical exposure (e.g., applied chemicals, food residues, occupational hazards) and lifestyle factors (e.g., physical activity, cosmetics, water source, smoking) with the majority (70% to 95%) of breast cancer risk associated with these factors.[56]

Organochlorine Compounds. Elevated levels of different organochlorine compounds (OCCs) have been found in the adipose tissue of breast cancer patients compared with controls. Chemicals such as dichlorodiphenyltrichloroethane (DDT), dichlorodiphenyldichloroethylene (DDE), polychlorinated biphenyls (PCBs), and hexachlorocyclohexane (HCH, a Lindane, a pesticide commonly used to treat lice infestations) are not only higher in breast cancer patients but are found in greater concentrations in the malignant tissue than in the adjacent healthy tissue.[57] Elevated serum levels of DDE can indicate a fourfold-increased risk of breast cancer compared with average risk.[58] Mothers who were exposed to DDT before the age of 14 showed a fivefold increase in risk of breast cancer, and the DDT association with breast cancer was only observed for women who were exposed before age 14 years.[59] Elevated maternal serum o,p'-DDT has not only been associated with an increase in the daughter's risk of breast cancer (OR = 3.7; 95% CI: 1.5–9) but is significantly, positively associated with advanced stage at diagnosis and with the occurrence of HER2-positive tumors.[60]

A 2015 systematic review examined the epidemiological evidence of a relationship between specific PCB congener exposure and breast cancer risk. The pooled odds ratios showed a significant increase in the risk of breast cancer in individuals with higher plasma/fat levels of PCB 99 (OR = 1.36; 95% CI: 1.02–1.80), PCB 183 (OR = 1.56; 95% CI: 1.25–1.95), and PCB 187 (OR = 1.18; 95% CI: 1.01–1.39).[61] Interestingly, breastfeeding decreases a woman's PCB levels, which likely helps explain why it reduces risk of breast cancer.[62]

Parabens. Parabens are present in many cosmetic products, including antiperspirants, and their estrogenic properties may be a cause for concern regarding breast cancer. Parabens have weak estrogenic activity and have been shown to induce the growth of MCF-7 human breast cancer cells *in vitro*.[63] In fact, these compounds have been found in breast cancer tissue in levels ranging from 20 ng/g tissue to 100 ng/g tissue.[64]

Colorectal Cancer

Water Chlorination. Men exposed to chlorinated surface water for 35 to 40 years had an increased risk of colon cancer compared with those exposed for < 10 years (OR = 1.53; 95% CI: 1.13–2.09).[65] In addition, men exposed to chlorination by-products (trihalomethanes) at levels of 75 µg/L for ≥ 35 years had two times the risk of those exposed for < 10 years.

DDT/DDE. Cell culture studies have shown that exposure low concentrations of p,p'-DDE induces colon cancer proliferation through the generation of ROS, activation of nicotinamide adenine dinucleotide phosphate (NADPH) oxidase, and the reduction of GSH content, superoxide dismutase, and catalase activities.[66] A 2004 study from China found the standardized incidence of colorectal cancer was significantly connected with the content of total DDT in rice (correlation coefficient = 0.636).[67]

Head and Neck Cancer

Aluminum. Higher concentrations of aluminum have been found in tissue biopsies along with elevated serum aluminum levels in patients with laryngeal papilloma and laryngeal cancer.[68]

Arsenic. A Chilean population of adults (age 30–49 years) who were *in utero* or ≤ 18 years of age when exposed to high concentrations of arsenic had an increased mortality rate (Standardized Mortality Ratio (SMR) = 8.1; 95% CI: 3.5–16.0) from laryngeal cancer.[69] Arsenic (72.4 ± 18.0 ng/g versus 43.1 ± 9.4 ng/g; p<0.001) and cobalt (68.7 ± 7.3 ng/g versus 39.6 ± 7.0; p<0.001) levels were found to be 60% higher in the tumors of patients with laryngeal cancer compared with the adjacent tissue.[70]

Tobacco and Alcohol. Tobacco and alcohol account for approximately 80% to 90% of all cancers of the head and neck.[71] Tobacco and alcohol increase the risk of head and neck cancer in a dose-dependent fashion and together develop a synergistic and multiplicative effect on the cancer risk.[72] In heavy smokers (> 60 pack-years), a relative risk of 23.4 (alcohol adjusted) for head and neck cancer has been calculated.[73] The attributable risk of oral cancer for alcohol consumption in men was estimated to be 23%.[74]

Liver Cancer

Hepatocellular carcinoma (HCC) is the sixth-most commonly occurring cancer in the world,[75] with more than 50% of HCCs occurring in China.[76]

DDT. Exposure to DDT may be a risk factor for liver cancer. In a study from Linxian, China, a fourfold-increased risk of HCC was found in conjunction with high serum levels of p,p'-DDT.[77] After adjusting for age, sex, area of residence, HBsAg, family history of HCC, history of acute hepatitis, smoking, alcohol, occupation (farmer versus other), and levels of p,p'-DDT or p,p'-DDE, the highest quintile of p,p'-DDT was associated with an increased risk of HCC (OR = 2.96; 95% CI: 1.19–7.40).[78] A 2012 study from China reported both p,p'-DDT and p,p'-DDE were independent risk factors of HCC with the highest risk of HCC among persons with high levels of p,p'-DDT and low levels of p,p'-DDE, suggesting that more recent exposure to p,p'-DDT might be necessary to increase risk of HCC.[79]

Pesticides. Animal studies have shown that exposure to the pyrethroid metofluthrin produced hepatocellular tumors through CYP2B induction, increased hepatocellular DNA replications, and increased hepatocyte proliferation.[80] However, further evaluation concluded that metofluthrin would not have any hepatocarcinogenic activity in humans.[81]

Vinyl Chloride. The relationship between rare hepatic angiosarcoma (HAS) and vinyl chloride was originally deduced by an alert plant physician who noted the oddly high occurrence of HAS in polyvinyl chloride production workers.[82] Epidemiological studies identified a monomer of vinyl chloride as the causative agent, and the calculated relative risk for HAS was approximately 5000, suggesting a strong causal relationship.[83]

Lung Cancer

Globally, lung cancer is the leading cause of cancer deaths in men and the second leading cause in women, killing an estimated 1,098,700 men and 491,200 women in 2012.[84] The most important cause of lung cancer is tobacco smoking.[85] Other risk factors for lung cancer include secondhand smoke,[86] indoor air pollution,[87] outdoor air pollution,[88] occupational chemical exposure,[89] radiation,[90] and exposure to arsenic, asbestos, silica dusts, and toxic elements.[91]

Smoking. In the United States the relative risk for the association between current smoking and lung cancer mortality in women increased from 2.7 in the 1960s to 12.7 in the 1980s and to 25.7 in cohorts conducted in the 2000s; corresponding relative risks for male current smokers, compared with men who had never smoked, were 12.22, 23.81, and 24.97.[92] In a group of lung cancer patients, 8-OHdG levels were significantly associated not only with smoking but also with the aggressiveness of the cancer.[93] Although marijuana smoke has been shown to contain carcinogenic compounds, studies between marijuana use and lung cancer has been inconclusive.[94]

Air Pollution. Various components of air pollution have been closely linked to increased rates and mortality from lung cancer.[95,96,97] Lung cancer risk for persons occupationally exposed to diesel exhaust is 19% to 68% higher than for those nonexposed and was more pronounced for the squamous- and large-cell subtypes.[98] Similar risk values were found in a Canadian population-based case-control study involving 857 male lung cancer patients, 553 population controls, and 1349 patients with other (nonlung) cancer types. After adjustments for potential confounders, when population controls were studied, those who had moderate exposure to diesel exhaust showed a 20% increased risk, whereas those with substantial diesel exposure showed a 60% risk.[99]

In subgroups of current, former, and never-smokers, the lung cancer risk associated with $PM_{2.5}$ was greatest for former smokers, 1.44 (95% CI: 1.04, 2.01); followed by never-smokers, 1.18 (95% CI: 1.00, 1.39); and then current smokers, 1.06 (95% CI: 0.97, 1.15).[100] Both nonsmoking men and women in California had higher rates of lung cancer with increasing levels of PM_{10} (5.21 for men and 1.21 for women) and SO_2 (2.66 for men and 2.14 for women). After PM_{10}, the second highest risk for developing lung cancer was found in men exposed to 100 PPB of ozone (Relative Risk (RR) = 3.56).[101]

Biomass Smoke. In nonsmoking women from India, the use of biomass fuel increased the risk of lung cancer (OR = 5.33; 95% CI: 1.7, 16.7).[102] A study of a Mexican population with no exposure to other carcinogens found 38.7% of the cases of lung cancer occurred in nonsmoking patients with long-term home exposure to biomass smoke.[103]

Radon. The Cancer Prevention Study-II observed that exposure to radon concentrations above the US Environmental Protection Agency (EPA) guideline value (148 Bq/m^3) represented an increase of 34% (95% CI: 7–68) in the risk of dying from lung cancer compared with those below the guideline value.[104]

Pesticides. Pesticide applicators in the highest quartile of chlorpyrifos lifetime exposure days (>56 days) had a relative risk of lung cancer 2.18 (95% CI 1.31–3.64) times that of those with no exposure.[105]

Arsenic. After adjusting for all appropriate confounders, persons consuming groundwater arsenic at levels above 20 µg/L (PPM) had an 83% increased risk of lung cancer, whereas those consuming water with arsenic levels just above the new US EPA standards (10 µg/L) had a 47% increased risk.[106] An increase in lung cancer risk associated with low levels of groundwater arsenic has also been found in a study done in the states of California and Nevada.[107]

Lymphohematopoietic Cancer

Pesticides. Non-Hodgkin's lymphoma (NHL) risk is higher in people occupationally exposed to OP compounds.[108] A study of farmers in Nebraska showed organophosphate exposure was significantly associated with NHL risk (OR = 1.9) and risk increased with days/years of use to OR = 3.1 for 21+ days.[109] Significantly elevated risks for leukemia have been observed with exposure to specific animal insecticides, including crotoxyphos (OR = 11.1), dichlorvos (OR = 2.0), and famphur (OR = 2.2).[110]

Pesticide exposures early in life appear to be more significant than later exposures in the development of childhood leukemias. A threefold-increased risk was found between use of no-pest strips in the home during the last 3 months of pregnancy and childhood leukemia.[111] The use of professional pest control services at any time from 1 year before birth to 3 years after was associated with a significantly increased risk of childhood leukemia (OR = 2.8; 95%CI: 1.4–5.7), and the exposure during year 2 was associated with the highest risk (OR = 3.6).[112]

Studies suggest that organochlorine pesticides may contribute to an increased risk of NHL. Immune system depression is considered to be one of the strongest risk factors for NHL,[113] and PCBs appear to have significant immunotoxic qualities.[114] It may be the quality of immunotoxicity that links both PCBs and non-PCB organochlorines to increased incidence of NHL, and when both are present, each independently contributes to the risk of NHL.[115] Elevated risks, with OR generally 1.5-fold or greater, have been found for personal handling, mixing, or application of chlordane, DDT, and lindane.[116] A strong dose-response relation was found between quartiles of total lipid-corrected serum PCB concentrations and risk of NHL (OR by quartile: 1.0; 1.3 [95% CI 0.5–3.3]; 2.8 [1.1–7.6]; and 4.5 [1.7–12.0]; p[trend] = 0.0008).[117]

A history of substantial previous exposure to organochlorine pesticides was found in patients with aplastic anemia.[118] The authors suggest that OC pesticide may become antigenic, thus inducing an autoimmune reaction responsible for the continuing marrow damage.

Benzene. Exposure to benzene results in increased levels of 8-OHdG, indicating that benzene induces DNA oxidative damage.[119] Epidemiological studies have shown a clear association between occupational exposure to benzene and acute leukemia in adults, especially acute nonlymphocytic leukemia.[120,121] Exposure of fathers to benzene and other solvents before conception and postnatally has been associated with increased risk of childhood leukemia.[122] Childhood leukemia and preconceptional exposure of fathers to benzene produced an OR of 5.81 (95% CI: 1.67–26.44).[123] A cumulative exposure relation with acute nonlymphocytic leukemia has been suggested when benzene concentrations were above about 20 to 50 PPM (64–164 µg/m³).[124] A metaanalysis examining a variety of occupational and household uses of benzenes and solvents, traffic density, and traffic-related air pollution demonstrated significant associations between childhood leukemias and each potential metric of benzene exposure.[125] In studies of occupational and household product exposure published from 1987 to 2014, the summary relative risk (sRR) for childhood leukemia was 1.96 (95% CI: 1.53–2.52); for studies of traffic density or traffic-related air pollution published from 1999 to 2014, the sRR was 1.48 (95% CI: 1.10–1.99); and in studies that involved detailed models of traffic pollution, the sRR was 1.70 (95% CI: 1.16–2.49).

Pancreatic Cancer

Smoking. Cigarette smoking is the most well-established environmental risk factor for pancreatic cancer worldwide.[126,127,128] Compared with the risk in nonsmokers, cigarette smokers have a 60% to 70% increased risk of pancreatic cancer.[129,130]

Cadmium. A study of persons living in South Louisiana specifically focused on pancreatic cancer risk in relation to cadmium burden.[131] In this study, urinary cadmium levels were presented in four quartiles with the following ranges: <0.5 µg/g, 0.5 to <1 µg/g, 1 to <1.5 µg/g, and 1.5+ µg/g creatinine. Persons with urinary cadmium levels in the second quartile (0.5 to <1.0 µg/g) had a 3.34 increased risk for pancreatic cancer, whereas those in the third quartile had an OR of 5.58, and those in the fourth quartile had a 7.70 increase in risk.

Arsenic. During the early summer of 1955, mass arsenic poisoning of bottle-fed infants occurred in the western part of Japan because of contaminated milk powder.[132] Follow-up studies of exposed populations found mortality rates (MR) of pancreatic cancer to be significantly elevated in adults aged 43 to 53 years (MR = 1.93; 95% CI: 1.07–3.47) and for the total of all ages (MR = 1.73; 95% CI: 1.23–2.61).[133,134] A 2008 study using estimated arsenic levels of participants of the Strong Heart Study from 1989 to 1991 found a corresponding hazard ratio of 2.46 (95% CI: 1.09–5.58) for pancreatic cancer after multivariate adjustment (region, age, sex, education, smoking status, alcohol, and BMI).[135] Another possible reason for the association of arsenic with pancreatic cancer might be that it also induces type 2 diabetes mellitus,[136] which is considered a risk factor for pancreatic cancer.[137]

Evidence suggests that concentrations of some OCCs in human tissues may be related to pancreatic cancer risk. Elevated risks for pancreatic cancer have been reported for DDT manufacturers (risk ratio for ever-exposed compared with never-exposed = 4.8; 95% CI: 1.3–17.6)[138] and for workers potentially exposed to PCBs.[139] An Australian study evaluating mortality of outdoor workers exposed to insecticides found mortality from pancreatic cancer was more frequent in subjects exposed to DDT (SMR = 5.27; 95% CI: 1.09–15.40 for subjects working < 3 years).[140]

K-ras mutations are the most frequent abnormality of oncogenes in human cancers. OCCs such as p,p'-DDT; p,p'-DDE; and some PCBs may play a role in the pathogenesis of exocrine pancreatic cancer through modulation of K-ras activation.[141] p,p'-DDT; p,p'-DDE; and PCB 138 have been associated with the two most prevalent K-ras mutations (Val and Asp).[142] Serum concentrations of p,p'-DDT were significantly higher in pancreatic cancer cases with a K-ras mutation than in cases without a mutation (OR for upper tertile = 8.7; 95% CI: 1.6–48.5), and the corresponding figures for p,p'-DDE showed an OR of 5.3 (1.1–25.5).[143]

Prostate Cancer
Smoking. Cigarette smoking may increase the risk of prostate cancer through exposure to carcinogens, and functional polymorphisms in genes involved in polycyclic aromatic hydrocarbons (PAHs) metabolism and detoxification may modify the effect.[144] Among Caucasians, heavy smoking increased prostate cancer risk nearly

twofold in those with the GSTM1 null genotype (OR = 1.73; 95% CI: 0.99–3.05).[145]

Arsenic. A dose-response relation was observed between arsenic levels in well water and prostate cancer.[146] In a population from Utah exposed to moderate arsenic levels in drinking water, the SMR for prostate cancer compared with the overall US population was 1.48 (95% CI: 1.07–1.91).[147]

Skin Cancer
Arsenic. Nonmelanoma skin cancer is the most common type of malignancy among Caucasians,[148] and the incidence rates of squamous cell carcinoma (SCC) and basal cell carcinoma (BCC) are increasing in the United States.[149] A study in New Hampshire reported an increased risk for SCC with exposure to arsenic levels common in US groundwater.[150] After adjustment for sex, age, BMI, education, smoking status, skin reaction to chronic sun exposure, and urinary creatinine, the OR of SCC was 1.33 for each 1 μg/L increase in urinary MMA (95% CI: 1.04, 1.70). Urinary ΣAs (1.03), iAS (1.26), and DMA (1.03) were also associated with increased odds of SCC.

Thyroid Cancer
Biocides. A population-based case-control study of 462 incident thyroid cancer cases in Connecticut showed that individuals who were occupationally ever exposed to biocides had an increased risk of thyroid cancer (OR = 1.65; 95% CI: 1.16–2.35).[151]

Hair Dye. A common component of permanent hair dye preparations, 2,4-diaminoanisole sulfate, when fed at high doses, caused a 58% increased incidence of thyroid neoplasms in male rats and 42% in female rats, compared with 7% to 8% in controls.[152,153]

Ionizing Radiation. Ionizing radiation during childhood is an established environmental risk factor for thyroid cancer.[154] Medical radiation exposure via diagnostic radiology has also been associated with an increased risk for thyroid cancer. The highest risk increase of well-differentiated thyroid microcarcinoma (tumor sizes ≤ 10 mm) occurred with nuclear medicine examinations (excluding cardiology tests and thyroid uptake studies; OR = 5.47), followed by chest CT scanning (OR = 4.30), head and neck CT scans (OR = 3.88), upper gastrointestinal series (OR = 3.56), lower gastrointestinal series (OR =

3.29), kidney radiography involving dye injection into a vein or artery (OR = 3.21), mammography (OR = 2.95), chest radiography (OR = 2.93), and abdomen CT scanning (OR = 2.54).[155]

ADDITIONAL FACTORS ASSOCIATED WITH CANCER

Chronic Infections

Leukocytes and other phagocytic cells combat bacteria, parasites, and virus-infected cells by destroying them with NO, H_2O_2, O_2^-, and HOCl.[156] Although these oxidants protect humans from immediately dying from infection, they cause oxidative damage to DNA and mutation.[157,158] Chronic hepatitis B and C viruses are a significant cause of hepatocellular carcinoma.[159,160] Schistosomiasis, a chronic infection caused by a parasitical worm, is associated with colorectal cancer, and with increasing density of ova nearer to the carcinoma.[161,162] *Schistosoma haematobium* is a well-known cause of SCC of the bladder with studies showing ova of *S. haematobium* in up to 85% of patients with bladder cancer.[163] The liver fluke, *Opisthorchis viverrini*, is known to have carcinogenic properties linked to cholangiocarcinoma.[164] *Helicobacter pylori* has been identified as a carcinogen accounting for 60% to 70% of gastric cancer globally.[165]

Alcohol

Acetaldehyde has been shown to promote cancer by interfering with the replication of DNA and by inhibiting the body's ability to repair damaged DNA.[166] Alcohol use increases the risk of developing a variety of cancers including colon, liver, breast, throat, mouth, and upper respiratory tract.[167]

Marijuana

The tar from a cannabis cigarette contains higher concentrations of the carcinogens benzanthracenes and benzopyrenes than tobacco smoke.[168] Marijuana smoke has been shown to be mutagenic in the Ames test and in tissue culture.[169] Smoking marijuana can lead to cancer of the mouth, jaw, tongue, and lung, and nonlymphoblastic leukemia in children of marijuana-smoking mothers.[170]

Cannabinoids have also been shown to have potential antitumor effects by modulating key cell-signaling pathways.[171] CBD, cannabigerol, cannabichromene, cannabidiol acid, and THC have all shown antitumor activities, with CBD being a potent inhibitor of breast cancer cell growth.[172] Cannabinoids have also shown promise in the treatment of skin cancer,[173] pancreatic cancer,[174] and lymphoma.[175]

BODY BURDEN

Cancer incidence increases with age and is driven by accumulation of mutations in the DNA as well as growing body load of environmental toxicants with half-lives measured in years and even decades. DNA mutation is a critical step in carcinogenesis and elevated levels of oxidative DNA lesions (8-hydroxyguanine, 8-OHdG) have been noted in various tumors. 8-OHdG is found in many tissues in the body and is released into the urine during DNA repair. In both nuclear and mitochondrial DNA, 8-OHdG is produced because of oxidative damage and has been used as a urinary marker for oxidative stress, carcinogenesis, and degenerative diseases.[176] Elevated 8-OHdG levels are found in breast cancer patients and are believed to be predictive of breast cancer risk.[177,178,179] Higher urinary levels of 8-OHdG are found in men with prostate cancer, and men treated with hormonal therapy for prostate cancer have reduced 8-OHdG levels.[180] 8-OHdG may be a valuable marker for several other cancers, including cervical cancer,[181] ovarian cancer,[182] nonsmall-cell lung cancer,[183,184] nasopharyngeal cancers,[185] acute myeloid leukemia,[186] gastric adenocarcinoma cases,[187] and in bladder cancer.[188]

INTERVENTION

The most essential action is to minimize exposure to endogenous and exogenous sources of oxidative stress by avoiding and, if possible, eliminating environmental carcinogens. Individuals who do not get adequate sleep, have chronic stress, consume excessive alcohol, have a diet filled with conventional and processed foods, and those exposed to pesticides, solvents, and toxic metals have an increased susceptibility to cancer. Therefore lifestyle patterns and targeted nutritional supplementation can have a significant effect on reducing cellular stress and optimizing cellular function.

Generally, antioxidants reduce the damaging effects of ROS, providing prevention as well as treatment benefits. However, antioxidant therapy should be used with caution in carcinogenesis as its effects depend on the stage at which it is introduced. For example, when used during the progression stage of cancer, antioxidants may stimulate the growth of tumor cells by enhancing their survival.[189] There is ample evidence on the use of antioxidants for cancer in general, as well as site-specific interventions. However, detailed interventions are too extensive for the limits of this chapter (more information in Chapter 2, Oxidative Damage and Inflammation).

REFERENCES

1. World Health Organization (WHO). (2017). *Databank. Cancer Fact Sheet.* https://whho.int/mediacentre/factsheets/fs297/en/. (Accessed 7 June 2017).
2. Hanahan, D., & Weinberg, R. A. (2000). The hallmarks of cancer. *Cell, 100*(1), 57–70. PubMed PMID: 10647931.
3. Vineia, P., Scatzkin, A., & Potter, J. D. (2010). Models of carcinogenesis: an overview. *Carcinogenesis, 31*(10), 1703–1709. PubMed PMID: 20430846.
4. National Toxicology Program. (2016). *14th Report on Carcinogens.* https://ntp.niehs.nih.gov/ntp/roc/content/introduction_508.pdf. (Accessed 8 June 2017).
5. Hoeijmakers, J. H. (2009). DNA damage, aging, and cancer. *The New England Journal of Medicine, 361*(19), 1914. PubMed PMID: 19812404.
6. Nakabeppu, Y. (2001). Regulation of intracellular localization of human MTH1, OGG1, and MYH proteins for repair of oxidative DNA damage. *Progress in Nucleic Acid Research and Molecular Biology, 68,* 75–94. PubMed PMID: 11554314.
7. Ohshima, H., Tatemichi, M., & Sawa, T. (2003). Chemical basis of inflammation-induced carcinogenesis. *Archives of Biochemistry and Biophysics, 417*(1), 3–11. PubMed PMID: 1291773.
8. Marnett, L. J., Hurd, H. K., et al. (1985). Naturally occurring carbonyl compounds are mutagens in Salmonella tester strain TA104. *Mutation Research, 148*(1–2), 25–34. PubMed PMID: 3881660.
9. Atherton, K. M., Williams, F. M., Egea González, F. J., et al. (2009). DNA damage in horticultural farmers: a pilot study showing an association with organophosphate pesticide exposure. *Biomarkers: Biochemical Indicators of Exposure, Response, and Susceptibility to Chemicals, 14*(7), 443–451. PubMed PMID: 19863182.
10. Yahia, D., Haruka, I., Kagashi, Y., & Tsuda, S. (2016). 8-hydroxy-2'-deoxyguanosine as a biomarker of oxidative DNA damage induced by perfluorinated compounds in TK6 cells. *Environmental toxicology, 31*(2), 192–200. PubMed PMID: 25113910.
11. Marczynski, B., Kraus, T., Rozynek, P., Raithel, H. J., & Baur, X. (2000). Association between 8-hydroxy-2'-deoxyguanosine levels in DNA of workers highly exposed to asbestos and their clinical data, occupational and non-occupational confounding factors, and cancer. *Mutation Research, 468*(2), 203–212. PubMed PMID: 10882897.
12. Yoshida, R., Ogawa, Y., Shioji, I., Yu, X., Shibata, E., Mori, I., et al. (2001). Urinary 8-oxo-7, 8-dihydro-2'-deoxyguanosine and biopyrrins levels among construction workers with asbestos exposure history. *Industrial Health, 39*(2), 186–188. PubMed PMID: 11341550.
13. Katanoda, K., Sobue, T., Satoh, H., et al. (2011). An association between long-term exposure to ambient air pollution and mortality from lung cancer and respiratory diseases in Japan. *Journal of Epidemiology, 21*(2), 132–143. PubMed PMID: 21325732.
14. Oh, S. M., Kim, H. R., Park, Y. J., Lee, S. Y., & Chung, K. H. (2011). Organic extracts of urban air pollution particulate matter (PM2.5)-induced genotoxicity and oxidative stress in human lung bronchial epithelial cells (BEAS-2B cells). *Mutation Research, 723*(2), 142–151. PubMed PMID: 21524716.
15. Mena, S., Ortega, A., & Estrela, J. M. (2009). Oxidative stress in environmental-induced carcinogenesis. *Mutation Research, 674*(1–2), 36–44. PubMed PMID: 18977455.
16. Ohshima, H., Tazawa, H., et al. (2005). Prevention of human cancer by modulation of chronic inflammatory processes. *Mutation Research, 591*(1–2), 110–122. PubMed PMID: 16083916.
17. Yang, C., & Frenkel, K. (2002). Arsenic-mediated cellular signal transduction, transcription factor activation, and aberrant gene expression: implications in carcinogenesis. *Journal of Environmental Pathology, Toxicology and Oncology, 21*(4), 331–342. PubMed PMID: 12510962.
18. Antoni, S., Ferlay, J., et al. (2017). Bladder cancer incidence and mortality: a global overview and recent trends. *European Urology, 71*(1), 96–108. PubMed PMID: 27370177.
19. IARC Working Group on the Evaluation of Carcinogenic Risks to Humans. (2012). Arsenic, metals, fibres, and dusts. *IARC Monographs on the Evaluation of Carcinogenic Risks to Humans, 100*(Pt. C), 11–465. PubMed PMID: 23189751.
20. Kitchin, K. T., & Ahmad, S. (2003). Oxidative stress as a possible mode of action for arsenic carcinogenesis. *Toxicology Letters, 137*(1–2), 3–13. PubMed PMID: 12505428.
21. Ren, X., Mn Hale, C. M., et al. (2011). An emerging role for epigenetic dysregulation in arsenic toxicity

and carcinogenesis. *Environmental Health Perspectives*, *119*(1), 11–19. PubMed PMID: 20682481.

22. Zhang, A., Feng, H., et al. (2007). Unventilated indoor coal-fired stoves in Guizhou province, China: cellular and genetic damage in villagers exposed to arsenic in food and air. *Environmental Health Perspectives*, *115*(4), 653–658. PubMed PMID: 17450239.

23. Chen, C. J., Kuo, T. L., & Wu, M. M. (1988). Arsenic and cancers. *Lancet*, *1*(8582), 414–415. PubMed PMID: 2893213.

24. Smith, A. H., Goycolea, M., et al. (1988). Marked increase in bladder and lung cancer mortality in a region of Northern Chile due to arsenic in drinking water. *American Journal of Epidemiology*, *147*(7), 660–669. PubMed PMID: 9554605.

25. Smith, A. H., Hopenhayn-Rich, C., et al. (1992). Cancer risks from arsenic in drinking water. *Environmental Health Perspectives*, *97*, 259–267. PubMed PMID: 1396465.

26. Baris, D., Waddell, R., Beane Freeman, L. E., et al. (2016). Elevated bladder cancer in northern New England: the role of drinking water and arsenic. *Journal of the National Cancer Institute*, *108*(9), pii: djw099. PubMed PMID: 27140955.

27. Saint-Jacques, N., Parker, L., Brown, P., & Dummer, T. J. (2014). Arsenic in drinking water and urinary tract cancers: a systematic review of 30 years of epidemiological evidence. *Environmental Health: A Global Access Science Source*, *13*, 44. PubMed PMID: 24889821.

28. Zhao, C. Q., Young, M. R., et al. (1997). Association of arsenic-induced malignant transformation with DNA hypomethylation and aberrant gene expression. *Proceedings of the National Academy of Sciences of the United States of America*, *94*(20), 10907–10912. PubMed PMID: 9380733.

29. Chen, Y. C., Su, H. J., et al. (2003). Arsenic methylation and bladder cancer risk in Taiwan. *Cancer Causes and Control*, *14*(4), 303–310. PubMed PMID: 12846360.

30. Kellen, E., Zeegers, M. P., et al. (2007). Blood cadmium may be associated with bladder carcinogenesis: the Belgian case-control study on bladder cancer. *Cancer Detection and Prevention*, *31*(1), 77–82. PubMed PMID: 17296271.

31. Somji, S., Zhou, X. D., et al. (2006). Urothelial cells malignantly transformed by exposure to cadmium (Cd(+2)) and arsenite (As(+3)) have increased resistance to Cd(+2) and As(+3)-induced cell death. *Toxicological Sciences*, *94*(2), 293–301. PubMed PMID: 16980690.

32. Sens, D. A., Park, S., et al. (2004). Inorganic cadmium- and arsenite-induced malignant transformation of human bladder urothelial cells. *Toxicological Sciences*, *79*(1), 56–63. PubMed PMID: 14976345.

33. King, W. D., & Marrett, L. D. (1996). Case-control study of bladder cancer and chlorination by-products in treated water (Ontario, Canada). *Cancer Causes and Control*, *7*(6), 596–604. PubMed PMID: 8932920.

34. D'Avanzo, B., La Vecchia, C., et al. (1995). Attributable risks for bladder cancer in Northern Italy. *Annals of Epidemiology*, *5*(6), 427–431. PubMed PMID: 8680604.

35. Baris, D., Karagas, M. R., et al. (2009). A case-control study of smoking and bladder cancer risk: emergent patterns over time. *Journal of the National Cancer Institute*, *101*(22), 1553–1561. PubMed PMID: 19917915.

36. Freedman, N. D., Silverman, D. T., et al. (2011). Association between smoking and risk of bladder cancer among men and women. *JAMA: The Journal of the American Medical Association*, *306*(7), 737–745. PubMed PMID: 21846855.

37. Burger, M., Catto, J. W., et al. (2013). Epidemiology and risk factors of urothelial bladder cancer. *European Urology*, *63*(2), 234–241. PubMed PMID: 22877502.

38. Ottaviani, G., & Jaffe, N. (2009). The epidemiology of osteosarcoma. *Cancer Treatment and Research*, *152*, 3–13. PubMed PMID: 20213383.

39. Moore, L. E., Lu, M., & Smith, A. H. (2002). Childhood cancer incidence and arsenic exposure in drinking water in Nevada. *Archives of Environmental Health*, *57*(3), 201–206. PubMed PMID: 12507173.

40. Sandhu, R., Lai, H., et al. (2011). Serum fluoride and sialic acid levels in osteosarcoma. *Biological trace element research*, *144*(1–3), 1–5. PubMed PMID: 19390788.

41. Kharb, S., Sandhu, R., & Kundu, Z. S. (2012). Fluoride levels and osteosarcoma. *South Asian journal of cancer*, *1*(2), 76–77. PubMed PMID: 24455518.

42. Young, N., Newton, J., et al. (2015). Community water fluoridation and health outcomes in England: a cross-sectional study. *Community Dentistry and Oral Epidemiology*, *43*(6), 550–559. PubMed PMID: 26153549.

43. Lee, W. J., Colt, J. S., Heineman, E. F., et al. (2005). Agricultural pesticide use and risk of glioma in Nebraska, United States. *Occupational and Environmental Medicine*, *62*(11), 786–792. PubMed PMID: 16234405.

44. Ruder, A. M., Carreon, T., Butler, M. A., et al. (2009). Exposure to farm crops, livestock, and farm tasks and risk of glioma: the Upper Midwest Health Study. *American Journal of Epidemiology*, *169*(12), 1479–1491. PubMed PMID: 19403843.

45. Davis, J. R., Brownson, R. C., Garcia, R., et al. (1993). Family pesticide use and childhood brain cancer. *Archives of Environmental Contamination and Toxicology, 24*(1), 87–92. PubMed PMID: 8466294.

46. Boffetta, P., Tredaniel, J., & Greco, A. (2000). Risk of childhood cancer and adult lung cancer after childhood exposure to passive smoke: a meta-analysis. *Environmental Health Perspectives, 108*(1), 73–82. PubMed PMID: 10620527.

47. Brooks, D. R., Mucci, L. A., Hatch, E. E., & Cnattingius, S. (2004). Maternal smoking during pregnancy and risk of brain tumors in the offspring. A prospective study of 1.4 million Swedish births. *Cancer Causes and Control, 15*(10), 997–1005. PubMed PMID: 15801484.

48. Barrington-Trimis, J. L., Searles Nielsen, S., et al. (2013). Parental smoking and risk of childhood brain tumors by functional polymorphisms in polycyclic aromatic hydrocarbon metabolism genes. *PLoS ONE, 8*(11), e79110. PubMed PMID: 24260161.

49. Wesseling, C., Pukkala, E., et al. (2002). Cancer of the brain and nervous system and occupational exposures in Finnish women. *Journal of Occupational and Environmental Medicine, 44*(7), 663–668. PubMed PMID: 12134530.

50. Rajaraman, P., Stewart, P. A., Samet, J. M., et al. (2006). Lead, genetic susceptibility, and risk of adult brain tumors. *Cancer Epidemiology, Biomarkers and Prevention: A Publication of the American Association for Cancer Research, Cosponsored by the American Society of Preventive Oncology, 15*(12), 2514–2520. PubMed PMID: 17164378.

51. [No authors listed]. (1979). Vinyl chloride, polyvinyl chloride and vinyl chloride-vinyl acetate copolymers. *IARC Monographs on the Evaluation of the Carcinogenic Risk of Chemicals to Humans, 19*, 377–438. PubMed PMID: 374232.

52. Wong, O., Whorton, M. D., et al. (1991). An industry-wide epidemiologic study of vinyl chloride workers, 1942-1982. *American Journal of Industrial Medicine, 20*(3), 317–334. PubMed PMID: 1928109.

53. Mundt, K. A., Dell, L. D., Austin, R. P., et al. (2000). Historical cohort study of 10,109 men in the North American vinyl chloride industry, 1942-72: update of cancer mortality to 31 December 1995. *Occupational and Environmental Medicine, 57*(11), 774–781. PubMed PMID: 11024202.

54. Ferlay, J., Soerjomataram, I., et al. (2015). Cancer incidence and mortality worldwide: sources, methods and major patterns in GLOBOCAN 2012. *International Journal of Cancer. Journal International du Cancer, 136*(5), E359–E386. PubMed PMID: 25220842.

55. Ghoncheh, M., Pournamdar, Z., & Salehiniya, H. (2016). Incidence and mortality and epidemiology of breast cancer in the world. *Asian Pacific Journal of Cancer Prevention: APJCP, 17*(S3), 43–46. PubMed PMID: 27165206.

56. Macon, M. B., & Fenton, S. E. (2013). Endocrine disruptors and the breast: early life effects and later life disease. *Journal of Mammary Gland Biology and Neoplasia, 18*(1), 43–61. PubMed PMID: 23417729.

57. Wassermann, M., Nogueira, D. P., et al. (1976). Organochlorine compounds in neoplastic and adjacent apparently normal breast tissue. *Bulletin of Environmental Contamination and Toxicology, 15*(4), 478–484. PubMed PMID: 816406.

58. Wolff, M. S., Toniolo, P. G., Lee, E. W., et al. (1993). Blood levels of organochlorine residues and risk of breast cancer. *Journal of the National Cancer Institute, 85*(8), 648–652. PubMed PMID: 8468722.

59. Cohn, B. A., Wolff, M. S., et al. (2007). DDT and breast cancer in young women: new data on the significance of age at exposure. *Environmental Health Perspectives, 115*(10), 1406–1414. PubMed PMID: 17938728.

60. Cohn, B. A., La Merrill, M., et al. (2015). DDT exposure in utero and breast cancer. *The Journal of Clinical Endocrinology and Metabolism, 100*(8), 2865–2872. PubMed PMID: 26079774.

61. Leng, L., Li, J., et al. (2016). Polychlorinated biphenyls and breast cancer: a congener-specific meta-analysis. *Environment International, 88*, 133–141. PubMed PMID: 26735351.

62. Bjermo, H., Darnerud, P. O., Lignell, S., et al. (2013). Fish intake and breastfeeding time are associated with serum concentrations of organochlorines in a Swedish population. *Environment International, 51*, 88–96. PMID: 23201820.

63. Byford, J. R., Shaw, L. E., Drew, M. G., et al. (2002). Oestrogenic activity of parabens in MCF7 human breast cancer cells. *The Journal of Steroid Biochemistry and Molecular Biology, 80*, 49–60.

64. Darbre, P. D., Aljarrah, A., Miller, W. R., et al. (2004). Concentrations of parabens in human breast tumours. *Journal of Applied Toxicology: JAT, 24*, 5–13.

65. King, W. D., Marrett, L. D., & Woolcott, C. G. (2000). Case-control study of colon and rectal cancers and chlorination by-products in treated water. *Cancer Epidemiology, Biomarkers and Prevention: A Publication of the American Association for Cancer Research, Cosponsored by the American Society of Preventive Oncology, 9*(8), 813–818. PubMed PMID: 10952098.

66. Song, L., Liu, J., Jin, X., et al. (2014). p,p'-dichlo rodiphenyldichloroethylene induces colorectal adenocarcinoma cell proliferation through oxidative

stress. *PLoS ONE, 9*(11), e112700. PubMed PMID: 25386960.

67. Chen, K., Zhao, Y. W., et al. (2004). Relationship between organochlorine pollution in soil and rice and the incidence of colorectal cancer in Jiashan county, Zhejiang province. *Zhonghua Liu Xing Bing Xue Za Zhi = Zhonghua Liuxingbingxue Zazhi, 25*(6), 479–483. PubMed PMID: 15231121.

68. Olszewski, J., Latusinski, J., et al. (2006). Comparative assessment of aluminum and lead concentrations in serum and tissue bioptates in patients with laryngeal papilloma or cancer. *B-ENT, 2*(2), 47–49. PubMed PMID: 16910286.

69. Smith, A. H., Marshall, G., et al. (2012). Mortality in young adults following in utero and childhood exposure to arsenic in drinking water. *Environmental Health Perspectives, 120*(11), 1527–1531. PubMed PMID: 22949133.

70. Collecchi, P., Esposito, M., et al. (1986). The distribution of arsenic and cobalt in patients with laryngeal carcinoma. *Journal of Applied Toxicology: JAT, 6*(4), 287–289. PubMed PMID: 3760455.

71. Rothman, K. J. (1978). Epidemiology of head and neck cancer. *The Laryngoscope, 88*(3), 435–438. PubMed PMID: 628297.

72. Maier, H., & Weidauer, H. (1995). Alcohol drinking and tobacco smoking are the chief risk factors for ENT tumors. Increased incidence of mouth cavity, pharyngeal and laryngeal carcinomas. *Fortschritte Der Medizin, 113*(11), 157–160. PubMed PMID: 7768477.

73. Maier, H., Dietz, A., Gewelke, U., et al. (1992). Tobacco and alcohol and the risk of head and neck cancer. *The Clinical Investigator, 70*(3–4), 320–327. PubMed PMID: 1521046.

74. Zheng, T. Z., Boyle, P., et al. (1990). Tobacco smoking, alcohol consumption, and risk of oral cancer: a case-control study in Beijing, People's Republic of China. *Cancer Causes and Control, 1*(2), 173–179. PubMed PMID: 2102288.

75. Jemal, A., Center, M. M., et al. (2010). Global patterns of cancer incidence and mortality rates and trends. *Cancer Epidemiology, Biomarkers and Prevention: A Publication of the American Association for Cancer Research, Cosponsored by the American Society of Preventive Oncology, 19*(8), 1893–1907. PubMed PMID: 20647400.

76. Parkin, D. M., Bray, F., Ferlay, J., & Pisani, P. (2005). Global cancer statistics, 2002. *CA: A Cancer Journal for Clinicians, 55*(2), 74–108. PubMed PMID: 15761078.

77. McGlynn, K. A., Abnet, C. C., et al. (2006). Serum concentrations of

1,1,1-trichlro-2,2-bis(p-chlorophenyl)ethane (DDT) and 1,1-dichloro-2,2-bis(p-chlorophenyl)ethylene (DDE) and risk of primary liver cancer. *Journal of the National Cancer Institute, 98*(14), 1005–1010. PubMed PMID: 16849683.

78. Persson, E. C., Graubard, B. I., Evans, A. A., et al. (2012). Dichlorodiphenyltrichloroethane and risk of hepatocellular carcinoma. *International Journal of Cancer. Journal International du Cancer, 131*(9), 2078–2084. PubMed PMID: 22290210.

79. Zhao, B., Shen, H., Liu, F., et al. (2012). Exposure to organochlorine pesticides is an independent risk factor of hepatocellular carcinoma: a case-control study. *Journal of Exposure Science and Environmental Epidemiology, 22*(6), 541–548. PubMed PMID: 21915153.

80. Deguchi, Y., Yamada, T., Hirose, Y., et al. (2009). Mode of action analysis for the synthetic pyrethroid metofluthrin-induced rat liver tumors: evidence for hepatic CYP2B induction and hepatocyte proliferation. *Toxicological Sciences, 108*(1), 69–80. PubMed PMID: 19176366.

81. Yamada, T., Uwagawa, S., Okuno, Y., et al. (2009). Case study: an evaluation of the human relevance of the synthetic pyrethroid metofluthrin-induced liver tumors in rats based on mode of action. *Toxicological Sciences, 108*(1), 59–68. PubMed PMID: 19176367.

82. Heath, C. W., Jr., Falk, H., & Creech, J. L., Jr. (1975). Characteristics of cases of angiosarcoma of the liver among vinyl chloride workers in the United States. *Annals of the New York Academy of Sciences, 246*, 231–236. PubMed PMID: 1054956.

83. Falk, H. (1987). Vinyl chloride-induced hepatic angiosarcoma. *Princess Takamatsu Symposia, 18*, 39–46. PubMed PMID: 3506545.

84. Islami, F., Torre, L. A., & Jemal, A. (2015). Global trends of lung cancer mortality and smoking prevalence. *Translational lung cancer research, 4*(4), 327–338. PubMed PMID: 26380174.

85. National Center for Chronic Disease Prevention and Health Promotion (US) Office on Smoking and Health. (2014). *The health consequences of smoking – 50 years of progress: a report of the surgeon general*. Atlanta, GA: Centers for Disease Control and Prevention. PubMed PMID: 24455788.

86. Oberg, M., Jaakkola, M. S., et al. (2011). Worldwide burden of disease from exposure to second-hand smoke: a retrospective analysis of data from 192 countries. *Lancet, 377*(9760), 139–146. PubMed PMID: 21112082.

87. Carazo Fernandez, L., Fernandez Alvarez, R., et al. (2013). Indoor air contaminants and their impact on

respiratory pathologies. *Archivos de bronconeumología*, *49*(1), 22–27. PubMed PMID: 22704531.

88. Raaschou-Nielsen, O., Beelen, R., et al. (2016). Particulate matter air pollution components and risk for lung cancer. *Environment International*, *87*, 66–73. PubMed PMID: 26641521.

89. De Matteis, S., Consonni, D., & Bertazzi, P. A. (2008). Exposure to occupational carcinogens and lung cancer risk. Evolution of epidemiological estimates of attributable fraction. *Acta bio-medica: Atenei Parmensis*, *79*(Suppl. 1), 34–42. PubMed PMID: 18924308.

90. IARC Working Group on the Evaluation of Carcinogenic Risks to Humans. (2012). Radiation. *IARC Monogr Eval Carcinog Risks Hum*, *100*(Pt. D), 7–303. PubMed PMID: 23189752.

91. Norseth, T. (1980). Asbestos and metals as carcinogens. *Journal of Toxicology and Environmental Health*, *6*(5–6), 1021–1028. PubMed PMID: 7463500.

92. Thun, M. J., Carter, B. D., Feskanich, D., et al. (2013). 50-year trends in smoking-related mortality in the United States. *The New England Journal of Medicine*, *368*(4), 351–364. PubMed PMID: 23343064.

93. Yano, T., Shoji, F., Baba, H., Koga, T., Shiraishi, T., Orita, H., et al. (2009). Significance of the urinary 8-OHdG level as an oxidative stress marker in lung cancer patients. *Lung Cancer*, *63*(1), 111–114. PubMed PMID: 18676055.

94. Hashibe, M., Morgenstern, H., Cui, Y., et al. (2006). Marijuana use and the risk of lung and upper aerodigestive tract cancers: results of a population-based case-control study. *Cancer Epidemiology, Biomarkers & Prevention: A Publication of the American Association for Cancer Research, cosponsored by the American Society of Preventive Oncology*, *15*(10), 1829–1834.

95. Reymão, M. S., Cury, P. M., Lichtenfels, A. J., et al. (1997). Urban air pollution enhances the formation of urethane-induced lung tumors in mice. *Environmental Research*, *74*(2), 150–158. PubMed PMID: 9339228.

96. Tokiwa, H., Nakanishi, Y., Sera, N., Hara, N., & Inuzuka, S. (1998). Analysis of environmental carcinogens associated with the incidence of lung cancer. *Toxicology Letters*, *99*, 33–41. PubMed PMID: 9801028.

97. Biggeri, A., Barbone, F., Iagazio, C., et al. (1996). Air pollution and lung cancer in Trieste, Italy: spatial analysis of risk as a function of distance from sources. *Environmental Health Perspectives*, *104*, 750–754. PubMed PMID: 8841761.

98. Velleneuve, P. J., Parent, M. E., Sahni, V., Johnson, K. C., & Canadian Cancer Registries Epidemiology Research Group. (2011). Occupational exposure to diesel and gasoline exhaust emissions and lung cancer in Canadian men. *Environmental Research*, *111*(5), 727–735. PubMed PMID: 21536265.

99. Parent, M. E., Rousseau, M. C., Boffetta, P., et al. (2007). Exposure to diesel and gasoline engine emissions and the risk of lung cancer. *American Journal of Epidemiology*, *165*(1), 53–62. PubMed PMID: 17062632.

100. Hamra, G. B., Guha, N., Cohen, A., et al. (2014). Outdoor particulate matter exposure and lung cancer: a systematic review and meta-analysis. *Environmental Health Perspectives*, *122*(9), 906–911. PubMed PMID: 24911630.

101. Beeson, W. L., Abbey, D. E., & Knutsen, S. F. (1998). Long-term concentrations of ambient air pollutants and incident lung cancer in California adults: results from the AHSMOG study. Adventist Health Study on Smog. *Environmental Health Perspectives*, *106*(12), 813–822. PubMed PMID: 9831542.

102. Behera, D., Belamugesh, T. (2005). Indoor air pollution as a risk factor for lung cancer in women. *The Journal of the Association of Physicians of India*, *53*, 190–192. PubMed PMID: 15926600.

103. Delgado, J., Martinez, L. M., et al. (2005). Lung cancer pathogenesis associated with wood smoke exposure. *Chest*, *128*(1), 124–131. PubMed PMID: 16002925.

104. Turner, M. C., Krewski, D., Chen, Y., et al. (2011). Radon and lung cancer in the American Cancer Society cohort. *Cancer Epidemiology, Biomarkers and Prevention: A Publication of the American Association for Cancer Research, Cosponsored by the American Society of Preventive Oncology*, *20*(3), 438–448. PubMed PMID: 21212062.

105. Lee, W. J., Blair, A., Hoppin, J. A., et al. (2004). Cancer incidence among pesticide applicators exposed to chlorpyrifos in the Agricultural Health Study. *Journal of the National Cancer Institute*, *96*(23), 1781–1789. PubMed PMID: 15572760.

106. D'Ippoliti, D., Santelli, E., De Sario, M., et al. (2015). Arsenic in drinking water and mortality for cancer and chronic diseases in central Italy, 1990-2010. *PLoS ONE*, *10*(9), e0138182. PubMed PMID: 26383851.

107. Dauphiné, D. C., Smith, A. H., Yuan, Y., et al. (2013). Case-control study of arsenic in drinking water and lung cancer in California and Nevada. *International Journal of Environmental Research and Public Health*, *10*(8), 3310–3324. PubMed PMID: 23917816.

108. Waddell, B. L., Zahm, S. H., Baris, D., et al. (2001). Agricultural use of organophosphate pesticides and the risk of non-Hodgkin's lymphoma among male farmers

(United States). *Cancer Causes and Control*, *12*(6), 509–517. PubMed PMID: 11519759.

109. Zahm, S. H., Weisenburger, D. D., Babbitt, R. C., et al. (1988). A case-control study of non-Hodgkin's lymphoma and agricultural factors in Eastern Nebraska. *American Journal of Epidemiology*, *128*, 901.

110. Brown, L. M., Blair, A., Gibson, R., et al. (1990). Pesticide exposure and other agricultural risk factors for leukemia among men in Iowa and Minnesota. *Cancer Research*, *50*(20), 6585–6591. PubMed PMID: 2208120.

111. Leiss, J. K., & Savitz, D. A. (1995). Home pesticide use and childhood cancer: a case-control study. *American Journal of Public Health*, *85*(2), 249–252. PubMed PMID: 7856787.

112. Ma, X., Buffler, P. A., Gunier, R. B., et al. (2002). Critical windows of exposure to household pesticides and risk of childhood leukemia. *Environmental Health Perspectives*, *110*(9), 955–960. PubMed PMID: 12204832.

113. Grulich, A. E., Vajdic, C. M., & Cozen, W. (2007). Altered immunity as a risk factor for non-Hodgkin lymphoma. *Cancer Epidemiology, Biomarkers and Prevention: A Publication of the American Association for Cancer Research, Cosponsored by the American Society of Preventive Oncology*, *16*(3), 405–408. PubMed PMID: 17337643.

114. Selgrade, M. K. (2007). Immunotoxicity: the risk is real. *Toxicological Sciences*, *100*(2), 328–332. PubMed PMID: 17878151.

115. De Roos, A. J., Hartge, P., et al. (2005). Persistent organochlorine chemicals in plasm and risk of non-Hodgkin's lymphoma. *Cancer Research*, *65*(23), 11214–11226. PubMed PMID: 16322272.

116. Cantor, K. P., Blair, A., et al. (1992). Pesticides and other agricultural risk factors for non-Hodgkin's lymphoma among men in Iowa and Minnesota. *Cancer Research*, *52*(9), 2447–2455. PubMed PMID: 1568215.

117. Rothman, N., Cantor, K. P., et al. (1997). A nested case-control study of non-Hodgkin lymphoma and serum organochlorine residues. *Lancet*, *350*(9073), 240–244. PubMed PMID: 9242800.

118. Rugman, F. P., & Cosstick, R. (1990). Aplastic anemia associated with organochlorine pesticide: case reports and review of evidence. *Journal of Clinical Pathology*, *43*(2), 98–101. PubMed PMID: 1690760.

119. Liu, L., Zhang, Q., Feng, J., et al. (1996). The study of DNA oxidative damage in benzene-exposed workers. *Mutation Research*, *370*(3–4), 145–150. PubMed PMID: 8917660.

120. Aksoy, M., Erdem, S., & DinCol, G. (1974). Leukemia in show-workers exposed chronically to benzene. *Blood*, *44*(6), 837–841. PubMed PMID: 4529630.

121. Decoufle, P., Blattner, W. A., & Blair, A. (1983). Mortality among chemical workers exposed to benzene and other agents. *Environmental Research*, *30*(1), 16–25. PubMed PMID: 6832104.

122. Colt, J. S., & Blair, A. (1998). Parental occupational exposures and risk of childhood cancer. *Environmental Health Perspectives*, *106*(Suppl. 3), 909–925. PubMed PMID: 9646055.

123. McKinney, P. A., Alexander, F. E., et al. (1991). Parental occupations of children with leukaemia in west Cumbria, north Humberside, and Gateshead. *BMJ (Clinical Research Ed.)*, *302*(6778), 681–687. PubMed PMID: 2021741.

124. Duarte-Davidson, R., Courage, C., Rushton, L., & Levy, L. (2001). Benzene in the environment: an assessment of the potential risks to the health of the population. *Occupational and Environmental Medicine*, *58*(1), 2–13. PubMed PMID: 11119628.

125. Carlos-Wallace, F. M., Zhang, L., et al. (2016). Parental, in utero, and early-life exposures to benzene and the risk of childhood leukemia: a meta-analysis. *American Journal of Epidemiology*, *183*(1), 1–14. PubMed PMID: 26589707.

126. Fuchs, C. S., Colditz, G. A., et al. (1996). A prospective study of cigarette smoking and the risk of pancreatic cancer. *Archives of Internal Medicine*, *156*(19), 2255–2260. PubMed PMID: 8885826.

127. Bonelli, L., Aste, H., et al. (2003). Exocrine pancreatic cancer, cigarette smoking, and diabetes mellitus: a case-control study in northern Italy. *Pancreas*, *27*(2), 143–149. PubMed PMID: 12883263.

128. Lee, C. T., Chang, F. Y., & Lee, S. D. (1996). Risk factors for pancreatic cancer in Orientals. *Journal of Gastroenterology and Hepatology*, *11*(5), 491–495. PubMed PMID: 8743923.

129. Hassan, M. M., Bondy, M. L., et al. (2007). Risk factors for pancreatic cancer: case-control study. *The American Journal of Gastroenterology*, *102*(12), 2696–2707. PubMed PMID: 17764494.

130. Silverman, D. T., Dunn, J. A., et al. (1994). Cigarette smoking and pancreas cancer: a case-control study based on direct interviews. *Journal of the National Cancer Institute*, *86*(20), 1510–1516. PubMed PMID: 7932805.

131. Luckett, B. G., Su, L. J., Rood, J. C., & Fontham, E. T. (2012). Cadmium exposure and pancreatic cancer in south Louisiana. *Journal of Environmental and Public Health*, *2012*, 180186. PubMed PMID: 23319964.

132. Dakeishi, M., Murata, K., & Grandjean, P. (2006). Long-term consequences of arsenic poisoning during infancy due to contaminated milk powder. *Environmental Health: A Global Access Science Source, 5,* 31. PubMed PMID: 17076881.

133. Yorifuji, T., Tsuda, T., et al. (2011). Cancer excess after arsenic exposure from contaminated milk powder. *Environmental Health and Preventive Medicine, 16*(3), 164–170. PubMed PMID: 21431798.

134. Yorifuji, T., Tsuda, T., & Grandjean, P. (2010). Unusual cancer excess after neonatal arsenic exposure from contaminated milk powder. *Journal of the National Cancer Institute, 102*(5), 360–361. PubMed PMID: 20068193.

135. Garcia-Esquinas, E., Pollan, M., et al. (2013). Arsenic exposure and cancer mortality in a US-based prospective cohort: the strong heart study. *Cancer Epidemiology, Biomarkers and Prevention: A Publication of the American Association for Cancer Research, Cosponsored by the American Society of Preventive Oncology, 22*(11), 1944–1953. PubMed PMID: 23800676.

136. Diaz-Villasenor, A., Burns, A. L., et al. (2007). Arsenic-induced alteration in the expression of genes related to type 2 diabetes mellitus. *Toxicology and Applied Pharmacology, 225*(2), 123–133. PubMed PMID: 17936320.

137. Lowenfels, A. B., & Maisonneuve, P. (2006). Epidemiology and risk factors for pancreatic cancer. *Best Practice & Research. Clinical Gastroenterology, 20*(2), 197–209. PubMed PMID: 16549324.

138. Garabrant, D. H., Held, J., et al. (1992). DDT and related compounds and risk of pancreatic cancer. *Journal of the National Cancer Institute, 84*(10), 764–771. PubMed PMID: 1573662.

139. Yassi, A., Tate, R., & Fish, D. (1994). Cancer mortality in workers employed at a transformer manufacturing plant. *American Journal of Industrial Medicine, 25*(3), 425–437. PubMed PMID: 8160660.

140. Beard, J., Sladden, T., et al. (2003). Health impacts of pesticide exposure in a cohort of outdoor workers. *Environmental Health Perspectives, 111*(5), 724–730. PubMed PMID: 12727601.

141. Lopez, T., Pumarega, J. A., Pollack, A. Z., et al. (2014). Adjusting serum concentrations of organochlorine compounds by lipids and symptoms: a causal framework for the association with K-ras mutations in pancreatic cancer. *Chemosphere, 114,* 219–225. PubMed PMID: 25113205.

142. Porta, M., Lopez, T., Pumarega, J., et al. (2009). In pancreatic ductal adenocarcinoma blood concentrations of some organochlorine compounds and coffee intake are independently associated with KRAS mutations. *Mutagenesis, 24*(6), 513–521. PubMed PMID: 19797353.

143. Porta, M., Malats, N., et al. (1999). Serum concentrations of organochlorine compounds and K-ras mutations in exocrine pancreatic cancer. PANKRAS II Study Group. *Lancet, 354*(9196), 2125–2129. PubMed PMID: 10609819.

144. Agalliu, I., Langeberg, W. J., Lampe, J. W., et al. (2006). Glutathione S-transferase M1, T1, and P1 polymorphisms and prostate cancer risk in middle-aged men. *The Prostate, 66*(2), 146–156. PubMed PMID: 16173036.

145. Nock, N. L., Liu, X., et al. (2006). Polymorphisms in polycyclic aromatic hydrocarbon metabolism and conjugation genes, interactions with smoking and prostate cancer risk. *Cancer Epidemiology, Biomarkers and Prevention: A Publication of the American Association for Cancer Research, Cosponsored by the American Society of Preventive Oncology, 15*(4), 756–761. PubMed PMID: 16614120.

146. Yang, C. Y., Chang, C. C., & Chiu, H. F. (2008). Does arsenic exposure increase the risk for prostate cancer? *Journal of Toxicology and Environmental Health. Part A, 71*(23), 1559–1563. PubMed PMID: 18923998.

147. Lewis, D. R., Southwick, J. W., et al. (1999). Drinking water arsenic in Utah: a cohort mortality study. *Environmental Health Perspectives, 107*(5), 359–365. PubMed PMID: 10210691.

148. Mudigonda, T., Pearce, D. J., et al. (2010). The economic impact of non-melanoma skin cancer: a review. *Journal of the National Comprehensive Cancer Network, 8*(8), 888–896. PubMed PMID: 20870635.

149. Rogers, H. W., Weinstock, M. A., et al. (2010). Incidence estimate of nonmelanoma skin cancer in the United States, 2006. *Archives of Dermatology, 146*(3), 283–287. PubMed PMID: 20231499.

150. Gilbert-Diamond, D., Li, Z., Perry, A. E., Spencer, S. K., et al. (2013). A population-based case-control study of urinary arsenic species and squamous cell carcinoma in New Hampshire, USA. *Environmental Health Perspectives, 121*(10), 1154–1160. PubMed PMID: 23872349. Erratum in: Environ Health Perspect. 2013;121(10):1159.

151. Zeng, F., Lerro, C., et al. (2017). Occupational exposure to pesticides and other biocides and risk of thyroid cancer. *Occupational and Environmental Medicine,* PubMed PMID: 28202579. Pii: oemed-2016-103931.

152. Ward, J. M., Stinson, S. F., et al. (1979). Neoplasms and pigmentation of thyroid glands in F344 rats exposed to 2,4-diaminoanisole sulfate, a hair dye component.

Journal of the National Cancer Institute, 62(4), 1067–1073. PubMed PMID: 285280.

153. Kitahori, Y., Ohshima, M., et al. (1989). Promoting effect of 2,4-diaminoanisole sulfate on rat thyroid carcinogenesis. *Cancer Letters, 45*(2), 115–121. PubMed PMID: 2731155.

154. Sinnott, B., Ron, E., & Schneider, A. B. (2010). Exposing the thyroid to radiation: a review of its current extent, risks, and implications. *Endocrine Reviews, 31*(5), 756–773. PubMed PMID: 20650861.

155. Zhang, Y., Chen, Y., Huang, H., et al. (2015). Diagnostic radiography exposure increases the risk for thyroid microcarcinoma: a population-based case-control study. *European Journal of Cancer Prevention, 24*(5), 439–446. PubMed PMID: 25932870.

156. Stamler, J. S., Singel, D. J., & Loscalzo, J. (1992). Biochemistry of nitric oxide and its redox-activated forms. *Science, 258*(5090), 1898–1902. PubMed PMID: 1281928.

157. Shacter, E., Beecham, E. J., et al. (1988). Activated neutrophils induce prolonged DNA damage in neighboring cells. *Carcinogenesis, 9*(12), 2297–2304. PubMed PMID: 2847879.

158. Cochrane, C. G. (1991). Cellular injury by oxidants. *The American Journal of Medicine, 91*(3C), 23S–30S. PubMed PMID: 1928208.

159. Gerber, M. A. (1993). Relation of hepatitis C virus to hepatocellular carcinoma. *Journal of Hepatology, 17*(Suppl. 3), S108–S111. PubMed PMID: 8389783.

160. Hayashi, P. H., & Zeldis, J. B. (1993). Molecular biology of viral hepatitis and hepatocellular carcinoma. *Comprehensive Therapy, 19*(5), 188–196. PubMed PMID: 8275664.

161. Matsuda, K., Masaki, T., et al. (1999). Possible associations of rectal carcinoma with *Shcistosoma japonicum* infection and membranous nephropathy: a case report with a review. *Japanese Journal of Clinical Oncology, 29*(11), 576–581. PubMed PMID: 10678562.

162. Ming-Chai, C., Chi-Yuan, C., et al. (1980). Evolution of colorectal cancer in schistosomiasis: transitional mucosal changes adjacent to large intestinal carcinoma in colectomy specimens. *Cancer, 46*(7), 1661–1675. PubMed PMID: 7417960.

163. Groeneveld, A. E., Marszalek, W. W., & Heyns, C. F. (1996). Bladder cancer in various population groups in the greater Durban area of KwaZulu-Natal, South Africa. *British Journal of Urology, 78*(2), 205–208. PubMed PMID: 8813914.

164. Khurana, S., Dubey, M. L., & Malla, N. (2005). Association of parasitic infections and cancers. *Indian Journal of Medical Microbiology, 23*(2), 74–79. PubMed PMID: 15928434.

165. Fock, K. M. (2014). Review article: the epidemiology and prevention of gastric cancer. *Alimentary Pharmacology and Therapeutics, 40*(3), 250–260. PubMed PMID: 24912650.

166. Seitz, H. K., & Becker, P. (2007). Alcohol metabolism and cancer risk. *Alcohol Research and Health: The Journal of the National Institute on Alcohol Abuse and Alcoholism, 30*(1), 38–47.

167. Bagnardi, V., Blangiardo, M., La Vecchia, C., & Corrao, G. (2001). Alcohol consumption and the risk of cancer: A meta-analysis. *Alcohol Research and Health: The Journal of the National Institute on Alcohol Abuse and Alcoholism, 25*(4), 263–270.

168. Wu, T. C., Scott, R., Burnett, S., et al. (1988). Pulmonary hazards of smoking marijuana as compared with tobacco. *The New England Journal of Medicine, 318*, 347–351.

169. Nahas, G., & Latour, C. (1992). The human toxicity of marijuana. *The Medical Journal of Australia, 156*(7), 495–497.

170. Robison, L. L., Buckley, J. D., Daigle, A. E., Wells, R., Benjamin, D., et al. (1989). Maternal drug use and risk of childhood nonlymphoblastic leukemia among offspring. An epidemiologic investigation implicating marijuana a report from the Children's Cancer Study Group). *Cancer, 63*(10), 1904–1911.

171. Bifulco, M., Laezza, C., Pisanti, S., & Gazzerro, P. (2006). Cannabinoids and cancer: pros and cons of an antitumor strategy. *British Journal of Pharmacology, 148*(2), 123–135.

172. Ligresti, A., Moriello, A. S., Starowicz, K., Matias, I., et al. (2006). Antitumor activity of plant cannabinoids with emphasis on the effect of cannabidiol on human breast carcinoma. *The Journal of Pharmacology and Experimental Therapeutics, 318*(3), 1375–1387. PubMed PMID: 16728591.

173. Blazquez, C., Carracedo, A., Barrado, L., Real, P. J., et al. (2006). Cannabinoid receptors as novel targets for the treatment of melanoma. *FASEB Journal: Official Publication of the Federation of American Societies for Experimental Biology, 20*(14), 2633–2635. PubMed PMID: 17065222.

174. Fogli, S., Nieri, P., Chicca, A., Adinolfi, B., et al. (2006). Cannabinoid derivatives induce cell death in pancreatic MIA PaCa-2 cells via a receptor-independent mechanism. *FEBS Letters, 580*(7), 1733–1739. PubMed PMID: 16500647.

175. Flygae, J., Gustafsson, K., Kimby, E., et al. (2005). Cannabinoid receptor ligands mediate growth inhibition and cell death in mantle cell lymphoma. *FEBS Letters, 579*(30), 6885–6889. PubMed PMID: 16337199.

176. Kasai, H. (1997). Analysis of a form of oxidative DNA damage, 8-hydroxy-2'-deoxyguanosine, as a marker of cellular oxidative stress during carcinogenesis. *Mutation Research*, *387*(3), 147–163. PubMed PMID: 9439711.

177. Pande, D., Negi, R., Karki, K., et al. (2012). Oxidative damage markers as possible discriminatory biomarkers in breast carcinoma. *Translational Research: The Journal of Laboratory and Clinical Medicine*, *160*(6), 411–418. PubMed PMID: 22885175.

178. Li, D., Zhang, W., Zhu, J., et al. (2001). Oxidative DNA damage and 8-hydroxy-2-deoxyguanosine DNA glycosylase/apurinic lyase in human breast cancer. *Molecular Carcinogenesis*, *31*(4), 214–223. PubMed PMID: 11536371.

179. Musarrat, J., Arezina-Wilson, J., & Wani, A. A. (1996). Prognostic and aetiological relevance of 8-hydroxyguanosine in human breast carcinogenesis. *European Journal of Cancer*, *32A*(7), 1209–1214. PubMed PMID: 8758255.

180. Miyake, H., Hara, I., Kamidono, S., & Eto, H. (2004). Oxidative DNA damage in patients with prostate cancer and its response to treatment. *The Journal of Urology*, *171*(4), 1533–1536. PubMed PMID: 15017214.

181. Romano, G., Sgambato, A., Mancini, R., et al. (2000). 8-hydroxy-2'-deoxyguanosine in cervical cells: correlation with grade of dysplasia and human papillomavirus infection. *Carcinogenesis*, *21*(6), 1143–1147. PubMed PMID: 10837002.

182. Pylväs, M., Puistola, U., Laatio, L., et al. (2011). Elevated serum 8-OHdG is associated with poor prognosis in epithelial ovarian cancer. *Anticancer Research*, *31*(4), 1411–1415. PubMed PMID: 21508394.

183. Peddireddy, V., Siva Prasad, B., Gundimeda, S. D., et al. (2012). Assessment of 8-oxo-7, 8-dihydro-2'-deoxyguanosine and malondialdehyde levels as oxidative stress markers and antioxidant status in non-small cell lung cancer. *Biomarkers: Biochemical Indicators of Exposure, Response, and Susceptibility to Chemicals*, *17*(3), 261–268. PubMed PMID: 22397584.

184. Calişkan-Can, E., Firat, H., Ardiç, S., et al. (2008). Increased levels of 8-hydroxydeoxyguanosine and its relationship with lipid peroxidation and antioxidant vitamins in lung cancer. *Clinical Chemistry and Laboratory Medicine*, *46*(1), 107–112. PubMed PMID: 18194082.

185. Huang, Y. J., Zhang, B. B., Ma, N., et al. (2011). Nitrative and oxidative DNA damage as potential survival biomarkers for nasopharyngeal carcinoma. *Medical Oncology*, *28*(1), 377–384. PubMed PMID: 20339958.

186. Zhou, F. L., Zhang, W. G., Wei, Y. C., et al. (2010). Involvement of oxidative stress in the relapse of acute myeloid leukemia. *The Journal of Biological Chemistry*, *285*(20), 15010–15015. PubMed PMID: 20233720.

187. Chang, C. S., Chen, W. N., Lin, H. H., Wu, C. C., & Wang, C. J. (2004). Increased oxidative DNA damage, inducible nitric oxide synthase, nuclear factor kappaB expression and enhanced antiapoptosis-related proteins in Helicobacter pylori-infected non-cardiac gastric adenocarcinoma. *World Journal of Gastroenterology*, *10*(15), 2232–2240. PubMed PMID: 15259072.

188. Soini, Y., Haapasaari, K. M., Vaarala, M. H., et al. (2011). 8-hydroxydeguanosine and nitrotyrosine are prognostic factors in urinary bladder carcinoma. *International Journal of Clinical and Experimental Pathology*, *4*(3), 267–275. PubMed PMID: 21487522.

189. Valko, M., Rhodes, C. J., Moncol, J., et al. (2006). Free radicals, metals and antioxidants in oxidative stress-induced cancer. *Chemico-Biological Interactions*, *160*(1), 1–40. PubMed PMID: 16430879.

52

Assessment

SUMMARY

- Questionnaires
  - Environmental exposure questionnaire, including residence and work/school chronology
  - Quick Environmental Exposure and Sensitivity Index
- Case history taking
  - Chronological history of health problems
  - Identify the classic presentation of environmental illness by noting the presence of signs and symptoms strongly associated with toxicant burden
- Identify the signs and symptoms associated with specific toxicant families
- Identify exposure to the toxicants that matches the presentation of the patient
- Determine that the timing of exposure matches the onset or exacerbation of the toxicant-associated signs and symptoms

The first section of this book reviewed the body burden of toxicants that all carry from breathing, eating, drinking, and using personal care products. In the Centers for Disease Control and Prevention (CDC) National Report on Human Exposure, 120 of the 246 toxicants assessed for were found in virtually all US residents.[1] So, the question is not if your client has a body burden of pollutants, as this fact is already established. Instead, the question is whether or not their toxicant load is a factor in causing their health problems or if it is an obstacle to cure. The third section of this book identified the signs, symptoms, and disease processes the ubiquitous toxicants have been associated with. The greatest health effects appear in the immune, neurological, endocrine, and cardiovascular systems, where these toxicants are found to be associated with, if not causal to, most, of the current epidemic of chronic diseases. Although pollutants such as vehicular exhaust are clearly associated with increased cardiovascular diseases,

not all cardiovascular diseases will have air pollution as a primary cause. So how does a clinician identify if toxicants are a factor in the patients' illness, and if so, which one(s) to deal with? Section III also makes it clear that many of the toxicants adversely affect multiple systems, organs, and tissues.

Physicians rarely take an environmental exposure history of their patients, even among patients working in industry.[2] The majority of primary care and pediatric physicians have no training to guide them in taking an environmental history, although most report a desire to be able to.[3,4,5] An easy-to-use environmental exposure questionnaire can be found in Appendix F. This questionnaire elicits information about biotransformation ability, chemical reactivity, and classic air, food, and water exposures (all of which have been covered in this book). It also gathers information that can easily be used to develop the residential and work/school timelines that are discussed later. The Agency for Toxic Substances and Disease Registry (ATSDR) also provides a very nice presentation on how to take an environmental history (https://www.atsdr.cdc.gov/csem/exphistory/docs/exposure_history.pdf).

The Quick Environmental Exposure and Sensitivity Index (QEESI) is a validated questionnaire that identifies those individuals with chemical sensitivity.[6,7,8] The QEESI has five self-rating scales of 10 questions each. The scale topics include chemical exposures, other exposures, symptoms, impact of sensitivities, and "masking index," which provides a measure of ongoing exposure. The chemical exposure and symptom scales are highly sensitive and specific for those with chemical sensitivities. The QEESI can be downloaded at http://drclaudiamiller.com/qeesitest/.

IDENTIFYING ENVIRONMENTAL ILLNESS

Physicians often want to run a laboratory test to identify those individuals who have environmentally-induced illness. Although such laboratory assessments can be quite helpful, they are the final step in identifying environmental illness, not the first. Doing toxicant testing before a proper environmental medicine history (as outlined later) is merely a fishing expedition and likely to be fruitless. Before laboratory testing, it must first be established that the individual has environmentally-induced health effects. Then the most likely toxins/toxicants need to be identified and clear exposure sources found. If laboratory tests exist for the suspected toxins/toxicants, then they can be used to confirm or deny the diagnostic hypothesis.

Step 1: Establish Environmental Illness and Toxicant Pictures

The first step in assessment is to identify if the patient's toxic burden has caused physiological or biochemical damage resulting in an adverse health effect (environmental illness). The diagnostic algorithm for Step 1 is illustrated in Figure 52.1. Every effect has a cause, and rarely (if ever) is the cause related to a deficiency of pharmaceutical agents. To help the patient regain health, the proper cause(s) of their illness must be identified and eliminated. Section III presented the health problems so strongly associated with pollutant overload that these problems are more likely than not caused by the individuals' total load. These problems include chemical sensitivity, asthma, allergies, autoimmunity, chronic infections,

reduced cognition (often termed "brain fog"), parkinsonism, infertility (male and female), type 2 diabetes, low testosterone in younger men, temperature dysregulation, and thrombocytopenia. If any of those are present in the patients' case history, then the patient is more likely than not environmentally ill. If they have a chief complaint other than any of those previously listed, then it must be determined whether their toxicant burden is a causative or exacerbating factor in those complaints.

Step 2: Identify the Pollutant(s) Most Responsible

The second step is to identify the pollutant(s) most responsible for the health problems. The diagnostic algorithm for Step 2 is illustrated in Figure 52.2. In Section II of this book, many of the ubiquitous toxicants are reviewed along with a synopsis of the signs, symptoms, and diseases associated with them. Although many of the pollutants cause similar problems, there are often some distinctive signs for each one. For example, mercury, lead, solvents, and pesticides are all neurotoxic and have many similar symptoms. But solvents often cause very severe brain fog and balance issues, whereas lead levels high enough to cause cognitive dysfunction are likely to also cause hypertension, gout, or parkinsonian-like problems. So the clinician must try to identify which compound, or class of compounds, is most likely causing the patients' health problems (Tables 52.1 and 52.2).

TABLE 52.1 Common Neurological Health Problems Associated with Solvents, Chlorinated Pesticides (OCP), Organophosphate Pesticides (OP), Lead (Pb), and Mercury (Hg)

Problem	Solvents	OCP	OP	Pb	Hg
ADHD			X	X	
Balance problems	X		X		
Depression	X	X	X	X	X
Fatigue	X	X	X	X	X
Headache	X		X		X
Insomnia				X	
Irritability/excitability	X				X
Memory problems	X	X		X	X
Parkinsonian-like presentation				X	
Poor cognition	X	X	X	X	X
Tremors			X		

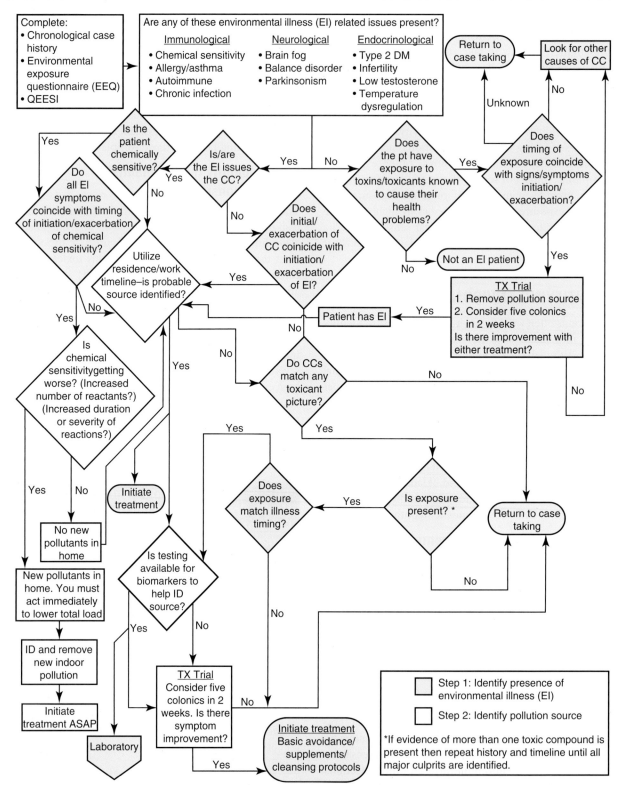

FIG. 52.1 Algorithm for diagnosing environmental illness.

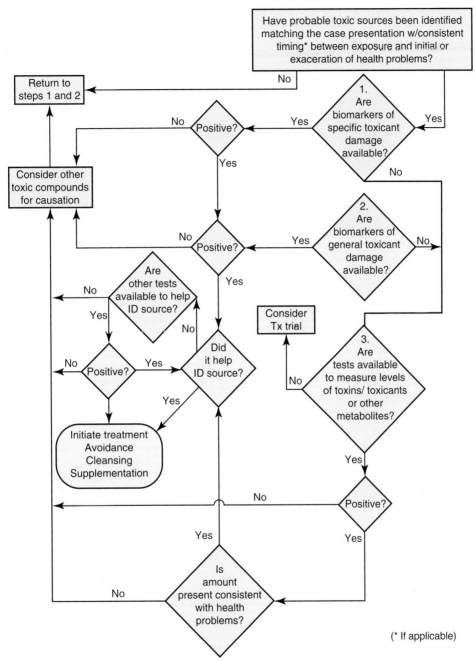

FIG. 52.2 Algorithm for diagnosing environmental illness.

Neuropsychological Testing. If cognitive dysfunction is the primary neurological presentation, utilizing neuropsychological (NP) testing may also be beneficial in helping spot the toxicant most likely to be causing these issues. NP is considered the most sensitive means of detecting neurological defects from toxicants.[9] NP assessment uses objective, standardized psychometric tests that measure and quantify aspects of psychological functioning such as intellectual level, memory, attention, language, planning, visuospatial, and verbal reasoning. NP testing

TABLE 52.2   Deficiencies in NP Testing According to Toxicant

NP Test Area	OP	PCB	VOC	PM$_{2.5}$ PAH	Ozone	Hg	Pb	Cd	As
Composite memory						X			
Verbal memory	X	PN / X	X	X		X	X		X
Visual memory	PN	PN / X	X		X	X	X		
Psychomotor speed	X		X						
Reaction time	X		X						
Complex attention					X			X	X
Processing speed			X		X		X		X
Executive function	X	PN				X	X		X
Working memory	X		X	X					
Sustained attention		PN		PN / X					
Simple attention		PN		PN / X		X			
Motor speed	PN	PN			X	X			

PN, Prenatal exposure.

has known reliability and validity, and compares the individuals' result with age-appropriate population samples. Having the ability to compare individual results to what is typically found in healthy persons of the same age group allows the testing to differentiate environmentally-induced central nervous system (CNS) dysfunction from age-related dysfunction.[10] This form of testing is done with a computer and can be done in office or online, making it readily available for clinicians and patients. It also has the benefit of being low cost and noninvasive, and gives quantitative results that can be used to compare with subsequent testing. Four of the most commonly used NP tests are as follows:

- The **Finger-Tapping Test** (also called simple reaction test time) uses a keyboard and prompts from the computer screen. The subject uses one finger first from the dominant hand and then the nondominant hand to hit the space bar as many times as they can in a set amount of time. This test shows psychomotor speed (also called visuomotor speed).
- The **Symbol Digit Substitution Test** (also called the Symbol Digit Coding Test) begins with a computer screen displaying two lines of boxes, one above the other. One set of boxes contains numbers, and either above or below that, another set contains symbols. When the computer screen prompts the beginning of the test, the subject must match the numbers to the appropriate symbols. This test reveals an individual's processing speed and several cognitive functions, including visual scanning, visual perception, visual memory, and motor function.

- The **Verbal Memory Test** uses a sequence of 15 words that are first shown one-at-a-time on the computer screen. They are then randomly repeated twice with 15 other distracter words with the subject needing to correctly identify the original 15. This test measures how well one can recognize, remember, and retrieve words (i.e., verbal memory).
- The **Continuous Performance Test** measures sustained attention, vigilance, and choice reaction time. For this test, the computer initially reveals a single letter. Then it reveals a random list of letters, including the original letter, one at a time, asking the subject to hit the space bar only when the original letter appears. This test measures sustained attention.

NP tests have revealed adverse neurological effects from a variety of common environmental toxicants including organophosphate pesticides, solvents, brominated flame retardants (polybrominated diphenyl ethers), air pollutants, and heavy metals.

Step 3: Identify Exposure Type

Step three is identifying clear exposure to the compound, or class of compounds, that you think are causing the individual's health problems. The patient may present with cognitive dysfunction, fatigue, and mood issues, and tell you that they are "poisoned by mercury," yet if they have no source of mercury exposure, that diagnosis is unlikely. In each of the chapters in Section II, other known markers indicating physiological or biological damage from the individual toxicant compounds are presented. Two of those markers for mercury included an elevated alanine transaminase (ALT) and the presence of precoproporphyrin and coproporphyrin in the urine. If the patient has the classic presentation of mercury (Table 52.3) and the laboratory markers, then the next step would be identifying the exposure source.

Because the greatest source of mercury exposure is fish consumption, it is easy enough to determine how often the patient is consuming fish. From the information presented in Chapter 14, it is clear that consuming fish just once weekly will result in a blood level of mercury consistent with the presence of health problems. The next most likely source of mercury is amalgam fillings. Although surface area of fillings is the most accurate assessment, current exposure is easily determined by counting the number of fillings. Counting the number of teeth with fillings, however, is not reliable for predicting body burden from fillings.

Mapping. The use of Google Earth can be quite beneficial in identifying large emitters of air pollutants that may be close to the patient's residence or workplace. Both Google Earth and MapQuest can also clearly identify proximity to busy roadways and airports. Information about pollution sources in each zip code can be found at the websites listed in Box 52.1. Scorecard.org contains information on industrial releases that were reported to the US Environmental Protection Agency (EPA) and published in the 2002 Toxic Release Inventory. Although old, many of the facilities continue to produce the same products and emissions. The World Air Quality Index

(www.aqicn.org) AQICN provides vehicular air pollution data for cities around the world. Local information on vehicular exhaust emissions can often be found at your county website (search under "air quality" or "ozone"). Information on fracking sites within the continental United States is available at earthjustice.org.

Step 4: Establish Timing of Exposure

Step four is to find out if the timing of the exposure matches the timing of the initiation or exacerbation of the pollutant-associated symptoms. This also requires knowledge of the half-life of suspected toxic compounds. For persistent toxicants such as cadmium, lead, chlorinated pesticides, or polychlorinated biphenyl (PCB), the onset of their related health problems may be insidious and not clearly found (e.g., hypertension). But if a host of persistent organic pollutant (POP)-related signs and symptoms occur during a time of significant weight loss (releasing high levels of POPs into the general circulation), then it may be more evident.[11] Lead-related symptoms are more commonly found in postmenopausal women from the baby boomer generation. As those with higher bone lead levels go into osteoporosis, their blood and soft-tissue lead levels increase, providing a "new" lead exposure source for those women.[12,13] Historical exposure to high levels of toxic compounds through work is commonly found but is almost never the cause of recent health problems.

Timing of exposure is not always possible to identify. We now know that there are a number of long-term health effects from *in utero* and perinatal exposures. Exposure during childhood to compounds associated with infertility in the offspring would be very hard to specifically identify, as the infertility will not be noticed for decades after the exposure. Because arsenic-related diseases typically occur after 40 years of exposure, coincidental timing would not apply to this toxicant either.

Create a Timeline. Timelines are the only means to identify progression of environmental illness. A timeline

TABLE 52.3 Signs, Symptoms, and Disease Associated with Nonoccupational Exposure to Mercury	
Classic Signs and Symptoms	**Classic Disease Presence**
Memory problems	Hypertension
Fatigue	Cardiovascular disease
Headache	Low thyroid
Cognitive difficulties	Autoimmune thyroiditis
Depression	Positive ANA
Musculoskeletal problems (diminished coordination, myalgia, tremors)	Blood sugar dysregulation (metabolic syndrome, insulin resistance, etc.)
Hair loss	NAFLD (elevated ALT)
Stomach issues	

BOX 52.1 Websites About Contamination by City or Zip Code

www.scorecard.org
http://aqicn.org
http://earthjustice.org/features/campaigns/fracking-across
   -the-united-states

- clarifies the dates of initiation and exacerbation of health problems,
- identifies association between exposure sources and health problems, and
- identifies which health problems are associated with the same exposures.

When timelines of health problems are compared with residential, work, and schooling timelines, the associations between exposure and illness often become unmistakable. Unfortunately, this requires the development of new case-taking skills, as health timelines are almost never done. The typical case history is a list of presenting symptoms with rough starting points and no associations with other health problems. A health timeline would include the beginning and exacerbation of symptoms along with initiation or worsening of other health problems. Residential, work, and schooling timelines are quite straightforward with start and stop dates. Once the residential, work, and schooling timeline has been elicited, it is easy to review the health timeline (use of the Environmental Exposure Questionnaire helps with this), and see how their residences and workplaces impacted their health. When patients are given an opportunity to think of their health problems in relation to where they lived or worked, a far more accurate health timeline is often produced.

When health problems occur in a certain residence, then more information on the residence must be elicited (Box 52.2).

BOX 52.2 **Necessary Details of Residences at Which Health Problems Began or Got Worse**

Type and age of dwelling	Garage–attached or detached
Chemicals stored in garage	Heat source
Last time furnace and AC vents were cleaned	Presence and age of carpeting
Frequency of furnace filter replacement	Pets in the home
Type and age of furnishings	Chemicals used in or around home
Pesticide use in or around home	History of remodeling
Any new furnishings	Water damage/mold presence
Hobbies done in the home	Scented products in the home

The most common cause of residence-related health problems is mold. Quite often, the resident will deny any water damage or mold presence. However, as discussed in Chapters 5 and 31, up to 50% of buildings in North America have water damage. The following questions have been found to be most effective in identifying moldy homes or workplaces.[14]

- Is there any visible mold?
- Is there a musty smell in any room?
- Have you received any insurance money for water damage in your home?
- Does the carpet ever get wet when it rains?
- Are there any water stains on the ceilings or walls?
- Does the roof leak?
- Has there ever been water in the basement?
- Has a pipe ever broken?
- Do the windows ever leak?
- Has water ever had to be cleared?

The timing of health problems may relate to new work, home, or schooling, necessitating potential exposures in all situations. Employees can also get material safety data sheets (MSDS) on all chemicals used in the workplace as well as finding out if there have been any previous or ongoing indoor air quality incidents. Talking to coworkers about their health can also be helpful. The proximity of a home or building to busy roadways with truck traffic or other industry or agriculture needs to be discovered. MapQuest and Google Earth can also be helpful here, as can scorecard.org (especially if they work at an industry listed on this site for their zip code).

PATIENT EXAMPLES

Example: Timing Is Key

Case 1. MH. MH is a 28-year-old male presenting with progressive numbness since age 16. Numbness began in the feet and slowly progressed up the body to his arms and hands. He had been diagnosed with multiple sclerosis and is reactive to perfumes. Recently his symptoms dramatically increased to the point that he is no longer ambulatory. He has increased tremors, numbness, loss of muscle mass, and was hunched over upon entry into the clinic. He complained of constant dry mouth, whole body pruritus that was worse in axilla and hands, fatigue, and constant sleepiness. Objectively, he had cognitive difficulties (brain fog) and spoke with a tremulous voice.

Current exacerbation began 5 months previously after doing a 2-day open house for his business. The business space he had rented was accessed through a hair-dressing salon and was frugally furnished with new furniture that was manufactured from pressboard material. He had just finished trade school, which was housed in a new building and had the classic "new building" odor. He had previously worked with concrete sealants for 7 years and had been around diesel vehicles since age 18.

The physician working with this individual felt that the exacerbation of the health problems was due to the 16 hours of "open house" in the new office. However, 5 months had elapsed since that exposure, and the patient's symptoms had not improved and were continuing to worsen. Once this fact was pointed out to the physician, she then elicited more information from the patient and found out that his bedroom had been remodeled 3 months before the open house. The remodeling included painting, new engineered wood flooring, and new bedroom furniture (all low-cost pressboard furniture).

With that information, the timing becomes clear. Although 90% of time is typically spent indoors, the greatest part of that is spent in the bedroom. He had been exposed to the off-gassing of building materials for a minimum of 8 hours daily for 3 to 4 months before the open house. When he spent 16 to 24 hours breathing those compounds for 2 consecutive days, his "barrel overflowed" and his symptoms began. As his disability increased, his time in his bedroom also increased, hence his continued physical deterioration. Had the "timing issue" not been taken into account, his health would have continued to deteriorate, as the source of exposure would not have been addressed.

Example: Putting it All Together

Case 2: MS. MS, a 46-year-old white male, presented to the clinic with chief complaints of repeated loss of consciousness (LOC), fatigue, bronchial pain, short-term memory loss, sexual dysfunction, irritability, and severe chemical sensitivity. He also has been experiencing tremors, paresthesias, poor hand-eye and foot-eye coordination, and temperature swings. His problems had been persistent and were continuing to worsen. He had been on disability from work for 12 months and had visited several doctors without any noticeable benefit. The repeated LOC was the most debilitating of all the health problems, occurring two to three times daily and lasting for up to 2 hours each if supplemental oxygen was started when prodromal symptoms first appeared. If he failed to start the oxygen in time, he could stay

unconscious for up to 6 hours. LOC could occur for no apparent reason but always occurred with exposure to any chemical fumes. He found that he had to set his clock to wake him up two to three times nightly to eat in order to prevent LOC during sleep. His adipose tissue was so burdened with toxicants that any lipolysis acted as an acute chemical exposure resulting in LOC. A complicated case, to be sure.

The first step in assessment is to identify the presence of environmental illness. In this case, the patient had chemical sensitivity, which is primarily caused by exposure to solvents or pesticides.[15, 16] The presence of chemical sensitivity also indicates immunotoxicity, glutathione depletion, the high probability of copy number variation in one or more of the glutathione transferases,[17,18,19] methylation single nucleotide polymorphism (SNP), possible paraoxonase 1 SNP, and magnesium deficiency. The presence of reactivity to foods also strongly indicated toxicant effect on his Th1/Th2 cytokine picture.[20]

The second step in assessment identified which toxicant(s) most closely fits his health presentation picture. The information contained in this textbook on toxicant pictures is compared with his symptom presentation in Table 52.4.

Based on Table 52.4, the two most likely classes of toxicants that could be at the root of his multiple health problems would be solvents and organophosphate pesticides (OCPs). OCPs are far less likely simply because ongoing exposure was of low probability.

Steps three and four look at exposure history and timing of exposures in relation to development of health problems. Doing timelines of illness, residences, and work will accomplish those two objectives. Simply listing his health problems by chronology instead of order of

TABLE 52.4 MS Case Presentation that May Be Associated with Solvents, Chlorinated Pesticides (OCP), Organophosphate Pesticides (OP), Lead (Pb), or Mercury (Hg)

Problem	Solvents	OCP	OP	Pb	Hg
Memory problems	X	X		X	X
Irritability	X	X	X	X	X
Fatigue	X	X	X	X	X
Chemical sensitivity	X		X		
Allergies	X	X	X		

importance, degree of morbidity, or by system revealed an interesting, and classic, progression.

1970 – Last felt well

1971 – Chronic tonsillitis began after leaving the US Navy

1978 – Tonsillectomy

- First "allergic" reaction to a food (by 1980, he was reactive to 20 foods)
- Began to experience recurrent bronchitis, upper respiratory infections (URIs), kidney stones, constipation

1984 – Eye-convergence problems began

1986 – Hearing problems began in left ear

- 35% hearing loss
- MRI showed calcium deposits in brainstem

1987 – Sores appeared on arms, neck, back, and face that took months to heal

- Severe morning fatigue began

1989 – Developed "walking pneumonia"

- Upper respiratory tract infection (URI)
- Initiation of presenting symptoms:
  - Debilitating fatigue
  - Bronchial pain
  - Short term memory loss
  - Sexual dysfunction
  - Irritability
  - Tremors
  - Paresthesias

- Coordination problems
- Temperature swings
- LOC

His health history information was placed on a timeline graph (Fig. 52.3). His immune problems are on the blue line, neurological on the green, endocrine on the red, and other problems on the brown line.

His residential and work history revealed that he was on active duty with the US Navy from 1968 to 1971, serving in Vietnam. He remembers being "accidentally" exposed to Agent Orange and experiencing a deep choking and gagging cough upon that exposure. In 1971, he moved to Los Angeles where he got a job with a large corporation. He lived in three different apartments and would "bug bomb" and repaint each one before taking occupancy. In 1978, he purchased a home that he painted as well. Upon moving in, he found that the home had termites and he proceeded to have routine spraying in the home using Dursban. In 1988, he was promoted and moved into an office with existing "grass-cloth wallpaper" which he had painted with exterior oil-based paint. The paint took months to cure, during which time he inhaled solvents throughout the entire workday. Fig. 52.4 shows the addition of his work and residential history to his timeline.

By reviewing Fig. 52.4, it becomes clear that his reduced cell-mediated immunity began after serving in the Navy and upon moving to Los Angeles, CA when he was living

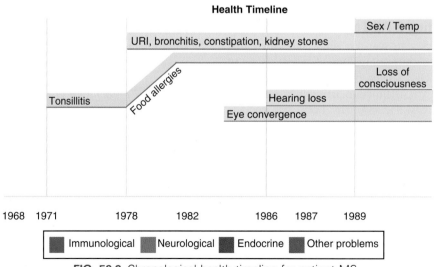

FIG. 52.3 Chronological health timeline for patient MS.

Health Timeline

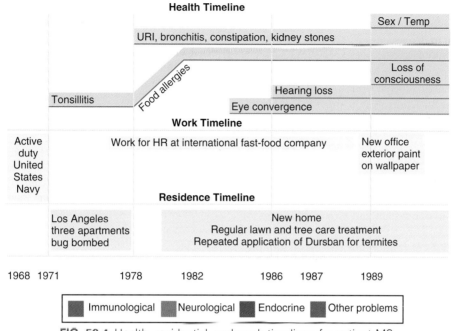

FIG. 52.4 Health, residential, and work timelines for patient MS.

in apartments and having them "bug bombed." When he moved into his new home, his immunotoxicity increased with the addition of food allergies and respiratory infections. Although he did not provide information on dates of Dursban spraying, he was clearly exposed to something else in 1984 and again in 1986 that initiated the onset of neurological problems with his vision and hearing. The onset of endocrine problems along with worsening of immune and neurological problems began after exposure to the oil-based paint in his office. Unfortunately, information on the initiation and exacerbation of his chemical reactivity was not gathered to add to this timeline.

THE DIAGNOSTIC OPPORTUNITY AFFORDED BY CHEMICAL SENSITIVITY

When any degree of chemical sensitivity is present, it provides the clinician with a clear picture of when health-damaging environmental exposures occurred. Quite often the initiation and exacerbation of chemical reactivity will coincide with the initiation and exacerbation of other seemingly unrelated health problems. When these issues occur simultaneously, it is more probable than not that the simultaneously occurring health problems are

due to the same toxicant overload causing the chemical reactivity.

When adverse physical, mental, or emotional reactions occur upon exposure to any chemical presence, the following information should be gathered.

1. When was chemical reactivity first noted? (This indicates timing of chemical overload.)
2. What was the first reaction triggered by? (This indicates which class of chemicals the person was most likely overloaded by.)
3. If they are now reactive to more compounds, find out when each of the other compounds became a problem. (This indicates new exposure and an increase in total load.)
4. If the intensity or duration of symptoms from these chemicals increased, find out the chronology of these exacerbations as well. (This indicates new or increased exposures and an increase in total load.)
5. Is the person's chemical reactivity currently:
   a. Getting better (their home is chemically safe)?
   b. Staying the same (their home is not chemically safe, but no new exposures have occurred)?
   c. Getting worse (their home has new exposure sources in it)?

6. What class of compounds is the person reacting to? (This will be the class that they were overexposed to, assisting you to design a proper avoidance and treatment protocol.)

The QEESI questionnaire has a sensitivity of 92% and a specificity of 95% in differentiating a chemically sensitive person from health controls and provides invaluable information to the clinician.[6]

CLASSIC PATTERNS

The progression of illness seen with MS (Case 2) is not uncommon. Manifestations of environmental illness typically begin in one system and progress for a period of time before another system is affected. In the case of MS, manifestations of immunotoxicity began and progressed for 12 years before neurological symptoms occurred. Problems in both of these systems then progressed for another 5 years before manifestations of endocrine toxicity began.

However, male or female infertility can often occur as a primary complaint without clear manifestations of pollutant interruption in other systems.

REFERENCES

1. Centers for Disease Control and Prevention: *National Report on Human Exposure to Environmental Chemicals: Updated Tables*, January 2017. Available at www.cdc.gov/exposurereport/. (Accessed 25 October 2017).

2. Nicotera, G., Nobile, C. G., Bianco, A., & Pavia, M. (2006). Environmental history-taking in clinical practice: knowledge, attitudes, and practice of primary care physicians in Italy. *Journal of Occupational and Environmental Medicine*, 48(3), 294–302. PubMed PMID: 16531834.

3. Hamilton, W. J., Ryder, D. J., Cooper, H. P., Jr., Williams, D. M., & Weinberg, A. D. (2005). Environmental health: a survey of Texas primary care physicians. *Texas Medicine*, 101(10), 62–70. PubMed PMID: 17094519.

4. Kilpatrick, N., Frumkin, H., Trowbridge, J., Escoffery, C., Geller, R., Rubin, L., et al. (2002). The environmental history in pediatric practice: a study of pediatricians' attitudes, beliefs, and practices. *Environmental Health Perspectives*, 110(8), 823–827. PubMed PMID: 12153766.

5. Trasande, L., Boscarino, J., Graber, N., Falk, R., Schechter, C., Galvez, M., et al. (2006). The environment in pediatric practice: a study of New York pediatricians' attitudes, beliefs, and practices towards children's environmental health. *Journal of Urban Health: Bulletin of the New York Academy of Medicine*, 83(4), 760–772. PubMed PMID: 16736113.

6. Miller, C. S., & Prihoda, T. J. (1999). The Environmental Exposure and Sensitivity Inventory (EESI): a standardized approach for measuring chemical intolerances for research and clinical applications. *Toxicology and Industrial Health*, 15(3–4), 370–385. PubMed PMID: 10416289.

7. Hojo, S., Kumano, H., Yoshino, H., Kakuta, K., & Ishikawa, S. (2003). Application of Quick Environment Exposure Sensitivity Inventory (QEESI) for Japanese population: study of reliability and validity of the questionnaire. *Toxicology and Industrial Health*, 19(2–6), 41–49. PubMed PMID: 15697173.

8. Skovbjerg, S., Berg, N. D., Elberling, J., & Christensen, K. B. (2012). Evaluation of the quick environmental exposure and sensitivity inventory in a Danish population. *Journal of Environmental and Public Health*, 2012, 304314. PubMed PMID: 22529872.

9. Ross, S. M., McManus, I. C., Harrison, V., & Mason, O. (2013). Neurobehavioral problems following low-level exposure to organophosphate pesticides: a systematic and meta-analytic review. *Critical Reviews in Toxicology*, 43(1), 21–44. PubMed PMID: 23163581.

10. Gualtieri, C. T., & Johnson, L. G. (2006). Reliability and validity of a computerized neurocognitive test battery, CNS Vital Signs. *Archives of Clinical Neuropsychology*, 21(7), 623–643. PubMed PMID: 17014981.

11. Cheikh Rouhou, M., Karelis, A. D., St-Pierre, D. H., & Lamontagne, L. (2016). Adverse effects of weight loss: Are persistent organic pollutants a potential culprit? *Diabetes & Metabolism*, 42(4), 215–223. PubMed PMID: 27321206.

12. Campbell, J. R., & Auinger, P. (2007). The association between blood lead levels and osteoporosis among adults – results from the third national health and nutrition examination survey (NHANES III). *Environmental Health Perspectives*, 115(7), 1018–1022. PubMed PMID: 17637916.

13. Machida, M., Sun, S. J., Oguma, E., & Kayama, F. (2009). High bone matrix turnover predicts blood levels of lead among perimenopausal women. *Environmental Research*, 109(7), 880–886. PubMed PMID: 19595303.

14. Bernazzani, D. (2016). *Mold in the indoor environment: remediation and legal issues related to health effects*. San Diego, CA: Environmental Health Symposium.

15. Caress, S. M., & Steinemann, A. C. (2003). A review of a two-phase population study of multiple chemical sensitivities. *Environmental Health Perspectives*, 111(12), 1490–1497. PubMed PMID: 12948889.

16. Miller, C. S., & Mitzel, H. C. (1995). Chemical sensitivity attributed to pesticide exposure versus remodeling. *Archives of Environmental Health*, *50*(2), 119–129. PubMed PMID: 7786048.

17. McKeown-Eyssen, G., Baines, C., Cole, D. E., Riley, N., Tyndale, R. F., Marshall, L., et al. (2004). Case-control study of genotypes in multiple chemical sensitivity: CYP2D6, NAT1, NAT2, PON1, PON2 and MTHFR. *International Journal of Epidemiology*, *33*(5), 971–978. PubMed PMID: 15256524.

18. Rea, W. J. (1992). *Chemical sensitivity* (Vol. 1). Boca Raton, FL: CRC Press.

19. Fujimori, S., Hiura, M., Yi, C. X., Xi, L., & Katoh, T. (2012). Factors in genetic susceptibility in a chemical sensitive population using QEESI. *Environmental Heatlh and Preventive Medicine*, *17*(5), 357–363. PubMed PMID: 22205546.

20. De Luca, C., Scordo, M. G., Cesareo, E., Pastore, S., Mariani, S., Maiani, G., et al. (2010). Biological definition of multiple chemical sensitivity from redox state and cytokine profiling and not from polymorphisms of xenobiotic-metabolizing enzymes. *Toxicology and Applied Pharmacology*, *248*(3), 285–292. PubMed PMID: 20430047.

53

Laboratory Assessment of Toxicant Levels

SUMMARY

- Identification of current exposure sources for prevention and preconception care
- Identify specific toxins/toxicants
- Assist in identifying exposure sources
- Determine effectiveness of avoidance and depuration methods
- Test blood or urine for markers of pollutants and their metabolites

INTRODUCTION

Of the 120 compounds found ubiquitously by the Centers for Disease Control and Prevention (CDC) in US residents,[1] less than half are commercially available for testing. However, available testing can still be used effectively to identify current exposures for prevention and preconception care. Such tests should never be used as the primary means of diagnosing environmental overload; instead, they should be used as confirmation. Once the toxic compound most likely to be causing disease has been identified with the assessment algorithm (Figure 52.1), testing (if available) can be used to confirm that hypothesis. Toxin or toxicant levels in the blood or urine can then also be compared with the ranges that have been associated with adverse health effects, as well as to national averages (if available). Such testing can also identify probable exposure sources, as well as other components of the individual's total load. Further, they can be used as a benchmark to measure the effectiveness of avoidance and depuration methods. If toxicant levels drop in alignment with their published half-life, then one could conclude that the exposure source was effectively addressed. Testing is also necessary to identify metals or persistent pollutants that necessitate specific protocol to reduce body burden.

To initiate treatment, protocols for different classes of toxicants (metals and persistent organic pollutants

REASONS TO TEST FOR POLLUTANTS AND METABOLITES

- Identify current exposures for prevention
- Confirm the conclusions reached from steps 1 to 4 (Chapter 52)
- Comparison to CDC ranges and to levels associated with adverse health problems
- Assistance in identifying pollutant source(s)
- Comparison with subsequent testing to assess effectiveness of avoidance or depuration techniques

[POPs]) require specific therapies. Toxicologists and occupational/industrial health physicians have used toxicant testing—available from national reference laboratories for decades—to identify acute or chronic poisonings. The reference values are typically based upon Occupational Safety and Health Administration (OSHA) industrial standards, with the detection limits based on no-observed-adverse-effect levels (NOAELs), typically higher than the values listed in the CDC 90th to 95th percentile ranges. Because adverse health effects have been documented at levels as low as the CDC 50th percentile (and some, like lead, have no apparent lower limit of measurable damage), these laboratory tests would fail to identify those at risk. Into this void has sprung up Clinical Laboratory Improvement Amendment (CLIA)-certified specialty labs that run a limited number of assays for toxic metals in blood and urine, serum testing for organochlorine pesticides (OCPs) and polychlorinated biphenyl (PCB), and urine testing for mycotoxins, metals, metabolites of organophosphate pesticides (OPs), glyphosate, phthalates, bisphenol A (BPA), parabens, and solvents.

NORMALIZING RESULTS

In the late 1980s, researchers found (initially with dioxins) that adjusting the levels of circulating POPs to the lipid present in the blood had a high correlation to adipose levels of POPs as measured by fat biopsies.[1] The POPs are released from the fat with lipids (mostly cholesterol), so performing this adjustment gives a much better sense of the level of toxicants in the adipose stores.

People with higher blood fats who have higher adipose POP burden will have higher ng/mL values, but those with less adipose POP burden may not. Before this revelation, it was virtually impossible with blood testing to determine whether body load was due to current exposure or past exposure being released from storage in fat. Making this distinction is also important to monitor the efficacy of cleansing on reducing adipose stores. For the vast majority of individuals, virtually all of the ng/mL in the serum come directly from lipid turnover.

Because of this research, the CDC now measures and publishes both ng/mL and ng/g lipid for their fat-soluble exposure reports. In addition, as POPs are fat soluble, those with elevated lipid levels will have higher levels of POPs in their blood. Adjusting for total lipids helps normalize this potential error.

PREVENTION AND PRECONCEPTION CARE

- Currently available toxicant and toxicant metabolite testing
  - Urinary metals
  - Urinary organophosphate pesticide metabolites
  - Urinary glyphosate metabolites
  - Urinary phthalate metabolites
  - Urinary BPA
  - Serum solvents and urinary solvent metabolites
  - Serum PCB
- Other important tests
  - Aromatic hydrocarbon exposure
  - Perfluorocarbons

The toxicant-related measurements offered by these CLIA-certified labs have levels of detection low enough to identify compounds present in the ranges typically found in the National Health and Nutritional Examination Survey (NHANES) and published by the CDC in their exposure report.[2] These tests can assist the clinician and patient in identifying exposure to certain toxic compounds that they may actually wish to avoid. This is a particularly important step in preconception care, which should become the standard for all wishing to conceive and have healthy children. Subsequent tests will be able to confirm whether or not the avoidance steps were successful. Theo Colburn's website, The Endocrine Disruption Exchange, provides an excellent source to easily see the numerous adverse health effects from fetal exposure to common toxicants.[2a]

IDENTIFICATION OF HEALTH-DAMAGING POLLUTANTS

After the assessment algorithm (Figure 52.1 – Chapter 52) has been followed and one has a better idea of which toxic compounds are causing the client's primary health problems, testing can be used to confirm the hypothesis and help identify the exposure source. The use of these tests before the assessment phase will typically be a huge waste of the client's time and money, unless their main interest lies in prevention.

Serum Testing

- Select OCPs
- Select PCBs
- Select aromatic and aliphatic hydrocarbons
- Metals

Serum testing usually identifies parent compounds. Serum values of chlorinated pesticides and PCBs are typically reported both in parts per billion (PPB) present in serum and as lipid-adjusted values (ng/g lipid). Adjusting the fat-soluble persistent toxicants to the amount of lipid in the blood provides an excellent representation for the level of those compounds in adipose storage (total body burden).[3] The CDC exposure report provides both parts per million (PPM) and ng/g lipid values for chlorinated pesticides and PPB and ng/g lipid for PCBs and lists them according to the mean, 50th, 75th, 90th, and 95th percentiles found in the US population.[1] These levels provide an excellent reference point to determine those with higher than "normal" amounts present. It must be kept in mind that higher POP levels can be found in persons undergoing weight loss.[4] The lipid-adjusted values provide a means of assessing the effectiveness of depuration protocol when done before and after treatment.

Persistent Organic Pollutants. Because the majority of the circulating OCPs and PCBs come from adipose stores, the patient's lipid-adjusted results will typically fall in a higher CDC percentile range than the PPB results (Table 53.1). One simply needs to calculate what percentage of the 95th percentile the patient's POP level is for serum and lipid adjusted, and compare the results.

Even though heptachlor epoxide is elevated, the serum levels are only 5.7-fold of the 95th percentile whereas the lipid-adjusted levels are 9.4-fold, indicating the serum content is coming primarily from adipose stores. Similarly, the dichlorodiphenyldichloroethylene (DDE) serum level is 3.6% of the 95th percentile, while the lipid adjusted is higher at 5.6%. This is the typical pattern for OCPs and PCBs. When the serum levels match or exceed the lipid-adjusted CDC percentile range, it indicates that current exposure sources are present (Table 53.2). In the following patient report, the serum PPB values for PCB 153 are 7.6-fold higher than the CDC's 95th percentile, while the lipid-adjusted values are only sixfold greater. In the absence of current exposure,

the only other possible cause would be serious weight loss.[5,6]

Solvents. Serum testing for volatile aromatic and aliphatic solvents is limited to benzene; ethylbenzene; styrene; toluene; m,p-xylene; o-xylene; n-hexane; 2-methylpentane; 3-methylpentane; and isooctane. Aromatic compounds have a short half-life and would not be expected to be detectable in the average person, unless currently exposed. In cases of consistent high current exposure and inadequate clearance, positive findings will occur. This is reflected in Table 53.3, showing that benzene, ethylbenzene, styrene, and o-xylene only show up 25% of the time.

Aliphatic compounds (n-hexane, 2-methylpentane, 3- methylpentane, and isooctane) are present in vehicular exhaust, and because they are slower to leave the body, low levels are typically found. Certain patterns of positive findings have become associated with specific exposure sources (Table 53.4).[7] Individuals who are living in urban areas and who have difficulty clearing solvents, most likely due to copy number variations of one or more glutathione transferase enzymes or depletion of the amino acids needed for conjugation, are often found to have ethylbenzene and xylene present along with the aliphatic compounds.

TABLE 53.1   **Patient with Elevated Heptachlor Epoxide Levels From Adipose Stores, Utilizing CDC Fourth Report Percentiles**

	PPB	95th Percentile	Lipid Adjusted (ng/g Lipid)	95th Percentile
DDE	0.44	12.10	104.83	1860
		(0.44/12.1 = 3.6% of the 95th percentile)	(104.83/1860 = 5.6% of 95th percentile)	
Heptachlor epoxide	7.42	0.13	1770.2	18.9
		(7.42/0.13 = 571% of 95th percentile)	(1770.2/18.9 = 936% of 95th percentile)	

TABLE 53.2   **Example of a Patient with Current Exposure to PCB 138, 153, and 180, Utilizing CDC Fourth Report Percentiles**

	PPB	95th Percentile	Lipid Adjusted (ng/g Lipid)	95th Percentile
PCB 138	0.27	0.48	33.4	75.3
		(0.27/0.48 = 56% of the 95th percentile)	(33.34/75.3 = 44.5% of the 95th percentile)	
PCB 153	4.73 ppb	0.62	584.04 μg/g	97.1
		(4.73/0.62 = 763% of 95th percentile)	(584/97.1 = 600% of 95th percentile)	
PCB 180	0.27	0.53	33.4	81.5
		(0.27/0.53 = 51% of 95th percentile)	(33.34/81.5 = 41% of 95th percentile)	

TABLE 53.3 Serum Solvent Levels in 2017 CDC Report

Solvent	Unit	Mean	75th %	90th %	95th %
Benzene	ng/mL	*	0.41	0.198	0.294
Ethylbenzene	ng/mL	*	0.038	0.038	0.122
Styrene	ng/mL	*	0.045	0.096	0.130
Toluene	ng/mL	0.110	0.170	0.280	0.400
M,p-xylene	ng/mL	0.079	0.130	0.231	0.343

TABLE 53.4 Typical Patterns of Detectable Solvents Indicating Exposure Sources, According to Percentile reference values

VOC	Urban Air Pollution W/Reduced Clearance Ability, %	Vehicular Exhaust Leak, %	Memory Foam Mattress or Pillow, %
Benzene		> 75th	> 75th
Ethylbenzene	> 75th	> 50th	
Styrene			> 75th
Toluene			
m,p-xylene	> 50th	> 50th	
o-xylene			
Hexane	50th	> 75th	50th
2-methylpentane	50th	> 75th	50th
3-methylpentane	50th	> 75th	50th
Isooctane	50th	> 75th	50th

TABLE 53.5 2017 CDC Fourth Report Blood Metal Levels (µg/L)

Metal	Mean	75th %	90th %	95th %
Cadmium	0.235	0.410	0.840	1.22
Lead	0.858	1.32	2.10	2.81
Mercury	0.683	1.29	2.65	4.36
Methyl Hg	0.434	1.09	2.62	4.28
Ethyl Hg	<LOD	<LOD	<LOD	<LOD
Inorg. Hg	*	<LOD	0.410	0.530

LOD – level of detection

Those exposed to a vehicular exhaust leak can be identified by the presence of both benzene and isooctane levels over the 75th percentile reference values. In these individuals, the other aliphatics (hexane and both methylpentanes) will also be higher, and it is likely that they will also have ethylbenzene and m,p-xylene present as well.

The finding of both benzene and styrene over the CDC 75th percentiles (without ethylbenzene, xylene, or toluene) has been noted in persons who are sleeping on mattresses or pillows containing memory foam.[8] Having them sleep on mattresses free of that specific type of foam typically results in clearance of these aromatic compounds from the blood.

Metals. Blood levels of mercury, lead and cadmium are all reflective of current exposure, with mercury levels predominately being methylmercury.[1] These levels can easily be compared with the published CDC population values to identify those with higher than normal toxicant levels (Table 53.5).

Urine Testing

- Select solvent metabolites
- Select organophosphate metabolites
- Glyphosate
- Select phthalates and parabens
- BPA
- Mycotoxins
- Metals

The presence of metabolites in the urine is indicative of both exposure and the ability to metabolize and excrete toxicants. Although a high level of pollutant metabolites will most often be due to excessive exposure, an induction of the biotransformation enzymes may also be present. Although low metabolite presence in the urine is typically interpreted to mean low exposure, there is a possibility that the patient may have a diminished toxicant clearance resulting in higher serum levels of the pollutant.

Solvent Metabolites. In the latest CDC Fourth Report update, solvent metabolites were measured and reported (Table 53.6). Some labs provide testing for a few of these compounds. With the ubiquitous nature of volatile organic

TABLE 53.6   Urinary Solvent Metabolites in 2017 CDC Fourth Report (NHANES 2011–2014)

Metabolite	Parent	Mean	75th %	90th %	95th %
N-acetyl-S-(phenyl)-L-cysteine	Benzene	*	1.29	2.10	3.03
N-acetyl-S-(3,4-dihyroxybutyl)-L-cysteine	1,3-butadiene	288	374	488	583
N-acetyl-S-(4-hydroxy-2-butenyl)-L-cysteine	"	11.8	18.2	60.4	108
N-acetyl-S-(N-methylcarbamoyl)-L-cysteine	N,N-dimethyl formamide	140	248	482	757
Phenylglyoxylic acid	Ethylbenzene styrene	202	285	401	518
N-acetyl-S-(phenyl-2-hydroxyethyl)-L-cysteine	Styrene	*	1.34	2.28	3.34
Mandelic acid	Styrene	167	232	363	513
N-acetyl-S-(benzyl)-L-cysteine	Toluene	7.39	.12.2	21.0	36.4
2-methylhippuric acid	Xylene	37.5	77.9	159	248
3 & 4-methylhippuric acid	Xylene	252	565	1050	1540

TABLE 53.7   Urinary Organophosphate and Pyrethroid Pesticide Metabolites (µg/g Creatinine) in CDC 2017 Update (NHANES 2011–2014)

Metabolite	Parent	Mean	75th %	90th %	95th %
para-nitrophenol	Parathion	0.473	0.923	1.87	2.62
3,5,6-trichloro-2-pyridinol	Chlorpyrifos	0.812	1.66	2.67	3.53
Diethylphosphate - DEP	OPs	*	3.20	8.86	15.7
Dimethylphosphate-DMP	"	*	9.10	20.0	33.6
Diethylthiophosphate - DETP	"	*	1.24	2.46	3.92
Dimethylthiophosphate - DMTP	"	2.34	5.91	17.5	33.7
3-phenoxybenzoic acid	Pyrethroids	0.438	1.01	2.88	5.44

compounds in urban air, a positive finding of urinary metabolites is probable but does not mean the solvents are also detectable in the blood. To date, sufficient studies relating health problems with levels of urinary solvent metabolites are lacking.

Organophosphate Pesticide Metabolites. Organophosphate pesticide metabolites (Table 53.7) are clearly associated with the consumption of nonorganic foods.[9,10] To date, sufficient studies relating health problems with urinary levels of OP metabolites are lacking, but the research that does exist (see Chapter 21) is alarming.

Glyphosate. Urine testing for glyphosate and its metabolite aminomethylphosphonic acid (AMPA) have recently become available, but neither national reference values or sufficient studies of adverse health effects are available to interpret the results.

Plastics. Only two phthalates have commercially available metabolite testing, the low-molecular-weight (LMW)

diethyl phthalate (DEP) and the high-molecular-weight (HMW) di(2-ethylhexyl) phthalate (DEHP), both of which also reflect fairly recent exposure.[11] Chapter 26 gives information on urinary phthalate levels in relation to health problems. BPA presence reflects exposure that can persist in higher levels for at least a week after exposure.[12,13] Chapter 25 gives information on urinary BPA levels in relation to health problems. Table 53.8 gives the NHANES 2011 to 2014 data for plastics.

Mycotoxins. Testing for urinary levels of macrocyclic trichothecenes, ochratoxin A, aflatoxin group (B1, B2, G1, G2), and gliotoxin is now available. The presence of these mycotoxins reflects current exposure to *Stachybotrys chartarum*, *Aspergillus*, and *Penicillium* species. Mold IgE antibody testing is also available through the standard national reference laboratories. The presence of IgE to the various molds indicates both recent exposure and immune activation. However, the absence of anti-mold antibodies does not rule out current exposure. In fact, only 25% of children exposed

TABLE 53.8 CDC Fourth Report 2017 Update (NHANES 2011–14) Urinary Phthalate, BPA, and Parabens (µg/g Creatinine)

Compound	Parent Compound	Mean	75th %	90th %	95th %
MEHP	DEHP	1.55	2.73	4.91	8.47
MEHHP	"	8.99	14.1	25.3	37.7
MEOHP	"	5.78	8.99	15.6	23.4
MECCP	"	14.7	22.7	38.9	59.8
MCNP	DiNP	2.83	4.59	9.36	14.6
MCOP	"	22.4	54.1	118	194
MiNP	"	*	2.69	7.88	17.6
MMP	"	1.32	2.84	6.13	11.0
MCPP	DMP	3.42	6.00	15.8	36.6
MBzP	DOP	5.15	9.49	17.4	26.7
MiBP	DiBP	6.83	11.6	19.4	27.5
MnBP	DnBP	8.66	15.8	27.9	41.2
MEP	DEP	43.2	94.2	263	541
Bisphenol A		1.28	2.12	3.88	5.09
Butylparaben		*	.250	3.50	10.0
Ethylparaben		*	5.41	36.6	99.3
Methylparaben		48.2	180	410	653
N propylparaben		5.74	36.7	124	222

in a moldy school building had detectable anti-mold antibodies.[14]

Metals. Urinary metal levels can be used to identify current exposure, and as such could be a part of all preventive assessments, including preconception care. When used properly, urine metal levels can aid in finding those with elevated body burdens of metals as well. Unfortunately, many well-intentioned clinicians run toxic metal testing as the first step in assessing environmental overload in hopes of finding a culprit. But because these metals will always be present, one is still left with the need to distinguish between presence and toxic effects. Hence, clinicians must first determine whether mercury, lead, cadmium, or arsenic fit the patient's disease picture and then identify exposure and consistent timing. Once the four basic steps of environmental illness assessment have concluded that one or more of the common toxic metals is involved in the patient's illness, metal testing can then be done for confirmation. This may include blood testing for current exposure to lead, methylmercury, or cadmium.

Metal levels found in a random or first morning urine sample should be compared with the CDC reference ranges (Table 53.9) and what is known about urine levels and adverse health effects, rather than the reference values provided by the laboratories. The chapters on arsenic, cadmium, lead, and mercury provide information of health effects associated with certain urine metal levels. Urine levels of arsenic, lead, and to some degree mercury, will provide information about current exposures to these compounds. Urine values over the CDC 75th percentile would indicate ongoing current exposure. Urinary levels of cadmium are indicative of total body load of cadmium.[1] An initial urinary concentration of lead ≥1 µg is indicative of an excessive body load of lead that would require chelation therapy.[15]

Arsenic does not bioaccumulate, but lifetime arsenic exposure can be estimated from the available data on water arsenic levels in the area the individual has resided and their current urine arsenic concentrations. To prevent contamination of the urine with nontoxic organic arsenicals, it is recommended that no seafood be consumed for the 4 days before sample collection. Toenail arsenic levels provide a more accurate representation of the long-term arsenic exposure,[16] but such testing is not commercially available at this time.

TABLE 53.9 2017 CDC Fourth Report Percentiles for Urinary and Blood Metal with Associated Health Problems for Urinary Arsenic and Cadmium—Urinary Toxic Metals (μg/g Creatinine)

Metal	Mean	75th %	90th %	95th %
Mercury Total	0.283	0.571	1.20	1.61
Lead	0.320	0.519	0.823	1.16
Arsenic Total	5.53	8.09	13.0	17.4
	Incr. glucose	Prediabetes	Genotoxicity	
		Cancer – liver, lung, prostate	SCC	
		CV mortality		
Cadmium	.144	.288	.563	.800
	Pancreatic CA	Osteoporosis		< Cognition
	Gestational diabetes	Cancer mortality		Learning disability
		CV mortality		Special education
		Hepatic inflammation		Diabetes
		NASH		Kidney damage
		Reduced FEV, FVC		

TABLE 53.10 Utilizing the Metal Mobilization Test for Mercury and Lead

Challenge Agent	Method	Positive Finding	Avoidance of False Negatives	Identifying Invalid MMT
CaEDTA & DMPS	IV	Pb > 60 μg/specimen	NA	NA
		Hg > 50 μg/specimen	GSH repletion before MMT	
DMSA	Oral	Pb > 25 μg/specimen	Insure proper absorption	If Hg increases <12-fold
		Hg > 25 μg/specimen	NAC and GSH repletion before MMT	Cd does not increase or drops

Metal Mobilization Testing

Metal mobilization testing (MMT) for mercury and lead provides the best estimation of body burden of these two metals. MMT utilizes urine metal assessment before and after the administration of a metal mobilizing agent. The total amount of metal in the pre- and postchallenge urine samples needs to be calculated as part of this method. Intravenous calcium edetate (CaEDTA) and oral 2,3-dimercaptosuccinic acid (DMSA) have both been used for lead mobilizations testing (Table 53.10);[17,18,19,20,21] 2,3-dimercaptopropane-1-sulfonate (DMPS) has been used for mercury mobilization testing, and DMSA can also be utilized.[22] Before the use of either of these compounds, it must be determined that kidney function is adequate and that the patient will have no adverse reaction to the compounds. Standard body-weight doses of these agents can only be used with patients who have

adequate kidney function. No chelation should be done when serum creatinine is ≥2.5 mg/dL, but half bodyweight dose chelation can be done with those whose creatinine is between 2.0 and 2.5 mg/dL no more than once weekly.[23] Previous uneventful exposure history or administration of a small dose of the intended metal mobilizing agent without reaction would provide evidence of nonreactivity. Protocols for utilizing intravenous and oral metal mobilizing tests can be found in Appendix D & E. Clinicians should avail themselves of proper training in intravenous and oral chelation protocols to insure safety and efficacy.

Ensuring an Accurate Result. If oral DMSA is used, then potential problems with absorption should be addressed before administration. Poor absorption will result in reduced excretion of either mercury or lead, which would result in a false negative MMT result. An assessment for elevated antigliadin antibodies would help differentiate those with probable absorption problems from those without. Elevated antigliadin antibodies have been found in individuals who exhibited poor absorption of DMSA.[24] Those with positive antigliadin antibodies would not be candidates for DMSA MMT.

Calculating Total Metal in Each Sample

$$total\ \mu g\ metal$$
$$= \frac{\mu g/g\ creatinine\ of\ metal \times creatinine\ level}{100,000}$$
$$\times total\ volume\ of\ urine\ collected$$

DMSA typically increases the mercury output by 12- to 70-fold,[25] so a post-DMSA increase in mercury of 12-fold or less would indicate malabsorption of DMSA. It has also been observed that a lack of increase in post-DMSA cadmium levels (and possibly even a reduction) have been noted only in those who do not properly absorb DMSA.[24]

The clearance of lead and mercury from the kidneys by DMSA is optimized by both N-acetyl cysteine (NAC) and glutathione. DMSA that has been conjugated with cysteine carries more metal than noncysteine-conjugated DMSA.[26] NAC itself has been shown to enhance the renal clearance of methylmercury.[27,28] All metals, whether attached to DMSA or not, need to be pumped into the proximal tubule by the phase 3 multidrug resistant associated protein (MRP) bound efflux pumps. MRPs require glutathione to properly pump any toxic compound out of the kidneys.[29,30] It would therefore be prudent to supplement with both NAC and liposomal glutathione for 2 weeks before the MMT.

Having taken the steps to insure a valid MMT, the total postchallenge μg concentration of both mercury and lead need to be calculated. If the total lead is < 60 μg, the total load would be considered insufficient to warrant chelation with EDTA.[17,18] Total post-DMSA lead values <10 μg would be considered insufficient to warrant chelation.[20,21] A total mercury of ≥50 μg would be considered a positive post-DMPS MMT. Because DMSA typically moves approximately 50% less mercury than DMPS, a positive post-DMSA MMT would therefore be ≥25 μg.

Breath Testing

The analysis of the exhaled breath for toxic exposure assessment is eliciting study by the scientific community, especially those in clinical medicine and occupational toxicology. In fact, it has been found to be more sensitive than blood-based analyses for volatile organic compound (VOC) quantification.[31] More than 200 compounds have been detected in the human breath,[32] and breath analysis is being investigated for the diagnosis of lung cancer, liver disease, myocardial infarction, and diabetes.[33,34,35,36] The benefits of this method of assessment are that it is less invasive than the acquisition of blood and much faster than a 24-hour urine collection; the exhaled breath is also a much simpler matrix than either the blood or urine. The challenge with breath is that excretion components are generally at much lower concentrations, and this requires some form of signal amplification to reach the detection limits of available equipment. One method is condensation of breath, and another method is the solid-phase microextraction (SPME) technique, which basically places a fiber of solid chromatographic media in a blow-tube. When the breath is passed through this tube, the VOC components of the breath adsorb to the media, which is then placed in a gas chromatograph/mass spectrometer (GCMS) and heated to desorb the breath components.[37] The GCMS then separates the components of the breath mixture and analyzes each for molecular weight and structure. The SPME technique allows the detection of substances in the nanomolar concentration range. This technique has been used to determine chlorinated solvent concentrations[38] and to measure organic alkanes and aromatics in the breath of lung cancer patients.[39] Investigators have undertaken similar analyses for other analytes.[40] These investigations have spawned a new field of study, dubbed "breathomics," in which the breath is dissected with a metabolomics approach to investigate health status and disease indicators such as oxidative stress.[41] Unfortunately, such testing is not currently available to most clinicians. Hopefully, this will change in the future along with the establishment of reference values for non-occupationally exposed individuals.

REFEREENCES

1. Patterson, D. G., Jr., Needham, L. L., Pirkle, J. L., et al. (1988). Correlation between serum and adipose tissue levels of 2,3,7,8-tetrachlorodibenzo-p-dioxin in 50 persons from Missouri. *Archives of Environmental Contamination and Toxicology*, 17(2), 139–143. PMID 3355228.
2. Centers for Disease Control and Prevention. (2017). *National Report on Human Exposure to Environmental*

Chemicals: Updated Tables. Available at www.cdc.gov/exposurereport/. Accessed October 25, 2017.

2a. http://endocrinedisruption.org/prenatal-origins-of-endocrine-disruption/critical-windows-of-development/timeline-test/.

3. Patterson, D. G., Jr., Needham, L. L., Pirkle, J. L., Roberts, D. W., Bagby, J., Garrett, W. A., et al. (1988). Correlation between serum and adipose tissue levels of 2,3,7,8-tetrachlorodibenzo-p-dioxin in 50 persons from Missouri. *Archives of Environmental Contamination and Toxicology, 17*(2), 139–143. PubMed PMID: 3355228.

4. Lim, J. S., Son, H. K., Park, S. K., Jacobs, D. R., Jr., & Lee, D. H. (2011). Inverse associations between long-term weight change and serum concentrations of persistent organic pollutants. *International Journal of Obesity (2005), 35*(5), 744–747. PubMed PMID: 20820170.

5. Walford, R. L., Mock, D., MacCallum, T., & Laseter, J. L. (1999). Physiologic changes in humans subjected to severe, selective calorie restriction for two years in biosphere 2: Health, aging, and toxicological perspectives. *Toxicological Sciences, 52*(2 Suppl.), 61–65. PubMed PMID: 10630592.

6. Imbeault, P., Chevrier, J., Dewailly, E., Ayotte, P., Després, J. P., Tremblay, A., et al. (2001). Increase in plasma pollutant levels in response to weight loss in humans is related to in vitro subcutaneous adipocyte basal lipolysis. *International Journal of Obesity and Related Metabolic Disorders: Journal of the International Association for the Study of Obesity, 25*(11), 1585–1591. PubMed PMID: 11753575.

7. Crinnion, W. J. Unpublished case studies.

8. Elgez, A. *Conditions Linked to Exposure in the Bedroom and How to Confirm Them.* 2016 Environmental Health Symposium, San Diego, CA.

9. Curl, C. L., Fenske, R. A., & Elgethun, K. (2003). Organophosphorus pesticide exposure of urban and suburban preschool children with organic and conventional diets. *Environmental Health Perspectives, 111*(3), 377–382. PubMed PMID: 12611667.

10. Lu, C., Barr, D. B., Pearson, M. A., & Waller, L. A. (2008). Dietary intake and its contribution to longitudinal organophosphorus pesticide exposure in urban/suburban children. *Environmental Health Perspectives, 116*(4), 537–542. PubMed PMID: 18414640.

11. Zota, A. R., Phillips, C. A., & Mitro, S. D. (2016). Recent Fast Food Consumption and Bisphenol A and Phthalates Exposures among the U.S. Population in NHANES, 2003-2010. *Environmental Health Perspectives, 124*(10), 1521–1528. PMID: 27072648.

12. Hartle, J. C., Navas-Acien, A., & Lawrence, R. S. (2016). The consumption of canned food and beverages and urinary Bisphenol A concentrations in NHANES 2003-2008. *Environmental Research, 150,* 375–382. PubMed PMID: 27362993.

13. Bae, S., & Hong, Y. C. (2015). Exposure to bisphenol A from drinking canned beverages increases blood pressure: Randomized crossover trial. *Hypertension, 65*(2), 313–319. PubMed PMID: 25489056.

14. Savilahti, R., Uitti, J., Laippala, P., Husman, T., Reiman, M., & Immunoglobulin, G. (2002). antibodies of children exposed to microorganisms in a water-damaged school. *Pediatric Allergy and Immunology: Official Publication of the European Society of Pediatric Allergy and Immunology, 13*(6), 438–442. PubMed PMID: 12485320.

15. Shannon, M., Grace, A., & Graef, J. (1989). Use of urinary lead concentration in interpretation of the EDTA mobilization test. *Veterinary and Human Toxicology, 31*(2), 140–142. PubMed PMID: 2494797.

16. Middleton, D. R., Watts, M. J., Hamilton, E. M., Fletcher, T., Leonardi, G. S., Close, R. M., et al. (2016). Prolonged exposure to arsenic in UK private water supplies: Toenail, hair and drinking water concentrations. *Environmental Science. Processes & Impacts, 18*(5), 562–574. PubMed PMID: 27120003.

17. Lin, J. L., Lin-Tan, D. T., Hsu, K. H., & Yu, C. C. (2003). Environmental lead exposure and progression of chronic renal diseases in patients without diabetes. *The New England Journal of Medicine, 348*(4), 277–286. PubMed PMID: 12540640.

18. Chen, K. H., Lin, J. L., Lin-Tan, D. T., Hsu, H. H., Hsu, C. W., Hsu, K. H., et al. (2012). Effect of chelation therapy on progressive diabetic nephropathy in patients with type 2 diabetes and high-normal body lead burdens. *American Journal of Kidney Diseases, 60*(4), 530–538. PubMed PMID: 22721929.

19. Markowitz, M. E., & Rosen, J. F. (1991). Need for the lead mobilization test in children with lead poisoning. *The Journal of Pediatrics, 119*(2), 305–310. PubMed PMID: 1907320.

20. Hoet, P., Buchet, J. P., Decerf, L., Lavalleye, B., Haufroid, V., & Lison, D. (2006). Clinical evaluation of a lead mobilization test using the chelating agent dimercaptosuccinic acid. *Clinical Chemistry, 52*(1), 88–96. PubMed PMID: 16239340.

21. Khan, D. A., Qayyum, S., Saleem, S., & Khan, F. A. (2009). Evaluation of lead body burden in occupational workers by lead mobilization test. *Journal of the Pakistan Medical Association, 59*(6), 350–354. PubMed PMID: 19534366.

22. Gonzalez-Ramirez, D., Maiorino, R. M., Zuniga-Charles, M., Xu, Z., Hurlbut, K. M., Junco-Munoz, P., et al. (1995). Sodium 2,3-dimercaptopropane-1-sulfonate

challenge test for mercury in humans: II. Urinary mercury, porphyrins and neurobehavioral changes of dental workers in Monterrey, Mexico. *The Journal of Pharmacology and Experimental Therapeutics, 272*(1), 264–274. PubMed PMID: 7815341.

23. Anderson, P., & Osborn, V. (2016). *Heavy metal toxicology. Clinical chelation: EDTA, DMPS, DMSA. IVNTP seminar.* Retrieved from www.ivnutritionaltherapy.com.

24. Crinnion, W. J. (2009). The benefit of pre- and post-challenge urine heavy metal testing: part 2. *Alternative Medicine Review: A Journal of Clinical Therapeutic, 14*(2), 103–108. PubMed PMID: 19594221.

25. Aposhian, H. V., Bruce, D. C., Alter, W., Dart, R. C., Hurlbut, K. M., & Aposhian, M. M. (1992). Urinary mercury after administration of 2,3-dimercaptopropane-1-sulfonic acid: Correlation with dental amalgam score. *FASEB Journal: Official Publication of the Federation of American Societies for Experimental Biology, 6*(7), 2472–2476. PubMed PMID: 1563599.

26. Flora, S. J., Pande, M., Kannan, G. M., & Mehta, A. (2004). Lead induced oxidative stress and its recovery following co-administration of melatonin or N-acetylcysteine during chelation with succimer in male rats. *Cellular and Molecular Biology, 50.* PubMed PMID: 15555419.

27. Aremu, D. A., Madejczyk, M. S., & Ballatori, N. (2008). N-acetylcysteine as a potential antidote and biomonitoring agent of methylmercury exposure. *Environmental Health Perspectives, 116*(1), 26–31. doi:10.1289/ehp.10383. PubMed PMID: 18197295.

28. Ballatori, N., Lieberman, M. W., & Wang, W. (1998). N-acetylcysteine as an antidote in methylmercury poisoning. *Environmental Health Perspectives, 106*(5), 267–271. PubMed PMID: 9520359.

29. Rius, M., Hummel-Eisenbeiss, J., Hofmann, A. F., & Keppler, D. (2006). Substrate specificity of human ABCC4 (MRP4)-mediated cotransport of bile acids and reduced glutathione. *American Journal of Physiology. Gastrointestinal and Liver Physiology, 290*(4), G640–G649. PubMed PMID: 16282361.

30. Zelcer, N., Reid, G., Wielinga, P., Kuil, A., van der Heijden, I., Schuetz, J. D., et al. (2003). Steroid and bile acid conjugates are substrates of human multidrug-resistance protein (MRP) 4 (ATP-binding cassette C4). *The Biochemical Journal, 371*(Pt. 2), 361–367. PubMed PMID: 12523936.

31. Lindstrom, A. B., & Pleil, J. D. (2002). A review of the USEPA's single breath canister (SBC) method for exhaled volatile organic biomarkers. *Biomarkers: Biochemical Indicators of Exposure, Response, and Susceptibility to Chemicals, 7*(3), 189–208.

32. Sanchez, J. M., & Sacks, R. D. (2003). GC analysis of human breath with a series-coupled column ensemble and a multibed sorption trap. *Analytical Chemistry, 75*(10), 2231–2236.

33. Buszewski, B., Kesy, M., Ligor, T., & Amann, A. (2007). Human exhaled air analytics: Biomarkers of diseases. *Biomedical Chromatography: BMC, 21*(6), 553–566.

34. Probert, C. S., Ahmed, I., Khalid, T., Johnson, E., Smith, S., & Ratcliffe, N. (2009). Volatile organic compounds as diagnostic biomarkers in gastrointestinal and liver diseases. *Journal of Gastrointestinal and Liver Diseases, 18*(3), 337–343.

35. Boots, A. W., Bos, L. D., van der Schee, M. P., van Schooten, F. J., & Sterk, P. J. (2015). Exhaled molecular fingerprinting in diagnosis and monitoring: Validating volatile promises. *Trends in Molecular Medicine, 21*(10), 633–644.

36. Fernández Del Río, R., O'Hara, M. E., Holt, A., Pemberton, P., Shah, T., Whitehouse, T., et al. (2015). Volatile biomarkers in breath associated with liver cirrhosis: Comparisons of pre- and post-liver transplant breath samples. *EBioMedicine, 2*(9), 1243–1250.

37. Grote, C., & Pawliszyn, J. (1997). Solid-phase microextraction for the analysis of human breath. *Analytical Chemistry, 69*(4), 587–596.

38. Guidotti, M., Onorati, B., Lucarelii, E., Blasi, G., & Ravaioli, G. (2001). Determination of chlorinated solvents in exhaled air, urine, and blood of subjects exposed in the workplace using SPME and GC-MS. *American Clinical Laboratory, 20*(4), 23–26.

39. Yu, H., Xu, L., & Wang, P. (2005). Solid phase microextraction for analysis of alkanes and aromatic hydrocarbons in human breath. *Journal of Chromatography. B, Analytical Technologies in the Biomedical and Life Sciences, 826*(1–2), 69–74.

40. Pleil, J. D., Smith, L. B., & Zelnick, S. D. (2000). Personal exposure to JP-8 jet fuel vapors and exhaust at air force bases. *Environmental Health Perspectives, 108*(3), 183–192.

41. Smolinska, A., Hauschild, A. C., Fijten, R. R., Dallinga, J. W., Baumbach, J., & van Schooten, F. J. (2014). Current breathomics–a review on data pre-processing techniques and machine learning in metabolomics breath analysis. *Journal of Breath Research, 8*(2), 027105.

54

Conventional Laboratory Tests to Assess Toxic Load

SUMMARY

- Presence in population: Conventional laboratory test results are modified in virtually the entire population in proportion to toxin load
- Major diseases: Virtually all chronic diseases

- Best measures: Gamma-glutamyl transferase (GGTP), alanine aminotransferase (ALT), uric acid, bilirubin, 8-OHdG

The incidence of chronic disease is increasing. Although medical apologists say this is because the population is aging, the harsh reality is that chronic disease is increasing in all age groups, including young people.[1] More than 50% of the US population now suffers from one or more diagnosed chronic diseases, and 25% of the population has two or more chronic conditions. In addition, at least 16% of the population describe themselves as chronically unwell with no specific disease diagnosis.

As the concentration and number of toxic compounds in the environment have increased, so has the incidence of ill health and chronic disease. Exposure to these toxins has consequences. A growing body of research indicates that exposure to endogenous and exogenous toxins is causing metabolic damage and physiological adaptation. This is reflected in changing "normal" values for standard laboratory tests, which are typically not considered measures of toxic exposure.

ASSESSMENT OF TOXIC LOAD

With toxic load becoming an increasing clinical problem, accurate assessment is essential not only for recognition of exposure but also for tracking efficacy of intervention. There are several accepted tests for metal toxicity that rely mostly on blood and urine. However, these are known to be useful only for acute exposure and are unreliable for body load. The typical standards for toxin load are population-based (i.e., unless a patient is in the top 5% of blood levels, they are usually not considered toxic). Although the top 5% is the standard to be considered toxic for most pollutants, there is sufficient reason to question its validity. One problem is the assumption that those with lower levels are healthy and are not being damaged by their toxic load. In addition, because the population has very high levels of ill health and diagnosed disease, normal is not actually healthy. Thus normal ranges of many standard laboratory tests now include the effects of physiological adaptation as well as actual damage. Several conventional laboratory tests within the supposed "normal" range show changes in proportion to the body load of specific toxins and toxicants.

DIRECT MEASURES OF TOXICANTS

Toxicants can be directly measured in urine, blood, breath, toenails, and adipose tissue. Blood levels of metals typically only reflect current exposure and are not very reliable in assessing total body load. Urine testing may be beneficial in examining the long-term, low-dose, chronic exposure to toxic compounds. But again, urine testing may not be reliable in assessing total body load. Direct measures of some toxicants are available and provide accurate and reliable current exposure levels. However, testing is expensive and is limited to only about 100 of the tens of thousands of toxicants in the environment. Direct measures of toxic load are covered in Chapter 53.

CONVENTIONAL LABORATORY TESTS

Although a detailed medical history, exposure assessment, and comprehensive physical examination are foundational in the diagnosis of toxicant exposure, conventional laboratory tests can be used to identify those who are suffering damage from toxicants and monitor treatment. Examples of conventional laboratory tests that change within the "normal" range in proportion to toxin load include:

- Complete blood count (CBC, e.g., red blood cell [RBC] count, white blood cell [WBC] count, platelet count, hemoglobin, basophilic stippling)
- Liver enzymes (e.g., ALT, GGTP)
- Inflammatory markers (e.g., C-reactive protein [CRP])
- Lipids (e.g., LDL, oxLDL, triglycerides)
- Thyroid hormones (e.g., T3, T4)
- Metabolites (e.g., bilirubin, uric acid, 8-OHdG)
- Blood sugar (e.g., insulin, fasting blood sugar [FBS], 2-hour postprandial [PP] blood glucose test)

Unfortunately, these tests generally do not indicate the specific toxicant but rather represent toxicant classes. Nonetheless, examining laboratory values in conjunction with detailed history and physical examination is useful in the recognition of toxic exposure. "Normal" is no longer "healthy."

Complete Blood Count

A CBC is one of the most common and least expensive laboratory tests ordered. It is not unusual for individuals to have laboratory values hovering at the low end of the normal reference range. Studies are now indicating that low normal values of platelets and total WBC count may be early indicators of toxic exposure. A study of paint workers exposed to a mixture of benzene-toluene-xylene showed a statistically significant macrocytosis, which may demonstrate an early manifestation of toxicant exposure.[2]

White Blood Cell Count. WBCs decrease in proportion to total body load of polychlorinated biphenyls (PCBs) and organochlorine pesticides (OCPs).[3] Although the values remained within the normal reference range, there was a 14% decrease in WBCs with exposure to PCBs and OCPs (Fig. 54.1). It should be noted that although total PCBs and OCPs correlate well, the correlation with specific chemicals in these classes is inconsistent.

Red Blood Cell Count. A long-term follow-up of individuals who participated in the Deepwater Horizon oil spill cleanup assessed the relationship between benzene, toluene, ethylbenzene, and xylene (BTEX) levels and RBC indices.[4] In this group of individuals, benzene was inversely associated with both hemoglobin levels and mean corpuscular hemoglobin concentrations, although it was positively correlated with red cell distribution width. A study of gas station workers showed a significant positive

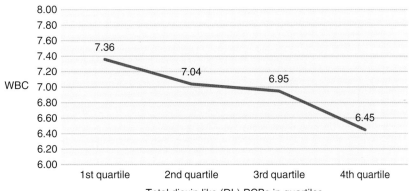

FIG. 54.1 Decrease in WBC in proportion to exposure to PCBs and OCPs. (Data from Serdar, B., LeBlanc, W. G., Norris, J. M., & Dickinson, L. M. [2014]. Potential effects of polychlorinated biphenyls [PCBs] and selected organochlorine pesticides [OCPs] on immune cells and blood biochemistry measures: A cross-sectional assessment of the NHANES 2003 to 2004 data. *Environmental Health, 13,* 114.)

association between toluene, ethylbenzene, and xylene, and abnormal WBC levels.[5]

Platelets. A study of auto repair workers showed subclinical abnormalities in platelet count with continuous low-level toluene exposure.[6] Even though the workers wore masks and protective gear, chronic low-level exposure to solvents decreased platelet count by 14% (216,000/mL versus 252,000/mL) compared with office workers in the same facility—who likely were exposed as well, though at lower levels. Researchers also noted a statistically significant relationship between neurological abnormalities (impairment of sympathetic and peripheral nerves) and a self-reported neuropsychiatric measurement (correlation coefficient (r) = 0.35–0.66). Although still within the normal range, the individuals exposed to the solvents clearly experienced measurable physiological effects. A study of 42 healthy, nonsmoking, gasoline-filling workers demonstrated that workers exposed to solvents for long periods of time (> 10 years) had a significant decrease in platelet levels compared with controls (Fig. 54.2).[7]

Basophilic Stippling. Basophilic stippling refers to a unique appearance of RBCs observed under a microscope in which the erythrocytes display small dots at the periphery. Stippling is a classic sign of lead poisoning as well as arsenic poisoning.

Liver Enzymes

The liver is one of the primary organs of detoxification. It activates nutrients, detoxifies harmful substances, makes blood clotting proteins, and performs many other vital functions. Eighty percent of the liver is made up of hepatocytes, which play a critical role in the metabolism of amino acids and ammonia, biochemical oxidation reactions, and detoxification of a variety of drugs, vitamins, hormones, and environmental toxicants. Enzymes located within the cells of the liver drive these chemical reactions and are induced as needed. Aspartate aminotransferase (AST), ALT, and gamma-glutamyltranspeptidase (GGT) are three of the most common enzymes tested. When liver cells are damaged or destroyed, the enzymes leak out into the blood where they can be measured. Several liver enzymes increase in proportionate response to the load of specific classes of toxicants—within the supposed normal range.

Gamma-Glutamyltransferase. Perhaps most useful is GGT, a key enzyme in glutathione (GSH) recycling. GGT is induced to provide more GSH, likely for phase II conjugation, as well as to neutralize oxidative stress. Cellular GGT metabolizes extracellular GSH, allowing precursor cysteine to be reutilized for *de novo* synthesis of intracellular GSH. Elevations of GGT within the "normal" range are strongly associated with several chronic diseases, including diabetes, coronary heart disease, hypertension, stroke, dyslipidemia, chronic kidney disease, and cancer.[8] Serum GGT levels within the normal range may also reflect the amounts of GSH conjugates formed during the metabolism of xenobiotics, and the association of serum GGT with type 2 diabetes reflects exposure to persistent organic pollutants (POPs). An increase in GGT

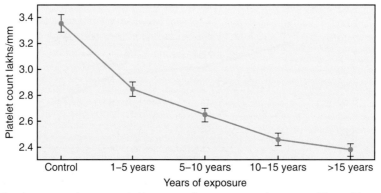

FIG. 54.2 Platelet count decreases with years of exposure to benzene. (From Uzma, N., Salar, B. M., Kumar, B. S., Aziz, N., David, M. A., & Reddy, V. D. [2008]. Impact of organic solvents and environmental pollutants on the physiological function in petrol filling workers. *International Journal of Environmental Research and Public Health, 5*[3], 139–146.)

concentration, within its physiological range, has been shown to be a sensitive biomarker for the development of diabetes with concentrations > 50 U/l, correlating with a 26-fold-increased risk of developing diabetes.[9] Compared with men with GGT levels below 15 U/l, the relative risk of all-cause mortality was two times greater for those with GGT levels between 30 to 49 U/l (Relative Risk (RR) = 2.09) and greater than three times (RR = 3.44) for men with GGT levels ≥ 50 U/l.[10] Elevations of GGT directly correlate with alcohol consumption (Fig. 54.3)[11] and, as shown in Figs. 54.4 and 54.5, toxic metal load (cadmium, lead, and mercury).[12,13] Serum GGT, within its reference range, is also associated with organochlorine pesticides and polycyclic aromatic hydrocarbons.[14]

Alanine Transaminase. ALT catalyzes the transfer of an amino group from L-alanine to α-ketoglutarate. The products of this transamination reaction are pyruvate and L-glutamate. Of the adult population in the United States, 10.4% has an elevated ALT, typically due to nonalcoholic fatty liver disease (NAFLD). For men aged 18 to 20, ALT values >37 IU/L are considered elevated, whereas the cutoff for men over the age of 21 is >48 IU/L. Women between the ages of 18 to 20 are elevated at an ALT of >30 IU/L; those above the age of 21 are

considered elevated >31 IU/L. ALT increases in a dose-dependent manner with body load of blood cadmium, lead, mercury, and PCBs within and above the normal range.[15] In the National Health and Nutritional Examination Survey (NHANES) 2003 to 2004 cohort, those with a blood mercury in the second quartile (25th–50th percentile) were twice as likely to have elevated ALT.[16] Data collected from the Korean National Health and Nutritional Examination Survey (KNHANES) showed that increasing blood mercury levels were associated with increases in AST, ALT, and elevated GGTP (>56 IU/L).[17,18]

Exposure to polycyclic aromatic hydrocarbons causes elevations in AST and ALT.[19] A study of 29 dry cleaner workers exposed to 16 parts per million (PPM) of perchloroethylene (PCE), far less than the permissible exposure limit of 100 PPM in the United States, showed dry cleaning operators had fatty infiltration, even though their serum aminotransferase levels were mostly normal.[20]

When serum log-perfluorooctanoic acid (PFOA; see Chapter 29) increases by one unit, serum ALT increases by 1.86 units (95% Confidence Interval (CI), 1.24–2.48; p = 0.005), and the serum log-GGT concentration is 0.08 units higher (95% CI, 0.05–0.11; p = 0.019).[21] Studies have also found AST, ALT and GGT increase with body load of PCBs and OCPs in

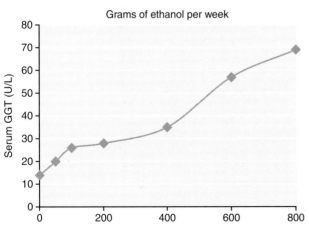

FIG. 54.3 GGT increases in proportion to alcohol consumption. (Data from Nagaya, T., Yoshida, H., Takahashi, H., Matsuda, Y., & Kawai, M. [1999]. Dose-response relationships between drinking and serum tests in Japanese men aged 40 to 59 years. *Alcohol, 17*[2], 133–138.)

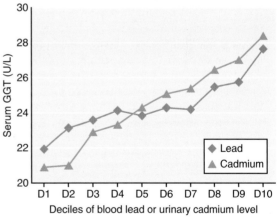

FIG. 54.4 GGT increases in proportion to cadmium and lead load. (From Lee, D. H., Lim, J. S., Song, K., Boo, Y., & Jacobs, D. R., Jr. [2006]. Graded associations of blood lead and urinary cadmium concentrations with oxidative-stress-related markers in the U.S. population: results from the third National Health and Nutrition Examination Survey. *Environmental Health Perspectives, 114*[3], 350–354.)

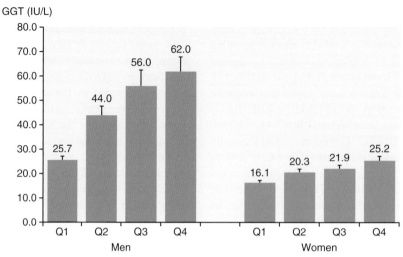

FIG. 54.5 GGT increases in proportion to mercury load. (From Seo, M. S,. Lee, H. R., Shim, J. Y., Kang, H. T., & Lee, Y. J. [2014]. Relationship between blood mercury concentrations and serum γ-glutamyltranspeptidase level in Korean adults using data from the 2010 Korean National Health and Nutrition Examination Survey. *Clinica Chimica Acta, 430,* 160–163.)

TABLE 54.1 Geometric Mean Levels (and 95% Confidence Intervals) of Liver Enzymes by Serum Organochlorine Pesticide Exposure Groups

		MIREX			
Blood Marker	**n**	**1**	**2**	**3**	**4**
Aspartate aminotransferase (AST) (U/L)	1951	23.2 (22.7, 23.6)	23.7 (22.3, 25.3)	24.3 (23.2, 25.5)	25[a] (23.6, 26.5)
Gamma glutamyltransferase (GGT) (U/L)	1951	18.8 (18.2, 19.4)	22.2[a] (20.2, 24.4)	22[a] (19, 25.3)	19.7 (16.6, 23.2)
		p,p'-DDE			
Alanine aminotransferase (ALT) (U/L)	1956	20.9 (20, 21.8)	22.9 (21.3, 24.5)	22.7[a] (21.7, 23.7)	22.5[a] (21.4, 23.6)
Gamma glutamyltransferase (GGT) (U/L)	1956	19 (18, 20)	21.1[a] (19.4, 22.9)	19.7 (17.8, 21.7)	18.9 (17.2, 20.7)
		p,p'-DDT			
Alanine aminotransferase (ALT) (U/L)	1965	20.4 (19.5, 21.3)	23.3[a] (22, 24.7)	22.8[a] (21.6, 24)	22.6[a] (21.6, 23.7)
Aspartate aminotransferase (AST) (U/L)	1965	22.6 (22, 23.2)	24.1[a] (23.1, 25.3)	23.8 (22.8, 24.7)	24[a] (23.3, 24.7)
Gamma glutamyltransferase (GGT) (U/L)	1965	18.1 (17, 19.2)	20.7[a] (18.9, 22.6)	20.3[a] (18.7, 22)	19.8 (17.8, 21.9)
		Trans-nonachlor			
Alanine aminotransferase (ALT) (U/L)	1955	19.3 (17.9, 20.8)	21 (20.2, 21.8)	23.1[a,b] (22.1, 24.1)	23.3[a,b] (21.9, 24.9)
Gamma glutamyltransferase (GGT) (U/L)	1955	15.4 (14.1, 16.9)	19[a] (18, 20)	20.4[a] (19, 21.9)	21.3[a] (18.9, 24)

TABLE 54.1   **Geometric Mean Levels (and 95% Confidence Intervals) of Liver Enzymes by Serum Organochlorine Pesticide Exposure Groups—cont'd**

Blood Marker	n	MIREX			
		1	2	3	4
		Oxychlordane			
Alanine aminotransferase (ALT) (U/L)	1978	20.1 (19.2, 21.1)	22[a] (20.9, 23.1)	23.7[a] (22.5, 25)	22[c] (20.7, 23.4)
Gamma glutamyltransferase (GGT) (U/L)	1978	16.1 (14.6, 17.9)	19.9[a] (18.6, 21.3)	21.4[a] (19.6, 23.3)	20.5[a] (18.2, 23.2)

[a]p < 0.05 when compared to geometric mean of the first group.
[b]p < 0.05 when compared to geometric mean of the second group.
[c]p < 0.05 when compared to geometric mean of the third group.
From Serdar, B., LeBlanc, W. G., Norris, J. M., & Dickinson, L. M. (2014). Potential effects of polychlorinated biphenyls (PCBs) and selected organochlorine pesticides (OCPs) on immune cells and blood biochemistry measures: a cross-sectional assessment of the NHANES 2003 to 2004 data. *Environmental Health*, 13, 114. Copyright © Serdar et al.; licensee BioMed Central. 2014. Reprinted under the terms and conditions of the Creative Commons Attribution (CC-BY) license (http://creativecommons.org/licenses/by/4.0/)

proportion to serum levels of these toxins (Table 54.1).[3] Obese, diabetic mice had increased levels of AST and ALT, enhanced steatosis, and elevated markers of oxidative stress after pulmonary exposure to diesel exhaust particles.[22]

Volatile organic compound (VOC) exposures, such as toluene, benzene, styrene, and xylene, have been associated with both normal liver and abnormal liver enzyme levels.[23] Seventy-five percent of household painters with VOC exposures and abnormal liver enzymes had fatty liver on biopsy,[24] and 100% of toluene-exposed printers with persistent mild liver enzyme elevation had hepatic steatosis.[25]

Alkaline Phosphatase. ALP is a hydrolase enzyme responsible for dephosphorylation. It is present in higher concentration in the liver, kidney, and bone. Chronic exposure of pesticides in agricultural workers was found to be associated with significantly higher activities of ALP compared with controls, and the number of years exposed to pesticides predicted higher activities of ALP.[26]

Inflammatory Markers

C-reactive protein (CRP) is a blood test marker used to detect inflammation. It is produced by the liver and is classified as an acute phase reactant, meaning that levels will rise in response to inflammation. Most environmental toxins are proinflammatory and increase oxidative stress

in the body. Data from NHANES 2003 to 2004 shows that exposure to polycyclic aromatic hydrocarbons (specifically 2-hydroxyphenanthrene and 9-hydroxyfluorine) is associated with elevated CRP levels (>3 mg/L), suggesting a role for OH-PAHs in the progression of atherosclerosis.[27] Fig. 54.6 demonstrates an association between CRP, body load of PCBs and OC pesticides, and an increased risk of metabolic syndrome.[28]

Lipids

An intriguing prospective study evaluated if POP levels could predict future cholesterol levels over time.[29] Results showed a huge variation, with some POPs having little effect whereas others had a substantial effect. As can be seen in Fig. 54.7, a single POP, PCB 194, showed the best correlation to elevation of LDL-cholesterol over a 5-year period. This is particularly interesting as most reports of POP levels in the blood standardize according to serum lipid levels. In a study of 525 White and African American residents of the United States, total pesticides were more strongly associated with elevations in serum lipids than were total PCBs, and the associations were stronger in African Americans.[30] Individuals in the highest quartile of PFOS exposure had total cholesterol levels that were 13.4 mg/dL (95% CI, 3.823.0) higher than those in the lowest quartile.[31] PFC exposure in adolescents is significantly associated with elevated total cholesterol and LDL cholesterol.[32] Considering, in most cases, cholesterol levels

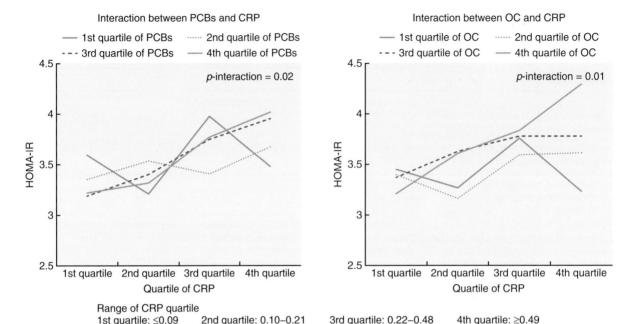

FIG. 54.6 Association between CRP, body load of PCBs and OC pesticides, and metabolic syndrome. (From Kim, K. S., Hong, N. S., Jacobs, D. R. Jr, & Lee, D. H. [2012]. Interaction between persistent organic pollutants and C-reactive protein in estimating insulin resistance among nondiabetic adults. *Journal of Preventive Medicine and Public Health, 45*[2], 62–69.)

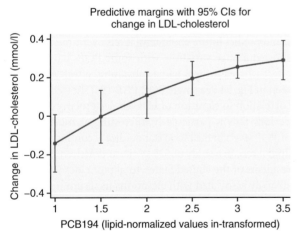

FIG. 54.7 PCB 194 predictive of LDL-cholesterol elevation. (From Penell, J., Lind, L., Salihovic, S., van Bavel, B., & Lind, P. M. [2014]. Persistent organic pollutants are related to change in circulating lipid levels during a 5-year follow-up. *Environmental Research, 134,* 190–197.)

increase with age, the research may underestimate actual body load.

Perhaps the most important aspect is that POPs oxidize cholesterol, and oxidized cholesterol is the most artery-damaging form. Studies also show a direct correlation between PCBs and the ratio of oxidized glutathione (GSSG) to GSH, a definitive measure of oxidative status. The sum of PCBs shows a strong, significant positive association with oxLDL and significant associations with GSH-related markers (GSSG and GSSG/GSH).[33]

Thyroid Hormones

PCB exposure has been associated with hypothyroidism. Studies show that PCBs decrease T4 and T3 production, and inhibit iodotyrosine deiodinase activity, leading to an overall decrease in thyroid hormone biosynthesis, as shown in Fig. 54.8.[34,35,36] Animal studies confirm that exposure to PCBs or dioxins results in reduction of serum thyroid hormone levels, especially T4.[37,38,39]

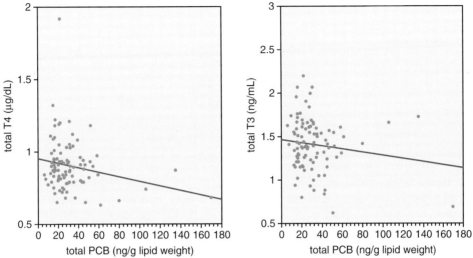

FIG. 54.8 T4 and T3 decrease in proportion to PCB body load. (From Kim, S., Park, J., Kim, H. J., Lee, J. J., Choi, G., Choi, S., Kim, S., Kim, S. Y., Moon, H. B., Kim, S., Choi, K. [2013]. Association between several persistent organic pollutants and thyroid hormone levels in serum among the pregnant women of Korea. *Environment International, 59,* 442–448.)

German children showed a significant positive correlation between PCB serum levels and elevation of TSH as well as a significant inverse correlation between serum PCB levels and FT4.[40] Elevated antithyroid antibodies, both antiperoxidase and antithyroglobulin, were found in workers in a PCB manufacturing plant, but no difference was found in the levels of T4 and TSH.[41]

Thyroid function decreases with PFOA levels but appears to occur only in older adults, suggesting that the toxicant effects are worse with aging.[42] Adolescents and adults in the 2007 to 2008 NHANES had a negative association between blood mercury levels and total T3 and T4.[43] Brominated flame retardants such as polybrominated diphenyl ethers (PBDEs), pentabromophenol (PBP), and tetrabromobisphenol A (TBBPA) have a structural resemblance to thyroxine (T4) and are potent competitors for T4 binding to TTR.[44] Statistical interactions suggest that concurrent exposure to PBDEs and PCBs elicited multiplicative effects on T3 levels in women, and that concurrent exposure to DDTs and PCBs elicited multiplicative effects of T4 in women and T3 in men.[45] Workers with higher occupational BPA exposure show higher FT3 concentrations as well as abnormal concentrations of FT4, TT3, TT4, and TSH.[46]

Metabolites

Uric Acid. Several metabolites can be used as an indirect measure of POPs. Serum uric acid increases in proportion to body load of perfluorinated hydrocarbons (PFOA and PFOS).[47] Fig. 54.9 demonstrates an interesting threshold effect where low levels of PFOA or PFOS show little effect initially, followed by rapid elevation in uric acid levels with odds ratios of hyperuricemia increasing by quintile of PFOA (ORs = 1.00, 1.33, 1.35, 1.47, and 1.47).[48]

Bilirubin. Bilirubin levels increase in proportion to the level of various PCBs, which is significant as bilirubin is considered the best prognostic measure of chronic liver dysfunction.[49,50] Direct bilirubin serves as a protective biomarker likely based on its endogenous antioxidant and cytoprotectant properties.[51] A wide range of liver-associated enzymes and molecules are associated with perfluorinated chemicals, with different measures responding to different chemicals (Fig. 54.10).[52]

Homocysteine. Homocysteine is an endogenous toxin that has been shown to reduce nitric oxide availability, increase levels of reactive oxygen species, and induce NF-κβ expression.[53,54] Lead levels have been positively

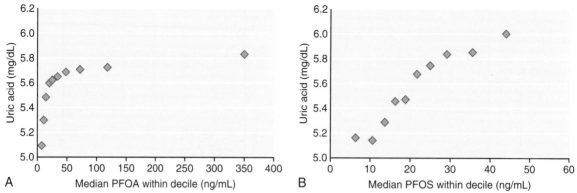

FIG. 54.9 Serum uric acid increases in proportion to body load of PFOA and PFOS. (From Steenland, K., Tinker, S., Shankar, A., & Ducatman, A. [2010]. Association of perfluorooctanoic acid (PFOA) and perfluorooctane sulfonate (PFOS) with uric acid among adults with elevated community exposure to PFOA. *Environmental Health Perspectives, 118,* 229–233.)

correlated with serum levels of homocysteine,[55] a biomarker associated with increased cardiovascular risk. Deficiencies in several B vitamins potentiate the damaging effects of lead on homocysteine (Fig. 54.11). Elevated homocysteine levels have been found among patients with Parkinson's disease, particularly in those taking L-dopa,[56] and the effect is accentuated in those with low folic acid levels.[57] Nutrient deficiencies accentuate the effects of toxins,[58] and the synergy between xenobiotics is often greater than additive effects. The combination of nutrient depletion, cofactor displacement, and high toxicant contamination in the food supply may be some of the main reasons the incidence of all chronic disease is increasing.

Blood Sugar Regulation

Considering that most POPs are insulin receptor site poisons, the greatest amount of research on potential disease causation is between toxic load and measures of blood sugar regulation: FBS, 2-hour PP sugar, HbA$_{1c}$, insulin levels, metabolic syndrome, and diabetes. Impaired insulin resistance is the most common mechanism of damage for all POPs, and these chemicals are also implicated in the obesity epidemic.[59,60,61,62] Fig. 54.12 shows the results of a 23-year prospective study examining levels of POPs in young adults and changes in glucose-related metabolism.[63] Several critical observations can be made from this study:

1. Until the age of 50, there is essentially no difference in blood sugar regulation measurements between those with the lowest and highest PCB levels. This suggests that the increasing toxic load has little effect in younger people.
2. In the youngest group, insulin production increases in response to toxin level. This is to be expected because the blocking of insulin receptor sites by PCBs requires more insulin. The ability to adapt decreases with aging.
3. At age 50, all the measures show very strong toxin-dose response, suggesting that the body's adaptive capabilities have become inadequate or are overwhelmed by ever-increasing toxic load.

Clinical Application

Recognizing and identifying toxic chemicals can present a difficult challenge for the clinician. A well-characterized methodology that is fully validated using both healthy and toxic individuals would be preferred. Examining the research, it appears that what is defined as "normal" is mostly toxic, with the body showing measurable signs of adaptation and metabolic dysfunction (Box 54.1). The optimal range for conventional laboratory tests is still to be determined. However, aside from the CBC and platelet count, a good starting place is to have patients in the lowest quartile of the range of each of these tests.

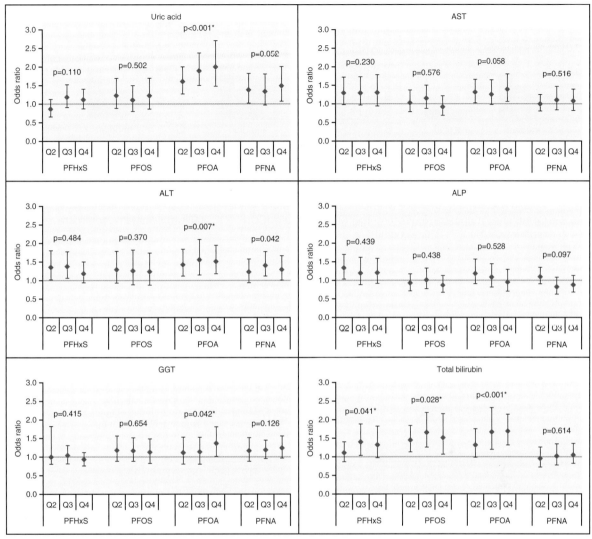

FIG. 54.10 Serum measures showing response to perfluorinated chemical exposure. (From Gleason, J. A., Post, G. B., & Fagliano, J. A. [2015]. Associations of perfluorinated chemical serum concentrations and biomarkers of liver function and uric acid in the U.S. population [NHANES], 2007 to 2010. *Environmental Research*, *136*, 8–14.)

BOX 54.1 Potential Laboratory Indications of High Body Toxic Load

- Gamma glutamyltransferase (GGT): > 25
- Uric acid: > 5.0 mg/dL
- Alanine aminotransferase (ALT): >30 U/L
- Bilirubin: >0.8 mg/dL
- Complete blood count (CBC): < 6,000
- Platelets: < 250,000
- Low T3 and/or T4

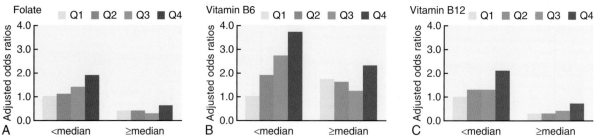

FIG. 54.11 Nutrient deficiencies accentuate effects of lead on homocysteine. (From Lee Y-M, Lee M-K, Bae S-G, Lee S-H, Kim S-Y, Lee D-H. Association of Homocysteine Levels With Blood Lead Levels and Micronutrients in the US General Population. Journal of Preventive Medicine and Public Health. 2012;45(6):387–393. doi:10.3961/jpmph.2012.45.6.387. Copyright © 2012 The Korean Society for Preventive Medicine. Reprinted under the terms and conditions of the Creative Commons Attribution-NonCommercial 3.0 Unported [CC BY-NC 3.0][https://creativecommons.org/licenses/by-nc/3.0/legalcode].)

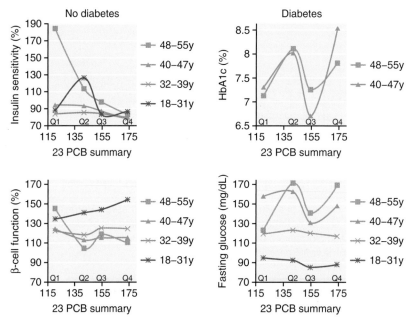

FIG. 54.12 23-year prospective study on effects of PCBs on blood sugar regulation. (From Suarez-Lopez, J. R., Lee, D. H., Porta, M., Steffes, M. W., & Jacobs, D. R., Jr. Persistent organic pollutants in young adults and changes in glucose related metabolism over a 23-year follow-up. *Environmental Research, 137,* 485–494.)

REFERENCES

1. Freed, V. M., Bernstein, A. B., & Bush, A. B. (2012). Multiple Chronic Conditions Among Adults Aged 45 and Over: Trends Over the Past 10 Years. NCHS Data Brief No. 100, July 2012. Available at: http://www.cdc.gov/nchs/data/databriefs/db100.htm. (Accessed 21 April 2016).

2. Haro-Garcia, L., Velez-Zamora, N., Aguilar-Madrid, G., et al. (2012). Blood disorders among workers exposed to a mixture of benzene-toluene-xylene (BTX) in a paint factory. *Revista Peruana de Medicina Experimental y Salud Pública, 29*(2), 181–187. PubMed PMID: 22858763.

3. Serdar, B., LeBlanc, W. G., Norris, J. M., & Dickinson, L. M. (2014). Potential effects of polychlorinated biphenyls (PCBs) and selected organochlorine pesticides (OCPs) on immune cells and blood biochemistry measures: A cross-sectional assessment of the NHANES 2003-2004 data. *Environmental Health: A Global Access Science Source, 13*, 114. PubMed PMID: 25515064.

4. Doherty, B. T., Kwok, R. K., Curry, M. D., et al. (2017). Associations between blood BTEXS concentrations and hematologic parameters among adult residents of the U.S. Gulf States. *Environmental Research, 156*, 579–587. PubMed PMID: 28448810.

5. Tunsaringkarn, T., Zapuang, K., & Rungsiyothin, A. (2013). Correlation between blood cell parameters and BTEX exposure among gasoline station workers. *Journal of Environmental and Occupational Science, 2*(1), 15–20.

6. Shih, H. T., Yu, C. L., Wu, M. T., et al. (2011). Subclinical abnormalities in workers with continuous low-level toluene exposure. *Toxicology and Industrial Health, 27*(8), 691–699. PubMed PMID: 21543466.

7. Uzma, N., Salar, B. M., Kumar, B. S., et al. (2008). Impact of organic solvents and environmental pollutants on the physiological function in petrol filling workers. *International Journal of Environmental Research and Public Health, 5*(3), 139–146. PubMed PMID: 19139531.

8. Lee, D. H., Steffes, M. W., & Jacobs, D. R., Jr. (2008). Can persistent organic pollutants explain the association between serum gamma-glutamyltransferase and type 2 diabetes? *Diabetologia, 51*(3), 402–407. PubMed PMID: 18071669.

9. Lee, D. H., Ha, M. H., Kim, J. H., et al. (2003). Gamma-glutamyltransferase and diabetes – a 4-year follow-up study. *Diabetologia, 46*(3), 359–364. PubMed PMID: 12687334.

10. Brenner, H., Rothenbacher, D., Arndt, V., et al. (1997). Distribution, determinants, and prognostic value of gamma-glutamyltransferase for all-cause mortality in a cohort of construction workers from southern Germany. *Preventive Medicine, 26*(3), 305–310. PubMed PMID: 9144754.

11. Nagaya, T., Yoshida, H., Takahashi, H., et al. (1999). Dose-response relationships between drinking and serum tests in Japanese men aged 40–59 years. *Alcohol, 17*(2), 133–138. PubMed PMID: 10064381.

12. Lee, D. H., Lim, J. S., Song, K., et al. (2006). Graded associations of blood lead and urinary cadmium concentrations with oxidative-stress-related markers in the U.S. population: Results from the third National Health and Nutrition Examination Survey. *Environmental Health Perspectives, 114*(3), 350–354. PubMed PMID: 16507456.

13. Seo, M. S., Lee, H. R., Shim, J. Y., et al. (2014). Relationship between blood mercury concentrations and serum γ-glutamyltranspeptidase level in Korean adults using data from the 2010 Korean National Health and Nutrition Examination Survey. *Clinica Chimica Acta, 430*, 160–163. PubMed PMID: 24508988.

14. Lee, D. H., & Jacobs, D. R. (2009). Is serum gamma-glutamyltransferase an exposure marker of xenobiotics? Empirical evidence with polycyclic aromatic hydrocarbon. *Clinical Chemistry and Laboratory Medicine, 47*(7), 860–862. PubMed PMID: 19575547.

15. Cave, M., Appana, S., Patel, M., et al. (2010). Polychlorinated biphenyls, lead, and mercury are associated with liver disease in American adults: NHANES 2003-2004. *Environmental Health Perspectives, 118*(12), 1735–1742. PubMed PMID: 21126940.

16. Lin, Y. S., Ginsberg, G., Caffrey, J. L., Xue, J., Vulimiri, S. V., Nath, R. G., et al. (2014). Association of body burden of mercury with liver function test status in the U.S. population. *Environment International, 70*, 88–94. PubMed PMID: 24908642.

17. Lee, H., Kim, Y., Sim, C. S., Ham, J. O., Kim, N. S., & Lee, B. K. (2014). Associations between blood mercury levels and subclinical changes in liver enzymes among South Korean general adults: Analysis of 2008-2012 Korean national health and nutrition examination survey data. *Environmental Research, 130*, 14–19. PubMed PMID: 24525240.

18. Seo, M. S., Lee, H. R., Shim, J. Y., Kang, H. T., & Lee, Y. J. (2014). Relationship between blood mercury concentrations and serum γ-glutamyltranspeptidase level in Korean adults using data from the 2010 Korean National Health and Nutrition Examination Survey. *Clinica Chimica Acta, 430*, 160–163. PubMed PMID: 24508988.

19. Min, Y. S., Lim, H. S., & Kim, H. (2015). Biomarkers for polycyclic aromatic hydrocarbons and serum liver

enzymes. *American Journal of Industrial Medicine, 58*(7), 764–772. PubMed PMID: 25940037.

20. Brodkin, C. A., Daniell, W., et al. (1995). Hepatic ultrasonic changes in workers exposed to perchloroethylene. *Occupational and Environmental Medicine, 52*(10), 679–685. PubMed PMID: 7489059.

21. Lin, C. Y., Lin, L. Y., Chiang, C. K., et al. (2010). Investigation of the associations between low-dose serum perfluorinated chemicals and liver enzymes in US adults. *The American Journal of Gastroenterology, 105*(6), 1354–1363. PubMed PMID: 20010922.

22. Tomaru, M., Takano, H., Inoue, K., et al. (2007). Pulmonary exposure to diesel exhaust particles enhances fatty change of the liver in obese diabetic mice. *International Journal of Molecular Medicine, 19*(1), 17–22. PubMed PMID: 17143543.

23. Brautbar, N., & Williams, J. (2002). Industrial solvents and liver toxicity: Risk assessment, risk factors and mechanisms. *International Journal of Hygiene and Environmental Health, 205*(6), 479–491. PubMed PMID: 12455270.

24. Dossing, M., Arlien-Soborg, P., et al. (1983). Liver damage associated with occupational exposure to organic solvents in house painters. *European Journal of Clinical Investigation, 13*(2), 151–157. PubMed PMID: 6409638.

25. Guzelian, P. S., Mills, S., & Fallon, H. J. (1988). Liver structure and function in print workers exposed to toluene. *Journal of Occupational Medicine, 30*(10), 791–796. PubMed PMID: 3230426.

26. Araoud, M., Neffeti, F., Douki, W., et al. (2012). Adverse effects of pesticides on biochemical and haematological parameters in Tunisian agricultural workers. *Journal of Exposure Science and Environmental Epidemiology, 22*(3), 243–247. PubMed PMID: 22377683.

27. Everett, C. J., King, D. E., Player, M. S., et al. (2010). Association of urinary polycyclic aromatic hydrocarbons and serum C-reactive protein. *Environmental Research, 110*(1), 79–82. PubMed PMID: 19836015.

28. Kim, K. S., Hong, N. S., Jacobs, D. R., Jr., & Lee, D. H. (2012). Interaction between persistent organic pollutants and C-reactive protein in estimating insulin resistance among non-diabetic adults. *Journal of Preventive Medicine and Public Health, 45*(2), 62–69. PubMed PMID: 22509446.

29. Penell, J., Lind, L., Salihovic, S., et al. (2014). Persistent organic pollutants are related to change in circulating lipid levels during a 5 year follow-up. *Environmental Research, 134*, 190–197. PubMed PMID: 25173051.

30. Aminov, Z., Haase, R., Olson, J. R., et al. (2014). Racial differences in levels of serum lipids and effects of exposure to persistent organic pollutants on lipid levels in residents of Anniston, Alabama. *Environment International, 73*, 216–223. PubMed PMID: 25160080.

31. Nelsen, J. W., Hatch, E. E., & Webster, T. F. (2010). Exposure to polyfluoroalkyl chemicals and cholesterol, body weight, and insulin resistance in the general U.S. population. *Environmental Health Perspectives, 118*(2), 197–202. PubMed PMID: 20123614.

32. Geiger, S. D., Xiao, J., Ducatman, A., et al. (2014). The association between PFOA, PFOS and serum lipid levels in adolescents. *Chemosphere, 98*, 78–83. PubMed PMID: 24238303.

33. Kumar, J., Monica Lind, P., Salihovic, S., et al. (2014). Influence of persistent organic pollutants on oxidative stress in population-based samples. *Chemosphere, 114*, 303–309. PubMed PMID: 25113216.

34. Kim, S., Park, J., Kim, H. J., et al. (2013). Association between several persistent organic pollutants and thyroid hormone levels in serum among the pregnant women of Korea. *Environment International, 59*, 442–448. PubMed PMID: 23928038.

35. Shimizu, R., Yamaguchi, M., Uramura, N., et al. (2013). Structure-activity relationships of 44 halogenated compounds for iodotyrosine deiodinase-inhibitory activity. *Toxicology, 314*(1), 22–29.

36. Schwacke, L. H., Zolman, E. S., Balmer, B. C., et al. (2012). Anaemia, hypothyroidism and immune suppression associated with polychlorinated biphenyl exposure in bottlenose dolphins (Tursiops truncatus). *Proceedings. Biological Sciences*, doi:10.1098/rspb.2011.0665.

37. Gauger, K. J., Kato, Y., Haraguchi, K., et al. (2004). Polychlorinated biphenyls (PCBs) exert thyroid hormone-like effects in the fetal rat brain but do not bind to thyroid hormone receptors. *Environmental Health Perspectives, 112*(5), 516–523. PubMed PMID: 15064154.

38. Hallgren, S., & Darnerud, P. O. (2002). Polybrominated diphenyl ethers (PBDEs), polychlorinated biphenyls (PCBs) and chlorinated paraffins (CPs) in rats-testing interactions and mechanisms for thyroid hormone effects. *Toxicology, 177*(2–3), 227–243. PubMed PMID: 12135626.

39. Martin, L., & Klaassen, C. D. (2010). Differential effects of polychlorinated biphenyl cogeners on serum thyroid hormone levels in rats. *Toxicological Sciences, 117*(1), 36–44. PubMed PMID: 20573785.

40. Osius, N., Karmaus, W., Kruse, H., & Witten, J. (1999). Exposure to polychlorinated biphenyls and levels of thyroid hormones in children. *Environmental*

Health Perspectives, 107, 843–849. PubMed PMID: 10504153.

41. Langer, P., Tajtakova, M., & Fodor, G. (1998). Increased thyroid volume and prevalence of thyroid disorders in a area heavily polluted by polychlorinated biphenyls. *European Journal of Endocrinology*, 139, 402–409. PubMed PMID: 9820616.

42. Shrestha, S., Bloom, M. S., Yucel, R., et al. (2015). Perfluoroalkyl substances and thyroid function in older adults. *Environment International*, 75, 206–214. PubMed PMID: 25483837.

43. Chen, A., Kim, S. S., Chung, E., & Dietrich, K. N. (2013). Thyroid hormones in relation to lead, mercury, and cadmium exposure in the National Health and Nutrition Examination Survey, 2007-2008. *Environmental Health Perspectives*, 121(2), 181–186. PubMed PMID: 23164649.

44. Meerts, I. A., van Zanden, J. J., Luijks, E. A., et al. (2000). Potent competitive interactions of some brominated flame retardants and related compounds with human transthyretin in vitro. *Toxicological Sciences*, 56(1), 95–104. PubMed PMID: 10869457.

45. Bloom, M. S., Jansing, R. L., Kannan, K., et al. (2014). Thyroid hormones are associated with exposure to persistent organic pollutants in aging residents of upper Hudson River communities. *International Journal of Hygiene and Environmental Health*, 217(4–5), 473–482. PubMed PMID: 24138783.

46. Wang, F., Hua, J., Chen, M., Xia, Y., et al. (2012). High urinary bisphenol A concentrations in workers and possible laboratory abnormalities. *Occupational and Environmental Medicine*, 69(9), 679–684. PubMed PMID: 22562051.

47. Geiger, S. D., Xiao, J., & Shankar, A. (2013). Positive association between perfluoroalkyl chemicals and hyperuricemia in children. *American Journal of Epidemiology*, 177(11), 1255–1262. PubMed PMID: 23552989.

48. Steenland, K., Tinker, S., Shankar, A., & Ducatman, A. (2010). Association of perfluorooctanoic acid (PFOA) and perfluorooctane sulfonate (PFOS) with uric acid among adults with elevated community exposure to PFOA. *Environmental Health Perspectives*, 118, 229–233. PubMed PMID: 20123605.

49. Dufour, D. R., Lott, J. A., Nolte, F. S., et al. (2000). Diagnosis and monitoring of hepatic injury. II. Recommendations for use of laboratory tests in screening, diagnosis, and monitoring. *Clinical Chemistry*, 46(12), 2050–2068. PubMed PMID: 11106350.

50. Kumar, J., Lind, L., Salihovic, S., et al. (2014). Persistent organic pollutants and liver dysfunction biomarkers in a population-based human sample of men and women. *Environmental Research*, 134, 251–256. PubMed PMID: 25173059.

51. Tian, J., Zhong, R., Liu, C., et al. (2016). Association between bilirubin and risk of nonalcoholic fatty liver disease based on a prospective cohort study. *Scientific Reports*, 6, 310006. PubMed PMID: 27484402.

52. Gleason, J. A., Post, G. B., & Fagliano, J. A. (2015). Associations of perfluorinated chemical serum concentrations and biomarkers of liver function and uric acid in the US population (NHANES), 2007-2010. *Environmental Research*, 136, 8–14. PubMed PMID: 25460614.

53. Weiss, N. (2005). Mechanisms of increased vascular oxidant stress in hyperhomocysteinemia and its impact on endothelial function. *Current Drug Metabolism*, 6(1), 27–36. PubMed PMID: 15720205.

54. Cheung, G. T., Siow, Y. L., & O, K. (2008). Homocysteine stimulates monocyte chemoattractant protein-1 expression in mesangial cells via NF-κβ activation. *Canadian Journal of Physiology and Pharmacology*, 86(3), 88–96. PubMed PMID: 18418435.

55. Schafer, J. H., Glass, T. A., Bressler, J., Todd, A. C., & Schwartz, B. S. (2005). Blood lead is a predictor of homocysteine levels in a population-based study of older adults. *Environmental Health Perspectives*, 113(1), 31–35. PubMed PMID: 15626644.

56. Zesiewicz, T. A., Wecker, L., Sullivan, K. L., et al. (2006). The controversy concerning plasma homocysteine in Parkinson disease patients treated with levodopa alone or with entacapone: Effects of vitamin status. *Clinical Neuropharmacology*, 29(3), 106–111. PubMed PMID: 16772808.

57. Dos Santos, E. F., Busanello, E. N., Miglioranza, A., et al. (2009). Evidence that folic acid deficiency is a major determinant of hyperhomocysteinemia in Parkinson's disease. *Metabolic Brain Disease*, 24(2), 257–269. PubMed PMID: 19294496.

58. Lee, Y. M., Lee, M. K., Bae, S. G., et al. (2012). Association of homocysteine levels with blood lead levels and micronutrients in the US general population. *Journal of Preventive Medicine and Public Health*, 45(6), 387–393. PubMed PMID: 23230469.

59. Remillard, R. B., Bunce, N. J., et al. (2002). Linking dioxins to diabetes: Epidemiology and biologic plausibility. *Environmental Health Perspectives*, 110(9), 853–858.

60. Tang, M., Chen, K., Yang, F., & Liu, W. (2014). Exposure to organochlorine pollutants and type 2 diabetes: a systematic review and meta-analysis. *PLoS ONE*, 9(10), e85556.

61. Weinhold, B. (2013). PCBs and diabetes: Pinning down mechanisms. *Environmental Health Perspectives, 121*(1), A32.

62. Grün, F., & Blumberg, B. (2007). Perturbed nuclear receptor signaling by environmental obesogens as emerging factors in the obesity crisis. *Reviews in Endocrine & Metabolic Disorders, 8*(2), 161–171.

63. Suarez-Lopez, J. R., et al. (2015). Persistent organic pollutants in young adults and changes in glucose related metabolism over a 23-year follow-up. *Environmental Research, 137*, 485–494.

55

8-Hydroxy-2'-deoxyguanosine and Other Nucleoside Metabolites

SUMMARY

- Presence in population: Ubiquitous in the urine of all persons, higher in those with greater oxidative stress
- Major diseases: Elevated levels of 8-hydroxy-2'-deoxyguanosine (8-OHdG) are found in all chronic diseases and can predict illness and outcome
- Primary sources: Hydroxyl radical damage to the DNA, associated with exposures to ubiquitous pollutants
- Best measure: Urinary 8-OHdG levels
- Best intervention: Avoidance of pollutants, whole food antioxidants

DESCRIPTION

Living organisms are continuously exposed to reactive oxygen species (ROS) as a consequence of biochemical reactions—especially mitochondrial adenosine triphosphate (ATP) production—as well as external factors. A variety of tests have been developed that measure lipid peroxidation, such as malondialdehyde (MDA), oxidized low-density lipoprotein (LDL), MDA-modified LDL, F2-isoprostane, and conjugated diene. Dityrosine and oxidized histidine have been used to determine protein oxidation. Among the bases in the nucleic acids, guanine is the most prone to oxidative damage. The hydroxylation of guanine by ROS leads to the misreading of the modified base, and repair is performed by the cell for survival.[1] Upon DNA repair, 8-OHdG is excreted in the urine.

Urinary 8-OHdG or urinary 8-oxo-7,8-dihydro-2'-deoxyguanosine (8-oxodG) is an oxidized nucleoside that appears in the urine secondary to DNA damage and is the most common biomarker of oxidative DNA damage. Urinary nucleoside metabolites not only measure DNA damage but also serve as indirect measures of oxidative stress and toxin load.[2] 8-oxodG is used to estimate exposure to cancer-causing agents, such as tobacco smoke, asbestos fibers, toxic metals, and polycyclic aromatic hydrocarbons, and is significantly increased by toxicant

exposure. 8-OHdG correlates with multiple cancers, mitochondrial damage, mercury levels, rate of aging, and smoking. 8-OHdG is also a fairly accurate predictor of chronic diseases such as atherosclerosis, diabetes, and cancer.[3] 8-OHdG may be most useful for monitoring toxic load and as a measure of treatment efficacy.

ASSESSMENT OF URINARY 8-OHdG

The quantification of 8-OHdG correlates well with high-performance liquid chromatography and electrochemical detection (HPLC-EC) and gas chromatography–mass spectrometry (GC-MS). However, these methods require prepurification and are not convenient for routine clinical analysis.[4,5] The use of enzyme-linked immunosorbent assay (ELISA) has garnered the most attention and has received widespread use. The benefits of ELISA are ease of use, the fact that no expensive equipment is required, potential application to numerous extracellular matrices (e.g., serum, plasma, urine, cerebrospinal fluid), the fact that no pretreatment of urine is required, and high throughput.[6] There is some evidence that ELISA overestimates 8-oxodG levels and may not be specific for accurate quantification.[7] This may be the result of ELISA detecting all oxidatively modified free bases and nucleosides carrying an 8-hydroxylated guanine base.

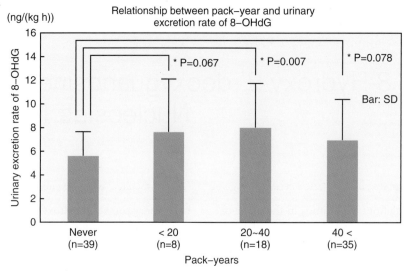

FIG. 55.1. Urinary 8-OHdg correlates with pack-years of smoking. (From Yano, T., Shoji, F., Baba, H., Koga, T., Shiraishi, T., Orita, H., Kohno, H. [2009]. Significance of the urinary 8-OHdG level as an oxidative stress marker in lung cancer patients. *Lung Cancer, 63*[1], 111–114.)

Several soluble oxidatively modified products have been found in urine, including 8-OHdG, 8-OHGua, thymine glycol, and 5-hydroxymethyluracil. One study found the total excretion of 8-OHGua species to be 212 nmol in 24 hours, with the oxidized base accounting for 64%, the ribonucleoside accounting for 23%, and the deoxynucleoside accounting for 13%, indicating substantial RNA oxidation in addition to DNA oxidation.[8] Nonetheless, ELISA continues to be the primary assay for urinary 8-OHdG.

SOURCES

Air Pollutants

- Smoking
- Particulate matter
- Perfluorocarbons
- Indoor building materials
- Solvents

Tobacco Smoke. Smokers have up to 300% more 8-oxodG than nonsmokers, and those living in polluted cities have almost twice the levels of those living in rural settings.[9] 8-OHdG increases in direct proportion to the number of cigarettes smoked,[10,11] and smokers excrete approximately 50% more 8-OHdG than nonsmokers.[12] Exposure to environmental tobacco smoke (secondhand

smoke) may be just as concerning. One study found that workplace employees exposed to environmental tobacco smoke had a statistically significant 63% increase in blood levels of 8-OHdG.[13] Benzene and styrene, both found in high levels in cigarette smoke, have independently been shown to increase 8-OHdG levels.[14,15]

As can be seen in Fig. 55.1, excretion of 8-OHdG increases directly with pack-years of smoking.[16] Those who have smoked the most have a slightly lower level, which may indicate that those with the highest levels have already died of lung cancer.

Urban Air Pollution. Exposure to particulate matter (PM), both PM_{10} and $PM_{2.5}$, has been found to increase urinary levels of 8-OHdG in several human studies. Each 1 mg/m^3 of $PM_{2.5}$ exposure resulted in an average urinary 8-OHdG increase of 1.67 mg/g cr.[17] Individuals who work in toll booths had urinary 8-OHdG levels almost twice those of non–toll-booth workers (13.6 µg/g cr vs. 7.3 µg/g cr).[18] Traffic policemen had higher urinary 8-OHdG levels than policemen who did not work traffic shifts.[19] Their level of the urinary marker for oxidative stress increased with the number of years they worked among traffic. Policemen with either the CYP1A1m1 SNP (resulting in increased induction by polycyclic aromatic hydrocarbons [PAHs]) or null GSTM1 polymorphism also had higher 8-OHdG levels. Interestingly, children with eczema had higher urinary 8-OHdG levels after exposure to $PM_{0.1}$ than children without atopic dermatitis.[20] Diesel exhaust, the prime source of $PM_{0.1}$ in the urban air, has been shown to increase 8-OHdG levels.[21] Fortunately, this increase in oxidative stress and urinary 8-OHdG could be blunted with supplementation of N-acetyl cysteine (NAC). Particulate matter (PM) from wood smoke also increases levels of this marker.[22]

Perfluorinated Compounds. Perfluorinated compounds, such as perfluorooctanoic acid (PFOA) and perfluorononanoic acid (PFNA), are suspected genotoxic agents responsible for oxidative DNA damage. An *in vitro* study showed that PFOA- and PFNA-induced DNA damage in human lymphoblastoid cell lines and levels of 8-OHdG were increased in a dose-dependent manner in both PFOA and PFNA exposure.[23]

Water-Damaged Buildings. For persons working in a water-damaged building, the levels of their sick building syndrome (SBS) symptoms were significantly associated with higher levels of urinary 8-OHdG (Table 55.1).[24] The mean urinary 8-OHdG level was higher in persons with SBS symptoms than in those without complaints (6.16 µg/g vs. 5.45 µg/g cr. [$p = .047$]). The most common presenting

SBS symptoms are headache; eye, nose and throat irritation; dizziness; disorientation; difficulty concentrating; and fatigue.[25] SBS is most often associated with the type of ventilation system, semivolatile organic compound (SVOC) and volatile organic compound (VOC) levels in buildings, moldiness, and stressors.[26,27,28,29] Four specific groups of VOCs—terpenes, aromatics, n-alkanes, and butanols—are significantly associated with the prevalence of chronic SBS symptoms.[30] Carpeting in home, schools, or workplaces has also been repeatedly associated with SBS.[30,31,32] Formaldehyde and ethylbenzene exposures are also associated with elevated 8-OHdG levels.[33,34] Both trichloroethylene (TCE) and tetrachloroethylene (PCE), common water contaminants and dry cleaning solvents, cause oxidative stress, resulting in increased 8-OHdG levels.[35]

Food Pollutants

- Cadmium
- Lead
- Mercury
- Organophosphate pesticides (OPs)

Cadmium. Enhanced oxidative stress and mitochondrial dysfunction from cadmium exposure has been documented along with an increased level of urinary 8-OHdG.[36,37]

Lead. Lead not only generates ROS but also causes a reduction in the activity of ROS-quenching enzymes, such as superoxide dismutase, catalase, and glutathione peroxidase, resulting in diminished antioxidant defense. In adults, lead-associated oxidative stress is associated with an increase in urinary 8-OHdG levels,[38] but such an increase has not been seen in children with similar blood lead levels (BLLs).[39]

Mercury. Mercury causes a great deal of oxidative damage throughout the body, including to the DNA. Hydroxyl radical damage to the DNA results in elevated levels of 8-OHdG in the urine, and urinary 8-OHdG correlates with toxic load. There are strong correlations with both blood and urine, as well as the occasional substantial outlier. Individuals without occupational exposure to mercury with mean blood and urine mercury levels of 0.91 µg/L and 0.95 µg/L had urinary 8-OHdG levels that averaged 2.08 ng/mg cr (range 0.95–4.7).[40] Mercury workers with far higher blood and urine mercury levels

TABLE 55.1   **Significant Associations ($p = .001$) With Exposures and 8-OHdG Levels in Persons with Sick Building Syndrome**

	≤3.79 µg/g	3.80–6.63 µg/g	>6.63 µg/g
Nonsmoker	132 (38%)	121 (35%)	91 (27%)
Smokers	0	7 (16%)	38 (84%)
No carpet	65 (45%)	34 (23%)	47 (32%)
Carpet	67 (28%)	94 (39%)	82 (34%)
CO_2 diff PPM[a]	483	770	781
TVOC - PPB	302	500	2580
Cotinine (µg/g cr)	1.95	3.15	6.22

[a]Difference in CO_2 levels between indoors and outdoors.
Data from Lu, C. Y., Ma, Y. C., Lin, J. M., Li, C. Y., Lin RS, & Sung FC. (2007). Oxidative stress associated with indoor air pollution and sick building syndrome-related symptoms among office workers in Taiwan. *Inhalation Toxicology*, 19(1), 57–65.

had correspondingly high urine 8-OHdG levels (mean 242.9 ng/mg cr). Women exposed to both MeHg and inorganic mercury with urinary mercury levels of 5.3 μg/g cr or higher also had elevated 8-OHdG levels.[41] Elevated 8-OHdG levels have been documented in children whose urinary mercury were in the second to fourth quartiles.[42] Children with a mean urinary mercury of 2.75 μg/g cr had mean 8-OHdG levels of 17.7 μg/g cr.

Organophosphate Pesticides. A positive correlation has been found between farmers exposed to OPs and oxidative stress biomarkers, including 8-OHdG.[43] Not only were the 8-OHdG levels positively associated with the amount of OPs sprayed monthly by the workers, but they were also significantly related to urinary OP metabolite levels (dimethylphosphate [DMP], diethylphthalate [DEP], and diethylthiophosphoric acid [DETP]). Urinary levels of 8-OHdG increased in Chinese children (with an average urinary 8-OHdG of 3.99 μg/g cr) along with their urinary OP metabolites.[44]

Water Pollutants

- Arsenic
- Chromium

The main mechanism by which monomethylarsonic acid (MMA) and inorganic arsenicals cause cellular and tissue damage is through oxidative stress.[45,46] Increases in urinary 8-OHdG levels have been found in those drinking groundwater high in arsenic as well as individuals who are occupationally exposed to arsenic.[47] The consumption of high-arsenic groundwater has been directly linked to an increase in urinary 8-OHdG levels in a population in West Bengal, India. However, when individuals from this area supplemented with 1 g of curcumin daily for 3 months, ROS generation and lipid peroxidation activity were reduced,[48] and the 8-OHdG level dropped, indicating a dramatic reduction in arsenic-induced DNA oxidative damage.[49]

Elevated levels of 8-OHdG have also been seen in workers exposed to hexavalent chromium, which now contaminates many water supplies in the United States (see Chapter 4).[50]

CLINICAL SIGNIFICANCE

- Cardiovascular disease
- Diabetes
- Neoplasia

Cardiovascular Disease

Oxidative DNA damage has been linked to an increased risk of coronary artery disease. ROS promote cell proliferation in atherosclerosis, oxidation of LDL, early plaque formation, and endothelial dysfunction.[51,52] One study observed increased immunoreactivity against 8-OHdG in carotid artery plaques in all cell types of the plaque (e.g., macrophages, smooth muscle cells, and endothelial cells), suggestive of increased oxidative DNA damage and repair.[53] Atherosclerotic plaques induced in rabbits fed a cholesterol-rich diet showed oxidative damage as manifested by elevated levels of 8-OHGua.[54] Interestingly, oxidative DNA damage and increased levels of DNA repair were strongly reversed with dietary lipid lowering. Carotid artery intima media thickness, a marker for atherosclerosis, is positively associated with plasma levels of 8-OHdG.[55] Individuals with coronary artery disease have higher 8-OHdG levels than persons without this problem.[56] It was noted that 8-OHdG levels increased along with the disease progression. 8-OhdG levels are also higher in persons who have experienced an acute myocardial infarction.[57]

Multiple studies of patients with heart failure found higher 8-OHdG levels compared with controls, with progressively increased levels associated with advancing New York Heart Association functional class.[58,59,60] Not only is 8-OHdG higher in individuals with congestive heart failure, but it also correlates with left ventricular ejection fraction.[61] 8-OHdG appears to be a useful biomarker for predicting cardiac events and evaluating treatment effectiveness.[62] 8-OHdG is also higher in persons who have had a stroke.[65]

Neoplasia

There is increasing evidence that malignant cells contain high levels of oxidized DNA lesions, and any lesions that are not repaired can lead to mutations and increase the risk of carcinogenesis.[63,64] ROS are associated with both tumor promotion and progression. 8-OHdG levels are elevated in breast cancer and are actually believed to be a predictive biomarker for this cancer.[65] In uterine myomas, increased levels of 8-OHdG were found to be associated with the size of the tumor.[66] The level of 8-OHdG in renal cell carcinoma compared with that in normal tissue was significantly associated with maximal tumor size, distant metastasis, pathological stage, microscopical venous invasion, and tumor grade.[67]

Elevated urinary 8-OHdG levels have also been found in patients with small cell lung carcinoma,[68] bladder cancer,[69] prostate cancers,[1,70] ovarian cancer,[71] nasopharyngeal cancer,[72] acute myeloid leukemia (AML),[73] and gastric cancer.[74] 8-OHdG appears to be predictive of cancer risk (occurrence), spread and aggression, improvement, and reoccurrence.

Diabetes

Oxidative stress can play a key role in the pathogenesis of diabetes, because elevations in glucose concentrations lead to an increased production of ROS by glucose oxidation, activation of nicotinamide adenine dinucleotide phosphate (NADPH) oxidase, and stimulation of the polyol pathway.[75] In individuals with type 2 diabetes who have poor glycemic control, urinary 8-OHdG levels were significantly higher than in normoglycemic subjects (5.03 ± 0.69 vs. 0.96 ± 0.15 pmol/mL), and hemoglobin A1C has been shown to be positively correlated with 24-hour urinary 8-OHdG excretions.[76] A significant difference of 24-hour urinary 8-OHdG excretions exists in diabetic nephropathy patients with macroalbuminuria compared with those with normoalbuminuria (19.2 ± 16.8 µg in 24 hours vs. 8.1 ± 1.7 µg in 24 hours; $p = 0.015$).[77] Elevated concentrations of 8-OHdG have also been found in urine, correlating with the severity of diabetic nephropathy and retinopathy, and can be used as a clinical marker to predict the development of diabetic complications.[78,79,80]

INTERVENTION

Among the most useful interventions to reduce 8-oxodG is a diet rich in colorful fruits and vegetables, particularly purple sweet potato leaves and almonds.[81] Adherence to the Mediterranean diet resulted in reduction of 8-OHdG levels in persons with metabolic syndrome.[82] Greater fruit and vegetable intake is independently associated with reduced 8-OHdG levels.[83] Polyphenol-rich vegetables, red wine, and fermented beverages also lowers this marker.[84] Quercitin, found highest in onions, is able to reduce DNA oxidative damage from methylmercury and lower 8-OHdG.[85] One study found that increasing fruits and vegetables to 12 servings a day decreased urinary 8-oxodG by 57% after only 2 weeks, with those eating the poorest diets beforehand improving the most.[86] Both the consumption of green tea and the practice of Tai Chi reduce 8-OHdG levels.[87] Antioxidants such as CoQ10,[88]

curcumin,[89] lycopene,[90] and green tea have all been shown to significantly reduce levels of 8-oxodG.[91]

Excess iron tends to generate ROS within cells, which increases mutagenic lesions. Iron-lowering treatments not only decrease elevated levels of 8-OHdG but also could prevent the development of hepatocellular carcinoma in chronic hepatitis C patients.[92]

REFERENCES

1. Chiou, C. C., Chang, P. Y., Chan, E. C., et al. (2003). Urinary 8-hydroxydeoxyguanosine and its analogs as DNA marker of oxidative stress: development of an ELISA and measurement in both bladder and prostate cancers. *Clinica Chimica Acta*, *334*(1–2), 87–94. PubMed PMID: 12867278.
2. Valavanidis, A., Vlachogianni, T., & Fiotakis, C. (2009). 8-hydroxy-2′–deoxyguanosine (8-OHdG): a critical biomarker of oxidative stress and carcinogenesis. *J Environ Sci Health C Environ Carcinog Ecotoxicol Rev.*, *27*(2), 120–139. PubMed PMID: 19412858.
3. Wu, L. L., Chiou, C. C., Chang, P. Y., et al. (2004). Urinary 8-OHdG: a marker of oxidative stress to DNA and a risk factor for cancer, atherosclerosis, and diabetes. *Clinica Chimica Acta*, *339*(1–2), 1–9. PubMed PMID: 14687888.
4. Ravanat, J. L., Guichard, P., Tuce, Z., & Cadet, J. (1999). Simultaneous determination of five oxidative DNA lesions in human urine. *Chemical Research in Toxicology*, *12*(9), 802–808. PubMed PMID: 10490501.
5. Degan, P., Shigenaga, M. K., Park, E. M., et al. (1991). Immunoaffinity isolation of urinary 8-hydroxy-2′-deoxyguanosine and 8-hydroxyguanine and quantitation of 8-hydroxy-2′-deoxyguanosine in DNA by polyclonal antibodies. *Carcinogenesis*, *12*(5), 865–871. PubMed PMID: 2029751.
6. Cooke, M. S., Olinski, R., & Loft, S. (2008). European Standards Committee on Urinary (DNA) Lesion Analysis. Measurement and meaning of oxidatively modified DNA lesions in urine. *Cancer Epidemiology, Biomarkers and Prevention: A Publication of the American Association for Cancer Research, Cosponsored by the American Society of Preventive Oncology*, *17*(1), 3–14. PubMed PMID: 18199707.
7. Cooke, M. S., Singh, R., Hall, G. K., Mistry, V., et al. (2006). Evaluation of enzyme-linked immunosorbent assay and liquid chromatography-tandem mass spectrometry methodology for the analysis of 8-oxo-7,8-dihydro-2′-deoxuguanosine in saliva and urine. *Free Radical Biology & Medicine*, *41*(12), 1829–1836. PubMed PMID: 17157185.

8. Weimann, A., Belling, D., & Poulsen, H. E. (2002). Quantification of 8-oxo-guanine and guanine as the nucleobase, nucleoside and deoxynucleoside forms in human urine by high-preformance liquid chromatography-electrospray tandem mass spectrometry. *Nucleic Acids Research*, *30*(2), E7. PubMed PMID: 11788733.

9. Buthbumrung, N., Mahidol, C., Navasumrit, P., et al. (2008). Oxidative DNA damage and influence of genetic polymorphisms among urban and rural schoolchildren exposed to benzene. *Chemico-Biological Interactions*, *172*(3), 185–194. PubMed PMID: 18282563.

10. Lu, C. Y., Ma, Y. C., Chen, P. C., Wu, C. C., & Chen, Y. C. (2014). Oxidative stress of office workers relevant to tobacco smoking and inner air quality. *International Journal of Environmental Research and Public Health*, *11*(6), 5586–5597. PubMed PMID:24865395.

11. Chiang, H. C., Huang, Y. K., Chen, P. F., Chang, C. C., Wang, C. J., Lin, P., et al. (2012). 4-(Methylnitrosamino)-1-(3-pyridyl)-1-butanone is correlated with 8-hydroxy-2'-deoxyguanosine in humans after exposure to environmental tobacco smoke. *The Science of the Total Environment*, *414*, 134–139. PubMed PMID: 22138374.

12. Loft, S., Vistisen, K., Ewertz, M., et al. (1992). Oxidative DNA damage estimated by 8-hydroxydeoxyguanosine excretion in humans: influence of smoking, gender and body mass index. *Carcinogenesis*, *13*(12), 2241–2247. PubMed PMID: 1473230.

13. Howard, D. J., Ota, R. B., Briggs, L. A., & Hampton, M. (1998). Pritsos CA. Environmental tobacco smoke in the workplace induces oxidative stress in employees, including increased production of 8-hydroxy-2'-deoxyguanosine. *Cancer Epidemiology, Biomarkers and Prevention: A Publication of the American Association for Cancer Research, Cosponsored by the American Society of Preventive Oncology*, *7*(2), 141–146. PubMed PMID: 9488589.

14. Liu, L., Zhang, Q., Feng, J., et al. (1996). The study of DNA oxidative damage in benzene-exposed workers. *Mutation Research*, *370*, 145–150. PMID: 8917660.

15. Marczynski, B., Rozynek, P., Elliehausen, H. G., et al. (1997). Detection of 8-hydroxydeooxyguanosine, a marker of oxidative DNA damage, in white blood cells of workers occupationally exposed to styrene. *Archives of Toxicology*, *71*, 496–500. PMID: 9248627.

16. Yano, T., et al. (2009). Significance of the urinary 8-OHdG level as an oxidative stress marker in lung cancer patients. *Lung Cancer (Amsterdam, Netherlands)*, *63*(1), 111–114. PubMed PMID: 18676055.

17. Kim, J. Y., Mukherjee, S., Ngo, L. C., & Christiani, D. C. (2004). Urinary 8-hydroxy-2'-deoxyguanosine as a biomarker of oxidative DNA damage in workers exposed to fine particulates. *Environmental Health Perspectives*, *112*(6), 666–671. PubMed PMID: 15121508.

18. Lai, C. H., Liou, S. H., Lin, H. C., et al. (2005). Exposure to traffic exhausts and oxidative DNA damage. *Occupational and Environmental Medicine*, *62*(4), 216–222. PubMed PMID: 15778253.

19. Prasad, S. B., Vidyullatha, P., Vani, G. T., et al. (2013). Association of gene polymorphism in detoxification enzymes and urinary 8-OHdG levels in traffic policemen exposed to vehicular exhaust. *Inhalation Toxicology*, *25*(1), 1–8. PubMed PMID: 23293967.

20. Song, S., Paek, D., Park, C., et al. (2013). Exposure to ambient ultrafine particles and urinary 8-hydroxyl-2-deoxyguanosine in children with and without eczema. *The Science of the Total Environment*, *458-460*, 408–413. PubMed PMID: 23685365.

21. Yamamoto, M., Singh, A., Sava, F., et al. (2013). MicroRNA expression in response to controlled exposure to diesel exhaust: attenuation by the antioxidant N-acetylcysteine in a randomized crossover study. *Environmental Health Perspectives*, *121*(6), 670–675. PubMed PMID: 23584289.

22. Commodore, A. A., Zhang, J. J., Chang, Y., et al. (2013). Concentrations of urinary 8-hydroxy-2'-deoxyguanosine and 8-isoprostane in women exposed to woodsmoke in a cookstove intervention study in San Marcos, Peru. *Environment International*, *60*, 112–122. PubMed PMID: 24041735.

23. Yahia, D., Haruka, I., Kagashi, Y., & Tsuda, S. (2016). 8-hydroxy-2'-deoxyguanosine as a biomarker of oxidative DNA damage induced by perfluorinated compounds in TK6 cells. *Environ Toxixol*, *31*(2), 192–200. PubMed PMID: 25113910.

24. Lu, C. Y., Ma, Y. C., Lin, J. M., et al. (2007). Oxidative stress associated with indoor air pollution and sick building syndrome-related symptoms among office workers in Taiwan. *Inhalation Toxicology*, *19*(1), 57–65. PubMed PMID: 17127643.

25. Middaugh, D. A., Pinney, S. M., & Linz, D. H. (1992). Sick building syndrome. Medical evaluation of two work forces. *Journal of Occupational Medicine*, *34*(12), 1197–1203. PubMed PMID: 1464788.

26. Seppänen, O., & Fisk, W. J. (2002). Association of ventilation system type with SBS symptoms in office workers. *Indoor Air*, *12*(2), 98–112. Review. PubMed PMID: 12216473.

27. Wolkoff, P., Wilkins, C. K., Clausen, P. A., & Nielsen, G. D. (2006). Organic compounds in office environments – sensory irritation, odor, measurements and the role of reactive chemistry. *Indoor Air*, *16*(1), 7–19. Review. PubMed PMID: 16420493.

28. Straus, D. C. (2009). Molds, mycotoxins, and sick building syndrome. *Toxicology and Industrial Health*, 25(9–10), 617–635. Review. doi:10.1177/0748233709348287. PubMed PMID: 19854820.

29. Ten Brinke, J., Selvin, S., Hodgson, A. T., et al. (1998). Development of new volatile organic compound (VOC) exposure metrics and their relationship to "Sick Building Syndrome" symptoms. *Indoor Air*, 8, 140–152.

30. Norbäck, D., Torgén, M., & Edling, C. (1990). Volatile organic compounds, respirable dust, and personal factors related to prevalence and incidence of sick building syndrome in primary schools. *British Journal of Industrial Medicine*, 47(11), 733–741. PubMed PMID: 2123116.

31. Kielb, C., Lin, S., Muscatiello, N., et al. (2015). Building-related health symptoms and classroom indoor air quality: a survey of school teachers in New York State. *Indoor Air*, 25(4), 371–380. PubMed PMID: 25196499.

32. Azuma, K., Ikeda, K., Kagi, N., Yanagi, U., & Osawa, H. (2015). Prevalence and risk factors associated with nonspecific building-related symptoms in office employees in Japan: relationships between work environment, Indoor Air Quality, and occupational stress. *Indoor Air*, 25(5), 499–511. PubMed PMID: 25244340.

33. Matsuoka, T., Takaki, A., Ohtaki, H., & Shioda, S. (2010). Early changes to oxidative stress levels following exposure to formaldehyde in ICR mice. *The Journal of Toxicological Sciences*, 35(5), 721–730. PubMed PMID: 20930466.

34. Chang, F. K., Mao, I. F., Chen, M. L., & Cheng, S. F. (2011). Urinary 8-hydroxydeoxyguanosine as a biomarker of oxidative DNA damage in workers exposed to ethylbenzene. *The Annals of Occupational Hygiene*, 55(5), 519–525. PubMed PMID: 21430133.

35. Toraason, M., Clark, J., Dankovic, D., et al. (1999). Oxidative stress and DNA damage in Fischer rats following acute exposure to trichloroethylene or perchloroethylene. *Toxicology*, 138(1), 43–53. PubMed PMID: 10566590.

36. Franken, C., Koppen, G., Lambrechts, N., et al. (2017). Environmental exposure to human carcinogens in teenagers and the association with DNA damage. *Environmental Research*, 152, 165–174. PubMed PMID: 27771571.

37. Huang, M., Choi, S. J., Kim, D. W., et al. (2009). Risk assessment of low-level cadmium and arsenic on the kidney. *Journal of Toxicology and Environmental Health. Part A*, 72(21–22), 1493–1498. PubMed PMID: 20077223.

38. Hong, Y. C., Oh, S. Y., Kwon, S. O., Park, M. S., Kim, H., Leem, J. H., et al. (2013). Blood lead level modifies the association between dietary antioxidants and oxidative stress in an urban adult population. *The British Journal of Nutrition*, 109(1), 148–154. PubMed PMID: 22464667.

39. Roy, A., Queirolo, E., Peregalli, F., Mañay, N., Martínez, G., & Kordas, K. (2015). Association of blood lead levels with urinary F_2-8α isoprostane and 8-hydroxy-2-deoxy-guanosine concentrations in first-grade Uruguayan children. *Environmental Research*, 140, 127–135. PubMed PMID: 25863186.

40. Chen, C., Qu, L., Li, B., Xing, L., Jia, G., Wang, T., et al. (2005). Increased oxidative DNA damage, as assessed by urinary 8-hydroxy-2′-deoxyguanosine concentrations, and serum redox status in persons exposed to mercury. *Clinical Chemistry*, 51(4), 759–767. PubMed PMID: 15695327.

41. Al-Saleh, I., Abduljabbar, M., Al-Rouqi, R., Elkhatib, R., Alshabbaheen, A., & Shinwari, N. (2013). Mercury (Hg) exposure in breast-fed infants and their mothers and the evidence of oxidative stress. *Biological Trace Element Research*, 153(1–3), 145–154. PubMed PMID: 23661328.

42. Al-Saleh, I., Al-Sedairi, Aa, & Elkhatib, R. (2012). Effect of mercury (Hg) dental amalgam fillings on renal and oxidative stress biomarkers in children. *The Science of the Total Environment*, 431, 188–196. PubMed PMID: 22683759.

43. Lee, K. M., Park, S. Y., Lee, K., et al. (2017). Pesticide metabolite and oxidative stress in male farmers exposed to pesticide. *Ann Occup Environ Med*, 29, 5. PubMed PMID: 28265414.

44. Ding, G., Han, S., Wang, P., et al. (2012). Increased levels of 8-hydroxy-2′-deoxyguanosine are attributable to organophosphate pesticide exposure among young children. *Environmental Pollution (Barking, Essex: 1987)*, 167, 110–114. PubMed PMID: 22561897.

45. Bernstam, L., & Nriagu, J. (2000). Molecular aspects of arsenic stress. *Journal of Toxicology and Environmental Health. Part B, Critical Reviews*, 3(4), 293–322. Review. PubMed PMID: 11055208.

46. Lambrou, A., Baccarelli, A., Wright, R. O., et al. (2012). Arsenic exposure and DNA methylation among elderly men. *Epidemiology (Cambridge, Mass.)*, 23(5), 668–676. PubMed PMID: 22833016.

47. Fujino, Y., Guo, X., Liu, J., et al. (2005). Japan Inner Mongolia Arsenic Pollution Study Group. Chronic arsenic exposure and urinary 8-hydroxy-2′-deoxyguanosine in an arsenic-affected area in Inner Mongolia, China. *Journal of Exposure Analysis and Environmental Epidemiology*, 15(2), 147–152. PubMed PMID: 15150536.

48. Biswas, J., Sinha, D., Mukherjee, S., Roy, S., Siddiqi, M., & Roy, M. (2010). Curcumin protects DNA damage in a chronically arsenic-exposed population of West Bengal. *Human and Experimental Toxicology, 29*(6), 513–524. PubMed PMID: 20056736.

49. Roy, M., Sinha, D., Mukherjee, S., & Biswas, J. (2011). Curcumin prevents DNA damage and enhances the repair potential in a chronically arsenic-exposed human population in West Bengal, India. *European Journal of Cancer Prevention, 20*(2), 123–131. PubMed PMID: 21332098.

50. Kuo, H. W., Chang, S. F., Wu, K. Y., & Wu, F. Y. (2003). Chromium (VI) induced oxidative damage to DNA: increase of urinary 8-hydroxydeoxyguanosine concentrations (8-OHdG) among electroplating workers. *Occupational and Environmental Medicine, 60*(8), 590–594. PubMed PMID: 12883020.

51. Warnholtz, A., Nickenig, G., Scholz, E., et al. (1999). Increased NADH-oxidase-mediated superoxide production in the early stages of atherosclerosis: evidence for involvement of the renin-angiotensin system. *Circulation, 99*(15), 2027–2033. PubMed PMID: 10209008.

52. Zalba, G., Beaumont, J., et al. (2000). Vascular oxidant stress: molecular mechanisms and pathophysiological implications. *Journal of Physiology and Biochemistry, 56*(1), 57–64. PubMed PMID: 10879682.

53. Martinet, W., Knaapen, M. W., DeMeyer, G. R., Herman, A. G., & Kockx, M. M. (2002). Elevated levels of oxidative DNA damage and DNA repair enzymes in human atherosclerotic plaques. *Circulation, 106*(8), 927–932. PubMed PMID: 12186795.

54. Martinet, W., Knaapen, M. W., et al. (2001). Oxidative DNA damage and repair in experimental atherosclerosis are reversed by dietary lipid lowering. *Circulation Research, 88*(7), 733–739. PubMed PMID: 11304497.

55. Ari, E., Kaya, Y., Demir, H., et al. (2011). Oxidative DNA damage correlates with carotid artery atherosclerosis in hemodialysis patients. *Hemodialysis International. International Symposium on Home Hemodialysis, 15*(4), 453–459. PubMed PMID: 22111813.

56. Xiang, F., Shuanglun, X., Jingfeng, W., et al. (2011). Association of serum 8-hydroxy-2'-deoxyguanosine levels with the presence and severity of coronary artery disease. *Coronary Artery Disease, 22*(4), 223–227. PubMed PMID: 21407076.

57. Ho, H. Y., Cheng, M. L., Chen, C. M., Gu, P. W., Wang, Y. L., Li, J. M., et al. (2008). Oxidative damage markers and antioxidants in patients with acute myocardial infarction and their clinical significance. *Biofactors (Oxford, England), 34*(2), 135–145. PubMed PMID: 19706979.

58. Di Minno, A., Turnu, L., Porro, B., et al. (2017). 8-hydroxy-2-deoxyguanosine levels and heart failure: a systematic review and meta-analysis of the literature. *Nutrition, Metabolism, and Cardiovascular Diseases, 27*(3), 201–208. PubMed PMID: 28065503.

59. Kroese, L. J., & Scheffer, P. G. (2014). 8-hydroxy-2'-deoxyguanosine and cardiovascular disease: a systematic review. *Current Atherosclerosis Reports, 16*(11), 452. PubMed PMID: 25252787.

60. Suzuki, S., Shishido, T., Ishino, M., et al. (2011). 8-hydroxy-2'-deoxyguanosine is a prognostic mediator for cardiac event. *European Journal of Clinical Investigation, 41*(7), 759–766. PubMed PMID: 21261617.

61. Kobayashi, S., Susa, T., Tanaka, T., et al. (2011). Urinary 8-hydroxy-2'-deoxyguanosine reflects symptomatic status and severity of systolic dysfunction in patients with chronic heart failure. *European Journal of Heart Failure, 13*(1), 29–36. PubMed PMID: 20965876.

62. Susa, T., Kobayashi, S., Tanaka, T., et al. (2012). Urinary 8-hydroxy-2'-deoxyguanosine as a novel biomarker for predicting cardiac events and evaluating the effectiveness of carvedilol treatment in patients with chronic systolic heart failure. *Circulation Journal, 76*(1), 117–126. PubMed PMID: 22008315.

63. Poulsen, H. E., Prieme, H., & Loft, S. (1998). Role of oxidative DNA damage in cancer initiation and promotion. *European Journal of Cancer Prevention, 7*(1), 9–16. PubMed PMID: 9511847.

64. Toyokuni, S., Okamoto, K., Yodoi, J., & Hiai, H. (1995). Persistent oxidative stress in cancer. *FEBS Letters, 358*(1), 1–3. PubMed PMID: 7821417.

65. Loft, S., Olsen, A., Møller, P., et al. (2013). Association between 8-oxo-7,8-dihydro-2'-deoxyguanosine excretion and risk of postmenopausal breast cancer: nested case-control study. *Cancer Epidemiology, Biomarkers and Prevention: A Publication of the American Association for Cancer Research, Cosponsored by the American Society of Preventive Oncology, 22*(7), 1289–1296. PubMed PMID: 23658396.

66. Foksinski, M., Kotzbach, R., Szymanski, W., & Olinski, R. (2000). The level of typical biomarker of oxidative stress 8-hydroxy-2'-deoxyguanosine is higher in uterine myomas than in control tissues and correlates with the size of the tumor. *Free Radical Biology & Medicine, 29*(7), 597–601. PubMed PMID: 11033411.

67. Miyake, H., Hara, I., Kamidono, S., & Eto, H. (2004). Prognostic significance of oxidative DNA damage evaluated by 8-hydroxy-2'-deoxyguanosine in patients undergoing radical nephrectomy for renal cell carcinoma. *Urology, 64*(5), 1057–1061. PubMed PMID: 15533518.

68. Erhola, M., Toyokuni, S., et al. (1997). Biomarker evidence of DNA oxidation in lung cancer patients: association of urinary 8-hydroxy-2'-deoxyguanosine excretion with radiotherapy, chemotherapy, and response to treatment. *FEBS Letters*, 409(2), 287–291. PubMed PMID: 9202163.

69. Soini, Y., Haapasaari, K. M., Vaarala, M. H., et al. (2011). 8-hydroxydeguanosine and nitrotyrosine are prognostic factors in urinary bladder carcinoma. *International Journal of Clinical and Experimental Pathology*, 4(3), 267–275. PubMed PMID: 21487522.

70. Miyake, H., Hara, I., Kamidono, S., & Eto, H. (2004). Oxidative DNA damage in patients with prostate cancer and its response to treatment. *The Journal of Urology*, 171(4), 1533–1536. PubMed PMID: 15017214.

71. Pylväs, M., Puistola, U., Laatio, L., et al. (2011). Elevated serum 8-OHdG is associated with poor prognosis in epithelial ovarian cancer. *Anticancer Research*, 31(4), 1411–1415. PubMed PMID: 21508394.

72. Huang, Y. J., Zhang, B. B., Ma, N., et al. (2011). Nitrative and oxidative DNA damage as potential survival biomarkers for nasopharyngeal carcinoma. *Medical Oncology*, 28(1), 377–384. PubMed PMID: 20339958.

73. Zhou, F. L., Zhang, W. G., Wei, Y. C., et al. (2010). Involvement of oxidative stress in the relapse of acute myeloid leukemia. *The Journal of Biological Chemistry*, 285(20), 15010–15015. PubMed PMID: 20233720.

74. Chang, C. S., Chen, W. N., Lin, H. H., et al. (2004). Increased oxidative DNA damage, inducible nitric oxide synthase, nuclear factor kappaB expression and enhanced antiapoptosis-related proteins in Helicobacter pylori-infected non-cardiac gastric adenocarcinoma. *World Journal of Gastroenterology*, 10(15), 2232–2240. PubMed PMID: 15259072.

75. Bonnefont-Rousselot, D. (2002). Glucose and reactive oxygen species. *Current Opinion in Clinical Nutrition and Metabolic Care*, 5(5), 561–568. PubMed PMID: 12172481.

76. Negishi, H., Ikeda, K., et al. (2001). The relation of oxidative DNA damage to hypertension and other cardiovascular risk factors in Tanzania. *Journal of Hypertension*, 19(3 Pt. 2), 529–533. PubMed PMID: 11327625.

77. Xu, G. W., Yao, Q. H., Weng, Q. F., Su, B. L., Zhang, X., & Xiong, J. H. (2004). Study of urinary 8-hydroxydeoxyguanosine as a biomarker of oxidative DNA damage in diabetic nephropathy patients. *Journal of Pharmaceutical and Biomedical Analysis*, 36(1), 101–104. PubMed PMID: 15351053.

78. Hinokio, Y., Suzuki, S., Hirai, M., et al. (2002). Urinary excretion of 8-oxo-7,8-dihydro-2'-deoxyguanosine as a predictor of the development of diabetic nephropathy. *Diabetologia*, 45(6), 877–882. PubMed PMID: 12107732.

79. Kanauchi, M., Nishioka, H., & Hashimoto, T. (2002). Oxidative DNA damage and tubulointerstitial injury in diabetic nephropathy. *Nephron*, 91(2), 327–329. PubMed PMID: 12053073.

80. Pan, H. Z., Chang, D., Feng, L. G., Xu, F. J., Kuang, H. Y., & Lu, M. J. (2007). Oxidative damage to DNA and its relationship with diabetic complications. *Biomedical and Environmental Sciences*, 20(2), 160–163. PubMed PMID: 17624192.

81. Chen, C. M., Lin Chen, C. Y., et al. (2008). Consumption of sweet potato leaves decreases lipid peroxidation and DNA damage in humans. *Asia Pacific Journal of Clinical Nutrition*, 17(3), 408–414. PubMed PMID: 18818160.

82. Mitjavila, M. T., Fandos, M., Salas-Salvadó, J., et al. (2013). The Mediterranean diet improves the systemic lipid and DNA oxidative damage in metabolic syndrome individuals. A randomized, controlled, trial. *Clinical Nutrition: Official Journal of the European Society of Parenteral and Enteral Nutrition*, 32(2), 172–178. PubMed PMID: 22999065.

83. Cocate, P. G., Natali, A. J., et al. (2014). Fruit and vegetable intake and related nutrients are associated with oxidative stress markers in middle-aged men. *Nutrition*, 30(6), 660–665. PubMed PMID: 24631385.

84. Pedret, A., Valls, R. M., Fernández-Castillejo, S., et al. (2012). Polyphenol-rich foods exhibit DNA antioxidative properties and protect the glutathione system in healthy subjects. *Molecular Nutrition & Food Research*, 56(7), 1025–1033. PubMed PMID: 22760977.

85. Barcelos, G. R., Grotto, D., Serpeloni, J. M., et al. (2011). Protective properties of quercetin against DNA damage and oxidative stress induced by methylmercury in rats. *Archives of Toxicology*, 85(9), 1151–1157. PubMed PMID: 21286687.

86. Thompson, H. J., Heimendinger, J., Haegele, A., et al. (1999). Effect of increased vegetable and fruit consumption on markers of oxidative cellular damage. *Carcinogenesis*, 20(12), 2261–2266. PubMed PMID: 10590217.

87. Qian, G., Xue, K., Tang, L., et al. (2012). Mitigation of oxidative damage by green tea polyphenols and Tai Chi exercise in postmenopausal women with osteopenia. *PLoS ONE*, 7(10), e48090. PubMed PMID: 23118932.

88. Niklowitz, P., Sonnenschein, A., et al. (2007). Enrichment of coenzyme Q10 in plasma and blood cells: defense against oxidative damage. *International Journal*

of Biological Sciences, 3(4), 257–262. PubMed PMID: 17479158.

89. Kowluru, R. A., & Kanwar, M. (2007). Effects of curcumin on retinal oxidative stress and inflammation in diabetes. *Nutrition & Metabolism [electronic resource], 4*, 8. PubMed PMID: 17437639.

90. Devaraj, S., Mathur, S., Basu, A., et al. (2008). A dose-response study on the effects of purified lycopene supplementation on biomarkers of oxidative stress. *Journal of the American College of Nutrition, 27*(2), 267–273. PubMed PMID: 18689558.

91. Hakim, I. A., Harris, R. B., Brown, S., et al. (2003). Effect of increased tea consumption on oxidative DNA damage among smokers: a randomized controlled study. *The Journal of Nutrition, 133*(10), 3303S–3309S. PubMed PMID: 14519830.

92. Kato, J., Kobune, M., et al. (2001). Normalization of elevated hepatic 8-hydroxy-2'-deoxyguanosine levels in chronic hepatitis C patients by phlebotomy and low iron diet. *Cancer Research, 61*(24), 8697–8702. PubMed PMID: 11751387.

Biotransformation and Elimination

SUMMARY

- Benefits: Breakdown and excretion of xenobiotic pollutants
- Primary mechanisms: Phase 1 and 2 biotransformation and phase 3 excretion
- Best interventions: High-protein, low-carb ohydrate diet, liposomal glutathione (GSH), magnesium, healthy microbiome, Mediterranean diet, Brassica family foods, curcumin, rooibos, green tea, N-acetyl cysteine, exercise
- Best measure: Case history

After entry to the body, most xenobiotic compounds undergo molecular changes, called *biotransformation*, before excretion from the body. Compounds that are lipid soluble are changed into more water-soluble molecules for easier excretion. However, for highly lipophilic compounds like persistent organic pollutants (POPs), this is largely unsuccessful; hence their persistence. Most of these processes occur in the liver, but all tissues, especially those that interface with the environment, have varying levels of the toxicant-metabolizing enzymes.

Biotransformation processes have been divided into two major phases (Fig. 56.1).

Phase 1: Functionalization, during which compounds are either completely neutralized (like caffeine by CYP1A2) or converted to more or less potent metabolites to facilitate phase 2 conjugation. This phase is inducible and typically responsible for the half-life ($t_{1/2}$) of most endogenous and exogenous compounds in the bloodstream.

Phase 2: Conjugation of metabolites—sometimes called "activated intermediates"—produced by phase 1 with endogenous molecules to become generally less toxic, more water soluble, and more easily excreted from the body (phase 3). Compounds going through methylation or acetylation attain some water solubility, whereas those going through glucuronidation, sulfonation, GSH conjugation, and amino acid conjugation are markedly more water-soluble.

The enzymes most responsible for phase 1 and to some degree in phase 2 can have their activity either induced or inhibited by environmental factors and can be polymorphic as well. A number of the enzymes are found to have single nucleotide polymorphisms (SNPs), which can either enhance or suppress their activity. Others, like the GSH transferase family, are prone to copy number variations (CNVs), which result in either a complete deletion of the gene or only one of the two being present. Finally, nutritional status, the condition of the microbiome, the levels of lipopolysaccharides present in the hepatic portal circulation, and the presence of various botanical and dietary flavonoids can also affect the activity of the biotransformation enzymes.

667

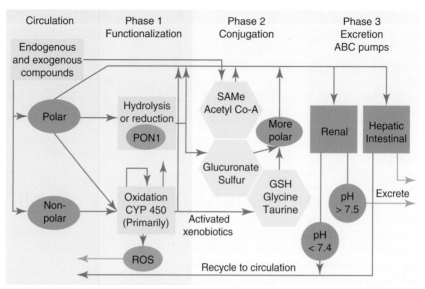

FIG. 56.1 Simplistic overview of biotransformation and elimination processes.

It is also important to note that although all xenobiotics have an optimal phase 1 and/or phase 2 enzymes that rapidly and safely processes them in large volume, several backup biotransformation pathways can also accommodate them. This is exemplified in Fig. 56.2, which shows the biotransformation pathways for toluene humans. In this figure, the arrows denote the pathways with the greatest ability to rapidly metabolize toluene. This high-volume pathway requires three phase 1 enzymes, first with cytochrome P450 (CYP), then both alcohol and aldehyde dehydrogenases, and then preferential conjugation with glycine to form hippuric acid. However, toluene can also be conjugated through GSH transferases, glucuronyl transferases, and N-acetyl transferases if the need arises.

FUNCTIONALIZATION (PHASE 1)

In phase 1, compounds undergo oxidation, reduction, or hydrolysis, attaching a functional group such as an –OH or an –O to compounds that are not already water soluble. The metabolites of phase 1 may be detoxified, undergo more phase 1 processes, be moved into the blood for use or excretion, be eliminated into the bile, or moved onto phase 2 for conjugation. The bulk of xenobiotic compounds undergo oxidation, with 90% being acted on by CYP-450 enzymes. Some compounds, like organophosphate pesticides (OP), are acted on by more than

one phase 1 process. OPs are initially activated into their more neurotoxic form by CYP3A4[1] and then inactivated through hydrolysis by paraoxonase (PON) 1. They do not require any phase 2 processing, because they are not lipophilic compounds. Table 56.1 provides an abbreviated list of phase 1 enzymes that facilitate the hydrolysis, reduction, or oxidation of commonly encountered toxicants.

Most xenobiotic compounds undergo oxidative biotransformation by one or more of three families of CYP-450 enzymes, CYP1, CYP2, and CYP3. Other families of CYPs are present in humans and are critical for health but do not affect toxic pollutants. These families are further divided by letters and numbers based on their preferred substrates and activations.

CYP-450 enzymes are found in high levels in all tissues that are first to contact xenobiotic pollutants (small intestines and the respiratory tract). CYPs in the small intestine begin the biotransformation of all xenobiotics that enter the body orally, known as *first-pass metabolism.* CYP3A4 comprises 80% of the total CYP content in the small intestines making it primarily responsible for all first-pass metabolism. This first-pass metabolism reduces the amount of many oral pharmaceutical agents entering circulation, especially those metabolized by CYP3A4.

The highest concentrations of xenobiotic-metabolizing enzymes are found in the liver and kidney, which are

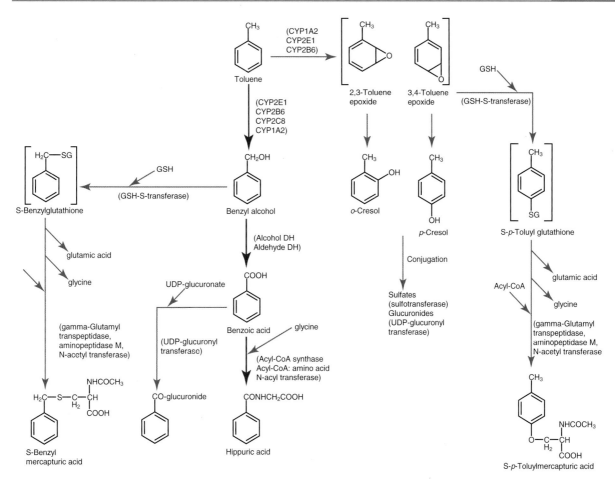

Proposed enzymes are noted in parentheses.

Sources: Angerer et al. 1998a; IARC 1999; Nakajima and Wang 1994; Nakajima et al. 1997; Tassaneeyakul et al. 1996

FIG. 56.2 Biotransformation of toluene in humans. (From Agency for Toxic Substances and Disease Registry. [2017]. *Toxicological profile for toluene.* Retrieved from https://www.atsdr.cdc.gov/toxprofiles/tp.asp?id=161&tid=29. Accessed 2 April 2018)

TABLE 56.1   Examples of Some of the Phase 1 Reactions Pertinent to Xenobiotics

Reaction	Enzyme	Function
Hydrolysis	Butyrylcholinesterase	Metabolizes aspirin, heroin, cocaine, etc.
	Paraoxonases (in plasma)	Detoxify organophosphate pesticides and act as antioxidants
	β-glucuronidase (in intestines)	Promotes enterohepatic recirculation of xenobiotic glucuronides
	Epoxide hydrolase	Metabolizes and detoxifies carcinogenic PAH metabolites
Reduction	Quinone reductase	Protects bone marrow from benzene damage, detoxifies vehicular exhaust
Oxidation	Alcohol dehydrogenase	Metabolizes alcohol into aldehyde
	Aldehyde dehydrogenase	Detoxifies aldehydes
	Cytochrome P450s	Anabolic and catabolic action on endogenous and exogenous compounds

---

BOX 56.1   **Requirements for CYP-P450 Oxidation**

1. CYP-450 enzymes
2. NADPH or NADH cytochrome P450 reductase
   a. NADPH
   b. Magnesium
   c. Niacin
3. Cytochrome b5 reductase
4. Oxygen
5. Intact phospholipid matrix
6. ATP

COMPOUNDS MADE MORE TOXIC BY PHASE 1

Acetaminophen
Aldrin
Aflatoxin B
Benzene
Benzopyrene
Cyclohexane
Heptachlor
Hexane
Saffrole
Styrene
Trichloroethylene
Vinyl chloride
Hexane

---

tasked with cleaning the blood. Hepatic CYP enzymes are primarily responsible for the normal $t_{1/2}$ of all chemical compounds in the bloodstream. In addition to the proper substrate and the proper CYP-450 enzyme, two different cytochrome reductases are needed along with nicotinamide adenine dinucleotide phosphate (NADPH), oxygen, an intact phospholipid membrane, and adenosine triphosphate (ATP) (Box 56.1).

Nutrition deficiencies and pollutant burden can easily affect the efficacy of CYP oxidation. Protein deficiency has long been linked to reduced hepatic levels of CYP-450, NADPH-cytochrome P450 reductase, cytochrome b5 reductase, hepatic GSH stores, an longer $t_{1/2}$ for a variety of compounds.[2,3,4,5] Protein deficiency predisposes to increased toxicity from malathion and hexachlorocyclohexane.[6] A high-carbohydrate, low-protein diet also inhibits drug metabolism.[7,8] In fact, a high sugar diet inhibits phase 1 drug clearance as effectively as cimetidine, a known CYP inhibitor.[9] Magnesium deficiency is associated with reduced levels of CYP-450, NADPH cytochrome reductase, and decreased biotransformation of aniline and aminopyrene.[10,11,12,13] ATP levels, vital for phases 1, 2, and 3, are often reduced by toxic xenobiotics (see Chapter 45).

All oxidation by CYP-450 enzymes produces oxygen radicals that will then need to be quenched to prevent increased oxidative stress. Some of these enzymes also produce metabolites that are more toxic than the parent compound. OPs are transformed by CYP3A4 into the oxon form, which is three times as toxic.[14] The common polycyclic aromatic hydrocarbon (PAH) benzo(a)pyrene, found in vehicular exhaust and cigarette smoke, is oxidized by the CYP1 series, forming the ultimate carcinogen benzo(a)pyrene 7,8-dihydrodiol-9,10-epoxide.[15]

CYP1A1, CYP1A2, and CYP1B1 act on PAHs from combustion. CYP1A1 is also found in the placenta, and when this enzyme is induced, it can increase the risk of preterm delivery.[16]

CYP2E1 metabolizes benzene, styrene, xylene, toluene, ethers, trichloroethylene, chloroform, CCL4, acetone, acetaminophen, methyl tert-butyl ethers, alcohols, halogenated anesthetics, fluoxetine, sulfadiazine, theophylline, and nitrosamines

CYP3A4 is the predominant CYP in the human liver, accounting for about 30% of total hepatic P450 content in liver microsomes.[17] This enzyme is responsible for metabolism of steroid hormones, immunosuppressants, and 25% of conventional drugs, such as cytotoxic agents and calcium-channel blockers.

Induction (Upregulation)

Consistent high exposure to CYP substrates can induce both specific and overall CYP function. The inducers, for the most part, are substrates of the CYP family that they induce (Table 56.2). For example, the aromatic hydrocarbons are metabolized by the CYP1 family for which they are powerful inducers.

CYP1A1 has a common SNP present in 33% of all Asians, 23% of African Americans, and 7% to 14% of whites, resulting in increased induction by PAHs.[18] Because PAHs going through CYP1A are made into carcinogenic epoxides, persons with this SNP have more DNA mutations and higher rates of lung cancer, especially when they also have a deletion of glutathione transferase (GST) M1.[19,20] Women with this SNP who had higher serum

TABLE 56.2 Common Inducers of CYP-450 Families		
CYP1	**CYP2**	**CYP3A4**
Benzopyrene	Phenobarbital	PCBs
3-methylcholanthrine	Phenytoin	Phthalates
Naphthoflavone	Carbamazepine	Glucocorticoids
2,3,7,8-TCDD	Ethanol	Pregnenolone
Chlorinated compounds		DHEA
Sulforaphanes (Brassica)		St. John's wort
		Multiple pharmaceuticals

From Tirona, R. G., & Kim, R. B. (2005). Nuclear receptors and drug disposition gene regulation. *Journal of Pharmaceutical Sciences, 94*(6), 1169–1186; Penning, T. M., & Drury, J. E. (2007). Human aldo-keto reductases: Function, gene regulation, and single nucleotide polymorphisms. *Archives of Biochemistry and Biophysics, 464*(2), 241–250.

levels of polychlorinated biphenyls (PCBs), also inducers of CYP1 series, have higher risks for breast cancer.[21]

Induction is mediated by a number of xenosensor receptors, including aryl hydrocarbon (AH), that stimulate epigenetic upregulation. This process takes time and requires regular and repeated exposure to the inducer. The induction of CYP3A4 is also typically accompanied by induction of CYP2A6, CYP2B6, CYP2C8, CYP2C9, and CYP2C19.

Inhibition (Downregulation)

Whereas upregulation requires consistent repeated exposure to an inducer over time, inhibition can occur with a single exposure. Inhibition of CYP function occurs from toxicants, trauma, endotoxicity, pharmaceutical agents, and flavonoids.

Mercury, lead, cadmium, and tributyl tin all reduce total hepatic CYP levels.[22,23,24,25,26] The four sulfhydryl-binding heavy metals, Pb, As, Hg, and Cd, also dose-dependently decreased PAH-stimulated induction of CYP1A1 and CYP1A2.[27] A number of OPs and the herbicide glyphosate are able to reduce the function of multiple CYP enzymes by more than 90%.[28] Trauma leads to a selective reduction of certain CYP 450s, and postsurgery patients are found to have 35% to 75% lower CYP function.[29,30]

A vast number of commonly used pharmaceutical agents, including antidepressants, antibiotics, oral contraceptives, antifungals, antihistamines, cardiovascular medication, proton pump inhibitors, H2 blockers, and many others, are potent inhibitors of hepatic CYP enzymes.[31] Cimetidine binds the heme molecule, causing nonspecific inhibition of all CYP isoforms.[32] The combined use of medications that inhibit CYP function can lead to serious problems. Individuals who were taking

BOX 56.2 Hepatic CYP-P450 Inhibitors	
Lipopolysaccharides	Glyphosate
Inflammation	Pharmaceuticals
Metals	Trauma
Pesticides	

a CYP3A4 inhibitor such as diltiazem, verapamil, or nitroimidazole at the same time they were taking erythromycin had a fivefold higher risk of sudden death.[33] For a full list of pharmaceutical inhibitors, inducers, and substrates, see http://medicine.iupui.edu/clinpharm/ddis/main-table/.

Several naturally occurring flavonoids are inhibitors of small intestinal CYP3A4 activity but do not appear to reduce hepatic CYP function. Grapefruit juice containing the furanocoumarins bergamottin, dihydroxybergamottin, and naringenin reduce intestinal 3A4.[34,35] The inhibition of intestinal 3A4 appears to be fairly complete and takes 3 days to recover from (after a single dose of 300 mL of single-strength grapefruit juice).[36] Grapefruit juice appears to have no effect on hepatic 3A4 activity, except when given in exceptionally high doses (three glasses of double-strength grapefruit juice daily for 3 days).[37,38] A very small dose of 2 mL of pomegranate juice inhibited intestinal 3A4, but showed no effect on hepatic 3A4.[39] Red wine also has some inhibition of intestinal 3A4 but not to the same extent as grapefruit juice.[40] Intestinal inhibition of CYP3A4 would lead to increased absorption of any drugs that are metabolized by that enzyme, resulting either in a reduction of the amount needed or a potential overdose.

Box 56.2 lists hepatic CYP inhibitors. Lipopolysaccharides (LPSs) and inflammation have both been shown to reduce hepatic CYP amount and activity.[41,42] LPSs are potent inducers of inflammation stimulating increased production of interleukin 6 (IL-6) and tumor necrosis factor (TNF)-α. Both TNF-α and LPS reduce CYP1A1, CYP2E1, and CYP3A2.[43] At the same time, the activity of NADPH-cytochrome c reductase and cytochrome b5 are also reduced, affecting all CYP oxidation processes.[44] However, LPSs are also able to reduce CYP levels independent of TNF-α.[45] Fortunately the inhibiting effects of LPS on 2E1 can be significantly reversed, and the inhibiting effect on 3A2 are fully blocked by curcumin (*Curcuma longa*).[46] Melatonin (10 mg/kg) was also shown to block the effect of LPS on hepatic CYP3A function and increase hepatic GSH levels.[47] Interestingly a maternal high-fat diet resulting in a higher endotoxin load has been associated with reduced hepatic CYP3A in the woman's offspring.[48]

Paraoxonase

PONs are important phase 1 enzymes with powerful antioxidant activity critical for health (Box 56.3). PONs are calcium-dependent enzymes containing a sulfhydryl (-SH) group, which renders them prone to inactivation by mercury, lead, cadmium, and arsenic.[49] Three different PONs are found in humans: PON1, which is critical in preventing neurotoxicity from OPs[50]; PON2; and PON3. PON1 is produced by the liver and then released into the plasma, where it is picked up by the HDL and carried through the body. PON1 is a powerful antioxidant enzyme and provides the HDL-associated cardiovascular protective action of quenching oxidized LDL.[51] PON1 levels and activity are directly linked to the degree of cardiovascular risk and atherosclerosis in an individual.[52] PON2 is mainly present in the mitochondria, where it is bound to Coenzyme Q_{10} and provides antioxidant protection to the mitochondrion.[53] PON3 is present in the liver, kidney, and plasma, where it catalyzes the hydrolysis of lovastatin and simvastatin.

Children younger than 2 years have lower levels of PON1 and are therefore more susceptible to the adverse effects of organophosphates.[54] Reduced PON1 activity is found in people with cardiovascular illness, type 1 and type 2 diabetes, and liver disorders, all of which are associated with toxicant overload.[55,56,57,58] The main cardioprotective actions of PON1, besides its powerful antioxidant ability, include both antiinflammatory and antifibrinolytic action.[59] HDL rich in PON1 can completely inhibit atheroma stimulation by LDL through blockage of monocyte chemotactic protein- 1. PON1 also prevents tissue damage from the superoxide radical and helps maintain GSH levels. PON1 is prone to polymorphic changes at positions 55 and 192, which can alter its function dramatically.[60]

Individuals with reduced PON1 function are at increased risk for neurotoxic damage from OPs and can develop neurological disorders strongly associated with neuroinflammation.[61] Individuals with either the PON1-192 G/A or G/G polymorphisms (both of which result in reduced activity) were more prone to neurotoxic effects of organophosphates than those with the same exposure who had experienced a traumatic brain injury.[62] Children with low PON1 activity who are residentially exposed to OPs are up to three times more likely to develop brain tumors.[63,64]

Although B-cell malignancies are already linked with environmental toxicants, individuals with the PON1-192 G/G (lowest activity) can have a fourfold increased risk of developing lymphoma.[65] Those with the PON1-55 M/M variant who were exposed to organophosphates were more than twice as likely to develop Parkinson's disease.[66] Reduced PON1 activity has also been linked to the development of dementia and Alzheimer's disease.[67,68] In fact, Mini Mental State Examination (MMSE) results show a positive correlation with PON activity. Low PON activity has also been associated with depression and bipolar disorders.[69]

Low PON1 activity predisposed sheep farmers exposed to OPs to develop a diffuse set of symptoms that evaded normal means of diagnosis until being labeled "dipper's

---

BOX 56.3   Paraoxonase and Health

- Two common function-reducing SNPs (192 and 55) increase risk for:
  - Cardiovascular disease
  - Diabetes
  - Parkinson's disease
  - Alzheimer's disease
  - Dementia
  - Neurotoxicity from pesticides
  - Childhood brain tumors
  - B-cell malignancies
- Paraoxonase detoxifies organophosphate pesticides
- Paraoxonase has antioxidant, antiinflammatory, and antifibrinolytic activity

TABLE 56.3 Pharmaceutical Agents That Reduce PON1 Activity

Anesthetics	Antibiotics	Antiseizure	Anticancer	Cardiovascular
Propofol	Teicoplanin	Carbamazepine	Cetuximab	Digoxin
Etomidate	Rifamycin	Valproic acid	Paclitaxel	Methylprednisolone
Ketamine	Tobramycin		Etoposide	Amiodarone
	Ceftriaxone Na		Docetaxel	Verapamil
	Cefuroxime Na		Ifosfamide	Dobutamine
	Ceftazidime			Metoprolol
	Ornidazole			Diltiazem
	Amikacin sulf.			Nifedipine
	Oxytetracycline			Nitrendipine
	Lincomycin			Isradipine
	Clindamycin			Amlodipine
	Streptomycin			
	Sulfonamides			

BOX 56.4 Enhancing PON1 Activity (Even With Low-Activity Single Nucleotide Polymorphisms)

Exercise	Anthocyans
Mediterranean diet	Quercitin
Olive oil	Walnuts
Fish oil	Aspirin
Coconut oil	

flu."[70,71,72] PON1 polymorphisms also increase an individual's risk for becoming chemically reactive to ambient levels of everyday compounds.[73]

In addition to SNPs and metals, reduced PON1 activity can be caused by a high-fat diet and a number of pharmaceutical agents, including several cardiovascular medicines (Table 56.3).[74,75,76,77,78,79,80]

A number of diet and lifestyle factors already associated with reducing cardiovascular risk increase PON1 activity, even in those with a low PON1 genotype, as summarized in Box 56.4. Regular aerobic and anaerobic exercise both increase PON1 activity.[81,82] The Mediterranean diet, long known to reduce cardiovascular risk,[83] also improves PON1 activity.[84] Fish oil, present in a Mediterranean diet from fish, has been shown to improve PON1 activity by itself.[85] Olive oil, another prime component of this diet, increases PON activity as well.[86] Anthocyans, the dark pigment in grapes, wine, and berries, has also demonstrated the ability to boost PON1 activity.[87,88] Quercetin,[89] high in

onions, walnuts,[90] and coconut oil,[91] are also effective in boosting the activity of this important enzyme. Interestingly, acetylsalicylic acid, commonly recommended to be taken daily for prevention of a heart attack, also increases PON1 activity (Table 56.4).[92]

CONJUGATION (PHASE 2)

Conjugation transforms xenobiotics to more polar compounds by the addition of a sulfur compound, certain amino acids, GSH, or a glucoronate. The addition of an acetyl or methyl group typically renders the compound nontoxic and allows for elimination as well. Most of these conjugations are done enzymatically and require energy in the form of ATP.

Acetylation

- Genetically rapid—increased cancer risk
- Genetically slow—increase autoimmunity risk

N-acetyl transferase (NAT) is one of the major enzymes in human breast tissue that help neutralize PAHs from cigarette smoke, air pollution, and well-done meat. NATs are also present in the liver and intestines and are commonly polymorphic, resulting in either increased (generally NAT1) or decreased (generally NAT2) activity. The two most common and health-affecting NAT1 SNPs are NAT1*10 and NAT1*11. Women with the NAT1*10 allele had a 30% greater risk of developing breast cancer, whereas those with the NAT1*11 allele had a fourfold elevated risk. Those with the NAT1*11 allele who ate

TABLE 56.4 PON1 Levels (U/L), Total Oxidant Status (TOS), and Oxidized LDL in Persons Before and After Taking 100 mg/day or 150 mg/day ASA (Aspirin)

	ASA Dose	Before ASA	ASA–30 days	ASA–60 days
Paraoxonase U/L	100 mg/d	187.2	192.52	213.6
	150 mg/d	187.0	195.43	206.01
TOS- Umol H_2O_2 equiv/L	100 mg/d	12.59	10.93	10.26
	150 mg/d	14.59	11.61	10.25
Oxidized LDL ng/mL	100 mg/d	190.61	141.73	116.29
	150 mg/d	187.94	174.99	126.83

red meat increased their risk to 6.1, whereas the risk for smokers rose to 13.2.[93]

The two most common slow metabolizer alleles are NAT2 191A and NAT2 481T, which are found in 50% of the US population, 5% to 10% of the Japanese, and 90% in Mediterranean countries. NAT2 slow acetylators have lower incidence of colorectal cancer but higher incidence of bladder cancer that increases with the lifetime dose of tobacco smoke.[94] Persons with the NAT2 defective alleles were 6.96 times more likely to have been afflicted with Spanish toxic syndrome from cooking with rapeseed oil that had been denatured with 2% aniline (meant for industrial purposes but illegally refined and sold for home use).[95] The most common finding in those who survived the poisoning was chronic autoimmunity. Persons with systemic lupus erythematosus (SLE) are also far more likely to be genetically slow acetylators.[96]

Amino Acid Conjugation With Glycine, Taurine, or (Less Often) Glutamine

- Reduced conjugation of solvents can result in balance disorder, cognitive problems, and reactivity to solvents

The amino acid conjugation process is not commonly affected by SNPs or CNVs that alter its activity. Amino acid conjugation is a prime method by which solvents are cleared to hippuric acids. The bioavailability of the amino acids taurine, glycine, and glutamine is a rate-limiting factor for this pathway. Individuals who are exposed to higher levels of solvents daily can rapidly run out of available stores of glycine and taurine, forcing the solvents to seek a different conjugation pathway. Supplementation with glycine and taurine as part of a comprehensive supplement protocol often results in clinically identifiable improvements.

Glucuronidation

- Inhibited by a high-carb ohydrate, low-protein diet, elevated blood glucose, or insulin
- Induced by green tea and watercress
- Reversed by intestinal β-glucuronidase

Uridine 5'-diphospho (UDP)-glucuronyl transferase combines UDP-glucuronate (this rate-limiting compound is supplied by glycogenolysis) or UDP-glucose to a metabolite of phase 1. When glycogenolysis is inhibited by glucose, fructose, or insulin, glucuronidation is inhibited (Fig. 56.3).[97] Depletion of hepatic glycogen stores, as seen with endurance athletes and the use of cannabis, also inhibits glucuronidation. Interestingly, glucuronidation is inhibited by a high-carbohydrate, low-protein diet[98] and reduced calorie intake.[99] The most common SNP is a low-activity UGT1A1 that causes Gilbert's syndrome, characterized by hyperbilirubinemia.

Glucuronidation is the prime phase 2 pathway for endogenous compounds like bilirubin, estrone, testosterone, progesterone, and thyroxine. Glucuronidation has a high capacity for xenobiotics but a low affinity, so only a few exogenous compounds like tetrahydrocannabinol, some aromatic hydrocarbons, and carbamate pesticides are glucuronidated. Activity of glucuronylsulfotransferase is increased by watercress[100] and green tea.[101] However, the glucuronides produced by this pathway can be acted on by β-glucuronidases in the intestines, allowing hepatic recirculation of these compounds.

Glutathione Conjugation

- Prone to CNV in GSTM1 more than in GSTT1
  - Deletion of GSTs results in increased risk for multiple cancers, solvent neurotoxicity, allergy, and asthma from vehicular exhaust
- Needs GSH
- Induced by Brassica, curcumin, green tea, rooibos

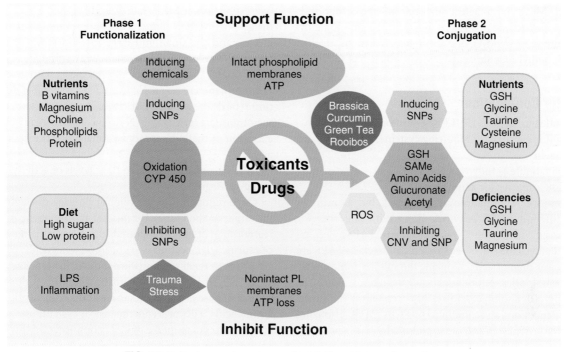

FIG. 56.3 Factors enhancing and inhibiting biotransformation.

GSH conjugation and amino acid conjugation are the primary phase 2 pathways for CYP-activated xenobiotics such as all PAHs, chlorinated products, and some solvents. Conjugation with GSH, typically mediated by transferases, forms mercapturic acids. This pathway requires sufficient GSH along with a functioning glutathione transferase (GST). There are four main GSTs that act on xenobiotic compounds, GSTM1, GSTT1, GSTP1, and GSTO1. GSTs are prone to CNVs; approximately 50% of whites 60% of Asians, and 30% of African Americans lack the GSTM1 gene.[18] GSTT1 is deleted in about 60% of Asians but only 20% of whites whereas GSTP1 is rarely null and GSTO1 never is. Fortunately, consumption of the Brassica family has been shown to enhance GST activity in persons with one of the null genotypes.[102] Several botanical compounds have also exhibited the ability to induce GST function, including curcumin,[103] green tea,[104] rosemary,[104] and rooibos.[105]

This pathway is also dependent on sufficient GSH, which has been shown to be depleted by all of the common pollutants, including mercury,[106] lead,[107] perfluorocarbons,[108] phthalates,[109] toluene and benzene,[110] PCBs,[111] chlorinated pesticides,[112] OPs,[113] particulate matter,[114] tobacco smoke,[115] and diesel exhaust particles.[116] GSH is also depleted by numerous pharmaceuticals, especially acetaminophen. Low GSH stores are also commonly found with aging, diabetes, cholestasis, alcoholic liver disease, cancer, neurodegenerative disease, and pulmonary fibrosis. GSH production is dependent on adequate cysteine levels and the proper function of the enzymes glutamate cysteine ligase (GCL) and glutathione synthase (GS),[117] a process dependent on sufficient cysteine, ATP, and magnesium.[118] Magnesium has been shown to replete GSH stores by itself.[119] GSH can also be repleted through reduction of oxidized glutathione (GSSG) by the enzyme GSH reductase.

Methylation

- S-adenosylmethionine (SAMe) is a required cofactor
- Can make arsenic more toxic or less toxic

Methylation is a common but minor pathway for xenobiotic clearance that actually decreases the polarity of some compounds. There are a number of methyl transferases, including catechol-O-methyltransferase (COMT), glycine-N-methyltransferase (GNMT), and arsenic (III) methyltransferase (AS3MT), all of which use SAMe as the cofactor. Inorganic arsenic compounds are methylated via AS3MT, resulting either in monomethyl arsenic acid (MMA), the most toxic form of arsenic, or dimethyl arsenic acid (DMA), which has far lower toxicity.

Sulfur Conjugation

- Sulfotransferases (SULT)—common SNPs
- Sulfonate cofactor requiring cysteine, vitamin C, and niacin
- Metabolite is fully water soluble
- Low capacity for xenobiotics

Xenobiotic sulfonation is catalyzed by a number of different SULT enzymes along with the cofactor 5-phosphoadenosine-5′-phosphosulfate (PAPS). Because cellular cysteine stores are limited, cell levels of PAPS are far lower than or GSH, reducing the sulfonation capacity for xenobiotics. Sulfonate conjugates are all nontoxic, highly water soluble, and readily excreted in the urine. SULT function can be inhibited by PCBs, PAHs, bisphenol A (BPA), triclosan, and other pollutants. SULTs have two common SNP variants:

SULT1A1: His (low-activity enzyme) was found in 41.6% of a study population.[120] Women with this variant have higher rates of breast cancer with increased estrogen exposure.

SULT1A1: Arg (normal activity level) showed increased rates of breast cancer with increased level of doneness of red meat.[121]

ROUTES OF EXCRETION (PHASE 3)

- Renal: ATP-binding cassette (ABC) family of membrane-bound efflux pumps
- Bile/intestinal: ABC family of membrane-bound efflux pumps
- GSH and ATP dependent
- Prone to both renal and hepatic recirculation

Once xenobiotic compounds have undergone transformation by phases 1 and 2, phase 3 is tasked with excreting these compounds from the body. The transport of chemical compounds across cell membranes is handled by protein pumps. Organic anion transporters (OAT) handle the transport of compounds into the cells, and the ABC transporters move compounds out. The primary ABC transporters for xenobiotic excretion are the GSH-dependent multidrug-resistant proteins (MRP) 1 to 5. MRPs pump chemicals out of cells, and overexpression of MRPs has caused resistance to certain drugs—hence their name. MRPs are found in the liver, kidney, and the small and large intestines, where they transport molecules conjugated with sulfonate, GSH, glucoronate, and taurine or glycine along with arsenic, cadmium, mercury, and platinum.[122,123,124,125] GSH depletion retards the action of MRPs, and repletion enhances their transport activity.[126,127] N-acetyl cysteine increases the excretion of methylmercury by renal MRP transporters as well.[128]

MRPs are polymorphic, so their levels of activity vary by up to 70-fold.[129]

Once pumped into the bile for passage through the intestines or the kidney tubules for release in the urine, reabsorption of these compounds can occur. All conjugates of taurine, glycine, and GSH become weak acids, which are prone to renal reabsorption if the urine is acidic (pH <7.4) (Fig. 56.4).[130,131] In the proximal tubules, γ-glutamyl transpeptidase is present to assist in the reabsorption of amino acids. This prevents the loss of cysteine and GSH and leads to the reuptake of GSH conjugates. In this area of the kidney, cadmium and lead are both reabsorbed and stored.

Compounds in the intestines that are still primarily lipophilic will be readily reabsorbed through some of the same ABC transporters, leading to hepatic recirculation.

With 94% to 97% of the bile being reabsorbed, most of the bile-bound xenobiotics undergo enterohepatic recirculation.[132] Compounds that have been ionized at intestinal pH are more likely to escape this recycling. Hepatic canalicular γ-glutamyl transpeptidase leads to a reuptake of GSH and GSH conjugates in this location as it does in the proximal tubules. Cholestasis results in retention and increased reabsorption of these compounds. Fecal clearance of lipophilic compounds can be stimulated by the consumption of nonabsorbable lipophilic substances (paraffin oil, rice bran fiber combined with cholestyramine and olestra).[133,134] Psyllium husks and cholestyramine also enhance increased fecal bile excretion.

Intestinal bacteria have metabolic actions that include reductases, hydrolase, demethylases, β-glucuronidases, and beta-glucosidases. PAHs are one class of compounds that are hydrolyzed and recirculated in a retoxified state. β-glucuronidases in the intestinal bacterial can deconjugate glucuronides and cause a release of carcinogenic aglycones and recirculation of estrogen.

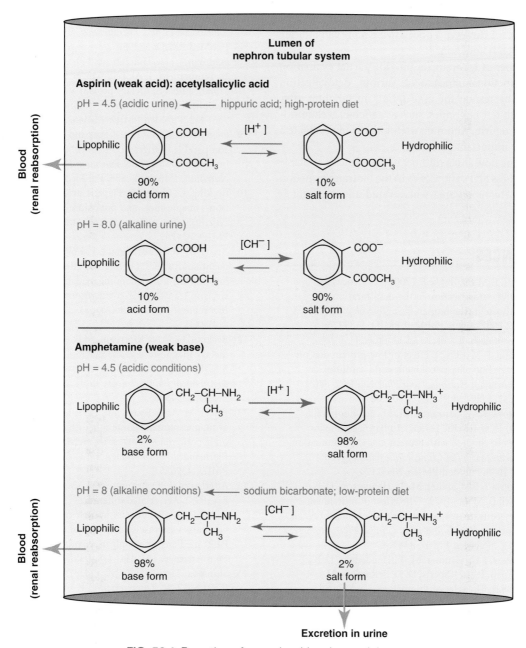

FIG. 56.4 Excretion of a weak acid and a weak base.

ASSESSMENT

A good case history will best identify individuals who have reduced biotransformation and excretion. Persons who need to take smaller doses of pharmaceuticals, because normal doses are too high, have inhibited phase 1 processes. Individuals who cannot consume caffeine in the afternoon without risking insomnia obviously have an inhibited CYP1A2. The erythromycin breath test can be used to assess CYP3A4 function,[135] and the caffeine clearance test can measure CYP1A2 activity.[136] Low HDL levels often indicate low PON1 activity, because HDL is the carrier for PON1, but currently no PON1 measurement is available.[61,62] However, a poor MMSE score can indicate reduced PON1 function.[72]

A number of laboratories provide partial evaluation of the functional efficacy of various detoxification pathways by testing for appropriate metabolites after dosing with test molecules, such as caffeine, acetaminophen, and aspirin. Although useful, they only evaluate a few of the important pathways.

There are now also a number of genetic tests available that can assess SNPs and CNVs in the biotransformation enzymes. This is an area where rapid advancement is expected.

REFERENCES

1. Buratti, F. M., & Testai, E. (2007). Evidences for CYP3A4 autoactivation in the desulfuration of dimethoate by the human liver. *Toxicology*, *241*(1–2), 33–46, 2007. Aug 6, PubMed PMID: 17897769.

2. El-Demerdash, E., Ali, A. A., El-Taher, D. E., & Hamada, F. M. (2012). Effect of low-protein diet on anthracycline pharmacokinetics and cardiotoxicity. *The Journal of Pharmacy and Pharmacology*, *64*(3), 344–352. PubMed PMID: 22309266.

3. Oshikoya, K. A., Sammons, H. M., & Choonara, I. (2010). A systematic review of pharmacokinetics studies in children with protein-energy malnutrition. *European Journal of Clinical Pharmacology*, *66*(10), 1025–1035. PubMed PMID: 20552179.

4. Mucklow, J. C., Caraher, M. T., Henderson, D. B., & Rawlins, M. B. (1979). The effect of individual dietary constituents on antipyrine clearance in Asian immigrants. *British Journal of Clinical Pharmacology*, *7*, 416–417. PubMed PMID: 444366.

5. Mucklow, J. C., Caraher, M. T., Henderson, D. B., Chapman, P. H., Roberts, D. F., & Rawlins, M. D. (1982). The relationship between individual dietary constituents and antipyrine metabolism in Indo-Pakistani immigrants to Britain. *British Journal of Clinical Pharmacology*, *13*(4), 481–486. PubMed PMID: 7066162.

6. Prabhakaran, S., Shameem, F., & Devi, K. S. (1993). Influence of protein deficiency on hexachlorocyclohexane and malathion toxicity in pregnant rats. *Veterinary and Human Toxicology*, *35*(5), 429–433. PubMed PMID: 7504364.

7. Fagan, T. C., Walle, T., Oexmann, M. J., Walle, U. K., Bai, S. A., & Gaffney, T. E. (1987). Increased clearance of propranolol and theophylline by high-protein compared with high-carbohydrate diet. *Clinical Pharmacology and Therapeutics*, *41*(4), 402–406. PubMed PMID: 3829577.

8. Feldman, C. H., Hutchinson, V. E., Pippenger, C. E., Blumenfeld, T. A., Feldman, B. R., & Davis, W. J. (1980). Effect of dietary protein and carbohydrate on theophylline metabolism in children. *Pediatrics*, *66*(6), 956–962. PubMed PMID: 7454487.

9. Demetriou, A. A. (1991). Diet and cimetidine induce comparable changes in theophylline metabolism in normal subjects. *JPEN Journal of Parenteral and Enteral Nutrition*, *15*(6), 687–688. PubMed PMID: 1766062.

10. Becking, G. C. (1976). Hepatic drug metabolism in iron-, magnesium- and potassium-deficient rats. *Federation Proceedings*, *35*(13), 2480–2485. PubMed PMID: 824159.

11. Archakov, A. I., Karuzina, I. I., Kokareva, I. S., & Bachmanova, G. I. (1973). The effect of magnesium ions on the dimethylaniline oxidation rate and electron transfer in liver microsomal fraction. *The Biochemical Journal*, *136*(2), 371–379. PubMed PMID: 4149444.

12. Becking, G. C., & Morrison, A. B. (1970). Role of dietary magnesium in the metabolism of drugs by NADPH-dependent rat liver microsomal enzymes. *Biochemical Pharmacology*, *19*(9), 2639–2644. PubMed PMID: 4394596.

13. Peters, M. A., & Fouts, J. R. (1970). The influence of magnesium and some other divalent cations on hepatic microsomal drug metabolism in vitro. *Biochemical Pharmacology*, *19*(2), 533–544. PubMed PMID: 4396251.

14. Atterberry, T. T., Burnett, W. T., & Chambers, J. E. (1997). Age-related differences in parathion and chlorpyrifos toxicity in male rats: Target and non-target esterase sensitivity and cytochrome P450-mediated metabolism. *Toxicology and Applied Pharmacology*, *147*, 411–418. PubMed PMID:9439736.

15. Shimada, T., Gillam, E. M., Oda, Y., Tsumura, F., Sutter, T. R., Guengerich, F. P., et al. (1999). Metabolism of benzo(a)pyrene to trans-7,8-dihydroxy-7,8-dihydrobenzo(a)pyrene by recombinant human cytochrome P450 1B1 and purified liver epoxide hydrolase. *Chemical Research in Toxicology*, *12*, 623–629. PubMed PMID: 10409402.

16. Huel, G., Campagna, D., Girard, F., Moreau, T., & Blot, P. (2000). Does selenium reduce the risk of threatened preterm delivery associated with placental cytochrome P4501A1 activity? *Environmental Research*, Section A. *84*, 228–233. PubMed PMID: 11097796.

17. Eaton, D. L. (2000). Biotransformation enzyme polymorphism and pesticide susceptibility.

Neurotoxicology, 21(1–2), 101–112. PubMed PMID: 10794390.

18. Crofts, F., Taioli, E., Trachman, J., Cosma, G. N., Currie, D., Toniolo, P., et al. (1994). Functional significance of different human CYP1A1 genotypes. *Carcinogenesis*, 15, 2961–2963. PubMed PMID: 8001264.

19. Pastorelli, R., Guanci, M., Cerri, A., Negri, E., La Vecchia, C., Fumagalli, F., et al. (1998). Impact of inherited polymorphisms in glutathione S-transferase M1, microsomal epoxide hydrolase, cytochrome P450 enzymes on DNA, and blood protein adducts of benzo(a)pyrene-diolperoxide. *Cancer Epidemiology, Biomarkers and Prevention*, 7, 703–709. PubMed PMID: 9718223.

20. Okada, T., Kawashima, K., Fukushi, S., Minakuchi, T., & Nishimura, S. (1994). Association between a Cytochrome P450 CYP1A1 genotype and incidence of lung cancer. *Pharamacogenetics*, 4, 333–340. PubMed PMID: 7704039.

21. Moysich, K. B., Shields, P. G., Freudenheim, J., Schisterman, E., Vena, J., Kostyniak, P., et al. (1999). Polychlorinated biphenyls, Cytochrome P4501A1 polymorphism, and postmenopausal breast cancer risk. *Cancer Epidemiology, Biomarkers and Prevention*, 8, 41–44. PubMed PMID: 9950238.

22. Iszard, M. B., Liu, J., & Klassen, C. D. (1995). Effects of several metallothionein inducers on oxidative stress defense mechanism in rats. *Toxicology*, 104, 25–33. PubMed PMID: 8560499.

23. Teare, F. W., Jasansky, P., Renaud, L., & Read, P. R. (1977). Acute effect of cadmium on hepatic drug-metabolizing enzymes in the rat. *Toxicology and Applied Pharmacology*, 41(1), 57–65. PubMed PMID: 898191.

24. Degawa, M., Arai, H., Miura, S., & Hashimoto, Y. (1993). Preferential inhibitions of hepatic P4501A2 expression and induction by lead nitrate in the rat. *Carcinogenesis*, 14, 1091–1094. PubMed PMID: 8508493.

25. Abbas-Ali, B. (1980). Effect of mercuric chloride on Microsomal enzyme system in mouse liver. *Pharmacology*, 21, 59–63. PubMed PMID: 7403256.

26. Rosenberg, D. W., & Kappas, A. (1989). Actions of orally administered organotin compounds on heme metabolism and cytochrome P-450 content and function in intestinal epithelium. *Biochemical Pharmacology*, 38(7), 1155–1161. PubMed PMID: 2706014.

27. Vakharia, D. D., Liu, N., Pause, R., Fasco, M., Bessette, E., Zhang, Q. Y., et al. (2001). Effects of metals on polycyclic aromatic hydrocarbon induction of CYP1A1 and CYP1A2 in human hepatocyte cultures. *Toxicology and Applied Pharmacology*, 170, 93–103. PubMed PMID: 11162773.

28. Abass, K., Turpeinen, M., & Pelkonen, O. (2009). An evaluation of the cytochrome P450 inhibition potential of selected pesticides in human hepatic microsomes. *Journal of Environmental Science and Health. Part. B, Pesticides, Food Contaminants, and Agricultural Wastes*, 44(6), 553–563. PubMed PMID: 20183062.

29. Haas, C. E., Kaufman, D. C., Jones, C. E., Burstein, A. H., & Reiss, W. (2003). Cytochrome P450 3A4 activity after surgical stress. *Critical Care Medicine*, 31(5), 1338–1346. PubMed PMID: 12771600.

30. Griffith, L. K., Rosen, G. M., & Rauckman, E. J. (1984). Effects of model traumatic injury on hepatic drug metabolism in the rat. III. Differential responses of Cytochrome p-450 subpopulations. *Drug Metabolism and Disposition*, 12(5), 588–592. PubMed PMID: 6149909.

31. He, N., Zhang, W. Q., Shockley, D., & Edeki, T. (2002). Inhibitory effects of H1-antihistamines on CYP2D6- and CYP2C9-mediated drug metabolic reactions in human liver microsomes. *European Journal of Clinical Pharmacology*, 57(12), 847–851. PubMed PMID: 11936702.

32. Furuta, S., Kamada, E., Suzuki, T., Sugimoto, T., Kawabata, Y., Shinozaki, Y., et al. (2001). Inhibition of drug metabolism in human liver microsomes by nizatidine, cimetidine and omeprazole. *Xenobiotica*, 31(1), 1–10. PubMed PMID: 11334262.

33. Ray, W. A., Murray, K. T., Meredith, S., Narasimhulu, S. S., Hall, K., & Stein, C. M. (2004). Oral erythromycin and the risk of sudden death from cardiac causes. *The New England Journal of Medicine*, 351(11), 1089–1096. PubMed PMID: 15356306.

34. Schmiedlin-Ren, P., Edwards, D. J., Fitzsimmons, M. E., He, K., Lown, K. S., Woster, P. M., et al. (1997). Mechanisms of enhanced oral availability of CYP3A4 substrates by grapefruit constituents. Decreased enterocyte CYP3A4 concentration and mechanism-based inactivation by furanocoumarins. *Drug Metabolism and Disposition: The Biological Fate of Chemicals*, 25(11), 1228–1233. PubMed PMID: 9351897.

35. Bailey, D. G., Dresser, G. K., Kreeft, J. H., Munoz, C., Freeman, D. J., & Bend, J. R. (2000). Grapefruit-felodipine interaction: Effect of unprocessed fruit and probable active ingredients. *Clinical Pharmacology and Therapeutics*, 68(5), 468–477. PubMed PMID: 11103749.

36. Greenblatt, D., von Moltke, L., & Harmatz, J. (2003). Time course of recovery of cytochrome p450 3A

function after single doses of grapefruit juice. *Clinical Pharmacology and Therapeutics, 74*(2), 121–129. PubMed PMID: 12891222.

37. Bailey, D. G., Dresser, G. K., & Bend, J. R. (2003). Bergamottin, lime juice, and red wine as inhibitors of cytochrome P450 3A4 activity: Comparison with grapefruit juice. *Clinical Pharmacology and Therapeutics, 73*(6), 529–537. PubMed PMID: 12811362.

38. Veronese, M. L., Gillen, L. P., Burke, J. P., Dorval, E. P., Hauck, W. W., Pequignot, E., et al. (2003). Exposure-dependent inhibition of intestinal and hepatic CYP3A4 in vivo by grapefruit juice. *Journal of Clinical Pharmacology, 43*(8), 831–839. PubMed PMID:12953340.

39. Hidaka, M., Okumura, M., Fujita, K., Ogikubo, T., Yamasaki, K., Iwakiri, T., et al. (2005). Effects of pomegranate juice on human cytochrome p450 3A (CYP3A) and carbamazepine pharmacokinetics in rats. *Drug Metabolism and Disposition: The Biological Fate of Chemicals, 33*(5), 644–648. PubMed PMID: 15673597.

40. Bailey, D. G., Dresser, G. K., & Bend, J. R. (2003). Bergamottin, lime juice, and red wine as inhibitors of cytochrome P450 3A4 activity: Comparison with grapefruit juice. *Clinical Pharmacology and Therapeutics, 73*(6), 529–537. PubMed PMID: 12811362.

41. Ke, S., Rabson, A. B., Germino, J. F., Gallo, M. A., & Tian, Y. (2001). Mechanism of suppression of cytochrome P-450 1A1 expression by tumor necrosis factor-alpha and lipopolysaccharide. *The Journal of Biological Chemistry, 276*(43), 39638–39644. PubMed PMID: 11470802.

42. Shedlofsky, S. I., Israel, B. C., McClain, C. J., Hill, D. B., & Blouin, R. A. (1994). Endotoxin administration to humans inhibits hepatic cytochrome P450-mediated drug metabolism. *The Journal of Clinical Investigation, 94*(6), 2209–2214. PubMed PMID: 7989576.

43. Roe, A. L., Warren, G., Hou, G., Howard, G., Shedlofsky, S. I., & Blouin, R. A. (1998). The effect of high dose endotoxin on CYP3A2 expression in the rat. *Pharmaceutical Research, 15*(10), 1603–1608. PubMed PMID: 9794504.

44. Morgan, E. (1989). Suppression of constitutive cytochrome P-450 gene expression in livers of rats undergoing and acute phase response to endotoxin. *Molecular Pharmacology, 36*(5), 699–707. PubMed PMID: 2511427.

45. Warren, G. W., Poloyac, S. M., Gary, D. S., Mattson, M. P., & Blouin, R. A. (1999). Hepatic cytochrome P-450 expression in tumor necrosis factor-alpha receptor (p55/p75) knockout mice after endotoxin administration. *The Journal of Pharmacology and Experimental Therapeutics, 288*(3), 945–950. PubMed PMID: 10027830.

46. Cheng, P., Wang, M., & Morgan, E. (2003). Rapid transcriptional suppression of rat cytochrome P450 genes by endotoxin treatment and its inhibition by curcumin. *The Journal of Pharmacology and Experimental Therapeutics, 307*(3), 1205–1212. PubMed PMID: 14557382.

47. Xu, D. X., Wei, W., Sun, M. F., et al. (2005). Melatonin attenuates lipopolysaccharide-induced down-regulation of pregnane X receptor and its target gene CYP3A in mouse liver. *Journal of Pineal Research, 38*(1), 27–34. PubMed PMID: 15617534.

48. Tajima, M., Ikarashi, N., Okaniwa, T., Imahori, Y., Saruta, K., Toda, T., et al. (2013). Consumption of a high-fat diet during pregnancy changes the expression of cytochrome P450 in the livers of infant male mice. *Biological and Pharmaceutical Bulletin, 36*(4), 649–657. PubMed PMID: 23358370.

49. Pollack, A. Z., Sjaarda, L., Ahrens, K. A., Mumford, S. L., Browne, R. W., Wactawski-Wende, J., et al. (2014). Association of cadmium, lead and mercury with paraoxonase 1 activity in women. *PLoS ONE, 9*(3), e92152. PubMed PMID: 24682159.

50. Costa, L. G., Richter, R. J., Li, W. F., Cole, T., Guizzetti, M., & Furlong, C. E. (2003). Paraoxonase (PON1) as a biomarker of susceptibility for organophosphate toxicity. *Biomarkers: Biochemical Indicators of Exposure, Response, and Susceptibility to Chemicals, 8*(1), 1–12. PubMed PMID: 12519632.

51. Devarajan, A., Shih, D., & Reddy, S. T. (2014). Inflammation, infection, cancer and all that…the role of paraoxonases. *Advances in Experimental Medicine and Biology, 824*, 33–41. PubMed PMID: 25038992.

52. Chistiakov, D. A., Melnichenko, A. A., Orekhov, A. N., & Bobryshev, Y. V. (2017). Paraoxonase and atherosclerosis-related cardiovascular diseases. *Biochimie, 132*, 19–27. PubMed PMID: 27771368.

53. Devarajan, A., Bourquard, N., Hama, S., Navab, M., Grijalva, V. R., Morvardi, S., et al. (2011). Paraoxonase 2 deficiency alters mitochondrial function and exacerbates the development of atherosclerosis. *Antioxidants & Redox Signaling, 14*(3), 341–351. PubMed PMID: 20578959.

54. Echobichon, J. D., & Stephens, D. S. (1973). Perinatal development of human blood esterases. *Clinical Pharmacology and Therapeutics, 14*(10), 41–47. PubMed PMID: 4734200.

55. Sun, T., Hu, J., Yin, Z., Xu, Z., Zhang, L., Fan, L., et al. (2016). Low serum paraoxonase1 activity levels predict

coronary artery disease severity. *Oncotarget*, 14305. doi:10.18632/oncotarget. PubMed PMID: 28038449.

56. Craciun, E. C., Leucuta, D. C., Rusu, R. L., David, B. A., Cret, V., & Dronca, E. (2016). Paraoxonase-1 activities in children and adolescents with type 1 diabetes mellitus. *Acta Biochimica Polonica*, 63(3), 511–515. PubMed PMID: 27337219.

57. Kedage, V., Muttigi, M. S., Shetty, M. S., Suvarna, R., Rao, S. S., Joshi, C., et al. (2010). Serum paraoxonase 1 activity status in patients with liver disorders. *Saudi Journal of Gastroenterology*, 16(2), 79–83. PubMed PMID: 20339175.

58. Patra, S. K., Singh, K., & Singh, R. (2013). Paraoxonase 1: A better atherosclerotic risk predictor than HDL in type 2 diabetes mellitus. *Diabetes & Metabolic Syndrome*, 7(2), 108–111. PubMed PMID: 23680251.

59. Macharia, M., Hassan, M. S., Blackhurst, D., Erasmus, R. T., & Matsha, T. E. (2012). The growing importance of PON1 in cardiovascular health: A review. *Journal of Cardiovascular Medicine (Hagerstown, Md)*, 13(7), 443–453. PubMed PMID: 22673025.

60. Searles Nielsen, S., Mueller, B. A., De Roos, A. J., Viernes, H. M., Farin, F. M., & Checkoway, H. (2005). Risk of brain tumors in children and susceptibility to organophosphorus insecticides: The potential role of paraoxonase (PON1). *Environmental Health Perspectives*, 113(7), 909–913. PubMed PMID: 16002382.

61. Costa, L. G., Giordano, G., Cole, T. B., Marsillach, J., & Furlong, C. E. (2013). Paraoxonase 1 (PON1) as a genetic determinant of susceptibility to organophosphate toxicity. *Toxicology*, 307, 115–122. PubMed PMID: 22884923.

62. Lee, B. W., London, L., Paulauskis, J., Myers, J., & Christiani, D. C. (2003). Association between human paraoxonase gene polymorphism and chronic symptoms in pesticide-exposed workers. *Journal of Occupational and Environmental Medicine*, 45(2), 118–122. PubMed PMID: 12625227.

63. Searles Nielsen, S., Mueller, B. A., De Roos, A. J., Viernes, H. M., Farin, F. M., & Checkoway, H. (2005). Risk of brain tumors in children and susceptibility to organophosphorus insecticides: The potential role of paraoxonase (PON1). *Environmental Health Perspectives*, 113(7), 909–913. PubMed PMID: 16002382.

64. Searles Nielsen, S., McKean-Cowdin, R., Farin, F. M., Holly, E. A., Preston-Martin, S., & Mueller, B. A. (2010). Childhood brain tumors, residential insecticide exposure, and pesticide metabolism genes. *Environmental Health Perspectives*, 118(1), 144–149. PubMed PMID: 20056567.

65. Conesa-Zamora, P., Ruiz-Cosano, J., Torres-Moreno, D., Español, I., Gutiérrez-Meca, M. D., Trujillo-Santos, J., et al. (2013). Polymorphisms in xenobiotic metabolizing genes (EPHX1, NQO1 and PON1) in lymphoma susceptibility: A case control study. *BMC Cancer*, 13, 228. PubMed PMID: 23651475.

66. Manthripragada, A. D., Costello, S., Cockburn, M. G., Bronstein, J. M., & Ritz, B. (2010). Paraoxonase 1, agricultural organophosphate exposure, and Parkinson disease. *Epidemiology (Cambridge, Mass)*, 21(1), 87–94. PubMed PMID: 19907334.

67. Wehr, H., Bednarska-Makaruk, M., Graban, A., Lipczyńska-Łojkowska, W., Rodo, M., Bochyńska, A., et al. (2009). Paraoxonase activity and dementia. *Journal of the Neurological Sciences*, 283(1–2), 107–108. PubMed PMID: 19268306.

68. Bednarska-Makaruk, M. E., Krzywkowski, T., Graban, A., Lipczyńska-Łojkowska, W., Bochyńska, A., Rodo, M., et al. (2013). Paraoxonase 1 (PON1) gene-108C>T and p.Q192R polymorphisms and arylesterase activity of the enzyme in patients with dementia. *Folia Neuropathologica*, 51(2), 111–119. PubMed PMID: 23821382.

69. Bortolasci, C. C., Vargas, H. O., Souza-Nogueira, A., Barbosa, D. S., Moreira, E. G., Nunes, S. O., et al. (2014). Lowered plasma paraoxonase (PON)1 activity is a trait marker of major depression and PON1 Q192R gene polymorphism-smoking interactions differentially predict the odds of major depression and bipolar disorder. *Journal of Affective Disorders*, 159, 23–30. PubMed PMID: 24679385.

70. Cherry, N., Mackness, M., Durrington, P., Povey, A., Dippnall, M., Smith, T., et al. (2002). Paraoxonase (PON1) polymorphisms in farmers attributing ill health to sheep dip. *Lancet*, 359(9308), 763–764. PubMed PMID: 11888590.

71. Cherry, N., Mackness, M., Mackness, B., Dippnall, M., & Povey, A. (2011). 'Dippers' flu' and its relationship to PON1 polymorphisms. *Occupational and Environmental Medicine*, 68(3), 211–217. PubMed PMID: 20921272.

72. Povey, A. C., Mackness, M. I., Durrington, P. N., Dippnall, M., Smith, A. E., Mackness, B., et al. (2005). Paraoxonase polymorphisms and self-reported chronic ill-health in farmers dipping sheep. *Occupational Medicine (Oxford, England)*, 55(4), 282–286. PubMed PMID: 15982977.

73. McKeown-Eyssen, G., Baines, C., Cole, D. E., Riley, N., Tyndale, R. F., Marshall, L., et al. (2004). Case-control study of genotypes in multiple chemical sensitivity: CYP2D6, NAT1, NAT2, PON1, PON2 and MTHFR.

International Journal of Epidemiology, 33(5), 971–978. PubMed PMID: 15256524.

74. Thomàs-Moyà, E., Gianotti, M., Proenza, A. M., & Lladó, I. (2007). Paraoxonase 1 response to a high-fat diet: Gender differences in the factors involved. *Molecular Medicine (Cambridge, Mass), 13*(3–4), 203–209. PubMed PMID: 17592556.

75. Alici, H. A., Ekinci, D., & Beydemir, S. (2008). Intravenous anesthetics inhibit human paraoxonase-1 (PON1) activity in vitro and in vivo. *Clinical Biochemistry, 41*(16–17), 1384–1390. PubMed PMID: 18640108.

76. Ekinci, D., & Beydemir, S. (2009). Evaluation of the impacts of antibiotic drugs on PON 1; a major bioscavenger against cardiovascular diseases. *European Journal of Pharmacology, 617*(1–3), 84–89. PubMed PMID: 19577563.

77. Dilek, E. B., Küfrevioğlu, Ö. İ., & Beydemir, Ş. (2013). Impacts of some antibiotics on human serum paraoxonase 1 activity. *Journal of Enzyme Inhibition and Medicinal Chemistry, 28*(4), 758–764. PubMed PMID: 22591317.

78. Işık, M., Demir, Y., Kırıcı, M., Demir, R., Şimşek, F., & Beydemir, Ş. (2015). Changes in the anti-oxidant system in adult epilepsy patients receiving anti-epileptic drugs. *Archives of Physiology and Biochemistry, 121*(3), 97–102. PubMed PMID: 26120045.

79. Alim, Z., & Beydemir, Ş. (2016). Some anticancer agents act on human serum paraoxonase-1 (hPON1) to reduce its activity. *Chemical Biology & Drug Design, 88*(2), 188–196. PubMed PMID: 26873069.

80. Türkeş, C., Söyüt, H., & Beydemir, S. (2014). Effect of calcium channel blockers on paraoxonase-1 (PON1) activity and oxidative stress. *Pharmacological Reports: PR, 66*(1), 74–80. PubMed PMID: 24905310.

81. Otocka-Kmiecik, A., Bortnik, K., Szkudlarek, U., Nowak, D., & Orłowska-Majdak, M. (2013). Effect of exercise on plasma paraoxonase1 activity in rugby players: Dependence on training experience. *Redox Report: Communications in Free Radical Research, 18*(3), 113–119. PubMed PMID: 23710701.

82. Turgay, F., Şişman, A. R., & Aksu, A. Ç. (2015). Effects of Anaerobic Training on Paraoxonase-1 Enzyme (PON1) Activities of High Density Lipoprotein Subgroups and Its Relationship with PON1-Q192R Phenotype. *Journal of Atherosclerosis and Thrombosis, 22*(4), 433–434. PubMed PMID: 25963585.

83. Kastorini, C. M., Panagiotakos, D. B., Chrysohoou, C., Georgousopoulou, E., Pitaraki, E., Puddu, P. E., et al. (2016). Metabolic syndrome, adherence to the Mediterranean diet and 10-year cardiovascular disease incidence: The ATTICA study. *Atherosclerosis, 246*, 87–93. PubMed PMID: 26761772.

84. Blum, S., Aviram, M., Ben-Amotz, A., & Levy, Y. (2006). Effect of a Mediterranean meal on postprandial carotenoids, paraoxonase activity and C-reactive protein levels. *Annals of Nutrition & Metabolism, 50*(1), 20–24. PubMed PMID: 16276071.

85. Ghorbanihaghjo, A., Kolahi, S., Seifirad, S., Rashtchizadeh, N., Argani, H., Hajialilo, M., et al. (2012). Effect of fish oil supplements on serum paraoxonase activity in female patients with rheumatoid arthritis: A double-blind randomized controlled trial. *Archives of Iranian Medicine, 15*(9), 549–552. PubMed PMID: 22924372.

86. Loued, S., Berrougui, H., Componova, P., Ikhlef, S., Helal, O., & Khalil, A. (2013). Extra-virgin olive oil consumption reduces the age-related decrease in HDL and paraoxonase 1 anti-inflammatory activities. *The British Journal of Nutrition, 110*(7), 1272–1284. PubMed PMID: 23510814.

87. Zhu, Y., Huang, X., Zhang, Y., Wang, Y., Liu, Y., Sun, R., et al. (2014). Anthocyanin supplementation improves HDL-associated paraoxonase 1 activity and enhances cholesterol efflux capacity in subjects with hypercholesterolemia. *The Journal of Clinical Endocrinology and Metabolism, 99*(2), 561–569. PubMed PMID: 24285687.

88. Farrell, N., Norris, G., Lee, S. G., Chun, O. K., & Blesso, C. N. (2015). Anthocyanin-rich black elderberry extract improves markers of HDL function and reduces aortic cholesterol in hyperlipidemic mice. *Food & Function, 6*(4), 1278–1287. PubMed PMID: 25758596.

89. Boesch-Saadatmandi, C., Egert, S., Schrader, C., Coumoul, X., Barouki, R., Muller, M. J., et al. (2010). Effect of quercetin on paraoxonase 1 activity – studies in cultured cells, mice and humans. *Journal of Physiology and Pharmacology, 61*(1), 99–105. Erratum in: J Physiol Pharmacol. 2011;62(1):131. PubMed PMID: 20228421.

90. Nus, M., Frances, F., Librelotto, J., Canales, A., Corella, D., Sánchez-Montero, J. M., et al. (2007). Arylesterase activity and antioxidant status depend on PON1-Q192R and PON1-L55M polymorphisms in subjects with increased risk of cardiovascular disease consuming walnut-enriched meat. *The Journal of Nutrition, 137*(7), 1783–1788. PubMed PMID: 17585031.

91. Arunima, S., & Rajamohan, T. (2013). Effect of virgin coconut oil enriched diet on the antioxidant status and paraoxonase 1 activity in ameliorating the oxidative

stress in rats - a comparative study. *Food & Function*, 4(9), 1402–1409. PubMed PMID: 23892389.

92. Kurban, S., & Mehmetoglu, I. (2010). Effects of acetylsalicylic acid on serum paraoxonase activity, Ox-LDL, coenzyme Q10 and other oxidative stress markers in healthy volunteers. *Clinical Biochemistry*, 43(3), 287–290. PubMed PMID: 19891963.

93. Zheng, W., Deitz, A. C., Campbell, D. R., Wen, W. Q., Cerhan, J. R., Sellers, T. A., et al. (1999). N-acetyltransferase 1 genetic polymorphism, cigarette smoking, well-done meat intake, and breast cancer risk. *Cancer Epidemiology, Biomarkers and Prevention: A Publication of the American Association for Cancer Research, Cosponsored by the American Society of Preventive Oncology*, 8(3), 233–239. PubMed PMID: 10090301.

94. Brockmoller, J., Cascorbi, I., Kerb, R., Sachse, C., & Roots, I. (1998). Polymorphism in xenobiotic conjugation and disease predisposition. *Toxicology Letters*, 102-103, 173–183. PubMed PMID: 10022251.

95. Ladona, M., Izquierdo-martinez, M., de la Paz, M. P., de la Torre, R., Ampurdanes, C., Segura, J., et al. (2001). Pharmacogenetic profile of xenobiotic enzyme metabolism in survivors of the Spanish Toxic Oil Syndrome. *Environmental Health Perspectives*, 109(4), 369–375. PubMed PMID: 11335185.

96. Santos, E. C., Pinto, A. C., Klumb, E. M., & Macedo, J. M. (2016). Polymorphisms in NAT2 (N-acetyltransferase 2) gene in patients with systemic lupus erythematosus. *Revista Brasileira De Reumatologia*, 56(6), 521–529. PubMed PMID: 27911600.

97. Banhegyi, G., Garzo, T., Antoni, F., & Mandl, J. (1988). Glycogenolysis and not gluconeogenesis is the source of UDP-glucuronic acid for glucuronidation. *Biochimica Et Biophysica Acta*, 967, 429–435. PubMed PMID: 3196758.

98. Pantuck, E. J., Pantuck, C. B., Kappas, A., Conney, A. H., & Anderson, K. E. (1991). Effects of protein and carbohydrate content of diet on drug conjugation. *Clinical Pharmacology and Therapeutics*, 50(3), 254–258. PubMed PMID: 1914359.

99. Sonne, J., Dragsted, J., Loft, S., Dossing, M., & Andreasen, F. (1989). Influence of a very low calorie diet on the clearance of oxazepam and antipyrine in man. *European Journal of Clinical Pharmacology*, 36, 407–409. PubMed PMID: 2737234.

100. Hecht, S. S., Carmella, S. G., & Murphy, S. E. (1999). Effects of watercress consumption on urinary metabolites of nicotine in smokers. *Cancer Epidemiology, Biomarkers and Prevention*, 8, 907–913. PubMed PMID: 10548320.

101. Bu Abbas, A., Clifford, M. N., Walker, R., & Ioannides, C. (1998). Contribution of caffeine and flavanols in the induction of hepatic phase II activities by green tea. *Food and Chemical Toxicology: An International Journal Published for the British Industrial Biological Research Association*, 36, 617–621. PubMed PMID: 9734711.

102. Lampe, J. W., & Peterson, S. (2002). Brassica, biotransformation and cancer risk: Genetic polymorphisms alter the preventive effects of cruciferous vegetables. *The Journal of Nutrition*, 132(10), 2991–2994. PubMed PMID: 12368383.

103. Polasa, K., & Krishnaswamy, K. (1993). Effect of turmeric on xenobiotic metabolising enzymes. *Plant Foods for Human Nutrition (Dordrecht, Netherlands)*, 44(1), 87–92. PubMed PMID: 8332589.

104. Sotelo-Félix, J. I., Martinez-Fong, D., Muriel, P., Santillán, R. L., Castillo, D., & Yahuaca, P. (2002). Evaluation of the effectiveness of Rosmarinus officinalis (Lamiaceae) in the alleviation of carbon tetrachloride-induced acute hepatotoxicity in the rat. *Journal of Ethnopharmacology*, 81(2), 145–154. PubMed PMID: 12065145.

105. Marnewick, J. L., Rautenbach, F., Venter, I., Neethling, H., Blackhurst, D. M., Wolmarans, P., et al. (2011). Effects of rooibos (Aspalathus linearis) on oxidative stress and biochemical parameters in adults at risk for cardiovascular disease. *Journal of Ethnopharmacology*, 133(1), 46–52. PubMed PMID: 20833235.

106. Strenzke, N., Grabbe, J., Plath, K. E. S., Rohwer, J., Wolff, H. H., & Gibbs, B. F. (2001). Mercuric chloride enhances immunoglobulin E-dependent mediator release from human basophils. *Toxicology and Applied Pharmacology*, 164, 257–263. PubMed PMID: 11485386.

107. Ahamed, M., Akhtar, M. J., Verma, S., Kumar, A., & Siddiqui, M. K. (2011). Environmental lead exposure as a risk for childhood aplastic anemia. *Bioscience Trends*, 5(1), 38–43. PubMed PMID: 21422599.

108. Hu, X. Z., & Hu, D. C. (2009). Effects of perfluorooctanoate and perfluorooctane sulfonate exposure on hepatoma Hep G2 cells. *Archives of Toxicology*, 83(9), 851–861. PubMed PMID: 19468714.

109. Zhou, D., Wang, H., Zhang, J., Gao, X., Zhao, W., & Zheng, Y. (2010). Di-n-butyl phthalate (DBP) exposure induces oxidative damage in testes of adult rats. *Systems Biology in Reproductive Medicine*, 56(6), 413–419. PubMed PMID: 20883123.

110. Wetmore, B. A., Struve, M. F., Gao, P., Sharma, S., Allison, N., et al. (2008). Genotoxicity of intermittent co-exposure to benzene and toluene in male CD-1

mice. *Chemico-Biological Interactions, 173*(3), 166–178. PubMed PMID: 18455711.

111. Hassoun, E. A., & Periandri-Steinberg, S. (2010). Assessment of the roles of antioxidant enzymes and glutathione in 3,3',4,4',5-Pentachlorobiphenyl (PCB 126)-induced oxidative stress in the brain tissues of rats after subchronic exposure. *Toxicological and Environmental Chemistry, 92*(2), 301. PubMed PMID: 20161674.

112. Jang, T. C., Jang, J. H., & Lee, K. W. (2016). Mechanism of acute endosulfan intoxication-induced neurotoxicity in Sprague-Dawley rats. *Arhiv Za Higijenu Rada I Toksikologiju, 67*(1), 9–17. PubMed PMID: 27092634.

113. Bebe, F. N., & Panemangalore, M. (2003). Exposure to low doses of endosulfan and chlorpyrifos modifies endogenous antioxidants in tissues of rats. *Journal of Environmental Science and Health. Part. B, Pesticides, Food Contaminants, and Agricultural Wastes, 38*(3), 349–363. PubMed PMID: 12716052.

114. Weichenthal, S., Crouse, D. L., Pinault, L., Godri-Pollitt, K., Lavigne, E., Evans, G., et al. (2016). Oxidative burden of fine particulate air pollution and risk of cause-specific mortality in the Canadian Census Health and Environment Cohort (CanCHEC). *Environmental Research, 146*, 92–99. PubMed PMID: 26745732.

115. Reddy, S., Finkelstein, E. I., Wong, P. S., Phung, A., Cross, C. E., & van der Vliet, A. (2002). Identification of glutathione modifications by cigarette smoke. *Free Radical Biology & Medicine, 33*(11), 1490–1498. PubMed PMID: 12446206.

116. Banerjee, A., Trueblood, M. B., Zhang, X., Manda, K. R., Lobo, P., et al. (2009). N-acetylcysteineamide (NACA) prevents inflammation and oxidative stress in animals exposed to diesel engine exhaust. *Toxicology Letters, 187*(3), 187–193. PubMed PMID: 19429263.

117. Lu, S. C. (2009). Regulation of glutathione synthesis. *Molecular Aspects of Medicine, 30*, 42–59. PubMed PMID: 18601945.

118. Gogos, A., & Shapiro, L. (2002). Large conformational changes in the catalytic cycle of glutathione synthase. *Structure (London, England: 1993), 10*(12), 1669–1676. PubMed PMID: 12467574.

119. El-Tanbouly, D. M., Abdelsalam, R. M., Attia, A. S., & Abdel-Aziz, M. T. (2015). Pretreatment with magnesium ameliorates lipopolysaccharide-induced liver injury in mice. *Pharmacological Reports : PR, 67*(5), 914–920. PubMed PMID: 26398385.

120. Daniels, J., & Kadlubar, S. (2013). Sulfotransferase genetic variation: From cancer risk to treatment response. *Drug Metabolism Reviews, 45*(4), 415–422. PubMed PMID: 24010997.

121. Zheng, W., Xie, D., Cerhan, J. R., Sellers, T. A., Wen, W., & Folsom, A. R. (2001). Sulfotransferase 1A1 polymorphism, endogenous estrogen exposure, well-done meat intake, and breast cancer risk. *Cancer Epidemiology, Biomarkers and Prevention, 10*, 89–94. PubMed PMID: 11219777.

122. Borst, P., de Wolf, C., & van de Wetering, K. (2007). Multidrug resistance-associated proteins 3, 4, and 5. *Pflugers Archiv: European Journal of Physiology, 453*(5), 661–673. PubMed PMID: 16586096.

123. Bridges, C. C., Joshee, L., van den Heuvel, J. J., Russel, F. G., & Zalups, R. K. (2013). Glutathione status and the renal elimination of inorganic mercury in the Mrp2(-/-) mouse. *PLoS ONE, 8*(9), e73559. PubMed PMID: 24039982.

124. Yuan, B., Yoshino, Y., Fukushima, H., Markova, S., Takagi, N., Toyoda, H., et al. (2016). Multidrug resistance-associated protein 4 is a determinant of arsenite resistance. *Oncology Reports, 35*(1), 147–154. PubMed PMID: 26497925.

125. Banerjee, M., Carew, M. W., Roggenbeck, B. A., Whitlock, B. D., Naranmandura, H., Le, X. C., et al. (2014). A novel pathway for arsenic elimination: Human multidrug resistance protein 4 (MRP4/ ABCC4) mediates cellular export of dimethylarsinic acid (DMAV) and the diglutathione conjugate of monomethylarsonous acid (MMAIII). *Molecular Pharmacology, 86*(2), 168–179. PubMed PMID: 24870404.

126. Rius, M., Hummel-Eisenbeiss, J., Hofmann, A. F., & Keppler, D. (2006). Substrate specificity of human ABCC4 (MRP4)-mediated cotransport of bile acids and reduced glutathione. *American Journal of Physiology. Gastrointestinal and Liver Physiology, 290*(4), G640–G649. PubMed PMID: 16282361.

127. Zelcer, N., Reid, G., Wielinga, P., Kuil, A., van der Heijden, I., Schuetz, J. D., et al. (2003). Steroid and bile acid conjugates are substrates of human multidrug-resistance protein (MRP) 4 (ATP-binding cassette C4). *The Biochemical Journal, 371*(Pt. 2), 361–367. PubMed PMID: 12523936.

128. Aremu, D. A., Madejczyk, M. S., & Ballatori, N. (2008). N-acetylcysteine as a potential antidote and biomonitoring agent of methylmercury exposure. *Environmental Health Perspectives, 116*(1), 26–31. PubMed PMID: 18197295.

129. Lang, T., Hitzl, M., Burk, O., Mornhinweg, E., Keil, A., Kerb, R., et al. (2004). Genetic polymorphisms in the multidrug resistance-associated protein 3 (ABCC3, MRP3) gene and relationship to its mRNA and protein expression in human liver. *Pharmacogenetics, 14*(3), 155–164. PubMed PMID: 15167703.

130. Proudfoot, A. T., Krenzelok, E. P., & Vale, J. A. (2004). Position Paper on urine alkalinization. *Journal of Toxicology. Clinical Toxicology, 42*(1), 1–26, Review. PubMed PMID: 15083932.

131. Sand, T. E., & Jacobsen, S. (1981). Effect of urine pH and flow on renal clearance of methotrexate. *European Journal of Clinical Pharmacology, 19*(6), 453–456. PubMed PMID: 7250179.

132. Birnbaum, L. S. (1985). The role of structure in the disposition of halogenated aromatic xenobiotics. *Environmental Health Perspectives, 61*, 11–20. PubMed PMID: 2998745.

133. Rohde, S., Moser, G. A., Päpke, O., & McLachlan, M. S. (1999). Clearance of PCDD/Fs via the gastrointestinal tract in occupationally exposed persons. *Chemosphere, 38*(14), 3397–3410. PubMed PMID: 10390849.

134. Geusau, A., Tschachler, E., Meixner, M., Sandermann, S., Päpke, O., Wolf, C., et al. (1999). Olestra increases faecal excretion of 2,3,7,8-tetrachlorodibenzo-p-dioxin. *Lancet, 354*(9186), 1266–1267. PubMed PMID: 10520643.

135. Rivory, L. P., Slaviero, K. A., Hoskins, J. M., & Clarke, S. J. (2001). The erythromycin breath test for the prediction of drug clearance. *Clinical Pharmacokinetics, 40*(3), 151–158. PubMed PMID: 11327195.

136. Shyu, J. K., Wang, Y. J., Lee, S. D., Lu, R. H., & Lo, K. J. (1996). Caffeine clearance test: A quantitative liver function assessment in patients with liver cirrhosis. *Zhonghua Yi Xue Za Zhi (Taipei), 57*(5), 329–334. PubMed PMID: 8768380.

57

Lung Excretion

SUMMARY

- Major route of elimination for low-molecular-weight compounds, especially those with low blood solubility and high membrane permeability
- Major diseases affecting this route of elimination include sarcoidosis, congestive heart failure, *cor pulmonale,* emphysema, asthma, scleroderma, asbestosis, cystic fibrosis, pulmonary fibrosis, and pulmonary edema (PE)
- Diffusion is proportional to the blood solubility of a compound and inversely proportional to the square root of its molecular weight
- The pulmonary system possesses biotransformation capability of considerable significance
- Analysis of exhaled breath for excreted substances is possible
- Excretion by this route is increased with elevated body temperature and decreased with PE

INTRODUCTION

The respiratory system is the primary interface for inhaled compounds and the center for gas exchange in the body. It is a site of pollutant ingestion, as has been covered in other chapters, but it is also a major pathway for xenobiotic elimination, even when these compounds were absorbed through other routes. Examples of this route of elimination include the smell of garlic in the breath after touching it or the measurement of blood alcohol content with a breathalyzer. Each of these depicts the lungs as an outlet for molecules taken into the body through different routes, although inhaled substances may also be eliminated through this pathway. New technologies are improving the utility of exhaled breath analysis, which is being used by both researchers and physicians for environmental exposure assessment and the evaluation of disease biomarkers.[1,2,3,4,5]

FUNCTION

Gas Exchange

The primary structure of gas exchange is the alveolus. Here, mixed venous blood is brought within close approximation with the outside world in the form of inspired atmospheric gas. For gas exchange to occur, the molecules must be capable of traversing three structures: the alveolar epithelium, the interstitial space, and the capillary endothelium. The movement across these structures is facilitated by a low molecular weight, a neutral charge, and a nonpolar charge distribution. The membranes in this area possess some xenobiotic transporters, such as multidrug-resistance–associated protein 1(MRP1) and multidrug-resistant protein 1 (MDR1); however, it is believed that the contribution of these to overall excretion rates is small compared with movement by simple diffusion. The propensity for simple diffusion is attributable to the massive surface area of the lungs, estimated to be 50 to 100 m^2 of contact surface area available for gas exchange between the pulmonary capillaries and the alveoli; 70 m^2 is thought to be perfused at rest, with each alveolus being about 200 to 250 μm in diameter.

Lung Excretion of Toxins. Compounds that have a propensity for excretion through the respiratory system are generally those with a high vapor pressure, and their excretion rate is inversely proportional to their solubility in blood.

The lungs act as a filter for many compounds present in the blood, similar to the kidneys. Because nearly the entirety of mixed venous blood must pass through the pulmonary capillaries, the pulmonary circulation has the ability to protect systemic circulation from various materials that may enter the blood. (Consider that intravenous [IV] nutrient solutions must pass through this system before arriving at their tissue target.) To fulfill this filtration/purification role, the pulmonary capillary bed contains lytic enzymes in the vascular endothelium and macrophages along with a prolific lymphatic system.

Excretion is based on the blood concentration of the toxin in relation to both ventilation and perfusion. If ventilation is reduced because of lung disease, such as asthma, or perfusion is decreased through a small vessel vasculitis, then excretion through this route may be impaired.

Because diffusion is the primary method of transport from the blood into the pulmonary airspace, limitations on pulmonary excretion appear as limitations in either diffusion or perfusion. Diffusion is proportional to the solubility of a compound and inversely proportional to the square root of its molecular weight. Important secondary factors that affect the solubility include the vapor pressure of the substance and any intermolecular interactions that may be present with different components of the blood, such as the binding of the molecule to plasma proteins like albumin. Because the binding to the plasma proteins sets up a second equilibrium that must be overcome for diffusion into the alveolar lumen, this limits the diffusibility of the substance. Methane gas does not bind to any plasma proteins and easily diffuses across the capillary-alveolar interface. The concentration difference between the amount of methane dissolved in the capillary blood and the concentration of methane in the alveolar gas should rapidly equilibrate. Therefore the excretion of methane is limited by the perfusion of the alveolar tissue. A person with a fibrotic alveolar-capillary barrier or one with interstitial edema may have decreased diffusability and hence reduced excretion. Conditions that may contribute to decreased diffusion capacity include sarcoidosis, scleroderma, asbestosis, emphysema, low cardiac output, or low pulmonary capillary volume.

Gas exchange is not the only factor when it comes to respiratory excretion as; there are multiple secretions involved in the function of the airways. The primary secretion is the production of pulmonary surfactant, which is synthesized by type II alveolar epithelial cells.

Although there are twice as many of the cuboidal type II cells covering the surface of the alveoli, they only account for 5% to 10% of the surface area; the squamous type I cells occupy most of the space. Pulmonary surfactant is a complex fluid composed of 85% to 90% lipids and 10% to 15% proteins. Phospholipids make up 85% of the lipid portion, and 75% of this is dipalmitoyl phosphatidyl choline. Protective components of the surfactant include the enzymes superoxide dismutase, catalase, and those associated with glutathione utilization and cycling along with transferrin, ceruloplasmin, and vitamin E. Some of this surfactant is taken up by type II cells to be processed and reexcreted, which can lead to further biotransformation of any solutes. Surfactant may exit the alveolar surface by absorption into the lymphatics, migration up the mucociliary escalator, or uptake by alveolar macrophages.

Many substances are released into the alveoli and airways through cellular secretion by specialized cells, such as goblet cells, submucosal-gland cells, Clara cells, and macrophages. These tracheobronchial secretions offer another potential route of excretion; however, they can also act as a potential barrier if they are found on the respiratory surfaces, because the diffusing substances would need to pass through these secretions to reach the alveolar lumen.

Biochemical Transformation

The respiratory tract is not generally considered a major contributor to biotransformation, but this deserves some reconsideration. The respiratory tract possesses a significant amount of cytochrome P450 capacity (CYP), roughly equaling one-tenth to one-third of the capacity of the liver.[6] Although this cytochrome activity is believed to be evolutionarily developed to reduce toxicity, similar to the liver it can also create more toxic species, and the lung activation of procarcinogens such as polycyclic aromatic hydrocarbons (PAH) and N-nitrosamines does occur.[7] Cytochrome enzymes CYP1A1, CYP1A2, CYP1B1, CYP2A3, CYP2A6, CYP2A10/11, CYP2A13, CYP2B1/4 CYP2B6, CYP2B7, CYP2E1, CYP2F1/2/4, CYP2J2, CYP2G1, CYP2S1, CYP3A4, CYP3A5, CYP3A7, and CYP4B1 have been found in lung cells by various researchers, with inconclusive results for CYP2Cs and CYP2D6.[8,9] Other phase I enzymes present in the lungs include epoxide hydrolases, flavin monooxygenases, prostaglandin-endoperoxide synthases, carbonyl reductases, and NAD(P) H:quinone oxidoreductase 1 (NQO1).[10] Lung cells also express phase II enzymes, including epoxide hydrolase, glucuronyl transferase (UGT1A), and glutathione S-transferase (GST).[7,11] (See Table 57.1 for examples of phase I and phase II enzymes found in pulmonary tissue.) In fact, pulmonary GST activity is approximately 30% of that of the liver, and polymorphisms in glutathione transferase genes have been associated with a possible increase in lung cancer risk.[6,12] Interestingly, many of these enzymes have different patterns of induction than in the liver.[6] The alveolar surface is yet another site of potential biochemical transformation. The phagocytic alveolar macrophage is a free-moving resident of the luminal lining of the alveolus found in varying numbers;

its role is to phagocytize inspired particles (particulate matter < 0.1 μm [$PM_{0.1}$]) and pathogens such as viruses and bacteria. It also contains aryl hydrocarbon hydroxylase, an enzyme that increases the water solubility of aryl hydrocarbons.[13]

Macrophages and the Mucociliary Escalator

Detoxification of inhaled PM is generally accomplished by macrophage uptake and destruction in their lysosome. This process is quite efficient for inhaled bacteria but proceeds exceedingly slowly for some particulates, like silica, asbestos, or beryllium. Ideally, macrophages that uptake this indigestible material should migrate to the mucociliary escalator by way of the pores of Kohn, to be removed through the airways. An alternative is for these macrophages to move into the septal interstitium and subsequently the lymphatic system. When these migratory patterns fail, macrophage death can redeposit the ingested particles onto the alveolar surface. Macrophage function and movement is inhibited by cigarette smoke.

The mucociliary escalator is a mechanism used in the excretion of large particles or when indigestible materials get caught in the lungs. It uses an estimated surface area of 0.5 m². The vehicle of transport is mucus composed of mucopolysaccharides, created by submucosal mucus glands, found near the supporting cartilage of the large airways. In certain pathological conditions like chronic bronchitis, the goblet cells of these glands may undergo hypertrophy, leading to increased mucous secretion but also increased mucus viscosity. The escalating movement of the escalator is based on the beating of cilia, which move the mucous lining toward the pharynx. Cigarette smoke inhibits the beating of these cilia, reducing the function of this excretion mechanism. Ultimately, expulsion may occur as the result of a sneeze or a cough—processes activated by the excitation of receptors in the nasopharynx or trachea respectively.

Further detoxification can happen through the action of surface enzymes and serum factors present in the airway secretions.

Other Considerations

Both the distribution of pollutants in the lung and their elimination from the lung may be affected by the patient's orientation with respect to gravity. When a person is standing, the blood flow to the apex of the lung is approximately 30% of the blood flow to the lower lung. When a person is lying down, this pattern of regional

TABLE 57.1　Phase I and II Enzymes and Representative Substrates Found in Pulmonary Tissue

Reaction Type	Representative Substrate
Oxidations	
Side Chain Oxidation	Pentobarbitone
Aromatic Hydroxylation	Benzo(a)pyrene
N-Dealkylation	Nortriptyline
N-Hydroxylation	N-Methylaniline
O-Dealkylation	Ethoxyresorufin
Epoxidation	Aldrin
Reduction	
Nitroreductase	Nitrazepam
Ketone Reductase	Acetophenone
N-Oxide Reductase	Imipramine N-oxide
Hydrolysis	
Acetylcholinesterase	Acetylcholine
Phase II	
Glucuronide Conjugation	4-Methylumbelliferone
Sulfate Conjugation	3-Hydroxybenzo(a)pyrene
N-Methyl Transferase	5-Hydroxytryptamine
O-Methyl Transferase	Phenol
S-Methyl Transferase	Mercaptoethanol
Catechol O-Methyl Transferase	Isoprenaline
Acetylation	Sulfanilamide
Glutathione Conjugation	Benz(a)anthracene 5,6-oxide

Modified from Cohen GM. Pulmonary metabolism of foreign compounds: its role in metabolic activation. Environmental Health Perspectives. 1990;85:31-41.

perfusion equalizes, with blood flow concentrating in the more gravity-dependent regions.

The elevation of body temperature increases the vapor pressure of any toxin to be excreted. The elevation of body temperature either through fever or the external application of heat with a sauna or other means increases the diffusability of toxins, promoting greater elimination.

Similarly, the conditioning of inspired air also plays a role in pulmonary elimination because this is not necessarily delegated purely to the upper airways. As respiration increases or the ambient air temperature decreases, greater portions of the tracheobronchial tree are needed for air conditioning. This moves the point at which inspired air reaches deeper into the lungs, and in some conditions, nonequilibrated air can reach airways down to 2 mm in diameter. Respiratory heat exchange may affect airway secretory processes, mucociliary transport, and the regulation of bronchial blood supply.[14,15,16]

Infections and toxic load may damage the integrity of the capillary endothelium or increase its permeability, leading to localized or generalized PE. Other causes of PE may include rapid administration of IV fluids and conditions that reduce pulmonary venous capacity. Extra fluid in the lungs will reduce the diffusability of toxic compounds. The lung has a large capacity to deal with fluid in the pulmonary interstitium, because pulmonary lymph flow may increase 10-fold under pathological conditions, so low-grade cases may be challenging to identify.

ANALYSIS

The analysis of the exhaled breath for toxic exposure assessment is eliciting study by the scientific community, especially those in clinical medicine and occupational toxicology. In fact, it has been found to be more sensitive than blood-based analyses for volatile organic compound (VOC) quantification.[17] More than 200 compounds have been detected in the human breath,[18] and breath analysis is being investigated for the evaluation of lung cancer, liver disease, myocardial infarction, and diabetes.[19,20,21,22] The benefits of this method of assessment are that it is less invasive than the acquisition of blood and much faster than a 24-hour urine collection; the exhaled breath is also a much simpler matrix than either the blood or urine. The challenge with the breath is that excretion components are generally at much lower concentrations,

and this requires some form of signal amplification to reach the detection limits of available equipment. One method is the condensation of the breath, and another method is the solid-phase microextraction (SPME) technique, in which a fiber of solid chromatographic media is placed in a blow-tube. When the breath is passed through this tube, the VOC components of the breath adsorb to the media, which is then placed in a gas chromatograph mass spectrometer (GCMS) and heated to desorb the breath components.[23] The GCMS then separates the components of the breath mixture and analyzes each for their molecular weight and structure. The SPME technique allows the detection of substances in the nanomolar concentration range. This technique has been used to determine chlorinated solvent concentrations[24] and to measure organic alkanes and aromatics in the breath of lung cancer patients.[25] Investigators have undertaken similar analyses for other analytes.[26] These investigations have spawned a new field of study, dubbed "breathomics," in which the breath is dissected with a metabolomics approach to investigate health status and disease indicators such as oxidative stress.[27]

SPECIFIC TOXICANTS

Mercury

Metallic mercury (Hg^0) is very lipophilic and has a substantial vapor pressure. Elimination through the pulmonary system is efficient, yet the blood half-life of mercury remains long. If the exposure to mercury vapor is short-term, one-third will be eliminated unchanged through exhalation.[28] Excretion through urine takes place, as does excretion into the digestive tract; however, oxidation of the mercury tends to occur in this pathway. Any oxidized mercury in the digestive tract that gets reduced through microbial biotransformation tends to return to circulation through diffusion across enterocytes.

Ethanol

Upon ingestion, ethanol is quickly absorbed, and breath alcohol content reaches a steady state after 9 minutes, meaning that the breath is no longer contaminated with alcohol being desorbed from the mucus membranes of the oral cavity.[29] The alcohol enters the bloodstream and begins to exit the body by way of pulmonary elimination. Pulmonary elimination increases until a second steady state is then reached in which the pulmonary elimination is proportional to the blood alcohol (ethanol) content (BAC). In most people, this steady-state is achieved 15 to 30 minutes after ingestion,[30] which is why the police are instructed to wait 15 minutes after contact before administering a breathalyzer. This waiting period allows the breath alcohol concentration (BrAC) to equilibrate with the BAC. The standard ratio of BAC:BrAC is roughly 2286:1, and most legal authorities use the value of 2100:1 to thus favor the defendant when screening automobile drivers for impairment.

Acetaldehyde

Acetaldehyde elimination is a good example of the complexities of pulmonary elimination of organic compounds. It has been investigated as an alternative approach for measuring the degree of intoxication from alcohol, because acetaldehyde is a metabolite of ethanol involving dehydrogenation. Like ethanol, acetaldehyde passes into multiple body compartments—easily crossing the blood-brain barrier. It can also be found tightly bound to common blood components such as hemoglobin, amino acids, and phospholipids. It has a much higher blood-air partition coefficient than ethanol at 190:1. This is likely, in part, because of the higher vapor pressure, which comes from the lower boiling point of 20.2°C (68.36°F) vs. the boiling point of ethanol at 78.37°C (173.1°F). Acetaldehyde is normally produced in the body by alcohol dehydrogenase and is normally metabolized by aldehyde dehydrogenase ($ALDH_2$). Genetic variation in the $ALDH_2$ enzyme can put a higher load on the pulmonary elimination of this molecule, because 40% to 50% of those from Asian descent have inherited an enzyme with a low K_m. Other pathways of metabolism and elimination also play a role, because smokers and "abstinent alcoholics" have been shown to have higher resting levels of the molecule.[31]

Perchloroethylene

To characterize the pharmacokinetics of inhaled perchloroethylene (PCE), direct measurements were made of the blood and breath of Sprague-Dawley rats while exposing them to either 50 or 500 parts per million (PPM) PCE by inhalation.[32] PCE in the exhaled breath increased rapidly to near steady state within 20 minutes and was directly proportional to the inhaled concentration. Uptake of PCE into blood was also rapid but continued to increase over the course of the 2-hour experiment. A physiology-based pharmacokinetic model was created that was able to account for similar levels of PCE and other VOCs in both rats and humans. It was able to simulate percentage and cumulative uptake of PCE over time and could predict systemically absorbed doses of PCE under a variety of exposure scenarios.

REFERENCES

1. Beauchamp, J. (2011). Inhaled today, not gone tomorrow: Pharmacokinetics and environmental exposure of volatiles in exhaled breath. *Journal of Breath Research*, 5(3), 037103.
2. Schmidt, K., & Podmore, I. (2015). Current Challenges in Volatile Organic Compounds Analysis as Potential Biomarkers of Cancer. *Journal of Biomarkers*, 2015, 981458.
3. Wang, Y., Hu, Y., Wang, D., Yu, K., Wang, L., Zou, Y., et al. (2012). The analysis of volatile organic compounds biomarkers for lung cancer in exhaled breath, tissues and cell lines. *Cancer Biomarkers: Section A of Disease Markers*, 11(4), 129–137.
4. Horváth, I., Lázár, Z., Gyulai, N., Kollai, M., & Losonczy, G. (2009). Exhaled biomarkers in lung cancer. *The European Respiratory Journal*, 34(1), 261–275.
5. Buszewski, B., Kesy, M., Ligor, T., & Amann, A. (2007). Human exhaled air analytics: Biomarkers of diseases. *Biomedical Chromatography : BMC*, 21(6), 553–566.
6. Buckpitt, A. R., & Cruikshank, M. K. (2013). Biochemical function of the respiratory tract: Metabolism of xenobiotics. In D. C. Klaassen (Ed.), *Casarett & Doull's toxicology the basic science of poisons* (8th ed.). New York: McGraw-Hill Education.
7. Castell, J. V., Donato, M. T., & Gomez-Lechon, M. J. (2005). Metabolism and bioactivation of toxicants in the lung. The in vitro cellular approach. *Experimental and Toxicologic Pathology*, 57 Suppl 1, 189–204.
8. Antilla, S., Raunio, H., & Hakkola, J. (2011). Cytochrome P450-mediated pulmonary metabolism of carcinogens: Regulation and cross-talk in lung carcinogenesis. *American Journal of Respiratory Cell and Molecular Biology*, 44(5), 583–590.
9. Hukkanen, J., Pelkonen, O., Hakkola, J., & Raunio, H. (2002). Expression and regulation of xenobiotic-metabolizing cytochrome P450 (CYP) enzymes in human lung. *Critical Reviews in Toxicology*, 32(5), 391–411.
10. Klaassen, C. D. (2013). *Casarett & Doull's toxicology the basic science of poisons* (8th ed.). New York: McGraw-Hill Education.
11. Cohen, G. M. (1990). Pulmonary metabolism of foreign compounds: Its role in metabolic activation. *Environmental Health Perspectives*, 85, 31–41.

12. Jourenkova-Mironova, N., Wikman, H., Bouchardy, C., et al. (1998). Role of glutathione S-transferase GSTM1, GSTM3, GSTP1 and GSTT1 genotypes in modulating susceptibility to smoking-related lung cancer. *Pharmacogenetics, 8*(6), 495–502.

13. Krohn, J., Taylor, F. A., & Prosser, J. (1996). *Natural Detoxification – The complete guide to clearing your body of toxins*. Point Roberts, WA: Hartley & Marks Publishers Inc.

14. McFadden, E. R., Jr. (1983). Respiratory heat and water exchange: Physiological and clinical implications. *Journal of Appllied Physiology: Respiratory, Environmental and Exercise Physiology, 54*(2), 331–336.

15. McFadden, E. R., Jr. (1992). Heat and water exchange in human airways. *The American Review of Respiratory Disease, 146*(5 Pt. 2), S8–S10.

16. Tsu, M. E., Babb, A. L., Ralph, D. D., & Hlastala, M. P. (1988). Dynamics of heat, water, and soluble gas exchange in the human airways: 1. A model study. *Annals of Biomedical Engineering, 16*(6), 547–571.

17. Lindstrom, A. B., & Pleil, J. D. (2002). A review of the USEPA's single breath canister (SBC) method for exhaled volatile organic biomarkers. *Biomarkers: Biochemical Indicators of Exposure, Response, and Susceptibility to Chemicals, 7*(3), 189–208.

18. Sanchez, J. M., & Sacks, R. D. (2003). GC analysis of human breath with a series-coupled column ensemble and a multibed sorption trap. *Analytical Chemistry, 75*(10), 2231–2236.

19. Buszewski, B., Kesy, M., Ligor, T., & Amann, A. (2007). Human exhaled air analytics: Biomarkers of diseases. *Biomedical Chromatography: BMC, 21*(6), 553–566.

20. Probert, C. S., Ahmed, I., Khalid, T., Johnson, E., Smith, S., & Ratcliffe, N. (2009). Volatile organic compounds as diagnostic biomarkers in gastrointestinal and liver diseases. *Journal of Gastrointestinal and Liver Diseases, 18*(3), 337–343.

21. Boots, A. W., Bos, L. D., van der Schee, M. P., van Schooten, F. J., & Sterk, P. J. (2015). Exhaled Molecular Fingerprinting in Diagnosis and Monitoring: Validating Volatile Promises. *Trends in Molecular Medicine, 21*(10), 633–644.

22. Fernández Del Río, R., O'Hara, M. E., Holt, A., Pemberton, P., Shah, T., Whitehouse, T., et al. (2015). Volatile biomarkers in breath associated with liver cirrhosis - comparisons of pre- and post-liver transplant breath samples. *EBioMedicine, 2*(9), 1243–1250.

23. Grote, C., & Pawliszyn, J. (1997). Solid-phase microextraction for the analysis of human breath. *Analytical Chemistry, 69*(4), 587–596.

24. Guidotti, M., Onorati, B., Lucarelii, E., Blasi, G., & Ravaioli, G. (2001). Determination of chlorinated solvents in exhaled air, urine, and blood of subjects exposed in the workplace using SPME and GC-MS. *American Clinical Laboratory, 20*(4), 23–26.

25. Yu, H., Xu, L., & Wang, P. (2005). Solid phase microextraction for analysis of alkanes and aromatic hydrocarbons in human breath. *Journal of Chromatography. B, Analytical Technologies in the Biomedical and Life Sciences, 826*(1–2), 69–74.

26. Pleil, J. D., Smith, L. B., & Zelnick, S. D. (2000). Personal exposure to JP-8 jet fuel vapors and exhaust at air force bases. *Environmental Health Perspectives, 108*(3), 183–192.

27. Smolinska, A., Hauschild, A. C., Fijten, R. R., Dallinga, J. W., Baumbach, J., & van Schooten, F. J. (2014). Current breathomics–a review on data pre-processing techniques and machine learning in metabolomics breath analysis. *Journal of Breath Research, 8*(2), 027105.

28. Lippmann, M. (2009). *Environmental Toxicants – Human exposures and their health effects* (3rd ed.). Hoboken, NJ: John Wiley & Sons Inc.

29. Fransson, M., Jones, A. W., & Andersson, L. (2005). Laboratory evaluation of a new evidential breath-alcohol analyser designed for mobile testing – the Evidenzer. *Medicine, Science, and the Law, 45*(1), 61–70.

30. Grubb, D., Rasmussen, B., Linnet, K., Olsson, S. G., & Lindberg, L. (2012). Breath alcohol analysis incorporating standardization to water vapour is as precise as blood alcohol analysis. *Forensic Science International, 216*(1–3), 88–91.

31. Jones, A. W. (1995). Measuring and reporting the concentration of acetaldehyde in human breath. *Alcohol and Alcoholism (Oxford, Oxfordshire), 30*(3), 271–285.

32. Dallas, C. E., Muralidhara, S., Chen, X. M., Ramanathan, R., Varkonyi, P., Gallo, J. M., et al. (1994). Use of a physiologically based model to predict systemic uptake and respiratory elimination of perchloroethylene. *Toxicology and Applied Pharmacology, 128*(1), 60–68.

58

Hair Excretion

SUMMARY

- A route of elimination for toxic metals, especially those that are thiophilic in nature (an affinity for sulfur)
- Metals and trace elements concentrate in the hair at levels that are 10 times that of the blood, urine, or serum
- Nutritional balance of the organism affects the concentrations of different toxicants in the hair

- Excretion by this route is based on the number of actively growing hairs and the rate of hair growth
- Hair analysis provides insight into tissue levels of toxins and is a proxy for recent, middle-term exposures
- Excretion by this route is optimized with adequate sulfur stores, protein, and blood flow

INTRODUCTION

The focus of this chapter is on the excretion of metals in the hair; clinical correlations for hair nutrients have been reviewed elsewhere.[1] Hair analysis for metals has been used by analytical chemists since the mid-20th century because of the bioaccumulation of these elements in this tissue. It has only been within the last 30 years that the analysis of organic substances in the hair has even been possible.[2] The development of better analytical tools has made possible the toxicological evaluation of many different substances that an individual has been exposed to in a period ranging from the previous week to previous few months. This includes substances that are rapidly cleared from the body that might not be properly assessed by any other method.

HAIR MINERAL ANALYSIS

Hair analysis has been applied to the evaluation of toxic exposure since the inception of modern environmental medicine, with references dating back to at least the early 1950s, which predates the use of blood or urine for a similar analysis.[3] However, there has been significant controversy recently about how well this form of measurement correlates to a patient's physiological state or body burden, and actionable levels are not well established. The challenge is to understand what constitutes the best method for establishing the body burden for a particular element or chemical.[4,5] Proponents argue that the interpretation of a hair mineral analysis (HMA) is fraught with intricacies that require years of study to understand the interrelationships and ratios necessary to deconvolute the complexities of this matrix, relating HMA to a "soft tissue mineral biopsy."[6]

The opponents of this mode of investigation cite issues with reproducibility, interlaboratory variability, and the lack of congruent reference intervals as discrediting evidence.[7,8,9,10] Some of this variance may be attributable to the particular washing method used by the laboratory,[6,11] but an in-depth discussion of the validity of HMA is beyond the scope of this chapter.

The fact that heavy metals and other toxins are excreted into the hair is beyond question. It is the standardization of the analysis and interpretation of the results that are currently debated.

highest sulfur proportions out of any hair studied. Cysteine accounts for 15.5% of the amino acids in human hair.[14]

EXCRETION OF MINERALS AND METALS

The excretion of metals in the hair can be explained by the composition of keratin previously discussed and the considerable affinity of certain metals for the element sulfur. The elements generally investigated in an HMA are electropositive in nature and can readily accept the available electron pair on a two-coordinate sulfur atom. This will form an interaction that will fall somewhere between an electrostatic attraction and a fully covalent bond. Some of the clinically used chelators (i.e., dimercaptosuccinic acid [DMSA] or alpha lipoic acid [ALA]) are based around the thiophilic nature of metals. The sulfur atoms in the cysteine molecules can occupy the bonding sphere of the metal, reducing its reactivity, chaperoning the molecule into the hair follicle and ultimately into the keratin structure.

The most standardized data for toxicant elimination through the hair is that for toxic metal excretion. Daily and yearly elimination data for each of the toxic metals typically screened for in clinical hair tests is compiled in Table 58.2 with a comparison to excretion by urine. It should be mentioned that this data is provided specifically for the scalp hair. There is potential for much greater elimination of these elements through the hair if the villus hair is taken into account. If the concentrations of the elements in this hair are consistent with the concentrations in scalp hair, the villus hair would provide roughly 22 times the excretion capacity of the scalp hair. However, defined calculations for this facet of hair excretion are not provided here because of the paucity of data available for corroboration.

Because the nails on the fingers and the toes are also composed of keratin, metals and other toxins can be excreted by this route similarly. Research examining these structures as biomarkers for exposure is available as well,[15,16,17,18] with some authors claiming that toenail arsenic could be the best method to assess the exposure to arsenic via drinking water.[19]

HAIR STATUS AND SYSTEMIC DISEASE

Hair is a nonessential product of metabolism. When the body is deficient in nutrients, the hair suffers; for instance,

Hair Growth

There are roughly 100,000 hairs on the average human scalp[12] (though obviously some have fewer). The scalp hairs in the active growing phase increase in length at a rate of 0.4 to 0.5 mm/day, which equates to 1.5 cm/month. At a density of 0.0054 mg/m, 239 mg of scalp hair is grown per day.[13] Hair growth statistics are summarized in Table 58.1.

Hair Composition

Hair emerges from the follicle as a cellular construct, which is why the HMA claims to be an intracellular gauge of mineral and metal status. The structure is made of three distinct zones that, understandably, grow simultaneously and concentrically. The most well-defined is the cuticle, which forms the hair surface and is composed of overlapping cornified squamous cells. The cortex consists of closely packed, elongated squamous cells that appear more cellular in nature, showing remnants of nuclei and melanosomes. The medulla is characterized by loosely aggregated cells that are often discontinuous, possessing even more cellular debris. Each of these cellular layers contains different types of keratin and different patterns of cornification.

Keratin. The structure of the hair is imparted by high concentrations of keratin protein, which is a general class that can be subdivided into the eukeratins and pseudokeratins. Keratins of a particular species have a conserved ratio of amino acids in their molecular structure. Eukeratins are differentiated by a consistent proportion of histidine to lysine to arginine of 112. Primate keratin has the characteristic of the highest cysteine and hence

TABLE 58.1 Hair Growth		
Total Number of Hairs 5,000,000	Hairs on Head 100,000	Hairs Not on Head 4,900,000
Growth rate (mm/day)	0.44	0.20
Millimeters of hair grown per day	44,000	980,000
Milligrams of hair grown per day	239	5,330
Grams of hair grown per day	0.24	5.33

TABLE 58.2   Metal Excretion via the Scalp Hair and Urine Based on Hair Growth Measurements and Reference Ranges According to Doctor's Data Inc.

Element	Reference Range (ug/g)	(ug/day)	Excretion by Urine (ug/day)	Excretion by Scalp Hair (ug/yr)	Excretion by Urine (ug/yr)
Aluminum	8.000	1.914	30.00	698.75	10,950.00
Antimony	0.066	0.016	0.30	5.76	109.50
Arsenic	0.080	0.019	150.00	6.99	54,750.00
Barium	0.750	0.179	8.00	65.51	2,920.00
Beryllium	0.020	0.005	1.00	1.75	365.00
Bismuth	2.000	0.479	5.00	174.69	1,825.00
Cadmium	0.070	0.017	1.50	6.11	547.50
Lead	1.000	0.239	2.50	87.34	912.50
Mercury	0.400	0.096	5.00	34.94	1,825.00
Platinum	0.005	0.001	0.20	0.44	73.00
Thallium	0.002	0.000	0.60	0.17	219.00
Thorium	0.002	0.000	0.03	0.17	10.95
Uranium	0.060	0.014	NA	5.24	NA
Nickel	0.200	0.048	NA	17.47	NA
Silver	0.140	0.034	NA	12.23	NA
Tin	0.300	0.072	6.00	26.20	2,190.00
Titanium	0.700	0.168	NA	61.14	NA

80% of children with marasmus or kwashiorkor have at least one sign of hair growth impairment; the most common is hypopigmentation and thinning.[20] Vitamin C can act as a natural chelator of metals while also assisting in promoting better redox balance through its antioxidant nature. Deficiency of vitamin C manifest as scurvy and can present with corkscrew hairs.[21] Telogen effluvium and alopecia areata have been associated with deficiencies of iron[22,23,24] and zinc,[25] and generalized hair loss occurs in conjunction with deficiencies in selenium, iron, biotin, and essential fatty acids.[26] Hair loss has also been found in heavy metal toxicity of a number of different metals,[27] including cadmium with bismuth,[28] selenium,[29] thallium,[30,31,32,33] mercury,[34,35] arsenic,[36] and cadmium.[37]

Hair anomalies accompany several forms of mucopolysaccharidosis (MPS), including MPS I, MPS II, MPS IIIA, and MPS IIIB, excluding MPS IVA, MPS IVB, and MPS VI (in these, the hair changes are minor if they are present at all). It is suggested that, because different glycosaminoglycans accumulate in the tissues of individuals with MPS, the accumulation of heparan sulfate rather than dermatan sulfate or keratan sulfate may be responsible for the changes of hair morphology in these patients.[38]

Although excessive hair growth, or hypertrichosis (HTC), is commonly attributed to congenital inheritance,[39] it can also arise as an acquired condition. A report has described this condition to be potentially associated with exposure to mercury; however, confounding factors were present.[40]

Hair regeneration is a process mediated by a two-step mechanism of stem cell activation. The hair follicle cycles between active growth, degeneration, and resting phases. During the telogen resting phase, the hair germ exists as a small cluster of cells between the dermal papilla and the "bulge," which contains the stem cells. In the late telogen phase, there is substantial metabolic activity in both the hair germ and the dermal papilla; however, the bulge provides the cell signaling necessary to maintain the process of regeneration.[41] The cell signaling involves the *wnt* pathway in the hair germ coupled to fibroblast growth factors and bone morphogenic protein (BMP) inhibitors from the dermal papilla. The science of hair stem cell signaling remains poorly understood. Interestingly, hair cells express the $Ca_v1.2$ calcium channel protein; however, they do not show signs of voltage-dependent calcium currents. $Ca_v1.2$ acts in a dominant-negative manner to delay anagen, and L-type channel blockers are able to induce anagen through inhibition of this channel. This is mediated by $Ca_v1.2$-regulation of the bulge-derived BMP inhibitor follistatin-like 1.[42] Because this area of research is still in its infancy, there is no data to implicate a role for heavy metals or organotoxicants in this process.

Cyclosporin is well known to induce HTC in patients who take it long term for immune suppression associated with organ transplants. In a study of 56 individuals with insulin-dependent diabetes who were on long-term therapy, 94.6% of them experienced unequivocal HTC. This has prompted advocacy for educating the patient regarding this socially challenging side effect before treatment.[43] The mechanism for this induction of HTC seems to be an increase in the mode-2 gating of the $Ca_v1.2$ calcium channel by the phosphorylation of S6 helices.[44]

EXCRETION OF NONELEMENTAL TOXINS AND TOXICANTS

Drugs of Abuse

Large strides are being made using hair analysis for the assessment of (intentional) exposure to drugs of abuse. The benefit of this method is that it allows assessment of exposure over time.[45,46,47,48]

Pesticides

The possibility of detecting pesticides in the hair has only been demonstrated over the past few years, and its validation as a biomarker for these compounds is still underway. A recent study using rats as a model found a linear relationship between exposure and hair concentration for the 19 pesticides tested. The authors conclude that, because the hair concentration is an average of short-term exposure, hair is a superior biological sample for epidemiological assessment in light of the fluctuations in fluid concentrations, especially for the nonpersistent compounds.[49]

Doxycycline

Pharmaceutical drugs are also excreted in the hair. Some have suggested that hair analysis of doxycycline can be a useful way to monitor patients for compliance during long-term antibiotic regimens.[50]

Mercury

Hair is an excellent marker for methylmercury (MeHg) levels. MeHg present in the circulating blood during hair formation is incorporated into the follicles. Total blood mercury and blood MeHg levels are linearly related to total mercury in the hair. With 80% of the total hair mercury being MeHg, hair mercury levels are an excellent marker of MeHg exposure during the time of hair growth (typically 1–1.5 cm/month). Hair mercury levels have been significantly correlated with mercury levels in the cerebrum, cerebellum, heart, spleen, liver, and kidneys.[51] In the 1999 to 2000 National Health and Nutritional Examination Survey (NHANES), levels of hair mercury were reported, providing the first national ranges available for comparison with individual findings (See Table 14.4 in Chapter 14).[52]

However, hair mercury levels can be artificially reduced in persons with certain polymorphisms. Glutathione (GSH), GSH-conjugating enzymes, and selenium all play important roles in clearing mercury from the body. Individuals with genotypically reduced activity of three GSH transferase enzymes (GSTT1, GSTP1–105, and GSTP1–114) are less able to clear mercury from the blood, resulting in lower urine and hair levels.[53] Similarly, those with a polymorphism in GSH synthase (GSS 5′) that reduces the production of GSH also exhibit reduced hair and urine mercury levels. A reduction of both urinary and hair mercury levels is also found in persons with polymorphisms in selenoprotein processing.

In the body, mercury is also bound by thiol-rich metallothionein (MT) proteins. Of the four common isoforms of MT, the presence of MT1M AA and MT2A CC both result in reduced urinary levels of mercury in dentists.[54] Those with either MT1A GA or GG and those with MT1M TT polymorphisms have less mercury in hair samples than should be present based on their blood MeHg levels.

AUTISM: ANALYSIS OF HAIR TESTING DATA WITH PATHOPHYSIOLOGICAL IMPLICATIONS

Autism is a condition that has been associated with environmental toxicity from many sources. Researchers have found associations with pesticides, phthalates, polychlorinated biphenyls (PCBs), solvents, toxic waste sites, air pollutants, and toxic metals. However, some studies have found negative correlations as well, and there is no singular factor that has been identified as a commonality for all individuals with autism.[55] The state of the science is moving beyond the idea that there is only one cause for autism and toward the question of what *may contribute* to autism. This field of inquiry yields more research and opens the door to a true environmental medicine approach.

Toxic Metals

At least 40 studies have been performed comparing the toxic metal burden of those with autism spectrum disorder (ASD) to control groups (CG) and, of these, at least 19 have assessed the concentration of metals in the hair. In most cases, there is some derangement in hair metal levels, finding hair metal levels either elevated or depressed. Notably, some populations have issues with mercury and others have issues with aluminum, lead, or cadmium, but overall the data is very heterogeneous. The consensus on the true keystone of this condition is far from settled, but it does seem to be related to the environmental medicine concept of total load with an idea that the higher the total load, the more likely the result will be autism. Research is moving toward an approach of investigating synergistic stressors that together are capable of producing the autistic phenotype. Many toxicants can create a physiological state similar to the ASD phenotype that consists of depleted GSH levels, increased oxidative stress, impaired cellular signaling, immune dysregulation, and impaired mitochondrial function.[56,57,58]

Mercury is toxic to cortical neurons through a mechanism likely mediated by activation of the N-methyl D-aspartate (NMDA) receptor, a major neuroexcitatory receptor.[59] The mechanism was found to be related to increased calcium influx into the neuron in response to NMDA activation, with intracellular calcium levels found to be increased up to fivefold in the rat neuron. One study looked at hair mercury levels in ASD as a function of age and concluded that 3 to 4 year olds had low hair levels of mercury, and 7 to 9 year olds had high hair levels of mercury compared with age-matched controls.[60] This result introduces the idea of a changing physiological regimen in the natural history of ASD; indeed, authors have stressed the importance of early intervention related to the knowledge of "critical periods (CPs)" of development.[61,62] These CPs are highly regulated events of neural plasticity governed by a sensitive balance of excitatory and inhibitory neurotransmission. Inflammation can disrupt development during these CPs, and interestingly for some processes, only males will show enduring consequences of their disruption.[63] This may help explain why four males are affected with ASD for every female.[64] From the perspective of this data, the results of the hair testing can be better understood. It may not be any one agent causing the ASD phenotype, but a trend toward a generalized inflammation or excitation-inhibition imbalance during one of these CPs.[65,66]

Trace Elements

The causative event may or may not continue to be present later into childhood or later into life and thus may not appear on environmental testing. For the best possible comparisons when this testing is undertaken, comparisons of more specific ages of cohorts or comparisons of environmental toxicants plotted as a function of the age of the participant are recommended. In fact, a second study substantiated this evidence, referring to the CP as the "infantile window."[67] It was found that the histogram of logarithmic hair zinc concentrations (graphed against age) in children with ASD was asymmetrical, with tailing in the lower range and an overall 29.7% having a zinc concentration of less than 2 standard deviations below the reference range. The incidence rate was calculated based on age group and subdivided by gender with 45.5%, 28.1%, and 3.3% of males, and 52.5%, 28.7%, and 3.5% of females being zinc-deficient at ages 0 to 3, 4 to 9, and 10 to 15 years of age, respectively.

Using a discriminant function analysis of 14 trace elements in an attempt to categorize patients as ASD or CG, a model found 100% success for identifying the ASD population and 90.5% success for the CG population. The authors found that the elements with the greatest discriminatory power were calcium, copper, zinc, chromium, and lithium, which allowed the correct classification of 85.7% of the CG population and 91.7% of the ASD population.[68] Considering that these are essential elements rather than toxic metals, this speaks to a nutritional component to the condition. The elements that stand out in this investigation are zinc and copper, with several studies investigating their role in ASD.[69,70,71,72,73]

A deficiency of zinc has a number of implications for ASD individuals. This deficiency affects many processes in both perinatal and postnatal development, including increased inflammation related to epithelial permeability and immune system abnormalities like the development of autoantibodies.[74] Inflammatory cytokines generated in the gastrointestinal (GI) system can affect the stress response in the hypothalamic-pituitary-adrenal (HPA) axis, leading to greater neuroexcitation in this condition.

In response to a deficiency of zinc, the body will upregulate MT in an effort to increase the GI uptake of zinc. The primary binding of metals to this protein is through the sulfhydryl groups of cysteine amino acids incorporated into the protein structure, with the overproduction of this protein leading to a potential deficiency of cysteine, which is necessary for GSH production.[75] Cysteine residues are important regulatory motifs for proteins, capable of acting as "molecular switches" to modulate the function of a large number of proteins in the brain and other organs; the ability for cysteine to do this is based on proper redox balance.[76] NMDA receptors are the primary neuroexcitatory receptors in the brain, responsible for neuronal development, synaptic plasticity, and memory; however, overactivation of these receptors leads to neuronal cell death, and this process has been implicated in both acute and chronic neurological disorders, so tight regulation is crucial for survival.[77] Zinc has been shown to be an important inhibitor of excessive NMDA excitation through binding to the sulfhydryl groups of the cysteine residues (or disulfide bonds between cysteine residues), serving as one safeguard against neuroexcitotoxicity. The redox state of these sulfhydryl groups further modulates the functional implications. One study found that individuals with ASD had significantly less protein in their hair than their CG counterparts and that the degree of deficiency was inversely proportional to their functional ability.[78]

Another consequence of inadequate dietary zinc is that MT facilitates absorption of copper, cadmium, and mercury (with current debates about whether this also applies to selenium and bismuth).[79] An increase in mercury in the body necessitates greater GSH, further stressing cysteine stores. Adequate GSH is necessary for numerous processes during neural development, including the maintenance of amino acid sulfhydryl redox states during protein synthesis,[80] cell cycle regulation, and cell differentiation (the importance of this was previously discussed).[81] Some researchers have found an association between antibodies to MT (anti-MT immunoglobulin G [IgG]) and both individuals with ASD who have GI disease[82] and family members of those with ASD.[83]

MT is a protein with a host of functions, attributing it a much more dynamic role in physiology than most clinicians would give it credit for. The MT proteins have been associated with gene expression regulation, homeostatic control of cellular metal metabolism, and cellular adaptations to stress, specifically including oxidative stress.[84] There are four isoforms of the protein MTI-MTIV, with MTI and MTII showing neuroprotective effects in central nervous system (CNS) pathology.[85] MTIII appears to be highly regulated in the body, and both elevated levels[86,87] and depressed levels[88,89] contribute to disease. In rat studies, aluminum was found to induce MT production in both the liver and the kidneys, causing a disruption of the normal tissue distribution of metals that interact with MT.[90,91] In contrast, aluminum has been shown to decrease the level of MT in the rat brain, and additional findings of dysregulated levels of iron, manganese, and zinc were found, with all of these effects ameliorated by providing exogenous zinc.[92] Considering this information, it would be challenging to create a hypothesis of increased or decreased MT in association with ASD at the serum level, but it seems likely that there is some dysfunction of activity of this class of proteins at the tissue level given the amount of transcription regulators that have been shown to be abnormal in this condition.

Genetics

Many agree that there is a strong genetic component to ASD[93]; however, the genetic polymorphisms found in ASD are heterogeneous, and this study is more complex than a single gene or constellation of single nucleotide polymorphisms (SNPs).[94,95,96,97,98] There have been many studies investigating the genetics of those with ASD,[99,100,101,102] and investigators in this field believe that the etiology of idiopathic ASD is strongly genetic, with oligogenic transmission being likely.[103] It is estimated that there are 10 to 15 "small-effect" alleles that commonly contribute to the phenotype and that different combinations of mutant alleles may be present in individuals expressing the phenotype. Some of the genes known to be associated with reduced toxicant clearance in ASD are PON1 (SNPs: C-108T, Q192R, and L55M), GSTM1, GSTP1, ALAD2,[104,105] SLC11A3, and MTF1. Individuals with ASD may have SNPs in one or many of these genes, which may affect their ability to excrete metals in their hair or through other pathways. No association was found between ASD and heavy metal regulatory genes MT1a, DMT1, LAT1, and MTF1.[106] There have been no definitive studies that show that an overwhelming proportion of individuals with ASD have any one gene mutation, defect, or SNP. The current state of the science goes back to the balance between total load and physiological susceptibility.

Timothy syndrome (TS) is a rare autosomal-dominant condition characterized by neurological and developmental defects, which include QT prolongation, heart arrhythmias, structural heart defects, syndactyly, and ASD.[107] There are two types, termed *classical* (type 1) and *atypical* (type 2), both of which are attributed to mutations in the gene encoding the $Ca_v1.2$ calcium channel previously mentioned. Beyond TS, $Ca_v1.2$ has been associated with severe learning deficits and psychiatric disorders, with experiments showing that knockout mice adapt to an outcome-based learning strategy rather than achieving success in the traditional way, implying a very specific effect of this channel on the learning process.[108] These channels have been implicated in synaptic plasticity, spatial memory, synaptic potentiation, and NMDA-independent long-term potentiation mediated through ERK activation.[109] Whether the $Ca_v1.2$ channel plays a role in mediating the effects of heavy metals on alopecia or ASD remains to be investigated; however, the possibility remains intriguing.

The previous discussion is meant to provide a scientific basis for the experimental results found when examining the elemental concentrations found in the hair of individuals with ASD. It should not be extrapolated to make inferences beyond this scope. ASD is a complex, multisystem illness and should be recognized as such.

REFERENCES

1. Pizzorno, J. E., & Murray, M. T. (2013). *Textbook of natural medicine.* Churchill Livingstone: Elsevier.
2. Villain, M., Cirimele, V., & Kintz, P. (2004). Hair analysis in toxicology. *Clinical Chemistry and Laboratory Medicine, 42*(11), 1265–1272. PMID: 15576289.
3. Griffon, H., & Barbaud, J. (1951). A method which can be used in toxicology for the detection of arsenic in hair, by the study of the radioactivity of this element induced in situ. *Annales Pharmaceutiques Francaises, 9*(9–10), 545–551. PMID: 14915273.
4. Skröder, H., Kippler, M., Nermell, B., Tofail, F., Levi, M., Rahman, S. M., et al. (2017). Major limitations in using element concentrations in hair as biomarkers of exposure to toxic and essential trace elements in children. *Environmental Health Perspectives, 125*(6), 067021. PMID: 28669939.
5. Wilhelm, M., & Idel, H. (1996). Hair analysis in environmental medicine. *Zentralblatt fur Hygiene Und Umweltmedizin, 198*(6), 485–501. PMID: 9353539.
6. Wilson, L. *Nutritional Balancing And Hair Mineral Analysis. L.D. Wilson Consultants, Inc. 05/12/16.*
7. Barrett, S. (1985). Commercial hair analysis. Science or scam? *JAMA: The Journal of the American Medical Association, 254*(8), 1041–1045. PMID: 4021042.
8. Seidel, S., Kreutzer, R., Smith, D., McNeel, S., & Gilliss, D. (2001). Assessment of commercial laboratories performing hair mineral analysis. *JAMA: The Journal of the American Medical Association, 285*(1), 67–72. PMID: 11150111.
9. Morley, N., & Ford, R. P. (2002). Hair-element analysis–still on the fringe. *Child: Care, Health and Development, 28*(Suppl. 1), 31–34. PMID: 12515436.
10. Drasch, G., & Roider, G. (2002). Assessment of hair mineral analysis commercially offered in Germany. *Journal of Trace Elements in Medicine and Biology: Organ of the Society for Minerals and Trace Elements (GMS), 16*(1), 27–31. PMID: 11878749.
11. Shamberger, R. J. (2002). Validity of hair mineral testing. *Biological Trace Element Research, 87*(1–3), 1–28. PMID: 12117220.
12. Oh, J. W. 1., Kloepper, J., Langan, E. A., Kim, Y., Yeo, J., Kim, M. J., et al. (2016). A Guide to Studying Human Hair Follicle Cycling In Vivo. *The Journal of Investigative Dermatology, 136*(1), 34–44. PMID: 26763421.
13. Legrand, M., Passos, C. J., Mergler, D., & Chan, H. M. (2005). Biomonitoring of mercury exposure with single human hair strand. *Environmental Science & Technology, 39*(12), 4594–4598. PMID: 16047797.
14. Block, R. J. (1939). The composition of keratins: The amino acid composition of hair, wool, horn, and other eukeratins. *The Journal of Biological Chemistry, 128*, 181–186.
15. Ab Razak, N. H., Praveena, S. M., & Hashim, Z. (2015). Toenail as a biomarker of heavy metal exposure via drinking water: A systematic review. *Reviews on Environmental Health, 30*(1), 1–7. PMID: 25332289.
16. Cottingham, K. L., Karimi, R., Gruber, J. F., Zens, M. S., Sayarath, V., Folt, C. L., et al. (2013). Diet and toenail arsenic concentrations in a New Hampshire population with arsenic-containing water. *Nutrition Journal, 12*, 149. PMID: 24237880.
17. Grashow, R., Zhang, J., Fang, S. C., Weisskopf, M. G., Christiani, D. C., & Cavallari, J. M. (2014). Toenail metal concentration as a biomarker of occupational welding fume exposure. *Journal of Occupational and Environmental Hygiene, 11*(6), 397–405. PMID: 24372360.
18. Slotnick, M. J., Meliker, J. R., & Nriagu, J. O. (2008). Intra-individual variability in toenail arsenic

concentrations in a Michigan population, USA. *Journal of Exposure Science and Environmental Epidemiology*, 18(2), 149–157. PMID: 17426735.

19. Marchiset-Ferlay, N., Savanovitch, C., & Sauvant-Rochat, M. P. (2012). What is the best biomarker to assess arsenic exposure via drinking water? *Environment International*, 39(1), 150–171. PMID: 22208756.

20. Diamanti, A., Pedicelli, S., D'Argenio, P., Panetta, F., Alterio, A., & Torre, G. (2011). Iatrogenic Kwashiorkor in three infants on a diet of rice beverages. *Pediatric Allergy and Immunology: Official Publication of the European Society of Pediatric Allergy and Immunology*, 22(8), 878–879. PMID: 22122793.

21. Magiorkinis, E., Beloukas, A., & Diamantis, A. (2011). Scurvy: Past, present and future. *European Journal of Internal Medicine*, 22(2), 147–152. PMID: 21402244.

22. St Pierre, S. A., Vercellotti, G. M., Donovan, J. C., & Hordinsky, M. K. (2010). Iron deficiency and diffuse nonscarring scalp alopecia in women: More pieces to the puzzle. *Journal of the American Academy of Dermatology*, 63(6), 1070–1076. PMID: 20888064.

23. Trost, L. B., Bergfeld, W. F., & Calogeras, E. (2006). The diagnosis and treatment of iron deficiency and its potential relationship to hair loss. *Journal of the American Academy of Dermatology*, 54(5), 824–844. PMID: 16635664.

24. Deloche, C., Bastien, P., Chadoutaud, S., Galan, P., Bertrais, S., Hercberg, S., et al. (2007). Low iron stores: A risk factor for excessive hair loss in non-menopausal women. *European Journal of Dermatology*, 17(6), 507–512. PMID: 17951130.

25. Saper, R. B., & Rash, R. (2009). Zinc: An essential micronutrient. *American Family Physician*, 79(9), 768–772. PMID: 20141096.

26. Daniells, S., & Hardy, G. (2010). Hair loss in long-term or home parenteral nutrition: Are micronutrient deficiencies to blame? *Current Opinion in Clinical Nutrition and Metabolic Care*, 13(6), 690–697. PMID: 20823774.

27. Castelo-Soccio, L. A. (2012). Hair manifestations of systemic disease. *Current Problems in Pediatric and Adolescent Health Care*, 42(8), 198–203. PMID: 22884026.

28. Bachanek, T., Staroslawska, E., Wolanska, E., & Jarmolinska, K. (2000). Heavy metal poisoning in glass worker characterised by severe. *Annals of Agricultural and Environmental Medicine*, 7(1), 51–53. PMID: 10865245.

29. Agarwal, P., Sharma, S., & Agarwal, U. S. (2016). Selenium toxicity: A rare diagnosis. *Indian Journal of Dermatology, Venereology and Leprology*, 82(6), 690–693. PMID: 27716724.

30. Hirata, M., Taoda, K., Ono-Ogasawara, M., Takaya, M., & Hisanaga, N. (1998). A probable case of chronic occupational thallium poisoning in a glass factory. *Industrial Health*, 36(3), 300–303. PMID: 9701911.

31. Moore, D., House, I., & Dixon, A. (1993). Thallium poisoning. Diagnosis may be elusive but alopecia is the clue. *BMJ (Clinical Research Ed.)*, 306(6891), 1527–1529. PMID: 8518684.

32. Lukács, M. (2003). Thallium poisoning induced polyneuropathy – clinical and electrophysiological data. *Ideggyogyaszati Szemle*, 56(11–12), 407–414. PMID: 14743595.

33. Mulkey, J. P., & Oehme, F. W. (1993). A review of thallium toxicity. *Veterinary and Human Toxicology*, 35(5), 445–453. PMID: 8249271.

34. Haas, N. S., Shih, R., & Gochfeld, M. (2003). A patient with postoperative mercury contamination of the peritoneum. *Journal of Toxicology. Clinical Toxicology*, 41(2), 175–180. PMID: 12733856.

35. Schrallhammer-Benkler, K., Ring, J., Przybilla, B., Meurer, M., & Landthaler, M. (1992). Acute mercury intoxication with lichenoid drug eruption followed by mercury contact allergy and development of antinuclear antibodies. *Acta Dermato-Venereologica*, 72(4), 294–296. PMID: 1357893.

36. Ghosh, A. (2013). Evaluation of chronic arsenic poisoning due to consumption of contaminated ground water in West Bengal, India. *International Journal of Preventive Medicine*, 4(8), 976–979. PMID: 24049627.

37. Pierard, G. E. (1979). Toxic effects of metals from the environment on hair growth and structure. *Journal of Cutaneous Pathology*, 6(4), 237–242. . PMID: 227944.

38. Malinowska, M., Jakóbkiewicz-Banecka, J., Kloska, A., Tylki-Szymańska, A., Czartoryska, B., Piotrowska, E., et al. (2008). Abnormalities in the hair morphology of patients with some but not all types of mucopolysaccharidoses. *European Journal of Pediatrics*, 167(2), 203–209. PMID: 17361416.

39. Wendelin, D. S., Pope, D. N., & Mallory, S. B. (2003). Hypertrichosis. *Journal of the American Academy of Dermatology*, 48(2), 161–179. PMID: 12582385.

40. Morand, J. J., Ly, F., Lightburn, E., & Mahé, A. (2007). Complications of cosmetic skin bleaching in Africa. *Medecine Tropicale: Revue Du Corps de Sante Colonial*, 67(6), 627–634. PMID: 18300529.

41. Greco, V., Chen, T., Rendl, M., Schober, M., Pasolli, H. A., Stokes, N., et al. (2009). A two-step mechanism for stem cell activation during hair regeneration. *Cell Stem Cell*, 4(2), 155–169. PMID: 19200804.

42. Yucel, G., Altindag, B., Gomez-Ospina, N., Rana, A., Panagiotakos, G., Lara, M. F., et al. (2013). State-dependent signaling by Cav1.2 regulates hair follicle stem cell function. *Genes & Development*, *27*(11), 1217–1222. PMID: 23752588.

43. Wysocki, G. P., & Daley, T. D. (1987). Hypertrichosis in patients receiving cyclosporine therapy. *Clinical and Experimental Dermatology*, *12*(3), 191–196. PMID: 3690882.

44. Erxleben, C., Liao, Y., Gentile, S., Chin, D., Gomez-Alegria, C., Mori, Y., et al. (2006). Cyclosporin and Timothy syndrome increase mode 2 gating of CaV1.2 calcium channels through aberrant phosphorylation of S6 helices. *Proceedings of the National Academy of Sciences of the United States of America*, *103*(10), 3932–3937. PMID: 16537462.

45. Flinders, B., Cuypers, E., Porta, T., Varesio, E., Hopfgartner, G., & Heeren, R. M. A. (2017). Mass spectrometry imaging of drugs of abuse in hair. *Methods in Molecular Biology*, *1618*, 137–147. PMID: 28523505.

46. Baciu, T., Borrull, F., Aguilar, C., & Calull, M. (2015). Recent trends in analytical methods and separation techniques for drugs of abuse in hair. *Analytica Chimica Acta*, *856*, 1–26. PMID: 25542354.

47. Wang, H., & Wang, Y. (2017). Matrix-assisted laser desorption/ionization mass spectrometric imaging for the rapid segmental analysis of methamphetamine in a single hair using umbelliferone as a matrix. *Analytica Chimica Acta*, *975*, 42–51. PMID: 28552305.

48. Flinders, B., Cuypers, E., Zeijlemaker, H., Tytgat, J., & Heeren, R. M. (2015). Preparation of longitudinal sections of hair samples for the analysis of cocaine by MALDI-MS/MS and TOF-SIMS imaging. *Drug Testing and Analysis*, *7*(10), 859–865. PMID: 25981643.

49. Appenzeller, B. M., Hardy, E. M., Grova, N., Chata, C., Faÿs, F., Briand, O., et al. (2016). Hair analysis for the biomonitoring of pesticide exposure: Comparison with blood and urine in a rat model. *Archives of Toxicology*, doi:10.1007/s00204-016-1910-9. PMID: 28011991.

50. Angelakis, E., Armstrong, N., Nappez, C., Richez, M., Chabriere, E., & Raoult, D. (2015). Doxycycline assay hair samples for testing long-term compliance treatment. *The Journal of Infection*, *71*(5), 511–517. PMID: 26299894.

51. Suzuki, T., Hongo, T., Yoshinaga, J., Imai, H., Nakazawa, M., Matsuo, N., et al. (1993). The hair-organ relationship in mercury concentration in contemporary Japanese. *Archives of Environmental Health*, *48*(4), 221–229. PubMed PMID: 8357270.

52. McDowell, M. A., Dillon, C. F., Osterloh, J., Bolger, P. M., Pellizzari, E., Fernando, R., et al. (2004). Hair mercury levels in U.S. children and women of childbearing age: Reference range data from NHANES 1999-2000. *Environmental Health Perspectives*, *112*(11), 1165–1171. PubMed PMID: 15289161.

53. Goodrich, J. M., Wang, Y., Gillespie, B., Werner, R., Franzblau, A., & Basu, N. (2011). Glutathione enzyme and selenoprotein polymorphisms associate with mercury biomarker levels in Michigan dental professionals. *Toxicology and Applied Pharmacology*, *257*(2), 301–308. PubMed PMID: 21967774.

54. Wang, Y., Goodrich, J. M., Gillespie, B., Werner, R., Basu, N., & Franzblau, A. (2012). An investigation of modifying effects of metallothionein single-nucleotide polymorphisms on the association between mercury exposure and biomarker levels. *Environmental Health Perspectives*, *120*(4), 530–534. PubMed PMID: 22233731. Erratum in: 2013 Jan;121(1):A13.

55. Rossignol, D. A., Genuis, S. J., & Frye, R. E. (2014). Environmental toxicants and autism spectrum disorders: A systematic review. *Translational Psychiatry*, *4*, e360. PMID: 24518398.

56. Rossignol, D. A., & Frye, R. E. (2012). A review of research trends in physiological abnormalities in autism spectrum disorders: Immune dysregulation, inflammation, oxidative stress, mitochondrial dysfunction and environmental toxicant exposures. *Molecular Psychiatry*, *17*(4), 389–401. PMID: 22143005.

57. Li, Z., Dong, T., Pröschel, C., & Noble, M. (2007). Chemically diverse toxicants converge on Fyn and c-Cbl to disrupt precursor cell function. *PLoS Biology*, *5*(2), e35. PMID: 17298174.

58. Shelton, J. F., Hertz-Picciotto, I., & Pessah, I. N. (2012). Tipping the balance of autism risk: Potential mechanisms linking pesticides and autism. *Environmental Health Perspectives*, *120*(7), 944–951. PMID: 22534084.

59. Xu, F., Farkas, S., Kortbeek, S., Zhang, F. X., Chen, L., Zamponi, G. W., et al. (2012). Mercury-induced toxicity of rat cortical neurons is mediated through N-Methyl-D-Aspartate receptors. *Molecular Brain*, *5*, 30. PMID: 22980357.

60. Majewska, M. D., Urbanowicz, E., Rok-Bujko, P., Namyslowska, I., & Mierzejewski, P. (2010). Age-dependent lower or higher levels of hair mercury in autistic children than in healthy controls. *Acta Neurobiologiae Experimentalis*, *70*(2), 196–208. PMID: 20628443.

61. LeBlanc, J. J., & Fagiolini, M. (2011). Autism: A "critical period" disorder? *Neural Plasticity*, *2011*, 921680. PMID: 21826280.

62. Ismail, F. Y., Fatemi, A., & Johnston, M. V. (2017). Cerebral plasticity: Windows of opportunity in the

developing brain. *European Journal of Paediatric Neurology*, 21(1), 23–48. PMID: 27567276.

63. Hoffman, J. F., Wright, C. L., & McCarthy, M. M. (2016). A critical period in purkinje cell development is mediated by local estradiol synthesis, disrupted by inflammation, and has enduring consequences only for males. *The Journal of Neuroscience: The Official Journal of the Society for Neuroscience*, 36(39), 10039–10049. PMID: 27683901.

64. James, S. J., Melnyk, S., Jernigan, S., Cleves, M. A., Halsted, C. H., Wong, D. H., et al. (2006). Metabolic endophenotype and related genotypes are associated with oxidative stress in children with autism. *American Journal of Medical Genetics. Part B, Neuropsychiatric Genetics: The Official Publication of the International Society of Psychiatric Genetics*, 141B(8), 947–956. PMID: 16917939.

65. Kenet, T., Froemke, R. C., Schreiner, C. E., Pessah, I. N., & Merzenich, M. M. (2007). Perinatal exposure to a noncoplanar polychlorinated biphenyl alters tonotopy, receptive fields, and plasticity in rat primary auditory cortex. *Proceedings of the National Academy of Sciences of the United States of America*, 104(18), 7646–7651. PMID: 17460041.

66. Xu, F., Farkas, S., Kortbeek, S., Zhang, F. X., Chen, L., Zamponi, G. W., et al. (2012). Mercury-induced toxicity of rat cortical neurons is mediated through N-Methyl-D-Aspartate receptors. *Molecular Brain*, 5, 30. PMID: 22980357.

67. Yasuda, H., & Tsutsui, T. (2013). Assessment of infantile mineral imbalances in autism spectrum disorders (ASDs). *International Journal of Environmental Research and Public Health*, 10(11), 6027–6043. PMCID: PMC3863885.

68. Wecker, L., Miller, S. B., Cochran, S. R., Dugger, D. L., & Johnson, W. D. (1985). Trace element concentrations in hair from autistic children. *Journal of Mental Deficiency Research*, 29(Pt. 1), 15–22. PMID: 4009700.

69. Bjorklund, G. (2013). The role of zinc and copper in autism spectrum disorders. *Acta Neurobiologiae Experimentalis*, 73(2), 225–236. PMID: 23823984.

70. Li, S. O., Wang, J. L., Bjørklund, G., Zhao, W. N., & Yin, C. H. (2014). Serum copper and zinc levels in individuals with autism spectrum disorders. *Neuroreport*, 25(15), 1216–1220. PMID: 25162784.

71. Faber, S., Zinn, G. M., Kern, J. C., 2nd, & Kingston, H. M. (2009). The plasma zinc/serum copper ratio as a biomarker in children with autism spectrum disorders. *Biomarkers: Biochemical Indicators of Exposure, Response, and Susceptibility to Chemicals*, 14(3), 171–180. PMID: 19280374.

72. Jackson, M. J., & Garrod, P. J. (1978). Plasma zinc, copper, and amino acid levels in the blood of autistic children. *Journal of Autism and Childhood Schizophrenia*, 8(2), 203–208. PMID: 670131.

73. Yasuda, H., Yoshida, K., Yasuda, Y., & Tsutsui, T. (2011). Infantile zinc deficiency: Association with autism spectrum disorders. *Scientific Reports*, 1, 129. doi:10.1038/srep00129. PMID: 22355646.

74. Vela, G., Stark, P., Socha, M., Sauer, A. K., Hagmeyer, S., & Grabrucker, A. M. (2015). Zinc in gut-brain interaction in autism and neurological disorders. *Neural Plasticity*, 2015, 972791. PMID: 25878905.

75. Hidalgo, J., Aschner, M., Zatta, P., & Vasák, M. (2001). Roles of the metallothionein family of proteins in the central nervous system. *Brain Research Bulletin*, 55(2), 133–145. PMID: 11470309.

76. Lipton, S. A., Choi, Y. B., Takahashi, H., Zhang, D., Li, W., Godzik, A., et al. (2002). Cysteine regulation of protein function – as exemplified by NMDA-receptor modulation. *Trends in Neurosciences*, 25(9), 474–480. PMID: 12183209.

77. Lipton, S. A., & Rosenberg, P. A. (1994). Excitatory amino acids as a final common pathway for neurologic disorders. *The New England Journal of Medicine*, 330(9), 613–622. PMID: 7905600.

78. Lakshmi Priya, M. D., & Geetha, A. (2011). A biochemical study on the level of proteins and their percentage of nitration in the hair and nail of autistic children. *Clinica Chimica Acta*, 412(11–12), 1036–1042. PMID: 21338594.

79. Nordberg, M., & Nordberg, G. F. (2000). Toxicological aspects of metallothionein. *Cellular and Molecular Biology (Noisy-Le-Grand, France)*, 46(2), 451–463. PMID: 10774933.

80. Jones, D. P. (2008). Radical-free biology of oxidative stress. *American Journal of Physiology. Cell Physiology*, 295(4), C849–C868. PMID: 18684987.

81. Shi, Z. Z., Osei-Frimpong, J., Kala, G., Kala, S. V., Barrios, R. J., Habib, G. M., et al. (2000). Glutathione synthesis is essential for mouse development but not for cell growth in culture. *Proceedings of the National Academy of Sciences of the United States of America*, 97(10), 5101–5106. PMID: 10805773.

82. Russo, A. J. (2009). Anti-metallothionein IgG and levels of metallothionein in autistic children with GI disease. *Drug, Healthcare and Patient Safety*, 1, 1–8. [Epub 2009 Jan 8]; PMID: 21701604.

83. Russo, A. F. (2008). Anti-metallothionein IgG and levels of metallothionein in autistic families. *Swiss Medical Weekly*, 138(5–6), 70–77. PMID: 18365350.

84. Aschner, M., & West, A. K. (2005). The role of MT in neurological disorders. *Journal of Alzheimer's Disease, 8*(2), 139–145, discussion 209-15. PMID: 16308482.

85. Stankovic, R. K., Chung, R. S., & Penkowa, M. (2007). Metallothioneins I and II: Neuroprotective significance during CNS pathology. *The International Journal of Biochemistry & Cell Biology, 39*(3), 484–489. PMID: 17097331.

86. Felizola, S. J., Nakamura, Y., Arata, Y., Ise, K., Satoh, F., Rainey, W. E., et al. (2014). Metallothionein-3 (MT-3) in the human adrenal cortex and its disorders. *Endocrine Pathology, 25*(3), 229–235. PMID: 24242700.

87. Pula, B., Tazbierski, T., Zamirska, A., Werynska, B., Bieniek, A., Szepietowski, J., et al. (2015). Metallothionein 3 expression in normal skin and malignant skin lesions. *Pathology Oncology Research, 21*(1), 187–193. PMID: 25015776.

88. Lee, S. J., Seo, B. R., & Koh, J. Y. (2015). Metallothionein-3 modulates the amyloid β endocytosis of astrocytes through its effects on actin polymerization. *Molecular Brain, 8*(1), 84. PMID: 26637294.

89. Byun, H. R., Choi, J. A., & Koh, J. Y. (2014). The role of metallothionein-3 in streptozotocin-induced beta-islet cell death and diabetes in mice. *Metallomics : Integrated Biometal Science, 6*(9), 1748–1757. PMID: 25054451.

90. Jeffery, E. H., Jansen, H. T., & Dellinger, J. A. (1987). In vivo interactions of aluminum with hepatic cytochrome P-450 and metallothionein. *Fundamental and Applied Toxicology, 8*(4), 541–548. PMID: 3609540.

91. Ghorbel, I., Chaabane, M., Elwej, A., Boudawara, O., Abdelhedi, S., Jamoussi, K., et al. (2016). Expression of metallothioneins I and II related to oxidative stress in the liver of aluminium-treated rats. *Archives of Physiology and Biochemistry, 122*(4), 214–222. PMID: 27230980.

92. Singla, N., & Dhawan, D. K. (2014). Zinc modulates aluminium-induced oxidative stress and cellular injury in rat brain. *Metallomics : Integrated Biometal Science, 6*(10), 1941–1950. PMID: 25141099.

93. Domingues, V. F., Nasuti, C., Piangerelli, M., Correia-Sá, L., Ghezzo, A., Marini, M., et al. (2016). Pyrethroid pesticide metabolite in urine and microelements in hair of children affected by autism spectrum disorders: A preliminary investigation. *International Journal of Environmental Research and Public Health, 13*(4), 388. PMID: 27482573.

94. De Rubeis, S., & Buxbaum, J. D. (2015). Genetics and genomics of autism spectrum disorder: Embracing complexity. *Human Molecular Genetics, 24*(R1), R24–R31. PMID: 26188008.

95. Hua, R., Wei, M., & Zhang, C. (2015). The complex genetics in autism spectrum disorders. *Science China. Life Sciences, 58*(10), 933–945. PMID: 26335739.

96. Hens, K., Peeters, H., & Dierickx, K. (2016). The ethics of complexity. Genetics and autism, a literature review. *American Journal of Medical Genetics. Part B, Neuropsychiatric Genetics: The Official Publication of the International Society of Psychiatric Genetics, 171B*(3), 305–316. PMID: 26870917.

97. de la Torre-Ubieta, L., Won, H. 1., Stein, J. L., & Geschwind, D. H. (2016). Advancing the understanding of autism disease mechanisms through genetics. *Nature Medicine, 22*(4), 345–361. PMID: 27050589.

98. Yin, J., & Schaaf, C. P. (2017). Autism genetics - an overview. *Prenatal Diagnosis, 37*(1), 14–30. PMID: 27743394.

99. Muhle, R., Trentacoste, S. V., & Rapin, I. (2004). The genetics of autism. *Pediatrics, 113*(5), e472–e486. PMID: 15121991.

100. International Molecular Genetic Study of Autism Consortium (IMGSAC). (2001). Further characterization of the autism susceptibility locus AUTS1 on chromosome 7q. *Human Molecular Genetics, 10*(9), 973–982. PMID: 11392322.

101. Yonan, A. L., Alarcón, M., Cheng, R., et al. (2003). A genomewide screen of 345 families for autism-susceptibility loci. *American Journal of Human Genetics, 73*(4), 886–897. PMCID: PMC1180610.

102. Hutcheson, H. B., Olson, L. M., Bradford, Y., Folstein, S. E., Santangelo, S. L., Sutcliffe, J. S., et al. (2004). Examination of NRCAM, LRRN3, KIAA0716, and LAMB1 as autism candidate genes. *BMC Medical Genetics, 5*, 12. PMID: 15128462.

103. Barrett, S. 1., Beck, J. C., Bernier, R., Bisson, E., Braun, T. A., Casavant, T. L., et al. (1999). An autosomal genomic screen for autism. Collaborative linkage study of autism. *American Journal of Medical Genetics, 88*(6), 609–615. PMID: 10581478.

104. Wetmur, J. G., Kaya, A. H., Plewinska, M., & Desnick, R. J. (1991). Molecular characterization of the human delta-aminolevulinate dehydratase 2 (ALAD2) allele: Implications for molecular screening of individuals for genetic susceptibility to lead poisoning. *American Journal of Human Genetics, 49*(4), 757–763. PMID: 1716854.

105. Sobin, C., Flores-Montoya, M. G., Gutierrez, M., Parisi, N., & Schaub, T. (2015). δ-Aminolevulinic acid dehydratase single nucleotide polymorphism 2 (ALAD2) and peptide transporter 2*2 haplotype (hPEPT2*2) differently influence neurobehavior in

low-level lead exposed children. *Neurotoxicology and Teratology*, *47*, 137–145. PMID: 25514583.

106. Owens, S. E., Summar, M. L., Ryckman, K. K., Haines, J. L., Reiss, S., Summar, S. R., et al. (2011). Lack of association between autism and four heavy metal regulatory genes. *Neurotoxicology*, *32*(6), 769–775. PMID: 21798283.

107. Splawski, I., Timothy, K. W., Sharpe, L. M., Decher, N., Kumar, P., Bloise, R., et al. (2004). Ca(V)1.2 calcium channel dysfunction causes a multisystem disorder including arrhythmia and autism. *Cell*, *119*(1), 19–31. PMID: 15454078.

108. Koppe, G., Mallien, A. S., Berger, S., Bartsch, D., Gass, P., Vollmayr, B., et al. (2017). CACNA1C gene regulates behavioral strategies in operant rule learning. *PLoS Biology*, *15*(6), e2000936. PMID: 28604818.

109. Moosmang, S., Haider, N., Klugbauer, N., Adelsberger, H., Langwieser, N., Müller, J., et al. (2005). Role of hippocampal Cav1.2 Ca2+ channels in NMDA receptor-independent synaptic plasticity and spatial memory. *The Journal of Neuroscience: The Official Journal of the Society for Neuroscience*, *25*(43), 9883–9892. PMID: 16251435.

59

Breast Milk Excretion

SUMMARY

- Significant route of elimination for lipophilic molecules
- Rate of elimination decreases with duration of lactation
- Reduction of body burden of toxicants appears to be significant
- This route of excretion is more important for lipophilic persistent organic pollutants (POPs) than heavy metals

INTRODUCTION

Breast milk is a complex colloid containing all of the nutrients needed by a newborn infant for its first 6 months of life. In addition to macronutrients and micronutrients, it also contains immune factors; each of these components affects the toxin/toxicant load of the milk in different ways. Breast milk is typically considered as a source of exposure for the infant; however, it should also be considered as a route of excretion for the mother. Both the presence of pregnancy and the act of nursing lower the total toxicant load of the mother. This leads to a substantial toxicant load on the infant, with the child's serum polychlorinated biphenyl (PCB) level equaling the mother's after 4 months of breastfeeding.[1] Increasing parity confers a decrease in breast cancer risk, with each additional birth providing a 10% risk reduction,[2] and women who have a child before the age of 20 years have a 50% reduction in lifetime breast cancer risk compared with nulliparous women.[3] This risk reduction is typically explained in terms of differential hormonal exposure or changes in cell development and cell subpopulations. However, this hypothesis has never been proven, and it is plausible that this risk reduction is more related to the reduction in toxicant levels of the mammary tissues. It should be stated that, even in recognition of the toxicity

of breast milk, breastfeeding is still recommended in cases of typical exposure.[4] Clinical action plans have been published to help decrease infant exposure to toxins and toxicants from breast milk.[5]

SYNTHESIS AND COMPOSITION OF BREAST MILK

The production of milk occurs in the mammary alveolar gland and involves the components of milk passing through a membrane located at the interface between the gland and the capillary vasculature. This process endows the milk with a composition of environmental chemicals comparable to the levels found in other fatty compartments of the body.[6,7] The most common mechanism for transport into the milk is passive diffusion, which allows for the movement of molecules with a molecular weight of less than 800 Da. This indicates that a lipophilic nature is of primary importance for this route of elimination. A component of this is the degree of ionization, which makes the pK_a of the molecule and the pH of the plasma worthy considerations. In general, molecules that act as weak bases are more likely to accumulate in the milk compared with those that act as weak acids.[8] A more in-depth discussion regarding acid-base modulation for the promotion of toxicant excretion can be found

TABLE 59.1   Composition of Milk Samples

		TIME OF COLLECTION	
	Average ± SD (n)	Summer (n)	Winter (n)
Energy (kcal/100 mL)	66.3 ± 13.3 (1180)	65.6 ± 13.2 (587)	66.9 ± 13.3 (593)
Solid matter (g/100 mL)	12.46 ± 1.56 (1180)	12.41 ± 1.59 (587)	12.50 ± 1.53 (593)
Ash (g/100 mL)	0.19 ± 0.06 (1180)	0.18 ± 0.05 (587)	0.19 ± 0.06 (593)
Total N (g/100 mL)	0.19 ± 0.04 (1180)	0.19 ± 0.04 (587)	0.19 ± 0.05 (593)
Lipids (g/100 mL)	3.46 ± 1.49 (1180)	3.39 ± 1.46 (587)	3.53 ± 1.51 (593)
Carbohydrates (g/100 mL)	7.58 ± 0.77 (1180)	7.62 ± 0.80 (587)	7.55 ± 0.75 (593)
Lactose (g/100 mL)	6.44 ± 0.49 (1172)	6.45 ± 0.49 (579)	6.43 ± 0.48 (593)
pH	6.5 ± 0.3 (1180)	6.5 ± 0.2 (587)	6.5 ± 0.3 (593)
Osmotic pressure (mOsm/kg·H_2O)	299 ± 14 (1179)	301 ± 12 (587)	298 ± 16 (592)
Cl (mg/100 mL)	35.9 ± 16.2 (1180)	38.7 ± 18.1 (587)	33.1 ± 13.5 (593)
Na (mg/100 mL)	13.5 ± 8.7 (1160)	13.8 ± 9.6 (567)	13.2 ± 7.7 (593)
Mg (mg/100 mL)	2.7 ± 0.9 (1170)	2.6 ± 0.9 (577)	2.7 ± 0.9 (593)
P (mg/100 mL)	15.0 ± 3.8 (1170)	14.6 ± 3.4 (577)	15.3 ± 4.1 (593)
K (mg/100 mL)	47.0 ± 12.1 (1167)	45.5 ± 11.9 (574)	48.5 ± 12.2 (593)
Ca (mg/100 mL)	25.0 ± 7.1 (1170)	23.7 ± 6.6 (577)	26.2 ± 7.4 (593)
Cr (mg/100 mL)	5.9 ± 4.7 (1166)	6.7 ± 3.9 (579)	5.1 ± 5.2 (587)
Mn (μg/100 mL)	1.1 ± 2.3 (1167)	0.9 ± 1.6 (580)	1.2 ± 2.9 (587)
Fe (μg/100 mL)	119 ± 251 (1155)	108 ± 252 (579)	129 ± 249 (576)
Cu (μg/100 mL)	35 ± 21 (1169)	36 ± 10 (582)	34 ± 29 (587)
Zn (μg/100 mL)	145 ± 135 (1165)	132 ± 127 (582)	159 ± 142 (583)
Se (μg/100 mL)	1.7 ± 0.6 (303)	1.8 ± 0.6 (169)	1.7 ± 0.7 (134)

From Yamawaki, N., Yamada, M., Kan-no, T., Kojima, T., Kaneko, T., & Yonekubo, A. (2005). Macronutrient, mineral and trace element composition of breast milk from Japanese women. *Journal of Trace Elements in Medicine and Biology, 19*(2–3), 171–181. doi:10.1016/j.jtemb.2005.05.001

elsewhere in this text. Additionally, small (<200 Da) water-soluble chemicals are able to cross the membrane with the bulk transfer of water. Toxicants that are larger than 800 Da and those bound to plasma proteins or erythrocytes are unlikely to enter the milk.[9]

Lactogenesis begins 40 hours after the birth of the child. The initial milk produced in the first 3 to 5 days is called colostrum, which is low in fat content (at around 2.9%). Over the next 2 to 6 weeks, the milk changes to become "transitional milk," increasing in fat concentration to 4%.[10] Breast milk contains about 3.5 g of fat per 100 mL, roughly half of the total energy content (Table 59.1).[11] The lipids are secreted in small droplets, increasing in concentration as the feeding progresses. It contains long-chain free fatty acids, such as docosahexaenoic acid and arachidonic acid, that are not typically found in other milks. The milk contains about 6.5 g of lactose and 0.9 g of protein per 100 mL. It contains less casein than other milks, and this casein has a different structure that forms more easily digested curds. Micronutrients include vitamins A, B1, B2, B6, B12, and D and many trace minerals.[12]

Analytical Considerations

Physical and chemical characteristics of toxicants determine their fractional excretion in the breast milk; these include lipid solubility, degree of ionization, and molecular weight. Because the breast milk has a much higher fat concentration than the other mobile phases of the body (i.e., blood, urine, saliva), the most likely compounds to be found in this form of elimination are those that are lipid soluble. As with any biological monitoring, the original chemical isn't necessarily the analyte of interest, but rather the primary metabolite can be the entity that is commonly observed. Good examples are dieldrin from aldrin exposure and dichlorodiphenyldichloroethylene (DDE) from dichlorodiphenyl-trichloroethane (DDT) exposure.[10] Complicating all efforts is the fact that breast milk is a heterogeneous mixture that changes in composition throughout the course of a single feeding, across a single day, and during the course of lactation as a whole. This lack of consistency makes data on collection of utmost importance, and unfortunately, this is lacking in most of the reports.

Depuration

In studying infant exposure to environmental toxicants in the breast milk, it is important to develop an understanding of depuration through the production of breast milk. This is most important for molecules with long half-lives in the body and those that are acquired through incidental environmental exposures. Factors that influence the elimination kinetics involved in this process are still poorly understood but likely involve the initial chemical concentration, the age of the mother, parity, the volume of milk produced, and properties of individual chemicals.[13] However, this route of depuration can be considerable, with a good correlation being shown between modeled and published values of 2,3,7,8-tetrachlorodibenzo-p-dioxin (TCDD) when assuming a 70% decline in levels of this substance after 6 months of daily breastfeeding.[14]

ANALYSIS

Usually the analysis of environmental chemicals in breast milk is referenced to the fat content of the sample. To do this, the fat content of the sample needs to be determined. The lipid-adjusted value allows for normalization for multiple samples from the same mother or samples between mothers. Organic compounds are typically quantified using either gas or liquid chromatograph (GC or LC, respectively) with verification using mass spectrometry (GCMS or LCMS). Metals are identified and quantified using atomic absorption spectroscopy (AAS) or inductively coupled plasma mass spectrometry (ICP-MS).[10]

Toxicants Excreted in Breast Milk

The following data needs to be viewed carefully knowing that there is considerable heterogeneity among the data sets presented on this topic.

Persistent Organic Pollutants.

PCBs, organochlorine compounds, and polybrominated biphenyls. Infants exposed to POPs through their mothers' milk will already have been exposed to these toxicants throughout their time *in utero*. Although subsequent neurological defects in children have been associated with *in utero* exposure, these problems are not associated with exposure through breast milk.[15] Studies of the breast milk from the mothers of 856 children found a decline in PCB and DDE levels of 20% after 6 months of breastfeeding; 43% of these women were primiparous, and the median time for breastfeeding was 29 weeks.[16,17] A study of 246 nursing women looked at the correlation between fish consumption and levels of omega-3 fatty acids and PCBs in breast milk found a direct increase of PCBs with omega-3 fatty acids.[18] They also looked at the effect of length of breastfeeding and found, as shown in Fig. 59.1, that the longer a woman breastfed, the lower the levels of many PCBs in breast milk, presumably related to depletion of fat stores.

In a study of 320 women, the cumulative length of previous lactations was negatively associated with concentrations of four classes of OCs—10 different organochlorine pesticides (OCPs), 8 PCB congeners, and 17 polychlorinated dibenzodioxin (PCDD) and polychlorinated dibenzofuran (PCDF).[19] The elimination kinetics of OCPs were studied at the onset of lactation using samples from 30 volunteers. The authors describe a rapid decrease in DDE of 80% over the first 10 days and linear decreases in the other OCPs studied; with the exception of heptachlor, many of these decreased in concentration by 50%.[20]

An analysis done on a mother nursing twins found a 92% decrease in hexachlorobenzene (HCB) and an 81% decrease in DDE over a period of 30 months of lactation.[21]

Other smaller, less-rigorous studies have shown no change in excretion or even increasing excretion over time, whereas others have shown conflicting results.[22,23]

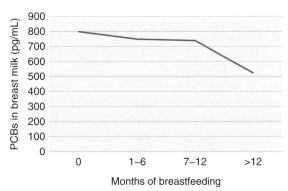

FIG. 59.1 Nursing decreases PCBs in breast milk.

Dioxins and Furans. In a study investigating dioxins and furans in the breast milk, the levels found in mothers breastfeeding their second child (74 samples) were 20% to 30% lower than those in the mothers breastfeeding their first child (79 samples).[24]

Toxic Metals. Toxic metals are found in smaller concentrations in the milk than the lipid-soluble chemicals. Levels of toxic metals are approximately 20% of those found in the blood of the mother.[25]

Aluminum and lead. The highest levels of metals have been shown to be found in early milk, declining in concentration with the duration of lactation. The greatest differences have been found with aluminum and lead, both of which decline by nearly 60% over the four stages of milk production.[26]

Mercury. In mature milk, associations have been found between mercury and both fish consumption and amalgam fillings,[27,28] but this association has not held true when transitional milk was investigated.[29]

Cadmium. Associations have been found between cigarette smoking and cadmium in the breast milk,[30] with one study finding an association between the number of cigarettes smoked by the mother and her breast milk cadmium levels.[31]

With these studies in mind, the infant's exposure to heavy metals, and thus the mother's elimination of such, tend to be more important with reference to vertical transfer through the placenta than by transmission via the breast milk.[32]

Other Toxicants. Other pollutants of significance found in breast milk include tetrachloroethene,[33] pharmaceuticals and drugs of abuse,[34,35] and antibiotics.[36]

REFERENCES

1. Patandin, S., Weisglas-Kuperus, N., de Ridder, M. A., et al. (1997). Plasma polychlorinated biphenyl levels in Dutch preschool children either breast-fed or formula-fed during infancy. *American Journal of Public Health*, 87(10), 1711–1714. PMID: 9357362.
2. Lambe, M., Hsieh, C. C., Chan, H. W., et al. (1996). Parity, age at first and last birth, and risk of breast cancer: a population-based study in Sweden. *Breast Cancer Research and Treatment*, 38(3), 305–311. PMID: 8739084.
3. Britt, K., Ashworth, A., & Smalley, M. (2007). Pregnancy and the risk of breast cancer. *Endocrine-Related Cancer*, 14(4), 907–933. PMID: 18045947.
4. LaKind, J. S., Berlin, C. M., & Mattison, D. R. (2008). The heart of the matter on breastmilk and environmental chemicals: essential points for healthcare providers and new parents. *Breastfeeding Medicine: The Official Journal of the Academy of Breastfeeding Medicine*, 3(4), 251–259. PMID: 19086828.
5. Condon, M. (2005). Breast is best, but it could be better: what is in breast milk that should not be? *Pediatric Nursing*, 31(4), 333–338. PMID: 16229133.
6. Jenness, R. (1979). The composition of human milk. *Seminars in Perinatology*, 3(3), 225–239. PMID: 392766.
7. Skaare, J. U., Tuveng, J. M., & Sande, H. A. (1988). Organochlorine pesticides and polychlorinated biphenyls in maternal adipose tissue, blood, milk, and cord blood from mothers and their infants living in Norway. *Archives of Environmental Contamination and Toxicology*, 17(1), 55–63. PMID: 3122671.
8. Miller, G. E., Banerjee, N. C., & Stowe, C. M., Jr. (1967). Diffusion of certain weak organic acids and bases across the bovine mammary gland membrane after systemic administration. *The Journal of Pharmacology and Experimental Therapeutics*, 157(1), 245–253. PMID: 6067597.
9. Atkinson, H. C., & Begg, E. J. (1988). The binding of drugs to major human milk whey proteins. *British Journal of Clinical Pharmacology*, 26(1), 107–109. PMID: 3203054.
10. Needham, L. L., & Wang, R. Y. (2002). Analytic considerations for measuring environmental chemicals in breast milk. *Environmental Health Perspectives*, 110(6), A317–A324. PMID: 12055062.
11. Yamawaki, N., Yamada, M., Kan-no, T., et al. (2005). Macronutrient, mineral and trace element composition of breast milk from Japanese women. *Journal of Trace Elements in Medicine and Biology: Organ of the Society for Minerals and Trace Elements (GMS)*, 19(2–3), 171–181. PMID: 16325533.
12. Ballard, O., & Morrow, A. L. (2013). Human milk composition: nutrients and bioactive factors. *Pediatric Clinics of North America*, 60(1), 49–74. PMID: 23178060.
13. LaKind, J. S., Berlin, C. M., & Naiman, D. Q. (2001). Infant exposure to chemicals in breast milk in the United States: what we need to learn from a breast milk monitoring program. *Environmental Health Perspectives*, 109(1), 75–88. PMID: 11171529.
14. Kreuzer, P. E., Csanády, G. A., Baur, C., et al. (1997). 2,3,7,8-Tetrachlorodibenzo-p-dioxin (TCDD) and congeners in infants. A toxicokinetic model of human lifetime body burden by TCDD with special emphasis

on its uptake by nutrition. *Archives of Toxicology, 71*(6), 383–400. PMID: 9195020.

15. Gascon, M., Verner, M. A., Guxens, M., et al. (2013). Evaluating the neurotoxic effects of lactational exposure to persistent organic pollutants (POPs) in Spanish children. *Neurotoxicology, 34*, 9–15. PubMed PMID: 23085522.

16. Rogan, W. J., & Gladen, B. C. (1985). Study of human lactation for effects of environmental contaminants: the North Carolina Breast Milk and Formula Project and some other ideas. *Environmental Health Perspectives, 60*, 215–221. PMID: 3928347.

17. Rogan, W. J., Gladen, B. C., McKinney, J. D., et al. (1986). Polychlorinated biphenyls (PCBs) and dichlorodiphenyl dichloroethene (DDE) in human milk: effects of maternal factors and previous lactation. *American Journal of Public Health, 76*(2), 172–177. PMID: 3080910.

18. Bjermo, H., Darnerud, P. O., Lignell, S., et al. (2013). Fish intake and breastfeeding time are associated with serum concentrations of organochlorines in a Swedish population. *Environment International, 51*, 88–96. PMID: 23201820.

19. Albers, J. M., Kreis, I. A., Liem, A. K., & van Zoonen, P. (1996). Factors that influence the level of contamination of human milk with poly-chlorinated organic compounds. *Archives of Environmental Contamination and Toxicology, 30*(2), 285–291. PMID: 8593086.

20. Klein, D., Dillon, J. C., Jirou-Najou, J. L., et al. (1986). Elimination kinetics of organochlorine compounds in the 1st week of breast feeding. *Food and Chemical Toxicology: An International Journal Published for the British Industrial Biological Research Association, 24*(8), 869–873. PMID: 2430874.

21. Schecter, A., Ryan, J. J., & Päpke, O. (1998). Decrease in levels and body burden of dioxins, dibenzofurans, PCBS, DDE, and HCB in blood and milk in a mother nursing twins over a thirty-eight month period. *Chemosphere, 37*(9–12), 1807–1816. PMID: 9828309.

22. LaKind, J. S., Berlin, C. M., & Naiman, D. Q. (2001). Infant exposure to chemicals in breast milk in the United States: what we need to learn from a breast milk monitoring program. *Environmental Health Perspectives, 109*(1), 75–88. PMID: 11171529.

23. LaKind, J. S., Amina Wilkins, A., & Berlin, C. M., Jr. (2004). Environmental chemicals in human milk: a review of levels, infant exposures and health, and guidance for future research. *Toxicology and Applied Pharmacology, 198*(2), 184–208. PMID: 15236953.

24. Fürst, P., Krüger, C., Meemken, H.-A., & Groebel, W. (1989). PCDD and PCDF levels in human milk—dependence on the period of lactation. *Chemosphere, 1*, 439–444.

25. Golding, J. (1997). Unnatural constituents of breast milk–medication, lifestyle, pollutants, viruses. *Early Human Development, 49*(Suppl.), S29–S43. PMID: 9363416.

26. Chao, H. H., Guo, C. H., Huang, C. B., et al. (2014). Arsenic, cadmium, lead, and aluminum concentrations in human milk at early stages of lactation. *Pediatrics and Neonatology, 55*(2), 127–134. PMID: 24231114.

27. Oskarsson, A., Palminger Hallén, I., & Sundberg, J. (1995). Exposure to toxic elements via breast milk. *The Analyst, 120*(3), 765–770. PMID: 7741226.

28. Oskarsson, A., Schültz, A., Skerfving, S., et al. (1996). Total and inorganic mercury in breast milk in relation to fish consumption and amalgam in lactating women. *Archives of Environmental Health, 51*(3), 234–241. PMID: 8687245.

29. Klemann, D., Weinhold, J., Strubelt, O., et al. (1990). Effects of amalgam fillings on the mercury concentrations in amniotic fluid and breast milk. *Deutsche Zahnärztliche Zeitschrift, 45*(3), 142–145. PMID: 2257818.

30. Hallén, I. P., Jorhem, L., Lagerkvist, B. J., & Oskarsson, A. (1995). Lead and cadmium levels in human milk and blood. *The Science of the Total Environment, 166*, 149–155. PMID: 7754354.

31. Radisch, B., Luck, W., & Nau, H. (1987). Cadmium concentrations in milk and blood of smoking mothers. *Toxicology Letters, 36*(2), 147–152. PMID: 3576645.

32. Massart, F., Gherarducci, G., Marchi, B., & Saggese, G. (2008). Chemical biomarkers of human breast milk pollution. *Biomark Insights, 3*, 159–169. PMID: 19578503.

33. Schreiber, J. S. (1993). Predicted infant exposure to tetrachloroethene in human breastmilk. *Risk Analysis, 13*(5), 515–524. PMID: 8259441.

34. Howard, C. R., & Lawrence, R. A. (1998). Breast-feeding and drug exposure. *Obstetrics and Gynecology Clinics of North America, 25*(1), 195–217. PMID: 9547767.

35. Arena, J. M. (1980). Drugs and chemicals excreted in breast milk. *Pediatric Annals, 9*(12), 452–457. PMID: 6256709.

36. Chung, A. M., Reed, M. D., & Blumer, J. L. (2002). Antibiotics and breast-feeding: a critical review of the literature. *Paediatric Drugs, 4*(12), 817–837. PMID: 12431134.

60

Avoidance

SUMMARY

- Air:
  - Removal of off-gassing materials and products from the home
  - Proper remediation of water-damaged, mold-containing material
  - Use of high-quality pleated electrostatic furnace and heating, ventilation, and air conditioning (HVAC) filters
  - Use of air purifiers
    - Electric
    - Plants
  - Use of personal masks and air filters
- Food:
  - Avoidance of commercial varieties of the most toxic fruits and vegetables
- Avoidance of regular consumption of fish with moderate to high mercury and farmed fish high in persistent organic pollutants (POPs)
- Avoidance of meats with high POP levels
- Water:
  - Water purification to remove water toxicants endemic to patient's area
- Personal care products:
  - Avoidance of toxicant-containing personal care products

INTRODUCTION

The absolute first treatment step for all environmentally ill individuals is avoidance. The predominant source(s) of toxicants that are causing, or preventing the cure of, the patient's major health problems must be eliminated. The unavoidable necessity of identifying and removing the exposure source is exemplified in an illustrative case study published in the *British Medical Journal*. A woman with elevated blood mercury was seen at a clinic in 2010 and treated with dimercaptosuccinic acid (DMSA), which successfully reduced total blood mercury from 90 µg/L to 2.5 µg/L.[1] In 2013, neuropsychological testing (see Chapter 42) revealed clear signs of severe dementia, which continued to progress. It was not until 2015 when she received a referral to a local hospital that it was discovered that she had been using a mercury-containing skin-lightening cream for years. The use of DMSA, although great at lowering body mercury load, could not compete with an ongoing mercury source. Only after the woman discontinued use of the skin-lightening cream did her neurological symptoms begin to abate.

Avoidance of common indoor pollutants is the highest-rated "treatment" for persons with severe chemical

TABLE 60.1 Rating of Treatment Efficacy for Reduction of Morbidity Associated With Chemical Intolerance in Percentages of Respondents—Listed by Help/Harm Ratio

Treatment	n	% Harmed	% No Effect	% Helped	Help/Harm Ratio
Chemical-free living space	820	0.6	4.5	94.8	155.2
Chemical avoidance	875	0.8	4.7	94.5	118.6
Prayer	609	1.4	34.4	64.2	48.3
Meditation	423	2.8	43.3	53.8	19.2
Acupressure	308	4.5	28.3	67.2	14.9
Touch for health	75	3.8	41.8	54.4	14.3
Air filter	786	6.0	11.8	82.1	13.7
Rotation diet	560	5.7	22.1	72.2	12.7
Acidophilus	661	4.1	44.0	52.0	12.7
Relocation	513	7.4	6.0	86.6	11.7
Reflexology	204	4.8	38.5	56.6	11.6
Personal oxygen	326	7.3	14.2	78.4	10.6

Modified from Gibson, P. R., Elms, A. N., & Ruding, L. A. (2003). Perceived treatment efficacy for conventional and alternative therapies reported by persons with multiple chemical sensitivity. *Environmental Health Perspectives, 111*(12), 1498–1504.

sensitivity (Table 60.1).[2] In a nationwide survey of individuals with severe chemical sensitivity, the two most effective treatments were having a chemical-free living space (helping 94.8% of respondents) and chemical avoidance (helping 94.5% of respondents). The results on Table 60.1 show that the next three most effective treatments were also methods to reduce chemical exposures: relocation (86.6%), air filters (82.1%), and personal oxygen (78.4%).

The sixth-most beneficial therapy (helping 72.2% of respondents) was a rotation diet, which avoids the most common food sensitivities.

Information has already been presented in this text to document toxicant body burden of persistent and nonpersistent pollutants and their major sources. Fortunately, the most majority of these exposure sources can be easily interdicted with simple techniques and lifestyle choices.

REDUCING EXPOSURE TO AIR POLLUTANTS

- Building less-toxic homes
- Proper mold remediation and prevention
- Removal of indoor air pollution sources
- Use of effective HVAC filters
- Use of electronic and botanical air purifiers
- Use of personal air filters

Construction Practices for Less-Toxic Homes and Offices

With the aim of reducing oil and natural gas consumption, energy-efficient materials and designs entered the construction trade in the early 1980s. Energy-efficient building methods emphasized a reduction of air exchange between the inside and outside air to minimize the energy needed to maintain indoor temperatures. Simultaneously with this "tighter" design came an influx of building materials containing a host of new chemical compounds. Building materials and furnishings now commonly contain (and off-gas) volatile organic compounds (VOCs) and semivolatile organic compounds (SVOCs), including plastics, flame retardants, and perfluocompounds. Benzene- and styrene-containing memory foam mattresses, mattress toppers, and pillows are now commonplace. Instead of building homes that can be adequately ventilated by a cross-breeze through open windows on opposite sides of the home, HVAC systems are installed. As might be expected, homes with natural ventilation via windows and doors have lower levels of indoor air pollutants than homes with HVAC systems.[3] Alarmingly, for those in areas with radon emissions, standard energy-efficient "tight" homes have higher indoor radon levels, predisposing their occupants to a greater risk for lung cancer.[4] Furthermore, many buildings have become water damaged through poor building practices, lack of preventive maintenance, and poor design.

BOX 60.1 Leadership in Energy and Environmental Design (LEED) Requirements Leading to Less-Toxic Environments

- High-efficiency gas hydronic heat and hot water
- Heat recovery ventilation that continuously exhausts air from bathrooms to capture and reuse heat loss for kitchen, bathroom, stairs, and hallways
- Green envelope (walls, insulation, doors, windows, etc.)
- Low VOC interior materials
- Nonsmoking policy

Green Buildings. The US Green Building Council* has established the Leadership in Energy and Environmental Design (LEED) certification program for constructing sustainable buildings. LEED provides a set of guidelines to be followed for buildings to receive different levels of their certification (Box 60.1). LEED standards can be used in new construction and renovations.

Green building design tends to result in improved health for those living in them.[5] However, it appears that rigorous adherence to green building practices are needed for this to occur. Low-income senior housing units that underwent a retrofit/remodel minimally conforming to LEED standards found reduced indoor formaldehyde levels but increased particulate matter <2.5 μm (PM2.5) (1.4- to 2-fold higher than outdoors for nonsmoker apartments).[6] Those residing in smoker apartments (not allowed in LEED certification) had $PM_{2.5}$ levels five to eight times higher than those that occurred outdoors. In new housing constructed to be more adherent to LEED standards, indoor $PM_{2.5}$ levels were reduced by 57%, whereas nitrous dioxide (NO_2) dropped 65% compared with conventional housing.[7] Those in green homes also reported a greater overall health rating and had dramatic reduction in sick building syndrome (SBS) symptoms. Lower respiratory symptoms were reduced by 48%, mucosal symptoms by 58%, neurological symptoms by 55%, and fatigue by 48%. Seniors who moved into green-renovated public housing scored better on the mental health index and reported more days of better mental health.[8] The

seniors who moved into green rather than conventional renovated units also had a 50% decrease in falls.

Remediation of Mold- and Water-Damaged Buildings

- Identify source
- Obtain professional remediation
  - Removal of all mold-contaminated building materials while controlling release of spores into the home air
  - Remediation of water intrusion source
  - Replacement with new building materials
- In the case of *Stachybotrys*, papers and fabrics present during mold presence may need to be completely replaced
- Topical antimold treatments should be avoided

Health problems associated with residences quite frequently turn out to be mold-related. The most common mycotoxins present in buildings include aflatoxin B1 from species of *Aspergillus;* ochratoxin from *Aspergillus* and *Penicillium* and trichothecene are primarily from *Stachybotrys chartarum* (toxic black mold) but are also produced by *Fusarium* and *Myrothecium.* Endotoxins, lipopolysaccharides from gram-negative bacterial cell walls, are also elevated in water-damaged buildings.[9] *Stachybotrys chartarum* requires both cellulose (abundant in wall board and lumber) and a constant moisture source to grow, as is often found in bathrooms, laundry rooms, and kitchens. Before mold can be eliminated from the home, the location of the mold growth needs to be identified. In some cases, the greatest mold growth will be hidden, but the Environmental Relative Moldiness Index (ERMI) test can determine which homes have higher mold counts and which rooms/areas are the most contaminated.[10,11,12]

The US Environmental Protection Agency (EPA) provides basic guidelines for remediation of mold intrusion into buildings.† Proper remediation should be done by a trained and licensed professional following established protocols to minimize the dispersal of mold spores throughout the building. All the contaminated building materials must be removed in sealed bags, the source of water intrusion discovered and remediated, and new building materials put into place. It is then best to have the ERMI test redone to ensure the source of indoor mold growth has been adequately addressed.

*http://www.usgbc.org

†https://www.epa.gov/mold/mold-remediation-schools-and-commercial-buildings-guide

Reduction of Sources of Indoor Air Pollution

- Smoking and combustion sources
- Carpeting
- Plastic products
- Nonstick pans
- Air fresheners and perfumed products

LEED standards include the use of low-VOC–containing building materials, but one must also be aware of the many SVOC compounds in building materials and furnishings and reduce their use as well. LEED also correctly made the call to require occupants in LEED-certified buildings to not smoke.

Smoking remains the greatest source of indoor air pollution and is fairly easily remedied by having persons stop smoking indoors. Smoking dramatically increases the levels of polycyclic aromatic hydrocarbons (PAHs), benzene, toluene, and styrene in the home.[13,14] Burning incense is the second-highest source of indoor PAHs after smoking. Elimination of those practices will immediately result in a reduction of indoor air pollutant levels.

Carpeting is the next greatest source of health-damaging indoor air pollutants in home, schools, or workplaces after smoking and incense.[15,16,17] Carpeting both emits a huge number of SVOCs in the home air and acts as a collector for other toxicants, including those tracked into the home. Organotins, organophosphate and pyrethroid pesticides, formaldehyde, and brominated flame retardants have all been identified in carpet samples.[18,19] Polybrominated diphenyl ethers (PBDEs) are also found in the most commonly used types of carpet padding.[20] Two different rubber- (styrene-butadiene rubber) backed carpet samples showed high emission levels of styrene and 4-phenylcyclohexene (4-PCH), which is responsible for the "new carpet odor."[21] Carpet with a polyvinyl chloride backing emitted formaldehyde, vinyl acetate, isooctane, 1,2-propanediol, and 2-ethyl-1-hexanol. Carpet with polyurethane backing primarily emitted butylated hydroxytoluene. Four other carpet samples consistently emitted high levels of the VOCs 4-PCH and 2,2-butyxyethoxy-ethanol (up to 170 and 320 $\mu g/m^3$), and lower levels of benzene, toluene, ethylbenzene, xylene, styrene, formaldehyde, and other carbonyl compounds.[22] Fortunately, carpet removal has repeatedly resulted in reduced SBS symptoms.[23,24]

High-molecular-weight phthalates are released from more solid materials such as shower curtains, toys, and vinyl flooring and are then carried by the dust.[25,26,27]

Low-molecular-weight phthalates are present in all perfumed products and in air fresheners, where they are accompanied by several solvents.[28,29] Taking showers without using a chlorine shower filter increases blood levels of chloroform and other disinfectant by-products.[30,31] Cooking with nonstick pans and having stain-resistant fabrics in the home increases the level of perfluorocarbons (PFCs) in the home dust and the occupant's blood.[32,33,34,35] The use of non-PFC-containing cookware is a fairly easy fix, whereas replacement of currently owned furnishings that contain PFC stain-resistant compounds is more challenging.

Removing Pollutants From the Indoor Air

- HVAC filters
- Air purifiers
  - Electric enclosed high efficiency particulate air (HEPA) and multifilter units
  - Masks (HEPA and ionic)
  - Houseplants

HVAC filters. Almost all homes built after the energy crisis in the late 1970s were built with an HVAC system of metal ducts that carry air throughout the home from a central point. This air is pulled through a filter, heated or cooled as needed, and then distributed through the ductwork. Dust, mold, or other foreign material present inside the ductwork is distributed throughout the home. For this reason, it is wise to have one of the many commercially available services regularly clean the ductwork. Once the ducts have been cleaned, the type of filter used can then have a great effect on the level of pollutants in the home air. Air filters are given a rating for Minimum Efficiency Reporting Value (MERV), with higher ratings providing greater removal of particle matter, as shown in Table 60.2.

When assessed for the most health-damaging ultrafine particles (UFP, or $PM_{0.1}$), standard 1-inch-thick MERV 6 and 11 have modest benefit with minimal drop in air pressure. However, standard 1-inch filters rated above MERV 12 or 13 are only marginally more effective and much more restrictive of airflow. Thus if limited to 1-inch-thick filters, a higher rating may not be practical.[36] If too high of a rating of MERV filter is used, the HVAC motor may be placed under a heavier load, which would likely shorten its service life.

The 5-inch-thick filters, which typically require a retrofit to the HVAC system, can reduce the UFP content in the air significantly. The authors of this study

TABLE 60.2 Efficiency of Ultrafine Particle (PM$_{0.1}$) Removal and Reduction in Pressure (Airflow) with Various 1- or 5-inch Filters in a Residential Home

Filter Ratings	UFP Removal	Pressure Drop
1-inch MERV 4	0%	4.4%
1-inch MERV 6	10%	6.9%
1-inch MERV 11	15%	11.8%
5-inch MERV 10	20%	10.5%
5-inch MERV 13	30% to 50%	13.8%
5-inch MERV 16	60% to 80%	16.6%

concluded: "In order to achieve substantial removal (>50%) of UFPs in real residential environments, much higher efficiency filters than are typically used in homes are likely required (MERV 13 or 16). Additionally, these particular deeper bed filters appear to achieve dual benefits of higher UFP removal with lower pressure drop, and thus should result in higher airflow rates in most residential HVAC systems."

For those living in an urban area within a mile of a major highway with truck traffic, the cost of such a retrofit and a year's supply of filters would be well worth the expenditure.

In an illustrative study, retrofitting of the HVAC system was done in three different urban schools with close proximity to the main freeway and one "control" school 2 km away from the freeway (Fig. 60.1).[37] Each school had their existing MERV 6 system upgraded with three prefilters, including another MERV 6, a MERV 15, and a gas-phase filter (Fig. 60.2). The existing MERV 6 filter was successful at removing black carbon (course particulate matter, not UFP) at an efficiency of 31% to 66%. Black carbon is often used as a marker for diesel exhaust and is known to contain benzene, 1,3-butadiene, and toluene. After the retrofit, the black carbon concentration inside the schools was reduced between 74% and 97% compared with outdoor levels. The schools with the retrofitted HVAC filtration had black carbon levels 49% to 96% lower than the ambient levels found in that urban area.

Air purifiers
- 40% to 60% reduction of PM$_{2.5}$
  - Room air purifiers containing replaceable MERV-rated HVAC filters
  - Room air purifiers with replaceable HEPA filter (not an HVAC filter)

- 80% to 96% reduction in PM$_{2.5}$
  - Large-square-foot air purifiers with two or more filters
    - Prefilter
    - HEPA
    - Charcoal
    - Gas phase
  - Combination of high MERV and stand-alone (SA) multifilter purifier

SA electric units containing a pleated electrostatic HVAC filter are available for rooms and have been studied for their effectiveness. A MERV 12–containing unit rated for 150 square feet was tested in dormitory rooms over 48 hours of continuous occupancy.[38] Not only did indoor PM$_{2.5}$ levels drop by 57%, but inflammatory markers dropped substantially and both systolic and diastolic blood pressure went down slightly (Table 60.3). Similar units were assessed in First Nation homes in Manitoba, the majority of which contained smokers, and produced a significant (>30 µg/m^3) reduction in mean levels of PM$_{0.1}$, PM$_{2.5}$, and PM$_{10}$.[39] In addition, the average forced expiratory volume in 1 second (FEV1) increased by 217 mL, systolic blood pressure dropped by 7.9 mm Hg, and diastolic blood pressure dropped by 4.5 mm Hg.

Even moderate-quality HEPA filters can have a dramatic effect in reducing indoor PM levels and improving health. The introduction of low-cost electric HEPA units that were only rated at 60% effectiveness into homes in an area with high levels of wood smoke was able to reduce indoor levels of PM$_{2.5}$.[40] After only 7 days of using the units, the residents of those homes had a 9.4% improvement in endothelial function and a 32.6% average drop in their high-sensitivity C-reactive protein (hs-CRP) levels.[41] Other commercially available HEPA units have reduced indoor PM$_{2.5}$ levels between 40% and 50%.[42,43] Such units have roughly the same effectiveness at clearing PM$_{2.5}$ as the units containing replaceable high-MERV furnace filters, which are far less expensive to replace.

Not surprisingly, units with multiple filters typically provide greater reduction in PM levels along with noticeable health improvements. Three schools in southern California that were in close proximity to busy highways and refineries had one of six different combinations of three methods of additional air filtration added to the existing MERV 7 filters.[44] High-performance panel filters (HP-PF), consisting of multilayered glass and synthetic fiber material (equivalent to MERV 16), could be used as a "prefilter" to the existing HVAC system. A register

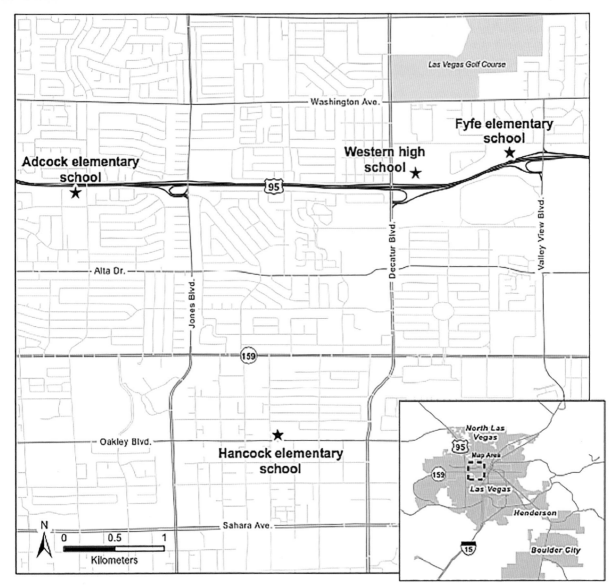

FIG. 60.1 Locations of schools where monitoring took place during the US 95 highway monitoring study. Inset map shows location of study as a dashed box within the greater Las Vegas metropolitan area. (From McCarthy, M. C., Ludwig, J. F., Brown, S. G., Vaughn, D. L., & Roberts, P. T. [2013]. Filtration effectiveness of HVAC systems at near-roadway schools. *Indoor Air, 23*[3], 196–207.)

system (RS) containing MERV 16 and gas-phase filter cartridges could be added to the vents delivering air to the rooms. An SA unit consisting of a MERV 16 HEPA filter, gas-phase cartridge filters, and a HEPA postfilter

was the third component.[‡] The various combinations of these methods reduced the black carbon, UPF, and $PM_{2.5}$ between 87% and 96% (Fig. 60.3). The baseline in this figure refers to the existing MERV 7 HVAC filtration system.

Masks. The use of high-efficiency respirator masks (not simple dust masks with thin stretchable elastic bands)

[‡]IQ Air GC Multigas units

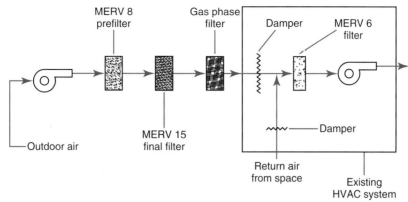

FIG. 60.2 Schematic diagram of filtration systems added to the Adock Elementary and Fyfe Elementary Schools. (From McCarthy, M. C., Ludwig, J. F., Brown, S. G., Vaughn, D. L., & Roberts, P. T. [2013]. Filtration effectiveness of HVAC systems at near-roadway schools. *Indoor Air, 23*[3], 196–207.)

TABLE 60.3 **Reduction in Blood Pressures and Inflammatory Markers After 48 Hours of Residence in a Room With a MERV 12 Filter Unit**	
Cardiovascular	**Biomarkers**
Systolic pressure–avg. 2.7 mm Hg drop	IL-1B–58% reduction Soluble CD40
Diastolic pressure–avg. 4.8% mm Hg drop	ligand–55% reduction Myeloperoxidase–33%
Exhaled nitrous oxide–17% drop	reduction Monocyte
	chemoattractant protein 1–17.5% reduction

have been shown to be effective against air pollution in Beijing.[45] Using 3M masks that were 97% effective in reducing $PM_{2.5}$ while walking a prescribed route daily resulted in improvement in multiple symptoms, less ST-segment depression, lower systolic blood pressure, and improved heart rate variability. The wearers reported improvements in headaches, dizziness, nausea, tiredness, cough, breathlessness, and irritation of the nose and throat.

Personal ionic air purifiers. Commonly available personal ionic air purifiers worn around the neck are 100% effective in reducing bioaerosol levels in an individual's personal breathing.[46] When SA units are used in a phone booth–sized enclosed space (2.6 m³), they can

be similarly effective. Alarmingly, the use of larger ionic air purifiers in a regular-sized room increases the concentrations of UFP, ozone, and formaldehyde.[47,48]

Indoor houseplants. Because of the high level of toxic out-gassing in materials used for spacecraft, the National Aeronautics and Space Administration (NASA) explored the possibility of using common houseplants to remove formaldehyde, benzene, and trichloroethylene from the air (Table 60.4).[49] In subsequent studies, two species of mother-in-law's tongue, *Sansevieria trifasciata* and *S. hyacinthoides,* were shown to reduce toluene and ethylbenzene levels.[50] *Chlorophytum comosum* (Spider plant) was also effective at decreasing ethylbenzene levels. Three or more *Dracaena deremensis* (Janet Craig) plants in an office setting reduced total VOC levels by 50% to 70%.[51] *Spathiphyllum* (Sweet chico) was also effective at lowering VOCs. When only six plants of Janet Craig, *Dracaena marginata,* Madagascar dragon tree, or Mauna Loa (peace lily) were placed in 52.5 m² classrooms for 9 weeks, the average CO_2 dropped from 2004 to 1121 parts per million (PPM), and total VOC dropped from 933 to 249 μg/m³.[52]

Formaldehyde off-gassing appears to be the most resistant to clearance by plants, despite the NASA findings. In offices with high formaldehyde off-gassing, 20 plants were needed to begin to reduce airborne formaldehyde levels.[51] Using 0 to 15 plants in that setting made no difference. When fewer than 10 plants were used in prefabricated "portable buildings" with high formaldehyde levels, no change was seen.[53] When 20 plants were used, formaldehyde concentrations only dropped 11%.

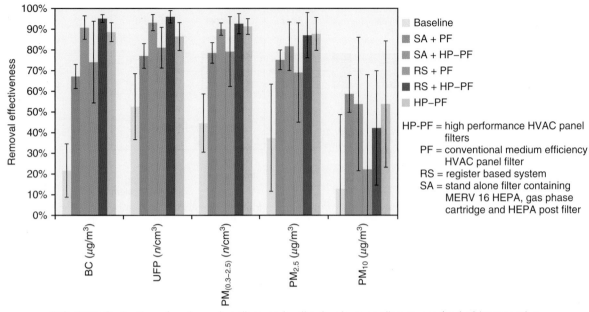

FIG. 60.3 Reduction of various air pollutants in all schools according to method of intervention. Polidori, A., Fine, P. M., White, V., & Kwon, P. S. (2013). Pilot study of high-performance air filtration for classroom applications. *Indoor Air*, 23(3), 185–195. PubMed PMID: 23137181.

TABLE 60.4   Percentage of Chemicals Removed From a Sealed Chamber by Houseplants in a 24-Hour Period in a NASA Study

Plant	Formaldehyde	Benzene	Trichloroethylene
Mass cane	70	21.4	12.5
Pot mum	61	53	41.2
Gerber daisy	50	67.7	35
Wernicke	50	52	10
Ficus	47.4	30	10.5
Leak control	2.8	5	10

From Wolverton, B. C., & Johnson, A. (1989). Interior landscape plants for indoor air abatement. *National Aeronautics and Space Administration*. Retrieved from https://ntrs.nasa.gov/archive/nasa/casi.ntrs.nasa.gov/19930073077.pdf

Reducing Exposure to Food Pollutants

- Avoid the fruits and vegetables with the highest chemical contamination
  - Replace with organic varieties
- Avoid tofu made from conventionally grown soy
- Avoid sardines and farmed salmon
- Avoid consumption of high-mercury fish
- Avoid regular consumption of fish with moderate levels of mercury
- Avoid food contamination with plasticizers

Avoiding the Most Toxic Fruits and Vegetables. As shown in Fig. 21.2, children who consumed diets consisting of 75% or more organic foods had a ninefold lower mean level (sixfold lower median level) of organophosphate pesticide (OP) residues in their urine than those whose diet was at least 75% nonorganic.[54]

A simple 5-day replacement with organic varieties of the foods normally consumed resulted in the virtual disappearance of urinary malathion and chlorpyrifos metabolites (Fig. 60.4).[55] The most commonly replaced foods were fresh fruits and vegetables, juices, processed fruits or vegetables (e.g., salsa), and wheat- or corn-based products (e.g., pasta, cereal, popcorn, or chips). Once the subjects returned to eating their normal conventional foods, five different OP metabolites reappeared in their urine. Results were similar when substitution was done in both the fall and winter.

Tofu made from conventionally grown soy is the greatest source of dietary cadmium, followed by cooked cereals and green leafy vegetables (both cooked and in salads).[56] "Tofu consumption" includes not just tofu but also tempeh and products such as soy hotdogs, soy cheese, and soy burgers. Once-weekly consumption of any of those products resulted in an average urinary cadmium of .11 µg/g (only 0.02 µg/g below levels found

in smokers). Ingestion of any of those products twice weekly or more increased the urinary cadmium burden to 0.30 µg/g, more than twice the increase found from smoking. It is probable that organic tofu will be similarly contaminated, because the soybeans appear to absorb cadmium from the soil.

Fish

- Avoid fish with moderate to high mercury levels
- Avoid consumption of fresh-water fish from the Great Lakes
- Avoid sardines and farmed salmon

The long half-life for mercury in fish (2 years) leads to substantial levels of mercury in the larger ocean fish (Table 3.9). With a 60-day half-life for methylmercury in humans,

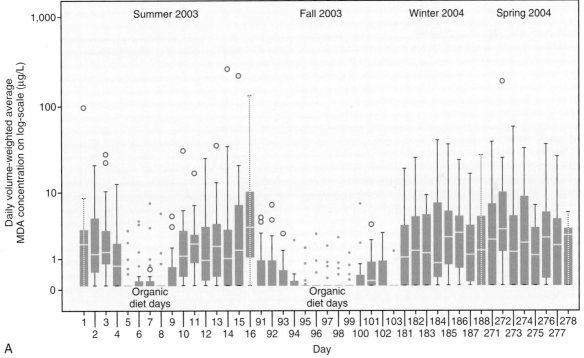

FIG. 60.4 One-year exposure profile of daily volume weighted averages of OP pesticide metabolite concentrations (µg/L) for Children's Pesticide Exposure Study (CPES) in Washington state CPES-WA children. Exposure data included urinary levels measured during the 5-day period in summer and fall 2003 when children consumed organic food items: (A) MDA; (B) TCPy. Days 5 to 9 and 95 to 99 were organic diet days. The horizontal lines in each plot represent 10th, 25th, 50th, 75th, and 90th percentiles, bottom to top. The concentration data on the y-axis is on the log-scale. The "o" and "*" symbols represent outliers and the extreme values, respectively. (From Lu, C., Barr, D. B., Pearson, M. A., & Waller, L. A. [2008]. Dietary intake and its contribution to longitudinal organophosphorus pesticide exposure in urban/suburban children. *Environmental Health Perspectives, 116*[4], 537–542.)

Continued

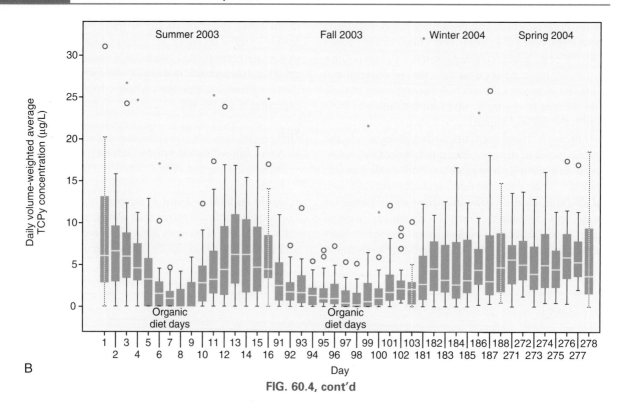

FIG. 60.4, cont'd

weekly intake of even fish with 0.1 PPM of mercury can result in elevated blood mercury levels. In addition, almost the entire eastern seaboard, much of the Gulf of Mexico, well over 1.2 million miles of freshwater rivers, and more than 16 million acres of freshwater lakes in the United States are under mercury advisories.[57] Unfortunately, the warnings to avoid consumption of locally caught fish from those waters are listed on the EPA website (https://www.epa.gov/fish-tech/national-listing-fish-advisories-2011-data) instead of in the bait shops, fish markets, and restaurants in those localities.

Consuming freshwater fish from the Great lakes and other areas of the country is a prime exposure source for POPs.[58,59,60] However, the consumption of farmed salmon is responsible for 97% of dietary POP exposure from fish.[61] More than two-thirds of all salmon consumed in North America is farmed, and salmon is one of the top three seafoods consumed in North America (the other two being shrimp and tuna).[62] The POP contaminants in farmed salmon come from the fish pellets used to feed them.[63] Although some grains have been added to these fish pellets to decrease the toxicity of farmed salmon,

their levels of the most health-damaging PCBs remains high.[64] Table 3.3 compares polychlorinated biphenyl (PCB) content between sardines, wild Alaskan salmon, farmed Atlantic salmon, and hamburger. Sardines had the highest concentration of the highly toxic PCBs 138, 153, and 180, followed closely by farmed salmon and then hamburger.

Because "wild caught" salmon commands a higher price, restaurants and fish markets have been found to "mislabel" their farmed salmon. Farmed salmon are often listed in menus as Norwegian Salmon, Chilean Salmon, British Columbia Salmon, or Scottish Salmon, all denoting the areas in which they were raised. Atlantic salmon *(Salmo salar)* is a different species than Pacific or Alaskan salmon *(Oncorhynchus),* which has several different salmon and trout genera. The most commonly consumed Alaskan salmon include *O. kitsutch*–Coho or silver salmon—*O. nerka*–Sockeye or red salmon—and *O. tshawytscha*–Chinook or King salmon. If in doubt, it is simple enough to ask the restaurant or fish market to identify exactly which "wild" salmon it is. If the reply is "it's just salmon," then they are likely selling farmed Atlantic *Salmo salar.*

Plastic Contamination

- Avoid high-fat foods stored in plastic
- Avoid foods heated in plastic or "microwave-safe" containers
- Avoid consuming food and drink stored in cans

Plastics migrate readily into foods with high fat content.[65] Their level in foods also goes up with length of time these materials are in contact with the food and dramatically increase if the food is heated.[66] Table 3.7 lists the foods with the highest content of the high-molecular-weight (HMW) phthalate di(2-ethylhexyl) phthalate (DEHP). High fat foods clearly top the list.

Individuals who participated in a 5-day Buddhist retreat that included a vegetarian diet (primarily grown at the monastery) experienced a 40% to 90% reduction in both low-molecular-weight (LMW) and HMW phthalates and antibiotic metabolites in their urine. They also had a 40% reduction in their malondialdehyde levels, indicating a reduction in oxidative stress.[67]

All but 0.2 ng of the total 12.6 ng/kg/day intake of bisphenol A (BPA) in US residents is from foods, primarily from canned foods.[68] Data from the National Health and Nutritional Examination Survey (NHANES) from 2005 to 2006 revealed that drinking soda pop and consuming school lunches and meals prepared outside of the home were the most significant sources of BPA.[69] On average, the consumption of one canned food item daily increased urinary BPA by 24%, whereas consuming two items increased urinary BPA by 54%.[70] However, not all canned foods increased urinary BPA to the same degree. Consumption of one canned soup increased urinary levels by 229%, canned pasta by 70%, and canned fruits and vegetables by 41%. Consuming one can of soup daily for 5 days has been shown to increase urinary BPA levels by more than 1000% (see Fig. 3.2).[71]

In one study, those who consumed fresh soup in the first week and canned soup in the second week ended up with slightly higher urinary BPA. However, those who consumed the canned soup in week 1 still had elevated urinary BPA a week later. In that study, bottled water and canned tuna were not found to be significant sources of this compound. Consumption of two glass-bottled soy milks resulted in an average urinary BPA level of 0.31 μg/L, yet drinking two cans of the same beverage increased urinary BPA to an average of 8.22 μg/L.[72]

Water

- Water purification to remove water toxicants endemic to the local area

Tap water is contaminated with a host of highly toxic compounds, including arsenic, lead, hexavalent chromium, methyl tert-butyl ether (MTBE), perchlorate, trichloroethylene, PFCs, herbicides (higher in spring and summer), and pharmaceuticals. Residents in areas with high groundwater arsenic levels can use reverse-osmosis (RO) filters to reduce up to 80% of their water arsenic.[73,74] RO units are also effective at removing chromate and perchlorate from tap water.[75] In fact, RO units remove 95% of all toxic compounds in the water, making them the most effective method for water decontamination.[76]

Personal Care Products

- Avoidance of toxicant-containing personal care products:
  - Body lotion
  - Perfumes and colognes
  - Shampoo and body wash
  - Deodorant
  - Antiaging facial creams

Significant reductions in urinary phthalate levels have been found in young girls when they reduced their frequency of handwashing, ceased drinking from plastic cups, and used less shower gel and shampoo.[77] The greatest reduction of phthalates is attainable by avoiding the use of body lotion, deodorant, perfume and colognes, antiaging facial creams, and bottled water.[78,79] The authors of *Slow Death by Rubber Duck* did a 2-day avoidance of all personal care products followed by 2 days of using normally applied products.[80] After the 2-day avoidance, the level of the LMW major excreted polypeptide (MEP, commonly found in personal care products) was 64 ng/L. After liberal use of personal care products for 2 days, the MEP urine level increased to 1410 ng/L.

REFERENCES

1. Zellner, T., Zellner, N., Felgenhauer, N., & Eyer, F. (2016). Dementia, epilepsy and polyneuropathy in a mercury-exposed patient: Investigation, identification of an obscure source and treatment. *BMJ Case Reports*, *2016*, PubMed PMID: 27793866.
2. Gibson, P. R., Elms, A. N., & Ruding, L. A. (2003). Perceived treatment efficacy for conventional and

alternative therapies reported by persons with multiple chemical sensitivity. *Environmental Health Perspectives, 111*(12), 1498–1504. PubMed PMID: 12948890.

3. Kumar, P., & Morawska, L. (2013). Energy-pollution nexus for urban buildings. *Environmental Science & Technology, 47*(14), 7591–7592. PubMed PMID: 23805849.

4. Arvela, H., Holmgren, O., Reisbacka, H., & Vinha, J. (2014). Review of low-energy construction, air tightness, ventilation strategies and indoor radon: Results from Finnish houses and apartments. *Radiation Protection Dosimetry, 162*(3), 351–363. PubMed PMID: 24243314.

5. Allen, J. G., MacNaughton, P., Laurent, J. G., Flanigan, S. S., Eitland, E. S., & Spengler, J. D. (2015). Green buildings and health. *Current Environmental Health Reports, 2*(3), 250–258. PubMed PMID: 26231502.

6. Frey, S. E., Destaillats, H., Cohn, S., Ahrentzen, S., & Fraser, M. P. (2015). The effects of an energy efficiency retrofit on indoor air quality. *Indoor Air, 25*(2), 210–219. PubMed PMID: 24920242.

7. Colton, M. D., MacNaughton, P., Vallarino, J., Kane, J., Bennett-Fripp, M., Spengler, J. D., et al. (2014). Indoor air quality in green vs conventional multifamily low-income housing. *Environmental Science & Technology, 48*(14), 7833–7841. PubMed PMID: 24941256.

8. Breysse, J., Dixon, S. L., Jacobs, D. E., Lopez, J., & Weber, W. (2015). Self-reported health outcomes associated with green-renovated public housing among primarily elderly residents. *Journal of Public Health Management and Practice: JPHMP, 21*(4), 355–367. PubMed PMID: 25679773.

9. Salonen, H., Duchaine, C., Létourneau, V., Mazaheri, M., Clifford, S., & Morawska, L. (2013). Endotoxins in indoor air and settled dust in primary schools in a subtropical climate. *Environmental Science & Technology, 47*(17), 9882–9890. PubMed PMID: 23927534.

10. Vesper, S., McKinstry, C., Haugland, R., Wymer, L., Bradham, K., Ashley, P., et al. (2007). Development of an Environmental Relative Moldiness index for US homes. *Journal of Occupational and Environmental Medicine, 49*(8), 829–833. PubMed PMID: 17693779.

11. Reponen, T., Singh, U., Schaffer, C., Vesper, S., Johansson, E., Adhikari, A., et al. (2010). Visually observed mold and moldy odor versus quantitatively measured microbial exposure in homes. *The Science of the Total Environment, 408*(22), 5565–5574. PubMed PMID: 20810150.

12. Vesper, S., & Wymer, L. (2016). The relationship between environmental relative moldiness index values and asthma. *International Journal of Hygiene and Environmental Health, 219*(3), 233–238. PubMed PMID: 26861576.

13. Wheeler, A. J., Wong, S. L., Khouri, C., & Zhu, J. (2013). Predictors of indoor BTEX concentrations in Canadian residences. *Health Reports, 24*(5), 11–17. PubMed PMID: 24258095.

14. Roberts, D., & Pontin, D. (2016). The health risks of incense use in the home: An underestimated source of indoor air pollution? *Community Practitioner: The Journal of the Community Practitioners' and Health Visitors' Association, 89*(3), 36–41. Review. PubMed PMID: 27111977.

15. Weschler, C. J., & Nazaroff, W. W. (2010). SVOC partitioning between gas phase and settled dust indoors. *Atmospheric Environment, 44*, 3609–3620.

16. Kielb, C., Lin, S., Muscatiello, N., Hord, W., Rogers-Harrington, J., & Healy, J. (2015). Building-related health symptoms and classroom indoor air quality: A survey of school teachers in New York State. *Indoor Air, 25*(4), 371–380. PubMed PMID: 25196499.

17. Norbäck, D., Björnsson, E., Janson, C., Widström, J., & Boman, G. (1995). Asthmatic symptoms and volatile organic compounds, formaldehyde, and carbon dioxide in dwellings. *Occupational and Environmental Medicine, 52*(6), 388–395. PubMed PMID: 7627316.

18. Allsopp, M., Santillo, D., & Johnson, P. (2001). *Hazardous chemicals in carpets.* Greenpeace Research Laboratories. http://www.greenpeace.to/publications/carpet.pdf. (Accessed 27 April 2017).

19. Roinestad, K. S., Louis, J. B., & Rosen, J. D. (1993). Determination of pesticides in indoor air and dust. *Journal of AOAC International, 76*(5), 1121–1126. PubMed PMID: 8241815.

20. DiGangi, J., & Strakova, J. (2011). *A survey of PBDEs in recycled carpet padding. IPEN.* http://ipen.org/sites/default/files/t/2011/04/POPs-in-recycled-carpet-padding-23-April-20111.pdf. (Accessed 27 April 2017).

21. Hodgson, A. T., Wooley, J. D., & Daisey, J. M. (1993). Emissions of volatile organic compounds from new carpets measured in a large-scale environmental chamber. *Journal of the Air and Waste Management Association (1995), 43*(3), 316–324. PubMed PMID: 8457318.

22. Katsoyiannis, A., Leva, P., & Kotzias, D. (2008). VOC and carbonyl emissions from carpets: A comparative study using four types of environmental chambers. *Journal of Hazardous Materials, 152*(2), 669–676. PubMed PMID: 17854990.

23. Azuma, K., Ikeda, K., Kagi, N., Yanagi, U., & Osawa, H. (2015). Prevalence and risk factors associated

with nonspecific building-related symptoms in office employees in Japan: Relationships between work environment, Indoor Air Quality, and occupational stress. *Indoor Air, 25*(5), 499–511. PubMed PMID: 25244340.

24. Norbäck, D., Torgén, M., & Edling, C. (1990). Volatile organic compounds, respirable dust, and personal factors related to prevalence and incidence of sick building syndrome in primary schools. *British Journal of Industrial Medicine, 47*(11), 733–741. PubMed PMID: 2123116.

25. Larsson, K., Lindh, C. H., Jönsson, B. A., Giovanoulis, G., Bibi, M., Bottai, M., et al. (2017). Phthalates, non-phthalate plasticizers and bisphenols in Swedish preschool dust in relation to children's exposure. *Environment International, 102*, 114–124. PubMed PMID: 28274486.

26. Jeon, S., Kim, K. T., & Choi, K. (2016). Migration of DEHP and DINP into dust from PVC flooring products at different surface temperature. *The Science of the Total Environment, 547*, 441–446. PubMed PMID: 26824397.

27. Sukiene, V., Gerecke, A. C., Park, Y. M., Zennegg, M., Bakker, M. I., Delmaar, C. J., et al. (2016). Tracking SVOCs' transfer from products to indoor air and settled dust with deuterium-labeled substances. *Environmental Science & Technology, 50*(8), 4296–4303. PubMed PMID: 27019300.

28. Kim, S., Hong, S. H., Bong, C. K., & Cho, M. H. (2015). Characterization of air freshener emission: The potential health effects. *The Journal of Toxicological Sciences, 40*(5), 535–550. PubMed PMID: 26354370.

29. Nørgaard, A. W., Kudal, J. D., Kofoed-Sørensen, V., Koponen, I. K., & Wolkoff, P. (2014). Ozone-initiated VOC and particle emissions from a cleaning agent and an air freshener: Risk assessment of acute airway effects. *Environment International, 68*, 209–218. PubMed PMID: 24769411.

30. Xu, X., & Weisel, C. P. (2005). Human respiratory uptake of chloroform and haloketones during showering. *Journal of Exposure Analysis and Environmental Epidemiology, 15*(1), 6–16. PubMed PMID: 15138448.

31. Lynberg, M., Nuckols, J. R., Langlois, P., et al. (2001). Assessing exposure to disinfection by-products in women of reproductive age living in Corpus Christi, Texans, and Cobb Count, Georgia: Descriptive results and methods. *Environmental Health Perspectives, 109*(6), 597–604.

32. Winkens, K., Koponen, J., Schuster, J., Shoeib, M., Vestergren, R., Berger, U., et al. (2017). Perfluoroalkyl acids and their precursors in indoor air sampled in children's bedrooms. *Environmental Pollution (Barking, Essex: 1987), 222*, 423–432. PubMed PMID: 28012670.

33. Fromme, H., Dreyer, A., Dietrich, S., Fembacher, L., Lahrz, T., & Völkel, W. (2015). Neutral polyfluorinated compounds in indoor air in Germany – the LUPE 4 study. *Chemosphere, 139*, 572–578. PubMed PMID: 26340371.

34. Ericson Jogsten, I., Nadal, M., van Bavel, B., Lindström, G., & Domingo, J. L. (2012). Per- and polyfluorinated compounds (PFCs) in house dust and indoor air in Catalonia, Spain: Implications for human exposure. *Environment International, 39*(1), 172–180. PubMed PMID: 22208757.

35. Huber, S., Haug, L. S., & Schlabach, M. (2011). Per- and polyfluorinated compounds in house dust and indoor air from northern Norway – A pilot study. *Chemosphere, 84*(11), 1686–1693. PubMed PMID: 21632089.

36. Brown, K. W., Minegishi, T., Allen, J. G., McCarthy, J. F., Spengler, J. D., & MacIntosh, D. L. (2014). Reducing patients' exposures to asthma and allergy triggers in their homes: An evaluation of effectiveness of grades of forced air ventilation filters. *The Journal of Asthma, 51*(6), 585–594. PubMed PMID: 24555523.

37. McCarthy, M. C., Ludwig, J. F., Brown, S. G., Vaughn, D. L., & Roberts, P. T. (2013). Filtration effectiveness of HVAC systems at near-roadway schools. *Indoor Air, 23*(3), 196–207. PubMed PMID: 23167831.

38. Chen, R., Zhao, A., Chen, H., Zhao, Z., Cai, J., Wang, C., et al. (2015). Cardiopulmonary benefits of reducing indoor particles of outdoor origin: A randomized, double-blind crossover trial of air purifiers. *Journal of the American College of Cardiology, 65*(21), 2279–2287. PubMed PMID: 26022815.

39. Weichenthal, S., Mallach, G., Kulka, R., Black, A., Wheeler, A., You, H., et al. (2013). A randomized double-blind crossover study of indoor air filtration and acute changes in cardiorespiratory health in a First Nations community. *Indoor Air, 23*(3), 175–184. PubMed PMID: 23210563.

40. McNamara, M. L., Thornburg, J., Semmens, E. O., Ward, T. J., & Noonan, C. W. (2017). Reducing indoor air pollutants with air filtration units in wood stove homes. *The Science of the Total Environment, 592*, 488–494. PubMed PMID: 28320525.

41. Allen, R. W., Carlsten, C., Karlen, B., Leckie, S., van Eeden, S., Vedal, S., et al. (2011). An air filter intervention study of endothelial function among healthy adults in a woodsmoke-impacted community. *American Journal of Respiratory and Critical Care Medicine, 183*(9), 1222–1230. PubMed PMID: 21257787.

42. Kajbafzadeh, M., Brauer, M., Karlen, B., Carlsten, C., van Eeden, S., & Allen, R. W. (2015). The impacts of traffic-related and woodsmoke particulate matter

on measures of cardiovascular health: A HEPA filter intervention study. *Occupational and Environmental Medicine, 72*(6), 394–400. PubMed PMID: 25896330.

43. Karottki, D. G., Spilak, M., Frederiksen, M., Gunnarsen, L., Brauner, E. V., Kolarik, B., et al. (2013). An indoor air filtration study in homes of elderly: Cardiovascular and respiratory effects of exposure to particulate matter. *Environmental Health: A Global Access Science Source, 12*, 116. PubMed PMID: 24373585.

44. Polidori, A., Fine, P. M., White, V., & Kwon, P. S. (2013). Pilot study of high-performance air filtration for classroom applications. *Indoor Air, 23*(3), 185–195. PubMed PMID: 23137181.

45. Langrish, J. P., Li, X., Wang, S., Lee, M. M., Barnes, G. D., Miller, M. R., et al. (2012). Reducing personal exposure to particulate air pollution improves cardiovascular health in patients with coronary heart disease. *Environmental Health Perspectives, 120*(3), 367–372. PubMed PMID: 22389220.

46. Grinshpun, S. A., Mainelis, G., Trunov, M., Adhikari, A., Reponen, T., & Willeke, K. (2005). Evaluation of ionic air purifiers for reducing aerosol exposure in confined indoor spaces. *Indoor Air, 15*(4), 235–245. PubMed PMID: 15982270.

47. Waring, M. S., & Siegel, J. A. (2011). The effect of an ion generator on indoor air quality in a residential room. *Indoor Air, 21*(4), 267–276. PubMed PMID: 21118308.

48. Alshawa, A., Russell A. R., & Nizkorodov SA.(2007). Kinetic analysis of competition between aerosol particle removal and generation by ionization air purifiers. *Environmental Science & Technology, 41*(7), 2498–2504. PubMed PMID: 17438806.

49. Wolverton, B. C., & Johnson, A. (1989). *Interior landscape plants for indoor air abatement*. National Aeronautics and Space Adminitration. John C Stennis Space Center. MS. https://ntrs.nasa.gov/search.jsp?R=19930073077. (Accessed 11 May 2017).

50. Sriprapat, W., Suksabye, P., Areephak, S., Klantup, P., Waraha, A., Sawattan, A., et al. (2014). Uptake of toluene and ethylbenzene by plants: Removal of volatile indoor air contaminants. *Ecotoxicology and Environmental Safety, 102*, 147–151. PubMed PMID: 24530730.

51. Dela Cruz, M., Christensen, J. H., Thomsen, J. D., & Müller, R. (2014). Can ornamental potted plants remove volatile organic compounds from indoor air? A review. *Environmental Science and Pollution Research International, 21*(24), 13909–13928. PubMed PMID: 25056742.

52. Pegas, P. N., Alves, C. A., Nunes, T., Bate-Epey, E. F., Evtyugina, M., & Pio, C. A. (2012). Could houseplants improve indoor air quality in schools? *Journal of Toxicology and Environmental Health. Part A, 75*(22–23), 1371–1380. PubMed PMID: 23095155.

53. Dingle, P., Tapsell, P., & Hu, S. (2000). Reducing formaldehyde exposure in office environments using plants. *Bulletin of Environmental Contamination and Toxicology, 64*(2), 302–308. PubMed PMID: 10656899.

54. Curl, C. L., Fenske, R. A., & Elgethun, K. (2003). Organophosphorus pesticide exposure of urban and suburban preschool children with organic and conventional diets. *Environmental Health Perspectives, 111*(3), 377–382. PubMed PMID: 12611667.

55. Lu, C., Barr, D. B., Pearson, M. A., & Waller, L. A. (2008). Dietary intake and its contribution to longitudinal organophosphorus pesticide exposure in urban/suburban children. *Environmental Health Perspectives, 116*(4), 537–542. PubMed PMID: 18414640.

56. Adams, S. V., Newcomb, P. A., Shafer, M. M., Atkinson, C., Bowles, E. J., Newton, K. M., et al. (2011). Sources of cadmium exposure among healthy premenopausal women. *The Science of the Total Environment, 409*(9), 1632–1637. PubMed PMID: 21333327.

57. U.S. Environmental Protection Agency: 2011 National Listing of Fish Advisories (NLFA). Available at https://www.epa.gov/sites/production/files/2015-06/documents/maps-and-graphics-2011.pdf. (Accessed 30 November 2017). (Accessed 1 May 2017).

58. Hanrahan, L. P., Falk, C., Anderson, H. A., Draheim, L., Kanarek, M. S., Olson, J., et al. (1999). Serum PCB and DDE levels of frequent Great Lakes sport fish consumers-a first look. The Great Lakes Consortium. *Environmental Research, 80*(2 Pt. 2), S26–S37. PubMed PMID: 10092417.

59. Newsome, W. H., & Andrews, P. (1993). Organochlorine pesticides and polychlorinated biphenyl cogeners in commercial fish from the Great Lakes. *Journal of AOAC International, 76*(4), 707–710. PubMed PMID: 8374320.

60. He, J. P., Stein, A. D., Humphrey, H. E., Paneth, N., & Courval, J. M. (2001). Time trends in sport-caught Great Lakes fish consumption and serum polychlorinated biphenyl levels among Michigan Anglers, 1973-1993. *Environmental Science & Technology, 35*(3), 435–440. PubMed PMID: 11351711.

61. van Leeuwen, S. P., van Velzen, M. J., Swart, C. P., van der Veen, I., Traag, W. A., & de Boer, J. (2009). Halogenated contaminants in farmed salmon, trout, tilapia, pangasius, and shrimp. *Environmental Science & Technology, 43*(11), 4009–4015. PubMed PMID: 19569323.

62. Knapp, G., et al. *The Great Salmon Run: Competition between wild and farmed salmon*. Available from http://www.iser.uaa.alaska.edu/Publications/2007_01-GreatSalmonRun.pdf. (Accessed 29 April 2017).

63. Carlson, D. L., & Hites, R. A. (2005). Polychlorinated biphenyls in salmon and salmon feed: Global differences and bioaccumulation. *Environmental Science & Technology, 39*(19), 7389–7395. PubMed PMID: 16245806.

64. Nøstbakken, O. J., Hove, H. T., Duinker, A., Lundebye, A. K., Berntssen, M. H., Hannisdal, R., et al. (2015). Contaminant levels in Norwegian farmed Atlantic salmon (Salmo salar) in the 13-year period from 1999 to 2011. *Environment International, 74*, 274–280. PubMed PMID: 25454244.

65. Page, B. D., & Lacroix, G. M. (1995). The occurrence of phthalate ester and di-2-ethylhexyl adipate plasticizers in Canadian packaging and food sampled in 1985-1989: A survey. *Food Additives and Contaminants, 12*(1), 129–151.

66. Castle, L., Nichol, J., & Gilbert, J. (1992). Migration of polyisobutylene from polyethylene/polyisobutylene films into foods during domestic and microwave oven use. *Food Additives and Contaminants, 9*(4), 315–330.

67. Ji, K., Lim Kho, Y., Park, Y., & Choi, K. (2010). Influence of a five-day vegetarian diet on urinary levels of antibiotics and phthalate metabolites: A pilot study with "Temple Stay" participants. *Environmental Research, 110*(4), 375–382. PubMed PMID: 20227070.

68. Lorber, M., Schecter, A., Paepke, O., Shropshire, W., Christensen, K., & Birnbaum, L. (2015). Exposure assessment of adult intake of bisphenol A (BPA) with emphasis on canned food dietary exposures. *Environment International, 77*, 55–62. PubMed PMID: 25645382.

69. Lakind, J. S., & Naiman, D. Q. (2011). Daily intake of bisphenol A and potential sources of exposure: 2005-2006 National Health and Nutrition Examination Survey. *Journal of Exposure Science and Environmental Epidemiology, 21*(3), 272–279. PubMed PMID: 20237498.

70. Hartle, J. C., Navas-Acien, A., & Lawrence, R. S. (2016). The consumption of canned food and beverages and urinary Bisphenol A concentrations in NHANES 2003-2008. *Environmental Research, 150*, 375–382. PubMed PMID: 27362993.

71. Carwile, J. L., Ye, X., Zhou, X., Calafat, A. M., & Michels, K. B. (2011). Canned soup consumption and urinary bisphenol A: A randomized crossover trial. *JAMA: The Journal of the American Medical Association, 306*(20), 2218–2220. PubMed PMID: 22110104.

72. Bae, S., & Hong, Y. C. (2015). Exposure to bisphenol A from drinking canned beverages increases blood pressure: Randomized crossover trial. *Hypertension, 65*(2), 313–319. PubMed PMID: 25489056.

73. George, C. M., Smith, A. H., Kalman, D. A., & Steinmaus, C. M. (2006). Reverse osmosis filter use and high arsenic levels in private well water. *Archives of Environmental and Occupational Health, 61*(4), 171–175. PubMed PMID: 17867571.

74. Walker, M., Seiler, R. L., & Meinert, M. (2008). Effectiveness of household reverse-osmosis systems in a Western U.S. region with high arsenic in groundwater. *The Science of the Total Environment, 389*(2–3), 245–252. PubMed PMID: 17919687.

75. Yoon, J., Amy, G., Chung, J., Sohn, J., & Yoon, Y. (2009). Removal of toxic ions (chromate, arsenate, and perchlorate) using reverse osmosis, nanofiltration, and ultrafiltration membranes. *Chemosphere, 77*(2), 228–235. PubMed PMID: 19679331.

76. Wimalawansa, S. J. (2013). Purification of contaminated water with reverse osmosis: Effective solution of providing clean water for human needs in developing countries. *International Journal of Emerging Technology and Advanced Engineering, 3*(12), 75–89.

77. Chen, C. Y., Chou, Y. Y., Lin, S. J., & Lee, C. C. (2015). Developing an intervention strategy to reduce phthalate exposure in Taiwanese girls. *The Science of the Total Environment, 517*, 125–131. PubMed PMID: 25725197.

78. Romero-Franco, M., Hernández-Ramírez, R. U., Calafat, A. M., Cebrián, M. E., Needham, L. L., Teitelbaum, S., et al. (2011). Personal care product use and urinary levels of phthalate metabolites in Mexican women. *Environment International, 37*(5), 867–871. PubMed PMID: 21429583.

79. Lewis, R. C., Meeker, J. D., Peterson, K. E., Lee, J. M., Pace, G. G., Cantoral, A., et al. (2013). Predictors of urinary bisphenol A and phthalate metabolite concentrations in Mexican children. *Chemosphere, 93*(10), 2390–2398. PubMed PMID: 24041567.

80. Smith, R., & Lourie, B. (2011). *Slow death by rubber duck: the secret danger of everyday things* Counterpoint press.

61

Sauna

SUMMARY

- Benefits: Improvements in cardiovascular, respiratory, immunological, and neurological health; increased excretion of persistent and nonpersistent pollutants
- Primary mechanisms: Increased production of growth hormone, nitric oxide, β-endorphins, prolactin, norepinephrine, heat shock protein, and catalase; reduced oxidative stress; enhanced toxicant mobilization
- Best sources: All forms of commercially available saunas show health benefits

OVERVIEW

Saunas have been used for hundreds of years, especially in the Scandinavian countries. Finland, with a population of 5 million persons, has close to 1 million saunas. Most Finns take a sauna bath weekly and grew up hearing the adage: "If the sauna, schnapps, and birch tar don't help, then death is near." There are several distinct types of saunas: Finnish sauna (Finnish steam bath), dry-heat sauna, infrared saunas, and far-infrared (FIR) saunas.

SAUNA TYPES

Radiant-Heat Saunas

When the term "sauna" is used in this textbook and throughout the medical literature without any modifiers (e.g., infrared), it generally refers to the Finnish steam sauna. This sauna uses a wood-paneled room with wooden benches and a radiant heater that keeps the temperature between 70° and 100°C (158°–212°F), with a face-level temperature of 80° to 90°C (176°–194°F). Steam is produced by pouring water over heated rocks. Generally, enough steam is produced to create a humidity of 50 to 60 g water vapor/m³. The standard length of a Finnish sauna is 5 to 20 minutes in the sauna, followed by cold immersion (swim or shower) and a period of room temperature recovery before repeating. In a single sauna session, this pattern is repeated two to three times.

Dry-Heat Saunas

Dry-heat saunas are essentially the same as Finnish steam saunas; however, no water is added to produce steam. Use of these saunas is also roughly the same as the protocol described for Finnish steam saunas.

Infrared Saunas (Infrared and Far-Infrared Saunas)

Infrared saunas use a different heating element and typically do not achieve the same temperatures as radiant-heat saunas. There are also no hot rocks to splash water on to provide humidity. There are two main types of infrared saunas: infrared and FIR. Infrared saunas use incandescent infrared heat lamps to produce heat. They emit primarily near-infrared wavelengths, with lesser amounts of middle-infrared and perhaps a tiny amount of FIR energy. They also emit a small amount of red, orange, and yellow visible light.

FIR saunas use ceramic or metallic elements for heating that mainly emit energy in the FIR range. Infrared wavelengths act primarily on cutaneous blood vessels and nerve receptors and despite common sales claims do not penetrate deeply into tissues. The existing studies on the use of FIR focuses primarily on cardiovascular benefits. To date, no standards have been set for temperature and duration for infrared saunas as they have for radiant-heat, Finnish saunas.

Wavelength Tissue Penetration. The infrared portion of the electromagnetic spectrum is divided into three regions or bands: near-, mid-, and far-infrared. Near-infrared (IR-A: 700–1400 nm) has the greatest tissue penetration of the three at up to 5 mm depth, whereas FIR (IR-C) has practically no penetration.[1,2] IR-A penetrates to the subcutaneous layer and provides the best dissipation of heat from the skin surface. Mid-infrared (IR-B: 1400–3000 nm) has the next deepest tissue penetration, but only to about 0.5 mm. IR-C (3,000 nm–1 mm) has the shallowest tissue penetration of about 0.1 mm. Near-infrared wavelengths not only provide the deepest penetration but also result in changes in mitochondrial signaling in skin cells.[3] Because of their penetrating ability, near-infrared wavelengths are being used for noninvasive blood glucose and hemoglobin testing.[4]

PHYSIOLOGICAL RESPONSE TO SAUNA THERAPY

Saunas produce thermal stress, resulting in a transient production of heat shock proteins.[5] The cardiovascular system responds to the thermal stress by increasing heart rate, with a 70% increase in cardiac output.[6,7] This is accompanied by a 40% decrease in peripheral resistance, resulting in increased peripheral circulation with a concomitant decreased circulation to muscles, kidneys, and viscera.[8] The increased peripheral blood flow allows for greater heat exchange through the skin that is increased with diaphoresis. With the reduction in peripheral resistance, the diastolic and arterial blood pressures decrease, whereas the systolic blood pressure typically remains unchanged for the duration of the sauna session.

There is a corresponding acute increase in metabolic rate and oxygen consumption, the overall effect being similar to moderate exercise.[8] In theory, this would be a benefit for those living in climates with limited exercise options during the winter months.

Sauna also reduces elevated erythrocyte thiobarbituric acid reactive substances (TBARS) and increases catalase activity reducing overall oxidative stress.[9] Regular sauna use also significantly reduces low density lipoprotein (LDL) cholesterol levels and provides a nonsignificant increase in high density lipoprotein (HDL) levels as well.[10]

The sympathetic nervous system and the hypothalamus-pituitary-adrenal axis also respond to help compensate for the thermal stress. Norepinephrine output increases in persons undergoing sauna baths, whereas the levels of epinephrine and cortisol typically do not, unless cold-water immersion is included in the protocol.[7,11] Plasma levels of growth hormone, β-endorphins, and prolactin also increase during a sauna session.[7,12] The increase in β-endorphins presumably accounts for some of the pleasure felt during and after a sauna session and may be the reason for the commonly noted pain relief. Growth hormone levels in young elite wrestlers increased from 1.52 ng/mL at rest to 7.50 ng/mL postsauna.[13]

Muscle relaxation also occurs, along with increased elastic properties of the tendons and joint capsule and reduced viscosity of synovial joint fluid.[14] There is a loss of water and electrolytes (sodium, potassium, and chlorine) through the skin during a sauna session; however, this loss is compensated by hormonal regulation via adrenal secretion of aldosterone.[7] Individuals with proper aldosterone secretion who have regular sauna baths do not experience excessive electrolyte loss. This is reflected in the fact that the traditional Finnish sauna protocol does not include electrolyte replacement.

Specific Benefits

Cardiovascular. Saunas are an effective but underused treatment for various forms of heart disease.

Myocardial infarction. Despite concerns to the contrary, saunas are not associated with increased mortality from sudden cardiac death or myocardial infarctions (MI) in countries that routinely use saunas. Only 1.7% of the 6175 sudden deaths in Finland occurred within 24 hours of taking a sauna.[15] In fact, Finnish men who regularly sauna have lower rates of sudden cardiac death, fatal coronary heart disease, and fatal cardiovascular disease (Table 61.1).[16] Taking a regular sauna session twice weekly reduced the risk of heart-related fatality, with greater reduction being achieved with increased sauna frequency. A total of 77 deaths occurred in saunas in Sweden during an 11-year period (1992–2003), of which 71% were directly related to elevated blood alcohol levels rather than cardiovascular factors.[17] The cardiovascular response to Finnish sauna in 69 men who had experienced an MI in the previous 4 to 6 weeks was compared with that of 32 healthy controls (non-MI).[18] All persons in the sauna group had increased cardiac output without problems, and the post-MI group showed no adverse

Sauna Frequency	Sudden Cardiac Death	Fatal Coronary Heart Disease	Fatal Cardiovascular Disease
1 time weekly	1	1	1
2–3 times weekly	0.71	0.71	0.68
4–7 times weekly	0.49	0.60	0.55
p trend	<0.008	<0.006	<0.001

TABLE 61.1   Hazard Ratios for 40- to 61-Year-Old Finnish Males Based on the Number of Weekly Finnish Sauna Sessions Typically Taken

Modified from Laukkanen, T., Khan, H., Zaccardi, F., & Laukkanen, J. A. (2015). Association between sauna bathing and fatal cardiovascular and all-cause mortality events. *JAMA Internal Medicine, 175*(4), 542–548.

effects from sitting in the sauna. Although the sauna increased cardiac workload similarly to brisk walking, only 8% of the men experienced cardiac dysrhythmias during a sauna, compared with 18% who experienced dysrhythmia during a submaximal exercise test. A 10-year observational study of 102 men who had experienced an MI 2 to 24 weeks earlier included 80 who then began regular saunas post-MI. Although 60% of the subjects reported angina during normal daily life, only 2% reported chest pains while in the sauna, a remarkable result considering the increased cardiac output during a sauna.[19] Daily 15-minute FIR sauna sessions for 3 weeks improved myocardial scintigraphy, treadmill exercise time, and flow-mediated dilation of the brachial artery in 24 patients with complete occlusion of one of the coronary arteries.[20]

Hypertension. As previously mentioned, sauna therapy is known to reduce peripheral resistance, which should reduce elevated blood pressure.[7] Sauna has also been shown to increase nitric oxide release, which is undoubtedly part of the mechanism for reduced peripheral resistance.[21] Both exercise and sauna, independently and together, were effective at reducing blood pressure in a group of untreated hypertensive adults.[22] A group of 114 hypertensive men who began biweekly saunas after receiving coronary bypass surgery experienced a nonsignificant reduction in blood pressure.[15] Biweekly saunas for 3 months provided 46 hypertensive males with an average blood pressure drop from 166/101 mm Hg to 143/92 mm Hg,[23] a decrease equivalent to that found with some antihypertensive medications. Reduction in blood pressure from Finnish sauna sessions appears to be more prevalent in older individuals.[24] FIR saunas at 60°C (140°F) for 15 minutes followed by 30 minutes of bed rest daily, now called *Waon therapy,* for 2 weeks

significantly reduced systolic blood pressure in individuals with at least one coronary risk factor.[25] Those who had a regimen of sauna and rest ended up with an average systolic pressure of 110 mm Hg, whereas those who just did the 30 minutes of rest averaged 122 mm Hg. Individuals using daily FIR sauna therapy also had lower urinary levels of 8-epi-PGF2-α, suggesting lower oxidative stress.

Congestive heart failure. Biweekly sauna sessions resulted in an 7% to 8% increased ventricular ejection fraction in men.[26] Waon-FIR sauna sessions provided a significant improvement in endothelial function, resulting in better brachial artery dilation in young men with cardiovascular risk.[27] That same Waon-FIR protocol has shown benefit for individuals with diagnosed congestive heart failure (CHF; New York Heart Association functional class II or III). Compared with a control group who was only treated with bed rest, the FIR sauna group experienced improvement in endothelial-dependent dilation of the brachial artery after only 10 sauna sessions.[28] Although the control group had no change in blood flow or CHF symptoms, 17 out of 20 in the sauna group reported an improvement of clinical symptoms. This same Waon-FIR protocol was also used for 2 weeks on 20 individuals with class II and III CHF who were experiencing at least 200 premature ventricular contractions (PVCs) in a 24-hour period.[29] As a control group, 10 other CHF patients with PVCs reclined on a bed in a 24°C (75.2°F) room for 45 minutes daily for 2 weeks. After 10 FIR sauna sessions, the treatment group experienced a reduction of PCVs from 3161 per 24 hours to an average of 848 per 24 hours, dramatically lower than the control group, who averaged 3097 PVCs every 24 hours. When this FIR protocol was done three times weekly for only 4 weeks, a trend toward improvement in the New York Heart Association classification and in the Minnesota Living with Heart Failure Questionnaire was noted in those who took part in the sauna and rest protocol over those who just had the rest regimen.[30] However, when it was done daily for 4 weeks, there were statistically significant reductions in systolic blood pressures, significant improvements in left ventricular ejection fraction, improved exercise tolerance, increased peak respiratory flow, and anaerobic threshold.[31] They also had a statistically significant reduction in their plasma epinephrine and had less hospitalization for CHF during the following year than those who did not sit in the sauna.

Neurological

Anorexia nervosa. A single case study reported that FIR sauna therapy helped improve anorexia nervosa in a teenage girl who did regular FIR sauna sessions in a home sauna unit.[32] According to the report, this individual gained weight, experienced a reduction in "hyper" activity, and regained emotional balance.

Bipolar disorder. An individual with solvent-induced bipolar disorder used avoidance, nutritional support, and sauna therapy to reduce total xenobiotic burden and enjoyed complete remission of his manic symptoms.[33]

Dementia. Regular use of Finnish sauna can dramatically reduce the risk of dementia and Alzheimer's disease.[34] Consistent with the studies previously discussed on cardiovascular fatalities, the more sauna sessions habitually done per week, the lower the risk of both forms of dementia. Those who had regular sauna baths four to seven times weekly were 65% less likely to develop Alzheimer's disease (Table 61.2). The mechanism by

which this dramatic protective effect happens has not been definitively proven. However, as previously discussed, saunas increase excretion of several neurotoxins and have been shown to increase the production of brain-derived neurotropic factor, which promotes brain regeneration.[35]

Depression. Twenty-eight patients with mild depression, general fatigue, and appetite loss took part in 20 FIR sauna sessions over a 4-week period. Each session lasted 15 minutes in a 60°C unit and was followed by 30 minutes of bed rest with a blanket; the controls only participated in the bed rest. Compared with the control group, the FIR sauna treatment group experienced statistically significant improvements in somatic complaints, hunger, and ability to relax.[36]

Pain. Forty-six patients hospitalized for chronic pain (of at least 6 months duration) used cognitive behavioral therapy, rehabilitation, and exercise therapy with or without 15 minutes of 60°C FIR sauna therapy 5 days weekly for 4 weeks. At the end of the treatment program, the sauna group exhibited diminished pain behaviors and had statistically lower anger scores.[37] A 2-year follow-up revealed that 77% of the sauna group were able to return to work, compared with only 50% of the nonsauna group. Eight weeks of thrice-weekly sauna sessions provided a reduction in tension headache pain but had no effect on duration of the headaches.[38]

Respiratory. Finnish saunas decrease pulmonary congestion and increase forced vital capacity (FVC), peak expiratory flow rate (PEF), and forced expiratory volume in one second (FEV_1).[39] Sauna therapy can help respiration in patients with asthma and bronchitis. Regular sauna therapy improved lung function in a group of 12 men from the Netherlands who had chronic obstructive pulmonary disease (COPD). None of these men experienced adverse effects from the sauna, but all experienced significant improvements in FEV_1 and FVC.[40] They also reported that they did not have to expend as much effort to breathe. Taking part in a Finnish sauna session twice a week for 6 months may even reduce the incidence of the common cold by 50%.[41] Repeated FIR sauna sessions improve peak nasal inspiratory flow in persons with allergic rhinitis and improve their FEV_1 as well.[42] One study recommended against saunas during the acute phase of a respiratory infection, whereas a more recent, controlled study showed statistically insignificant improvement in symptom duration and statistically significant

TABLE 61.2 Hazard Ratios of Finnish Males (Aged 42–60 Years of Age at Beginning of Study) for Dementia and Alzheimer's Disease Based on Their Sauna Frequency Over 20+ Years Follow-Up		
Disease	**Sauna 1× Weekly**	**Sauna 2–3× Weekly**	**Sauna 4–7× Weekly**
Dementia	1	0.78	0.34
Alzheimer's	1	0.80	0.35

Data from Laukkanen, T., Kunutsor, S., Kauhanen, J., & Laukkanen, J. A. (2017). Sauna bathing is inversely associated with dementia and Alzheimer's disease in middle-aged Finnish men. *Age and Ageing, 46*(2), 245–249.

decreases in medication use and severity of symptoms and higher patient perception of efficacy.[43,44]

Autoimmunity. After 20 Waon-FIR sauna sessions, an individual with Sjörgren's syndrome and class II-III CHF reported "dramatic" improvements in symptoms of xerostomia and arthritis.[45] Her levels of human leukocyte antigen (HLA)-A, HLA-B, and HLA-C, which had been 3.4 times higher than normal, dropped to the high end of normal after the sessions.

Seventeen patients with rheumatoid arthritis (RA) and another 17 patients with ankylosing spondylitis participated in 4 weeks of twice-weekly Waon-FIR saunas.[46] All participants experienced a reduction in fatigue, pain, and stiffness, and those with RA showed nonsignificant ($p = 0.06$) improvements in pain, stiffness, and fatigue.

Chronic Fatigue. Two women with severe chronic fatigue resistant to prednisolone treatment began with 30 Waon-FIR sauna sessions 5 days weekly for 6 weeks, with subsequent once- or twice-weekly sessions for the following 11 months.[47] Both women reported dramatic improvements in fatigue, pain, sleep disturbances, and low-grade fevers.

Depuration (Excretion of Toxicants)

Mercury. Sauna therapy is often recommended as a means of increasing mercury excretion, but very little on this topic is found in the literature. The ratio of sweat versus urine mercury in mercury workers varied from the sweat carrying 75% of that found in urine (μg/L) to more than twofold that in the urine. The highest sweat mercury levels were consistently found in those who sweated the most.[48] This finding would appear to indicate that the more one sweats, the more effective sweat becomes at mobilizing toxicants. The blood, urine, sweat (BUS) study found the average concentration of urinary mercury to be 0.65 μg/L, whereas that of sweat was 0.86 μg/L in the participants.[49] Thus, although sweat is one avenue for mercury clearance, a measure of liters of sweat daily would be needed to compare to the regular daily mercury excretion through diuresis.

Lead. Lead is found in lower concentrations in sweat than in either blood or urine. Sweat from individuals with elevated blood lead levels averaging 8.62 μg/dL only averaged 5.2 μg/L, which was only about 25% of the concentration found in the urine.[50] Lead found in sweat

(and saliva) appears to be primarily from lead absorbed through the skin (rather than the lungs or gastrointestinal [GI] system).[51] However, a study on the toxicokinetics of lead revealed that soft tissue, not blood, is the source for lead in sweat, making sauna a potential part of any protocol to control soft tissue lead levels in osteoporotic individuals.[52]

Cadmium, Nickel, and Antimony. Cadmium and nickel are present in higher concentrations in sweat than they are in urine.[53] Sweating has also been explored as a method for reducing antimony levels in persons with high exposure.[54]

Bisphenol A and Phthalates. Sweating as a method of mobilizing toxicants was assessed in a small group of patients with chronic illness and an equal number of healthy controls. Serum and urine samples were taken within a 7-day period, during which these individuals collected sweat samples. FIR saunas were used by 10, standard Finnish steam sauna by 7, and exercise alone by 3. Both bisphenol A (BPA) and phthalates were documented in sweat and urine from individuals in the BUS study who used either FIR or Finnish saunas (Table 61.3).[55,56] BPA and di(2-ethylhexyl) phthlate (DEHP) were both found to be present in the sweat of individuals who did not have these toxicants present in their serum. This would indicate that both BPA and DEHP have some degree of storage in the subcutaneous fat pads. Mono-ethylhexyl phthalic acid (MEHP) was found in the sweat at concentrations double that in the urine. Five polybrominated diphenyl ether (PBDE) flame retardants found in the serum of these individuals were also mobilized into their sweat with sauna use.[57] As with both BPA and phthalates, some PBDE congeners were present in the sweat but not present in the serum.

Chlorinated Pesticides and Polychlorinated Biphenyls. Multiple chlorinated pesticides, including dichlorodiphenyl-trichloroethane (DDT), dichlorodiphenyldichloroethylene (DDE), methoxychlor, endrin, and endosulfan sulfate were also mobilized in the sweat through both types of sauna. In these individuals, the chlorinated pesticides were found more often in sweat than in urine or serum, with some compounds only being found in the sweat.[58] Sweat samples also contained polychlorinated biphenyls (PCBs) that were not in the serum but did not contain perfluorocarbons (PFCs) that

TABLE 61.3 PBDE Congeners Present in Sweat Samples Induced by Exercise, FIR, or Finnish Steam Sauna

Type of Intervention	Overall Mean Blood/Sweat Ratio				
	BDE 28	BDE 47	BDE 99	BDE 100	BDE 153
Exercise (n = 3)	137.2	25.5	4.8	16.9	26.9
Infrared sauna (n = 8)	17.9	32.1	3.25	94.6	71.8
Steam sauna (n = 6)	69.5	26.3	5.6	2.4	121.2

Insufficient perspiration samples are not included.
From Genuis, S. K., Birkholz, D., & Genuis, S. J. (2017). Human excretion of polybrominated diphenyl ether flame retardants: Blood, urine, and sweat study. *BioMed Research International, 2017*, 3676089. Copyright © 2017 Shelagh K. Genuis et al. Reprinted under the terms and conditions of the Creative Commons Attribution (CC-BY) license (http://creativecommons.org/licenses/by/4.0/).

TABLE 61.4 Mean Total PCB Levels in Adipose and Serum in 10 Electrical Workers and 10 Controls

Group	Prepurification Average Levels	Postpurification Average Levels	12-Month Follow-Up Average Levels
Group A Adipose mg/kg	20.9	14.5	16.7
Group A Serum	139.4	80.3	168.8
Group B Adipose mg/kg	40.9	37.0	38.2
Group B Serum	284.8	292.6	287.1
Control Adipose mg/kg	22.4	23.1	27.4
Control Serum	139.8	179.4	183.8

Data from Tretjak, Z., Root, D. E., Tretjak, A., Slivnik, R., Edmondson, E., & Graves, R., et al. (1990). Xenobiotic reduction and clinical improvements in capacitor workers: A feasible method. *Journal of Environmental Science and Health, A25*(7), 731–751.

were present in the serum.[59] There were no significant differences in toxicant mobilization between types of sauna (Table 61.3). Sweating, either induced by radiant-heat or FIR heating units, is effective at mobilizing adipose stores of both persistent and nonpersistent toxicants, except for PFCs.

Protocols. Various depuration programs, often including nutritional and other components along with sauna sessions, have been used to reduce the burden of persistent pollutants in humans.

Hubbard Method. One of the earliest published methods was the Hubbard Purification Rundown (also called the Hubbard Method), designed by L. Ron Hubbard, founder of the Church of Scientology.[60] The components of the 3- to 6-week Hubbard protocol are as follows:
- Physical exercise for 20 to 30 minutes daily
- Radiant dry-heat saunas, 140° to 180°F, done in 30-minute sessions, for a total of 2.5 to 5 hours daily
- A daily multiple vitamin/mineral
- Daily increasing doses of niacin
- Water, sodium, and potassium replacement to replace fluids and electrolytes lost during sauna therapy
- 1 to 8 tablespoons of vegetable oil daily
- Balanced meals and adequate sleep

This protocol was used with a group of 10 electrical workers who had been exposed to PCBs, with another 10 workers serving as controls.[61] Based on initial PCB levels in blood and gluteal adipose tissue, the six cases with the lowest total PCB average were designated as group A, and those having higher starting values were designated as group B. The adipose levels in both groups A and B were found to be lower 12 months after the treatment, whereas the control group had higher adipose PCB stores (Table 61.4).

A small group of 9/11 Trade Center rescue workers who used this protocol also achieved a reduction in their serum levels of polychlorinated dibenzodioxins (PCDDs), polychlorinated dibenzofurans (PCDFs), and PCBs.[62]

The use of the Hubbard protocol provided symptomatic improvements for a group of firefighters who became ill after responding to an exploded PCB-containing transformer.[63] The firemen rapidly began to experience symptoms of extreme fatigue, headache, muscle weakness, arthralgias, memory loss, and reduced concentration after this incident. After completing 2 to 3 weeks of the Hubbard protocol, significant improvements were noted on neurocognitive testing for memory, vision, cognition, and motor function. Interestingly, no correlation was found between PCB levels in the firemen and their measurable neurological deficits. Utah police officers who became ill after exposure to methamphetamine had statistically significant improvements in overall health and neurological health (measured by the short form (SF)-36) after completing the Hubbard protocol (Fig. 61.1).[64]

Means at treatment enrollment compared with those at completion produced significance at $p < 0.001$ for all subscales, using the paired two-tailed Student's t-test.[63]

Rea Protocol. William Rea, MD, Director of Environmental Health Center, Dallas (EHC-D), has also

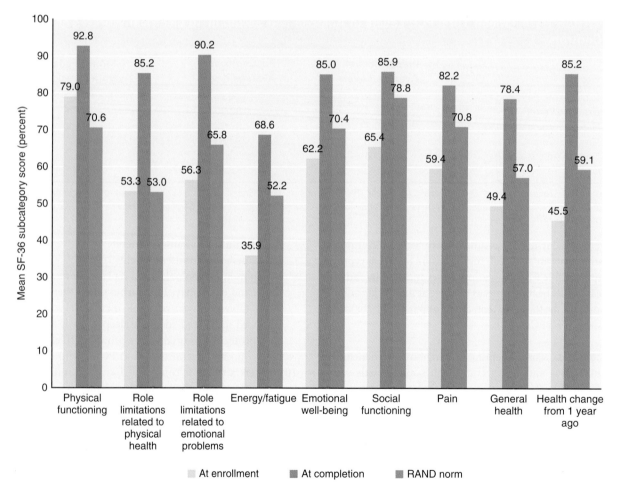

FIG. 61.1 Meth Cops RAND 36-item Short Form Health Survey (SF-36) health status before and after detoxification therapy, in comparison with RAND population norms. (From Ross, G. H., & Sternquist, M. C. [2012]. Methamphetamine exposure and chronic illness in police officers: Significant improvement with sauna-based detoxification therapy. *Toxicology & Industrial Health*, *28*[8], 758–768.)

documented the benefit of thermal chambers as a component of a more comprehensive protocol in his practice. His method consisted of the following:

- Living in chemical-free living facilities
- Two hours daily of radiant dry-heat sauna (set between 140° and 160° F)
- 15 to 30 minutes of exercise daily
- 20 to 30 minutes of massage daily
- Niacin, up to 3 g daily
- Vitamins, minerals, and amino acids given orally and intravenously
- IV vitamin C (15 g daily) with another 2 to 8 g orally
- Other vitamins and minerals per physician recommendation

The use of this protocol on 210 chemically sensitive individuals resulted in 86% of the participants reporting a reduction in their chemical reactivity.[65] In addition, 57% of subjects with abnormal balance and 31% of subjects with autonomic nervous system disorders, as measured via an iriscorder, improved. Serum levels of aromatic and aliphatic solvents were reduced in 63% of individuals at the end of the program.

A second group of 69 chemically sensitive individuals were treated either as outpatients (n = 56) or as inpatients in a chemical-free "nontoxic" hospital unit (n = 13), where all the air, food, and water was purified.[66] Of the 56 outpatients, 15 completed the sauna protocol along with lifestyle modifications designed to reduce their daily air- and food-borne toxicant exposures, whereas the remainder just did lifestyle modification. Blood tests for circulating solvents were conducted before and after these modifications on all participants. All of the participants in the inpatient program had improvement in signs and symptoms by the time of discharge (average stay 3.8 months), and 70% of the outpatients noted improvement with avoidance techniques after an average of 8.8 months. However, 80% of the outpatients who used sauna therapy experienced improvement after an average duration of only 7 weeks. The amount of solvent clearance from the blood of the individuals undergoing sauna therapy was similar to that of individuals in the inpatient environmental unit but was achieved in less than half the time.

Crinnion Naturopathic Protocol. Sauna therapy was also used as part of a naturopathic depuration protocol that was done 5 days weekly for a minimum of 3 weeks and included the following:

- Physical exercise was conducted on a rebounder or exercycle for 15 to 20 minutes daily.
- Radiant dry thermal chambers at 120° to 130° F were used for three 61-minute sessions, 5 days per week, with cool-down time in between.
- Glass-bottled spring water and electrolyte replacement were made available for use in each sauna session.
- Ginger or yarrow tea was made available as an optional diaphoretic in the first sauna session of the day.
- No niacin was given.
- Constitutional hydrotherapy (alternating hot and cold towels covering first the ventral surface and then the dorsal surface of the body) as described by Boyle and Seine[67] was done after the sauna and before the colonic irrigations.
- One capsule daily of an herbal combination (consisting of *Chelidonium majus, Chionanthus virginicus, Arctium lappa, Taraxacum officinale, Urtica dioica, Uva ursi, Silybum marianum*) was given to encourage bile production and release.
- Colonic irrigations (50 minutes) were performed with purified water.
- Consumption of adverse food reactors was avoided.
- Fruits and vegetables with high amounts of pesticide residues (United States Department of Agriculture pesticide data program) were avoided.
- Dietary avoidance of red meats.
- Consumption of sugar was avoided.

A retrospective chart review and anonymous questionnaire follow-up of 112 individuals who used this protocol revealed that more than 80% of the participants reported "good" to "great" results (Table 61.5).[68] All participants had serious enough morbidity to motivate them to take a minimum of 3 weeks out of their lives for this full-time cleansing program (8 hours in-office daily, 5 days weekly). Multiple chemical sensitivity (MCS) was the most common presenting complaint (25 of 112 participants), and 84% of that subgroup reported good to great improvement. All 16 of those whose chief complaint was some form of autoimmune disease reported good or great improvement, with 75% of them reporting their improvement as "great."

CONTRAINDICATIONS FOR SAUNA THERAPY

Very few contraindications for sauna therapy exist. Published recommendations suggest that persons with

TABLE 61.5   Results of 15 or More Sessions of the Crinnion Cleansing Program Listed by Complaint and Patient-Assessed Degree of Improvement

Complaints	Worse	No Change	Slight	Good	Great	Total
MCS	0	2	1	8	13	25
Autoimmune	0	0	0	4	12	16
Neurological	0	3	2	4	6	15
Fatigue	0	1	0	6	7	14
Neoplasia	0	2	0	2	4	8
Allergies	0	0	1	5	1	7
General cleansing	0	0	2	5	0	7
Musculoskeletal	0	0	2	2	1	5
Dermatological	0	0	0	3	1	4
Respiratory	0	0	0	0	3	3
GI/Liver	0	0	0	1	2	3
General debility	0	1	1	0	1	3
HIV/AIDS	0	0	1	1	0	2
Addictions	0	0	0	0	1	1
Totals	0	9	10	41	52	112
Percent	0	8	9	36.6	46.4	

From Crinnion, W. J. (1997). Results of a decade of naturopathic treatment for environmental illnesses. *Journal of Naturopathic Medicine, 7*(2), 21–27.

aortic stenosis, unstable angina, severe orthostatic hypotension, or any history of recent MI avoid sauna therapy.[19,69] However, men who used Finnish saunas as soon as 6 weeks after an MI experienced a reduced risk of a subsequent MI.[18,19] Some researchers have recommended that persons with fevers and certain skin conditions (cholinergic urticaria, abrasions, and oozing rashes) avoid saunas.[53,70]

Use of saunas during pregnancy remains an area of controversy. A study of women in the Boston, MA, area found an association between exposure to high heat during their first 2 months of pregnancy by fevers, hot tubs, or sauna and risk of having a child with neural tube defects such as anencephaly or spina bifida.[71] However, these findings must be compared with Finland, where 95% to 99% of pregnant women engage in regular sauna sessions, which has the lowest rates of anencephaly in the world.[72,73] In contrast, Ireland, where saunas are not part of the cultural experience, has rates of anencephaly among the highest in the world. Pregnant Finnish women engaging in regular sauna baths show no adverse health outcomes for themselves or their children.[74,75] No increased risk of childhood epilepsy was found with maternal sauna use during pregnancy, but maternal fevers during pregnancy did increase risk.[76] With the exception of complicated pregnancies, such as in the presence of toxemia, sauna appears to present no harm to the fetus or the mother when the woman is used to taking regular sauna baths.[77] However, women who are not regular sauna users should be recommended to avoid sauna and hot tub use during pregnancy.

REFERENCES

1. Alander, J., Autere, A., Kannianinen, O., Koljonen, J., Nordling, T. E. M., & Valisuo, P. (2008). Near infrared wavelength relevance detection of ultraviolet radiation-induced erythema. *Journal of Near Infrared Spectroscopy, 16*, 233–241.
2. Bachem, A., & Reed, C. I. (1930). The penetration of light through human skin. *The American Journal of Physiology, 97*(1), 86–91.
3. Schroeder, P., Lademann, J., Darvin, M. E., Stege, H., Marks, C., Bruhnke, S., et al. (2008). Infrared radiation-induced matrix metalloproteinase in human skin: implications for protection. *The Journal of Investigative Dermatology, 128*(10), 2491–2497. PubMed PMID: 18449210.
4. Troy, T. L., & Thennadil, S. N. (2001). Optical properties of human skin in the near infrared wavelength range of 1000 to 2200 nm. *Journal of*

Biomedical Optics, 6(2), 167–176. PubMed PMID: 11375726.

5. Krause, M., Ludwig, M. S., Heck, T. G., & Takahashi, H. K. (2015). Heat shock proteins and heat therapy for type 2 diabetes: pros and cons. *Current Opinion in Clinical Nutrition and Metabolic Care*, 18(4), 374–380. PubMed PMID: 26049635.

6. Kauppinen, K. (1989). Sauna, shower, and ice water immersion. Physiological responses to brief exposures to heat, cool, and cold. Part II. Circulation. *Arctic Medical Research*, 48(2), 64–74. PubMed PMID: 2736002.

7. Kukkonen-Harjula, K., Oja, P., Laustiola, K., Vuori, I., Jolkkonen, J., Siitonen, S., et al. (1989). Haemodynamic and hormonal responses to heat exposure in a Finnish sauna bath. *European Journal of Applied Physiology and Occupational Physiology*, 58(5), 543–550. PubMed PMID: 2759081.

8. Vuori, I. (1988). Sauna bather's circulation. *Annals of Clinical Research*, 20(4), 249–256. PubMed PMID: 3218896.

9. Sutkowy, P., Woźniak, A., Boraczyński, T., Mila-Kierzenkowska, C., & Boraczyński, M. (2014). The effect of a single Finnish sauna bath after aerobic exercise on the oxidative status in healthy men. *Scandinavian Journal of Clinical and Laboratory Investigation*, 74(2), 89–94. PubMed PMID: 24304490.

10. Gryka, D., Pilch, W., Szarek, M., Szygula, Z., & Tota, Ł. (2014). The effect of sauna bathing on lipid profile in young, physically active, male subjects. *International Journal of Occupational Medicine and Environmental Health*, 27(4), 608–618. PubMed PMID: 25001587.

11. Kauppinen, K., Pajari-Backas, M., Volin, P., & Vakkuri, O. (1989). Some endocrine responses to sauna, shower and ice water immersion. *Arctic Medical Research*, 48(3), 131–139. PubMed PMID: 2789570.

12. Jezová, D., Kvetnanský, R., & Vigas, M. (1994). Sex differences in endocrine response to hyperthermia in sauna. *Acta Physiologica Scandinavica*, 150(3), 293–298. PubMed PMID: 8010136.

13. Kiyici, R., & Ucan, I. (2014). The comparison of the wrestlers' status of some physical, physiological and growth hormone status after resting, competition and sauna sessions. *Procedia, Social and Behavioral Sciences*, 116, 19–22.

14. Hasan, J., Karvonen, M. J., & Piironen, P. (1967). Special review. II. Physiological effects of extreme heat. As studied in the Finnish "sauna" bath. *American Journal of Physical Medicine*, 46(2), 1226–1246. PubMed PMID: 5337808.

15. Luurila, O. J. (1978). Cardiac arrhythmias, sudden death and the Finnish sauna bath. *Advances in Cardiology*, 25, 73–81. PubMed PMID: 707206.

16. Laukkanen, T., Khan, H., Zaccardi, F., & Laukkanen, J. A. (2015). Association between sauna bathing and fatal cardiovascular and all-cause mortality events. *JAMA Internal Medicine*, 175(4), 542–548. PubMed PMID: 25705824.

17. Rodhe, A., & Eriksson, A. (2008). Sauna deaths in Sweden, 1992-2003. *The American Journal of Forensic Medicine and Pathology*, 29(1), 27–31. PubMed PMID: 19749613.

18. Luurila, O. J. (1980). Arrhythmias and other cardiovascular responses during Finnish sauna and exercise testing in healthy men and post-myocardial infarction patients. *Acta Medica Scandinavica. Supplementum*, 641, 1–60. PubMed PMID: 6933826.

19. Eisalo, A., & Luurila, O. J. (1988). The Finnish sauna and cardiovascular diseases. *Annals of Clinical Research*, 20(4), 267–270. PubMed PMID: 3218899.

20. Sobajima, M., Nozawa, T., Ihori, H., Shida, T., Ohori, T., Suzuki, T., et al. (2013). Repeated sauna therapy improves myocardial perfusion in patients with chronically occluded coronary artery-related ischemia. *International Journal of Cardiology*, 167(1), 237–243. PubMed PMID: 22244482.

21. Ikeda, Y., Biro, S., Kamogawa, Y., Yoshifuku, S., Eto, H., Orihara, K., et al. (2005). Repeated sauna therapy increases arterial endothelial nitric oxide synthase expression and nitric oxide production in cardiomyopathic hamsters. *Circulation Journal*, 69(6), 722–729. PubMed PMID: 15914953.

22. Gayda, M., Paillard, F., Sosner, P., Juneau, M., Garzon, M., Gonzalez, M., et al. (2012). Effects of sauna alone and postexercise sauna baths on blood pressure and hemodynamic variables in patients with untreated hypertension. *Journal of Clinical Hypertension (Greenwich, Conn.)*, 14(8), 553–560. PubMed PMID: 22863164.

23. Siewert, C., Siewert, H., Winterfeld, H. J., & Strangfeld, D. (1994). [The behavior of central and peripheral hemodynamics in isometric and dynamic stress in hypertensive patients treatment with regular sauna therapy]. *Zeitschrift fur Kardiologie*, 83(9), 652–657. German. PubMed PMID: 7801668.

24. Sawatari, H., Chishaki, A., Miyazono, M., Hashiguchi, N., Maeno, Y., Chishaki, H., et al. (2015). Different physiological and subjective responses to the hyperthermia between young and older adults: basic study for thermal therapy in cardiovascular diseases. *The Journals of Gerontology. Series A, Biological Sciences and Medical Sciences*, 70(7), 912–916. PubMed PMID: 25528016.

25. Masuda, A., Miyata, M., Kihara, T., Minagoe, S., & Tei, C. (2004). Repeated sauna therapy reduces urinary

8-epi-prostaglandin F(2alpha). *Japanese Heart Journal*, 45(2), 297–303. PubMed PMID: 15090706.

26. Winterfeld, H. J., Siewert, H., Strangfeld, D., Warnke, H., Aurisch, R., Kruse, J., et al. (1988). [Use of walking and sauna therapy in the rehabilitation of hypertensive patients with ischemic heart disease following aortocoronary venous bypass operation with special reference to hemodynamics]. *Zeitschrift fur Kardiologie*, 77(3), 190–193. German. PubMed PMID: 3260059.

27. Imamura, M., Biro, S., Kihara, T., Yoshifuku, S., Takasaki, K., Otsuji, Y., et al. (2001). Repeated thermal therapy improves impaired vascular endothelial function in patients with coronary risk factors. *Journal of the American College of Cardiology*, 38(4), 1083–1088. PubMed PMID: 11583886.

28. Kihara, T., Biro, S., Imamura, M., Yoshifuku, S., Takasaki, K., Ikeda, Y., et al. (2002). Repeated sauna treatment improves vascular endothelial and cardiac function in patients with chronic heart failure. *Journal of the American College of Cardiology*, 39(5), 754–759. PubMed PMID: 11869837.

29. Kihara, T., Biro, S., Ikeda, Y., Fukudome, T., Shinsato, T., Masuda, A., et al. (2004). Effects of repeated sauna treatment on ventricular arrhythmias in patients with chronic heart failure. *Circulation Journal*, 68(12), 1146–1151. PubMed PMID: 15564698.

30. Basford, J. R., Oh, J. K., Allison, T. G., Sheffield, C. G., Manahan, B. G., Hodge, D. O., et al. (2009). Safety, acceptance, and physiologic effects of sauna bathing in people with chronic heart failure: a pilot report. *Archives of Physical Medicine and Rehabilitation*, 90(1), 173–177. PubMed PMID: 19154844.

31. Miyamoto, H., Kai, H., Nakaura, H., Osada, K., Mizuta, Y., Matsumoto, A., et al. (2005). Safety and efficacy of repeated sauna bathing in patients with chronic systolic heart failure: a preliminary report. *Journal of Cardiac Failure*, 11(6), 432–436. PubMed PMID: 16105634.

32. Gutierrez, E., & Vazquez, R. (2001). Heat in the treatment of patients with anorexia nervosa. *Eating and Weight Disorders*, 6(1), 49–52. PubMed PMID: 11300546.

33. Sprouse, A., Curtis, L., & Bartlik, B. (2013). Organic solvent-induced bipolar disorder: a case report. *Advances in Mind-Body Medicine*, 27(3), 19–23. PubMed PMID: 23784607.

34. Laukkanen, T., Kunutsor, S., Kauhanen, J., & Laukkanen, J. A. (2016 Dec 7). Sauna bathing is inversely associated with dementia and Alzheimer's disease in middle-aged Finnish men. *Age and Ageing*, [Epub ahead of print], PubMed PMID: 27932366.

35. Goekint, M., Roelands, B., Heyman, E., Njemini, R., & Meeusen, R. (2011). Influence of citalopram and environmental temperature on exercise-induced changes in BDNF. *Neuroscience Letters*, 494(2), 150–154. PubMed PMID: 21385602.

36. Masuda, A., Nakazato, M., Kihara, T., Minagoe, S., & Tei, C. (2005). Repeated thermal therapy diminishes appetite loss and subjective complaints in mildly depressed patients. *Psychosomatic Medicine*, 67(4), 643–647. PubMed PMID: 16046381.

37. Masuda, A., Koga, Y., Hattanmaru, M., Minagoe, S., & Tei, C. (2005). The effects of repeated thermal therapy for patients with chronic pain. *Psychotherapy and Psychosomatics*, 74(5), 288–294. PubMed PMID: 16088266.

38. Kanji, G., Weatherall, M., Peter, R., Purdie, G., & Page, R. (2015). Efficacy of regular sauna bathing for chronic tension-type headache: a randomized controlled study. *Journal of Alternative and Complementary Medicine (New York, N.Y.)*, 21(2), 103–109. PubMed PMID: 25636135.

39. Kiss, D., Popp, W., Wagner, C., Zwick, H., & Sertl, K. (1994). Effects of the sauna on diffusing capacity, pulmonary function and cardiac output in healthy subjects. *Respiration; International Review of Thoracic Diseases*, 61(2), 86–88. PubMed PMID: 8008993.

40. Cox, N. J., Oostendorp, G. M., Folgering, H. T., & van Herwaarden, C. L. (1989). Sauna to transiently improve pulmonary function in patients with obstructive lung disease. *Archives of Physical Medicine and Rehabilitation*, 70(13), 911–913. PubMed PMID: 2596966.

41. Ernst, E., Pecho, E., Wirz, P., & Saradeth, T. (1990). Regular sauna bathing and the incidence of common colds. *Annals of Medicine*, 22(4), 225–227. PubMed PMID: 2248758.

42. Kunbootsri, N., Janyacharoen, T., Arrayawichanon, P., Chainansamit, S., Kanpittaya, J., Auvichayapat, P., et al. (2013). The effect of six-weeks of sauna on treatment autonomic nervous system, peak nasal inspiratory flow and lung functions of allergic rhinitis Thai patients. *Asian Pacific Journal of Allergy and Immunology*, 31(2), 142–147. PubMed PMID: 23859414.

43. Laitinen, L. A., Lindqvist, A., & Heino, M. (1988). Lungs and ventilation in sauna. *Annals of Clinical Research*, 20(4), 244–248. PubMed PMID: 3218895.

44. Pach, D., Knöchel, B., Lüdtke, R., et al. (2010). Visiting a sauna: does inhaling hot dry air reduce common cold symptoms? A randomised controlled trial. *The Medical Journal of Australia*, 193(11–12), 730–734. PubMed PMID: 21143077.

45. Tei, C., Orihara, F. K., & Fukudome, T. (2007). Remarkable efficacy of thermal therapy for Sjögren syndrome. *Journal of Cardiology*, 49(5), 217–219. PubMed PMID: 17552286.

46. Oosterveld, F. G., Rasker, J. J., Floors, M., Landkroon, R., van Rennes, B., Zwijnenberg, J., et al. (2009). Infrared sauna in patients with rheumatoid arthritis and ankylosing spondylitis. A pilot study showing good tolerance, short-term improvement of pain and stiffness, and a trend towards long-term beneficial effects. *Clinical Rheumatology*, 28(1), 29–34. PubMed PMID: 18685882.

47. Masuda, A., Kihara, T., Fukudome, T., Shinsato, T., Minagoe, S., & Tei, C. (2005). The effects of repeated thermal therapy for two patients with chronic fatigue syndrome. *Journal of Psychosomatic Research*, 58(4), 383–387. PubMed PMID: 15992574.

48. Lovejoy, H. B., Bell, Z. G., Jr., & Vizena, T. R. (1973). Mercury exposure evaluations and their correlation with urine mercury excretions. 4. Elimination of mercury by sweating. *Journal of Occupational Medicine*, 15(7), 590–591. PubMed PMID: 4711652.

49. Genius, S. J., Birkholz, D., Rodushkin, I., & Beesoon, S. (2010). Blood, urine, and sweat (BUS) study: monitoring and elimination of bioaccumulated toxic elements. *Archives of Environmental Contamination and Toxicology*, PubMed PMID: 21057782.

50. Omokhodion, F. O., & Crockford, G. W. (1991). Lead in sweat and its relationship to salivary and urinary levels in normal healthy subjects. *The Science of the Total Environment*, 103(2–3), 113–122. PubMed PMID: 1882227.

51. Lilley, S. G., Florence, T. M., & Stauber, J. L. (1988). The use of sweat to monitor lead absorption through the skin. *The Science of the Total Environment*, 76(2–3), 267–278. PubMed PMID: 3238426.

52. Rabinowitz, M. B., Wetherill, G. W., & Kopple, J. D. (1976). Kinetic analysis of lead metabolism in healthy humans. *The Journal of Clinical Investigation*, 58(2), 261–270. PubMed PMID: 783195.

53. Cohn, J. R., & Emmett, E. A. (1978). The excretion of trace metals in human sweat. *Annals of Clinical and Laboratory Science*, 8(4), 270–275. PubMed PMID: 686643.

54. Fuzaïlov, IuM. (1992). [The role of the sweat glands in excreting antimony from the body in people living in the biogeochemical provinces of the Fergana Valley]. *Gigiena Truda I Professional'nye Zabolevaniia*, 5, 13–15. Russian. PubMed PMID: 1427342.

55. Genuis, S. J., Beesoon, S., Birkholz, D., & Lobo, R. A. (2012). Human excretion of bisphenol A: blood, urine, and sweat (BUS) study. *Journal of Environmental and Public Health*, 2012, 185731. PubMed PMID: 22253637.

56. Genuis, S. J., Beesoon, S., Lobo, R. A., & Birkholz, D. (2012). Human elimination of phthalate compounds:

blood, urine, and sweat (BUS) study. *The Scientific World Journal*, 2012, 615068. PubMed PMID: 23213291.

57. Genuis, S. K., Birkholz, D., & Genuis, S. J. (2017). Human Excretion of Polybrominated Diphenyl Ether Flame Retardants: Blood, Urine, and Sweat Study. *BioMed Research International*, 2017, 3676089. PubMed PMID: 28373979.

58. Genuis, S. J., Lane, K., & Birkholz, D. (2016). Human Elimination of Organochlorine Pesticides: Blood, Urine, and Sweat Study. *BioMed Research International*, 2016, 1624643. PubMed PMID: 27800487.

59. Genuis, S. J., Beesoon, S., & Birkholz, D. (2013). Biomonitoring and elimination of perfluorinated compounds and polychlorinated biphenyls through perspiration: blood, urine, and sweat study. *ISRN Toxicology*, 2013, 483832. PubMed PMID: 24083032.

60. Schnare, D. W., Denk, G., Shields, M., & Brunton, S. (1982). Evaluation of a detoxification regimen for fat stored xenobiotics. *Medical Hypotheses*, 9(3), 265–282. PubMed PMID: 7144634.

61. Tretjak, Z., Root, D. E., Tretjak, A., Slivnik, R., et al. (1990). Xenobiotic reduction and clinical improvements in capacitor workers: a feasible method. *Journal of Environment and Health Sciences*, A25(7), 731–751.

62. Dahlgren, J., Cecchini, M., Takhar, H., & Paepke, O. (2007). Persistent organic pollutants in 9/11 world trade center rescue workers: reduction following detoxification. *Chemosphere*, 69(8), 1320–1325. [Epub 2007 Jan 17]; PubMed PMID: 17234251.

63. Kilburn, K. H., Warsaw, R. H., & Shields, M. G. (1989). Neurobehavioral dysfunction in firemen exposed to polychlorinated biphenyls (PCBs): possible improvement after detoxification. *Archives of Environmental Health*, 44(6), 345–350. PubMed PMID: 2514627.

64. Ross, G. H., & Sternquist, M. C. (2012). Methamphetamine exposure and chronic illness in police officers: significant improvement with sauna-based detoxification therapy. *Toxicology and Industrial Health*, 28(8), 758–768. PubMed PMID: 22089658.

65. (1996). Reduction of chemical sensitivity by means of heat depuration, physical therapy and nutritional supplementation in a controlled environment. *Journal of Nutritional & Environmental Medicine*, 6, 141–148.

66. Rea, W. J., Pan, Y., & Johnson, A. R. (1991). Clearing of toxic volatile hydrocarbons from humans. *Boletín de la Asociación Médica de Puerto Rico*, 83(1), 321–324.

67. Boyle, W., & Seine, A. (1988). *Lecturers in naturopathic hydrotherapy*. Eclectic Medical Pub. Sandy, OR.

68. Crinnion, W. J. (1997). Results of a decade of naturopathic treatment for environmental illnesses. *Journal of Naturopathic Medicine, l7*(2), 21–27.

69. Luurila, O. J. (1992). The sauna and the heart. *Journal of Internal Medicine, 231*(4), 319–320. PubMed PMID: 1588253.

70. Hannuksela, M., & Väänänen, A. (1988). The sauna, skin and skin diseases. *Annals of Clinical Research, 20*(4), 276–278. PubMed PMID: 3218900.

71. Milunsky, A., Ulcickas, M., Rothman, K. J., Willett, W., Jick, S. S., & Jick, H. (1992). Maternal heat exposure and neural tube defects. *JAMA: The Journal of the American Medical Association, 268*(7), 882–885. PubMed PMID: 1640616.

72. Rapola, J., Saxén, L., & Granroth, G. (1978). Anencephaly and the sauna. *Lancet, 1*(8074), 1162. PubMed PMID: 77458.

73. Waldenstrom, U. (1994). Warm tub bath and sauna in early pregnancy: risk of malformation uncertain. *Acta Obstetricia et Gynecologica Scandinavica, 73*, 449–451. PubMed PMID: 8042454.

74. Vähä-Eskeli, K., Erkkola, R., Irjala, K., Uotila, P., Poranen, A. K., & Säteri, U. (1992). Responses of placental steroids, prostacyclin and thromboxane A2 to thermal stress during pregnancy. *European Journal of Obstetrics, Gynecology, and Reproductive Biology, 43*(2), 97–103. PubMed PMID: 1563566.

75. Vähä-Eskeli, K., Erkkola, R., & Seppänen, A. (1991). Is the heat dissipating ability enhanced during pregnancy? *European Journal of Obstetrics, Gynecology, and Reproductive Biology, 39*(3), 169–174. PubMed PMID: 2032587.

76. Sun, Y., Vestergaard, M., Christensen, J., & Olsen, J. (2011). Prenatal exposure to elevated maternal body temperature and risk of epilepsy in childhood: a population-based pregnancy cohort study. *Paediatric and Perinatal Epidemiology, 25*(1), 53–59. PubMed PMID: 21133969.

77. Vaha-Eskeli, K., & Erkkola, R. (1988). The sauna and pregnancy. *Annals of Clinical Research, 20*, 79–82.

62

Gastrointestinal and Renal Elimination

SUMMARY

- Benefits: Reduction in overall body burden of environmental pollutants
- Primary mechanisms: Reduction of renal and hepatic recycling, enhancement of the clearance of fat-soluble compounds
- Best sources: Dietary measures to alkalinize urine, probiotics, rice bran fiber (RBF), bile sequestrants, chlorophyll, green and black tea, retrograde colonic irrigations, saponin-containing botanicals

OVERVIEW

The elimination of xenobiotic pollution from a person's body can be labeled as decontamination, cleansing, or depuration. The terms "detox" and "detoxification" mean either 1) to remove a harmful substance (as a poison or toxin) or the effect of such from, or 2) to render (a harmful substance) harmless, and these terms are often erroneously used to describe the process of reducing total toxicant body burden. The term "detox" is also commonly used for drug and alcohol treatment, a more accurate application.

Chapter 56 reviewed the processes by which xenobiotic pollutants are eliminated through the urine and stool. Excreted pollutants that are still highly fat soluble are readily reabsorbed via passive diffusion in both the intestines and proximal tubules of the kidneys. These lipophilic compounds can also be actively transported with bile salts back into the bloodstream. However, even water-soluble toxicant metabolites can be reabsorbed into the kidneys, especially when the urine is acidic (a common occurrence in environmentally burdened individuals and those who consume the typical acid-inducing diet—see Chapter 56).

After avoidance, the next step in reducing the body burden of pollutants is to reduce both hepatic and renal recycling, optimizing the normal clearance processes. The

following step would then seek to increase clearance even more from that point.

REDUCING HEPATIC AND RENAL RECYCLING (REABSORPTION)

- Alkalinizing the urine
- Balancing the microbiome with whole food fibers and probiotic supplements

Renal Recycling

Compounds excreted in the urine are at least partly ionized or disassociated based on their dissociation constant (Ka) and the urine pH. The more the compound is ionized, the less it diffuses back into the tubules. Because pKa is a logarithmic function, a small change in urine pH can have a large effect on whether the compound is reabsorbed. Xenobiotics conjugated in phase II liver pathways with glycine, taurine, or glutathione are weak acids and are less prone to ionization in acidic urine, which increases their renal reuptake. Conversely, a more alkaline urine enhances the ionization, resulting in greater elimination. A great example of this is dimercaptosuccinic acid (DMSA)-bound cadmium. Although DMSA has a higher affinity for cadmium than for lead or mercury, a DMSA challenge typically moves very little cadmium in a normal acidic urine. At a urinary pH of 5.5, the cadmium is almost

737

completely released from the DMSA, but at a pH of 7.4, it is almost completely bound.[1] Forced alkalinization of the urine, achieving a pH of 7.5 or higher has been used to reverse potentially fatal poisonings by compounds like the herbicide 2,4-D (a main component of Agent Orange).[2] Forced alkalinization is accomplished through intravenous administration of sodium bicarbonate and is recommended as a treatment for chemical poisoning.[3]

Fortunately, urinary alkalinization can be accomplished by enhancing the intake of whole foods (alkaline ash) and reducing the intake of proteins with high sulfur-containing amino acids. It can also be accomplished using oral alkalinizing agents such as citrates and using high-bicarbonate, low-sulfur mineral water.[4] Several companies have urinary alkalinizing products available over the counter for use; some even provide pH strips to measure the effectiveness of their product. Although these methods will rarely raise the pH above 7.5, it will often reach 7. Because pKa is logarithmic, any increase in pH will reduce renal reuptake.

Hepatic Recycling

Microbiome. The microbiome, now known to have a huge effect on health, can either encourage or discourage recycling of certain compounds. The microbiome associated with Western diets appears to produce more beta-glucuronidase, leading to the release of compounds that have been bound to glucoronate by phase II, many of which are highly carcinogenic.[5] Restoring microbiome balance using whole food fibers, including almonds and black currents, reduces beta-glucuronidase activity.[6,7] Beta-glucuronidase inhibition can also be enhanced with licorice (*Glycyrrhiza glabra*),[8] milk thistle (*Silybum marianum*),[9] and calcium d-glucarate.[10,11]

Lactobacillus sp. are able to break down aldehydes through enhancement of the enzyme aldehyde dehydrogenase.[12] In addition, both *Lactobacillus sp.* and *Propionibacterium sp.* are able to bind aflatoxin B1 in the intestine, preventing it from causing damage to the liver and other organs.[13] In animal studies, *Lactobacillus rhamnosus* LGG demonstrated the ability to bind a sizeable amount of aflatoxin B1.[14] A 90-person human study in China reported on the effects of taking 20 to 50 billion colony forming units (CFU) of a 1:1 mixture of *Lactobacillus rhamnosus* LC705 and *Propionibacterium freudenreichii* daily for 5 weeks. Participants in the probiotic group had a 36% decrease in aflatoxin levels in the third week and a 55% decrease by week 5,[15] demonstrating

a potential for these bacteria to provide protection from hepatocellular carcinoma in those who are exposed to aspergillus.

Although these probiotics have demonstrated the ability to bind toxins, they also appear to have benefit for chemical toxicants. More than 900 people with debilitating chemical sensitivity were surveyed about which medical or health treatment made them better or worse. Of all the therapies tried, the supplement with the highest help-to-harm ratio (harm was reported by only 4.1% of respondents, no effect was experienced in another 44%, and clear help was noted by 52%) was acidophilus.[16]

Intestinal Binding Agents

- Cholestyramine
- Colestimide
- Activated charcoal
- RBF
- Chlorophyll

Cholestyramine. Cholestyramine, which effectively binds bile acids and prevents their recirculation, has been used to treat individuals with environmental overload. It has increased fecal excretion of the biologically persistent perfluorocarbons that are not mobilized by sweat and has been used to treat persons with mycotoxin-induced illnesses.[17,18,19] In animal models, it has demonstrated the ability to reduce the toxicity of the chlorinated pesticide lindane[20] but in humans was not able to significantly increase polychlorinated biphenyl (PCB) excretion.[21] However, a different cholesterol-lowering agent, colestimide, was able to increase PCB excretion in humans.[21]

Activated charcoal. Activated charcoal (AC) is used to adsorb chemical poisons in the intestines, preventing their movement into the circulation. AC is effective for some, but not all, pharmaceuticals[22] and has also shown benefit for pesticides,[23] although overall it appears to be less effective than cholestyramine. Although metals are not well adsorbed by AC, it has been used in cases of both mercury[24,25] and thallium poisoning.[26]

Fibers. In 1968, PCB-contaminated rice bran cooking oil poisoned a great number of Japanese in what came to be called "Yusho disease" (oil poisoning). This poisoning stimulated a great deal of research in methods that would increase the excretion of biologically persistent PCBs from the body. Results of these studies showed that RBFs and chlorophyll-containing compounds top the list of effective natural agents.

RBF has demonstrated the ability to bind PCBs and other toxicants, including the combustion by-product benzo(a)pyrene.[27] When measured against other fibers, RBF dramatically reduced the reabsorption of PCBs from the intestines in animals,[28] whereas wheat bran showed no benefit.[29] In PCB-exposed animals, RBF increased fecal PCB excretion 6.6 times and spinach fiber 4.1 times.[30] A 10% RBF diet increased the excretion of toxic furans 4.5 times more than placebo in another animal study.[31] Yusho patients who consumed 7 to 10 g of fermented RBF three times daily (after each meal) for a year experienced 81% greater elimination of furans and 74% greater elimination of dioxins over those not consuming the fiber.[32] Interestingly, the highest amount of PCB excretion in both animals and humans came from a combination of RBF and cholestyramine (which had minimal effect on its own).[33,34]

Chlorophyll. Chlorophyll has long been considered a blood purifier, and recent studies have documented its effectiveness at helping clear persistent chemical pollutants from the body. The chlorophyll-containing seaweed nori increased the fecal excretion of two different dioxins by a factor of 5.5 and 6 times over controls when present as 10% of the total animal diet.[35] Animals given chlorella had increased dioxin excretion varying from 30% to more than 300% greater than the control group.[36] The higher the content of chlorophyll in the diet, the greater the excretion of these fat-soluble persistent toxicants in the feces became.[37] The ranges of chlorophyll went from a low of 0.1% to a high of 0.5% in the diet. A diet with 0.1% chlorophyll is roughly equivalent to consuming 10% of diet as spinach or 20% as seaweed. In the 0.1% group, the fecal excretion of the various toxicants ranged from 40% to 80% greater than the control group. At the end of the study, all the animals that were given the chlorophyll had lower total body burden of these persistent pollutants than their counterparts. Pregnant Japanese women who consumed chlorophyll-rich chlorella during pregnancy had 30% less dioxin in their milk than controls.[38] The women consuming chlorella also had significantly less PCBs in their breast milk and a nonsignificant decrease in their adipose levels of dioxins and PCBs.

Diets containing green vegetables also enhance the excretion of persistent pollutants in proportion to their chlorophyll content.[39] The vegetables with the smallest increase in fecal dioxin excretion (60% to 300% increase) are Chinese cabbage, broccoli, onion, Welsh onion, cabbage, and celery. The vegetables with the next highest dioxin excretion (330% to 480% increase) are kale, Chinese chive, Shungiku, Chingetsuai, green lettuce, and sweet peppers. The group that tops the charts, with an increased dioxin excretion of 760% to 1160%, includes the darkest green vegetables: Komatsuna, mitsuba, spinach, and perilla.

Fecal Fat Enhancement

- Olestra (no longer available)
- Orlistat
- Saponin-containing botanicals
- Green and black tea
- *Lactobacillus sp.*

Through passive diffusion, fat-soluble toxicants cross the intestinal mucosa to enter lipids in the feces. By increasing the amount of fat in the stool, the level of fat-soluble toxicants leaving the body automatically increases. The daily consumption of 25 g of Olestra, a nonabsorbable fat, increased the fecal excretion of various fat-soluble toxicants by a factor of 1.5 to 11-fold.[40] Two women with acute toxicity from 2,3,7,8-tetrachlorodibenzo-p-dioxin (TCDD) successfully lowered their dioxin burden with Olestra but also experienced fat-soluble vitamin deficiencies as a result.[41] Olestras' main side effect, referred to as "anal leakage," is uncontrollable loose bowel movements caused by the fecal fat content. Olestra was also used on an overweight man with type 2 diabetes in Australia who was severely poisoned with PCBs.[42] He had chloracne, a common symptom of PCB overload, along with headaches and numbness in his lower body that got worse with any weight loss. He consumed seven potato chips containing only 16 g of Olestra daily for 2 years without any adverse bowel effects. At the end of those 24 months, he was 40 pounds lighter, had normal cholesterol, no longer had diabetes, and had a dramatic drop in his adipose PCB stores from 3200 to 56 mg/kg (Table 62.1). He was able to do all this without other dietary changes and without experiencing any chloracne. Residents of Anniston, AL, who were contaminated with PCBs from adjacent industry significantly reduced their body burden of PCBs by consuming 15 g of Olestra daily.[43] Unfortunately, the only commercial source of Olestra (fat-free Pringles) was recently removed from the market, making this depuration method currently unavailable.

Pancreatic Lipase Inhibitors

For dietary fats and oils to be absorbed, they must first be hydrolyzed by pancreatic lipase. The inhibition of the

TABLE 62.1   Effects of 2 Years of 16 g of Olestra Daily

	Before Olestra (8/2001)	After Olestra (8/2003)
Adipose PCB (Arochlor 1254)	3200 mg/kg	56 mg/kg
Body weight (kg)	101	83
Body mass index (kg/m²)	33.0	27.1
Cholesterol (mmol/L)	8.6	3.7
Triglycerides (mmol/L)	11.8	1.4
Blood glucose (mmol/L)	17	5.3

From Redgrave, T. G., Wallace, P., Jandacek, R. J., & Tso, P. (2005). Treatment with a dietary fat substitute decreased Arochlor 1254 contamination in an obese diabetic male. *Journal of Nutritional Biochemistry, 16*(6), 383–384.

pancreatic lipases results in diminished fat absorption and increased levels of fecal fat. Orlistat, a potent inhibitor of pancreatic lipase, dramatically increases fecal fat levels and is available as a weight loss product.[44] Orlistat users are warned to stay on a low-fat diet to prevent anal leakage. Although orlistat could be used to enhance the excretion of persistent pollutants, botanicals containing saponins and polyphenols can also be used.

Botanical pancreatic lipase inhibitors including wild yam *(Dioscorea)*, ginseng, and tea *(Camellia sinensis)* contain high levels of saponins. Saponins are complex compounds that have a soapy nature and are found in many plants. The saponins dioscin and diosgenin from *Dioscorea* inhibited pancreatic lipase and dramatically reduced weight gain in rats fed a diet high in beef fat.[45] Saponins from Japanese ginseng were tested in mice alongside orlistat and proved equally effective in preventing weight gain from a high-fat diet while doubling fecal fat excretion.[46] Tea is better known for its polyphenol concentration, but the theasaponins and saponins from *Camellia sinensis* can also inhibit lipase, prevent weight gain in animals on a high-fat diet, and increase fecal fat content.[47] Although saponins are not found in high amounts in a cup of green tea, they are high in the seeds and other parts of the plant.

Both epigallocatechin gallate (EGCG) from green tea and polyphenols from oolong tea inhibit pancreatic lipase activity.[48] This inhibition is different from the inhibition by orlistat, which directly inhibits the production of lipase. Lipase action on lipids can also be inhibited by altering lipid droplet size and surface area (fat emulsion properties), preventing the attachment of lipase. Tea catechins[49] and theaflavins[50] have both demonstrated this ability, which is likely the reason that both green and black teas have been associated with weight loss.[51] Tea polyphenols increase fecal fat, and therefore the excretion of persistent pollutants, from 5.5 to 6.9 g in 3 days.[52] In volunteers consuming a higher-fat diet, those who also consumed "polyphenol-rich oolong tea" had more than twice the amount of fecal fat excretion as those who drank a placebo liquid without polyphenols.[53] PCB-exposed animals who consumed 4 g of matcha tea daily had more than four times the PCB excretion as the placebo group.[54] Thus sufficient quantities of properly prepared extracts of green teas can be very helpful in clearing persistent toxicants from the body in addition to aiding in weight loss.

Probiotics, including *Lactobacillus gasseri*, are able to inhibit pancreatic lipase action and enhance fecal fat in both animals and humans.[55] This inhibition is via the same mechanism of altering fat emulsion properties as is found with green tea. *L. gasseri* also has previously been shown to stimulate fat loss in humans.[56]

Several different lactobacillus species, along with streptococcus, altered fat droplet size and increased fecal fat (Figs. 62.1 and 62.2). Fig. 62.1 shows the dramatic effect that different lactobacillus species have on fat droplet size. It is interesting to note that even with the differences between certain strains of *L. gasseri*, all of them alter fat emulsion properties. Fig. 62.2 shows the difference in fecal fat excretion in persons consuming only 5 billion CFU of *L. gasseri* 2055 in fermented milk for a week.

Bowel Cleansing

More active xenobiotic decontamination is possible through bowel cleansing. Whole bowel irrigation, through the administration of polyethylene glycol, has been used on individuals acutely poisoned by lead,[57] iron,[58] and mercury.[59] It can also be effective for individuals who have overdosed on time-release or enteric-coated drugs.[60]

Retrograde Colonic Irrigation. Retrograde colonic irrigation (RCI) has proven useful for individuals with defecation disorders after bowel and rectal surgeries[61] and for those with fecal incontinence or constipation.[62,63,64] RCIs primarily differ from colonic irrigations available to the general public by the amount of water used. RCI treatments typically use 500 to 1000 mL of water, whereas standard colonic irrigations can use 30 to 50 L. The use

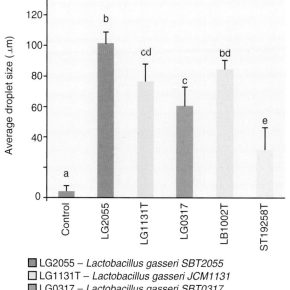

■ LG2055 – *Lactobacillus gasseri SBT2055*
☐ LG1131T – *Lactobacillus gasseri JCM1131*
■ LG0317 – *Lactobacillus gasseri SBT0317*
☐ LB1002T – *Lactobacillus delbrueckii bulgaricus JCM1002*
☐ ST19258T – *Streptococcus thermophiles ATCC19258*

FIG. 62.1 Suppressive effect of lactic acid bacteria on pancreatic lipase–mediated hydrolysis of triolein in an emulsion. (From Ogawa, A., Kobayashi, T., Sakai, F., Kadooka, Y., & Kawasaki, Y. [2015]. *Lactobacillus gasseri* SBT2055 suppresses fatty acid release through enlargement of fat emulsion size *in vitro* and promotes fecal fat excretion in healthy Japanese subjects. *Lipids in Health and Disease, 14*, 20.) Copyright © Ogawa et al.; licensee BioMed Central. 2015. Reprinted under the terms and conditions of the Creative Commons Attribution [CC-BY] license [http://creativecommons.org/licenses/by/4.0/]

of antegrade colonic irrigation (Fig. 62.3) has also recently come into use for patients who have postsurgical incontinence problems. This method introduces water through an appendicostomy, which then flushes through the rest of the colon.[65,66,67]

Colonic Irrigation. Colonic irrigations are widely derided in the medical community but have proved surprisingly beneficial for individuals with environmentally induced illnesses. A handful of articles critical of colonic irrigations have appeared in the medical literature, all of which include references to articles discussing enemas or botanical medicines rather than colonic irrigations.[68,69,70] Such oversights only work to further obscure the facts about colonic irrigations.

The documented adverse effects of colonic irrigations include an outbreak of amebiasis among clients receiving colonic irrigation from a chiropractor in Colorado who failed to follow standards for disinfection and sterile procedures.[71] There are also two published articles describing a total of four patients who experienced bowel perforation during colonic irrigations.[72,73] However, a quick review of PubMed for bowel perforation and rectal perforation revealed 28 articles reporting numerous rectal perforation cases as a result of barium enemas, 1 article on perforation from proctosigmoidoscopy, and 18 from the use of enemas (both self- and medically administered). The sole study on the safety and effectiveness of colonic irrigations covered 38 practitioners and 242 of their clients in the United Kingdom.[74] The clients, with a mean age of 44 years, completed an average of 35 colonics each (range 1–2500), with a total of 8470 procedures. The authors reported that the practitioners appeared well-trained and that many had medical backgrounds. No serious side effects were reported for any of those 8470 colonic irrigations.

Colonic irrigations have also been assessed as an option to polyethylene glycol (PEG-ES) and aqueous sodium phosphate (ASP) for colonoscopy prep.[75] In one study, 53 patients had colonic irrigations, 52 took ASP, and 55 used PEG-ES to prepare for the procedure. The physicians doing the procedure rated the bowel cleansing effectiveness of the colonic irrigations at 92%, whereas ASP was rated at 62% and PEG-ES only 49% effective. Furthermore, the patients who used colonic hydrotherapy rated it the highest for comfort, and 96% wanted to use it again, far higher than either of the other methods were rated. In this small group, no adverse side effects were noted.

Colonic irrigations have been found to increase the number of circulating lymphocytes and neutrophils, indicating an enhancement of the immune response.[76] One of the oft-repeated claims against colonic irrigation (besides toxic megacolon, infection, or bowel perforation) is that healthy bowel flora would be somehow washed out of the body. It was found that repeated colonic irrigations did not cause dysbiosis or electrolyte loss but did provide symptomatic improvement for allergies, relief of constipation, and a reduction in ovarian cysts size.[77] This last study also provided pictures of the cloudy nonfecal releases that occur during colonic irrigations that can vary in color from yellow through orange, green, gray, and black. Therapists often refer to these as

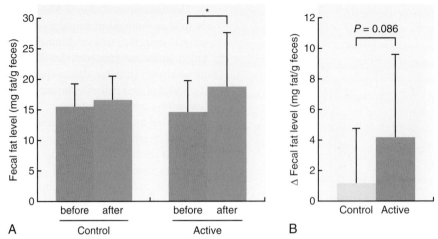

FIG. 62.2 Effects of intake of fermented milk containing *Lactobacillus gasseri SBT2055* on fecal fat excretion in humans. Statistical analysis was performed using paired Student's t-test (A) and unpaired Student's t-test (B).

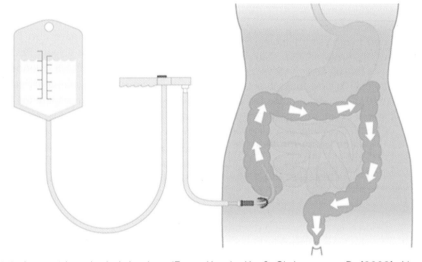

FIG. 62.3 Antegrade colonic irrigation. (From Krogh, K., & Christensen, P. [2009]. Neurogenic colorectal and pelvic floor dysfunction. *Best Practice & Research: Clinical Gastroenterology, 23*[4], 53–543.)

"bile releases," which might be accurate, because rectal distention is known to stimulate gallbladder emptying.[78] It has been observed that while clients are having these types of releases, they can experience a variety of unpleasant symptoms, including vasovagal-type responses. Samples taken of these "bile releases" in two breast cancer patients who had detectable levels of chlorinated pesticides in their blood revealed 0.5 parts per billion (PPB) of gamma-chlordane in one sample.[79]

Colon therapists also occasionally note what appears to be grains of sand moving slowly along the bottom of the exit tube. Samples taken of this material confirm that it contains numerous metals (Table 62.2).[80]

Colonic irrigations have been used as a part of depuration/decontamination programs in clinical settings.

TABLE 62.2 Mineral Analysis of Colonic Sand from Three Individuals Undergoing Colonic Irrigations

	Zn	Al	Cu	Ni	Pb	Sn	As	Cd	Sb	Ur	Th	Be
1	625	65	63	3.1	2.0	.96	.26	.20	.13	.19	.044	.015
2	22	23	6.0	.31	2.4	.15	.69	.005	.34	.005	.005	<dL
3	47	112	23	2.7	1.7	.17	.14	.35	.018	.069	.012	.007

Participants in a 1-week spa program including at least four colonic irrigations, yoga, and dietary changes were assessed for symptomatic and physiological effects.[81] At the end of the 7 days, the 15 participants had an average weight loss of 7 pounds, a reduction of diastolic blood pressure (from 73.7 to 68.00 mm Hg), reductions in serum sodium and chloride, and an increase in hemoglobin. Statistically significant improvements in depression, anxiety, tension, and vigor were also recorded.

Colonic irrigations were a major component in a 5 day per week naturopathic depuration protocol that lasted a minimum of 3 weeks. Up to three 1-hour sauna sessions preceded the colonic irrigations and were followed by constitutional hydrotherapy.[82]

A retrospective chart review and anonymous follow-up questionnaire of 112 individuals who used this protocol revealed that more than 80% of the participants reported "good" to "great" results (Table 61.5).[83] All participants had serious enough morbidity to motivate them to take a minimum of 3 weeks out of their lives for this full-time cleansing program (8 hours in-office daily, 5 days weekly). Multiple chemical sensitivity (MCS) was the most common presenting complaint (25 of 112 participants), and 84% of that subgroup reported good to great improvement. All 16 of those whose chief complaint was some form of autoimmune disease reported good or great improvement, with 75% of them reporting their improvement as "great." It should also be noted that out of a total of 1680 colonic irrigations all 112 of these individuals received during the course of their cleansing none reported any adverse events.

After this study was completed, it was concluded that persons complaining of either chemical sensitivity or autoimmunity continued to enjoy great improvement with colon therapy alone.[83]

Contraindications for colonic irrigations include renal or heart failure, severe hemorrhoids or rectal prolapse, bowel resection, previous abdominal surgery, and pregnancy.

REFERENCES

1. Fang, X., Hua, F., & Fernando, Q. (1996). Comparison of rac- and meso-2,3-dimercaptosuccinic acids for chelation of mercury and cadmium using chemical speciation models. *Chemical Research in Toxicology, 9*(1), 284–290. PubMed PMID: 8924605.
2. Jearth, V., Negi, R., Chauhan, V., & Sharma, K. (2015). A rare survival after 2,4-D (ethyl ester) poisoning: Role of forced alkaline diuresis. *Indian Journal of Critical Care Medicine: Peer-Reviewed, Official Publication of Indian Society of Critical Care Medicine, 19*(1), 57–58. PubMed PMID: 25624656.
3. Proudfoot, A. T., Krenzelok, E. P., & Vale, J. A. (2004). Position paper on urine alkalinization. *Journal of Toxicology. Clinical Toxicology, 42*(1), 1–26. Review. PubMed PMID: 15083932.
4. Roux, S., Baudoin, C., Boute, D., Brazier, M., De La Guéronniere, V., & De Vernejoul, M. C. (2004). Biological effects of drinking-water mineral composition on calcium balance and bone remodeling markers. *The Journal of Nutrition, Health and Aging, 8*(5), 380–384. PubMed PMID: 15359356.
5. Nowak, A., Śliżewska, K., Błasiak, J., & Libudzisz, Z. (2014). The influence of Lactobacillus casei DN 114 001 on the activity of faecal enzymes and genotoxicity of faecal water in the presence of heterocyclic aromatic amines. *Anaerobe, 30*, 129–136. PubMed PMID: 25280921.
6. Liu, Z., Lin, X., Huang, G., Zhang, W., Rao, P., & Ni, L. (2014). Prebiotic effects of almonds and almond skins on intestinal microbiota in healthy adult humans. *Anaerobe, 26*, 1–6. PubMed PMID: 24315808.
7. Molan, A. L., Liu, Z., & Plimmer, G. (2014). Evaluation of the effect of blackcurrant products on gut microbiota and on markers of risk for colon cancer in humans. *Phytotherapy Research: PTR, 28*(3), 416–422. PubMed PMID: 23674271.
8. Shim, S. B., Kim, N. J., & Kim, D. H. (2000). Beta-glucuronidase inhibitory activity and hepatoprotective effect of 18 beta-glycyrrhetinic acid from the rhizomes of Glycyrrhiza uralensis. *Planta Medica, 66*(1), 40–43. PubMed PMID: 10705732.

9. Kim, D. H., Jin, Y. H., Park, J. B., & Kobashi, K. (1994). Silymarin and its components are inhibitors of beta-glucuronidase. *Biological and Pharmaceutical Bulletin, 17*(3), 443–445. PubMed PMID: 8019514.

10. Walaszek, Z., Hanausek, M., Narog, M., Raich, P. C., & Slaga, T. J. (2004). Mechanisms of lung cancer chemoprevention by D-glucarate. *Chest, 125*(5 Suppl.), 149S–150S. PubMed PMID: 15136472.

11. (2002). Calcium-D-glucarate. *Alternative Medicine Review: A Journal of Clinical Therapeutic, 7*(4), 336–339. PubMed PMID: 12197785.

12. Nosova, T., Jousimies-Somer, H., Jokelainen, K., Heine, R., & Salaspuro, M. (2000). Acetaldehyde production and metabolism by human indigenous and probiotic Lactobacillus and Bifidobacterium strains. *Alcohol and Alcoholism (Oxford, Oxfordshire), 35*(6), 561–568. PubMed PMID: 11093962.

13. Gratz, S., Mykkänen, H., & El-Nezami, H. (2005). Aflatoxin B1 binding by a mixture of Lactobacillus and Propionibacterium: In vitro versus ex vivo. *Journal of Food Protection, 68*(11), 2470–2474. PubMed PMID: 16300092.

14. Gratz, S., Täubel, M., Juvonen, R. O., Viluksela, M., Turner, P. C., Mykkänen, H., et al. (2006). Lactobacillus rhamnosus strain GG modulates intestinal absorption, fecal excretion, and toxicity of aflatoxin B(1) in rats. *Applied and Environmental Microbiology, 72*(11), 7398–7400. PubMed PMID: 16980432.

15. El-Nezami, H. S., Polychronaki, N. N., Ma, J., Zhu, H., Ling, W., Salminen, E. K., et al. (2006). Probiotic supplementation reduces a biomarker for increased risk of liver cancer in young men from Southern China. *The American Journal of Clinical Nutrition, 83*(5), 1199–1203. PubMed PMID: 16685066.

16. Gibson, P. R., Elms, A. N., & Ruding, L. A. (2003). Perceived treatment efficacy for conventional and alternative therapies reported by persons with multiple chemical sensitivity. *Environmental Health Perspectives, 111*(12), 1498–1504. PubMed PMID: 12948890.

17. Genuis, S. J., Birkholz, D., Ralitsch, M., & Thibault, N. (2010). Human detoxification of perfluorinated compounds. *Public Health, 124*(7), 367–375. PubMed PMID: 20621793.

18. Hope, J. (2013). A review of the mechanism of injury and treatment approaches for illness resulting from exposure to water-damaged buildings, mold, and mycotoxins. *TheScientificWorldJournal, 2013*, 767482. PubMed PMID: 23710148.

19. Hudnell, H. K. (2005). Chronic biotoxin-associated illness: Multiple-system symptoms, a vision deficit, and effective treatment. *Neurotoxicology and Teratology, 27*(5), 733–743. Review. PubMed PMID: 16102938.

20. Kassner, J. T., Maher, T. J., Hull, K. M., & Woolf, A. D. (1993). Cholestyramine as an adsorbent in acute lindane poisoning: A murine model. *Annals of Emergency Medicine, 22*(9), 1392–1397. PubMed PMID: 7689801.

21. Mochida, Y., Fukata, H., Matsuno, Y., & Mori, C. (2007). Reduction of dioxins and polychlorinated biphenyls (PCBs) in human body. *Fukuoka Igaku Zasshi, 98*(4), 106–113. Review. PubMed PMID: 17533984.

22. (1999). Position statement and practice guidelines on the use of multi-dose activated charcoal in the treatment of acute poisoning. American Academy of Clinical Toxicology; European Association of Poisons Centres and Clinical Toxicologists. *Journal of Toxicology. Clinical Toxicology, 37*(6), 731–751. Review. PubMed PMID: 10584586.

23. Tuncok, Y., Gelal, A., Apaydin, S., Guven, H., Fowler, J., & Gure, A. (1995). Prevention of oral dichlorvos toxicity by different activated charcoal products in mice. *Annals of Emergency Medicine, 25*(3), 353–355. PubMed PMID: 7864476.

24. McKinney, P. E. (1999). Elemental mercury in the appendix: An unusual complication of a Mexican-American folk remedy. *Journal of Toxicology. Clinical Toxicology, 37*(1), 103–107. PubMed PMID: 10078167.

25. Ly, B. T., Williams, S. R., & Clark, R. F. (2002). Mercuric oxide poisoning treated with whole-bowel irrigation and chelation therapy. *Annals of Emergency Medicine, 39*(3), 312–315. PubMed PMID: 11867987.

26. Rusyniak, D. E., Furbee, R. B., & Kirk, M. A. (2002). Thallium and arsenic poisoning in a small midwestern town. *Annals of Emergency Medicine, 39*(3), 307–311. PubMed PMID: 11867986.

27. Sera, N., Morita, K., Nagasoe, M., Tokieda, H., Kitaura, T., & Tokiwa, H. (2005). Binding effect of polychlorinated compounds and environmental carcinogens on rice bran fiber. *The Journal of Nutritional Biochemistry, 16*, 50–58. PubMed PMID: 15629241.

28. Kimura, Y., Nagat, Y., & Buddington, R. (2004). Some dietary fibers increase elimination of orally administered polychlorinated biphenyls but not that of retinol in mice. *The Journal of Nutrition, 134*, 135–142. PubMed PMID: 14704306.

29. De Vos, S., & De Schrijver, R. (2005). Polychlorinatedbiphenyl distribution and faecal excretion in rats fed wheat bran. *Chemosphere, 61*, 374–382. PubMed PMID: 16182854.

30. Morita, K., Hamamura, K., & Iida, T. (1995). Binding of PCB by several types of dietary fiber in vivo and in vitro. *Fukuoka Igaku Zasshi, 86*, 212–217. PubMed PMID: 7628811.

31. Morita, K., Hirakawa, H., Matsueda, T., Iida, T., & Tokiwa, H. (1993). Stimulating effect of dietary fiber on fecal excretion of polychlorinated dibenzofuans (PCDF) and polychlorinated dibenzo-p-dioxins (PCDD) in rats. *Fukuoka Igaku Zasshi, 84*, 273–281. PubMed PMID: 8392484.

32. Nagayama, J., Takasuga, T., Tsuji, H., et al. (2003). Active elimination of causative PCDFs/DDs congeners of Yusho by one year intake of FEBRA in Japanese people. *Fukuoka Igaku Zasshi, 94*, 118–125.

33. Takenaka, S., Morita, K., Tokiwa, H., & Takahashi, K. (1991). Effects of rice bran fibre and cholestyramine on the faecal excretion of Kanechlor 600 (PCB) in rats. *Xenobiotica, 21*(3), 351–357. PubMed PMID: 1907420.

34. Iida, T., Nakagawa, R., Hirakawa, H., Matsueda, T., Morita, K., Hamamura, K., et al. (1995). Clinical trial of a combination of rice bran fiber and cholestyramine for promotion of fecal excretion of retained polychlorinated dibenzofuran and polychlorinated biphenyl in Yu-Cheng patients. *Fukuoka Igaku Zasshi, 86*(5), 226–233. PubMed PMID: 7628813.

35. Morita, K., & Tobiishi, K. (2002). Increasing effect of nori on the fecal excretion of dioxin by rats. *Bioscience, Biotechnology, and Biochemistry, 66*, 2306–2313. PubMed PMID: 12506965.

36. Morita, K., Matsueda, T., Iida, T., & Hasegawa, T. (1999). Chlorella accelerates dioxin excretion in rats. *The Journal of Nutrition, 129*, 1731–1736. PubMed PMID: 10460212.

37. Morita, K., Ogata, M., & Hasegawa, T. (2001). Chlorophyll derived from chlorella inhibits dioxin absorption from the gastrointestinal tract and accelerates dioxin excretion in rats. *Environmental Health Perspectives, 109*, 289–294. PubMed PMID: 11333191.

38. Nakano, S., Noguchi, T., Takekoshi, H., Suzuki, G., & Nakano, M. (2005). Maternal-fetal distribution and transfer of dioxins in pregnant women in Japan, and attempts to reduce maternal transfer with Chlorella (Chlorella pyrenoidosa) supplements. *Chemosphere, 61*(9), 1244–1255. PubMed PMID: 15985279.

39. Morita, K., Matsueda, T., & Iida, T. (1999). Effect of green vegetables on digestive tract absorption of polychlorinated dibenzo-p-dioxins and polychlorinated dibenzofurans in rats. *Fukuoka Igaku Zasshi = Hukuoka Acta Medica, 90*, 171–183. PubMed PMID: 10396873.

40. Moser, G. A., & McLachlan, M. S. (1999). A non-absorbable dietary fat substitute enhances elimination of persistent lipophylic contaminants in humans. *Chemosphere, 39*, 1513–1521. PubMed PMID: 10481251.

41. Geusau, A., Schmaldienst, S., Derfler, K., Papke, O., & Abraham, K. (2002). Severe 2,3,7,8-tetrac hlorodibenzo-p-dioxins (TCDD) intoxication: Kinetics and trials to enhance elimination in two patients. *Archives of Toxicology, 76*, 316–325. PubMed PMID: 12107649.

42. Redgrave, T. G., Wallace, P., Jandacek, R. J., & Tso, P. (2005). Treatment with a dietary fat substitute decreased Arochlor 1254 contamination in an obese diabetic male. *The Journal of Nutritional Biochemistry, 16*(6), 383–384. PubMed PMID: 15936651.

43. Jandacek, R. J. (2016). Intervention to reduce PCBs: Learnings from a controlled study of Anniston residents. *Environmental Science and Pollution Research International, 23*(3), 2022–2026. PubMed PMID: 25721531.

44. Ahnen, D. J., Guerciolini, R., Hauptman, J., Blotner, S., Woods, C. J., & Wargovich, M. J. (2007). Effect of orlistat on fecal fat, fecal biliary acids, and colonic cell proliferation in obese subjects. *Clinical Gastroenterology and Hepatology, 5*(11), 1291–1299. PubMed PMID: 17920338.

45. Kwon, C. S., Sohn, H. Y., Kim, S. H., Kim, J. H., Son, K. H., Lee, J. S., et al. (2003). Anti-obesity effect of Dioscorea nipponica Makino with lipase-inhibitory activity in rodents. *Bioscience, Biotechnology, and Biochemistry, 67*(7), 1451–1456. PubMed PMID: 12913286.

46. Han, L. K., Zheng, Y. N., Yoshikawa, M., Okuda, H., & Kimura, Y. (2005). Anti-obesity effects of chikusetsusaponins isolated from Panax japonicus rhizomes. *BMC Complementary and Alternative Medicine, 5*, 9. PubMed PMID: 15811191.

47. Han, L. K., Kimura, Y., Kawashima, M., et al. (2001). Teasaponins and fat absorption. *International Journal of Obesity and Related Metabolic Disorders: Journal of the International Association for the Study of Obesity, 25*, 1459–1464. PubMed PMID: 11729639.

48. Nakai, M., Fukui, Y., Asami, S., Toyoda-Ono, Y., Iwashita, T., Shibata, H., et al. (2005). Inhibitory effects of oolong tea polyphenols on pancreatic lipase in vitro. *Journal of Agricultural and Food Chemistry, 53*(11), 4593–4598. PubMed PMID: 15913331.

49. Shishikura, Y., Khokhar, S., & Murray, B. S. (2006). Effects of tea polyphenols on emulsification of olive oil in a small intestine model system. *Journal of Agricultural and Food Chemistry, 54*(5), 1906–1913. PubMed PMID: 16506852.

50. Glisan, S. L., Grove, K. A., Yennawar, N. H., & Lambert, J. D. (2017). Inhibition of pancreatic lipase by black tea theaflavins: Comparative enzymology and in silico modeling studies. *Food Chemistry, 216*, 296–300. PubMed PMID: 27596423.

51. Gilardini, L., Pasqualinotto, L., Di Pierro, F., Risso, P., & Invitti, C. (2016). Effects of Greenselect Phytosome® on weight maintenance after weight loss in obese women: A randomized placebo-controlled study. *BMC Complementary and Alternative Medicine*, 16, 233. PubMed PMID: 27450231.

52. Ashigai, H., Taniguchi, Y., Suzuki, M., Ikeshima, E., Kanaya, T., Zembutsu, K., et al. (2016). Fecal lipid excretion after consumption of a black tea polyphenol containing beverage-randomized, placebo-controlled, double-blind, crossover study. *Biological and Pharmaceutical Bulletin*, 39(5), 699–704. PubMed PMID: 26887502.

53. Hsu, T. F., Kusumoto, A., Abe, K., Hosoda, K., Kiso, Y., Wang, M. F., et al. (2006). Polyphenol-enriched oolong tea increases fecal lipid excretion. *European Journal of Clinical Nutrition*, 60(11), 1330–1336. PubMed PMID: 16804556.

54. Morita, K., Matsueda, T., & Iida, T. (1997). Effect of green tea (matcha) on gastrointestinal tract absorption of polychlorinated biphenyls, polychlorinated dibenzofuans and polychlorinated dibenzo-p-dioxins in rats. *Fukuoka Igaku Zasshi*, 88, 162–168. PubMed PMID: 9194336.

55. Ogawa, A., Kobayashi, T., Sakai, F., Kadooka, Y., & Kawasaki, Y. (2015). Lactobacillus gasseri SBT2055 suppresses fatty acid release through enlargement of fat emulsion size in vitro and promotes fecal fat excretion in healthy Japanese subjects. *Lipids in Health and Disease*, 14, 20. PubMed PMID: 25884980.

56. Kadooka, Y., Sato, M., Ogawa, A., Miyoshi, M., Uenishi, H., Ogawa, H., et al. (2013). Effect of Lactobacillus gasseri SBT2055 in fermented milk on abdominal adiposity in adults in a randomised controlled trial. *The British Journal of Nutrition*, 110(9), 1696–1703. PubMed PMID: 23614897.

57. Roberge, R. J., & Martin, T. G. (1992). Whole bowel irrigation in an acute oral lead intoxication. *The American Journal of Emergency Medicine*, 10(6), 577–583. Review. PubMed PMID: 1388389.

58. Everson, G. W., Bertaccini, E. J., & O'Leary, J. (1991). Use of whole bowel irrigation in an infant following iron overdose. *The American Journal of Emergency Medicine*, 9(4), 366–369. PubMed PMID: 1675852.

59. Ly, B. T., Williams, S. R., & Clark, R. F. (2002). Mercuric oxide poisoning treated with whole-bowel irrigation and chelation therapy. *Annals of Emergency Medicine*, 39(3), 312–315. PubMed PMID: 11867987.

60. Thanacoody, R., Caravati, E. M., Troutman, B., Höjer, J., Benson, B., Hoppu, K., et al. (2015). Position paper update: Whole bowel irrigation for gastrointestinal decontamination of overdose patients. *Clinical Toxicology (Philadelphia, Pa.)*, 53(1), 5–12. PubMed PMID: 25511637.

61. Koch, S. M., Uludağ, O., El Naggar, K., van Gemert, W. G., & Baeten, C. G. (2008). Colonic irrigation for defecation disorders after dynamic graciloplasty. *International Journal of Colorectal Disease*, 23(2), 195–200. [Epub 2007 Sep 21]; PubMed PMID: 17896111.

62. Gosselink, M. P., Darby, M., Zimmerman, D. D., Smits, A. A., van Kessel, I., Hop, W. C., et al. (2005). Long-term follow-up of retrograde colonic irrigation for defaecation disturbances. *Colorectal Disease: The Official Journal of the Association of Coloproctology of Great Britain and Ireland*, 7(1), 65–69. PubMed PMID: 15606588.

63. Briel, J. W., Schouten, W. R., Vlot, E. A., Smits, S., & van Kessel, I. (1997). Clinical value of colonic irrigation in patients with continence disturbances. *Diseases of the Colon and Rectum*, 40(7), 802–805. PubMed PMID: 9221856.

64. Cazemier, M., Felt-Bersma, R. J., & Mulder, C. J. (2007). Anal plugs and retrograde colonic irrigation are helpful in fecal incontinence or constipation. *World Journal of Gastroenterology*, 13(22), 3101–3105. PubMed PMID: 17589927.

65. Worsøe, J., Christensen, P., Krogh, K., Buntzen, S., & Laurberg, S. (2008). Long-term results of antegrade colonic enema in adult patients: Assessment of functional results. *Diseases of the Colon and Rectum*, 51(10), 1523–1528. doi:10.1007/s10350-008-9401-6. [Epub 2008 Jul 12]; PubMed PMID: 18622642.

66. Patton, V., & Lubowski, D. Z. (2015). Clinical outcome and efficacy of antegrade colonic enemas administered via an indwelling cecostomy catheter in adults with defecatory disorders. *Diseases of the Colon and Rectum*, 58(4), 457–462. PubMed PMID: 25751803.

67. Haugen, V., Rothenberger, D. A., & Powell, J. (2008). Antegrade irrigations of a surgically reconstructed Hartmann's pouch to treat intractable diversion colitis. *Journal of Wound, Ostomy, and Continence Nursing*, 35(2), 231–232. PubMed PMID: 18344801.

68. Acosta, R. D., & Cash, B. D. (2009). Clinical effects of colonic cleansing for general health promotion: A systematic review. *The American Journal of Gastroenterology*, 104(11), 2830–2836. PubMed PMID: 19724266.

69. Seow-Choen, F. (2009). The physiology of colonic hydrotherapy. *Colorectal Disease: The Official Journal of the Association of Coloproctology of Great Britain and Ireland*, 11(7), 686–688. PubMed PMID: 19508546.

70. Mishori, R., Otubu, A., & Jones, A. A. (2011). The dangers of colon cleansing. *The Journal of Family Practice*, 60(8), 454–457. PubMed PMID: 21814639.

71. Centers for Disease Control (CDC). (1981). Amebiasis associated with colonic irrigation – Colorado. *MMWR. Morbidity and Mortality Weekly Report*, 30(9), 101–102. PubMed PMID: 6789134.

72. Tan, M. P., & Cheong, D. M. (1999). Life-threatening perineal gangrene from rectal perforation following colonic hydrotherapy: A case report. *Annals of the Academy of Medicine, Singapore*, 28(4), 583–585. PubMed PMID: 10561777.

73. Handley, D. V., Rieger, N. A., & Rodda, D. J. (2004). Rectal perforation from colonic irrigation administered by alternative practitioners. *The Medical Journal of Australia*, 181(10), 575–576. PubMed PMID: 15540974.

74. Taffinder, N. J., Tan, E., Webb, I. G., & McDonald, P. J. (2004). Retrograde commercial colonic hydrotherapy. *Colorectal Disease: The Official Journal of the Association of Coloproctology of Great Britain and Ireland*, 6(4), 258–260. PubMed PMID: 15206969.

75. Fiorito, J., Culpepper-Morgan, J., Estabrook, S., Scofield, P., Usatii, V., & Cuomo, J. *Hydrotherapy compared with PEG-ES and aqueous sodium phosphate as bowel preparation for elective colonoscopy: A prospective randomized single-blinded trial*. Presented at the 2006 American College of Gastroenterology annual scientific meeting.

76. Uchiyama-Tanaka, Y. (2009). Colon irrigation causes lymphocyte movement from gut-associated lymphatic tissues to peripheral blood. *Biomedical Research (Tokyo, Japan)*, 30(5), 311–314. PubMed PMID: 19887728.

77. Uchiyama-Tanaka, Y. *The influence of colonic irrigation on human intestinal microbiota*. New Advances in the Basic and Clinical Gastroenterology. Thomas Brzozowski ed. https://www.intechopen.com/books/new-advances-in-the-basic-and-clinical-gastroenterology. (Accessed 22 April 2017).

78. van Hoek, F., Mollen, R. M., Hopman, W. P., Kuijpers, H. H., & Jansen, J. B. (2000). Effect of rectal distension on gallbladder emptying and circulating gut hormones. *European Journal of Clinical Investigation*, 30(11), 988–994. PubMed PMID: 11114961.

79. Crinnion, W. J. Unpublished research.

80. Crinnion, W. J. Unpublished research.

81. Wintering, N. A., Wilson, J. C., & Newberg, A. B. (2012). A pilot study to evaluate the physiological effects of a spa retreat that uses caloric restriction and colonic hydrotherapy. *Integrative Medicine*, 11(6), 26–32.

82. Boyle, W., & Seine, A. (1988). *Lecturers in naturopathic hydrotherapy*. Sandy, OR: Eclectic Medical Publishing.

83. Crinnion, W. J. (1997). Results of a decade of naturopathic treatment for environmental illnesses. *Journal of Naturopathic Medicne*, 17(2), 21–27.

63

Microbiome

SUMMARY

- Benefits: Antiinflammatory (including antineuroinflammation), antiallergy, antiobesity, antidiabetes, anticancer, improved xenobiotic biotransformation and excretion, reduction of xenobiotic toxicity
- Primary mechanisms: Balancing of Th cytokine levels, reduction of nuclear factor kappa B (NFκB)
and proinflammatory cytokines, improved cytochrome levels and function, improved glutathione production, enhanced methylation, butyric acid production
- Best sources: Whole foods diet, blueberry skins, probiotics, and prebiotic supplementation

OVERVIEW

There are more than 1000 different species of bacteria in the human intestines, with 100,000,000,000 (100 billion) bacterial organisms in just 1 g of stool. These bacteria include primarily the following:

- Firmicutes phyla (primarily gram-positive microbes, including *Enterococcus, Bacillus, Lactobacillus* [with 120 species], and *Clostridium* spp.)
- Bacteroidetes phyla (primarily gram-negative microbes), the dominant microbe in the elderly (67%)
- Actinobacteria phyla (gram-positive), including 29 different species of bifidobacteria

HEALTH PROPERTIES OF PROBIOTICS[1]

- Prevention and reduction of endotoxicity
- Utilization of fiber for growth
- Synthesis of B_{12}
- Manufacture of organic short-chain fatty acids (SCFAs) of acetate, propionate, and butyrate from dietary fiber,[2] which has the following benefits:
  - Reduced cancer risk (butyrate)
  - Reduced cholesterol levels (propionate)

- Improved cellular integrity of all enterocytes (butyrate)
- Improved mucosal barrier and tight junctions (butyrate)
- Reduced intestinal and systemic inflammation (butyrate)
- Improved antipathogen environment
- Enhanced anticandida and immune enhancement[3] (butyrate)
  - Inhibition of candida biofilm formation
- Improved calcium and magnesium absorption (related to lowered pH)[4-6]
- Reduction of beta-glucuronidase
- Inhibition or exclusion of intestinal pathogens
- Synthesis of B-galactosidase
- Deconjugation of bile acids
- Production of antimicrobial substances
- Balanced Th1/Th2 cytokine levels
  - Reduced allergic reactivity
  - Reduced autoimmunity
  - Improved cell-mediated immunity (CMI)
- Promotion and maintenance of mucosal barrier integrity
- Improved lactose tolerance

- Improved glucose balance and risk of metabolic syndrome
  - Weight balance (antiobesity)
  - Antidiabetes
- Improved mood and mental function
  - Reduction of neuroinflammation

ENDOTOXEMIA

Endotoxins are lipopolysaccharides (LPSs) from the cell walls of gram-negative bacteria (bacteroidetes) that can pass through the intestine into the portal circulation and cause inflammation, neuroinflammation, obesity, insulin resistance, metabolic syndrome, diabetes mellitus, acute pancreatitis, and steatohepatitis, along with renal and cardiovascular diseases (Box 63.1).[7] High-fat diets in both animal and human models alter the microflora (reduction of *Bifidobacterium* spp., *Eubacterium rectale* [a clostridium], and *Bacteroides*) and predispose to endotoxemia, obesity, and type 2 diabetes mellitus (T2DM). In situations of fatty liver disease, the increased fat content provides a high number of chylomicron carriers that readily transport the LPS into the general circulation and across the blood-brain barrier, causing inflammation throughout the body.[8] Bifidobacterium counts in the intestines and LPS levels in the portal circulation are inversely correlated. High-fat diets also increase the activation of mast cells and the release of tumor necrosis factor alpha (TNF-α, all of which increase gut permeability and LPS movement into the bloodstream.[9]

LPS adversely affects the biotransformation (phases 1 and 2) of xenobiotic compounds in the liver. LPSs suppress CYP450 messenger RNA and reduce levels of both nicotinamide adenine dinucleotide phosphate (NADPH)-cytochrome c-reductase and cytochrome b5, two of the three critical components needed for production of all cytochromes.[10] LPSs reduce sex-specific cytochromes by 17% (female) and 35% (male) of normal function. LPS exposure results in a general reduction of all cytochrome levels and has been specifically linked to reduced activity of the 1A, 2B, 2E, 3A, and 4A families.[11,12] LPS inhibition of CYP3A2 can be prevented by the supplementation of either curcumin or melatonin.[13,14] High circulating levels of maternal LPS have also been linked to reduced hepatic CYP3A4 levels in fetal livers.[15] LPS downregulates glutamyl-cysteine ligase, one of the two critical enzymes for glutathione synthesis, resulting in lower levels of available glutathione. LPS also reduces the effectiveness of phase 2 glutathione transferase activity, preventing the rapid clearance of xenobiotics from the circulation. In addition, LPS reduces the production of S-adenosylmethionine necessary for proper methylation.[16]

FACTORS THAT ALTER THE MICROBIOME

Dietary choices affect the microbiome more than any other factor. Diets that provide high levels of the plant fibers that are the preferred fuel of healthy bacteria will shift the microbiome dramatically.[17]

> **NOTE** Standard American Diet = Standard American Microbiome

Adding or changing plant fibers in the diet, even by using supplemental fiber, will alter the gut flora populations with health-promoting increases in *Lactobacillus* and *Bifidobacterium* spp.[18] The microbiome is also influenced by which vegetable family is being consumed, like the Brassica family: broccoli, cabbage, cauliflower, that have a high sulfur content, thus predisposing to sulfur-loving bacteria.[19] Ancient human microbiome signatures, like those seen in Otzi the 5200-year-old iceman found in the Italian Alps, are quite similar to those seen in individuals consuming a plant-based diet today.[20]

Although the dietary fibers influence the growth of certain bacteria, so does the total amount of dietary fat. Bile acids are released into the gut in proportion to the amount of fat in consumed food. The high amount of bile acids present in the intestines of those who consume

> ### BOX 63.1 Diseases Associated With Microbiome Imbalance
>
> - Obesity
> - Diabetes types 1 and 2
> - Irritable bowel syndrome (IBS)
> - Inflammatory bowel disease (IBD)
> - Neuroinflammation
> - Colon cancer
> - Abnormal immune response
>
> Data from Xu, X., Xu, P., Ma, C., Tang, J., & Zhang, X. (2013). Gut microbiota, host health, and polysaccharides. *Biotechnology Advances, 31*(2), 318–337.

a high-fat diet shifts the microbiome toward greater numbers of bile acid–resistant organisms (*Alistipes, Bilophila,* and *Bacteroides*) while destroying those bacteria that are not resistant.[21] When mice were switched from a low-fat, polysaccharide-rich (high plant content) diet to a high-fat, high-sugar (Standard American Diet—SAD), their microbiome began to change within a day.[22] The different microbiome pictures seen in these animals fed two different diets were also found in children raised with either plant-based or traditional Western diets.[23] A high-fat diet promotes a proobesity microbiome characterized by higher levels of *Firmicutes* and lower levels of *Bifidobacterium* and *Bacteroidetes* after only 4 weeks.[24] However, after gastric bypass surgery, the microbiome reverts back to higher *Bifidobacteria* levels, just as one would see by increasing prebiotic levels or by going on a diet.[25] In a primate model, it was found that a high-fat maternal diet resulted in the same gut dysbiosis in the offspring and that the dysbiosis was not entirely fixed by the offspring going on a low-fat diet.[26] Lower numbers of butyrate-producing bacteria, are also commonly found in persons with diabetes, whereas nondiabetics have higher levels of butyrate production.[27]

Xenobiotics. Antibiotic use rapidly changes the microbiome,[28] with alterations of the microbial balance persisting for weeks after antibiotic use.[29] Corticosteroids also rapidly change the microbiome.[30] The ingestion of toxic chemicals and metals can also cause an imbalance of the microbiome. Animals exposed to a small amount of the organophosphate pesticide chlorpyrifos for 30 days were found to have increased levels of *Bacteroides,* lower levels of *Bifidobacterium,* and very low levels of *Lactobacillus.*[31] Diazinon, a commonly used organophosphate insecticide present in commercially grown produce, causes similar results.[32] Mice fed drinking water with 10 parts per million (PPM) of arsenic (the current US standard exceeded in many areas of the United States and the world) for 4 weeks displayed a dramatic shift in the microbiome, predisposing the mice to diabetes, obesity, and other health problems.[33] Low-level cadmium exposure results in a microbiome shift favoring inflammation and endotoxemia.[34] Bisphenol A, found in soup and other canned products, caused microbiome shifts in animals similar to those seen in animals with both high-fat and high-sugar diets.[35] Persistent organic pollutants, often found in farmed salmon, also shift the microbiome.[36]

SPECIFIC BENEFITS

Gastrointestinal Health

Two of the most abundant and researched families of bowel organisms are *Lactobacillus* and *Bifidobacterium.* Both of these families are anaerobic (although they are oxygen tolerant), gram-positive bacteria that play major roles in intestinal immunity. Pathogenic bacteria can only cause problems within the gastrointestinal (GI) tract by first adhering to the mucosal barrier, where they then cause inflammation. To prevent this binding action, the intestine has a constant peristaltic action, secretes copious amounts of mucus to prevent adhesion, and produces secretory immunoglobulin A (SIgA) to provide an immune response to pathogen presence. *Lactobacillus* and *Bifidobacteria* assist these mechanisms by producing other chemical compounds that further prevent adhesion and the growth of pathogenic bacteria in the intestinal tract.[37,38]

SIgA holds the primary role in intestinal immunity, prevents intestinal permeability, and is a central player in preventing adverse food reactions. Its levels are reduced with chronic emotional or physical stressors, trauma, burns, and intestinal inflammatory conditions.[39-41] Multiple studies have shown that supplementation with *Lactobacillus* and *Bifidobacterium* spp. increase intestinal SIgA levels in both animals[42,43] and humans.[44,45] The product VSL3 (containing a combination of *Lactobacillus* and *Bifidobacterium; Lactobacillus acidophilus, casei* and *bulgaricus;* and *Bifidobacterium lactis Bb12* and *longum*) has been shown to increase SIgA levels. *Saccharomyces boulardii* supplementation increases both SIgA and interleukin-10 (IL-10).[46] The presence of IL-10 stimulates a T-helper cell 1 (Th1) response that is antiallergy, antiautoimmunity, and procellular immunity, rather than a proallergy Th2 response.

Immune Function

The probiotics previously mentioned have also been shown to improve general immune function,[47,48] reduce episodes of upper respiratory tract infections (colds), and decrease the need for antibiotics.[49]

In genetically altered mice with no commensal intestinal flora, the general immune system remains undeveloped and incapable of proper immune response.[50] The overriding imbalance in such animals is a reduction of Th1-stimulating chemical messengers (cytokines) and an enhanced level of Th2-promoting cytokines. This Th1/

Th2 imbalance is manifested by the presence of allergies, asthma, chronic infections, and autoimmunity, as discussed in Chapter 43. A small group of healthy adults took 500 million colony forming units (CFU) of each of the following daily for 8 weeks: *L. rhamnosus, L. plantarum, L. salivarius, B. bifidum,* for a total of 2 billion CFU daily.[51] At the end of 8 weeks, those who took the probiotics showed significant increases in their levels of circulating phagocytic monocytes and neutrophils, indicating greater cellular immune function.

Allergy

IgE-mediated food reactions, known as "food allergies," are becoming more common and are directly linked to a Th1/Th2 imbalance. Although healthy subjects do not exhibit atopy, allergic reactions are commonly found in mice without proper bowel bacteria. Once these mice have been inoculated with either *Eschericia coli* or *Bifidobacterium,* their oral tolerance to foods is restored.[52] Supplementing neonatal mice with either *Lactobacillus rhamnosus GG* or *Bifidobacterium lactis Bb-12* from birth to 8 weeks of age provided complete suppression of egg-induced allergic sensitization of their airways.[53] The animals given the probiotics exhibited a rebalancing of their immune system, correcting the Th2 dominance. The potential for the same rebalancing and reversal of food allergies in children has been proposed as well.[54]

Babies who developed allergies by 2 years of age had insufficient enterococci at 1 month of age and low bifidobacteria at their first birthday.[55] Children with allergies typically have higher levels of clostridia and lower levels of bifidobacteria; nonallergic children have higher levels of both lactobacilli and bifidobacteria.[56] Probiotic therapy has been used to reduce the overall allergic reactivity in children, which is accomplished by increasing Th1 activity and reducing Th2 function.[57]

Infants who developed eczema from drinking cow's milk were given whey protein, which could easily trigger their reaction, along with *Lactobacillus rhamnosus GG* for a month. Amazingly, they had a reduction in both their eczema and their intestinal inflammation, yet the control group did not.[58] In a multigenerational human study, expectant mothers were given 4.8 billion CFU of probiotics (a combination of 1.6 billion CFU of *Bifidobacterium bifidum BGN4,* 1.6 billion CFU of *Bifidobacterium lactis AD011,* and 1.6 billion CFU of *Lactobacillus acidophilus AD031*) once daily from 8 weeks before to 6 months after delivery.[59] The children were exclusively breastfed during their first 3 months and were monitored until they were a year old. The children whose mothers took the probiotics had 50% fewer cases of eczema than the children whose mothers did not take the probiotics.

Individuals with Japanese cedar pollinosis who participated in a double-blind study were given fermented milk with either placebo yogurt or a combination of *Lactobacillus GG/Lactobacillus gasseri.* After 9 weeks, those taking the probiotic mixture exhibited a significant reduction in allergic symptoms.[60] Those consuming the probiotic-containing fermented milk for 10 weeks were also rewarded with a microbiome shift (increased bacteroides and reduced firmicutes).[61] A 13-week double-blind trial with *Bifidobacterium longum (BB536)* on another group of Japanese adults with cedar pollinosis revealed that BB536 relieved allergic symptoms and suppressed elevation of cedar-specific IgE.[62] A second study with BB536 on Japanese adults with cedar pollinosis confirmed the benefit of this probiotic to reduce allergic symptoms and allergy medication use.[63] The daily use of *Lactobacillus plantarum* in fermented citrus juice for 8 weeks in another group of cedar allergy suffers gave very similar results, showing that at least three different probiotics can be beneficial for reducing pollen allergies.[64]

Inflammation

Saccharomyces boulardii has been shown to be beneficial in reducing inflammation in Crohn's disease (CD), ulcerative colitis (UC), and irritable bowel syndrome (IBS). It is also helpful in the eradication of *Helicobacter pylori*[65] and several other gut pathogens (*Clostridium difficile, E. coli,* and cholera) by producing enzymes that cleave the pathogen or disable their toxins. *Saccharomyces boulardii* also prevents the ability of pathogens to adhere to the mucosa and colonize; it modulates local and systemic immune responses, stabilizes the mucosal barrier, and aids in the absorption of nutrients.

Butyrates are the major health-promoting SCFA produced from the fermentation of vegetable fibers by intestinal bacteria. Proper levels of butyric acids in the intestines prevent the development of cancer cells and speed the death of any cancer cells that may be present in the colon.[66] The production of butyrates from indigestible food fibers appear to be the reason high-fiber diets have been linked to lower rates of colon cancer, but only with the fibers that result in butyrate production. Butyrates are the main energy source for the colonocytes[67] and act to dramatically reduce and prevent inflammation and oxidative stress and help maintain healthy tissue, including prevention of "leaky gut."[68] To have good levels of butyrates in the bowel, one must have enough of the whole food fibers necessary to promote and sustain a healthy population of butyrate-forming bacteria. Individuals with inflammatory bowel disease have fewer bifidobacteria and lower levels of butyric acids.[69] Individuals with UC typically have lower levels of lactobacilli and bifidobacteria with increased numbers of *Clostridium* species (Enterobacteriaceae).[70,71]

Repletion with bifidobacteria has demonstrated a powerful antiinflammatory effect at least partly related to their inhibition of NFκB stimulated by LPSs.[72] *B. bifidum* NCC189, S16, and S17, and *B. lactis* NCC362 had the greatest effect on suppressing or reducing the LPS-induced production of NFκB, thereby preventing mucosal inflammation. However, they did nothing to prevent NFκB stimulation from TNF-α. When different bifidobacteria were given to mice with bowel inflammation, *B. bifidum S17* exhibited the greatest antiinflammatory activity against LPS-induced inflammation. Of the bifidobacteria tested, this was also the one with the greatest ability to adhere to the mucosal membrane and implant itself in the colon.[73] Bifidobacteria also decreased the level of beta-glucuronidase in the cecum,[74,75] preventing toxicant recycling and allowing the compounds that have been bound to glucuronate to pass through the intestines and exit the body. Beta-glucuronidase activity is also correlated with colon cancer risk. Even patients with acute pancreatitis who were given a moderate dose of probiotics (2.5 billion, four times over 7 days) showed a significant reduction of C-reactive protein levels, indicating a powerful antiinflammatory effect.[76]

A double-blind randomized controlled trial of 18 persons with UC revealed that 30 consecutive daily doses of 200 billion CFU of *Bifidobacterium longum* along with a prebiotic provided significant improvement in inflammation. Both TNF-α and IL-1a were significantly reduced, as were the levels of inflammation in mucosal epithelial tissues.[77] A group of 20 individuals with UC who could not take standard medications were given 1.5 trillion CFU of a proprietary probiotic combination (VSL3) daily for a year (5×10^{11} three times daily) with checkups every 2 months. By the end of the study, 15 of the 20 (75%) had achieved clinical remission of their UC.[78]

In a double-blind study, 9 of 18 UC patients received a twice-daily supplement of only 20 billion *Bifidobacteria*

longum cells, along with an oligosaccharide prebiotic. After only 4 weeks of therapy, the probiotic group had reduced bowel inflammation, growth of new healthy cells lining the bowel, and lower levels of the inflammatory cytokines TNF-α and IL-1.[79] Comparing these results with the previously reported study indicates that greater benefit is possible with lower CFU of probiotics when combined with adequate prebiotic levels. This only makes sense, as the administered probiotics will not thrive in a system without their preferred fuel. Further supporting this idea that sufficient prebiotic fiber potentiates the probiotic benefit is a small study of 10 individuals with CD. The patients were given only 75 billion CFUs of a combination lactobacillus and bifidobacteria (as opposed to 1.5 trillion CFU of VSL-3) along with 9.9 g of psyllium (a fiber that bacteria use to produce butyric acid) daily for an average of 13 months. The probiotics were *B. breve* (30 billion CFU), *L. casei* (30 billion CFU), and *B. longum* (10 billion CFU; no specific strains were reported). At the end of the study, 7 of the 10 (70%) were in remission from the CD.[80] Four of the ten subjects stopped taking the psyllium because of bloating, but one of these had achieved remission before stopping.

A group of Swedish researchers published three papers on a probiotic combination of *Lactobacillus* bacteria (*L. crispatus* DSM 16743, *L. gasseri* DSM 16737 typically dominant in healthy vaginal tissue, and *L. plantarum*, dominant bacteria in lactic acid-fermented foods and plant material) and one *Bifidobacterium* (*B. infantis* DSM 15158 found primarily in breastfed infants), along with blueberry skins as a prebiotic.[81] Blueberry skins alone succeeded in doubling the butyric acid levels over the control diet with no additional probiotics. However, when blueberry skins were given with the bifidobacteria, the butyric acid increased fivefold. The combination of lactobacilli and blueberry skins tripled the butyric acid level.

After finding that the combination of blueberry skin and probiotics increased butyric acid levels, researchers assessed the combined effect on chemical-induced severe colitis in animals. They used a probiotic combination of *L. crispatus*, *L. gasseri*, and *B. infantis* with either rye bran or blueberry skins. All of the combinations provided improvement for the disease index, but the combination of blueberry skins and the probiotics gave the greatest improvement.[82] Levels of Enterobacteriaceae dropped along with the disease index ratings. Blueberry skins with probiotics also reduced bacterial translocation to the liver and levels of oxidative stress and inflammatory markers (myeloperoxidase, malondialdehyde, and serum IL-12). The findings showed that intestinal inflammation was reduced along with intestinal permeability and liver endotoxin overload. The decrease in malondialdehyde corresponded with the rise in colon levels of the healthy SCFAs: acetic and butyric acids.

Neuroinflammation

Traumatic brain injury, autism, cognitive decline, and mood imbalance are all linked with neuroinflammation, as presented in Chapter 42. Probiotic supplementation has proven to be beneficial in each of these situations, although some of the research presented later in this chapter did not measure neuroinflammatory markers.

Traumatic Brain Injury. A group of traumatic brain injury comatose patients were administered 1 billion CFU of a combination of generic strains of *B. longum, L. bulgaricus,* and *Streptococcus thermophiles* via gastric tube for 21 days.[83] At the end of 3 weeks of supplementation, the cytokine picture improved, showing Th1/Th2 balance and reduced inflammation.

Autism. Microflora imbalances are found in autistic children and may play a huge role in their intestinal and neurological problems. Autistic children have higher levels of gram-negative *Desulfovibrio, Bacteroides vulgatus,* and *Clostridium,* along with lower levels of *Bacteroides fragilis. Clostridium* reduces sulfates and ferments amino acids to produce exotoxins and propionate, both of which worsen autism spectrum disorder (ASD) behavior in children. Clostridia also produce p-cresol that depletes glutathione,[84] a critical antioxidant thiol deficient in autistic children. In mouse models of ASD, where the same neurological and GI problems are present as in human ASD subjects, treatment with *Bacteroides fragilis* corrected intestinal permeability, improved microbial composition, and ameliorated deficits in communication and ASD behaviors.[85]

Recently 18 children with the diagnosis of ASD underwent a 10-week trial of microbiome alteration with an 8-week follow-up.[86] The children were first given 14 days of vancomycin to clear any possible pathogenic bacteria. Then they began 8 weeks of oral probiotic replacement (standard human gut microbiota) along with Prilosec to prevent stomach acid from causing a reduction in probiotic numbers. By the end of the 8 weeks of microbiome replacement the adverse GI symptoms of the ASD children dropped by 82%. Only 2 of the 18 children were the improvements of the GI symptoms rated less than 50%. By the end of the 8 weeks of follow-up the GI symptomatic improvements remained at 77%. More importantly the neurologic ASD presentations in all the children improved significantly with no reduction of improvement noted at the 8-week follow-up visit. The researchers noted that after the trial the bacterial diversity of the children increased significantly and did not drop at the follow-up visit either. The children also experienced a four-fold increase in the levels of bifidobacteria, to amounts similar to those found in neurotypical children.

Cognition. Minimal hepatic encephalopathy (MHE) is found in patients with cirrhosis and leads to cognitive abnormalities that affect activities of daily living. It is directly associated with the high circulating amount of ammonia in the bloodstream in cirrhotic patients. It is also the stepping-stone to overt hepatic encephalopathy. A group of patients with MHE were given either a placebo or a daily sachet of 10 billion CFU of *pediococcus pentosaceus,* Leuconostoc mesenteroides, L. paracasei, and *L. plantarum* along with 10 g of prebiotics (inulin, beta glucan, pectin, and starch) daily for 30 days.[87] This 30-day treatment resulted in a rebalanced microbiome, reduced endotoxemia and ammonia, and reversed MHE for 50% of the study group.

Persons with alcohol-induced cirrhosis also benefited from a serving of VSL-3 three times daily for 3 months.[88] None of the 160 participants had full-blown hepatic encephalopathy (HE) before starting the VSL-3, and after 3 months of supplementation, 50% fewer of those taking the probiotic developed HE than the controls. Additionally, those on the probiotic had significantly reduced levels of blood ammonia and small intestinal bacterial overgrowth (SIBO).

Mood. Healthy women drinking milk with 10 billion CFU of *Bifidobacterium lactis CNCM* and 1 billion CFU of *L. bulgaricus* and *S. thermophilus* for 4 weeks showed a modulation of their emotional responses to negative stimuli. This brain "balancing" effect was also seen in mice given *B. longum NCC3001,* who experienced a reduction in anxiety when given this probiotic.[89] This effect was also seen in 66 individuals who took 3 billion CFU of *L. helveticus R0052* and *B. longum R0175* for 30 days and experienced a decrease in global scores of anxiety and depression.[90,91]

Gastrointestinal Inflammation and Function

Gluten intolerance and celiac disease. Bifidobacteria have also demonstrated the ability to reduce small intestinal inflammation that occurs from gluten. Bifidobacteria levels are lower in patients with celiac disease (CD), yet Enterobacteriaceae (*Bacteroides* and *E. coli*) were higher.[92,93] A nonspecific strain of *Bifidobacteria lactis* prevented and reduced cellular damage to epithelial cells from gliadin and prevented increased intestinal permeability. The authors speculated that it might be related to protease activity in the bifidobacteria that is able to break down the gliadin proteins.[94]

In a laboratory setting, *B. longum IATA* ES1 successfully hydrolyzed gliadin proteins, producing peptides that were typically of far lower molecular mass (2500 Daltons instead of 30,000 Daltons). Bifidobacteria also prevented inflammation of intestinal cells from gliadin. The cultures with bifidobacteria produced approximately 20% less NFκB, 40% less TNF-α, and 100% less IL-1β.[95] NFκB is the main trigger for inflammation and is aided in pro-inflammation by both TNF-α and IL-1β. The fact that bifidobacteria downregulate all three proinflammatory compounds shows the antiinflammatory power of this probiotic. *B. longum CECT 7347* was also able to alleviate the toxic reactions of gliadin to the intestinal lining.[96]

Individuals consuming a gluten-free diet (GFD) for 1 month experienced significant changes in their microbiome, but not as one would hope. The levels of beneficial bifidobacteria, *B. longum,* and lactobacilli actually decreased, whereas the level of Enterobacteriaceae increased in accordance with the reduction in polysaccharides entering the intestines.[97] Unfortunately, this imbalance is similar to what is found in active celiac disease and does not predispose to gut healing after cessation of gluten intake. This may explain why a GFD does not always result in rapid intestinal healing. It would also indicate that anyone on a GFD should be on a combination of prebiotics and probiotics to optimize their microbiome and intestinal health.

Endotoxemia. Improvements in fatty liver, which will then attenuate endotoxicity, have been observed with oligosaccharide prebiotic stimulation of *Bifidobacterium* growth.[98] Nonalcoholic steatohepatitis (NASH) subjects receiving 16 g daily of oligosaccharides for 8 weeks experienced a significant reduction of insulin resistance,

alanine transaminase (ALT), and aspartate transaminase (AST). Among a group of 66 alcoholics hospitalized for alcohol psychoses, those receiving a combination of 0.9×10^8 CFU of *B. bifidum* and 0.9×10^9 of *L. plantarum* for only 5 days experienced a significant reduction of ALT AST, and gamma-glutamyl transpeptidase (GGTP) and an improved microbial balance.[99] The alcoholics started with lower levels of bifidobacteria and lactobacilli, which were improved with the probiotic supplementation.

A double-blind, randomized trial of people with nonalcoholic fatty liver disease (NAFLD) reported that those who took a tablet containing only a 500 million count of *L. bulgaricus* (nonspecific strain) and *S. thermophiles* (nonspecific strain) displayed a reduction of both AST and ALT levels with 3 months of probiotic treatment.[100] A metaanalysis of the studies on probiotics and NAFLD revealed that probiotics significantly decreased the following:

- ALT
- AST
- Total cholesterol
- HDL levels
- TNF-α
- Homeostatic model assessment (HOMA) levels (insulin resistance)[101]

Biotransformation and Excretion. The production of glutathione requires a supply of l-cysteine, the presence of magnesium, and the functioning of both glutamyl-cysteine ligase and glutathione synthase. Magnesium is commonly deficient in the population in general and in environmentally ill persons in particular. A 5-week study of postmenopausal women revealed that those who took 10 g/day of a prebiotic (fructooligosaccharides [FOSs]) along with 87.5 mg of supplemental magnesium absorbed more than 12% more of the magnesium and had higher body magnesium stores.[102] A similar study with calcium only showed improved absorption in women who were at least 6 years postmenopausal.[103]

Lactobacillus spp. are able to break down aldehydes in the body through enhancement of the enzyme aldehyde dehydrogenase.[104] In addition, both lactobacilli and propionibacteria are able to bind a portion of aflatoxin B1 in the intestine, preventing it from causing damage to the liver and other organs.[105] In animal studies, *Lactobacillus rhamnosus LGG* demonstrated the ability to bind a sizeable amount of aflatoxin B1.[106] A 90-person human study in an area of China with high aspergillus counts reported on the effects of taking 20 to 50 billion CFU of a 1:1 mixture of *L. rhamnosus LC705* and *Propionibacterium freudenreichii* daily for 5 weeks. Participants on the probiotic group experienced a 36% decrease in aflatoxin levels in the third week and a 55% decrease by week 5,[107] demonstrating a potential for these bacteria to provide protection from hepatocellular carcinoma in those exposed to aspergillus.

Although these probiotics have demonstrated a fantastic ability to bind toxins, they also appear to have benefit for chemical toxicants as well. More than 900 people with debilitating chemical sensitivity were surveyed about which medical or health treatment made them better or worse. Of all the therapies tried, the supplement with the highest help-to-harm ratio (clear help was noted by 52%, harm was reported by only 4.1% of respondents, and no effect was perceived in another 44%) was acidophilus.[108]

Probiotics, including *L. rhamnosus* and propionibacteria, are able to bind cadmium and lead present in foods, preventing their absorption.[109] *L. plantarum* supplementation was able to prevent cadmium toxicity in animals exposed to potentially toxic levels of this heavy metal.[110] This same bacteria has been able to reverse lead and aluminum toxicity in animals, including rebalancing of glutathione levels.[111,112] Protection against the toxic effects of mercury and the chlorinated pesticide endosulfan has also been afforded by *L. plantarum*.[113,114]

SUPPORT

Diet

Mediterranean Diet. As previously mentioned, dietary choices including whole food fibers and avoidance of high-fat diets have rapid and dramatic effects on the microbiome. One of the healthiest and most time-honored diet plans, the Mediterranean diet (MD), has demonstrated the ability to positively affect the microbiome for those who adhere to its tenets.[115] It is therefore not surprising that the MD is able to reduce the risk of cardiovascular disease, diabetes, obesity, and a host of other health problems that are common in those persons consuming a Western diet.

Berries. As mentioned previously, blueberry skins have demonstrated the ability to dramatically increase butyrate levels when given with probiotics and have even

out-performed beta-glucan from oats in this regard.[82,83] Humans who were supplemented for a month with black current extract exhibited a decrease in clostridia and bacteroidetes, increased numbers of lactobacilli and bifidobacteria, and decreased in beta-glucuronidase.[116] Several of the berries have also exhibited powerful antimicrobial activity against intestinal pathogens such as *H. pylori, Campylobacter jejuni, Candida albicans,* and salmonella.[117,118] Polyphenols from red wine, chocolate, and green tea, when taken in dietary doses, can moderately reduce intestinal inflammation induced by LPSs.[119]

Botanical Medicines. Two commonly used botanical agents (berberine and green tea) also have a powerful effect on the microbiota balance. Berberine is the main active alkaloid in the common herbs goldenseal (*Hydrastis canadensis*) and barberry (*Berberis vulgaris*) and provides most of the antibacterial activity of both. Berberine has recently been shown to reverse the common dysbiosis in animals fed a high-fat diet,[120] prevent obesity and insulin resistance, and modulate SCFA production. This may be the mechanism by which berberine affects weight and glucose metabolism.[121]

The other common botanical with the ability to kill off intestinal pathogens is green tea (*Camellia sinensis*). Green tea inhibits the growth of a number of clostridial species, including *C. difficile,* and stimulates the growth of bifidobacteria.[122,123] The polyphenols in green tea have a wide range of antimicrobial activity, may be helpful in preventing caries, and can help reverse the antibiotic resistance of methicillin-resistant *Staphylococcus aureus* (MRSA).[124] In both animals and humans, green tea also alters the chemistry of the stool, reducing the amount of ammonia and foul-smelling phenols and increasing both moisture content and the amount of organic acids.[125,126] Green tea significantly decreases the amount of beta-glucuronidase in the intestines, thereby reducing the risk of colon cancer.[127]

Probiotics. Table 63.1 provides a summary of probiotic benefit by species and strain.

Prebiotics. Prebiotics are defined as "a nondigestible food ingredient that beneficially affects the host by selectively stimulating the growth and/or activity of one or a limited number of bacteria in the colon, and thus improves host health."[128] Lactobacilli and bifidobacteria feed on dietary plant fibers, allowing them to have strong

TABLE 63.1	**Summary of Probiotic Benefit by Species and Strain**	
Organism	**Strain**	**Benefit**
Lactobacillus spp.	Various	Increase in intestinal S IgA, reduction of CRP, treatment for NASH, NAFLD, aldehyde breakdown, butyrate production
L. rhamnosus	GG	Suppression of allergic reactivity, rebalanced Th1/Th2 ratios, reduction in eczema and intestinal inflammation, antidiarrhea, binds aflatoxin
L. bulgaricus		Treatment for NASH and NAFLD, reduction of HOMA, improvement in emotional stability
L. paracasei		Reversal of MHE
L. plantarum		Reversal of MHE
Bifidobacteria spp.	Various	Increase in intestinal S IgA, reduction of levels of B-glucuronidase, reduction of CRP, prevention and reduction of damage from gliadin, inhibition of NFκB, TNF-α, IL-1, liver healing, brain balancing, treatment for NASH and NAFLD, butyrate production
B. bifidus	NCC189	Rebalanced Th1/Th2 ratios, antiinflammatory by reducing NFκB, antidiarrhea, gluten antiinflammatory
	S-16, S-17	Antiinflammatory by reducing NFκB, best mucosal adherence and antiinflammatory activity
B. lactis	Bb-12	Suppression of allergic reactivity, rebalanced Th1/Th2 ratios, gluten antiinflammatory
	NCC362	Antiinflammatory by reducing NFκB
B. longum		Rebalanced Th1/Th2 ratios, antiinflammatory (reduced TNF-α and IL-1), suppression of colon and breast tumors, gluten antiinflammatory, gluten digestion
	R0175	Improvement in anxiety and depression
B. brevis		Antiinflammatory
Streptococcus thermophiles		Rebalanced Th1/Th2 ratios, treatment for NASH and NAFLD, reduction of HOMA
Saccharomyces Boulardii		Increase in intestinal S IgA, IL-10 (promoting Th1 dominance), reduction in inflammation in Crohn's, UC, and IBS, antidiarrhea
Bacteroidetes fragilis		Autism

populations and produce a tremendous amount of organic acids with far-reaching health benefits for the human body. However, most Western diets do not contain enough dietary fiber necessary to maintain a healthy microbial balance. For this reason, there are several fibers used to encourage the growth of these healthy microbes. Unfortunately, probiotics products that also contain prebiotics only have a few hundred milligrams of prebiotics, which is completely insufficient for the task (5–20 grams).

Dietary plant fibers that are resistant to human digestion and provide fuel for these healthy bacteria and that are also used as prebiotics are listed in the following section.[129] The percent that is fiber is noted. However, there is substantial variation in the research reports on the amounts of the various types of fiber. This is likely related to normal variance in natural products, different

subspecies, different growing conditions, variations in time of harvest, variations in measurement technologies, and other factors. For example, the inulin content of chicory ranges from 8% to 85%. The listed values are a best estimate of the median. The James Duke Ethnobotany database[129] is an extremely useful resource for those who want to delve more deeply.

1. Fructans (fibers with fructosyl-fructose linkages)—soluble fibers
   a. Levans (linear fructans)
   b. Inulin
      i. Chicory *(Cichorium intybus)* root—58%
      ii. Burdock *(Arctium lappa)* root—50%
      iii. Elecampane *(Inula helenium)* root—44%
      iv. Taraxacum officinale root—40%
   c. Oligofructose

d. Short-chain fructose oligosaccharides (glucose linked to fructose)

The typical daily consumption of fructans in the United States ranges between 1 and 4 g per day (75% from wheat, 10% to 18% from onions, 4% from bananas).[130] FOSs are highest in garlic (16%), Jerusalem artichoke (17% to 21%), and onions (1% to 8%).

Fructans are the preferred fuel for nine different bifidobacteria, and for many *Bacteroides* species, they have a bifidogenic effect. An intake of 15 g/day of either inulin or FOS resulted in significant increases in bifidobacteria levels.[131] FOS supplementation also enhances the absorption of calcium and magnesium from the large intestine in animals and humans.[4-6] An intake of 5 to 20 g of fructans has been recommended to improve bowel flora.[132]

2. Galactooligosaccharides (GOS) are a commercially prepared prebiotic used in the food industry and for infant nutrition. They stimulate the growth of both lactobacilli and bifidobacteria. GOS also inhibit the mucosal adherence of pathogenic bacteria.[133]
   a. Tomatillo (*Physalis ixocarpa*) has 4% oligosaccharides.
   b. Soybean (*Glycine max*) has 12% polysaccharides.
3. Lactulose is a disaccharide manufactured from lactose that is poorly absorbed in the intestines and is highly bifidogenic. It has been used as a prebiotic since the 1950s.[133]
4. Resistant starches from food sources—soluble fiber, high amylose starches, and amylopectins—are all strongly bifidogenic.[133]
   a. Beta-glucans (from oats, barley, and other grains) are resistant starches that increase levels of both bifidobacteria and lactobacillius. Both *in vitro* and *in vivo* testing confirms that the amount of beta-glucan in the diet directly affects the levels of SCFAs and lactic acid in the bowel.
   b. Pectin-containing plants
      i. Marshmallow (*Althea off*) root—35%
      ii. Calabash gourd (*Lagenaria siceraria*) fruit—21%
      iii. Carrot (*Daucus carota*) root—18%
      iv. Hops (*Humulus lupulus*) fruit—14%
      v. Apple (*Malus domestica*) fruit—6%

The most common prebiotics in use today are either inulins from chicory or acacia gums. However, some novel polysaccharides are now showing up in the medical literature and may play multiple roles in health when they are applied.

REFERENCES

1. Lee, Y. K., & Salminen, S. (2009). *Handbook of probiotics and prebiotics* (2nd ed.). Hoboken, NJ: Wiley & Sons, Publ.
2. Zhang, X., Zhao, Y., Zhang, M., Pang, X., Xu, J., Kang, C., et al. (2012). Structural changes of gut microbiota during berberine-mediated prevention of obesity and insulin resistance in high-fat diet-fed rats. *PLoS ONE*, 7(8), e42529. PubMed PMID: 22880019.
3. Nguyen, L. N., Lopes, L. C., Cordero, R. J., & Nosanchuk, J. D. (2011). Sodium butyrate inhibits pathogenic yeast growth and enhances the functions of macrophages. *The Journal of Antimicrobial Chemotherapy*, 66(11), 2573–2580. PubMed PMID: 21911344.
4. Fukushima, A., Ohta, A., Sakai, K., & Sakuma, K. (2005). Expression of calbindin-D9k, VDR and Cdx-2 messenger RNA in the process by which fructooligosaccharides increase calcium absorption in rats. *Journal of Nutritional Science and Vitaminology*, 51(6), 426–432. PubMed PMID: 16521702.
5. Tahiri, M., Tressol, J. C., Arnaud, J., Bornet, F. R., Bouteloup-Demange, C., Feillet-Coudray, C., et al. (2003). Effect of short-chain fructooligosaccharides on intestinal calcium absorption and calcium status in postmenopausal women: a stable-isotope study. *The American Journal of Clinical Nutrition*, 77(2), 449–457. PubMed PMID:12540407.
6. Tahiri, M., Tressol, J. C., Arnaud, J., Bornet, F., Bouteloup-Demange, C., Feillet-Coudray, C., et al. (2001). Five-week intake of short-chain fructo-oligosaccharides increases intestinal absorption and status of magnesium in postmenopausal women. *Journal of Bone and Mineral Research*, 16(11), 2152–2160. PubMed PMID: 11697813.
7. Kelly, C. J., Colgan, S. P., & Frank, D. N. (2012). Of microbes and meals: the health consequences of dietary endotoxemia. *Nutrition in Clinical Practice*, 27(2), 215–225. PubMed PMID: 22378797.
8. Pugazhenthi, S., Qin, L., & Reddy, P. H. (2016). Common neurodegenerative pathways in obesity, diabetes, and Alzheimer's disease. *Biochimica et Biophysica Acta*, pii: S0925-4439(16)30097-7. PubMed PMID: 27156888.
9. Piya, M. K., Harte, A. L., & McTernan, P. G. (2013). Metabolic endotoxaemia: is it more than just a gut feeling? *Current Opinion in Lipidology*, 24(1), 78–85. PubMed PMID: 23298961.
10. Morgan, E. T. (1989). Suppression of constitutive cytochrome P-450 gene expression in livers of rats

undergoing an acute phase response to endotoxin. *Molecular Pharmacology, 36*(5), 699–707. PubMed PMID: 2511427.

11. Tajima, M., Ikarashi, N., Okaniwa, T., Imahori, Y., Saruta, K., Toda, T., et al. (2013). Consumption of a high-fat diet during pregnancy changes the expression of cytochrome P450 in the livers of infant male mice. *Biological and Pharmaceutical Bulletin, 36*(4), 649–657. PubMed PMID: 23358370.

12. Warren, G. W., Poloyac, S. M., Gary, D. S., Mattson, M. P., & Blouin, R. A. (1999). Hepatic cytochrome P-450 expression in tumor necrosis factor-alpha receptor (p55/p75) knockout mice after endotoxin administration. *The Journal of Pharmacology and Experimental Therapeutics, 288*(3), 945–950. PubMed PMID: 10027830.

13. Roe, A. L., Warren, G., Hou, G., Howard, G., Shedlofsky, S. I., & Blouin, R. A. (1998). The effect of high dose endotoxin on CYP3A2 expression in the rat. *Pharmaceutical Research, 15*(10), 1603–1608. PubMed PMID: 9794504.

14. Cheng, P. Y., Wang, M., & Morgan, E. T. (2003). Rapid transcriptional suppression of rat cytochrome P450 genes by endotoxin treatment and its inhibition by curcumin. *The Journal of Pharmacology and Experimental Therapeutics, 307*(3), 1205–1212. PubMed PMID: 14557382.

15. Li, X. Y., Zhang, C., Wang, H., Ji, Y. L., Wang, S. F., Zhao, L., et al. (2008). Tumor necrosis factor alpha partially contributes to lipopolysaccharide-induced downregulation of CYP3A in fetal liver: its repression by a low dose LPS pretreatment. *Toxicology Letters, 179*(2), 71–77. PubMed PMID: 18501536.

16. Ko, K., Yang, H., Noureddin, M., Iglesia-Ara, A., Xia, M., Wagner, C., et al. (2008). Changes in S adenosylmethionine and GSH homeostasis during endotoxemia in mice. *Laboratory Investigation: A Journal of Technical Methods and Pathology, 88*(10), 1121–1129. PubMed PMID: 18695670.

17. Flint, H. J. (2012). The impact of nutrition on the human microbiome. *Nutrition Reviews, 70*(Suppl. 1), S10–S13. PubMed PMID:22861801.

18. Hooda, S., Boler, B. M., Serao, M. C., Brulc, J. M., Staeger, M. A., Boileau, T. W., et al. (2012). 454 pyrosequencing reveals a shift in fecal microbiota of healthy adult men consuming polydextrose or soluble corn fiber. *The Journal of Nutrition, 142*(7), 1259–1265. PubMed PMID:22649263.

19. Li, F., Hullar, M. A., Schwarz, Y., & Lampe, J. W. (2009). Human gut bacterial communities are altered by addition of cruciferous vegetables to a controlled fruit- and vegetable-free diet. *The Journal of Nutrition, 139*(9), 1685–1691. PubMed PMID: 19640972.

20. Levy, S. (2013). Ancient gut microbiomes shed light on modern disease. *Environmental Health Perspectives, 121*(4), A118. PubMed PMID: 23548507.

21. David, L. A., Maurice, C. F., Carmody, R. N., Gootenberg, D. B., Button, J. E., Wolfe, B. E., et al. (2014). Diet rapidly and reproducibly alters the human gut microbiome. *Nature, 505*(7484), 559–563. PubMed PMID: 24336217.

22. Turnbaugh, P. J., Ridaura, V. K., Faith, J. J., Rey, F. E., Knight, R., & Gordon, J. I. (2009). The effect of diet on the human gut microbiome: a metagenomic analysis in humanized gnotobiotic mice. *Science Translational Medicine, 1*(6), 6ra14. PubMed PMID.

23. De Filippo, C., Cavalieri, D., Di Paola, M., Ramazzotti, M., Poullet, J. B., Massart, S., et al. (2010). Impact of diet in shaping gut microbiota revealed by a comparative study in children from Europe and rural Africa. *Proceedings of the National Academy of Sciences of the United States of America, 107*(33), 14691–14696. PubMed PMID: 20679230.

24. Kelder, T., Stroeve, J. H., Bijlsma, S., Radonjic, M., & Roeselers, G. (2014). Correlation network analysis reveals relationships between diet-induced changes in human gut microbiota and metabolic health. *Nutr Diabetes, 4*, e122. PubMed PMID: 24979151.

25. Osto, M., Abegg, K., Bueter, M., le Roux, C. W., Cani, P. D., & Lutz, T. A. (2013). Roux-en-Y gastric bypass surgery in rats alters gut microbiota profile along the intestine. *Physiology and Behavior, 119*, 92–96. PubMed PMID: 23770330.

26. Ma, J., Prince, A. L., Bader, D., Hu, M., Ganu, R., Baquero, K., et al. (2014). High-fat maternal diet during pregnancy persistently alters the offspring microbiome in a primate model. *Nature Communications, 5*, 3889. PubMed PMID: 24846660.

27. Qin, J., Li, Y., Cai, Z., Li, S., Zhu, J., Zhang, F., et al. (2012). A metagenome-wide association study of gut microbiota in type 2 diabetes. *Nature, 490*(7418), 55–60. PubMed PMID: 23023125.

28. Maurice, C. F., Haiser, H. J., & Turnbaugh, P. J. (2013). Xenobiotics shape the physiology and gene expression of the active human gut microbiome. *Cell, 152*(1–2), 39–50. PubMed PMID: 23332745.

29. Pérez-Cobas, A. E., Gosalbes, M. J., Friedrichs, A., Knecht, H., Artacho, A., Eismann, K., et al. (2013). Gut microbiota disturbance during antibiotic therapy: a multi-omic approach. *Gut, 62*(11), 1591–1601. PubMed PMID: 23236009.

30. Huang, E. Y., Inoue, T., Leone, V. A., Dalal, S., Touw, K., Wang, Y., et al. (2015). Using corticosteroids to reshape

the gut microbiome: implications for inflammatory bowel diseases. *Inflammatory Bowel Diseases*, 21(5), 963–972. PubMed PMID: 25738379.

31. Joly, C., Gay-Quéheillard, J., Léké, A., Chardon, K., Delanaud, S., Bach, V., et al. (2013). Impact of chronic exposure to low doses of chlorpyrifos on the intestinal microbiota in the Simulator of the Human Intestinal Microbial Ecosystem (SHIME)and in the rat. *Environmental Science and Pollution Research International*, 20(5), 2726–2734. PubMed PMID: 23135753.

32. Gao, B., Bian, X., Mahbub, R., & Lu, K. (2017). Sex-specific effects of organophosphate diazinon on the gut microbiome and its metabolic functions. *Environmental Health Perspectives*, 125(2), 198–206. PubMed PMID: 27203275.

33. Lu, K., Abo, R. P., Schlieper, K. A., Graffam, M. E., Levine, S., Wishnok, J. S., et al. (2014). Arsenic exposure perturbs the gut microbiome and its metabolic profile in mice: an integrated metagenomics and metabolomics analysis. *Environmental Health Perspectives*, 122(3), 284–291. PubMed PMID: 24413286.

34. Zhang, S., Jin, Y., Zeng, Z., Liu, Z., & Fu, Z. (2015). Subchronic exposure of mice to cadmium perturbs their hepatic energy metabolism and gut microbiome. *Chemical Research in Toxicology*, 28(10), 2000–2009. PubMed PMID: 26352046.

35. Lai, K. P., Chung, Y. T., Li, R., Wan, H. T., & Wong, C. K. (2016). Bisphenol A alters gut microbiome: Comparative metagenomics analysis. *Environmental Pollution (Barking, Essex: 1987)*, 218, 923–930. PubMed PMID: 27554980.

36. Zhang, L., Nichols, R. G., Correll, J., Murray, I. A., Tanaka, N., Smith, P. B., et al. (2015). Persistent organic pollutants modify gut microbiota-host metabolic homeostasis in mice through aryl hydrocarbon receptor activation. *Environmental Health Perspectives*, 123(7), 679–688. PubMed PMID: 25768209.

37. Jack, R. W., Tagg, J. R., & Ray, B. (1995). Bacteriocins of gram-positive bacteria. *Microbiological Reviews*, 59(2), 171–200. PubMed PMID: 7603408.

38. Kaila, M., Isolauri, E., Soppi, E., Virtanen, E., Laine, S., & Arvilommi, H. (1992). Enhancement of the circulating antibody secreting cell response in human diarrhea by a human Lactobacillus strain. *Pediatric Research*, 32(2), 141–144. PubMed PMID: 1324462.

39. Engeland, C. G., Hugo, F. N., Hilgert, J. B., Nascimento, G. G., Junges, R., Lim, H. J., et al. (2016). Psychological distress and salivary secretory immunity. *Brain, Behavior, and Immunity*, 52, 11–17. PubMed PMID: 26318411.

40. Ng, V., Koh, D., Mok, B., Lim, L. P., Yang, Y., & Chia, S. E. (2004). Stressful life events of dental students and salivary immunoglobulin A. *International Journal of Immunopathology and Pharmacology*, 17(2 Suppl.), 49–56. PubMed PMID: 15345192.

41. Harmatz, P. R., Carter, E. A., Sullivan, D., Hatz, R. A., Baker, R., Breazeale, E., et al. (1989). Effect of thermal injury in the rat on transfer of IgA protein into bile. *Annals of Surgery*, 210(2), 203–207. PubMed PMID: 2757421.

42. Thang, C. L., Boye, J. I., & Zhao, X. (2013). Low doses of allergen and probiotic supplementation separately or in combination alleviate allergic reactions to cow β-lactoglobulin in mice. *The Journal of Nutrition*, 143(2), 136–141. PubMed PMID: 23236021.

43. Castillo, N. A., de Moreno de LeBlanc, A., M Galdeano, C., & Perdigón, G. (2013). Comparative study of the protective capacity against Salmonella infection between probiotic and nonprobiotic Lactobacilli. *Journal of Applied Microbiology*, 114(3), 861–876. PubMed PMID: 23163296.

44. Holscher, H. D., Czerkies, L. A., Cekola, P., Litov, R., Benbow, M., Santema, S., et al. (2012). Bifidobacterium lactis Bb12 enhances intestinal antibody response in formula-fed infants: a randomized,double-blind, controlled trial. *JPEN. Journal of Parenteral and Enteral Nutrition*, 36(1 Suppl.), 106S–17S. PubMed PMID: 22237870.

45. Kabeerdoss, J., Devi, R. S., Mary, R. R., Prabhavathi, D., Vidya, R., Mechenro, J., et al. (2011). Effect of yoghurt containing Bifidobacterium lactis Bb12® on faecal excretion of secretory immunoglobulin A and human beta-defensin 2 in healthy adult volunteers. *Nutrition Journal*, 10, 138. PubMed PMID: 22196482.

46. Generoso, S. V., Viana, M. L., Santos, R. G., Arantes, R. M., Martins, F. S., Nicoli, J. R., et al. (2011). Protection against increased intestinal permeability and bacterial translocation induced by intestinal obstruction in mice treated with viable and heat-killed Saccharomyces boulardii. *European Journal of Nutrition*, 50(4), 261–269. PubMed PMID: 20936479.

47. Chiang, B. L., Sheih, Y. H., Wang, L. H., Liao, C. K., & Gill, H. S. (2000). Enhancing immunity by dietary consumption of a probiotic lactic acid bacterium (Bifidobacterium lactis HN019): optimization and definition of cellular immune responses. *European Journal of Clinical Nutrition*, 54(11), 849–855. PubMed PMID: 11114680.

48. Sheih, Y. H., Chiang, B. L., Wang, L. H., Liao, C. K., & Gill, H. S. (2001). Systemic immunity-enhancing effects in healthy subjects following dietary consumption of the lactic acid bacterium Lactobacillus

rhamnosus HN001. *Journal of the American College of Nutrition, 20*(2 Suppl.), 149–156. PubMed PMID: 11349938.

49. Hao, Q., Lu, Z., Dong, B. R., Huang, C. Q., & Wu, T. (2011). Probiotics for preventing acute upper respiratory tract infections. *The Cochrane Database of Systematic Reviews*, (9), CD006895, PubMed PMID: 21901706.

50. Macpherson, A. J., & Harris, N. L. (2004). Interactions between commensal intestinal bacteria and the immune system. *Nature Reviews. Immunology, 4*(6), 478–485. PubMed PMID:15173836.

51. Berman, S., Eichelsdoerfer, P., Yim, D., Elmer, G., & Wenner, C. (2006). Daily ingestion of a nutritional probiotic supplement enhances innate immune function in healthy adults. *Nutrition Research, 26,* 454–459.

52. Tanaka, K., & Ishikawa, H. (2004). Role of intestinal bacterial flora in oral tolerance induction. *Histology and Histopathology, 19*(3), 907–914. PubMed PMID:15168353.

53. Feleszko, W., Jaworska, J., Rha, R. D., Steinhausen, S., Avagyan, A., et al. (2007). Probiotic-induced suppression of allergic sensitization and airway inflammation is associated with an increase of T regulatory-dependent mechanisms in a murine model of asthma. *Clinical and Experimental Allergy: Journal of the British Society for Allergy and Clinical Immunology, 37*(4), 498–505. PubMed PMID: 17430345.

54. Canani, R. B., & Di Costanzo, M. (2013). Gut microbiota as potential therapeutic target for the treatment of cow's milk allergy. *Nutrients, 5*(3), 651–662. PubMed PMID: 23455693.

55. Björkstén, B., Sepp, E., Julge, K., Voor, T., & Mikelsaar, M. (2001). Allergy development and the intestinal microflora during the first year of life. *The Journal of Allergy and Clinical Immunology, 108*(4), 516–520. PubMed PMID: 11590374.

56. Ozdemir, O. (2010). Various effects of different probiotic strains in allergic disorders: an update from laboratory and clinical data. *Clinical and Experimental Immunology, 160*(3), 295–304. PubMed PMID: 20345982.

57. Savilahti, E., Kuitunen, M., & Vaarala, O. (2008). Pre and probiotics in the prevention and treatment of food allergy. *Current Opinion in Allergy and Clinical Immunology, 8*(3), 243–248. PubMed PMID: 18560300.

58. Majamaa, H., & Isolauri, E. (1997). Probiotics: a novel approach in the management of food allergy. *The Journal of Allergy and Clinical Immunology, 99*(2), 179–185. PubMed PMID: 9042042.

59. Kim, J. Y., Kwon, J. H., Ahn, S. H., Lee, S. I., Han, Y. S., et al. (2010). Effect of probiotic mix (Bifidobacterium bifidum, Bifidobacterium lactis, Lactobacillus acidophilus) in the primary prevention of eczema: a double-blind, randomized, placebo-controlled trial. *Pediatric Allergy and Immunology : Official Publication of the European Society of Pediatric Allergy and Immunology, 21*(2 Pt. 2), e386–e393. PubMed PMID: 19840300.

60. Kawase, M., He, F., Kubota, A., Hiramatsu, M., Saito, H., Ishii, T., et al. (2009). Effect of fermented milk prepared with two probiotic strains on Japanese cedar pollinosis in a double-blind placebo-controlled clinical study. *International Journal of Food Microbiology, 128*(3), 429–434. PubMed PMID: 18977549.

61. Harata, G., Kumar, H., He, F., Miyazawa, K., Yoda, K., Kawase, M., et al. (2016). Probiotics modulate gut microbiota and health status in Japanese cedar pollinosis patients during the pollen season. *European Journal of Nutrition*, PubMed PMID: 27412706.

62. Xiao, J. Z., Kondo, S., Yanagisawa, N., Takahashi, N., Odamaki, T., Iwabuchi, N., et al. (2006). Probiotics in the treatment of Japanese cedar pollinosis: a double-blind placebo-controlled trial. *Clinical and Experimental Allergy: Journal of the British Society for Allergy and Clinical Immunology, 36*(11), 1425–1435. PubMed PMID: 17083353.

63. Xiao, J. Z., Kondo, S., Yanagisawa, N., Miyaji, K., Enomoto, K., Sakoda, T., et al. (2007). Clinical efficacy of probiotic Bifidobacterium longum for the treatment of symptoms of Japanese cedar pollen allergy in subjects evaluated in an environmental exposure unit. *Allergology International, 56*(1), 67–75. PubMed PMID: 17259812.

64. Harima-Mizusawa, N., Iino, T., Onodera-Masuoka, N., Kato-Nagaoka, N., Kiyoshima-Shibata, J., Gomi, A., et al. (2014). Beneficial Effects of Citrus Juice Fermented with Lactobacillus plantarum YIT 0132 on Japanese Cedar Pollinosis. *Biosci Microbiota Food Health, 33*(4), 147–155. PubMed PMID: 25379362.

65. Kelesidis, T., & Pothoulakis, C. (2012). Efficacy and safety of the probiotic Saccharomyces boulardii for the prevention and therapy of gastrointestinal disorders. *Therapeutic advances in gastroenterology, 5*(2), 111–125. PubMedPMID: 22423260.

66. Wollowski, I., Rechkemmer, G., & Pool-Zobel, B. L. (2001). Protective role of probiotics and prebiotics in colon cancer. *The American Journal of Clinical Nutrition, 73*(2 Suppl.), 451S–455S. PMID: 11157356.

67. Donohoe, D. R., Garge, N., Zhang, X., Sun, W., O'Connell, T. M., Bunger, M. K., et al. (2011). The microbiome and butyrate regulate energy metabolism

and autophagy in the mammalian colon. *Cell Metabolism*, 13(5), 517–526. PubMed PMID: 21531334.

68. Hamer, H. M., Jonkers, D., Venema, K., Vanhoutvin, S., Troost, F. J., & Brummer, R. J. (2008). Review article: the role of butyrate on colonic function. *Alimentary Pharmacology and Therapeutics*, 27(2), 104–119. PMID: 17973645.

69. Takaishi, H., Matsuki, T., Nakazawa, A., Takada, T., et al. (2008). Imbalance in intestinal microflora constitution could be involved in the pathogenesis of inflammatory bowel disease. *International Journal of Medical Microbiology*, 298(5–6), 463–472. PMID: 17897884.

70. Bullock, N. R., Booth, J. C., & Gibson, G. R. (2004). Comparative composition of bacteria in the human intestinal microflora during remission and active ulcerative colitis. *Current Issues in Intestinal Microbiology*, 5(2), 59–64. PubMed PMID: 15460067.

71. Noor, S. O., Ridgway, K., Scovell, L., Kemsley, E. K., Lund, E. K., Jamieson, C., et al. (2010). Ulcerative colitis and irritable bowel patients exhibit distinct abnormalities of the gut microbiota. *BMC Gastroenterology*, 10, 134. PubMed PMID: 21073731.

72. Riedel, C. U., Foata, F., Philippe, D., Adolfsson, O., Eikmanns, B. J., & Blum, S. (2006). Anti-inflammatory effects of bifidobacteria by inhibition of LPS-induced NF-kappaB activation. *World Journal of Gastroenterology*, 12(23), 3729–3735. PMID: 16773690.

73. Preising, J., Philippe, D., Gleinser, M., Wei, H., Blum, S., Eikmanns, B. J., et al. (2010). Selection of bifidobacteria based on adhesion and anti-inflammatory capacity in vitro for amelioration of murine colitis. *Applied and Environmental Microbiology*, 76(9), 3048–3051. PMID: 20228095.

74. Park, H. Y., Bae, E. A., Han, M. J., Choi, E. C., & Kim, D. H. (1998). Inhibitory effects of Bifidobacterium spp. isolated from a healthy Korean on harmful enzymes of human intestinal microflora. *Archives of Pharmacal Research*, 21(1), 54–61. PubMed PMID: 9875515.

75. Gmeiner, M., Kneifel, W., Kulbe, K. D., Wouters, R., De Boever, P., Nollet, L., et al. (2000). Influence of a synbiotic mixture consisting of Lactobacillus acidophilus 74-2 and a fructooligosaccharide preparation on the microbial ecology sustained in a simulation of the human intestinal microbial ecosystem (SHIME reactor). *Applied Microbiology and Biotechnology*, 53(2), 219–223. PubMed PMID: 10709985.

76. Sharma, B., Srivastava, S., Singh, N., Sachdev, V., Kapur, S., & Saraya, A. (2011). Role of probiotics on gut permeability and endotoxemia in patients with acute pancreatitis: a double-blind randomized controlled trial. *Journal of Clinical Gastroenterology*, 45(5), 442–448. PubMed PMID: 21135704.

77. Furrie, E., Macfarlane, S., Kennedy, A., Cummings, J. H., Walsh, S. V., O'neil, D. A., et al. (2005). Synbiotic therapy (Bifidobacterium longum/Synergy 1) initiates resolution of inflammation in patients with active ulcerative colitis: a randomized controlled pilot trial. *Gut*, 54(2), 242–249. PubMed PMID:15647189.

78. Venturi, A., Gionchetti, P., Rizzello, F., Johansson, R., et al. (1999). Impact on the composition of the faecal flora by a new probiotic preparation: preliminary data on maintenance treatment of patients with ulcerative colitis. *Alimentary Pharmacology and Therapeutics*, 13(8), 1103–1108. PMID:10468688.

79. Furrie, E., Macfarlane, S., Kennedy, A., Cummings, J. H., Walsh, S. V., O'neil, D. A., et al. (2005). Synbiotic therapy (Bifidobacterium longum/Synergy 1) initiates resolution of inflammation in patients with active ulcerative colitis: a randomised controlled pilot trial. *Gut*, 54(2), 242–249. PMID: 15647189.

80. Fujimori, S., Tatsuguchi, A., Gudis, K., Kishida, T., et al. (2007). High dose probiotic and prebiotic cotherapy for remission induction of active Crohn's disease. *Journal of Gastroenterology and Hepatology*, 22(8), 1199–1204. PMID: 17688660.

81. Bränning, C., Håkansson, A., Ahrné, S., Jeppsson, B., Molin, G., & Nyman, M. (2009). Blueberry husks and multi-strain probiotics affect colonic fermentation in rats. *The British Journal of Nutrition*, 101(6), 859–870. PubMedPMID: 18680631.

82. Håkansson, A., Bränning, C., Adawi, D., Molin, G., Nyman, M., & Jeppsson, B. (2009). Ahrné S. Blueberry husks, rye bran and multi-strain probiotics affect the severity of colitis induced by dextran sulphate sodium. *Scandinavian Journal of Gastroenterology*, 44(10), 1213–1225. PMID: 19670079.

83. Tan, M., Zhu, J. C., Du, J., Zhang, L. M., & Yin, H. H. (2011). Effects of probiotics on serum levels of Th1/Th2 cytokine and clinical outcomes in severe traumatic brain-injured patients: a prospective randomized pilot study. *Critical Care: The Official Journal of the Critical Care Forum*, 15(6), R290. PubMed PMID: 22136422.

84. Kang, D. W., Park, J. G., Ilhan, Z. E., Wallstrom, G., Labaer, J., Adams, J. B., et al. (2013). Reduced incidence of Prevotella and other fermenters in intestinal microflora of autistic children. *PLoS ONE*, 8(7), e68322. PubMed PMID: 23844187.

85. Hsiao, E. Y., McBride, S. W., Hsien, S., Sharon, G., Hyde, E. R., McCue, T., et al. (2013). Microbiota modulate behavioral and physiological abnormalities

associated with neurodevelopmental disorders. *Cell*, 155(7), 1451–1463. PubMed PMID: 24315484.

86. Kang, D. W., Adams, J. B., Gregory, A. C., et al. (2017). Microbiota Transfer Therapy alters gut ecosystem and improves gastrointestinal and autism symptoms: an open-label study. *Microbiome*, 5(1), 10. doi:10.1186/s40168-016-0225-7. PubMed PMID: 28122648.

87. Liu, Q., Duan, Z. P., Ha, D. K., Bengmark, S., Kurtovic, J., & Riordan, S. M. (2004). Synbiotic modulation of gut flora: effect on minimal hepatic encephalopathy in patients with cirrhosis. *Hepatology (Baltimore, Md.)*, 39(5), 1441–1449. PubMed PMID: 15122774.

88. Lunia, M. K., Sharma, B. C., Sharma, P., Sachdeva, S., & Srivastava, S. (2014). Probiotics prevent hepatic encephalopathy in patients with cirrhosis: a randomized controlled trial. *Clinical Gastroenterology and Hepatology*, 12(6), 1003–1008, e1. PubMed PMID: 24246768.

89. Bercik, P., Park, A. J., Sinclair, D., Khoshdel, A., Lu, J., Huang, X., et al. (2011). The anxiolytic effect ofnBifidobacterium longum NCC3001 involves vagal pathways for gut-brain communication. *Neurogastroenterology and Motility*, 23(12), 1132–1139. PubMed PMID: 21988661.

90. Messaoudi, M., Lalonde, R., Violle, N., Javelot, H., Desor, D., Nejdi, A., et al. (2011). Assessment of psychotropic-like properties of a probiotic formulation (Lactobacillus helveticus R0052 and Bifidobacterium longum R0175) in rats and human subjects. *The British Journal of Nutrition*, 105(5), 755–764. PubMed PMID: 20974015.

91. Messaoudi, M., Violle, N., Bisson, J. F., Desor, D., Javelot, H., & Rougeot, C. (2011). Beneficial psychological effects of a probiotic formulation (Lactobacillus helveticus R0052 and Bifidobacterium longum R0175) in healthy human volunteers. *Gut Microbes*, 2(4), 256–261. PubMed PMID:21983070.

92. De Palma, G., Nadal, I., Medina, M., Donat, E., Ribes-Koninckx, C., Calabuig, M., et al. (2010). Intestinal dysbiosis and reduced immunoglobulin-coated bacteria associated with coeliac disease in children. *BMC Microbiology*, 10, 63. PubMed PMID: 20181275.

93. Nadal, I., Donat, E., Ribes-Koninckx, C., Calabuig, M., & Sanz, Y. (2007). Imbalance in the composition of the duodenal microbiota of children with coeliac disease. *Journal of Medical Microbiology*, 56(Pt. 12), 1669–1674. PubMed PMID:18033837.

94. Lindfors, K., Blomqvist, T., Juuti-Uusitalo, K., Stenman, S., Venäläinen, J., Mäki, M., et al. (2008). Live probiotic Bifidobacterium lactis bacteria inhibit the toxic effects induced by wheat gliadin in epithelial cell

culture. *Clinical and Experimental Immunology*, 152(3), 552–558. PubMed PMID: 18422736.

95. Laparra, J. M., & Sanz, Y. (2010). Bifidobacteria inhibit the inflammatory response induced by gliadins in intestinal epithelial cells via modifications of toxic peptide generation during digestion. *Journal of Cellular Biochemistry*, 109(4), 801–807. PMID: 20052669.

96. Olivares, M., Laparra, M., & Sanz, Y. (2012). Oral administration of Bifidobacterium longum CECT 7347 modulates jejunal proteome in an in vivo gliadin-induced enteropathy animal model. *Journal of Proteomics*, 77, 310–320. PubMed PMID: 23023000.

97. Sanz, Y. (2010). Effects of a gluten-free diet on gut microbiota and immune function in healthy adult humans. *Gut Microbes*, 1(3), 135–137. PubMed PMID: 21327021.

98. Daubioul, C. A., Horsmans, Y., Lambert, P., Danse, E., & Delzenne, N. M. (2005). Effects of oligofructose on glucose and lipid metabolism in patients with nonalcoholic steatohepatitis: results of a pilot study. *European Journal of Clinical Nutrition*, 59(5), 723–726. PubMed PMID: 15770222.

99. Kirpich, I. A., Solovieva, N. V., Leikhter, S. N., Shidakova, N. A., Lebedeva, O. V., et al. (2008). Probiotics restore bowel flora and improve liver enzymes in human alcohol-induced liver injury: a pilot study. *Alcohol (Fayetteville, N.Y.)*, 42(8), 675–682. PMID: 19038698.

100. Aller, R., De Luis, D. A., Izaola, O., Conde, R., Gonzalez Sagrado, M., et al. (2011). Effect of a probiotic on liver aminotransferases in nonalcoholic fatty liver disease patients: a double blind randomized clinical trial. *European Review for Medical and Pharmacological Sciences*, 15(9), 1090–1095. PubMed PMID: 22013734.

101. Ma, Y. Y., Li, L., Yu, C. H., Shen, Z., Chen, L. H., & Li, Y. M. (2013). Effects of probiotics on nonalcoholic fatty liver disease: a meta-analysis. *World Journal of Gastroenterology*, 19(40), 6911–6918. PubMed PMID:24187469.

102. Tahiri, M., Tressol, J. C., Arnaud, J., Bornet, F., Bouteloup-Demange, C., Feillet-Coudray, C., et al. (2001). Five-week intake of short-chain fructo-oligosaccharides increases intestinal absorption and status of magnesium in postmenopausal women. *Journal of Bone and Mineral Research*, 16(11), 2152–2160. PubMed PMID: 11697813.

103. Tahiri, M., Tressol, J. C., Arnaud, J., Bornet, F., Bouteloup-Demange, C., Feillet-Coudray, C., et al. (2001). Five-week intake of short-chain fructo-oligosaccharides increases intestinal absorption and status of magnesium in postmenopausal women.

Journal of Bone and Mineral Research, 16(11), 2152–2160. PubMed PMID: 11697813.

104. Nosova, T., Jousimies-Somer, H., Jokelainen, K., Heine, R., & Salaspuro, M. (2000). Acetaldehyde production and metabolism by human indigenous and probiotic Lactobacillus and Bifidobacterium strains. *Alcohol and Alcoholism (Oxford, Oxfordshire)*, 35(6), 561–568. PubMed PMID: 11093962.

105. Gratz, S., Mykkänen, H., & El-Nezami, H. (2005). Aflatoxin B1 binding by a mixture of Lactobacillus and Propionibacterium: in vitro versus ex vivo. *Journal of Food Protection*, 68(11), 2470–2474. PubMed PMID: 16300092.

106. Gratz, S., Täubel, M., Juvonen, R. O., Viluksela, M., Turner, P. C., Mykkänen, H., et al. (2006). Lactobacillus rhamnosus strain GG modulates intestinal absorption, fecal excretion, and toxicity of aflatoxin B(1) in rats. *Applied and Environmental Microbiology*, 72(11), 7398–7400. PubMed PMID: 16980432.

107. El-Nezami, H. S., Polychronaki, N. N., Ma, J., Zhu, H., Ling, W., Salminen, E. K., et al. (2006). Probiotic supplementation reduces a biomarker for increased risk of liver cancer in young men from Southern China. *The American Journal of Clinical Nutrition*, 83(5), 1199–1203. PubMed PMID: 16685066.

108. Gibson, P. R., Elms, A. N., & Ruding, L. A. (2003). Perceived treatment efficacy for conventional and alternative therapies reported by persons with multiple chemical sensitivity. *Environmental Health Perspectives*, 111(12), 1498–1504. PubMed PMID: 12948890.

109. Ibrahim, F., Halttunen, T., Tahvonen, R., & Salminen, S. (2006). Probiotic bacteria as potential detoxification tools: assessing their heavy metal binding isotherms. *Canadian Journal of Microbiology*, 52(9), 877–885. PubMed PMID: 17110980.

110. Zhai, Q., Wang, G., Zhao, J., Liu, X., Narbad, A., Chen, Y. Q., et al. (2014). Protective effects of Lactobacillus plantarum CCFM8610 against chronic cadmium toxicity in mice indicate routes of protection besides intestinal sequestration. *Applied and Environmental Microbiology*, 80(13), 4063–4071. PubMed PMID: 24771031.

111. Tian, F., Zhai, Q., Zhao, J., Liu, X., Wang, G., Zhang, H., et al. (2012). Lactobacillus plantarum CCFM8661 alleviates lead toxicity in mice. *Biological Trace Element Research*, 150(1–3), 264–271. PubMed PMID: 22684513.

112. Yu, L., Zhai, Q., Liu, X., Wang, G., Zhang, Q., Zhao, J., et al. (2016). Lactobacillus plantarum CCFM639 alleviates aluminium toxicity. *Applied Microbiology and Biotechnology*, 100(4), 1891–1900. PubMed PMID: 26610803.

113. Majlesi, M., Shekarforoush, S. S., Ghaisari, H. R., Nazifi, S., Sajedianfard, J., & Eskandari, M. H. (2017). Effect of probiotic bacillus coagulans and lactobacillus plantarum on alleviation of mercury toxicity in rat. *Probiotics Antimicrob Proteins*, PubMed PMID: 28084611.

114. Bouhafs, L., Moudilou, E. N., Exbrayat, J. M., & Lahouel, M. (2015). Idoui T. Protective effects of probiotic Lactobacillus plantarum BJ0021 on liver and kidney oxidative stress and apoptosis induced by endosulfan in pregnant rats. *Renal Failure*, 37(8), 1370–1378. PubMed PMID: 26287934.

115. Gutiérrez-Díaz, I., Fernández-Navarro, T., Sánchez, B., Margolles, A., & González, S. (2016). Mediterranean diet and faecal microbiota: a transversal study. *Food Funct*, 7(5), 2347–2356. PubMed PMID: 27137178.

116. Molan, A. L., Liu, Z., & Plimmer, G. (2014). Evaluation of the effect of blackcurrant products on gut microbiota and on markers of risk for colon cancer in humans. *Phytotherapy Research : PTR*, 28(3), 416–422. PubMed PMID:23674271.

117. Nohynek, L. J., Alakomi, H. L., Kähkönen, M. P., Heinonen, M., Helander, I. M., Oksman-Caldentey, K. M., et al. (2006). Berry phenolics: antimicrobial properties and mechanisms of action against severe human pathogens. *Nutrition and Cancer*, 54(1), 18–32. PubMed PMID: 16800770.

118. Puupponen-Pimiä, R., Nohynek, L., Hartmann-Schmidlin, S., Kähkönen, M., Heinonen, M., Määttä-Riihinen, K., et al. (2005). Berry phenolics selectively inhibit the growth of intestinal pathogens. *Journal of Applied Microbiology*, 98(4), 991–1000. PubMed PMID: 15752346.

119. Nicod, N., Chiva-Blanch, G., Giordano, E., Dávalos, A., Parker, R. S., & Visioli, F. (2014). Green tea, cocoa, and red wine polyphenols moderately modulate intestinal inflammation and do not increase high-density lipoprotein (HDL) production. *Journal of Agricultural and Food Chemistry*, 62(10), 2228–2232. PMID: 24559192.

120. Xie, W., Gu, D., Li, J., Cui, K., & Zhang, Y. (2011). Effects and action mechanisms of berberine and Rhizoma coptidis on gut microbes and obesity in high-fat diet-fed C57BL/6J mice. *PLoS ONE*, 6(9), e24520. PubMed PMID: 21915347.

121. Zhang, X., Zhao, Y., Zhang, M., Pang, X., Xu, J., Kang, C., et al. (2012). Structural changes of gut microbiota during berberine-mediated prevention of obesity and insulin resistance in high-fat diet-fed rats. *PLoS ONE*, 7(8), e42529. PubMed PMID: 22880019.

122. Ahn, Y.-J., Sakanaka, S., Kim, M.-J., Kawamura, T., Fujisawa, T., & Mitsuoka, T. (1990). Effect of green tea

extract on growth of intestinal bacteria. *Microb Ecol Health Dis, 3,* 335–338.

123. Molan, A. L., Liu, Z., & Tiwari, R. (2010). The ability of green tea to positively modulate key markers of gastrointestinal function in rats. *Phytotherapy Research: PTR, 24*(11), 1614–1619. PubMed PMID: 21031617.

124. Taylor, P. W., Hamilton-Miller, J. M., & Stapleton, P. D. (2005). Antimicrobial properties of green tea catechins. *Food science and technology bulletin, 2,* 71–81. PubMed PMID: 19844590.

125. Hara, H., Orita, N., Hatano, S., Ichikawa, H., Hara, Y., Matsumoto, N., et al. (1995). Effect of tea polyphenols on fecal flora and fecal metabolic products of pigs. *The Journal of Veterinary Medical Science / The Japanese Society of Veterinary Science, 57*(1), 45–49. PubMed PMID: 7756423.

126. Goto, K., Kanaya, S., Ishigami, T., & Hara, Y. (1999). The effects of tea catechins on fecal conditions of elderly residents in a long-term care facility. *Journal of Nutritional Science and Vitaminology, 45*(1), 135–141. PubMed PMID: 10360248.

127. Molan, A., Liu, Z., & Tiwari, R. (2010). The ability of green tea to positively modulate key markers of gastrointestinal function in rats. *Phytotherapy Research: PTR, 24*(11), 1614–1619. PubMed PMID 21031617.

128. Gibson, G. R., & Roberfroid, M. B. (1995). Dietary modulation of the human colonic microbiota: introducing the concept of prebiotics. *The Journal of Nutrition, 125*(6), 1401–1412. PubMed PMID: 7782892.

129. *James Duke's Ethnobotany database*: https://phytochem.nal.usda.gov (accessed 9/2/2014 and 7/16/17).

130. van Loo, J., Coussement, P., de Leenheer, L., Hoebregs, H., & Smits, G. (1995). On the presence of inulin and oligofructose as natural ingredients in the western diet. *Critical Reviews in Food Science and Nutrition, 35*(6), 525–552. Review. PubMed PMID: 8777017.

131. Gibson, G. R., Beatty, E. R., Wang, X., & Cummings, J. H. (1995). Selective stimulation of bifidobacteria in the human colon by oligofructose and inulin. *Gastroenterology, 108*(4), 975–982. PubMed PMID: 7698613.

132. Tuohy, K. M., Probert, H. M., Smejkal, C. W., & Gibson, G. R. (2003). Using probiotics and prebiotics to improve gut health. *Drug Discovery Today, 8*(15), 692–700. PubMed PMID: 12927512.

133. Cho, S. S., & Finocchiaro, E. T. (2010). *Handbook of prebiotics and probiotic ingredients. Health benefits and food applications.* Boca Raton: CRC press.

64

Chelation (Oral and Intravenous)

SUMMARY

- Major diseases: Acute metal toxicity, neurodegenerative conditions, cardiovascular disease
- Primary sources: Diet (food and water)
- Best intervention: 2,3-dimercapto-1-propanesulfonic acid (DMPS), 2,3-dimercaptosuccinic acid (DMSA),

2-[2-[bis(carboxymethyl)amino]ethyl-(carboxymethyl)amino]acetic acid (EDTA), deferoxamine (DFO), N-acetyl cysteine (NAC)

DESCRIPTION

Toxic metals are considered major environmental pollutants and are a common underlying factor in most cases of toxicant overload. In some individuals, metals are the primary toxicants present. The toxic metals and metalloids most prevalent in and toxic to humans are lead, mercury, cadmium, and arsenic. These metals are damaging to several organ systems, the most sensitive of which are the kidneys, liver, brain, and immune system (see Section III: Systemic Effects of Toxins). Toxic metals have multiple and overlapping mechanisms of toxicity, including increasing free radical production, enzyme poisoning, direct DNA damage, endocrine disruption, and mitochondrial or cell wall damage. Considering their toxicity, the Centers for Disease Control and Prevention (CDC) ranks arsenic, lead, and mercury as the three worst toxicants present at Superfund sites, with cadmium as the seventh.

With a few interesting exceptions, the standard of assessment for metal "poisoning" is whole blood levels, with reference ranges based on Occupational Safety and Health Administration (OSHA) workplace standards. The problem with this method is that blood primarily indicates current exposure and does not at all consider total body load of these metals or the huge variation in individual susceptibility to specific toxicants. Before

initiating chelation therapy or metal mobilization testing, it is prudent for the physician to ensure the patient is not allergic or chemically intolerant to the agent and that the patient has sufficient creatinine clearance to handle the toxic metal flushing.

There remains significant scientific debate regarding metal mobilization testing (see Chapter 53), and the decision to treat subacute levels of metal poisoning requires careful assessment of patient risk versus benefit. There is no scientific disagreement about the use of chelating agents to increase the excretion of toxic metals. Indeed, the removal of toxic metals from the human body can be a useful tool in avoiding the onset or progression of many diseases associated with metal intoxication. The primary way to remove accumulated toxic metals from human organs is to bind these metals to chelating agents with the goal of forming complexes that can be excreted in the urine. Chelation therapy is considered the best treatment against metal poisoning.

Pharmaceutical chelators are small organic molecules that typically form coordination complexes involving sulfur (DMSA, DMPS) or oxygen and nitrogen atoms (EDTA). There are numerous chelating drugs used as antidotes to metal toxicity, including dimercaprol (also called *British anti-Lewisite,* abbreviated BAL); succimer (meso-DMSA); 2,3-dimercapto-1-propanesulfonic acid (also called *unithiol* and abbreviated DMPS);

TABLE 64.1 Overview of Chelation Drugs			
Chemical Name (Common Names, Abbreviations)	**Activation Metabolism**	**Coordination (Binding) Groups**	**Elements Chelated**
2,3-bis(sulfanyl)butanedioic acid (dimercaptosuccinic acid; succimer; DMSA; chemet)	Excretion via urine > 90% as DMSA-cysteine disulfide conjugates	Oxygen and sulfhydryl	Lead Arsenic Mercury Cadmium Silver Tin Copper
Sodium 2,3-bis(sulfanyl) propane-1-sulfonate (sodium dimercaptopropanesulfonate; DMPS; unithiol)	84% of IV dose excreted through urine	Oxygen and sulfhydryl	Mercury Arsenic Lead Cadmium Tin Silver Copper Selenium Zinc Magnesium
2-[2-[bis(carboxymethyl)amino] ethyl-(carboxymethyl)amino]acetic acid (ethylenediaminetetraacetic acid; edetic acid; EDTA; edrate; sequestrol; endathamil)	Not metabolized; excreted unchanged, generally bound with a different cation	Oxygen	Lead Cadmium Zinc
(2S)-2-amino-3-methyl-3-sulfanylbutanoic acid (3-sulfanyl-D-valine; penicillamine; mercaptyl; D-penicillamine; cuprimine)	Rarely excreted unchanged; excreted mainly as disulfides	Oxygen, hydroxyl, sulfhydryl, and amine	Copper Arsenic Zinc Mercury Lead
2,3-bis(sulfanyl)propan-1-ol (dimercaprol; British anti-Lewisite; BAL; 2,3-dimercaptopropanol; dicaptol)	Excreted unchanged in urine	Sulfhydryl and hydroxyl	Arsenic Gold Mercury Lead (BAL in combination with CaNa$_2$EDTA)

Modified from Sears, M. E. (2013). Chelation: Harnessing and enhancing heavy metal detoxification—A review. *Scientific World Journal, 2013*(219840), 1–13.

D-penicillamine (DPA); N-acetyl-D penicillamine (NAPA); calcium disodium ethylenediaminetetraacetate (CaNa$_2$EDTA); calcium trisodium or zinc trisodium diethylenetriaminepentaacetate (CaNa$_3$DTPA, ZnNa$_3$DTPA); deferoxamine (DFO); deferipone (L1); triethylenetetramine (trientine); NAC; and Prussian blue (PB). In addition, several synthetic homologues of these agents have been designed and tested, including polyaminopolycarboxylic acids (EDTA and DTPA), derivatives of BAL (DMPS, DMSA, and monoalkylesters and dialkylesters of DMSA), and carbodithioates. The

therapeutic selection of an effective chelating agent is based on the toxicokinetics and chemical considerations of the metal involved and the chelating agent. The most commonly used chelating agents in humans intoxicated with toxic metals are summarized in Table 64.1 and further reviewed later.

CHELATING AGENTS

The agents listed in this section are presented in alphabetical order (primarily by abbreviation), not by clinical order.

Desferrioxamine or Deferoxamine

DFO is a high-molecular-weight, highly hydrophilic chelator that was first introduced in the 1960s in short-term studies of iron-loaded patients.[1] DFO is poorly absorbed orally and rapidly metabolized in plasma[2,3] and therefore requires prolonged parenteral infusions (12 hours) to reach plateau plasma concentrations.[4] DFO is an iron chelator that prevents iron-catalyzed free radical reactions. DFO is effective at lowering serum ferritin and hepatic iron levels[5,6] and preventing endocrine complications,[7] and long-term therapy is associated with a reduction in cardiac complications.[8]

DFO has also been used in aluminum toxicity because of its high affinity for aluminum and the high stability of the DFO-Al complex.[9] In animal studies, DFO reduced tissue aluminum concentrations,[10] reversed aluminum-induced lipid peroxidation (LPO),[11] and partially reversed aluminum-induced neurofibrillary degeneration.[12]

2,3-Dimercaptopropane-1-Sulfonate

DMPS was developed in 1951 and patented under the name Dimaval by Heyl Chem-Fabrik G (Berlin) for the treatment of mercury overload. DMPS is not currently approved by the US Food and Drug Administration (FDA) for metal treatment, although it has been used to treat acute arsenic poisoning.[13] However, the FDA does approve it to be used by compounding pharmacists. DMPS is a water-soluble dithiol, with an oral bioavailability of the parent drug of approximately 39%. After intravenous (IV) administration, DMPS is rapidly transformed to disulfide forms, and the metabolites (acyclic and cyclic disulfide chelates) are excreted in the urine. The elimination half-life of total DMPS is 20 hours.[14] DMPS increases urinary excretion of arsenic, cadmium, lead, and mercury and has been shown to also to cause a minor increase in excretion of essential trace metals (copper, selenium, zinc, magnesium), necessitating supplementation before and after treatment.[15]

Standard oral dosing of DMPS is 10 mg/kg, whereas IV DMPS is 3 mg/kg; both are typically given once or twice monthly. Transdermal application of DMPS has shown no evidence of absorption into the blood or enhanced mercury excretion.[16]

2,3-Dimercaptosuccinic Acid

DMSA is an sulfhydryl-containing, water-soluble, chelating agent developed in the 1950s as an alternative to more toxic chelating agents. After oral administration, DMSA is absorbed quite rapidly. It has a half-life of 2 to 3 hours in the blood and is equally excreted through urine and bile.[17] DMSA accumulates in the kidney, where it is extensively metabolized in humans to mixed disulfides of cysteine.[18] Approximately 10% to 25% of an orally administered dose of DMSA is excreted in urine, the majority (>90%) as DMSA-cysteine disulfide conjugates. Urinary excretion of the unaltered (not metabolized) drug peaks at about 2 hours and is essentially complete by 9 hours, whereas urinary excretion of altered DMSA peaks at about 4 hours and is not complete for 24 to 48 hours.[19] In up to 60% of patients treated at full dosages with DMSA, there is a transient modest rise (typically 14%) in transaminase activity during treatment. Skin reactions occur in approximately 6% of treated patients.

The sulfhydryl group binds tightly to metals located on kidney tissue surfaces and carries them out of the body. Hundreds of articles have been published showing the effectiveness of DMSA in the binding and excretion of toxic metals. DMSA increases urinary excretion of arsenic, cadmium, lead, and mercury. DMSA is FDA approved for the treatment of lead, and although it has demonstrated the ability to reduce mercury levels, it is not FDA approved for mercury toxicity.[20]

The full body-weight dose for DMSA is 30 mg/kg/day given in three divided doses of 10 mg/kg each. Dividing the daily dose into three considers the DMSA peak in both the blood and urine that occurs 4 hours after consumption.[21] DMSA is typically given for 5 days, followed by a 9-day rest period, with follow-up metal mobilization testing done every five cycles. When used with lead-burdened individuals, the blood lead level (BLL) rebounds close to pre-DMSA levels within 2 weeks of DMSA cessation.[22] If one of the therapeutic goals is reduction of BLLs, then a rest of less than 14 days between cycles is recommended. There is no single established protocol for DMSA in the treatment of lead that is universally accepted and followed. The dosing is based either on body weight or body surface area. The use of body-weight doses of DMSA has been shown to be safe in children as young as 12 months of age.[23] No harm was observed even after a DMSA overdose (185 mg/kg) in a 3-year-old child.[24] The following protocols have all been used

- 10 mg/kg every 8 hours for a total of 30 mg/kg/day for 5 days, followed by 10 mg/kg twice daily for another 14 days

- 1050 mg/m^2(body size)/day for 7 days, then 700 mg/m^2/day for 19 days
- 10 mg/kg every other day for a month
- 30 mg/kg divided into three daily doses (during waking hours) for 5 days, wait 9 days, and then repeat
- 30 mg/kg divided into three daily doses (during waking hours) for 2 days, wait 5 days, and then repeat. This protocol is used in persons who begin to experience increased symptoms from mercury mobilization on day 3 of DMSA.

Using one of these protocols, a study of Chinese children with BLLs between 10 and 25 μg/dL examined the efficacy of DMSA at the 10/mg/kg level every other day for a month.[25] One of the treatment groups received concurrent daily doses of 1250 mg calcium and 200 mg of ascorbic acid in addition to the DMSA. The combination of DMSA and nutrients proved to be more efficacious in reducing BLLs, rebalancing ALAD levels, and reducing bone lead levels.

A randomized, double-blind controlled trial of children with autism showed reductions in measures of the severity of autism associated with the difference in urinary excretion of toxic metals before and after treatment with DMSA.[26] Regression analysis found that the body burden of toxic metals was significantly related to the variations in the severity of autism. The metals of greatest influence were lead, antimony, mercury, tin, and aluminum. DMSA was shown to be safe and effective in removing toxic metals (especially lead) and dramatically effective at normalizing red blood cell (RBC) glutathione in children with autism.[27]

Within the integrative medicine community, typically lower dosages are used for longer periods of time to decrease adverse drug reactions (ADRs). The protocol used by JP is 250 mg of DMSA every third night, in conjunction with fiber and NAC. WC pioneered the use of 10 mg/kg three times a day for either 5 days on and 9 days off or 2 days on and 5 days off as part of a comprehensive nutritional protocol. Full protocols are provided in Chapter 65.

2-[2-[Bis(carboxymethyl)amino]ethyl-(carboxymethyl)amino]acetic Acid

EDTA is often used to chelate metals because it has high formation constants with several of them.[28] Table 64.2 provides a list of the logarithm values of formation constants of deprotonated EDTA with some metal ions. The formation constant for mercury (Hg^{2+}) is more than

TABLE 64.2 Metal Ion Formation Constants for EDTA

METAL ION FORMATION CONSTANTS	
Ion	Formation Constant ($\log_{10} K_f$)
Fe^{3+}	25.10
Hg^{2+}	21.70
Cu^{2+}	18.80
Pb^{2+}	18.04
Zn^{2+}	16.50
Cd^{2+}	16.40
Al^{3+}	16.30
Fe^{2+}	14.32
Ca^{2+}	10.69
Mg^{2+}	8.79
Na$^+$	1.66
K$^+$	0.80
20° C, 0.1M ion	

10 orders of magnitude greater than that for calcium (Ca^{2+}), and the formation constant for lead (Pb^{2+}) is about 10 orders of magnitude greater than magnesium (Mg^{2+}). However, when used in humans and animals, EDTA does not appreciably mobilize mercury. Considering the formation constants are generally greater for toxic metals compared with essential minerals lends a significant safety factor to long-term EDTA use. Close monitoring for adverse effects and mineral imbalances is necessary, and oral supplementation with trace minerals (copper, zinc, calcium, and magnesium) is appropriate to avoid deficiencies.

CaNa$_2$EDTA is not metabolized, and EDTA chelates are excreted rapidly in the urine. EDTA binds lead and cadmium strongly and may bind to mercury if other minerals are depleted. The typical dose of IV CaEDTA is 50 mg/kg with saline to proper osmolarity delivered over 20 minutes. In animal studies, the lowest dose of EDTA reported to cause toxicity was 750 mg/kg/day, which is equivalent to 45 g per day for a 60-kg person.[29]

Several studies have found that EDTA-chelatable lead correlated with renal dysfunction,[30,31] neurobehavioral dysfunction,[32] or declines in function of the peripheral nervous system.[33] However, CaEDTA has been associated with increased gastrointestinal absorption of lead and increased brain lead concentrations. CaEDTA primarily pulls lead from the trabecular bone and secondarily from the kidneys, but although doing so may temporarily increase soft tissue stores of lead in persons with a very high lead burden.[34] Tissue analysis of rats exposed to lead acetate in drinking water for 3 to 4 months and then injected with CaEDTA indicated that lead was mobilized from bone and redistributed to both brain and liver.[35]

Individuals with renal disease who did not have diabetes and who had a high body lead burden (at least 80 µg but less than 600 µg) received either IV CaEDTA or a placebo weekly for up to 48 months.[36] After the first 3 months of weekly CaEDTA treatment, it was noted that both the BLLs and the total body lead levels dropped dramatically. As the body lead burden levels dropped, the renal function improved, as evidenced by reduced serum creatinine and improved glomerular filtration rate. It was estimated that ongoing chelation therapy could delay the need for dialysis by several years.

N-Acetyl Cysteine

NAC is a nontoxic N-acetyl derivative of cysteine containing a thiol group. NAC is widely available, relatively inexpensive, easily administered, and well tolerated by patients. It is distributed mainly to extracellular water and is rapidly eliminated in urine, with approximately one-third excreted during the first 12 hours after administration.[37] In humans, the half-life of NAC in blood plasma is approximately 2 hours. In urine, NAC is excreted as the symmetrical disulfide, the mixed disulfide with cysteine, and as the free thiol.[38]

NAC is a potent antioxidant and detoxicant that does not alter tissue distribution of essential trace metals (calcium, magnesium, iron, zinc, and copper).[39] NAC produces a transient, dose-dependent increase in urinary excretion of methylmercury that is proportional to the body burden and can decrease brain and fetal levels of methylmercury.[40] The typical oral dose of NAC is 30 mg/kg daily.

Other

Studies show that supplementation of antioxidants along with a chelating agent proves to be a better treatment regimen than monotherapy with chelating agents. Several nutrients, including alpha-lipoic-acid,[41,42] probiotics, vitamin E, melatonin, and fiber, used concurrently with DMSA not only provided greater reversal of lead-induced biochemical and physiological damage but significantly increased the excretion of lead itself.[43] Coadministration of NAC with DMSA provided greater lead excretion, likely because cysteine-conjugated DMSA carries the greatest amount of lead from the body.[44] Alpha-lipoic-acid has also been shown to prevent neuronal damage from mercury, as well as increase its excretion. Unfortunately, most of the data are from animal studies where the antioxidant substances were injected into the animals, and therefore little to no data exists on the most beneficial doses of these agents for humans.

Spirulina platensis has been found to protect against toxic metal-induced organ damage and to prevent anemia, leukopenia, and the deposition of metals in the brain. Forty-one patients with chronic arsenic poisoning were randomly treated orally by either placebo or spirulina extract (250 mg) plus zinc (2 mg) twice daily for 16 weeks. There was a sharp increase in urinary excretion of arsenic (138 µg/L) at 4 weeks after spirulina plus zinc administration, and the effect was continued for another 2 weeks. Spirulina extract plus zinc removed 47.1% of arsenic from scalp hair.[45]

Products containing modified citrus pectin plus alginate have been reported to reduce lead and mercury (74% average decrease) in case studies.[46] However, virtually all the data has been from one group of researchers and does not hold up under closer scrutiny.[47]

CHELATABLE TOXICANTS

Aluminum

Aluminum has been shown to accumulate in several mammalian tissues, including the brain, bones, liver, and kidneys. The brain appears to be the most vulnerable to the toxic effects of aluminum, and a potential link has been observed between aluminum and Alzheimer's disease, amyotrophic lateral sclerosis (ALS), and autism spectrum disorders.[48] Aluminum is certainly a potential contributor to the onset, progression, and aggressiveness of neurological disease.[49] Although a causal link has not been proven, several studies have positive outcomes using chelation in the treatment of conditions associated with aluminum overload.

DFO is a trivalent ion chelator that can remove excess iron and/or aluminum from the body. A small-cohort, 2-year, single-blind study of patients with Alzheimer's disease treated with DFO (125 mg intramuscularly twice daily, 5 days per week, for 24 months) demonstrated a significant reduction in the rate of decline of daily living skills in the DFO-treated group compared with the placebo or no-treatment groups.[50] Among hemodialysis patients with aluminum overload, treatment with DFO at both the standard dose (5 mg/kg/week) and low dose (2.5 mg/kg/week) offered similar therapeutic effects and successful treatment response rates.[51]

Lead

Chronic low-level lead exposure is associated with a number of adverse health conditions. No threshold for safety exists. Cumulative lead burden in adults, via bone lead assessment, has been associated with the risk of developing parkinsonism,[52,53] Alzheimer's disease,[54] and decreased cognition.[55] Several studies link childhood learning disorders and neurodevelopmental damage to low-level lead exposure, with some evidence showing decreased IQ in children with supposedly safe (<5 µg/dL) blood concentrations of lead.[56,57,58]

Oral DMSA and oral and parenteral sodium calcium edetate are both effective chelators of lead, and BLLs drop with the use of either CaEDTA or DMSA. CaEDTA and DMSA have been shown to mobilize lead from different compartments, with EDTA primarily mobilizing lead from the trabecular bone, and DMSA primarily mobilizing lead from soft tissue (primarily the kidneys).[59] Studies using DMSA have repeatedly shown that the BLLs rise within 2 weeks of DMSA cessation.[60] The regular release of bone lead into the bloodstream from normal bone turnover daily restores both blood and soft tissue lead levels. For this reason, short-term intermittent use of DMSA is ineffective at reversing neurological dysfunction.[61] Based on this homeostatic balance, the most effective means of achieving long-term reduction of both blood and soft tissue lead levels may be ongoing, rather than intermittent, DMSA therapy.

DMSA is FDA approved as a treatment for lead toxicity. Based on efficacy and safety, DMSA may be the most appropriate oral chelator as a treatment for lead toxicity in children and adults.[62,63] In a case series of 17 lead-poisoned adults, DMSA therapy increased lead excretion on average by a factor of 12.[64] Although DMSA may not have a significant effect on lead in bone, it has been shown to reduce hippocampal lead, which may be more directly relevant to changes in health over time.[65] A combination of both EDTA and DMSA may be more effective than either alone. After controlling for blood lead and weight, lead-exposed workers who received EDTA before DMSA excreted, on average, 1068 µg more lead after DMSA than did workers who did not receive EDTA before the DMSA ($p = 0.0002$).[66]

EDTA chelates lead by displacement of the central calcium ion with lead. Repeated chelation therapy (CaEDTA weekly for 24 months) improved renal function and slowed the progression of renal insufficiency in patients with nondiabetic chronic renal disease and high-normal body lead burdens (at least 80 µg but less than 600 µg).[67] Subjects in this study were included or excluded based on the lead mobilization test. Although chelation with EDTA and DMSA both lowered BLLs, children with acute lead intoxication treated with EDTA appeared, on average, to have 6.47 mg/dL ($p < 0.05$; 95% CI, 0.821–12.12) lower BLL than those treated with DMSA.[68]

Mercury

Mercury is a ubiquitous environmental pollutant and potent neurotoxin. Concerns regarding mercury exposure have increased as sources affecting the general population have also increased. Dental amalgams, fish, air, water, and vaccinations all contain various levels of mercury. Considering mercury is toxic at any level, the cumulative effect of these sources increases the potential for mercury toxicity.

Mercury is often chelated with either DMSA or DMPS. DMSA and DMPS contain two sulfhydryl groups each and possess the critical ability to bind mercury tighter than it is bound to extracellular and intracellular thiols. DMSA is the typical agent of choice because it is less toxic and can be given orally. DMSA primarily moves mercury from the kidneys, which contain the highest mercury concentration in the body,[69] but does not mobilize mercury from amalgams.[70]

Several studies have shown DMSA to be effective at increasing mercury excretion. One study looked at urinary excretion of mercury at various lengths of time after cessation of occupational exposure to mercury vapor. Researchers found a clear correlation between exposure to mercury vapor and mercury levels before and after DMSA.[71] A small study looked at blood and urinary mercury levels associated with fish consumption. Researchers found an increase in blood mercury in proportion to amount of fish eaten, but no difference in baseline between those who ate no fish, those who ate one to two servings a week, and those who ate three or more servings per week. However, they did find significant differences after introduction of DMSA at 30 mg/kg in all groups, with a significantly larger increase in proportion to fish consumption (Fig. 64.1).[72]

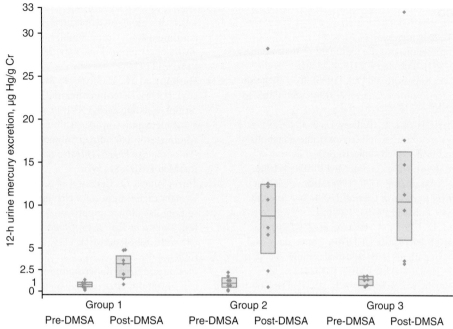

FIG. 64.1 Results of challenge testing according to amount of fish eaten. (From Ruha, A. M., Curry, S. C., Gerkin, R. D., Osterloh, J. D., & Wax, P. M. [2009]. Urine mercury excretion following meso-dimercaptosuccinic acid challenge in fish eaters. *Archives of Pathology & Laboratory Medicine*, *133*[1], 87–92. © 2010 College of American Pathologists.)

A case report of a patient who manifested neurological symptoms 10 years after he was administered mercurials for the treatment of syphilis demonstrated complete resolution of symptoms after long-term EDTA treatment.[73]

NAC used in conjunction with hemodialysis of methylmercury-contaminated human blood was quite effective at enhancing methylmercury clearance from blood.[74] In animal studies, NAC supplementation exhibited a 5- to 10-fold increase in urinary methylmercury excretion compared with controls.[75]

Animal studies have shown DMSA, DMPS, and NAC significantly decrease the mercury levels in placental and fetal tissues of pregnant rats and increase urinary excretion of mercury.[76,77] Renal clearance of DMPS-, DMSA- and NAC-mercury conjugates are all mediated through MRP2 export proteins in the proximal tubules,[78,79] and elimination of mercury is dependent on adequate thiol stores.

DMPS, DMSA, and NAC are similar in their mercury-mobilizing effects. When given separately, DMSA increased urinary mercury excretion by 163%, DMPS by 135%, and NAC by 131%.[80] Neither DMSA or DMPS directly removes central nervous system (CNS) mercury, and both

chelate several trace minerals, although deficiencies have not been noted.[81,82]

DMPS increases the urinary excretion of mercury and reduces mercury concentrations in the kidneys, blood, and brain.[83] DMPS has also shown benefit at reversing mercury-associated symptoms, including tremors, memory loss, insomnia, and metallic taste in the mouth, and demonstrated objective improvements in neurocognitive testing and in rombergism.[84,85]

Arsenic and Cadmium

For both arsenic and cadmium chelation, DMSA is quite useful for acute exposure, but it is unlikely to remove intracellular levels of these toxic metals. In animal studies, the DMSA derivative monoisoamyl dimercaptosuccinic acid (MiADMSA) has been shown to remove arsenic from blood and soft tissue when given with DMSA.[86] However, because arsenic does not bioaccumulate, the need for chelation is small. Similarly, the DMSA derivatives mono-methyl DMSA (MmDMSA) and monocyclohexyl DMSA (MchDMSA) have been shown to reduce total body cadmium with no redistribution of brain cadmium.[87]

REFERENCES

1. Olivieri, N. F., & Brittenham, G. M. (1997). Iron-chelating therapy and the treatment of thalassemia. *Blood*, *89*(7), 2621. PubMed PMID: 9028304.

2. Callender, S. T., & Weatherall, D. J. (1980). Iron chelation with oral desferrioxamine. *Lancet*, *2*(8196), 689. PubMed PMID: 6106796.

3. Summers, M. R., Jacobs, A., Tudway, D., et al. (1979). Studies in desferrioxamine and ferrioxamine metabolism in normal and iron-loaded subjects. *British Journal of Haematology*, *42*(4), 547–555. PubMed PMID: 476006.

4. Hershko, C., & Weatherall, D. J. (1988). Iron-chelating therapy. *Critical Reviews in Clinical Laboratory Sciences*, *26*(4), 303–345. PubMed PMID: 3077034.

5. Cappellini, M. D., Cohen, A., Piga, A., et al. (2006). A phase 3 study of deferasirox (ICL670), a once-daily oral iron chelator, in patients with beta-thalassemia. *Blood*, *107*(9), 3455–3462. PubMed PMID: 16352812.

6. Cohen, A., Martin, M., & Schwartz, E. (1984). Depletion of excessive liver iron stores with desferrioxamine. *British Journal of Haematology*, *58*(2), 369–373. PubMed PMID: 6477838.

7. Brittenham, G. M., Griffith, P. M., Nienhuis, A. W., et al. (1994). Efficacy of deferoxamine in preventing complications of iron overload in patients with thalassemia major. *The New England Journal of Medicine*, *331*(9), 567–573. PubMed PMID: 8047080.

8. Borgna-Pignatti, C., Rugolotto, S., De Stephano, P., et al. (2004). Survival and complications in patients with thalassemia major treated with transfusion and deferoxamine. *Haematologica*, *89*(10), 1187–1193. PubMed PMID: 15477202.

9. Ackrill, P., & Day, J. P. (1985). Desferrioxamine in the treatment of aluminum overload. *Clinical Nephrology*, *24*(Suppl. 1), S94–S97. PubMed PMID: 3842106.

10. Melograna, J. M., & Yokel, R. A. (1984). Effects of subchronic desferrioxamine infusion on aluminum toxicity in rabbits. *Research Communications in Chemical Pathology and Pharmacology*, *44*(3), 411–422. PubMed PMID: 6463364.

11. Julka, D., & Gill, K. D. (1996). Effect of aluminum on regional brain antioxidant defense status in Wistar rats. *Research in Experimental Medicine. Zeitschrift fur Die Gesamte Experimentelle Medizin Einschliesslich Experimenteller Chirurgie*, *196*(3), 187–194. PubMed PMID: 8875705.

12. Savory, J., Herman, M. M., Erasmus, R. T., et al. (1994). Partial reversal of aluminum-induced neurofibrillary degeneration by desferrioxamine in adult male rabbits. *Neuropathology and Applied Neurobiology*, *20*(1), 31–37. PubMed PMID: 8208339.

13. Wax, P. M., & Thornton, C. A. (2000). Recovery from severe arsenic-induced peripheral neuropathy with 2,3-dimercapto-1-propanesulphonic acid. *Journal of Toxicology. Clinical Toxicology*, *38*(7), 777–780. PubMed PMID: 11192465.

14. Hurlbut, K. M., Maiorino, R. M., Mayersohn, M., et al. (1994). Determination and metabolism of dithiol chelating agents XVI: Pharmacokinetics of 2,3-dimercapto-1-propanesulfonate after intravenous administration to human volunteers. *Journal Pharmacology Expert Therapeutics*, *268*(2), 662–668. PubMed PMID: 8113976.

15. Torres-Alanis, O., Garza-Ocanas, L., et al. (2000). Urinary excretion of trace elements in humans after sodium 2,3-dimercaptopropane-1-sulfonate challenge test. *Journal of Toxicology. Clinical Toxicology*, *38*(7), 697–700. PubMed PMID: 11192456.

16. Cohen, J. P., Ruha, A. M., Curry, S. C., et al. (2013). Plasma and urine dimercaptopropanesulfonate concentrations after dermal application of transdermal DMPS (TD-DMPS). *Journal of Medical Toxicology: Official Journal of the American College of Medical Toxicology*, *9*(1), 9–15. PubMed PMID:23143832.

17. Aposhian, H. V., Maiorino, R. M., Rivera, M., et al. (1992). Human studies with the chelating agents, DMPS and DMSA. *Journal of Toxicology. Clinical Toxicology*, *30*(4), 505–528. PubMed PMID: 1331491.

18. Bradberry, S., & Vale, A. (2009). Dimercaptosuccinic acid (succimer; DMSA) in inorganic lead poisoning. *Clinical Toxicology (Philadelphia, Pa.)*, *47*(7), 617–631. PubMed PMID: 19663612.

19. Aposhian, H. V., Maiorino, R. M., Dart, R. C., & Perry, D. F. (1989). Urinary excretion of meso-2,3-dimercaptosuccinic acid in human subjects. *Clinical Pharmacology and Therapeutics*, *45*(5), 520–526. PubMed PMID: 2541962.

20. Graziano, J. H. (1986). Role of 2,3-dimercaptosuccininc acid in the treatment of heavy metal poisoning. *Medical Toxicology*, *1*, 155–162. PubMed PMID:3023784.

21. Aposhian, H. V., Maiorino, R. M., Rivera, M., Bruce, D. C., Cart, R. C., Hurlburt, K. M., et al. (1992). Human studies with the chelating agents DMPS and DMSA. *Clinical Toxicology*, *30*(4), 505–528. PubMed PMID: 1331491.

22. Chisolm, J. J., Jr. (2000). Safety and efficacy of meso-2,3-dimercaptosuccinic acid (DMSA) in children with elevated blood lead concentrations. *Journal of Toxicology. Clinical Toxicology*, *38*(4), 365–375. PubMed PMID: 10930052.

23. Forman, J., Moline, J., Cernichiari, E., et al. (2000). A cluster of pediatric metallic mercury exposure cases treated with meso-2,3-dimercaptosuccinic acid (DMSA).

Environmental Health Perspectives, 108(6), 575–577. PubMed PMID: 10856034.

24. Sigg, T., Burda, A., Leikin, J. B., et al. (1998). A report of pediatric SUCCIMER overdose. *Veterinary and Human Toxicology, 40*(2), 90–91. PubMed PMID: 9554061.

25. Jin, Y., Yu, F., Liao, Y., et al. (2011). Therapeutic efficiency of succimer used with calcium and ascorbic acid in the treatment of mild lead-poisoning. *Environmental Toxicology and Pharmacology, 31*(1), 137–142. PubMed PMID: 21787678.

26. Adams, J. B., Baral, M., Geis, E., et al. (2009). The severity of autism is associated with toxic metal body burden and red blood cell glutathione levels. *Journal Toxicology, 2009*, 532640. PubMed PMID: 20107587.

27. Adams, J. B., Baral, M., Geis, E., et al. (2009). Safety and efficacy of oral DMSA therapy for children with autism spectrum disorders: Part A – medical results. *BMC Clinical Pharmacology, 9*, 16. PubMed PMID: 19852789.

28. Martin, B. L. (1999). Development of a scale for the comparison of metals in enzyme action. *Journal of Inorganic Biochemistry, 75*(4), 245–254. PubMed PMID: 10532851.

29. Lanigan, R. S., & Yamarik, T. A. (2002). Final report on the safety assessment of EDTA, calcium disodium EDTA, diammonium EDTA, dipotassium EDTA, disodium EDTA, TEA-EDTA, tetrasodium EDTA, tripotassium EDTA, trisodium EDTA, HEDTA, and trisodium HEDTA. *International Journal of Toxicology, 21*(Suppl. 2), 95–142. PubMed PMID: 12396676.

30. Wedeen, R. P., D'Haese, P., Van de Vyver, F. L., et al. (1986). Lead nephropathy. *American Journal of Kidney Diseases, 8*(5), 380–383. PubMed PMID: 3098095.

31. Craswell, P. W., Price, J., Boyle, P. D., et al. (1986). Chronic lead nephropathy in Queensland: Alternative methods of diagnosis. *Australian and New Zealand Journal of Medicine, 16*(1), 11–19. PubMed PMID: 3085647.

32. Yokoyama, K., Araki, S., & Aono, H. (1988). Reversibility of psychological performance in subclinical lead absorption. *Neurotoxicology, 9*(3), 405–410. PubMed PMID: 3200509.

33. Araki, S., Murata, K., & Aono, H. (1986). Subclinical cervico-spino-bulbar effects of lead: A study of short-latency somatosensory evoked potentials in workers exposed to lead, zinc, and copper. *American Journal of Industrial Medicine, 10*(2), 164–175. PubMed PMID: 3019134.

34. Weiss, B., Cory-Slechta, D. A., & Cox, C. (1990). Modification of lead distribution by diethyldithiocarbamate. *Fundamental and Applied Toxicology, 15*(4), 791–799. PubMed PMID: 1964918.

35. Cory-Slechta, D. A., Weiss, B., & Cox, C. (1987). Mobilization and redistribution of lead over the course of calcium disodium ethylenediamine tetraacetate chelation therapy. *The Journal of Pharmacology and Experimental Therapeutics, 243*(3), 804–813. PubMed PMID: 3121845.

36. Lin-Tan, D. T., Lin, J. L., Yen, T. H., et al. (2007). Long-term outcome of repeated lead chelation therapy in progressive non-diabetic chronic kidney diseases. *Nephrology, Dialysis, Transplantation, 22*(10), 2924–2931. PubMed PMID: 17556414.

37. Borgstrom, L., Kagedal, B., & Paulsen, O. (1986). Pharmakokinetics of N-acetylcysteine in man. *European Journal of Clinical Pharmacology, 31*(2), 217–222. PubMed PMID: 3803419.

38. Hannestad, U., & Sorbo, B. (1979). Determination of 3-mercaptolactate, mercaptoacetate and N-acetylcysteine in urine by gas chromatography. *Clinica Chimica Acta, 95*(2), 189–200. PubMed PMID: 527218.

39. Hjortso, E., Fomsgaard, J. S., Fogh-Andersen, N., & Does, N. (1990). acetylcysteine increase the excretion of trace metals (calcium, magnesium, iron, zinc, and copper) when given orally? *European Journal of Clinical Pharmacology, 39*(1), 29–31. PubMed PMID: 2276385.

40. Aremu, D. A., Madejczyk, M. S., & Ballatori, N. (2008). N-acetylcysteine as a potential antidote and biomonitoring agent of methylmercury exposure. *Environmental Health Perspectives, 116*(1), 26–31. PubMed PMID: 18197295.

41. Pande, M., & Flora, S. J. (2002). Lead induced oxidative damage and its response to combined administration of alpha-lipoic acid and succimers in rats. *Toxicology, 177*(2–3), 187–196. PubMed PMID: 12135622.

42. Sivaprasad, R., Nagaraj, M., & Varalakshmi, P. (2004). Combined efficacies of lipoic acid and 2,3-dimercaptosuccinic acid against lead-induced lipid peroxidation in rat liver. *The Journal of Nutritional Biochemistry, 15*(1), 18–23. PubMed PMID: 14711456.

43. Flora, S. J., Pande, M., & Mehta, A. (2003). Beneficial effect of combined administration of some naturally occurring antioxidants (vitamins) and thiol chelators in the treatment of chronic lead intoxication. *Chemico-Biological Interactions, 145*(3), 267–280. PubMed PMID: 12732454.

44. Flora, S. J., Pande, M., Kannan, G. M., & Mehta, A. (2004). Lead induced oxidative stress and its recovery following co-administration of melatonin or N-acetylcysteine during chelation with succimer in male rats. *Cellular and Molecular Biology (Noisy-Le-Grand, France), 50*, PubMed PMID: 15555419.

45. Misbahuddin, M., Islam, A. Z., Khandker, S., et al. (2006). Efficacy of spirulina extract plus zinc in patients of chronic arsenic poisoning: A randomized placebo-controlled study. *Clinical Toxicology (Philadelphia, Pa.), 44*(2), 135–141. PubMed PMID: 16615668.

46. Eliaz, I., Weil, E., & Wilk, B. (2007). Integrative medicine and the role of modified citrus pectin/alginates in heavy metal chelation and detoxification – five case reports. *Forsch Komplementmed, 14*(6), 358–364. PubMed PMID: 18219211.

47. Crinnion, W. (2008). Is modified citrus pectin an effective mobilizer of heavy metals in humans? *Alternative Medicine Review: A Journal of Clinical Therapeutic, 13*(4), 283–286. PubMed PMID: 19238763.

48. Shaw, C. A., & Tomljenovic, L. (2013). Aluminum in the central nervous system (CNS): Toxicity in humans and animals, vaccine adjuvants, and autoimmunity. *Immunologic Research, 56*(2–3), 304–316. PubMed PMID: 23609067.

49. Exley, C. (2014). What is the risk of aluminum as a neurotoxin? *Expert Review of Neurotherapeutics, 14*(6), 589–591. PubMed PMID: 24779346.

50. Crapper McLachlan, D. R., Dalton, A. J., et al. (1991). Intramuscular desferrioxamine in patients with Alzheimer's disease. *Lancet, 337*(8757), 1618. PubMed PMID: 1674295.

51. Kan, W. C., Chien, C. C., Wu, C. C., et al. (2010). Comparison of low-dose deferoxamine versus standard-dose deferoxamine for treatment of aluminum overload among haemodialysis patients. *Nephrology, Dialysis, Transplantation, 25*(5), 1604–1608. PubMed PMID: 19948879.

52. Coon, S., Stark, A., Peterson, E., Gloi, A., et al. (2006). Whole-body lifetime occupational lead exposure and risk of Parkinson's disease. *Environmental Health Perspectives, 114*(12), 1872–1876. PubMed PMID: 17185278.

53. Weisskopf, M. G., Weuve, J., Nie, H., et al. (2010). Association of cumulative lead exposure with Parkinson's disease. *Environmental Health Perspectives, 118*(11), 1609–1613. PubMed PMID: 20807691.

54. Bakulski, K. M., Rozek, L. S., Dolinoy, D. C., Paulson, H. L., & Hu, H. (2012). Alzheimer's disease and environmental exposure to lead: The epidemiologic evidence and potential role of epigenetics. *Current Alzheimer Research, 9*(5), 564–573. PubMed PMID: 22272628.

55. Shih, R. A., Glass, T. A., Bandeen-Roche, K., Carlson, M. C., Bolla, K. I., Todd, A. C., et al. (2006). Environmental lead exposure and cognitive function in community-dwelling older adults. *Neurology, 67*(9), 1556–1562. PubMed PMID: 16971698.

56. Tuthill, R. (1996). Hair lead levels related to children's classroom attention deficit behavior. *Archives of Environmental Health, 51*(3), 214–220. PubMed PMID: 8687242.

57. Needleman, H., Schell, A., Bellinger, D., et al. (1990). The long-term effects of exposure to low doses of lead in childhood. *The New England Journal of Medicine, 322*(2), 83–88. PubMed PMID: 2294437.

58. Iqbal, S., Muntner, P., Batuman, V., & Rabito, F. A. (2008). Estimated burden of blood lead levels 5 μg/dl in 1999-2002 and declines from 1988 to 1994. *Environmental Research, 107*(3), 305–311. PubMed PMID: 18339369.

59. Bradberry, S., & Vale, A. (2009). A comparison of sodium calcium edetate (edetate calcium disodium) and succimer (DMSA) in the treatment of inorganic lead poisoning. *Clinical Toxicology (Philadelphia, Pa.), 47*(9), 841–858. PubMed PMID: 19852620.

60. Chisolm, J. J., Jr. (2000). Safety and efficacy of meso-2,3-dimercaptosuccinic acid (DMSA) in children with elevated blood lead concentrations. *Journal of Toxicology. Clinical Toxicology, 38*(4), 365–375. PubMed PMID: 10930052.

61. Dietrich, K. N., Ware, J. H., Salganik, M., et al. (2004). Treatment of Lead-Exposed Children Clinical Trial Group. Effect of chelation therapy on the neuropsychological and behavioral development of lead-exposed children after school entry. *Pediatrics, 114*(1), 19–26. PubMed PMID: 15231903.

62. Chisolm, J. J., Jr. (2000). Safety and efficacy of meso-2, 3-dimercaptosuccinic acid (DMSA) in children with elevated blood lead concentrations. *Journal of Toxicology. Clinical Toxicology, 38*(4), 365–375. PubMed PMID: 10930052.

63. Fournier, L., Thomas, G., Garner, R., et al. (1988). 2, 3-dimercaptosuccinic acid treatment of heavy metal poisoning in humans. *Medical Toxicology and Adverse Drug Experience, 3*(6), 499–504. PubMed PMID: 2851085.

64. Bradberry, S., Sheehan, T., & Vale, A. (2009). Use of oral dimercaptosuccinic acid (succimer) in adult patients with inorganic lead poisoning. *QJM: Monthly Journal of the Association of Physicians, 102*(10), 721–732. PubMed PMID: 19700440.

65. Zhang, J., Wang, X. F., Lu, Z. B., et al. (2004). The effects of meso-2,3-dimercaptosuccinic acid and oligomeric procyanidins on acute lead neurotoxicity in rat hippocampus. *Free Radical Biology & Medicine, 37*(7), 1037–1050. PubMed PMID: 15336320.

66. Lee, B. K., Schwartz, B. S., Stewart, W., & Ahn, K. D. (1995). Provocative chelation with DMSA and EDTA: Evidence for differential access to lead storage sites. *Occupational and Environmental Medicine, 52*(1), 13–19. PubMed PMID: 7697134.

67. Lin, J. L., Lin-Tan, D. T., Hsu, K. H., & Yu, C. C. (2003). Environmental lead exposure and progression of chronic renal diseases in patients without diabetes. *The New England Journal of Medicine, 348*(4), 277–286. PubMed PMID: 12540640.

68. Tantanasrikul, S., Chaivisuth, B., Siriratanapreuk, S., et al. (2002). The management of environmental lead exposure in the pediatric population: Lessons from Clitty Creek, Thailand. *Journal of the Medical Association of Thailand, 85*(Suppl. 2), S762–S768. PubMed PMID: 12403258.

69. Roels, H. A., Boeckx, M., Ceulemans, E., & Lauwerys, R. R. (1991). Urinary excretion of mercury after occupational exposure to mercury vapour and influence of the chelating agent meso-2,3-dimercaptosuccinic acid (DMSA). *British Journal of Industrial Medicine, 48*(4), 247–253. PubMed PMID: 1851035.

70. Aposhian, H. V., Bruce, D. C., Alter, W., et al. (1992). Urinary mercury after administration of 2,3-dimercaptopropane-1-sulfonic acid: Correlation with dental amalgam score. *FASEB Journal : Official Publication of the Federation of American Societies for Experimental Biology, 6*(7), 2472–2476. PubMed PMID: 1563599.

71. Roels, H. A., Boeckx, M., Ceulemans, E., & Lauwerys, R. R. (1991). Urinary excretion of mercury after occupational exposure to mercury vapour and influence of the chelating agent meso-2,3-dimercaptosuccinic acid (DMSA). *British Journal of Industrial Medicine, 48*(4), 247–253. PubMed PMID: 1851035.

72. Ruha, A. M., Curry, S. C., Gerkin, R. D., et al. (2009). Urine mercury excretion following meso-dimercaptosuccinic acid challenge in fish eaters. *Archives of Pathology & Laboratory Medicine, 133*(1), 87–92. 19123743.

73. Corsello, S., Fulgenzi, A., Vietti, D., & Ferrero, M. E. (2009). The usefulness of chelation therapy for the remission of symptoms caused by previous treatment with mercury-containing pharmaceuticals: A case report. *Cases Journal, 2*, 199. PubMed PMID: 19946446.

74. Lund, M. E., Banner, W., Jr., Clarkson, T. W., et al. (1984). Treatment of acute methylmercury ingestion by hemodialysis with N-acetylcysteine (Mucomyst) infusion and 2,3-dimercaptopropane sulfonate. *Journal of Toxicology. Clinical Toxicology, 22*(1), 31–49. PubMed PMID: 6492229.

75. Ballatori, N., Lieberman, M. W., & Wang, W. (1998). N-acetylcysteine as an antidote in methylmercury poisoning. *Environmental Health Perspectives, 106*(5), 267–271. PubMed PMID: 9520359.

76. Bridges, C. C., Joshee, L., & Zalups, R. K. (2008). MRP2 and the DMPS- and DMSA-mediated elimination of mercury in TR(-) and control rats exposed to thiol S-conjugates of inorganic mercury. *Toxicological Sciences, 105*(1), 211–220. PubMed PMID: 18511429.

77. Bridges, C. C., Joshee, L., & Zalups, R. K. (2009). Effect of DMPS and DMSA on the placental and fetal disposition of methylmercury. *Placenta, 30*(9), 800–805. PubMed PMID: 19615742.

78. Zalups, R. K., & Bridges, C. C. (2009). MRP2 involvement in renal proximal tubular elimination of methylmercury mediated by DMPS or DMSA. *Toxicology and Applied Pharmacology, 235*(1), 10–17. PubMed PMID: 19063911.

79. Zalups, R. K., & Bridges, C. C. (2012). Relationships between the renal handling of DMPS and DMSA and the renal handling of mercury. *Chemical Research in Toxicology, 25*(9), 1825–1838. PubMed PMID: 22667351.

80. Hibberd, A. R., Howard, M. A., & Hunnisett, A. G. (1998). Mercury from dental amalgam fillings: Studies on oral chelating agents for assessing and reducing mercury burdens in humans. *Journal of Nutritional & Environmental Medicine, 8*, 219–231.

81. Aposhian, H. V. (1983). DMSA and DMPS-water soluble antidotes for heavy metal poisoning. *Annual Review of Pharmacology and Toxicology, 23*, 193–215. PubMed PMID: 6307120.

82. Flora, S. J., Mittal, M., & Mehta, A. (2008). Heavy metal induced oxidative stress and its possible reversal by chelation therapy. *The Indian Journal of Medical Research, 128*(4), 501–523. PubMed PMID: 19106443.

83. Pingree, S. D., Simmonds, P. L., & Woods, J. S. (2001). Effects of 2,3-dimercapto-1-propanesulfonic acid (DMPS) on tissue and urine mercury levels following prolonged methylmercury exposure in rats. *Toxicological Sciences, 61*(2), 224–233. PubMed PMID: 11353131.

84. Böse-O'Reilly, S., Drasch, G., Beinhoff, C., et al. (2003). The Mt. Diwata study on the Philippines 2000-treatment of mercury intoxicated inhabitants of a gold mining area with DMPS (2,3-dimercapto-1-propane-sulfonic acid, Dimaval). *The Science of the Total Environment, 307*(1–3), 71–82. PubMed PMID:12711426.

85. Bradberry, S. M., Sheehan, T. M., Barraclough, C. R., & Vale, J. A. (2009). DMPS can reverse the features of severe mercury vapor-induced neurological damage. *Clinical Toxicology (Philadelphia, Pa.), 47*(9), 894–898. PubMed PMID:19852623.

86. Bhadauria, S., & Flora, S. J. S. (2007). Response of arsenic-induced oxidative stress, DNA damage, and metal imbalance to combined administration of DMSA and monoisoamyl-DMSA during chronic arsenic poisoning in rats. *Cell Biology and Toxicology*, *23*(2), 91–104. PubMed PMID: 17086449.

87. Jones, M. M., Singh, P. K., Gale, G. R., et al. (1992). Cadmium mobilization in vivo by intraperitoneal or oral administration of mono alkyl esters of meso 2,3-dimercaptosuccinic acid in the mouse. *Pharmacology and Toxicology*, *70*(5 Pt. 1), 336–343. PubMed PMID: 1319053.

65

Nutritional Supplementation for Environmental Toxins and Toxicants

SUMMARY

- Supplementation to enhance biotransformation and excretion
- Supplementation to ameliorate toxicant-induced damage
- Enhancing antioxidant activity
- Supplementation to repair tissue damage and enhance organ function

OVERVIEW

Proper avoidance techniques and depuration protocols will successfully reduce the total body burden of toxic environmental compounds. In addition to those approaches, supplementation is necessary to help restore cellular and tissue function. All of the common pollutants are powerful prooxidants that cause oxidative damage to tissues and cells, and most appear to also be antiantioxidants through reduction of cellular antioxidants and antioxidant enzyme levels. Compounds that enhance glutathione (GSH) production or GSH enzyme function and that protect against toxicant-induced depletion of the these elements are most effective at blocking or reversing cell and tissue damage from environmental contaminants. A number of compounds that are protective against a host of pollutants are known to be powerful antioxidants, inducers of biotransformation function, and enhancers of antioxidant enzyme activity. Many of these same natural compounds have shown to be highly effective at preventing the common toxicant-induced illnesses that are covered in Section III of this book. Polyphenols commonly found in many traditional diets appear to be some of the most active antitoxicant compounds. Individuals with higher levels of polyphenols in their urine have lower levels of oxidized glutathione (GSSG) and less oxidative damage to their DNA reflected by lower urinary 8-hydroxy-2′-deoxyquanosine (8-OHdG)

levels.[1] The food groups most significantly associated with these benefits were fruits, chocolate, and vegetables. The intake of Brassica family vegetables is inversely related to urinary F2-isoprostane levels, a marker for tissue lipid peroxidation damage.[2]

MOST COMMON NATURAL ANTITOXICANT COMPOUNDS

- Antioxidant nutrients—vitamins C and E, selenium
- N-acetyl cysteine (NAC) and magnesium
- Green tea—*Camelia sinensis*
- Curcumin—*Turmeric longa*
- Anthocyanins (dark berries)
- Brassica family of vegetables
- *Ginkgo biloba*
- Quercetin
- Omega-3 oils

A fairly small number of common food, spices, and nutrients provide powerful protection against the toxic tissue damage from ubiquitous pollutants (Fig. 56.3). Virtually all of these compounds are already well known among naturopathic and alternative medical practitioners as potent antioxidants. NAC, a stable form of cysteine, is known to have a wide range of health-promoting and disease-reversing actions for a variety of tissues and organs in the human body. NAC is one of the prime antioxidant nutrients that has been proven effective against some of the most commonly encountered pollutants. Magnesium, a mineral normally only associated with blood pressure reduction and muscular and neurological relaxation, is also found to be quite beneficial for protection against a number of toxic compounds, as are vitamins C and E. However, the most versatile and powerful antitoxicant compounds are the commonly consumed Brassica family of vegetables, green tea, and curcumin. All of these botanicals contain compounds that have both antioxidant action and the ability to enhance biotransformation and excretion of toxic pollutants.

ENHANCEMENT OF BIOTRANSFORMATION AND EXCRETION

Phase 1: CYP and Other Common Oxidase Enzymes

- High-protein, low-carbohydrate, low-fat diet
- Magnesium

Nutrition and pollutant burden can easily affect the basic requirements for cytochrome (CYP) function. Protein deficiency has long been linked to reduced hepatic levels of CYP-450, nicotinamide adenine dinucleotide phosphate (NADPH)-cytochrome P450 reductase, cytochrome b5 reductase, hepatic GSH stores, and longer half-life for a variety of compounds.[3,4,5,6] Protein deficiency predisposes to increased toxicity from malathion and hexachlorocyclohexane,[7] whereas a high-protein diet, with lower fat and carbohydrate intake, improves phase 1 function.[8,9] A high-sugar diet inhibits phase 1 drug clearance as effectively as cimetidine, a known CYP inhibitor.[10] Magnesium deficiency is associated with reduced levels of CYP-450 and NADPH-cytochrome reductase and decreased biotransformation of aniline and aminopyrene.[11,12,13,14] Adenosine triphosphate (ATP) levels, vital for phases 1, 2, and 3, are often reduced by toxic xenobiotics (see Chapter 45)

Phase 1: Paraoxonase

- Components of the Mediterranean diet
- Anthocyanins
- Quercitin
- Exercise

A number of diet and lifestyle factors already associated with reducing cardiovascular risk also increase PON1 activity, even in those with a low PON1 genotype. Regular aerobic and anaerobic exercise both increase PON1 activity.[15,16] The Mediterranean diet, long known

to reduce cardiovascular risk,[17] also improves paraoxonase 1 (PON1) activity.[18] Omega-3 oils, present in the Mediterranean diet through fish consumption, has been shown to improve PON1 activity by itself.[19] Olive oil, another prime component of this diet, increases paraoxonase activity as well.[20] Anthocyanins, the dark pigment in grapes, wine, and berries, have also demonstrated the ability to boost PON1 activity.[21,22] Quercetin,[23] high in onions, along with walnuts[24] and coconut oil,[25] are also effective in boosting the activity of this important enzyme. Interestingly, acetylsalicylic acid, commonly recommended to be taken daily for prevention of a heart attack, also increases PON1 activity.[26]

ENHANCING PON1 ACTIVITY (EVEN WITH LOW-ACTIVITY PON1 SNPS)	
Exercise	Anthocyanins
Mediterranean diet	Quercetin
Olive oil	Walnuts
Fish oil	Aspirin
Coconut oil	

Phase 2: Conjugation

Amino acid conjugation, glucuronidation, and GSH conjugation are the three phase 2 pathways that are most active in clearing environmental pollutants from the body.

Amino Acid Conjugation

- Glycine
- Taurine

Amino acid conjugation is the main pathway by which solvents are cleared from the body. The primary amino acids used in this pathway are glycine and taurine. Supplementation with these is often needed for individuals with daily exposure to solvents (including all urban dwellers who are exposed daily to vehicular exhaust).

Glucuronidation

- Glucuronates (high in *Brassica* sp.)
- Enhanced by high-protein, low-carb diet
- *Brassica* sp., green tea, and quercetin induce uridine diphosphate glucuronyltransferase (UDPGT) activity
- *Bifidobacteria longum* and *Lactobacillus rhamnosus* reduce β-glucuronidase activity in the intestines

Glucuronidation is the prime phase 2 pathway for endogenous compounds like bilirubin, estrone, testosterone, progesterone, and thyroxine. Glucuronidation has a

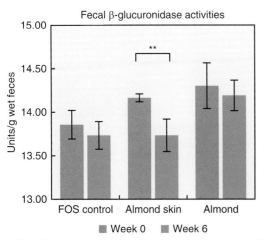

FIG. 65.1 β-glucuronidase levels before (purple) and after (teal) treatment in persons receiving FOS, almond skins, or roasted almonds daily for 6 weeks. (From Liu, Z., Lin, X., Huang, G., Zhang, W., Rao, P., & Ni, L. [2014]. Prebiotic effects of almonds and almond skins on intestinal microbiota in healthy adult humans. *Anaerobe, 26*, 1–6.)

high capacity for xenobiotics but a low affinity, so only a few exogenous compounds like tetrahydrocannabinol, some aromatic hydrocarbons, and carbamate pesticides are glucuronidated. Activity of glucuronyl transferases (UDPGT) is increased by *Brassica* sp.[27,28] and quercetin.[29]

Supplementation with yogurt,[30] *Lactobacillus rhamnosus*,[31] and *Bifidobacterium longum*[32] individually have all reduced intestinal β-glucuronidase levels, potentially conferring a degree of cancer protection. Adults who consumed either 8 g of fructooligosaccharides, 10 g of almond skins, or 56 g of almonds daily all experienced an increase in bifidobacteria and lactobacilli populations and a reduction in β-glucuronidase levels, with the almond skins showing the greatest benefit (Fig. 65.1).[33] Silymarin,[34] extracts of chokeberry, honeysuckle,[35] and purple rice[36] have all successfully reduced β-glucuronidase levels. Calcium glucuronate supplements have been used widely in the alternative medicine community for this purpose as well.[37] The Brassica family, known to induce UDPGT activity, is also naturally high in calcium glucuronates and would be an excellent first choice to enhance the activity of this system.

Glutathione

- NAC
- Magnesium
- Liposomal GSH
- Curcumin
- Green tea
- Other botanicals

Exposure to virtually all of the environmental toxins and toxicants results in a decrease in cellular and tissue levels of GSH. Fortunately, numerous supplements have proven an ability to increase GSH levels, even in the face of toxicant exposures (Fig. 65.2). NAC, a powerful antioxidant in its own right, provides cysteine, the preferred substrate for *de novo* synthesis of GSH. Supplementation of NAC to individuals with functioning glutamyl cysteine ligase (GCLC) and GSH synthase (GS) results in a significant increase in GSH levels.[38] Magnesium is necessary for both steps in *de novo* GSH synthesis, and a deficiency of magnesium is associated with low GSH levels,[39] whereas magnesium supplementation increases GSH.[40] The use of liposomal GSH supplementation has proven highly effective in humans to increase GSH levels and rebalance cytokine levels.[41]

A number of the most commonly used antitoxicant botanicals have all been shown to enhance the function of the GSH synthesizing enzymes to increase GSH levels. Included in these are curcumin,[42,43] rosemary,[44] green tea polyphenols,[45] and milk thistle.[46] Ginkgo,[47] *Bacopa moneira*,[48] and quercetin[49] also increase GSH levels through mechanisms that are not yet clear.

After GSH is synthesized, it can be used in a number of ways. It is a powerful quencher of free radicals that can act on its own or with glutathione peroxidase (whose cofactor is selenium). Once GSH has become oxidized (GSSG), it can be recycled to reduce GSH via GSH reductase enzyme, which does not work well when there is high oxidative stress. GSH can also be conjugated with phase 1 metabolites by any of the different glutathione transferase (GST) enzymes (M1, P1, T1, O1), forming mercapturic acids. Numerous botanical agents, full of powerful antioxidant compounds, have beneficial effects on many of the GSH enzymes simultaneously (Table 65.1).

AMELIORATION OF SPECIFIC TOXICANT-INDUCED DAMAGE

Metals

- Methyl donors
  - S-adenosyl-L-methionine (SAMe), methylfolate, folate, methylcobalamin, L-methionine

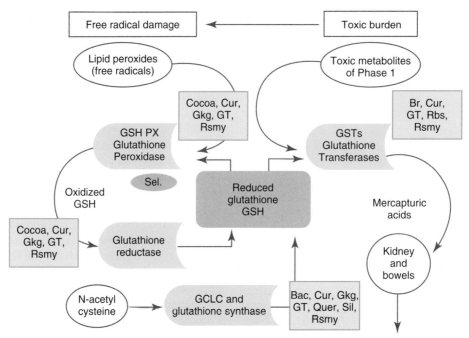

FIG. 65.2 Glutathione pathways, enzymes, cofactors, and botanical agents that increase enzyme functions: Bacopa moneira *(Bac)*, *Brassica* sp. *(Br)*, curcumin *(Cur)*, ginkgo *(Gkg)*, green tea *(GT)*, quercitin *(Quer)*, silymarin *(Sil)*, rooibos *(Rbs)*, and rosemary *(Rsmy)*.

TABLE 65.1	Botanical Agents that Enhance Glutathione Enzymatic Functions		
GCLC + GS	**Glutathione Peroxidase**	**Glutathione Reductase**	**Glutathione Transferases**
• Bacopa[48]	• Cocoa[175]	• Cocoa[180]	• Broccoli family[185]
• Curcumin[42,43]	• Curcumin[176]	• Curcumin[181]	• Curcumin[186]
• Ginkgo[47]	• Ginkgo[177]	• Green tea[182]	• Green tea[187]
• Green tea[45]	• Green tea[178]	• Rooibos[183]	• Rooibos[188]
• Milk thistle[46]	• Rosemary[179]	• Rosemary[184]	• Rosemary[189]
• Rosemary[44]			

- Vitamins C and E
- Lean protein
- Brassica family
- Curcumin
- Green and black teas

Arsenic. A number of natural supplements improve the methylation and excretion of inorganic arsenic and prevent or reverse arsenic-related tissue damage. SAMe, folate, methylfolate, methylcobalamin, and L-methionine all enhance the methylation of inorganic arsenic.[50] In an animal model, supplementation with vitamins C and E prevented almost all arsenic-induced oxidative damage, in part by maintaining intracellular GSH stores.[51] Mexican women consuming higher levels of those vitamins along with zinc, selenium, and vitamin C have lower levels of monomethylarsonous acid (+3) (MMA), more dimethylarsinous acid (+3) (DMA), and less toxicity from arsenic (Chapter 9).[52] Methylcobalamin and GSH are able to nonenzymatically enhance double methylation of inorganic arsenic, dramatically reducing its toxicity.[53] Daily folic acid supplementation at a dose of 800 μg daily has been shown in volunteers to significantly lower blood arsenic levels.[54]

Several common dietary components have demonstrated benefit in dealing with arsenic, including protein, Brassica-family vegetables, and some botanical agents. A good quality-protein level in the diet demonstrated effectiveness at increasing the excretion of inorganic arsenicals.[5] Members of the Brassica family of vegetables, rich sources of sulforaphane compounds, appear to prevent cellular damage from arsenic.[55,56] One of the most commonly used dietary spices is turmeric *(Curcuma longa)*, which contains the flavonoid curcumin. Curcumin has multiple beneficial effects against arsenic, including enhancing the double methylation and excretion of inorganic arsenic and reversing arsenic-induced cellular damage.[57,58,59] DNA damage from arsenic is a marker of genotoxicity and results in elevated urinary levels of 8-OHdG. The consumption of high-arsenic groundwater has been directly linked to an increase in urinary 8-OHdG levels in a population in West Bengal, India. However, when individuals from this area supplemented with 1 g of curcumin daily for 3 months, the 8-OHdG level dropped, indicating a dramatic reduction in arsenic-induced DNA oxidative damage.[60] Daily intake of green and black teas have also been shown to reverse arsenic-induced cytotoxicity and genotoxicity.[61,62] Green tea, and to a lesser extent vitamin C, prevent neurological damage from arsenic.[63] This benefit seems to be related to both the epigallocatechin gallate (EGCG) and theaflavin contents of these teas. Both *Aloe vera* and *Centella asiatica* have demonstrated the ability to ameliorate arsenic-induced oxidative damage as well.[64,65]

Cadmium

- NAC
- α-lipoic acid (ALA)
- Selenium
- Magnesium
- Carnosine
- Garlic, onions, nutmeg
- Quercetin
- Blueberries, anthocyanins

NAC and ALA reverse cadmium-induced oxidative damage. ALA restores cadmium-induced depletion of GSH in the liver and throughout the body by enhancing GCLC the enzyme primarily responsible for making GSH.[66] ALA is equally effective as intravenous GSH in restoring cadmium-induced hematological imbalances[67] and oxidative damage in renal tissues.[68] ALA and selenium were both effective at reversing testicular damage from

cadmium and restoring testosterone levels.[69] Furthermore, the combination of ALA and melatonin exert a synergistic effect against cadmium-induced cardiotoxicity.[70]

Both magnesium and carnosine are effective at preventing and reversing cadmium-induced cellular and tissue damage. Magnesium supplementation helps lower cadmium tissue levels and restores cadmium-induced GSH loss.[71] Carnosine prevented hepatotoxicity from cadmium in mice through preventing GSH depletion and reversing the cadmium-induced increase in myeloperoxidase and caspace-3 activities.[72]

Anthocyan-containing botanical agents like grape skins and grape juice are protective against multiple parameters of cadmium toxicity.[73,74,75,76] Blueberries are also quite high in polyphenolic compounds and have demonstrated effectiveness against cadmium-induced cytotoxicity.[77] When given concurrently with cadmium exposure, blueberry extract prevented increases in oxidative stress and maintained antioxidant enzyme activity in a dose-dependent manner. Onion extract along with quercetin (onions being the highest dietary source of this flavonoid) have both demonstrated the ability to reverse cadmium-induced toxicity and dyslipidemia.[78,79] More recently, a spice mixture containing garlic, ginger, and nutmeg at levels used in cooking was able to protect rats from cadmium-induced hepatic and renal damage.[80]

Mercury

- NAC
- Zinc, selenium, vitamin E
- Curcumin
- *Brassica* sp.

NAC acts on the phase 3 membrane-bound efflux pumps in the kidneys to increase the excretion of methylmercury (MeHg) from the body.[81,82] NAC has demonstrated both protection against and reversal of mercury-induced cellular and tissue damage throughout the body, especially when used in combination with selenium and zinc.[83,84] Both zinc[85] and selenium[86] have shown benefit by themselves in blocking mercury-induced hepatic and neurological damage, as has vitamin E.[87] The benefits of NAC includes restoration of GSH levels and antioxidant enzyme activities along with reducing elevated levels of alanine transaminase (ALT). MeHg neurotoxicity via reduced DNA synthesis and apoptotic activity have both been blocked and reversed by NAC supplementation.[88] It also offers protection to the neurons and astrocytes by repleting the GSH content in those cells.[89] NAC has demonstrated effectiveness at protecting both the kidneys and pancreatic beta cells from mercury-induced oxidative damage.[90,91,92] NAC appears to be a highly valuable supplement for mercury-exposed persons.

Curcumin has exhibited multiple benefits against mercury. At a dose of 80 mg/kg, it was shown to reduce peroxide levels; increase GSH; and restore the activity of catalase, GSH peroxidase, and superoxide dismutase.[93] Both before and after mercury exposure, consumption of curcumin reduced levels of mercury in the liver, kidney, and brain, making this botanical a possible safe alternative for persons who cannot take the sulfhydryl-containing DMSA or DMPS. *Ginkgo biloba* was able to restore depleted GSH levels and reduce malondialdehyde levels and myeloperoxidase activity in animals exposed to mercury.[94]

Methionine has shown benefit in reducing MeHg transport into the brain,[95] and several studies have shown the benefit of selenium supplementation.[96,97,98] ALA has been shown to ameliorate the neural oxidative damage caused by mercury.[99] However, controversy around the use of ALA with mercury exists because of an animal study that used both intravenous MeHg and intravenous ALA.[100] In this study, the lowest dose of ALA (37.5 μmol/kg) doubled the excretion of MeHg, but each doubling of the ALA dose caused a marked reduction of MeHg excretion, with the highest dose (300 μmol/kg) effectively blocking MeHg release. Upon autopsy, the MeHg-exposed animals who were also given ALA had higher MeHg concentrations in their brain tissue.

Dietary factors that ameliorate mercury toxicity include the sulforaphanes from the Brassica family, which may be able to prevent mercury-induced neurotoxicity.[101] Tea polyphenols can also prevent neurotoxicity from methylmercury to some degree.[102]

Lead

- NAC
- ALA
- Vitamins C and E
- SAMe
- L-methionine
- Zinc
- Curcumin and garlic

In addition to the benefit of reducing the total body lead burden, CaEDTA therapy has also been shown to reverse the prooxidant effects of lead.[103] These effects included a restoration of superoxide dismutase (SOD) and catalase

levels, a reduction of malondialdehyde levels, improved PON1 function, and a reversal of the depression of acetylcholinesterase activity.

The use of antioxidant compounds as stand-alone agents (not in conjunction with DMSA or CaEDTA) has demonstrated effectiveness in reversing lead-induced damage.[104] Because lead can never be completely cleared from the body, the ability to prevent and reverse cellular and tissue damage from lead becomes a critical point for persons with lead-associated health problems. This should be kept in mind when working with any Boomer-generation adult who is experiencing increased bone turnover. Both dietary-based antioxidants and antioxidant supplementation appear to be effective in this regard.[105] The best documented of these nutrients is N-acetyl cysteine (NAC), which powerfully reverses the oxidative stress after lead exposures. This compound has repeatedly shown benefit in improving biochemical and physiological markers in lead workers and has been successful in lowering blood lead levels (BLLs).[106] Oral NAC doses of only 400 and 800 mg daily in lead workers resulted in statistically significant reductions in BLLs.[107] Other antioxidants that have demonstrated effectiveness at reversing cellular and tissue damage from lead include vitamins C and E, L-methionine, zinc, melatonin, and ALA. The most impressive results were found with SAMe, which was able to improve cognition and learning in lead-poisoned animals.[108] Higher serum vitamin C levels are independently associated with decreased prevalence of elevated BLLs.[109] Lead workers (average BLL of 73 μg/dL) consuming only 1000 mg of vitamin C and 400 IU of vitamin E daily experienced a significant reduction of oxidative damage even with high lead exposure.[110] Smokers who took either placebo or 200 mg of vitamin C daily had no change in their blood or urine lead levels, but those taking 1000 mg of vitamin C daily had an 81% reduction in their BLLs.[111]

Common dietary components have also demonstrated benefit against lead burden. In animal models, both garlic (*Allium sativum*) and black cumin (*Nigella sativa*) were shown to significantly reduce tissue lead levels.[112,113] Curcumin is able to bind lead and other heavy metals,[114] reduce lead levels in animals, and reverse the lead-induced oxidative stress.[115] The lead reduction activity of curcumin appears to be dose related, with more bioavailable forms of curcumin providing greater reduction of tissue lead levels.[116] In animal studies, lead content in the liver, kidneys, and brain were all reduced with curcumin, along with dramatic reversal of the oxidative stress caused by lead. Curcumin also reversed cognitive defects in lead-poisoned animals that were challenged to find their way through a water maze. The animals given curcumin not only had higher levels of GSH in their brains, but they retained better spatial memory and had faster escape times from the maze.[117]

Polycyclic Aromatic Hydrocarbons

- Vitamins C and E
- NAC
- Omega-3
- *Brassica* sp.
- Curcumin
- Green tea
- Quercitin

Polycyclic aromatic hydrocarbons (PAHs) are produced by combustion of fuels (cigarettes, natural gas, diesel, wood, volcano, etc.) and are omnipresent in the environment. The Centers for Disease Control and Prevention (CDC) Fourth Report lists 10 PAH metabolites that are found ubiquitously in the urine of all US residents. Benzo(a)pyrene (BaP), found in high amounts in diesel exhaust and cigarette smoke, is metabolized by the CYP1 series into the highly carcinogenic benzo(a)pyrene 7,8-dihydrodiol 9,10 epoxide that forms DNA adducts.[118] PAH damage to the DNA results in increased levels of 8-OHdG and is associated with all chronic diseases, as well as low-birth-weight babies in exposed mothers.[119] However, women who consume more fruits and vegetables have lower levels of DNA adducts and are less likely to have low-birth-weight babies even with high PAH exposure. Persons with higher serum levels of the common antioxidant vitamins C and E are not as likely to have increased asthma or chronic obstructive pulmonary disease (COPD) events when the ambient level of $PM_{2.5}$ increases.[120] Female smokers taking only 500 mg of vitamin C and 400 IU of vitamin E daily had a 31% drop in BaP DNA adducts.[121] Smokers who had intact GSTM1 genes and took the antioxidant vitamins had a 43% reduction in DNA adducts.

Individuals with the CYP1A1*2A single nucleotide polymorphism (SNP), which leads to greater CYP induction from PAH exposure, who also have a null GST genotype have far higher rates of lung cancer, because they are producing more BaP epoxides than phase 2 in the liver can clear.[122] Diesel exhaust particles (DEP), high in BaP levels, reduce intracellular GSH levels, and reduce

the function of GSH transferase and other antioxidant enzymes.[123] Nebulized GSH may be beneficial for protection against PAHs.[124] NAC, a low-cost and effective way to boost GSH levels, blocks oxidative damage and airway reactivity from diesel exhaust.[125,126]

Fish is one of the common components of the Mediterranean diet. When fish oil capsules were given to elderly nursing home residents in Mexico City, the typical polycylic aromatic hydrocarbon (PAH)-induced depletion of reduced glutathione (GSH) levels and superoxide dismutase activity was greatly diminished.[127] A dose of 3 g of fish oil daily was also found to block the adverse cardiac effects of PAHs in a group of middle-aged adults.[128] Although even small elevations in $PM_{2.5}$ levels can affect heart-rate variability, 2 g of fish oil daily were able to attenuate that effect in elderly individuals.[129]

Onions are also common components of the Mediterranean and many other traditional diets. Quercitin has demonstrated the ability to reduce the amount of PAH-DNA adducts and prevent cellular toxicity.[130,131] The protective actions of quercetin include reversing GSH depletion and reducing the action of antioxidant enzyme activity that occurs from PAH exposure. However, the main mechanism by which DNA protection (and therefore cancer protection) is conferred appears to be through GST induction, the main pathway for clearance of PAH-epoxides from the circulation. Feeding quercetin to pregnant mice throughout their pregnancy resulted in a genetic upregulation of their CYP1A1, CYP1B1, GST, NADPH quinone oxidoreductase, and glucuronyl transferase enzymes.[29] Interestingly, the offspring had epigenetic upregulation of the activity of all those biotransformation enzymes that persisted throughout adulthood, resulting in fewer PAH-DNA adducts in those animals.

Many traditional diets are also high in members of the Brassica family, which includes broccoli, Brussels sprouts, cabbage, kale, and cauliflower, all of which contain sulfur-containing glucoraphanins and sulforaphanes. The consumption of a broccoli-sprout beverage, with a set amount of glucoraphanins and sulforaphanes, was provided to 291 persons in the highly polluted Yangtze Valley region in China.[132] It was found that those who consumed the beverage increased their excretion of the PAH acrolein by 50%, whereas benzene excretion almost doubled, even in those with null GST genotypes.

In addition to increasing hepatic metabolism of PAHs, sulforaphanes increase phase 2 enzyme function in upper airways,[133] reduce the inflammatory response,[134] and reduce the oxidative stress and inflammation from diesel exhaust that typically leads to increased allergic reactivity.[135] Broccoli intake reduces DNA damage in smokers by 41%,[136] and, not surprisingly, sulforaphane intake is also associated with a reduction of lung cancer incidence of up to 22%.[137]

Curcumin is able to prevent the powerful prooxidant effects of BaP and enhance levels of GSH and the activity of GSH peroxidase, GSH reductase, GSH transferase, superoxide dismutase, and catalase.[138] These actions result in lower BaP-DNA adducts in the animals given curcumin (Fig. 65.3). The beneficial effect of curcumin was even greater for animals given piperine (from black pepper), which increases the absorbability of curcumin.

Curcumin also prevents nicotine-induced oxidative stress[139] and cellular and tissue damage caused by the combination of tobacco smoke and alcohol.[140]

Green tea, consumed by millions of people for millennia, contains catechins with powerful antioxidant compounds known to increase apoptosis rates for numerous types of cancer cells, as well as maintaining mental function and improving the intestinal microbiome. The application of green or black tea to ground meat before cooking prevented the production of mutagenic PAH compounds that normally occur with cooking.[141] Heavy smokers with present GSTT1 and GSTM1 genes who consumed four cups of decaffeinated green tea daily had significant drops in their urinary 8-OHdG levels, whereas all the other groups had an increase in DNA oxidative damage.[142] Those with null genotypes for GSTM1 received benefit, whereas those with GSTT1 null did not. Only those with the GSTT1 null genotype received a reduction in 8-OHdG levels with black tea consumption (Table 65.2).

TABLE 65.2 Unadjusted Means of Urinary 8-OHdG (ug/g cr) in Heavy Smokers According to Beverage Consumed and GST Genotype

Group	Timing	Water	Black Tea	Green Tea
GSTM1 +	Baseline	9.6	12.1	9.1
	Month 4	11.2	14.9	7.4
GSTM1 -	Baseline	8.3	9.3	12.1
	Month 4	11.1	11.9	8.5
GSTT1 +	Baseline	8.8	10.9	9.6
	Month 4	11.6	14.2	7.3
GSTT1 -	Baseline	8.8	10.3	9.1
	Month 4	11.4	8.5	10.4

Modified from Hakim, I. A., Harris, R. B., Chow, H. H., Dean, M., Brown, S., & Ali, IU. (2004). Effect of a 4-month tea intervention on oxidative DNA damage among heavy smokers: Role of glutathione S-transferase genotypes. *Cancer Epidemiology, Biomarkers & Prevention, 13*(2), 242–249.

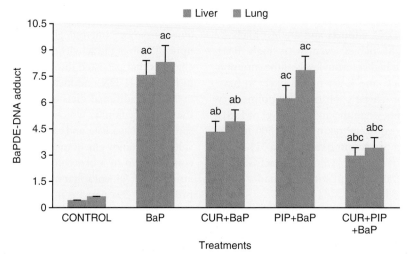

FIG. 65.3 BaP-DNA adducts in animals given BaP, curcumin and BaP, piperine and BaP, or curcumin and piperine with BaP. (From Sehgal, A., Kumar, M., Jain, M., & Dhawan, D. K. (2013). Modulatory effects of curcumin in conjunction with piperine on benzo(a)pyrene-mediated DNA adducts and biotransformation enzymes. *Nutrition and Cancer, 65*(6), 885–890.)

Other polyphenol-containing food and botanical agents that have demonstrated the ability to reduce the toxic effect of PAHs include *Ginkgo biloba*,[143] clove *(Syzygium aromaticum)*,[144] raspberries,[145] and *Withania somnifera*.[146]

Solvents

- NAC
- Glycine and taurine
- Curcumin
- Green tea
- Silymarin

Individuals who were exposed to high amounts of solvents daily through working in the paint industry were protected from chromosomal aberrations by daily consumption of selenium and vitamins A, C, and E.[147] Pump workers who were exposed to benzene daily who consumed six cups of green tea daily for 6 months did not experience the GSH reduction that non–tea drinkers did.[148] In addition, the green tea drinkers had near-normal levels of antioxidant enzyme function, along with reduced urinary levels of both benzene and phenol. The powerful hepatotoxic action of carbon tetrachloride can be effectively blocked by several natural compounds. Silymarin *(Silybum marianum)*, curcumin, picroliv *(Picrorhiza kurroa)*, and ellagic acid (grapes, strawberries, black currents, and raspberries) extracts given before carbon tetrachloride (CCL4) exposure prevented hepatoxicity in animals (Table 65.3)[149]

It can be seen in Table 65.3 that the lowest levels of malondialdehyde (MDA) in the CCL$_4$-exposed animals

TABLE 65.3 Effect of Pretreatment with 50 mg/kg of Individual Botanical Extracts on Oxidative Stress Markers in CCL$_4$-Exposed Mice (units per mg of protein)

Group	MDA (umol/mg)	GSH (µg/mg)	Catalase (k/mg)
Control	31.87	27.29	1.37
CCL$_4$	100.10	7.81	1.00
Silymarin + CCL$_4$	44.32	19.19	1.29
Picroliv + CCL$_4$	44.86	17.83	1.19
Curcumin + CCL$_4$	52.79	22.59	1.55
Ellagic acid + CCL$_4$	53.74	16.72	1.56

Modified from Girish, C., & Pradhan, S. C. (2012). Hepatoprotective activities of picroliv, curcumin, and ellagic acid compared with silymarin on carbon-tetrachloride-induced liver toxicity in mice. *Journal of Pharmacology & Pharmacotherapeutics, 3*(2), 149–155.

was achieved with silymarin, the best-known liver-protecting botanical agent. However, the highest levels of GSH and catalase were achieved with curcumin. All botanicals were equally effective at reducing elevated liver enzymes (Fig. 65.4).

Curcumin, ALA, and NAC are also able to protect CCL$_4$-exposed rats from developing liver fibrosis.[150]

Other botanicals that have proved effective at protecting the liver from CCL$_4$ hepatotoxicity include rosemary *(Rosemarinus officinalis)*,[151] *Ginkgo biloba*,[152] rooibos *(Aspalathus linearis)*,[153] licorice *(Glycyrrhiza glabra)*,[154] and goji berry *(Lycium chinense)*.[155] All of these are commonly used botanicals known for their health benefits and powerful antioxidant activity.

Pesticides and Antimicrobials

- Magnesium
- NAC
- Brassica (sulforaphane)
- Curcumin
- Green tea

Although chlorinated pesticides are no longer used in many countries, they are persistent in the environment, and humans continue to be exposed to them. In addition to agricultural use, the chlorinated pesticide lindane was also used topically for scabies and head lice, often in children. Lindane exposure reduces GSH levels along with the activity of SOD, catalase, GST, GSH peroxidase (GPx), GSH reductase (GR), and NADPH quinine reductase. Curcumin, given either before or after lindane exposure, was able to reverse those effects, with the greatest reversal occurring with pretreatment (Table 65.4).[156] Curcumin is also effective at reversing the oxidative stress caused by 2,3,7,8-tetrachlorodibenzo-p-dioxin, one of the most toxic environmental pollutants.[157]

Triclocarban is a chlorinated compound (very similar to triclosan) used in antimicrobial household and personal care products, including hand sanitizers. Triclocarban is found in about 25% of the total US population that participated in the 2013 to 2014 National Health and Nutritional Examination Survey (NHANES) but was found ubiquitously in the non-Hispanic blacks in that cohort.[158] Triclocarban has been shown to stimulate noncancerous breast cells to become premalignant, but curcumin was able to effectively block that progression.[159]

Both magnesium and NAC have been successfully used adjunctively with atropine for acute organophosphate

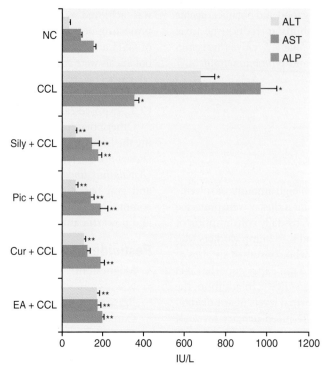

FIG. 65.4 The effect of pretreatment with 50 mg/kg of botanical agents for 7 days on liver enzymes of mice exposed to CCL$_4$. (Modified from Girish, C., & Pradhan, S. C. [2012]. Hepato-protective activities of picroliv, curcumin, and ellagic acid compared with silymarin on carbon-tetrachloride-induced liver toxicity in mice. *Journal of Pharmacology & Pharmacotherapeutics, 3*[2], 149–155.)

(OP) poisonings. All acute OP poison cases entering a hospital in Bangladesh were given atropine and prali-doxime to treat muscarinic symptoms. In addition, some were then given a bolus of either 4, 8, 12, or 16 g of MgSO$_4$.[160] Sixty percent of the control group (standard atropine and pralidoxime treatment) died. None of the patients who got 16 g of MgSO$_4$ died, while only 19% of those receiving 4 g, 25% of those receiving 8 grams, and 12.5% of those receiving 12 g died. Intravenous NAC (600 mg three times daily for 3 days) helped improve oxidative stress markers and reduce atropine dosage in acute OP poisoned cases in Egypt but made no significant change in mortality rates or duration of hospital stays.[161] An animal model of fenthion (a common OP) poisoning showed that an intravenous dose of 150 mg/kg NAC improved survival rate up to 80%, whereas atropine provided 100% survival. Unfortunately this study did have a treatment group that received both atropine and

intravenous NAC.[162] Several studies in China have docu-mented the effectiveness of adjunctive use of crude rhubarb for patients with acute OP poisoning.[163]

Curcumin (200 mg/kg) was able to prevent neurotoxic-ity from parathion in animals, no small feat for such a potent neurotoxic pesticide.[164] Both curcumin and sul-foraphane were effective at blocking the hepatotoxic effects of malathion in animals.[165] Both curcumin and sulfora-phane reduced malondialdehyde levels and increased GSH and nitric oxide levels after malathion intoxication. A combination of curcumin and vitamin E demonstrated the ability to prevent chlorpyriphos (an OP)-induced lung damage in animals.[166]

Individuals who were poisoned by aluminum phos-phide fumigant and who were given intravenous NAC had improvement in their oxidative stress markers, shorter hospitalization (2.7 vs. 8.5 days), less need for intubation and ventilation (45.4% vs. 73.3%), and less mortality

TABLE 65.4   Effect of 30 mg/kg Lindane and 200 mg/kg Curcumin on Lipid Peroxides (LPO), GSH, and Antioxidant Enzyme Function in the Liver of Wistar Rats (units µmol/min/mg protein)

Parameter	Control	Lindane	Cur Pretx	Cur Posttx
LPO	4.23	6.89	4.68	4.96
GSH	2.11	1.30	2.04	1.92
SOD	68.39	36.12	67.36	66.72
CAT	29.60	16.62	28.67	27.73
GST	661.85	407.09	614.77	570.22
GPx	22.89	14.47	21.90	21.09
GR	38.31	22.40	36.20	33.27
NADPH quinone reductase	81.98	47.71	78.70	75.05

Modified from Singh, R., & Sharma, P. (2011). Hepatoprotective effect of curcumin on lindane-induced oxidative stress in male Wistar rats. *Toxicology International*, 18(2), 124–129.

(36% vs. 60%) than those receiving conventional treatment alone.[167]

Mycotoxins

- Green tea
- Silymarin

The best-known example of an effective natural treatment for mycotoxin poisoning is the use of *Silybum marianum* for acute amanitin poisoning. Milk thistle is so effective for amanitin toxicity that an intravenous preparation of this herb (Legalon) has become a standard of care for amanitin poisoning.[168] Green tea polyphenols are able to reduce DNA-aflatoxin adduct levels in a time- and dose-dependent manner in persons chronically exposed to aspergillus.[169] Green tea also increased the GSH conjugation and excretion of aflatoxin in those consuming the polyphenol extract. Urinary levels of 8-OHdG, a marker for oxidative damage to the DNA, was also reduced by the intake of green tea extract in persons chronically exposed to aspergillus.[170] Green tea extract intake also reduced urinary markers of sphingolipid disruption in persons chronically exposed to fumonisin B1 in their diets, providing potential neuroprotection.[171] Curcumin reduced the amount of DNA-aflatoxin adducts in animals[172] and prevented hepatic and renal damage from occurring.[173,174]

REFERENCES

1. Pedret, A., Valls, R. M., Fernández-Castillejo, S., Catalán, Ú., Romeu, M., et al. (2012). Polyphenol-rich foods exhibit DNA antioxidative properties and protect the glutathione system in healthy subjects. *Molecular Nutrition & Food Research*, 56(7), 1025–1033. PubMed PMID: 22760977.
2. Fowke, J. H., Morrow, J. D., Motley, S., Bostick, R. M., & Ness, R. M. (2006). Brassica vegetable consumption reduces urinary F2-isoprostane levels independent of micronutrient intake. *Carcinogenesis*, 27(10), 2096–2102. PubMed PMID: 16704986.
3. El-Demerdash, E., Ali, A. A., El-Taher, D. E., & Hamada, F. M. (2012). Effect of low-protein diet on anthracycline pharmacokinetics and cardiotoxicity. *The Journal of Pharmacy and Pharmacology*, 64(3), 344–352. PubMed PMID: 22309266.
4. Oshikoya, K. A., Sammons, H. M., & Choonara, I. (2010). A systematic review of pharmacokinetics studies in children with protein-energy malnutrition. *European Journal of Clinical Pharmacology*, 66(10), 1025–1035. PubMed PMID: 20552179.
5. Mucklow, J. C., Caraher, M. T., Henderson, D. B., & Rawlins, M. B. (1979). The effect of individual dietary constituents on antipyrine clearance in Asian immigrants. *British Journal of Clinical Pharmacology*, 7, 416–417. PubMed PMID: 444366.
6. Mucklow, J. C., Caraher, M. T., Henderson, D. B., et al. (1982). The relationship between individual dietary constituents and antipyrine metabolism in Indo-Pakistani immigrants to Britain. *British Journal of Clinical Pharmacology*, 13(4), 481–486. PubMed PMID: 7066162.
7. Prabhakaran, S., Shameem, F., & Devi, K. S. (1993). Influence of protein deficiency on hexachlorocyclohexane and malathion toxicity in pregnant rats. *Veterinary and Human Toxicology*, 35(5), 429–433. PubMed PMID: 7504364.
8. Fagan, T. C., Walle, T., Oexmann, M. J., et al. (1987). Increased clearance of propranolol and theophylline by high-protein compared with high-carbohydrate diet. *Clinical Pharmacology and Therapeutics*, 41(4), 402–406. PubMed PMID: 3829577.
9. Feldman, C. H., Hutchinson, V. E., Pippenger, C. E., et al. (1980). Effect of dietary protein and carbohydrate on theophylline metabolism in children. *Pediatrics*, 66(6), 956–962. PubMed PMID: 7454487.

10. Demetriou, A. A. (1991). Diet and cimetidine induce comparable changes in theophylline metabolism in normal subjects. *JPEN. Journal of Parenteral and Enteral Nutrition, 15*(6), 687–688. PubMed PMID: 1766062.

11. Becking, G. C. (1976). Hepatic drug metabolism in iron-, magnesium- and potassium-deficient rats. *Federation Proceedings, 35*(13), 2480–2485. PubMed PMID: 824159.

12. Archakov, A. I., Karuzina, I. I., Kokareva, I. S., & Bachmanova, G. I. (1973). The effect of magnesium ions on the dimethylaniline oxidation rate and electron transfer in liver microsomal fraction. *The Biochemical Journal, 136*(2), 371–379. PubMed PMID: 4149444.

13. Becking, G. C., & Morrison, A. B. (1970). Role of dietary magnesium in the metabolism of drugs by NADPH-dependent rat liver microsomal enzymes. *Biochemical Pharmacology, 19*(9), 2639–2644. PubMed PMID: 4394596.

14. Peters, M. A., & Fouts, J. R. (1970). The influence of magnesium and some other divalent cations on hepatic microsomal drug metabolism in vitro. *Biochemical Pharmacology, 19*(2), 533–544. PubMed PMID: 4396251.

15. Otocka-Kmiecik, A., Bortnik, K., Szkudlarek, U., et al. (2013). Effect of exercise on plasma paraoxonase1 activity in rugby players: Dependence on training experience. *Redox Report: Communications in Free Radical Research, 18*(3), 113–119. PubMed PMID: 23710701.

16. Turgay, F., Şişman, A. R., & Aksu, A. Ç. (2015). Effects of anaerobic training on paraoxonase-1 enzyme (PON1) activities of high density lipoprotein subgroups and its relationship with PON1-Q192R phenotype. *Journal of Atherosclerosis and Thrombosis, 22*(4), 433–434. PubMed PMID: 25963585.

17. Kastorini, C. M., Panagiotakos, D. B., Chrysohoou, C., et al. ATTICA Study Group. (2016). Metabolic syndrome, adherence to the Mediterranean diet and 10-year cardiovascular disease incidence: The ATTICA study. *Atherosclerosis, 246*, 87–93. PubMed PMID: 26761772.

18. Blum, S., Aviram, M., Ben-Amotz, A., & Levy, Y. (2006). Effect of a Mediterranean meal on postprandial carotenoids, paraoxonase activity and C-reactive protein levels. *Annals of Nutrition & Metabolism, 50*(1), 20–24. PubMed PMID: 16276071.

19. Ghorbanihaghjo, A., Kolahi, S., Seifirad, S., et al. (2012). Effect of fish oil supplements on serum paraoxonase activity in female patients with rheumatoid arthritis: A double-blind randomized controlled trial. *Archives of Iranian Medicine, 15*(9), 549–552. PubMed PMID: 22924372.

20. Loued, S., Berrougui, H., Componova, P., et al. (2013). Extra-virgin olive oil consumption reduces the age-related decrease in HDL and paraoxonase 1 anti-inflammatory activities. *The British Journal of Nutrition, 110*(7), 1272–1284. PubMed PMID: 23510814.

21. Zhu, Y., Huang, X., Zhang, Y., et al. (2014). Anthocyanin supplementation improves HDL-associated paraoxonase 1 activity and enhances cholesterol efflux capacity in subjects with hypercholesterolemia. *The Journal of Clinical Endocrinology and Metabolism, 99*(2), 561–569. PubMed PMID: 24285687.

22. Farrell, N., Norris, G., Lee, S. G., Chun, O. K., & Blesso, C. N. (2015). Anthocyanin-rich black elderberry extract improves markers of HDL function and reduces aortic cholesterol in hyperlipidemic mice. *Food & Function, 6*(4), 1278–1287. PubMed PMID: 25758596.

23. Boesch-Saadatmandi, C., Egert, S., Schrader, C., et al. (2010). Effect of quercetin on paraoxonase 1 activity–studies in cultured cells, mice and humans. *Journal of Physiology and Pharmacology, 61*(1), 99–105. Erratum in: J Physiol Pharmacol. 2011;62(1):131. PubMed PMID: 20228421.

24. Nus, M., Frances, F., Librelotto, J., et al. (2007). Arylesterase activity and antioxidant status depend on PON1-Q192R and PON1-L55M polymorphisms in subjects with increased risk of cardiovascular disease consuming walnut-enriched meat. *The Journal of Nutrition, 137*(7), 1783–1788. PubMed PMID: 17585031.

25. Arunima, S., & Rajamohan, T. (2013). Effect of virgin coconut oil enriched diet on the antioxidant status and paraoxonase 1 activity in ameliorating the oxidative stress in rats – a comparative study. *Food & Function, 4*(9), 1402–1409. PubMed PMID: 23892389.

26. Kurban, S., & Mehmetoglu, I. (2010). Effects of acetylsalicylic acid on serum paraoxonase activity, Ox-LDL, coenzyme Q10 and other oxidative stress markers in healthy volunteers. *Clinical Biochemistry, 43*(3), 287–290. PubMed PMID: 19891963.

27. Walters, D. G., Young, P. J., Agus, C., et al. (2004). Cruciferous vegetable consumption alters the metabolism of the dietary carcinogen 2-amino-1-methyl-6-phenylimidazo[4,5-b]pyridine (PhIP) in humans. *Carcinogenesis, 25*(9), 1659–1669. PubMed PMID: 15073045.

28. Hecht, S. S., Carmella, S. G., & Murphy, S. E. (1999). Effects of watercress consumption on

urinary metabolites of nicotine in smokers. *Cancer Epidemiology, Biomarkers and Prevention*, 8, 907–913. PubMed PMID: 10548320.

29. Vanhees, K., van Schooten, F. J., Moonen, E. J., et al. (2012). Maternal intake of quercetin during gestation alters ex vivo benzo[a]pyrene metabolism and DNA adduct formation in adult offspring. *Mutagenesis*, 27(4), 445–451. PubMed PMID: 22334599.

30. de Moreno de LeBlanc, A., & Perdigón, G. (2005). Reduction of beta-glucuronidase and nitroreductase activity by yoghurt in a murine colon cancer model. *Biocell*, 29(1), 15–24. PubMed PMID: 15954463.

31. Dominici, L., Villarini, M., Trotta, F., et al. (2014). Protective effects of probiotic Lactobacillus rhamnosus IMC501 in mice treated with PhIP. *Journal of Microbiology and Biotechnology*, 24(3), 371–378. PubMed PMID: 24346468.

32. Rowland, I. R., Rumney, C. J., Coutts, J. T., & Lievense, L. C. (1998). Effect of Bifidobacterium longum and inulin on gut bacterial metabolism and carcinogen-induced aberrant crypt foci in rats. *Carcinogenesis*, 19(2), 281–285. PubMed PMID: 9498277.

33. Liu, Z., Lin, X., Huang, G., et al. (2014). Prebiotic effects of almonds and almond skins on intestinal microbiota in healthy adult humans. *Anaerobe*, 26, 1–6. PubMed PMID: 24315808.

34. Kohno, H., Tanaka, T., Kawabata, K., et al. (2002). Silymarin, a naturally occurring polyphenolic antioxidant flavonoid, inhibits azoxymethane-induced colon carcinogenesis in male F344 rats. *International Journal of Cancer. Journal International du Cancer*, 101(5), 461–468. PubMed PMID: 12216075.

35. Frejnagel, S., & Juskiewicz, J. (2011). Dose-dependent effects of polyphenolic extracts from green tea, blue-berried honeysuckle, and chokeberry on rat caecal fermentation processes. *Planta Medica*, 77(9), 888–893. PubMed PMID: 21240841.

36. Summart, R., & Chewonarin, T. (2014). Purple rice extract supplemented diet reduces DMH-induced aberrant crypt foci in the rat colon by inhibition of bacterial β-glucuronidase. *Asian Pacific Journal of Cancer Prevention : APJCP*, 15(2), 749–755. PubMed PMID: 24568490.

37. Dwivedi, C., Heck, W. J., Downie, A. A., et al. (1990). Effect of calcium glucuronate on beta-glucuronidase activity and glucuronate content of certain vegetables and fruits. *Biochemical Medicine and Metabolic Biology*, 43(2), 83–92. PubMed PMID: 2346674.

38. Atkuri, K. R., Mantovani, J. J., Herzenberg, L. A., & Herzenberg, L. A. (2007). N-Acetylcysteine – a safe antidote for cysteine/glutathione deficiency. *Current Opinion in Pharmacology*, 7(4), 355–359. PubMed PMID: 17602868.

39. Mills, B. J., Lindeman, R. D., & Lang, C. A. (1986). Magnesium deficiency inhibits biosynthesis of blood glutathione and tumor growth in the rat. *Proceedings of the Society for Experimental Biology and Medicine*, 181(3), 326–332. PubMed PMID: 3945642.

40. Bede, O., Nagy, D., Surányi, A., et al. (2008). Effects of magnesium supplementation on the glutathione redox system in atopic asthmatic children. *Inflammation Research*, 57(6), 279–286. PubMed PMID: 18516713.

41. Ly, J., Lagman, M., Saing, T., et al. (2015). Liposomal glutathione supplementation restores TH1 cytokine response to mycobacterium tuberculosis infection in HIV-infected individuals. *Journal of Interferon and Cytokine Research*, 35(11), 875–887. PubMed PMID: 26133750.

42. Biswas, S. K., McClure, D., Jimenez, L. A., et al. (2005). Curcumin induces glutathione biosynthesis and inhibits NF-kappaB activation and interleukin-8 release in alveolar epithelial cells: Mechanism of free radical scavenging activity. *Antioxidants & Redox Signaling*, 7(1–2), 32–41. PubMed PMID: 15650394.

43. Sankar, P., Telang, A. G., & Manimaran, A. (2012). Protective effect of curcumin on cypermethrin-induced oxidative stress in Wistar rats. *Experimental and Toxicologic Pathology*, 64(5), 487–493. PubMed PMID: 21130633.

44. Shibata, S., Ishitobi, H., Miyaki, S., et al. (2016). Carnosic acid protects starvation-induced SH-SY5Y cell death through Erk1/2 and Akt pathways, autophagy, and FoxO3a. *International Journal of Food Sciences and Nutrition*, 67(8), 977–982. PubMed PMID: 27435046.

45. Kumar, M., Sharma, V. L., Sehgal, A., & Jain, M. (2012). Protective effects of green and white tea against benzo(a)pyrene induced oxidative stress and DNA damage in murine model. *Nutrition and Cancer*, 64(2), 300–306. PubMed PMID: 22243054.

46. Lucena, M. I., Andrade, R. J., de la Cruz, J. P., et al. (2002). Effects of silymarin MZ-80 on oxidative stress in patients with alcoholic cirrhosis. Results of a randomized, double-blind, placebo-controlled clinical study. *International Journal of Clinical Pharmacology and Therapeutics*, 40(1), 2–8. PubMed PMID: 11841050.

47. Sener, G., Omurtag, G. Z., Sehirli, O., et al. (2006). Protective effects of ginkgo biloba against acetaminophen-induced toxicity in mice. *Molecular and Cellular Biochemistry*, 283(1–2), 39–45. PubMed PMID: 16444584.

48. Singh, M., Murthy, V., & Ramassamy, C. (2012). Standardized extracts of Bacopa monniera protect against MPP+- and paraquat-induced toxicity by modulating mitochondrial activities, proteasomal functions, and redox pathways. *Toxicological Sciences, 125*(1), 219–232. PubMed PMID: 21972102.

49. Granado-Serrano, A. B., Martín, M. A., Bravo, L., et al. (2012). Quercetin modulates Nrf2 and glutathione-related defenses in HepG2 cells: Involvement of p38. *Chemico-Biological Interactions, 195*(2), 154–164. PubMed PMID: 22197970.

50. Heck, J. E., Nieves, J. W., Chen, Y., Parvez, F., et al. (2009). Dietary intake of methionine, cysteine, and protein and urinary arsenic excretion in Bangladesh. *Environmental Health Perspectives, 117*(1), 99–104. PubMed PMID: 19165394.

51. Mondal, R., Biswas, S., Chatterjee, A., et al. (2016). Protection against arsenic-induced hematological and hepatic anomalies by supplementation of vitamin C and vitamin E in adult male rats. *Journal of Basic and Clinical Physiology and Pharmacology, 27*(6), 643–652. PubMed PMID: 27464034.

52. López-Carrillo, L., Gamboa-Loira, B., Becerra, W., et al. (2016). Dietary micronutrient intake and its relationship with arsenic metabolism in Mexican women. *Environmental Research, 151*, 445–450. PubMed PMID: 27565879.

53. Zahkaryan, R., & Aposhian, V. (1999). Arsenite methylation by methylvitamin B12 and glutathione does not require an enzyme. *Toxicology and Applied Pharmacology, 154*, 287–291. PMID: 9931288.

54. Peters, B. A., Hall, M. N., Liu, X., et al. (2015). Folic acid and creatine as therapeutic approaches to lower blood arsenic: A randomized controlled trial. *Environmental Health Perspectives, 123*(12), 1294–1301. PubMed PMID:25978852.

55. Zheng, Y., Tao, S., Lian, F., Chau, B. T., et al. (2012). Sulforaphane prevents pulmonary damage in response to inhaled arsenic by activating the Nrf2-defense response. *Toxicology and Applied Pharmacology, 265*(3), 292–299. PubMed PMID: 22975029.

56. Shinkai, Y., Sumi, D., Fukami, I., Ishii, T., & Kumagai, Y. (2006). Sulforaphane, an activator of Nrf2, suppresses cellular accumulation of arsenic and its cytotoxicity in primary mouse hepatocytes. *FEBS Letters, 580*(7), 1771–1774. PubMed PMID: 16516206.

57. Biswas, J., Sinha, D., Mukherjee, S., et al. (2010). Curcumin protects DNA damage in a chronically arsenic-exposed population of West Bengal. *Human and Experimental Toxicology, 29*(6), 513–524. PubMed PMID: 20056736.

58. Gao, S., Duan, X., Wang, X., et al. (2013). Curcumin attenuates arsenic-induced hepatic injuries and oxidative stress in experimental mice through activation of Nrf2 pathway, promotion of arsenic methylation and urinary excretion. *Food and Chemical Toxicology: An International Journal Published for the British Industrial Biological Research Association, 59*, 739–747. PubMed PMID: 23871787.

59. El-Demerdash, F. M., Yousef, M. I., & Radwan, F. M. (2009). Ameliorating effect of curcumin onsodium arsenite-induced oxidative damage and lipid peroxidation in different rat organs. *Food and Chemical Toxicology: An International Journal Published for the British Industrial Biological Research Association, 47*(1), 249–254. PubMed PMID: 19049818.

60. Roy, M., Sinha, D., Mukherjee, S., & Biswas, J. (2011). Curcumin prevents DNA damage and enhances the repair potential in a chronically arsenic-exposed human population in West Bengal, India. *European Journal of Cancer Prevention, 20*(2), 123–131. PubMed PMID: 21332098.

61. Sinha, D., Roy, M., Dey, S., et al. (2003). Modulation of arsenic induced cytotoxicity by tea. *Asian Pacific Journal of Cancer Prevention: APJCP, 4*(3), 233–237. PubMed PMID: 14507244.

62. Sinha, D., Roy, M., Siddiqi, M., & Bhattacharya, R. K. (2005). Arsenic-induced micronuclei formation in mammalian cells and its counteraction by tea. *Journal of Environmental Pathology, Toxicology and Oncology, 24*(1), 45–56. PubMed PMID: 15715508.

63. Sárközi, K., Papp, A., Horváth, E., et al. (2016). Green tea and vitamin C ameliorate some neuro-functional and biochemical signs of arsenic toxicity in rats. *Nutritional Neuroscience, 19*(3), 102–109. PubMed PMID: 25211010.

64. Gupta, R., & Flora, S. J. (2006). Effect of Centella asiatica on arsenic induced oxidativestress and metal distribution in rats. *Journal of Applied Toxicology: JAT, 26*(3), 213–222. PubMed PMID: 16389662.

65. Gupta, R., & Flora, S. J. (2005). Protective value of Aloe vera against some toxic effects of arsenic in rats. *Phytotherapy Research: PTR, 19*(1), 23–28. PubMed PMID: 15799004.

66. Xu, Y., Zhou, X., Shi, C., Wang, J., & Wu, Z. (2015). α-Lipoic acid protects against the oxidative stress and cytotoxicity induced by cadmium in HepG2 cells through regenerating glutathione regulated by glutamate-cysteine ligase. *Toxicology Mechanisms and Methods, 25*(8), 596–603. PubMed PMID: 26365678.

67. Nikolić, R., Krstić, N., Jovanović, J., et al. (2015). Monitoring the toxic effects of Pb, Cd and Cu on hematological parameters of Wistar rats and potential

protective role of lipoic acid and glutathione. *Toxicology and Industrial Health*, *31*(3), 239–246. PubMed PMID: 23293128.

68. Veljkovic, A. R., Nikolic, R. S., Kocic, G. M., et al. (2012). Protective effects of glutathione and lipoic acid against cadmium-induced oxidative stress in rat's kidney. *Renal Failure*, *34*(10), 1281–1287. PubMed PMID: 23009295.

69. El-Maraghy, S. A., & Nassar, N. N. (2011). Modulatory effects of lipoic acid and selenium against cadmium-induced biochemical alterations in testicular steroidogenesis. *Journal of Biochemical and Molecular Toxicology*, *25*(1), 15–25. PubMed PMID: 20957662.

70. Mukherjee, R., Banerjee, S., Joshi, N., et al. (2011). A combination of melatonin and alpha lipoic acid has greater cardioprotective effect than either of them singly against cadmium-induced oxidative damage. *Cardiovascular Toxicology*, *11*(1), 78–88. Erratum in: *Cardiovasc Toxicol*. 2011 Mar;11(1):89-90. PubMed PMID: 21046280.

71. Djukić-Cosić, D., Ninković, M., Malicević, Z., et al. (2007). Effect of magnesium pretreatment on reduced glutathione levels in tissues of mice exposed to acute and subacute cadmium intoxication: A time course study. *Magnesium Research*, *20*(3), 177–186. PubMed PMID: 17972460.

72. Fouad, A. A., Qureshi, H. A., Yacoubi, M. T., & Al-Melhim, W. N. (2009). Protective role of carnosine in mice with cadmium-induced acute hepatotoxicity. *Food and Chemical Toxicology: An International Journal Published for the British Industrial Biological Research Association*, *47*(11), 2863–2870. PubMed PMID: 19748544.

73. Pires, V. C., Gollücke, A. P., Ribeiro, D. A., et al. (2013). Grape juice concentrate protects reproductive parameters of male rats against cadmium-induced damage: A chronic assay. *The British Journal of Nutrition*, *110*(11), 2020–2029. PubMed PMID: 23656754.

74. de Moura, C. F., Ribeiro, F. A., Handan, B. A., et al. (2016). Grape juice concentrate protects rat liver against cadmium intoxication: Histopathology, cytochrome C and metalloproteinases expression. *Drug Research*, *66*(7), 339–344. PubMed PMID: 27056637.

75. de Moura, C. F., Ribeiro, F. A., de Jesus, G. P., et al. (2014). Antimutagenic and antigenotoxic potential of grape juice concentrate in blood and liver of rats exposed to cadmium. *Environmental Science and Pollution Research International*, *21*(22), 13118–13126. PubMed PMID: 24996944.

76. Lamas, C. A., Gollücke, A. P., & Dolder, H. (2015). Grape juice concentrate (G8000(®)) intake mitigates

77. Gong, P., Chen, F. X., Wang, L., et al. (2014). Protective effects of blueberries (Vaccinium corymbosum L.) extract against cadmium-induced hepatotoxicity in mice. *Environmental Toxicology and Pharmacology*, *37*(3), 1015–1027. PubMed PMID: 24751684.

78. Ige, S. F., & Akhigbe, R. E. (2013). Common onion (Allium cepa) extract reverses cadmium-induced organ toxicity and dyslipidaemia via redox alteration in rats. *Pathophysiology*, *20*(4), 269–274. PubMed PMID: 23727273.

79. Morales, A. I., Vicente-Sánchez, C., Sandoval, J. M., et al. (2006). Protective effect of quercetin on experimental chronic cadmium nephrotoxicity in rats is based on its antioxidant properties. *Food and Chemical Toxicology: An International Journal Published for the British Industrial Biological Research Association*, *44*(12), 2092–2100. PubMed PMID: 16962696.

80. Ugwuja, E. I., Erejuwa, O. O., & Ugwu, N. C. (2016). Spices Mixture Containing Garlic, Ginger and Nutmeg Has Protective Effects on the Kidneys and Liver of Cadmium Exposed Rats. *Advanced Pharmaceutical Bulletin*, *6*(2), 271–274. PubMed PMID: 27478792.

81. Aremu, D. A., Madejczyk, M. S., & Ballatori, N. (2008). N-acetylcysteine as a potential antidote and biomonitoring agent of methylmercury exposure. *Environmental Health Perspectives*, *116*(1), 26–31. PubMed PMID: 18197295.

82. Ballatori, N., Lieberman, M. W., & Wang, W. (1998). N-acetylcysteine as an antidote in methylmercury poisoning. *Environmental Health Perspectives*, *106*(5), 267–271. PubMed PMID: 9520359.

83. Joshi, D., Mittal, D. K., Shukla, S., et al. (2014). N-acetyl cysteine and selenium protects mercuric chloride-induced oxidative stress and antioxidant defense system in liver and kidney of rats: A histopathological approach. *Journal of Trace Elements in Medicine and Biology: Organ of the Society for Minerals and Trace Elements (GMS)*, *28*(2), 218–226. PubMed PMID: 24485406.

84. Joshi, D., Mittal, D., Shrivastav, S., et al. (2011). Combined effect of N-acetyl cysteine, zinc, and selenium against chronic dimethylmercury-induced oxidative stress: A biochemical and histopathological approach. *Archives of Environmental Contamination and Toxicology*, *61*(4), 558–567. PubMed PMID: 21424224.

85. Afonne, O. J., Orisakwe, O. E., Ndubuka, G. I., et al. (2000). Zinc protection of mercury-induced toxicity

in mice. *Biological and Pharmaceutical Bulletin, 23*(3), 305–308. PubMed PMID: 10726883.

86. Meinerz, D. F., de Paula, M. T., Comparsi, B., et al. (2011). Protective effects of organoselenium compounds against methylmercury-induced oxidative stress in mouse brain mitochondrial-enriched fractions. *Brazilian Journal of Medical and Biological Research = Revista brasileira de pesquisas medicas e biologicas / Sociedade Brasileira de Biofisica ... [et al.], 44*(11), 1156–1163. PubMed PMID: 22002094.

87. Kalender, S., Uzun, F. G., Demir, F., et al. (2013). Mercuric chloride-induced testicular toxicity in rats and the protective role of sodium selenite and vitamin E. *Food and Chemical Toxicology: An International Journal Published for the British Industrial Biological Research Association, 55*, 456–462. PubMed PMID: 23369933.

88. Falluel-Morel, A., Lin, L., Sokolowski, K., et al. (2012). N-acetyl cysteine treatment reduces mercury-induced neurotoxicity in the developing rat hippocampus. *Journal of Neuroscience Research, 90*(4), 743–750. PubMed PMID: 22420031.

89. Kaur, P., Aschner, M., & Syversen, T. (2006). Glutathione modulation influences methyl mercury induced neurotoxicity in primary cell cultures of neurons and astrocytes. *Neurotoxicology, 27*(4), 492–500. PubMed PMID: 16513172.

90. Ekor, M., Adesanoye, O. A., & Farombi, E. O. (2010). N-acetylcysteine pretreatment ameliorates mercuric chloride-induced oxidative renal damage in rats. *African Journal of Medicine and Medical Sciences, 39*(Suppl.), 153–160. PubMed PMID: 22416658.

91. Girardi, G., & Elias, M. M. (1991). Effectiveness of N-acetylcysteine in protecting against mercuric chloride-induced nephrotoxicity. *Toxicology, 67*(2), 155–164. PubMed PMID: 1674384.

92. Chen, Y. W., Huang, C. F., Yang, C. Y., et al. (2010). Inorganic mercury causes pancreatic beta-cell death via the oxidative stress-induced apoptotic and necrotic pathways. *Toxicology and Applied Pharmacology, 243*(3), 323–331. PubMed PMID: 20006636.

93. Agarwal, R., Goel, S. K., & Behari, J. R. (2010). Detoxification and antioxidant effects of curcumin in rats experimentally exposed to mercury. *Journal of Applied Toxicology : JAT, 30*(5), 457–468. PubMed PMID: 20229497.

94. Sener, G., Sehirli, O., Tozan, A., et al. (2007). Ginkgo biloba extract protects against mercury(II)-induced oxidative tissue damage in rats. *Food and Chemical Toxicology : An International Journal Published for the British Industrial Biological Research Association, 45*(4), 543–550. PubMed PMID: 17267089.

95. Mokrzan, E. M., Kerper, L. E., Ballatori, N., & Clarkson, T. W. (1995). Methylmercury-thiol uptake into cultured brain capillary endothelial cells on amino acid system L. *The Journal of Pharmacology and Experimental Therapeutics, 272*(3), 1277–1284. PubMed PMID: 7891344.

96. Ganther, H. E. (1978). Modification of methylmercury toxicity and metabolism by selenium and vitamin E: Possible mechanisms. *Environmental Health Perspectives, 25*, 71–76. PubMed PMID: 720304.

97. Drasch, G., Wanghofer, E., Roider, G., & Strobach, S. (1996). Correlation of mercury and selenium in the human kidney. *Journal of Trace Elements in Medicine and Biology: Organ of the Society for Minerals and Trace Elements (GMS), 10*(4), 251–254. PubMed PMID: 9021677.

98. Høl, P. J., Vamnes, J. S., Gjerdet, N. R., et al. (2001). Dental amalgam and selenium in blood. *Environmental Research, 87*(3), 141–146. PubMed PMID: 11771928.

99. Anuradha, B., & Varalakshmi, P. (1999). Protective role of DL-alpha-lipoic acid against mercury-induce neural lipid peroxidation. *Pharmacological Research, 39*, 67–80.

100. Gregus, Z., Stein, A. F., Varga, F., & Klaasen, C. D. (1992). Effect of lipoic acid on biliary excretion of glutathione and metals. *Toxicology and Applied Pharmacology, 114*, 88–96.

101. Feng, S., Xu, Z., Wang, F., et al. (2017). Sulforaphane prevents methylmercury-induced oxidative damage and excitotoxicity through activation of the Nrf2-ARE pathway. *Molecular Neurobiology, 54*(1), 375–391. PubMed PMID: 26742517.

102. Liu, W., Xu, Z., Yang, T., et al. (2014). The protective role of tea polyphenols against methylmercury-induced neurotoxic effects in rat cerebral cortex via inhibition of oxidative stress. *Free Radical Research, 48*(8), 849–863. PubMed PMID: 24821269.

103. Čabarkapa, A., Borozan, S., Živković, L., et al. (2015). CaNa2EDTA chelation attenuates cell damage in workers exposed to lead–a pilot study. *Chemico-Biological Interactions, 242*, 171–178. PubMed PMID: 26460059.

104. Caylak, E., Aytekin, M., & Halifeoglu, I. (2008). Antioxidant effects of methionine, alpha-lipoic acid, N-acetylcysteine and homocysteine on lead-induced oxidative stress to erythrocytes in rats. *Experimental and Toxicologic Pathology, 60*(4–5), 289–294. PubMed PMID: 18407480.

105. Patrick, L. (2006). Lead toxicity part II: The role of free radical damage and the use of antioxidants in the pathology and treatment of lead toxicity. *Alternative Medicine Review: A Journal of Clinical*

Therapeutic, 11(2), 114–127. PubMed PMID: 16813461.

106. Kasperczyk, S., Dobrakowski, M., Kasperczyk, A., et al. (2014). Effect of treatment with N-acetylcysteine on non-enzymatic antioxidant reserves and lipid peroxidation in workers exposed to lead. *Annals of Agricultural and Environmental Medicine, 21*(2), 272–277. PubMed PMID: 24959775.

107. Kasperczyk, S., Dobrakowski, M., Kasperczyk, A., et al. (2013). The administration of N-acetylcysteine reduces oxidative stress and regulates glutathione metabolism in the blood cells of workers exposed to lead. *Clinical Toxicology (Philadelphia, Pa.), 51*(6), 480–486. PubMed PMID: 23731375.

108. Cao, X. J., Huang, S. H., Wang, M., Chen, J. T., & Ruan, D. Y. (2008). S-adenosyl-L-methionine improves impaired hippocampal long-term potentiation and water maze performance induced by developmental lead exposure in rats. *European Journal of Pharmacology, 595*(1–3), 30–34. PMID: 18713624.

109. Simon, J. A., & Hudes, E. S. (1999). Relationship of ascorbic acid to blood lead levels. *JAMA: The Journal of the American Medical Association, 281*(24), 2289–2293. PubMed PMID: 10386552.

110. Rendón-Ramírez, A. L., Maldonado-Vega, M., Quintanar-Escorza, M. A., et al. (2014). Effect of vitamin E and C supplementation on oxidative damage and total antioxidant capacity in lead-exposed workers. *Environmental Toxicology and Pharmacology, 37*(1), 45–54. PubMed PMID: 24560336.

111. Dawson, E. B., Evans, D. R., Harris, W. A., et al. (1999). The effect of ascorbic acid supplementation on the blood lead levels of smokers. *Journal of the American College of Nutrition, 18*(2), 166–170. PubMed PMID: 10204833.

112. Massadeh, A. M., Al-Safi, S. A., Momani, I. F., et al. (2007). Garlic (Allium sativum L.) as a potential antidote for cadmium and lead intoxication: Cadmium and lead distribution and analysis in different mice organs. *Biological Trace Element Research, 120*(1–3), 227–234. PubMed PMID: 17916975.

113. Massadeh, A. M., Al-Safi, S. A., Momani, I. F., et al. (2007). Analysis of cadmium and lead in mice organs: Effect of Nigella sativa L. (Black Cumin) on the distribution and immunosuppressive effect of cadmium-lead mixture in mice. *Biological Trace Element Research, 115*(2), 157–167. PubMed PMID: 17435259.

114. Gupta, S. C., Prasad, S., Kim, J. H., Patchva, S., et al. (2011). Multitargeting by curcumin as revealed by molecular interaction studies. *Natural Product Reports, 28*(12), 1937–1955. PubMed PMID: 21979811.

115. Shukla, P. K., Khanna, V. K., Khan, M. Y., & Srimal, R. C. (2003). Protective effect of curcumin against lead neurotoxicity in rat. *Human and Experimental Toxicology, 22*(12), 653–658. PubMed PMID: 14992327.

116. Flora, G., Gupta, D., & Tiwari, A. (2013). Preventive efficacy of bulk and nanocurcumin against lead-induced oxidative stress in mice. *Biological Trace Element Research, 152*(1), 31–40. PubMed PMID:23292317.

117. Dairam, A., Limson, J. L., Watkins, G. M., Antunes, E., & Daya, S. (2007). Curcuminoids, curcumin, and demethoxycurcumin reduce lead-induced memory deficits in male Wistar rats. *Journal of Agricultural and Food Chemistry, 55*(3), 1039–1044. PubMed PMID: 17263510.

118. Shimada, T., Gillam, E. M., Oda, Y., et al. (1999). Metabolism of benzo(a)pyrene to trans-7,8-dihydroxy-7,8-dihydrobenzo(a)pyrene by recombinant human cytochrome P450 1B1 and purified liver epoxide hydrolase. *Chemical Research in Toxicology, 12*, 623–629. PubMed PMID: 10409402.

119. Pedersen, M., Schoket, B., Godschalk, R. W., et al. (2013). Bulky dna adducts in cord blood, maternal fruit-and-vegetable consumption, and birth weight in a European mother-child study (NewGeneris). *Environmental Health Perspectives, 121*(10), 1200–1206. PubMed PMID: 23906905.

120. Canova, C., Dunster, C., Kelly, F. J., et al. (2012). PM10-induced hospital admissions for asthma and chronic obstructive pulmonary disease: The modifying effect of individual characteristics. *Epidemiology (Cambridge, Mass.), 23*(4), 607–615. PubMed PMID: 22531667.

121. Mooney, L. A., Madsen, A. M., Tang, D., et al. (2005). Antioxidant vitamin supplementation reduces benzo(a)pyrene-DNA adducts and potential cancer risk in female smokers. *Cancer Epidemiology, Biomarkers and Prevention: A Publication of the American Association for Cancer Research, Cosponsored by the American Society of Preventive Oncology, 14*(1), 237–242. PubMed PMID: 15668500.

122. Shah, P. P., Singh, A. P., Singh, M., et al. (2008). Interaction of cytochrome P4501A1 genotypes with other risk factors and susceptibility to lung cancer. *Mutation Research, 639*(1–2), 1–10. PubMed PMID: 18082227.

123. Al-Humadi, N. H., Siegel, P. D., Lewis, D. M., et al. (2002). Alteration of intracellular cysteine and glutathione levels in alveolar macrophages and lymphocytes by diesel exhaust particle exposure. *Environmental Health Perspectives, 110*(4), 349–353. PubMed PMID: 11940452.

124. Allen, J. (2008). Inhaled glutathione for the prevention of air pollution-related health effects: A brief review. *Alternative Therapies in Health and Medicine, 14*(3), 42–44. PubMed PMID: 18517105.

125. Yamamoto, M., Singh, A., Sava, F., et al. (2013). MicroRNA expression in response to controlled exposure to diesel exhaust: Attenuation by the antioxidant N-acetylcysteine in a randomized crossover study. *Environmental Health Perspectives, 121*(6), 670–675. PubMed PMID: 23584289.

126. Carlsten, C., MacNutt, M. J., Zhang, Z., et al. (2014). Anti-oxidant N-acetylcysteine diminishes diesel exhaust-induced increased airway responsiveness in person with airway hyper-reactivity. *Toxicological Sciences, 139*(2), 479–487. PubMed PMID: 24814479.

127. Romieu, I., Garcia-Esteban, R., Sunyer, J., et al. (2008). The effect of supplementation with omega-3 polyunsaturated fatty acids on markers of oxidative stress in elderly exposed to PM(2.5). *Environmental Health Perspectives, 116*(9), 1237–1242. PubMed PMID: 18795169.

128. Tong, H., Rappold, A. G., Diaz-Sanchez, D., et al. (2012). Omega-3 fatty acid supplementation appears to attenuate particulate air pollution-induced cardiac effects and lipid changes in healthy middle-aged adults. *Environmental Health Perspectives, 120*(7), 952–957. PubMed PMID: 22514211.

129. Romieu, I., Téllez-Rojo, M. M., Lazo, M., et al. (2005). Omega-3 fatty acid prevents heart rate variability reductions associated with particulate matter. *American Journal of Respiratory and Critical Care Medicine, 172*(12), 1534–1540. PubMed PMID: 16210665.

130. Kang, Z. C., Tsai, S. J., & Lee, H. (1999). Quercetin inhibits benzo[a]pyrene-induced DNA adducts in human Hep G2 cells by altering cytochrome P-450 1A1 gene expression. *Nutrition and Cancer, 35*(2), 175–179. PubMed PMID: 10693172.

131. Jin, N. Z., Zhu, Y. P., Zhou, J. W., et al. (2006). Preventive effects of quercetin against benzo[a] pyrene-induced DNA damages and pulmonary precancerous pathologic changes in mice. *Basic and Clinical Pharmacology and Toxicology, 98*(6), 593–598. PubMed PMID: 16700823.

132. Egner, P. A., Chen, J. G., Zarth, A. T., et al. (2014). Rapid and sustainable detoxication of airborne pollutants by broccoli sprout beverage: Results of a randomized clinical trial in China. *Cancer Prevention Research, 7*(8), 813–823. PubMed PMID: 24913818.

133. Riedl, M. A., Saxon, A., & Diaz-Sanchez, D. (2009). Oral sulforaphane increases Phase II antioxidant enzymes in the human upper airway. *Clinical Immunology (Orlando, Fla.), 130*(3), 244–251. PubMed PMID: 19028145.

134. Ritz, S. A., Wan, J., & Diaz-Sanchez, D. (2007). Sulforaphane-stimulated phase II enzyme induction inhibits cytokine production by airway epithelial cells stimulated with diesel extract. *American Journal of Physiology. Lung Cellular and Molecular Physiology, 292*(1), L33–L39. PubMed PMID: 16905640.

135. Heber, D., Li, Z., Garcia-Lloret, M., et al. (2014). Sulforaphane-rich broccoli sprout extract attenuates nasal allergic response to diesel exhaust particles. *Food & Function, 5*(1), 35–41. PubMed PMID: 24287881.

136. Riso, P., Martini, D., Møller, P., et al. (2010). DNA damage and repair activity after broccoli intake in young healthy smokers. *Mutagenesis, 25*(6), 595–602. PubMed PMID: 20713433.

137. Lam, T. K., Gallicchio, L., Lindsley, K., et al. (2009). Cruciferous vegetable consumption and lung cancer risk: A systematic review. *Cancer Epidemiology, Biomarkers and Prevention: A Publication of the American Association for Cancer Research, Cosponsored by the American Society of Preventive Oncology, 18*(1), 184–195. PubMed PMID: 19124497.

138. Sehgal, A., Kumar, M., Jain, M., & Dhawan, D. K. (2013). Modulatory effects of curcumin in conjunction with piperine on benzo(a)pyrene-mediated DNA adducts and biotransformation enzymes. *Nutrition and Cancer, 65*(6), 885–890. PubMed PMID: 23909733.

139. Kalpana, C., & Menon, V. P. (2004). Curcumin ameliorates oxidative stress during nicotine-induced lung toxicity in Wistar rats. *The Italian Journal of Biochemistry, 53*(2), 82–86. PubMed PMID: 15646012.

140. Vanisree, A. J., & Sudha, N. (2006). Curcumin combats against cigarette smoke and ethanol-induced lipid alterations in rat lung and liver. *Molecular and Cellular Biochemistry, 288*(1–2), 115–123. PubMed PMID: 16691314.

141. Weisburger, J. H., Veliath, E., Larios, E., et al. (2002). polyphenols inhibit the formation of mutagens during the cooking of meat. *Mutation Research, 516*(1–2), 19–22. PubMed PMID: 11943606.

142. Hakim, I. A., Harris, R. B., Chow, H. H., et al. (2004). Effect of a 4-month tea intervention on oxidative DNA damage among heavy smokers: Role of glutathione S-transferase genotypes. *Cancer Epidemiology, Biomarkers and Prevention: A Publication of the American Association for Cancer Research, Cosponsored by the American Society of Preventive Oncology, 13*(2), 242–249. PubMed PMID: 14973088.

143. Tozan, A., Sehirli, O., Omurtag, G. Z., et al. (2007). Ginkgo biloba extract reduces naphthalene-induced

oxidative damage in mice. *Phytotherapy Research: PTR,* *21*(1), 72–77. PubMed PMID: 17094175.

144. Banerjee, S., Panda, C. K., & Das, S. (2006). Clove (Syzygium aromaticum L.), a potential chemopreventive agent for lung cancer. *Carcinogenesis,* *27*(8), 1645–1654. PubMed PMID: 16501250.

145. Hecht, S. S., Huang, C., Stoner, G. D., et al. (2006). Identification of cyanidin glycosides as constituents of freeze-dried black raspberries which inhibit anti-benzo[a]pyrene-7,8-diol-9,10-epoxide induced NFkappaB and AP-1 activity. *Carcinogenesis, 27*(8), 1617–1626. PubMed PMID: 16522666.

146. Senthilnathan, P., Padmavathi, R., Banu, S. M., & Sakthisekaran, D. (2006). Enhancement of antitumor effect of paclitaxel in combination with immunomodulatory Withania somnifera on benzo(a)pyrene induced experimental lung cancer. *Chemico-Biological Interactions, 159*(3), 180–185. PubMed PMID: 16375880.

147. El Safty, A., Metwally, F. M., Mohammed Samir, A., et al. (2015). Studying the effect of antioxidants on cytogenetic manifestations of solvent exposure in the paint industry. *Toxicology and Industrial Health, 31*(12), 1087–1094. PubMed PMID: 23625906.

148. Emara, A. M., & El-Bahrawy, H. (2008). Green tea attenuates benzene-induced oxidative stress in pump workers. *Journal of Immunotoxicology, 5*(1), 69–80. PubMed PMID: 18382860.

149. Girish, C., & Pradhan, S. C. (2012). Hepatoprotective activities of picroliv, curcumin, and ellagic acid compared to silymarin on carbon-tetrachloride-induced liver toxicity in mice. *Journal of Pharmacology & Pharmacotherapeutics, 3*(2), 149–155. PubMed PMID: 22629090.

150. Morsy, M. A., Abdalla, A. M., Mahmoud, A. M., et al. (2012). Protective effects of curcumin, α-lipoic acid, and N-acetylcysteine against carbon tetrachloride-induced liver fibrosis in rats. *Journal of Physiology and Biochemistry, 68*(1), 29–35. PubMed PMID: 21986891.

151. Sotelo-Félix, J. I., Martinez-Fong, D., Muriel, P., et al. (2002). Evaluation of the effectiveness of Rosmarinus officinalis (Lamiaceae) in the alleviation of carbon tetrachloride-induced acute hepatotoxicity in the rat. *Journal of Ethnopharmacology, 81*(2), 145–154. PubMed PMID: 12065145.

152. He, S. X., Luo, J. Y., Wang, Y. P., et al. (2006). Effects of extract from Ginkgo biloba on carbon tetrachloride-induced liver injury in rats. *World Journal of Gastroenterology, 12*(24), 3924–3928. PubMed PMID: 16804984.

153. Ulicná, O., Greksák, M., Vancová, O., et al. (2003). Hepatoprotective effect of rooibos tea (Aspalathus linearis) on CCl4-induced liver damage in rats. *Physiological Research, 52*(4), 461–466. PubMed PMID: 12899659.

154. Jeong, H. G., You, H. J., Park, S. J., et al. (2002). Hepatoprotective effects of 18beta-glycyrrhetinic acid on carbon tetrachloride-induced liver injury: Inhibition of cytochrome P450 2E1 expression. *Pharmacological Research, 46*(3), 221–227. PubMed PMID: 12220964.

155. Ha, K. T., Yoon, S. J., Choi, D. Y., et al. (2005). Protective effect of Lycium chinense fruit on carbon tetrachloride-induced hepatotoxicity. *Journal of Ethnopharmacology, 96*(3), 529–535. PubMed PMID: 15619574.

156. Singh, R., & Sharma, P. (2011). Hepatoprotective effect of curcumin on lindane-induced oxidative stress in male wistar rats. *Toxicology International, 18*(2), 124–129. PubMed PMID: 21976817.

157. Ciftci, O., Ozdemir, I., Tanyildizi, S., et al. (2011). Antioxidative effects of curcumin, β-myrcene and 1,8-cineole against 2,3,7,8-tetrachlorodibenzo-p-dioxin-induced oxidative stress in rats liver. *Toxicology and Industrial Health, 27*(5), 447–453. PubMed PMID: 21245202.

158. Centers for Disease Control and Prevention. (2017). *National Report on Human Exposure to Environmental Chemicals: Updated Tables.* Available at www.cdc.gov/exposurereport/. (Accessed 25 October 2017).

159. Sood, S., Choudhary, S., & Wang, H. C. (2013). Induction of human breast cell carcinogenesis by triclocarban and intervention by curcumin. *Biochemical and Biophysical Research Communications, 438*(4), 600–606. PubMed PMID: 23942114.

160. Basher, A., Rahman, S. H., Ghose, A., et al. (2013). Phase II study of magnesium sulfate in acute organophosphate pesticide poisoning. *Clinical Toxicology (Philadelphia, Pa.), 51*(1), 35–40. PubMed PMID: 23311540.

161. El-Ebiary, A. A., Elsharkawy, R. E., Soliman, N. A., et al. (2016). N-acetylcysteine in acute organophosphorus pesticide poisoning: A randomized, clinical trial. *Basic and Clinical Pharmacology and Toxicology, 119*(2), 222–227. PubMed PMID: 26786042.

162. Yurumez, Y., Cemek, M., Yavuz, Y., et al. (2007). Beneficial effect of N-acetylcysteine against organophosphate toxicity in mice. *Biological and Pharmaceutical Bulletin, 30*(3), 490–494. PubMed PMID: 17329844.

163. Wang, L., & Pan, S. (2015). Adjuvant treatment with crude rhubarb for patients with acute

organophosphorus pesticide poisoning: A meta-analysis of randomized controlled trials. *Complementary Therapies in Medicine*, 23(6), 794–801. PubMed PMID: 26645518.

164. Canales-Aguirre, A. A., Gomez-Pinedo, U. A., Luquin, S., et al. (2012). Curcumin protects against the oxidative damage induced by the pesticide parathion in the hippocampus of the rat brain. *Nutritional Neuroscience*, 15(2), 62–69. PubMed PMID: 22333997.

165. Alp, H., Aytekin, I., Hatipoglu, N. K., et al. (2012). Effects of sulforophane and curcumin on oxidative stress created by acute malathion toxicity in rats. *European Review for Medical and Pharmacological Sciences*, 16(Suppl. 3), 144–148. PubMed PMID: 22957429.

166. Hassani, S., Sepand, M. R., Jafari, A., et al. (2015). Protective effects of curcumin and vitamin E against chlorpyrifos-induced lung oxidative damage. *Human and Experimental Toxicology*, 34(6), 668–676. PubMed PMID: 25233897.

167. Tehrani, H., Halvaie, Z., Shadnia, S., et al. (2013). Protective effects of N-acetylcysteine on aluminum phosphide-induced oxidative stress in acute human poisoning. *Clinical Toxicology (Philadelphia, Pa.)*, 51(1), 23–28. PubMed PMID: 23148565.

168. Mengs, U., Pohl, R. T., & Mitchell, T. (2012). Legalon® SIL: The antidote of choice in patients with acute hepatotoxicity from amatoxin poisoning. *Current Pharmaceutical Biotechnology*, 13(10), 1965–1970, Review. PubMed PMID: 22352731.

169. Tang, L., Tang, M., Xu, L., et al. (2008). Modulation of aflatoxin biomarkers in human blood and urine by green tea polyphenols intervention. *Carcinogenesis*, 29(2), 411–417. PubMed PMID: 18192689.

170. Luo, H., Tang, L., Tang, M., et al. (2006). Phase IIa chemoprevention trial of green tea polyphenols in high-risk individuals of liver cancer: Modulation of urinary excretion of green tea polyphenols and 8-hydroxydeoxyguanosine. *Carcinogenesis*, 27(2), 262–268. PubMed PMID: 15930028.

171. Xue, K. S., Tang, L., Cai, Q., et al. (2015). Mitigation of fumonisin biomarkers by green tea polyphenols in a high-risk population of hepatocellular carcinoma. *Scientific Reports*, 5, 17545. PubMed PMID:26626148.

172. Poapolathep, S., Imsilp, K., Machii, K., et al. (2015). The effects of curcumin on aflatoxin b1- induced toxicity in rats. *Biocontrol Science*, 20(3), 171–177. PubMed PMID: 26412696.

173. Alm-Eldeen, A. A., Mona, M. H., Shati, A. A., & El-Mekkawy, H. I. (2015). Synergistic effect of black tea and curcumin in improving the hepatotoxicity induced by aflatoxin B1 in rats. *Toxicology and Industrial Health*, 31(12), 1269–1280. PubMed PMID: 23796760.

174. El-Mahalaway, A. M. (2015). Protective effect of curcumin against experimentally induced aflatoxicosis on the renal cortex of adult male albino rats: A histological and immunohisochemical study. *International Journal of Clinical and Experimental Pathology*, 8(6), 6019–6030. PubMed PMID: 26261479.

175. Martín, M. A., Serrano, A. B., Ramos, S., et al. (2010). Cocoa flavonoids up-regulate antioxidant enzyme activity via the ERK1/2 pathway to protect against oxidative stress-induced apoptosis in HepG2 cells. *The Journal of Nutritional Biochemistry*, 21(3), 196–205. PubMed PMID: 19195869.

176. Bala, K., Tripathy, B. C., & Sharma, D. (2006). Neuroprotective and anti-ageing effects of curcumin in aged rat brain regions. *Biogerontology*, 7(2), 81–89. PubMed PMID: 16802111.

177. Ilhan, A., Gurel, A., Armutcu, F., et al. (2004). Ginkgo biloba prevents mobile phone-induced oxidative stress in rat brain. *Clinica Chimica Acta*, 340(1–2), 153–162. PubMed PMID: 14734207.

178. Teng, Y. S., & Wu, D. (2017). Anti-fatigue effect of green tea polyphenols (-)-epigallocatechin-3-gallate (EGCG). *Pharmacognosy Magazine*, 13(50), 326–331. PubMed PMID: 28539729.

179. Xiang, Q., Liu, Z., Wang, Y., et al. (2013). Carnosic acid attenuates lipopolysaccharide-induced liver injury in rats via fortifying cellular antioxidant defense system. *Food and Chemical Toxicology: An International Journal Published for the British Industrial Biological Research Association*, 53, 1–9. PubMed PMID: 23200889.

180. Martín, M. A., Serrano, A. B., Ramos, S., et al. (2010r). Cocoa flavonoids up-regulate antioxidant enzyme activity via the ERK1/2 pathway to protect against oxidative stress-induced apoptosis in HepG2 cells. *The Journal of Nutritional Biochemistry*, 21(3), 196–205. PubMed PMID: 19195869.

181. Marnewick, J. L., Rautenbach, F., Venter, I., et al. (2011). Effects of rooibos (Aspalathus linearis) on oxidative stress and biochemical parameters in adults at risk for cardiovascular disease. *Journal of Ethnopharmacology*, 133(1), 46–52. PubMed PMID: 20833235.

182. Khan, G., Haque, S. E., Anwer, T., Ahsan, M. N., Safhi, M. M., & Alam, M. F. (2014). Cardioprotective effect of green tea extract on doxorubicin-induced cardiotoxicity in rats. *Acta Poloniae Pharmaceutica*, 71(5), 861–868. PubMed PMID: 25362815.

183. Ajuwon, O. R., Katengua-Thamahane, E., Van Rooyen, J., et al. (2013). Protective effects of rooibos (Aspalathus linearis) and/or red palm oil

(Elaeis guineensis) supplementation on tert-butyl hydroperoxide-induced oxidative hepatotoxicity in Wistar rats. *Evidence-based Complementary and Alternative Medicine, 2013*, 984273. PubMed PMID: 23690869.

184. El-Demerdash, F. M., Abbady, E. A., & Baghdadi, H. H. (2016). Oxidative stress modulation by Rosmarinus officinalis in creosote-induced hepatotoxicity. *Environmental Toxicology, 31*(1), 85–92. PubMed PMID: 25044495.

185. Steinkellner, H., Rabot, S., Freywald, C., Nobis, E., Scharf, G., Chabicovsky, M., et al. (2001). Effects of cruciferous vegetables and their constituents on drug metabolizing enzymes involved in the bioactivation of DNA-reactive dietary carcinogens. *Mutation Research, 480-481*, 285–297, Review. PubMed PMID:11506821.

186. Polasa, K., & Krishnaswamy, K. (1993). Effect of turmeric on xenobiotic metabolizing enzymes. *Plant Foods for Human Nutrition (Dordrecht, Netherlands), 44*(1), 87–92. PubMed PMID: 8332589.

187. Srinivasan, P., Suchalatha, S., Babu, P. V., et al. (2008). Chemopreventive and therapeutic modulation of green tea polyphenols on drug metabolizing enzymes in 4-Nitroquinoline 1-oxide induced oral cancer. *Chemico-Biological Interactions, 172*(3), 224–234. PubMed PMID: 18336807.

188. Marnewick, J. L., Joubert, E., Swart, P., et al. (2003). Modulation of hepatic drug metabolizing enzymes and oxidative status by rooibos (Aspalathus linearis) and Honeybush (Cyclopia intermedia), green and black (Camellia sinensis) teas in rats. *Journal of Agricultural and Food Chemistry, 51*(27), 8113–8119. PubMed PMID: 14690405.

189. Debersac, P., Vernevaut, M. F., Amiot, M. J., et al. (2001). Effects of a water-soluble extract of rosemary and its purified component rosmarinic acid on xenobiotic-metabolizing enzymes in rat liver. *Food and Chemical Toxicology: An International Journal Published for the British Industrial Biological Research Association, 39*(2), 109–117. PubMed PMID: 11267703.

Dimercaptosuccinic Acid Metal Mobilization Protocol
Two Days On and Five Days Off

To reduce the burden of heavy metals in your body, you need to do the following:

1. Avoid any further heavy metal exposure.
   a. Avoid the consumption of large ocean fish (swordfish, shark, halibut, tuna, Atlantic or farmed salmon, etc.) and *any* freshwater fish (trout, catfish, etc.).
   b. Avoid cigarette smoke.
2. Use dimercaptosuccinic acid (DMSA) to pull heavy metals from your body tissues and out through your kidneys.
   a. **DMSA**—Divide total daily body-weight dose into three daily doses, 2 days on and then 5 days off. This is done for 10-week sessions, often for up to 12 months. The urine test is repeated on the first day of taking DMSA on every tenth week. When retesting the urine, you will need to repeat the testing protocol that you have already completed (taking the full daily dose of DMSA in the morning on an empty stomach after voiding your bladder, and then collecting all of your urine for 6 hours). **Do not use DMSA if you react to it**.
   b. On the evenings of the days you are taking DMSA, take 2 capsules of **activated charcoal.**
   c. If you experience adverse gastrointestinal (GI) symptoms (gas, bloating, etc.) from taking DMSA, you can take 1 capsule of **ITI Mentharil** each time you take the DMSA. This will help calm your intestines.
   d. **Thorne Heavy Metal Support**—Three capsules daily on the 5 days *when you are not taking DMSA*. This will replenish the micronutrients that are cleared from your body by DMSA *and* will help protect your kidneys during this time. (DMSA increases the heavy metal movement through the kidneys.)
3. Take the following supplements listed here daily to help the heavy metals move out easily.
   a. **Thorne Basic Detox Nutrients**—Four capsules three times daily to help the body handle the cleansing.
   b. **Thorne Magnesium Citrate**—Two capsules twice daily. Magnesium is typically deficient in those with who are heavy metal burdened. When chelation is being done, the need for magnesium increases.
   c. **Thorne Buffered C Powder**—One teaspoon in water twice daily, in the morning and again in the evening. This will help alkalinize the urine and increase the excretion of cadmium and mercury in the urine.
   d. **Whey protein powder**—Two tablespoons daily to help move out mercury (unless you react to whey or dairy, in which case **do not take this**). This can be mixed with milk or juice as a "smoothie."
   e. **Thorne Fibermend**—One scoop three times daily. This is very effective at binding toxins and helping them leave the body.
4. Colonic irrigations once weekly with DMSA to clear toxins from bowel.

What to do in case of a bad reaction to moving out the heavy metals:

If you have any adverse reactions from the movement of heavy metals out of your body after the DMSA, do the following:

1. Let your clinician know immediately.
2. Have a colonic irrigation immediately, and then plan on doing colonics after each DMSA round. It is best to do hydrotherapy and colonic irrigations weekly to continue to move the heavy metals out of your body.
3. Take three capsules of activated charcoal to help absorb the heavy metals that are in your intestines.

© 2017 www.crinnionopinion.com

Dimercaptosuccinic Acid Metal Mobilization Protocol
Five Days On and Nine Days Off

To reduce the burden of heavy metals in your body, you need to do the following:

1. Avoid any further heavy metal exposure.
   a. Avoid the consumption of large ocean fish (swordfish, shark, halibut, tuna, Atlantic or farmed salmon) and *any* freshwater fish (trout, catfish, etc.).
   b. Avoid cigarette smoke.
2. Use dimercaptosuccinic acid (DMSA) to pull heavy metals from your body tissues and out through your kidneys.
   a. **DMSA**—Divide total daily body-weight dose into three daily doses, 5 days on and then 9 days off. This is done for 10-week sessions, often for up to 12 months. The urine test is repeated on the first day of taking DMSA on every tenth week. When retesting the urine, you will need to repeat the testing protocol that you have already completed (taking the full daily dose of DMSA in the morning on an empty stomach after voiding your bladder, and then collecting all of your urine for 6 hours). **Do not use DMSA if you have any adverse reaction.**
   b. On the evenings of the days you are taking DMSA, take two capsules of **activated charcoal.**
   c. If you experience adverse gastrointestinal (GI) symptoms (gas, bloating, etc.) from taking DMSA, you can take one capsule of **ITI Mentharil** each time you take the DMSA. This will help calm your intestines.
   d. **Thorne Heavy Metal Support**—Three capsules daily on the 9 days *when you are not taking DMSA*. This will replenish the micronutrients that are cleared from your body by DMSA *and* will help protect your kidneys during this time. (DMSA increases the heavy metal movement through the kidneys.)
3. Take the following supplements listed here daily to help the heavy metals move out easily.
   a. **Thorne Basic Detox Nutrients**—Four capsules three times daily to help the body handle the cleansing.
   b. **Thorne Magnesium Citrate**—Two capsules twice daily. Magnesium is typically deficient in those who are heavily metal burdened. When chelation is being done, the need for magnesium increases.
   c. **Thorne Buffered C Powder**—One teaspoon in water twice daily, in the morning and again in the evening. This will help alkalinize the urine and increase the excretion of cadmium and mercury in the urine.
   d. **Whey protein powder**—Two tablespoons daily to help move out mercury (unless you react to whey or dairy, in which case **do not take this**). This can be mixed with milk or juice as a "smoothie."
   e. **Thorne Fibermend**—One scoop three times daily. This is very effective at binding toxins and helping them leave the body.
4. Colonic irrigations once weekly with DMSA to clear toxins from bowel.

What to do in case of a bad reaction to moving out the heavy metals:

If you have any adverse reactions from the movement of heavy metals out of your body after the DMSA, do the following:

1. Let your clinician know immediately.
2. Have a colonic irrigation immediately, and then plan on doing them after each DMSA round. It is best to do hydrotherapy and colonic irrigations weekly to continue to move the heavy metals out of your body.
3. Take three capsules of activated charcoal to help absorb the heavy metals that are in your intestines.

© 2017 www.crinnionopinion.com

CaEDTA/DMPS IV Metal Mobilization Protocol

To reduce the burden of heavy metals in your body, you need to do the following:

1. Avoid any further heavy metal exposure:
   a. Avoid the consumption of large ocean fish (swordfish, shark, halibut, tuna, Atlantic or farmed salmon) and *any* freshwater fish (trout, catfish, etc.).
   b. Avoid cigarette smoke.
2. Use calcium disodium edetate (CaEDTA)/ 2,3-dimercaptopropane-1-sulfonate (DMPS) chelation to pull heavy metals from your body tissues and out through your kidneys.
   a. Return to clinic once every 2 weeks for an intravenous (IV) infusion of CaEDTA and DMPS.
   b. Two hours prior to every CaEDTA/DMPS IV, take **2000 mg of L-glycine**. This will help increase the flushing of heavy metals.
   c. **Take** Divide total daily body-weight dose into three daily doses for the 4 days following the IV. This will help mobilize more lead from the soft tissues that may have increased after CaEDTA mobilized lead from the bone.
   d. **Thorne Heavy Metal Support**—Take three capsules daily on the days between each chelation. This will replenish the micronutrients that are cleared from your body by chelation *and* will help protect your kidneys during this time. (Chelation increases the heavy metal movement through the kidneys.)
   e. The week after each chelation return to the clinic for a **nutrient IV**.
      i. Ascorbic Acid—4 mL
      ii. B complex— mL
      iii. Hydroxycobalamin—1 mL
      iv. B6—1 mL
      v. Magnesium sulfate—2 mL
      vi. Calcium gluconate—2 mL
      vii. Glutathione—15 mL
      viii. Selenium—1 mL
      ix. Sodium bicarb—1 cc
      x. Sterile water—22 cc
3. Take the following supplements listed here daily to help the heavy metals move out easily.
   a. **Thorne Basic Detox Nutrients**—Four capsules three times daily to help the body handle the cleansing. This is a multivitamin/mineral that is specially designed for a person who has a toxic burden.
   b. **Thorne Magnesium Citrate**—Two capsules twice daily. Magnesium is typically deficient in those who are heavily metal-burdened. When chelation is being done, the need for magnesium increases. If you take more magnesium than you can absorb, you can begin to experience loose stools. If this occurs, please reduce the dose.
   c. **Whey protein powder**—Two tablespoons daily to help move out mercury. Do not take this product if you react to whey or dairy. This can be mixed with milk or juice as a "smoothie."
   d. **Fiber**—One scoop three times daily to bind the heavy metal toxins that are being excreted through the bowel, preventing them from all being reabsorbed.
   e. **N-acetyl cysteine**—1500 mg daily to help boost glutathione levels. This and alpha lipoic acid help the brain dramatically while lead is being mobilized.
   f. **Alpha lipoic acid**—300 mg caps once daily to help protect your brain from the lead.
4. Colonic irrigations after each chelation IV to clear toxins from bowel.

What to do in case of a bad reaction to moving out the heavy metals:

If you have any adverse reactions from the movement of heavy metals out of your body after the chelation, do the following:

1. Let your clinician know immediately.
2. Have a colonic irrigation immediately, and then plan on doing colonics after each chelation round. It is best to do hydrotherapy and colonic irrigations weekly to continue to move the heavy metals out of your body.
3. Take three capsules of activated charcoal to help absorb the heavy metals that are in your intestines.

© 2017 www.crinnionopinion.com

D | APPENDIX

Intravenous Metal Mobilization Testing

The purpose of this assay is to identify current exposure to toxic metals and to gauge the approximate body load of mercury and lead. This test will also provide baseline data to use for comparison during chelation therapy. Two urine tests will be done, one before and one after you take an agent (dimercaptosuccinic acid [DMSA]) to mobilize heavy metals. By comparing the two tests we can determine the validity of the test and tell if you have a lot of **stored** heavy metals in your body, reflecting chronic buildup.

To prepare for the test:

Do not eat any shellfish for the week prior to the test.

On the day of the test:

1. For the first urine sample, you have two options:
   a. **BEST** option: Collect your first morning urine as the "pre-flush" sample (put this in the pre-flush container that you received from the lab). Be sure to record the total volume of urine collected (this will need to be noted in the laboratory request form).
   b. Collect your urine immediately prior to getting the IV at the office.
2. Receive the proper bodyweight dose of intravenous CaEDTA/DMPS. IV glutathione may also be added.
3. Collect your urine for the next 6 hours (in a container that you receive from the lab marked post-flush), and return the container to the lab. Please be sure to record the total volume of urine collected so that it can be noted on the lab request form. Refrigerate the sample if you cannot return the sample to the lab on the same day as the test.

© 2017 www.crinnionopinion.com

Oral Metal Mobilization Testing

The purpose of this assay is to identify current exposure to toxic metals and to gauge the approximate body load of mercury and lead. This test will also provide baseline data to use for comparison during chelation therapy. Two urine tests will be done, one before and one after you take an agent (dimercaptosuccinic acid [DMSA]) to mobilize heavy metals. By comparing the two tests we can determine the validity of the test and tell if you have a lot of **stored** heavy metals in your body, reflecting chronic buildup.

To prepare for the test:

Do not eat any shellfish for the week prior to the test.

On the day of the test:

1. Collect your first morning urine as the "pre-flush" sample (put this in the pre-DMSA container that you received from the lab). Be sure to record the total volume of urine collected (this will need to be noted in the laboratory request form).
2. Then, with an empty stomach and an empty bladder take the full recommended bodyweight dose of DMSA with water. You can then proceed with your normal morning routine, including eating at your normal time.
3. Collect your urine for the next 6 hours (in a container that you receive from the lab marked post-DMSA), and return the container to the lab. Please be sure to note the total volume of urine collected so that it can be noted on the lab request form. Refrigerate the sample if you cannot return the sample to the lab on the same day as the test.

© 2017 www.crinnionopinion.com

F | APPENDIX

Environmental Exposure Questionnaire

Name:_____   Date:_____

A. METABOLISM OF POLLUTANTS:

1. Have you often had to lower the regular dose of prescription, over-the-counter medication, or herbal supplements because you were too sensitive to normal doses?   □ Yes   □ No
2. Do you avoid caffeine in the afternoon or altogether because it can keep you up at night?   □ Yes   □ No
3. Have you ever experienced adverse reactions to medications?   □ Yes   □ No
   a) If so, what happened with which medicine?

B. TOXICANT-RELATED HEALTH PROBLEMS:

1. Do you have a sudden onset of physical, mental, or emotional symptoms (headaches, skin rashes, nausea, fatigue, shortness of breath, etc.) upon exposure to chemical odors (cleaners, perfumes, new materials, cigarette smoke, diesel exhaust, etc.)?   □ Yes   □ No
   a) When did you first notice any such reaction? (age you were when it began)
   b) What was the chemical you first reacted to?
   c) In the last 6 months, are your chemical reactions getting
      □   Better
      □   Worse
      □   Staying the same
   d) Do you experience unpleasant symptoms when you walk down the soap aisle in the grocery store, or do you find yourself avoiding the soap aisle altogether?   □ Yes   □ No
   e) List the chemicals that you react to and the approximate age you were when it began:

Age
- □   Cleaners
- □   Perfumes
- □   Cigarette smoke
- □   Vehicular exhaust
- □   Paints

Age
- □   New carpet or fabric
- □   Plastics
- □   Pesticides or other agricultural chemicals
- □   Other (list)_____
  _____

2. For any of the following illnesses that you have had, please note the age at which it began:

Age

☐ _____ Asthma
☐ _____ Allergies
☐ _____ Rheumatoid arthritis
☐ _____ Lupus
☐ _____ Sjogren's syndrome
☐ _____ Autoimmune thyroiditis
☐ _____ Any other auto immune illness
☐ _____ Balance disorder
☐ _____ Brain fog—diminished cognition
☐ _____ Memory loss
☐ _____ Depression or anxiety

Age

☐ _____ Parkinsonism
☐ _____ Tremors
☐ _____ Adult onset diabetes
☐ _____ Infertility
☐ _____ Low testosterone
☐ _____ Hypothyroid
☐ _____ Gout
☐ _____ Gestational diabetes
☐ _____ Gestational hypertension
☐ _____ Overweight
_____

C. POLLUTANT EXPOSURE:

Air Pollution

	1–5	5–10	10–20	20–30	More Than 30	Don't Know
1. How many minutes-drive is it from your house to the closest highway/freeway?	☐	☐	☐	☐	☐	☐
2. How many minutes-drive is it from your house to a busy street or boulevard?	☐	☐	☐	☐	☐	☐
3. How many minutes-drive is it from your house to the closest agricultural area?	☐	☐	☐	☐	☐	☐
4. How many minutes-drive is it from your house to the closest industrial area where you see smokestacks?	☐	☐	☐	☐	☐	☐
5. How many minutes-drive is it from your house to the closest golf course?	☐	☐	☐	☐	☐	☐
6. How many minutes-drive is it from your house to the closest landfill?	☐	☐	☐	☐	☐	☐
7. How many years have you lived in a city, town, or state that is known for its air pollution (such as Los Angeles or Salt Lake City)?	☐	☐	☐	☐	☐	☐

8. How often can you "see the air" in your area? ☐ 1–4 times monthly ☐ Most of the time ☐ All of the time ☐ Rarely

9. Do you have air purifiers in your home? ☐ Yes ☐ No
   ☐ Ozone
   ☐ Ion generator
   ☐ HEPA
   ☐ IQ Air, Blue Air, Austin Air, Aller Air, or similar multifilter purifier

10. Are shoes worn inside your home? ☐ Yes ☐ No
11. Do you have an attached garage that your car is parked in? ☐ Yes ☐ No
12. Do you drive a diesel vehicle? ☐ Yes ☐ No
13. Does your vehicle have an exhaust leak? ☐ Yes ☐ No ☐ Unknown
14. What is the approximate year or decade your current home was built?

15. Type of appliances (stove and hot water heater):
    - ☐ Electric
    - ☐ Natural gas
16. Type of heating:
    - ☐ Electric
    - ☐ Gas
    - ☐ Oil
    - ☐ Wood
    - ☐ Diesel
17. When were your air ducts last cleaned out?
18. When was your furnace filter last replaced?
    - ☐ Within the last month
    - ☐ Within the last 3 months
    - ☐ Don't know
19. Are pesticides used in your home or yard? ☐ Yes ☐ No
20. How often do you have clothes dry cleaned? ☐ Weekly ☐ Monthly
    ☐ Every 3–6 months ☐ Rarely/Never
21. How often do you get hair coloring? ☐ Monthly ☐ Every 3–6 months ☐ Rarely/Never
22. How often are you in a salon in which acrylic nail service is provided? ☐ Weekly ☐ Monthly
    ☐ Every 3–6 months ☐ Rarely/Never
23. Do you sleep on any of the following?
    - ☐ Pillow-top mattress
    - ☐ Memory foam mattress
    - ☐ Memory foam pillow
24. Do you use spray or plug-in air fresheners in your home? ☐ Yes ☐ No
25. Have you ever worked at a job, or did schooling, that brought you in contact with industrial chemicals? ☐ Yes ☐ No
    a) How many years? ☐ 1–5 ☐ 5–10 ☐ 10–20 ☐ 20–30
    ☐ More than 30
    b) What chemicals?
26. Have you lived in a new home or a recently remodeled home? ☐ Yes ☐ No
    a) What was your age when living there?
27. What are the newest pieces of furniture you have purchased for your home?
    a) When were they purchased?
    b) Are any upholstery or drapes in the home treated with Scotchguard (stain resistance)? ☐ Yes ☐ No
28. Does your current home have wall-to-wall carpeting? ☐ Yes ☐ No
    a) How old is the carpeting? ☐ 1–5 years ☐ 5–10 years ☐ More than 10 years
    b) Is it treated with Scotchguard (stain resistance)? ☐ Yes ☐ No
29. Are nonstick Teflon pans used for cooking in your home? ☐ Yes ☐ No
30. Do you have any hobbies that require the use of solvents, paints, gasoline, or lead? ☐ Yes ☐ No
If so, list them here
31. Do you have pets in your home that you apply anti-flea or tick products to? ☐ Yes ☐ No
    a) If so, how often? ☐ Daily ☐ Weekly ☐ Monthly
    ☐ Less than once a month

Food Pollution

	Rarely/ Never	Less Than Once Weekly	Once Weekly	Twice or More Weekly
1. How often do you consume the following?				
a) Tuna	☐	☐	☐	☐
b) Salmon (Chilean, Norwegian, BC, or "just plain salmon")	☐	☐	☐	☐
c) Alaskan salmon (one or more of the following: King, Coho, Sockeye, Red, or Pink)	☐	☐	☐	☐
d) Swordfish	☐	☐	☐	☐
e) Chilean Sea Bass	☐	☐	☐	☐
f) Orange Roughy	☐	☐	☐	☐
g) Sardines	☐	☐	☐	☐
2. How often do you consume (eating or juicing) commercial varieties (nonorganic) of any of the following:				
a) Apples	☐	☐	☐	☐
b) Celery	☐	☐	☐	☐
c) Cherry tomatoes	☐	☐	☐	☐
d) Cucumber	☐	☐	☐	☐
e) Grapes (Imported)	☐	☐	☐	☐
f) Nectarines	☐	☐	☐	☐
g) Peaches	☐	☐	☐	☐
h) Potatoes	☐	☐	☐	☐
i) Snap peas	☐	☐	☐	☐
j) Spinach	☐	☐	☐	☐
k) Strawberries	☐	☐	☐	☐
l) Sweet bell peppers (any color)	☐	☐	☐	☐
3. How often do you consume canned soup?	☐	☐	☐	☐
4. How often do you make prepackaged "microwave-safe meals"?	☐	☐	☐	☐
5. How often do you microwave food in Styrofoam or nonceramic "microwave-safe" plastics?	☐	☐	☐	☐
6. How often do you consume dark green leafy vegetables?	☐	☐	☐	☐

Metals

1. Were you raised in a smoking household? ☐ Yes ☐ No
2. Have you ever smoked? ☐ Yes ☐ No
   a) How many packs a day? ☐ Less than 1 ☐ 1 ☐ More than 1
   b) How many years? ☐ 1–5 ☐ 5–10 ☐ 10–20 ☐ 20–30
   ☐ More than 30
3. Have you lived in a home that was built before 1978? ☐ Yes ☐ No
4. Have you remodeled a home that was built before 1978? ☐ Yes ☐ No
5. Have you ever had silver amalgams in your teeth? ☐ Yes ☐ No
   a) Total number: ☐ 1–3 ☐ 4–6 ☐ 7 or more
   b) How many years have they been in your mouth? ☐ 1–5 ☐ 5–10 ☐ 10–20 ☐ 20–30

c) How many years ago was the most recent amalgam put into your mouth? ☐ 1–5 ☐ 5–10 ☐ 10–20 ☐ 20–30

d) Do you grind your teeth at night? ☐ Yes ☐ No ☐ Unknown

6. How often do you consume tofu? ☐ Rarely/never ☐ Less than once weekly ☐ Once weekly ☐ Twice or more weekly

7. Do you use filtered water for drinking and cooking? ☐ Yes ☐ No
   - ☐ Brita (or similar charcoal filter device)
   - ☐ Under-counter multicartridge filter
   - ☐ R/O
   - ☐ Alkaline
   - ☐ Other (list)

Mycotoxins

1. Have you had any of the following in your current or past residence?

	Current Residence		Past Residence	
a) A roof leak?	☐ Yes	☐ No	☐ Yes	☐ No
b) Water in the basement?	☐ Yes	☐ No	☐ Yes	☐ No
c) Broken water pipe?	☐ Yes	☐ No	☐ Yes	☐ No
d) Window leaks?	☐ Yes	☐ No	☐ Yes	☐ No
e) Does your carpet ever get wet when it rains?	☐ Yes	☐ No	☐ Yes	☐ No
f) Any water stains on ceilings or walls?	☐ Yes	☐ No	☐ Yes	☐ No
g) Ever received insurance money for water in the home?	☐ Yes	☐ No	☐ Yes	☐ No
h) Ever needed assistance to clear water from your home?	☐ Yes	☐ No	☐ Yes	☐ No
i) Any rooms in the home that smell musty?	☐ Yes	☐ No	☐ Yes	☐ No
j) Do you suspect that your home has mold in it?	☐ Yes	☐ No	☐ Yes	☐ No
k) Do you have a front-loading washer?	☐ Yes	☐ No	☐ Yes	☐ No
l) Is any amount of mold visible around the shower/tub or sinks in your home?	☐ Yes	☐ No	☐ Yes	☐ No

2. Is your home water supply from a well or cistern? ☐ Yes ☐ No

Lifestyle Pollutants

1. Do you have any silicone-containing implants? ☐ Yes ☐ No
   a) How many years ago were the implants put in? ☐ 1–5 ☐ 5–10 ☐ 10–20 ☐ 20–30

2. Do you have any implants of other materials (Teflon, stainless steel, etc.)? ☐ Yes ☐ No

3. How often do you use the following personal care products?

	Rarely/ Never	Less than once weekly	Daily	More than once daily
a) Skin lotion	☐	☐	☐	☐
b) Sunscreen	☐	☐	☐	☐
c) Scented deodorant	☐	☐	☐	☐
d) Cologne or perfume	☐	☐	☐	☐

4. In your home, do you have any of the following:
   - ☐ Wifi routers
   - ☐ Bluetooth appliances
   - ☐ Smart meter
   - ☐ Cordless phones

ENVIRONMENTAL TOXIC EXPOSURE / RESIDENCE HISTORY

Name:_____ Date:_____

Fill in the table below listing all residences in which you have lived. Start with the present and go back as far as you can remember. Ask family members and parents, if alive, for additional information. In the Known Exposures column, use the appropriate letters for each exposure as listed below.

Residence Location (City, County, State)	Dates From–to (mo. & yr.)	City, Suburb, Rural	Amount of traffic (hi–med–lo)	Age of Home at the Time	Known Exposures (Choose From the List Below)	Did You Have to Move Out for Health Reasons? If so, Why?

A. House built pre-1978
B. Commercial business nearby
C. Agricultural area
D. Within 5 min. drive of roadway with truck traffic
E. Dry-cleaned clothes kept in bedroom closet
F. Pets sprayed, dipped, or collared for fleas or ticks
G. Use of air fresheners
H. Regular use of chemicals (i.e., paints, cleaners; think of hobbies in each location)

I. Unfinished pressure-treated lumber (outdoor play sets, decking, patio furniture)
J. Pesticide/herbicide use—yours or your neighbors: lawns, house bugs, gardens
K. Family members bringing home contaminants on clothes
L. Major power lines over or near the home
M. Attached garage
N. Storage of gasoline, solvents, etc., in garage

O. Tobacco smoke (you or someone in the house smoked)
P. New construction, remodeling
Q. Mobile home
R. New furniture
S. Wall-to-wall carpet
T. Natural gas or oil heat
U. Gas stove, wood stove, fireplace
V. Water damage in home

ENVIRONMENTAL TOXIC EXPOSURE / OCCUPATIONAL HISTORY

Name:_____ Date:_____

Fill in the table below listing all jobs at which you have worked, including short-term, seasonal, and part-time employment. Start with your present job and go back to the first. Use additional paper if necessary.

Workplace (Name, City, County, State)	Dates Worked from–to (mo. & yr.)	Full Time? (yes/no)	Type of Industry (Describe)	Describe Your Job Duties	Known Health Hazards in Workplace (i.e., dusts/solvents)	Protective Equipment Used	Were You Ever Off Work for a Health Problem or Injury?

Environmental Exposure Questionnaire
Interpretation Guide

A. METABOLISM OF POLLUTANTS:

1. Yes: **Phase one is slow.**
2. Yes: **CYP1A2 is low and will have difficulty clearing PAH (combustion by-products).**
3. Yes: **They likely have poor phase 2.**

B. TOXICANT-RELATED HEALTH PROBLEMS:

1. Yes: a) **They are environmentally ill. b) They are immunotoxic. c)They are deficient in GSH & Mg. d) They are chemically overburdened. e) They likely have null GSTM1 and a PON1 SNP.**
   a) **Age they were first chemically overloaded.**
   b) **Chemical class they were first overburdened by.**
   c) In the last 6 months, are your chemical reactions getting
      ☐ Better – **House is environmentally safe.**
      ☐ Worse – **New toxicants present in home.**
      ☐ Staying the same – **No new toxicants in home.**
   d) Yes: **They are chemically reactive –** see B. 1.
   e) **Age they were overburdened with each of the following:**

Age		Age	
☐ _____	Cleaners	☐ _____	New carpet or fabric
☐ _____	Perfumes	☐ _____	Plastics
☐ _____	Cigarette smoke	☐ _____	Pesticides or other agricultural chemicals
☐ _____	Vehicular exhaust	☐ _____	Other (list)
☐ _____	Paints	_____	

2. **All of the below are considered "Environmental Illnesses." Indicate the patient's age at the initiation or exacerbation of each condition or disorder.**

Age		Age	
☐ _____	Asthma	☐ _____	Parkinsonism
☐ _____	Allergies	☐ _____	Tremors
☐ _____	Rheumatoid arthritis	☐ _____	Adult onset diabetes
☐ _____	Lupus	☐ _____	Infertility

810

Age			Age	
☐ _____	Sjogren's syndrome		☐ _____	Low testosterone
☐ _____	Autoimmune thyroiditis		☐ _____	Hypothyroid
☐ _____	Any other auto immune illness		☐ _____	Gout
☐ _____	Balance disorder		☐ _____	Gestational diabetes
☐ _____	Brain fog—diminished cognition		☐ _____	Gestational hypertension
☐ _____	Memory loss		☐ _____	Overweight
☐ _____	Depression or anxiety		_____	

3. **Illnesses coinciding with chemical reactivity above will identify causative agents.**

C. POLLUTANT EXPOSURE:

Air Pollution

Shows Proximity to These Toxicant Sources.	1–5	5–10	10–20	20–30	More Than 30	Don't Know
1. How many minutes-drive is it from your house to the closest highway/freeway?	☐	☐	☐	☐	☐	☐
2. How many minutes-drive is it from your house to a busy street or boulevard?	☐	☐	☐	☐	☐	☐
3. How many minutes-drive is it from your house to the closest agricultural area?	☐	☐	☐	☐	☐	☐
4. How many minutes-drive is it from your house to the closest industrial area where you see smokestacks?	☐	☐	☐	☐	☐	☐
5. How many minutes-drive is it from your house to the closest golf course?	☐	☐	☐	☐	☐	☐
6. How many minutes-drive is it from your house to the closest landfill?	☐	☐	☐	☐	☐	☐
7. How many years have you lived in a city, town, or state that is known for its air pollution (like Los Angeles or Salt Lake City)?	☐	☐	☐	☐	☐	☐

8. How often can you "see the air" in your area?   ☐ 1–4 times monthly   ☐ Most of the time
☐ All of the time   ☐ Rarely

Shows outdoor air pollutant burden.
9. Do you have air purifiers in your home?
   - ☐ Ozone (**indicates increased oxidative stress, poor air quality**)
   - ☐ Ion generator (**indicates increased oxidative stress, poor air quality**)
   - ☐ HEPA (**indicates fair air purification quality**)
   - ☐ IQ Air, Blue Air, Austin Air, Aller Air, or similar multifilter purifier (**indicates best air purification quality**)
10. Are shoes worn inside your home?   ☐ Yes: **Enhanced indoor air pollution.**
11. Do you have an attached garage that your car is parked in?   ☐ Yes: **Enhanced indoor air pollution.**
12. Do you drive a diesel vehicle?   ☐ Yes: **Enhanced exposure.**

Shows Proximity to These Toxicant Sources.

	1–5	5–10	10–20	20–30	More Than 30	Don't Know

13. Does your vehicle have an exhaust leak? ☐ Yes: **Exposure to benzene.**

14. Approximate year or decade current home was built? **Prior to 1978 indicates increased Pb exposure.**

15. Type of appliances (stove and hot water heater):
    - ☐ Electric: **No potential exposure source.**
    - ☐ Natural gas: **Potential exposure source.**

16. Type of heating:
    - ☐ Electric: **No toxic exposure source.**
    - ☐ Gas: **Potential exposure source.**
    - ☐ Oil: **Potential exposure source.**
    - ☐ Wood: **Increased risk of asthma.**
    - ☐ Diesel: **Potential exposure source.**

17. When were your air ducts last cleaned out? **Lack of cleaning increases potential for higher indoor air pollution load.**

18. When was your furnace filter last replaced?
    - ☐ Within the last month: **Good.**
    - ☐ Within the last 3 months: **OK.**
    - ☐ Don't know: **Terrible–high indoor pollution risk.**

19. Are pesticides used in your home or yard? ☐ Yes: **Look for OP and Pyrethroid pesticide symptoms picture.**

20. How often do you have clothes dry cleaned? ☐ Weekly/ Every 3–6 months: **High solvent exposure potential.**

21. How often do you get hair coloring? ☐ Monthly/ Every 3–6 months: **High exposure source, high autoimmune potential.**

22. How often are you in a salon in which acrylic nail service is provided? ☐ Weekly/Monthly: **Regular toluene exposure.**

23. Do you sleep on any of the following? **High exposure to benzene and styrene.**
    - ☐ Pillow-top mattress
    - ☐ Memory foam mattress
    - ☐ Memory foam pillow

24. Do you use spray or plug-in air fresheners in your home? ☐ Yes: **Exposure to solvents.**

25. Have you ever worked at a job, or did schooling, that brought you in contact with industrial chemicals? ☐ Yes: **Exposure.**
    a) How many years? ☐ 1–5 ☐ 5–10 ☐ 10–20 ☐ 20–30 ☐ More than 30

    b) What chemicals?

26. Have you lived in a new home or a recently remodeled home? ☐ Yes: **High exposure to building chemicals.**
    a) What was your age when living there? **Correlate with age illnesses began or became exacerbated.**

27. What are the newest pieces of furniture you have purchased for your home? **Look for pressboard furniture**
    a) When were they purchased? **Correlate with age illnesses began**
    b) Are any upholstery or drapes in the home treated with Scotchguard (stain resistance)? ☐ Yes: **Exposure to perflourocarbons**

Shows Proximity to These Toxicant Sources.	1–5	5–10	10–20	20–30	More Than 30	Don't Know

28. Does your current home have wall-to-wall carpeting? ☐ Yes: **Exposure to numerous chemicals Correlate with age illnesses began.**
    a) How old is the carpeting?
    b) Is it treated with Scotchguard (stain resistance)? ☐ Yes: **Exposure to perflourocarbons.**
29. Are nonstick Teflon pans used for cooking in your home? ☐ Yes: **Exposure to perflourocarbons.**
30. Do you have any hobbies that requires the use of solvents, ☐ Yes: **Solvent exposure sources.**
    paints, gasoline, or lead?
    If so, list them here
31. Do you have pets in your home that you apply anti-flea ☐ Yes: **Neonicotinoid exposure.**
    or tick products to?
    a) If so, how often: ☐ Daily/ Weekly: **High neonicotinoid exposure.**

Food Pollution

	Rarely/ Never	Less Than Once Weekly	Once Weekly	Twice or More Weekly
1. How often do you consume the following?				
a) Tuna: **Mercury exposure**	☐	☐	**High Hg**	**Very high Hg**
b) Farmed salmon: **Exposure to PCBs/Hg**	☐	☐	**High PCB/Hg**	**High PCB/Hg**
c) Alaskan salmon: **No significant exposure, possible Hg**	☐	☐	☐	**Possible Hg**
d) Swordfish	☐	☐	**High Hg**	**Very high Hg**
e) Chilean Sea Bass	☐	☐	**High Hg**	**Very high Hg**
f) Orange Roughy	☐	☐	**High Hg**	**Very high Hg**
g) Sardines	☐	☐	**High PCB**	**High PCB**
2. How often do you consume (eating or juicing) commercial varieties (nonorganic) of any of the following:				
a) Apples	☐	☐	**High OP**	**Very High OP**
b) Celery	☐	☐		
c) Cherry tomatoes	☐	☐		
d) Cucumber	☐	☐		
e) Grapes (Imported)	☐	☐		
f) Nectarines	☐	☐		
g) Peaches	☐	☐		
h) Potatoes	☐	☐		
i) Snap peas	☐	☐		
j) Spinach	☐	☐		
k) Strawberries	☐	☐		
l) Sweet bell peppers (any color)	☐	☐		
3. How often do you consume canned soup?	☐	☐	**BPA**	**Very High BPA**
4. How often do you make prepackaged "microwave-safe meals"?	☐	☐	**Plastics**	**Plastics**
5. How often do you microwave food in Styrofoam or nonceramic "microwave-safe" plastics?	☐	☐	**Styrene Plastics**	**Styrene Plastics**

	Rarely/ Never	Less Than Once Weekly	Once Weekly	Twice or More Weekly
6. How often do you consume dark green leafy vegetables?	☐	☐	**Low Cd/ Thallium**	**Cd/Thallium**

Metals

1. Were you raised in a smoking household?   ☐ Yes: **Pb, Cd, As.**
2. Have you ever smoked?   ☐ Yes: **Pb, Cd, As.**
   a) How many packs a day?   **Increasing amounts of Pb, Cd, As.**
   b) How many years?   **Increasing amounts of Pb, Cd, As.**
3. Have you lived in a home that was built before 1978?   ☐ Yes: **Pb exposure.**
4. Have you remodeled a home that was built before 1978?   ☐ Yes: **Pb exposure.**
5. Have you ever had silver amalgams in your teeth?   ☐ Yes: **Hg exposure.**
   a) Total number: **4–7: Higher Hg kidney burden, lower Se.**
   b) How many years have they been in your mouth?   **Increasing exposure.**
   c) How many years ago was the most recent amalgam put into your mouth?   **More recent: Greater Hg release.**
   d) Do you grind your teeth at night?   ☐ Yes: **Increased Hg exposure.**
6. How often do you consume tofu?   **Once or more weekly–High Cd burden.**
7. Do you use filtered water for drinking and cooking?   **No: Exposure to inorganic arsenic–relative**
   ☐   Brita (or similar charcoal filter device)   **groundwater As level in their geographic area.**
   ☐   Under counter multicartridge filter   **RO filter prevents As exposure.**
   ☐   R/O
   ☐   Alkaline
   ☐   Other (list)

Mycotoxins

1. Have you had any of the following in your current or past residence?   **Current residence**   **Past residence**
   a) A roof leak?   **Yes: Mold exposure**   **Yes: Mold exposure**
   b) Water in the basement?
   c) Broken water pipe?
   d) Window leaks?
   e) Does your carpet ever get wet when it rains?
   f) Any water stains on ceilings or walls?
   g) Ever received insurance money for water in the home?
   h) Ever needed assistance to clear water from your home?
   i) Any rooms in the home that smell musty?
   j) Do you suspect that your home has mold in it?
   k) Do you have a front-loading washer?
   l) Is any amount of mold visible around the shower/tub or sinks in your home?
2. Is your home water supply from a well or cistern?   ☐ Yes: **Potential mycotoxin exposure.**

Lifestyle Pollutants

1. Do you have any silicone-containing implants?
   a) How many years ago were the implants put in?

   ☐ **Yes: Potential silicone-related autoimmune disorder. Correlate with date of any AI connective tissue problem.**

2. Do you have any implants of other materials (Teflon, stainless steel, etc.)?

   ☐ Yes: **Potential AI**

3. How often do you use the following personal care products?

	Rarely/ Never	Less than once weekly	Daily	More than once daily
a) Skin lotion	☐	☐	**Phthalate exposure**	
b) Sunscreen	☐	☐		
c) Scented deodorant	☐	☐		
d) Cologne or perfume	☐	☐		

4. In your home, do you have any of the following: EMF exposure
   ☐ Wifi routers
   ☐ Bluetooth appliances
   ☐ Smart meter
   ☐ Cordless phones

INDEX

Page numbers followed by "*f*" indicate figures, "*t*" indicate tables, and "*b*" indicate boxes.